Oral Cancer

Tadaaki Kirita • Ken Omura
Editors

Oral Cancer

Diagnosis and Therapy

Springer

Editors
Tadaaki Kirita
Department of Oral and Maxillofacial Surgery
Nara Medical University
Nara, Japan

Ken Omura
Oral Cancer Center
Tokyo General Hospital
Tokyo, Japan

ISBN 978-4-431-54937-6 ISBN 978-4-431-54938-3 (eBook)
DOI 10.1007/978-4-431-54938-3
Springer Tokyo Heidelberg New York Dordrecht London

Library of Congress Control Number: 2015930257

Printed on acid-free paper

Springer is part of Springer Science+Business Media (www.springer.com)

Preface

The oral and pharyngeal region represents the sixth leading site of cancer in the world, and oral cancer is widely accepted to have a higher incidence in people older than 50 years, primarily due to the relationship with chronic exposures to tobacco, alcohol, and other carcinogenic products. Particularly in India, Bangladesh, Pakistan, and Sri Lanka, oral cancer is the most common, accounting for about one third of all cancers. Recently, the incidence of this cancer in young adults (age <40 years) has appeared to be increasing in many Western countries.

Oral cancers can be treated curatively in the early stages by surgery or radiotherapy; however, locoregionally advanced disease continues to be a major clinical problem due to poor prognosis, poor appearance, and post-therapeutic functional impairment. It is not a tribute to professionals or public health authorities that an area of the body that is so easily accessible for examination and a lesion that is so easily diagnosed can still result in so many deaths. Early diagnosis of a lesion during the localized early stage, combined with adequate treatment, thus appears to be the most effective way to further improve oral cancer control. Prevention of oral cancer is also obviously important for the high-risk population of tobacco-smoking, alcohol-drinking males with poor oral hygiene and nutrition.

Therapy for oral cancer has improved significantly over the last 25 years. Chemotherapy has been added to surgical approaches and megavoltage radiation. Chimeric monoclonal antibody has also been applied in treatment with radiation and platinum-based chemotherapy. The increasing application of microvascular surgery for free tissue transfer has produced new dimensions in reconstructive techniques for oral cancer surgery. A combined therapeutic team approach is now the rule, with authoritative voices in all specialties joining their talents and experience for the benefit of the patient. Prompt implementation of multidisciplinary treatment based on the latest knowledge and clinical data will further contribute to the progression of oral cancer treatment.

The purpose of this publication is to present a wealth of information on oral cancers in one source. This book is composed of excellent contributions from well-established and distinguished specialists who have been working on topics related to the epidemiology, pathology, and treatment of oral cancer. The contributors have written their respective chapters based on their professional knowledge for target readers, including cancer researchers, oncologists, molecular biologists, pathologists, and clinicians in oral cancer. The editors are grateful to all the contributors for their excellent efforts in making their chapters accessible to these readers.

It is hoped that this book will allow a more intelligent understanding of oral cancer, resulting in skillful, excellent treatment to maximize the patient's chance of cure and preserve the highest quality of life.

Nara, Japan — Tadaaki Kirita
Tokyo, Japan — Ken Omura

Contents

Epidemiology of the Oral Cancer

1

Nobuharu Yamamoto and Takahiko Shibahara

Abstract

Oral cancer is a malignant neoplasm that occurs in the oral cavity. Squamous cell carcinoma accounts for over 90 % of the oral cancers in Japan, and others include adenocarcinoma derived from minor salivary gland, sarcoma, malignant lymphoma, and metastatic cancer. A number of cohort studies and case–control studies have been conducted as epidemiological technique to elucidate oral cancers. The number of oral cancer patients in Japan was 2,100 in 1975 and 6,900 in 2005 and further is estimated to be 10,000 patients by 2015, which is 1.6 times higher than the current number. Age-adjusted male-to-female ratio is 3:2, which is higher in males than in females, and the incidence of oral cancers decreases with the aging of the population in developed countries with the exception of Japan, in which the ratio is increasing. Of oral cancers, tongue carcinoma is the most common and accounts for 40 % of oral cancers. The oral cavity, an entrance of the digestive system, is exposed to chemical stimuli such as smoking, drinking, and food as well as to mechanical stimuli including caries and ill-fitting prosthetic appliance and characterized by the existence of multiple circumstances in particular and risk factors associated with carcinogenesis. Examination of oral cancers can be easily conducted because these cancers can be confirmed directly by visual observation and palpation. The significance of oral cancer examination is early diagnosis and early treatment of not only oral cancers but also premalignant lesions, including leukoplakia and erythroplakia, and precancerous conditions, including lichen planus. It is reported that the detection rate of oral cancers and premalignant lesions is 0.99 % in oral cancer screening and that the prevalence of precancerous lesions is 2.5 % in Japanese. Some patients with oral cancer may synchronously or metachronously develop double cancers. In patients with head and neck cancer including oral cancer, 60–70 % of double cancers are found in the upper gastrointestinal tract or lung.

Keywords

Epidemiology • Japanese • Oral cancer • Prevention • Squamous cell carcinoma

1.1 Introduction: Oral Cancer in Japan

The number of death from cancer has been increasing to 340,000 yearly in Japan (30.3 % of the total deaths). This number corresponds to the number of deaths from car accidents of 60 years. It is estimated that half of the people of Japan are affected with cancer in their life regardless of sex. Cancer is a national disease, and it is no doubt that Japan is a

N. Yamamoto (✉) • T. Shibahara
Department of Oral and Maxillofacial Surgery,
Tokyo Dental College, 2-9-18 Misaki-cho, Chiyoda-ku,
Tokyo 101-0061, Japan
e-mail: nyamamot@tdc.ac.jp

T. Kirita and K. Omura (eds.), *Oral Cancer: Diagnosis and Therapy*,
DOI 10.1007/978-4-431-54938-3_1, © Springer Japan 2015

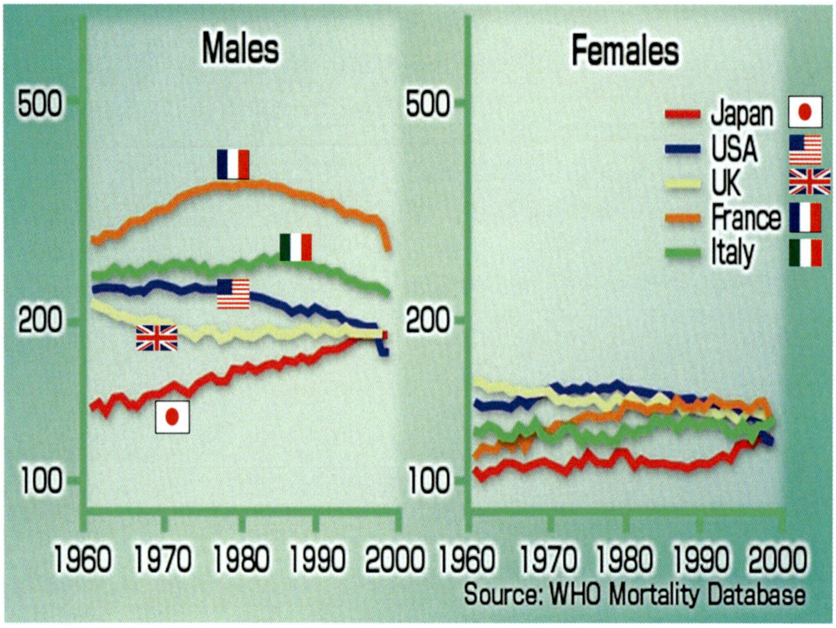

Fig. 1.1 Number of deaths due to oral and pharyngeal cancers by developed country (per 100,000 population). Increase is observed only in Japan among developed countries and this is a disturbing fact

major cancer-affected country. According to the Revised Policy Statement of the Federation Dentaire Internationale (FDI) in 2000, the number of death from oral cancers including pharyngeal cancer was 318,000 throughout the world (2002). On the other hand, it is thought that the number of death from breast cancers in the same year was 477,000. When taking account of 1–2 % of incidence rate of oral cancers of the entire tumors, it is shown how high the incidence of oral cancer rate is [1].

The number of death from oral cancers (6,000 patients/year) and incidence of oral cancers as well as total cancers demonstrate an upward trend [2]. The number of patients with oral cancer was 2,100 in 1975 and increased to 6,900 in 2005 and is estimated to become 10,000 patients, which is 1.6 times higher than the present number, by 2015 in Japan [2–4]. In addition, such increase is observed only in Japan among developed countries and this is a disturbing fact. Actual number of death from oral cancer and incidence rate of oral cancer in the USA, the UK, and Italy are higher than in Japan, but annual changes of the rate are obviously decreasing in those countries. These decreases would reflect the results of countermeasures against cancers (Fig. 1.1) [5]. It is known that the medical services in Japan provide the latest equipment and maintain state-of-the-art standard; however, these services seem to fail reducing the cancers. This may reflects a tendency of the current medical system emphasizing on treatment but not prevention.

Clinical statistics obtained in our department and measures for prevention of oral cancer that we addressed are presented, as well as epidemiology is discussed in this article.

1.2 Frequency of Oral Cancer

The number of cancer patients as well as patients with oral cancers is increasing with the advent of a super-aging society in Japan. The incidence rates of oral cancer are different by ethnic, country, region, lifestyle, and practice.

Although an exact nationwide survey on oral cancers has not been conducted yet, the numbers of death from oropharyngeal cancers per 100,000 of population in males and females were 2.4 and 1.3, 5.1 and 2.9 in 1975 and 1995, respectively, and are estimated to increase to 8.6 and 5.2 by 2015 according to the Annual Report on Health and Welfare [2]. Treatment performance has also been improved during these years; however, the increase of death from cancers largely exceeds the treatment performance. This means the development of cancers also increases. The incidence of oral cancers in Japan is as described in the above section [2–4], and this number corresponds to about 1 % of the total cancer number and 40 % of the total number of head and neck cancers. Therefore, it is considered that such steady increase was caused by an increase of super-aging people [6–13].

Age-adjusted prevalence of oral cancer is highest in 60's similar to other cancers, and the male-to-female ratio is 3:2, which is higher in males than in females. According to nationwide statistics of Japanese Society of Oral and Maxillofacial Surgeons on oral cancers in 2002 [14], of 1777 patients, male patients were 1,051 (59.1 %) and female patients were 726 (40.9 %). By age groups, 50s patients were 323 (18.1 %), 60s patients were 471 (26.5 %), and 70's

Table 1.1 Oral cancer patient characteristics in our department (2003/1–2012/12, $n=348$)

Patient characteristics	$n=348$
Age, mean (range)	62.9 (21–94)
Sex, men/women	188/160
Performance status	0–2
Primary site (%)	
Tongue	183 (52.6)
Mandibular gingiva	68 (19.5)
Maxillary gingiva	38 (10.9)
Buccal mucosa	26 (7.5)
Oral floor	22 (6.3)
Palate	9 (2.6)
Others	2 (0.6)
Histology (%)	
Well	102 (29.3)
Moderate	36 (10.3)
Poor	8 (2.3)
Early	36 (10.3)
Unknown	166 (47.7)
Mean follow-up, month (range)	46.3 (4.4–123.2)
T-stage (%)	
1	113 (32.5)
2	151 (43.4)
3	36 (10.4)
4	48 (13.8)
N-stage (%)	
0	209 (60.1)
1	77 (22.1)
2a	8 (2.3)
2b	33 (9.4)
2c	21 (6.0)
Stage (%)	
I	103 (26.5)
II	94 (24.2)
III	74 (19.1)
IV	77 (19.8)

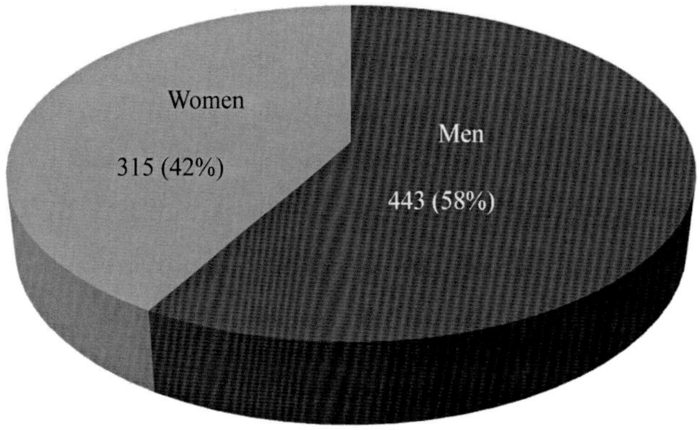

Fig. 1.2 The incidence according to the men and women with oral squamous cell carcinoma in our department. The male-to-female ratio is 3:2, which is higher in males than in females

patients were 517 (29.1 %), and patients of 50 years old and older account for 80 % of the total patients. In the present day seeing the super-aged society, it is estimated that the number of old–old patients would increase furthermore. Although it was previously considered that the development of oral cancer in 30's and younger is rare, increase in 20's patients is reported in these years. Effects of lifestyle, living environment, chemical factors, viruses, and bacteria are considered. Clinical characteristics with recently 10-year oral cancer patients in our department are shown in Table 1.1 and Figs. 1.2, 1.3, and 1.4.

The incidence of oral cancers is high in countries with a higher rate of both smoking and drinking habit [10, 15], especially high in south Asian countries. It is considered that a habit of chewing tobacco such as betel nut highly contributes to this tendency, and it is estimated that the incidence rate of oral cancer is 0.5–5 % and the number of patients with oral cancer reaches 2.5 million in India [16–19]. Mortality rate from oropharyngeal cancer in Japan is lower than France and Italy, and this is considered because this is largely affected by food and life habitat [5].

Cancer registry is increasingly becoming popular, but still inadequate. Establishment of nationwide cancer registry in consideration of the Private Information Protection Law would be required.

1.3 Favorite Site

Favorite site of oral cancer is different depending on the race and lifestyle. We describe about frequency of oral cancer occurrence by sites in Japan in this section. The frequency of oral cancer occurrence by sites is different depending on the ethnic, country, region, lifestyle, and practice. According to a tally by the Japanese Society of Oral and Maxillofacial Surgeons in 2002, the occurrence frequency of oral cancer ($n=1,784$) by sites was highest in the tongue and accounted for 40 % of the entire oral cancers [14], followed by the mandibular gingiva (20.3 %), maxillary gingiva (12.0 %), buccal mucosa (10.3 %), oral floor (9.2 %), maxillary antrum, and palate in Japan [5]. In the USA, the frequencies were reported as the tongue (35.2 %), oral floor (28.0 %), mandibular and maxillary gingiva (10.4 %), hard palate (8.9 %), and buccal mucosa (2.9 %) [10]. Eighty percent of tongue cancer tends to occur at the lingual border, and it is exceptionally rare to occur at the apex or back of tongue. For gingiva, research has still not shown that the occurrence frequencies are different between the maxilla and mandible. The occurrence frequency in our department was also in the order of the tongue, mandibular gingiva, oral floor, buccal mucosa, maxillary gingiva, palate, and lips, in which percentages almost

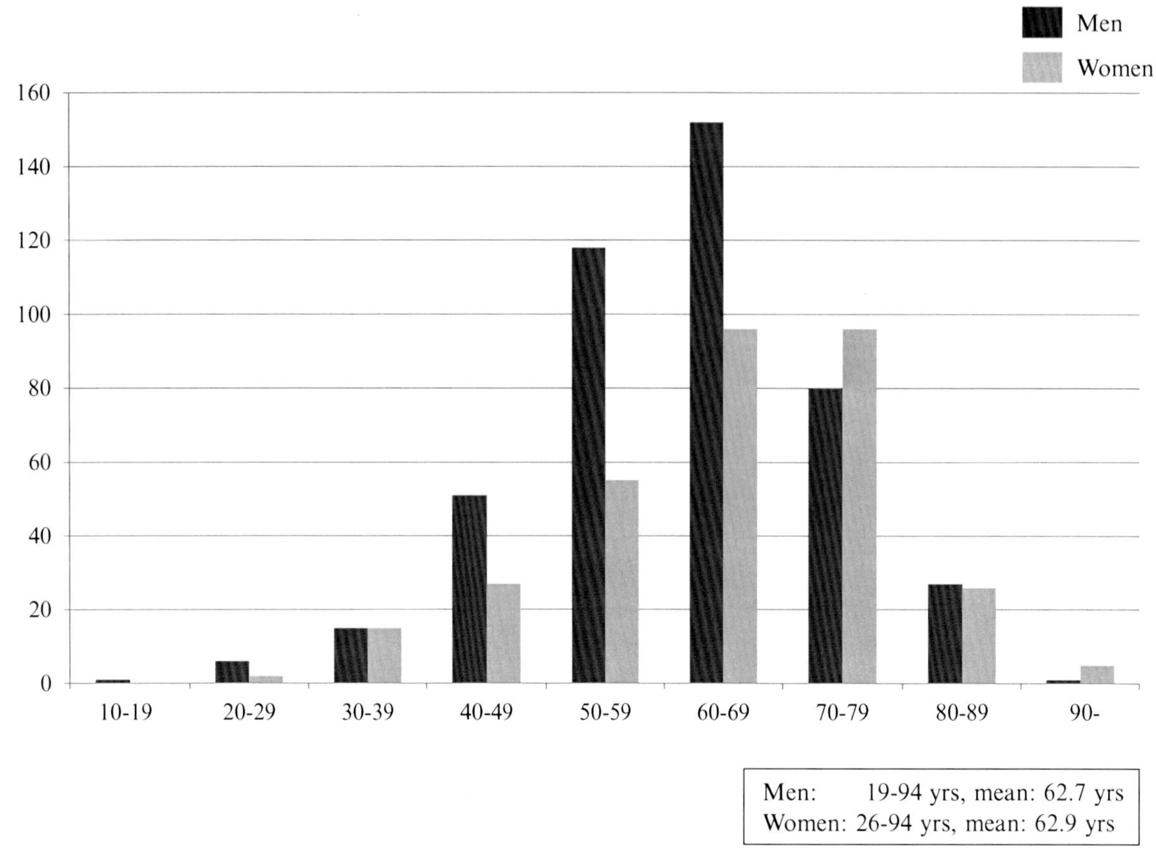

Fig. 1.3 The age distribution according to the men and women with oral squamous cell carcinoma in our department. Age-adjusted prevalence of oral cancer is highest in the 1960s similar to other cancers

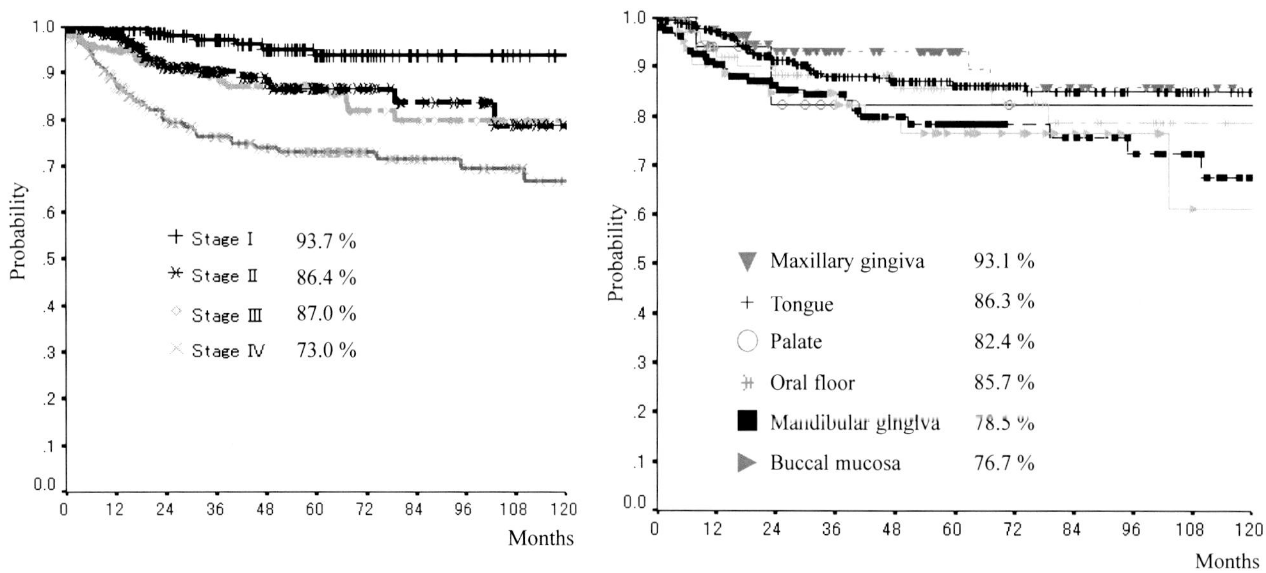

Fig. 1.4 The 5-year survival rate according to stage and site of the oral squamous cell carcinoma in our department

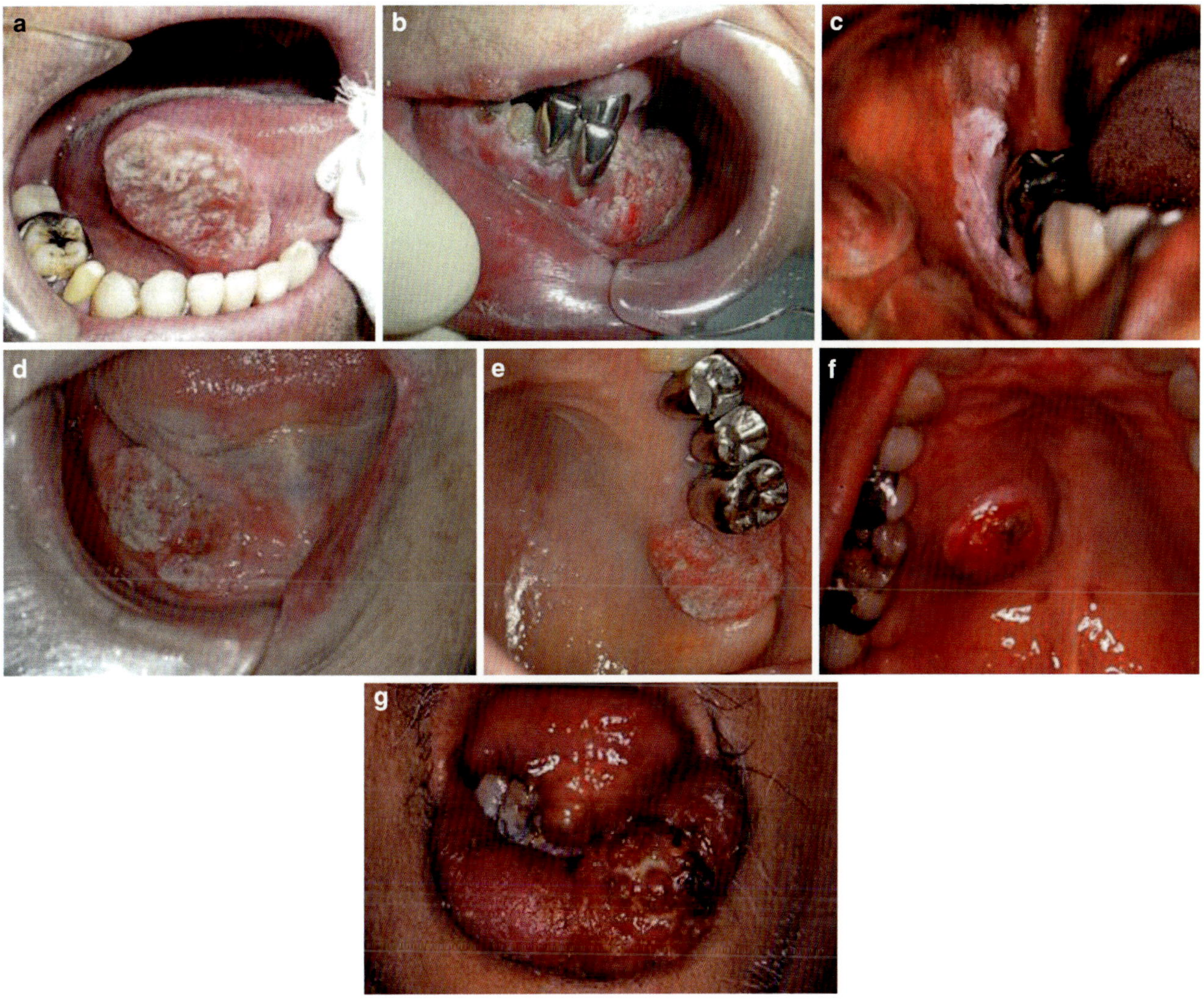

Fig. 1.5 Favorite site of oral cancer. (**a**) Tongue cancer. (**b**) Mandibular gingival cancer. (**c**) Buccal mucosa cancer. (**d**) Oral floor cancer. (**e**) Maxillary gingival cancer. (**f**) Palate cancer. (**g**) Lower lip cancer

corresponded to the statistics published from other facilities (Table 1.1). Characteristics by sites of occurrence are summarized as below:

1. Tongue cancer (Fig. 1.5a)
   (a) Tongue cancer accounts for 40 % of the entire oral cancers and makes up the majority of the oral cancers.
   (b) Tongue cancer occurs more commonly at the lingual border or inferior surface of tongue and occurs only infrequently at the apex or back of tongue.
   (c) Advanced tongue cancer spreads over the oral floor and tongue base and causes adhesion, lingual movement disorder, dysmasesis, dysphagia, dysarthria, and trismus, and it results in respiratory distress when it progresses to the pharyngeal region.
2. Mandibular gingival cancer (Fig. 1.5b)
   (a) Mandibular gingival cancer accounts for 20 % of the oral cancers and occurs in the next highest number after tongue cancer.
   (b) It is often detected through symptoms such as inadaptation of denture, swelling or ulcer formation of gingiva, or tooth movement.
   (c) It is often treated with misdirected therapy including tooth extraction, anti-inflammation treatment, and adjustments to denture without aim based on the diagnosis of periodontal diseases and stomatitis.
   (d) Mandibular gingival cancer is likely to cause destruction and absorption of the mandibular bone in relatively early stage because the tumor becomes infiltrated along the periosteum. Infiltration is categorized into three types, pressure type, invasive type, and moth-eaten type based on its characteristics.
3. Buccal mucosa cancer (Fig. 1.5c)
   (a) The frequency of buccal mucosa cancer is only about 10 % in Japan, but is highest, about 50 %, in India. It is believed that the reason of such a high rate in India is caused by betel nut and chewing tobacco, which are key carcinogenic factors.

(b) Buccal mucosa cancer occurs more commonly in buccal mucosal surface facing to the molar tooth region and in the distomolar region.
(c) Most of the cancers are well-differentiated type and often associated with leukoplakia.

4. Oral floor cancer (Fig. 1.5d)
(a) The frequency of oral floor cancer is about 10 % and relatively low. Patients become aware of mass formation associated with ulcer and induration of the oral floor in many cases.
(b) Oral floor cancer infiltrates into the opening or duct of the submandibular gland and may be associated with excretory disturbance of saliva or swelling of the submandibular gland.
(c) Oral floor cancer can spread to the tongue and gingiva or adhere to periosteum of the jawbone or infiltrate into suprahyoid muscles, which form the oral floor, relatively early in the course because the oral floor is close to the tongue, gingiva, and mandible.
(d) Patients have marked pain and a feeling of strangeness during eating and talking and also easily develop inadaptation of denture.

5. Maxillary gingival cancer (Fig. 1.5e) and maxillary sinus cancer
(a) Maxillary cancer consists of maxillary gingival cancer, which develops from the gingiva, and maxillary sinus cancer, which occurs primarily in the maxillary sinus mucosa. The frequency of oral floor cancer is about 10 % and relatively low.
(b) Subjective symptoms of maxillary gingival cancer include swelling, ulcer, and pain, but few tooth pain occurs. When advanced, the cancer infiltrates and destroys the buccal and palatine mucosa, as well as the nasal cavity and maxillary sinus floor.
(c) Subjective symptoms of maxillary sinus cancer are mainly nasal symptoms, such as nasal congestion, rhinorrhea, and nasal bleeding; oral symptoms, such as tooth pain, tooth movement, and swelling of the palate; and swelling of the cheek. If the cancer spreads into the orbit, exophthalmos, double vision, and visual impairment occur.

6. Palate cancer (Fig. 1.5f)
(1) The frequency of palate cancer is about 2 % and low. The site of onset is the hard palate by gingiva in general; however, the cancer crosses over the midline or results in absorption and destruction of the soft palate, gingiva, or palatal bone in advanced cases.
(b) Subjective symptoms are mainly swelling of the palate region and followed by ulcer and pain.

7. Lip cancer (Fig. 1.5g)
(a) The frequency of lip cancer is about 1 % and lowest.
(b) Lip cancer occurs more commonly in the lower lip and develops ulcers and swelling relatively early in the course.

1.4 Risk Factors and Prevention of Oral Cancer

1. Risk factors of oral cancer
A number of risk factors of oral cancer have been reported [21, 22]. Risk factors of oral cancer reported up to the present are summarized in Fig. 1.6. Surprisingly, however, only few factors have been epidemiologically or experimentally established. In addition, it is widely recognized as an underlying concept that oral cancer is very unlikely to develop with single factor and is caused by overlapping several factors in multistages. Especially smoking and drinking are representative risk factors of oral cancer, which are epidemiologically and experimentally established.

1 Smoking
2 Drinking
3 Physical stimuli (tilted tooth, caries, poor fillings, poorly-fitting denture)
4 Chemical stimuli (spices, high-salt food etc.)
5 Mucosal damage due to inflammation (periodontitis, maxillary sinusitis)
6 Virus infection (hepatitis viruses, HPV etc.)
7 Age

Fig. 1.6 Risk factors of oral cancer

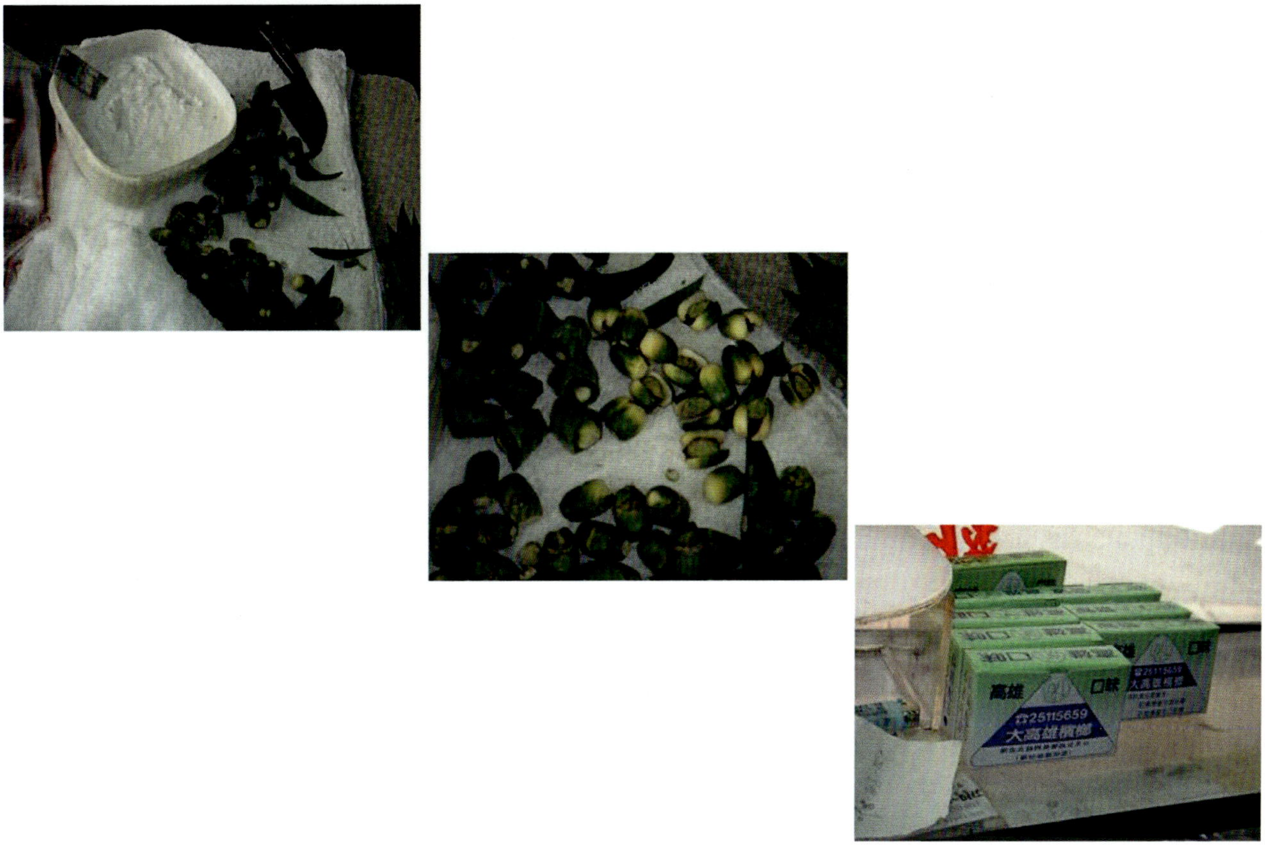

Fig. 1.7 Chewing tobacco and betel nut in Taiwan. Betel nut and chewing tobacco, which are key carcinogenic factors in buccal mucosa cancer

2. Smoking and oral cancer
   There are no other risk factors like smoking in which causal association with cancer has been clearly established. Now, tobacco could be said to be an enemy of every disease to put it in extreme terms. Smoking is a luxury item, which also has the highest causal relation with carcinogenesis in oral cancer.

   The occurrence frequency of oral cancer is extremely high in Sri Lanka, India, or Taiwan as compared with Japan, and about 30 % of the entire cancer is oral cancer. It has been epidemiologically shown that such high occurrence of oral cancer is caused by a habit of chewing tobacco and betel nut (Fig. 1.7) [21]. The Declaration of Opposition to Smoking is adopted by about 40 academic societies including the Japanese Society of Oral and Maxillofacial Surgeons at the present day and supports promotion of the antismoking movement in Japan. It is indisputable that smoking is the largest factor for the prevention of oral cancer. A number of studies on carcinogenicity of smoking have been conducted since the mid-1900s, and it has been demonstrated that there are a number of substances that act as initiators or promoters in the carcinogenic process in about 4,000 kinds of chemical substances contained in cigarette smoke [23]. About 40 substances including benzopyrene and nitrosamines have been identified as carcinogenesis-related substances to date [23]. In addition, it is considered that oral cancer, pharyngeal cancer, laryngeal cancer, esophageal cancer, gastric cancer, pancreatic cancer, liver cancer, kidney cancer, bladder cancer, and uterine cancer are associated with smoking. Recently, smoking rate of Japanese is on a declining trend. However, it is pointed out that an increasing tendency is observed in only young females.
3. Drinking and oral cancer
   Drinking is a factor, which causation with oral cancer has been demonstrated similar to smoking. Different from tobacco, alcohol (= ethanol) itself has no carcinogenicity. However, it has been clarified in many studies that alcohol is indirectly associated with carcinogenesis. Moreover, a synergistic effect due to concomitant exposure to drinking and smoking often becomes a problem. Drinking and smoking cause exposure of carcinogenic factors to all pharynx, larynx, esophagus, and stomach in addition to the oral cavity at the same time (field cancerization); therefore, this is also related to the development of double cancer. According to our department, double cancers with upper digestive tract cancer were observed in 10.4 % of the entire oral cancer patients [24].

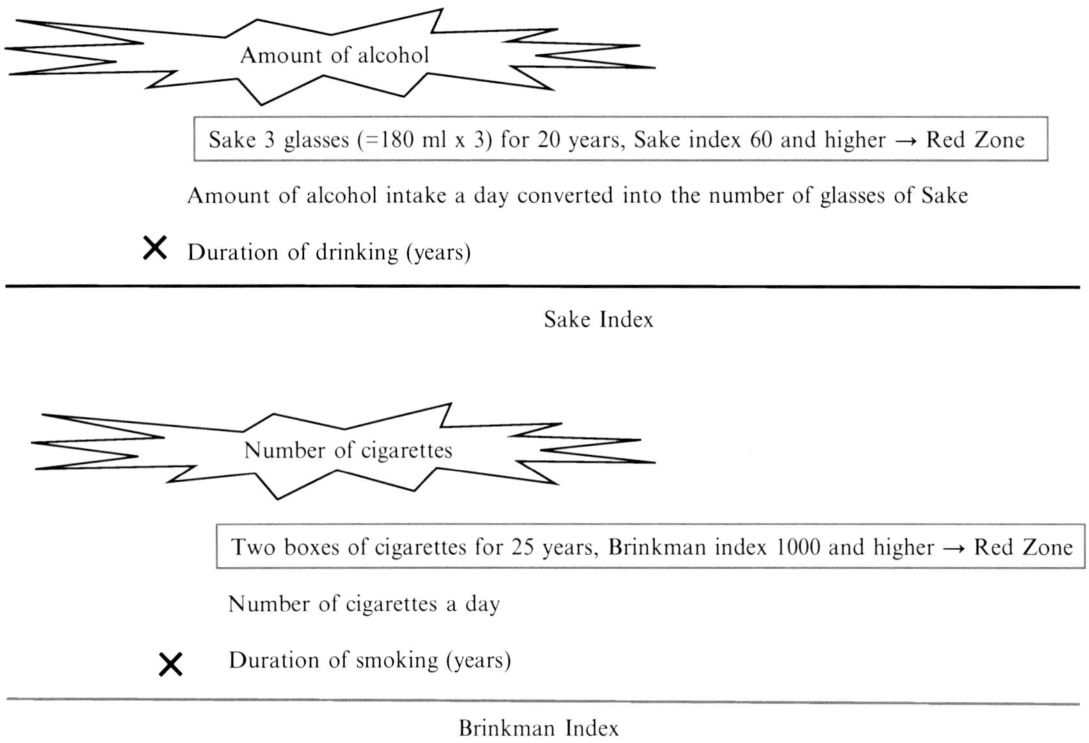

Fig. 1.8 Oral cancer risk and Sake and Brinkman indices. Sake index that is 60 or higher and Brinkman index that is 1,000 or higher are defined as the risk zones

The carcinogenic mechanism of alcohol was poorly understood until recently in contrast to tobacco. There is no report of carcinogenesis induced by only alcohol administration in animal experiments. However, International Agency for Research on Cancer (IARC) recognized alcohol as a carcinogen because acetaldehyde, which is a metabolic product of alcohol, has carcinogenicity [25]. In other words, the carcinogenic mechanism may directly or indirectly interact with biological reactions. As direct interaction, metabolic enzymes localizing in the oral mucosa degrade alcohol, and it causes exposure of the mucosa to acetaldehyde. Homann et al. [26] reported that bacteria existing inside the oral cavity increase carcinogenic risk of oral cancer by degradation of alcohol to acetaldehyde. As indirect interaction, it is considered that effects of alcohol include effect of acetaldehyde metabolized in the liver on local mucosa, effect as a solvent of carcinogens derived from tobacco and others, decrease of metabolic function of the liver, decrease of immunological capacity due to alcohol ingestion, and lowering of nutritional status.

4. Epidemiology of smoking and drinking

As the results of a meta-analysis of reports on a large-scale epidemiological studies, IARC concluded that smoking and drinking are distinct risk factors of oral cancer [25]. Of course, the more daily consumption of as well as longer exposure time to smoking and drinking result in increase of carcinogenic risk. Accordingly, an index that takes account of them has an important implication. Brinkman index and Sake index shown in Fig. 1.8 are widely used to express relationship between the amount and duration of smoking and drinking with oral cancer. Sake index that is 60 or higher and Brinkman index that is 1,000 or higher are defined as the risk zones (Fig. 1.8). However, pack-years is used as a new smoking index instead of Brinkman index in recent years. This index is calculated by dividing Brinkman index by 20.

Based on the above findings, we conducted a case–control study in 191 patients with oral cancer and 121 healthy subjects with no oral mucosal diseases who visited our department [27]. The results of multiple logistic analysis on risk for the development of oral cancer are shown in Table 1.4. Risk of developing oral cancer (odds ratio) by smoking alone was 2.5, but it elevated to 4.3 in heavy smokers with Brinkman index 1,000 or higher. In addition, odds ratio of drinking alone was 4.5; however, it elevated to 10.4 in heavy drinker with Sake index 60 or higher. When subjects have a habit of smoking and drinking, the risk of developing oral cancer resulted in 4.8, which was higher than smoking or drinking alone. In other words, it is considered that the risk of oral cancer is high in people with Brinkman index 1,000 or higher and Sake index 60 or higher and especially high in people who have both smoking and drinking habits.

Table 1.2 Oral cancer risk in smoking and drinking-related metabolic genes

	Odds ratio (95 % confidence interval)
Patients with GSTM1 defect	2.5 (1.6–5.4)
Patients with ALDH2 hetero defect	2.9 (1.1–7.8)

Table 1.3 The risk of developing oral cancer in smoking and drinking

	Odds ratio (95 % confidence interval)
Smoking	2.5 (1.1–5.6)
B.I. 1,000〜	4.3 (1.6–11.5)
Drinking	4.5 (2.5–8.1)
S.I. 60〜	10.4 (3.6–29.4)
Smoking + drinking	4.8 (1.8–13.0)

B.I. Brinkman index, *S.I.* Sake index

5. Genotypic analysis of metabolic enzymes related to smoking and drinking
Carcinogens accumulate in the body through tobacco use or alcohol ingestion and then are metabolized and detoxified. Recently, it is revealed that there are differences in individual's metabolic capability due to genetic variant of metabolic enzymes. In other words, it is speculated that the same loading from smoking and/or drinking may cause different degrees of carcinogenic risk in individuals because metabolic and detoxification capabilities against carcinogens vary considerably from individual to individual. Accordingly, we conducted an analysis of genes related to smoking and drinking in 127 patients with oral cancer and 33 healthy subjects with smoking and drinking habits, who preliminarily gave informed consent (Table 1.2) [27]. As a smoking-related enzyme, gene polymorphism of glutathione S-transferase M1 (GSTM1), which is an enzyme degrading benzopyrene in tobacco, was identified and analyzed with a multiple logistic analysis (Table 1.3) [27]. As a result, the risk of developing oral cancer in smokers with GSTM1 gene mutation was 2.5 times higher. Then aldehyde dehydrogenase 2 (ALDH2), which is an enzyme that degrades acetaldehyde, was identified and analyzed with a multiple logistic analysis. As a result, the risk of developing oral cancer in individuals with drinking habit with ALDH2 gene mutation (hetero deletion) was 2.9 times higher. Furthermore, an Italian research team recently conducted a meta-analysis of papers on ALDH2 gene polymorphism, including our report, and concluded that carcinogenic factor of drinking-related head and neck cancers is acetaldehyde [28]. Moreover, they also reported that higher alcohol consumption causes higher carcinogenic risk in ALDH2-deleted individuals [28].

   As mentioned above, the polymorphism pattern of metabolism-related genes may contribute to the identification of risk factors of oral cancer because the polymorphism pattern varies from individual to individual. New biomarkers would be discovered in the future, and the development of tailor-made prevention may be expected in this area.

6. Virus infection and oral cancer
Several types of carcinogenesis caused by virus infection have been reported. For example, it is famous that hepatitis B virus and hepatitis C virus cause liver cancer and is also well known that adult T-cell leukemia (ATL) is caused by RNA virus (retrovirus). In the head and neck region, EB virus belonging to herpesvirus group causes Burkitt's lymphoma. In addition, it is reported that human papillomavirus (HPV) is associated with the development of oral cancer [29]. Recently HPV is watched with interest as the cause of oral cancer especially in young individuals with no risk factors of smoking and drinking.
7. Age and oral cancer
Japan is becoming an unprecedented aging society with a falling birthrate in the world with progress of super-aging society and lowering of birthrate in these years. It is reported that oral cancer appears most frequently at 50 years old and older. However, it is considered that recent increasing tendency is due to the increasing number of the elderly.
8. Oral cancers in high-risk females (Figs. 1.9, 1.10, and 1.11)
In general, it is believed that oral cancers are often found in middle-aged males and less frequent in females. It is presumed that this is greatly associated with having much stress from work in addition to lifestyle habits such as smoking and drinking. However, increase of female patients is recently being seen as a problem. There are more than a small number of female patients with no smoking/drinking history and no clear carcinogenic cause. There is a report that HPV, which is a cause of cervical cancer, is associated with carcinogenesis; however, concrete conclusion is still not obtained. Especially female patients need attention to aesthetic recovery in addition to functional aspect sufficiently taking into account the social background and living environment.

   We compared treatment results of males and females with oral cancer in recent two decades (the first 10 years and later 10 years were analyzed separately) in our department (Fig. 1.9). As a result, 5-year survival rate was lower in females (Fig. 1.10) than males (Fig. 1.11), and it was noted that the number of recurrence and metastasis was increased in females diagnosed with early cancer.

9. Young patients and oral cancer
It has been known that oral cancer often occurs in males of 60 years and older; however, recently it is pointed out that the rate of oral cancer in young individuals and females is increasing [30–32]. There is no

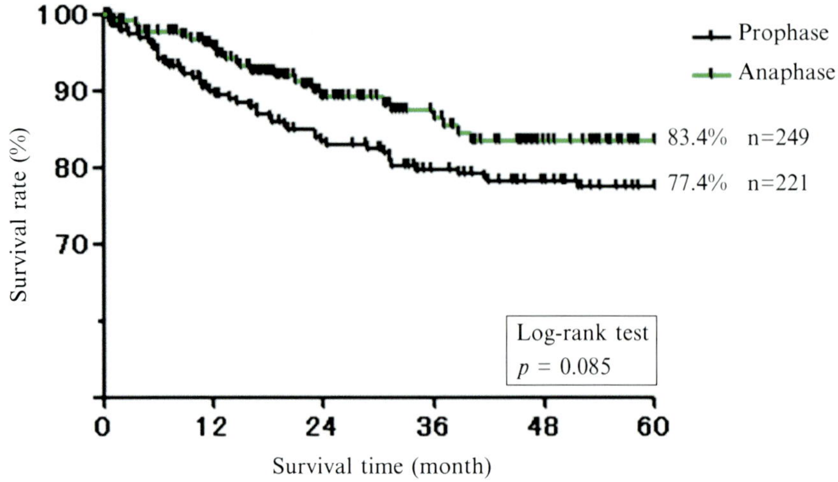

Fig. 1.9 Five-year survival rate (whole men and women). The first 10 years and later 10 years were analyzed separately

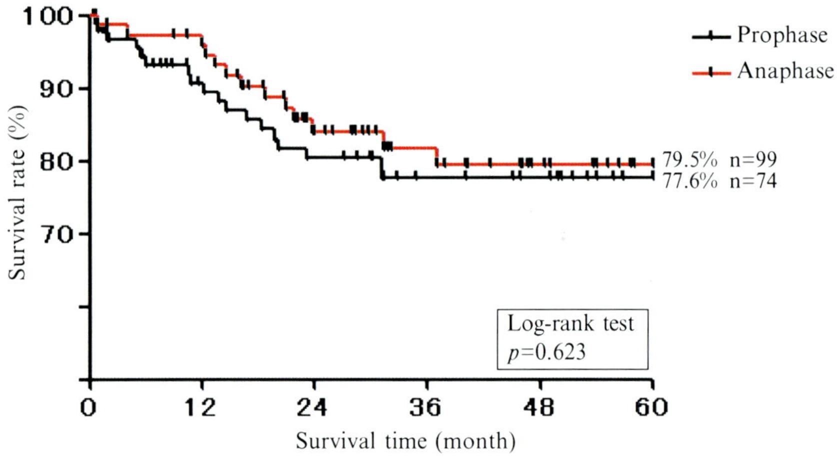

Fig. 1.10 Five-year survival rate (women). Five-year survival rate was lower in females than males

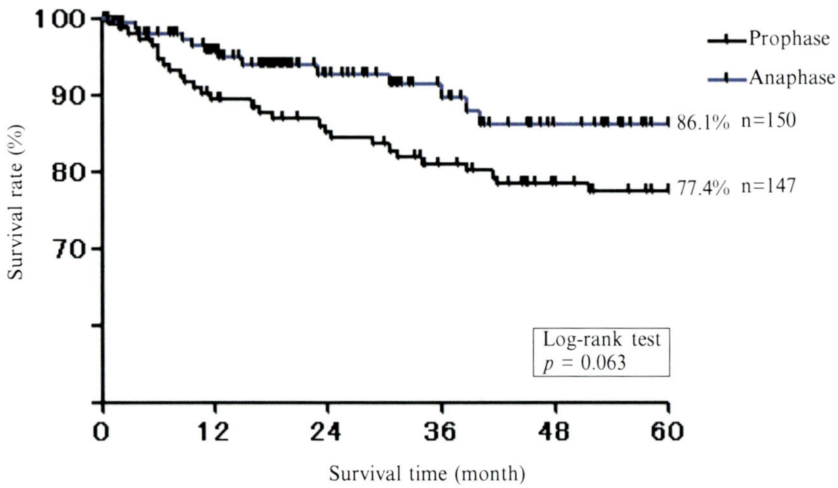

Fig. 1.11 Five-year survival rate (men). Five-year survival rate was lower in females than males

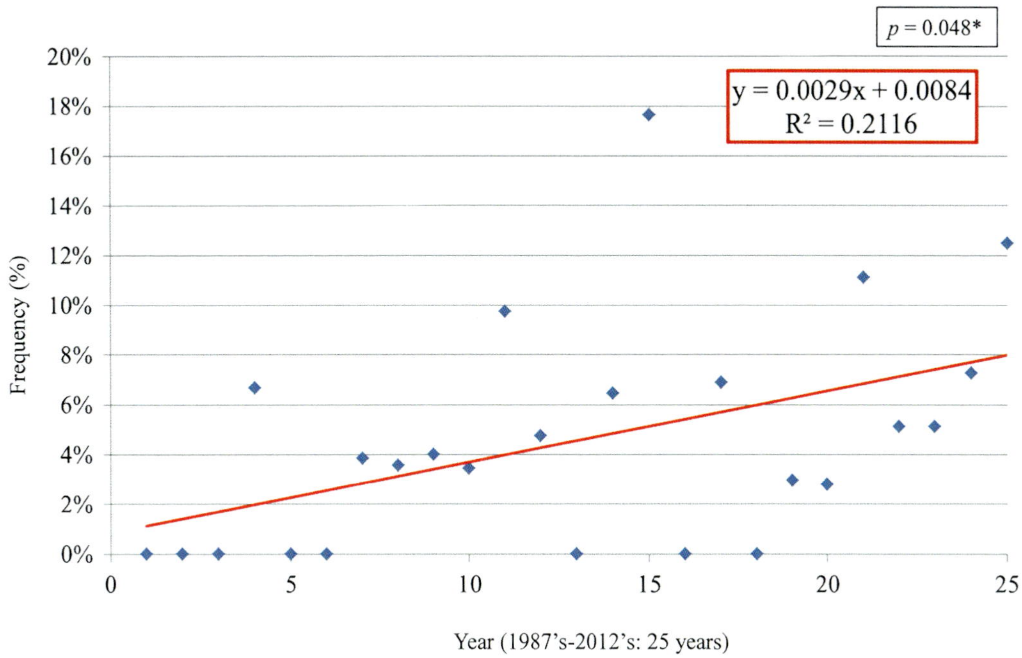

Fig. 1.12 Annual change in the rate of cancer in young patients (under 40 years old). Statistically significant increase was observed in annual changes in the rate of cancer in young individuals (below 40 years old) ($p = 0.048$)

strict definition of "young individuals," but many reports use 40 years old as a benchmark [30–36]. Our university has also examined for 25 years from 1987 to 2012, and the rate of oral cancer in young individuals below 40 years old was 37/758 cases (5.0 %), which was almost the same rate as reported from other facilities. On the other hand, statistically significant increase was observed in annual changes in the rate of cancer in young individuals (below 40 years old) (Fig. 1.12).

Critical causes include age, sex, smoking, alcohol consumption, virus, and mechanical factors such as poorly fitted prosthesis and sectorial tooth, and genetic abnormality. However, critical causes for young individuals are still unclear [32–34]. Many of the patients in our university had no smoking/drinking history; therefore, it was considered that mechanical factors including odontoparallaxis and malposition of a tooth might cause the cancers.

In addition, it has been known that male-to-female ratios of oral cancer in young individuals come closer to 1 [34]. The majority of primary sites were the tongue [30–34], and well-differentiated squamous cell cancers are often observed in terms of pathological appearance [32]. The male-to-female ratio in our university was 1.38, and a decrease in age was also observed as compared with a group of 40 years and older. Furthermore, the rate of primary sites was significantly high in the tongue, 76.3 %. For the degree of differentiation, the rate of well-differentiated cancers was 39.5 % (Table 1.4).

Table 1.4 Characteristics of young patients with oral cancer in our department (1987/1–2012/12, $n = 38$)

Patient characteristics	Young (under 40 years) $n = 38$
Age, median (range)	34 (19–40)
Sex, men/women (sex ratio)	22/16 (1.38)
Primary site (%)	
Tongue	29 (76.3)
Maxillary gingiva	5 (13.2)
Mandibular gingiva	1 (2.6)
Others	3 (7.9)
Follow-up median month (range)	35.8 (3.2–268.8)
Differentiation (%)	
Well	15 (39.5)
Others	23 (60.5)
Stage (%)	
I	11 (28.9)
II	9 (23.7)
III	9 (23.7)
IV	9 (23.7)

For prognosis in young individuals, there is not yet a unified view: some reports concluded that it was better in young individuals [34–36], some other reports concluded that it was almost the same [30, 32], and others concluded that it was poor in young individuals [33]. Results in our university indicated that young individuals had good outcome: 5-year overall survival rate was 94.3 %; 5-year relapse-free survival rate was 88.2 %. However, there was no statistically significant difference

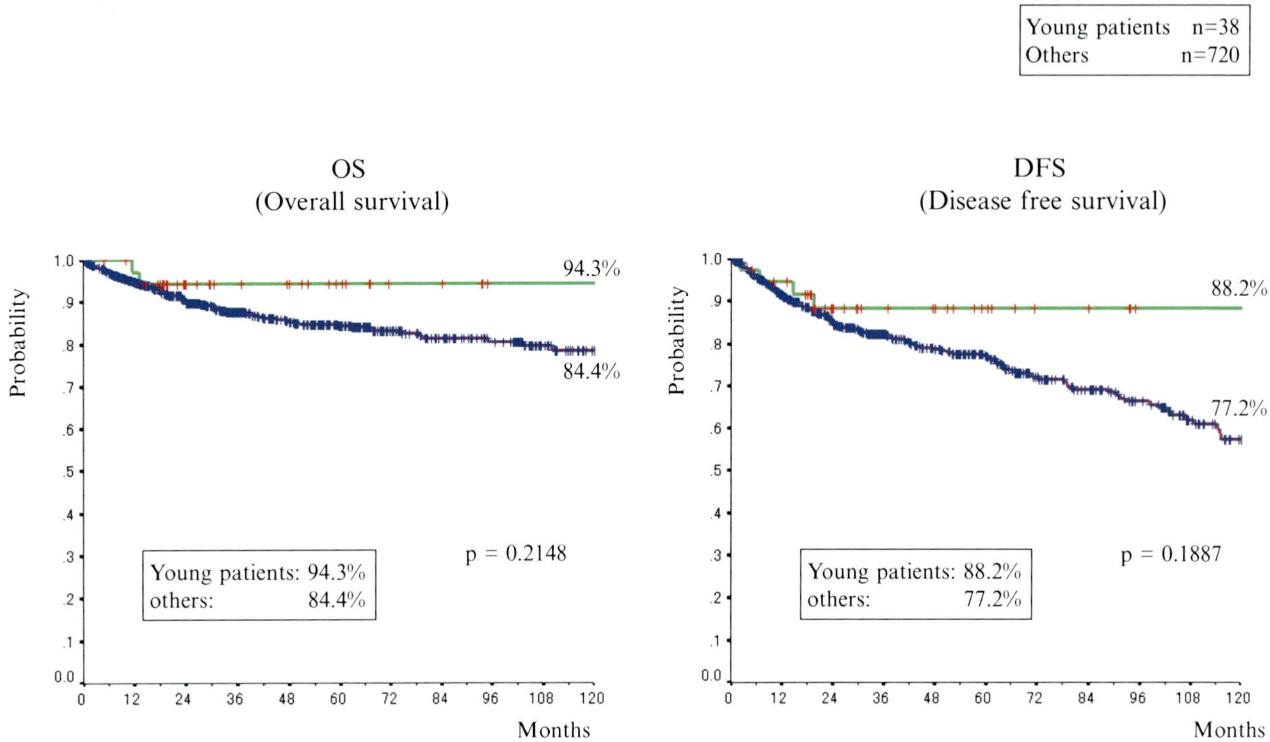

Fig. 1.13 The comparison between survival rates with young patients and others (1987/1–2012/12: 25 years). Five-year overall survival rate was 94.3 %; 5-year relapse-free survival rate was 88.2 %. However, there was no statistically significant difference as compared with a group of 40 years and older, and the rates were equivalent

as compared with a group of 40 years and older, and the rates were equivalent (Fig. 1.13). It is anticipated that pathogenic mechanism would be understood in the future.

10. Oral cancer and prevention
    (a) Three steps for cancer prevention
    A concept, which is adopted from the concept of natural disease prevention proposed by Leavell and Clark for cancer prevention, is the following:
    Primary prevention: To prevent the onset of cancer by reducing and eliminating risk factors of health issues
    Secondary prevention: To implement early detection and early treatment of cancer
    Tertiary prevention: To conduct rehabilitation to promote early return to society without increasing in severity of the cancer as much as possible and to prevent recurrence
    (b) Eight items for cancer prevention (Fig. 1.14)
    The National Cancer Center proposed "Evidence-based cancer prevention" in 2005. This is developed based on past enormous amount of statistics and experimental data and based on scientific evidence. This proposal concluded that about 60 % of the entire cancers (30 % by tobacco cessation and further 30 % by devices of dietary habits and others) could be prevented by implementing these eight items. This is beneficial information for us oral surgeons and also results in enlightenment of patients.
    (c) Summary of prevention
    Measures against smoking, drinking, diet, and infectious diseases are important for the primary prevention of oral cancer, that is to say, to avoid becoming oral cancer. Now, most of the patients with cancer and their families, or more widely the people, are increasingly demanding for cancer care. Therefore, it is most important to achieve the target of oral cancer prevention through cooperation among the following three bodies: (a) patients with cancer, their families, and people; (b) healthcare professionals; and (c) government and politics.

1.5 Precancerous Lesion

Leukoplakia is considered as a typical precancerous lesion because some of oral leukoplakia cases become malignant, and some cases diagnosed as leukoplakia have already become cancerous. Malignant transformation rate of oral leukoplakia is discussed in this section.

1. Stop smoking if you are a smoker. If you are not a smoker, avoid second-hand smoking wherever possible.
2. Moderate alcohol intake. More specifically, do not exceed 1 glass (180 ml) of Sake (a large bottle of beer) a day. If you have a low tolerance for alcohol, do not try to drink immoderately.
3. Try to take at least 400 g of vegetables and fruits a day. For example, take vegetables at every meal, and take fruits everyday.
4. Minimize intake of salt cured food products and salt. More specifically, limit your salt intake to less than 10 g a day. Limit intake of high salinity foods like salted fish guts and sea urchin eggs less than once a week.
5. Continuation of regular exercise. For example, moderate physical activities such as walking for about 60 minutes in total almost everyday, and intense exercise that makes you sweaty about once a week.
6. Maintain your body weight during adulthood (Do not become obese, do not become too thin.). More specifically, maintain your BMI between 20 and 27.

- BMI = body weight (kg) ÷ [body height(m)]^2

7. Minimize intake of hot food and hot beverage. For example, drink hot beverage after cooling.
8. Confirm the presence or absence of hepatitis virus infection, and take measures to treat (infected person) or prevent (uninfected person) the infection.

Fig. 1.14 "Evidence-based cancer prevention" proposed by the National Cancer Center

Precancerous lesion is defined as a tissue that underwent morphological changes, which is obviously likely to develop cancer as compared with normal tissues. Clinically it includes leukoplakia and erythroplakia, and histopathologically it includes epithelial dysplasia. Oral leukoplakia is a pathological white spot lesion due to hyperkeratosis of the oral mucosa and defined as a "significant white lesion of the oral mucosa, which cannot be characterized as any other diseases" [37].

Histopathologically, leukoplakia includes hyperkeratosis of epithelia (hyperorthokeratosis, acanthosis, or hyperparakeratosis), lesions associated with epithelial dysplasia, as well as carcinomas in situ and invasive cancers [38]. However, lesions diagnosed as carcinoma in situ or invasive cancer are not included in leukoplakia.

Malignant transformation rate of oral leukoplakia differs depending on race, lifestyle habits including smoking, treatment, and duration of observation period (duration of symptoms) in addition to the unclear definition of leukoplakia. The rate is reported as 0.13–17.5 % overseas [39, 40] and 3.1–16.3 % in Japan [41, 42]. The rate of malignant transformation becomes higher when an observation period becomes longer, and it is reported that 5-year cumulative malignant transformation rate was 1.2–14.5 %, and 10-year cumulative malignant transformation rate was 2.4–29.0 % [43]. Malignant transformation is affected by age, clinical types, sites, critical forms, and the presence or absence of epithelial dysplasia. Leukoplakia is more easily becoming cancerous in female patients as well as in patients of 50 years and older. It is considered that verrucous leukoplakia, nodular leukoplakia, ulcerous leukoplakia, and non-homogenous leukoplakia, which is an erythema mixed type, as well as other leukoplakias occurred in the movable mucosal tissues, especially in the tongue, buccal mucosa, and mouth floor, multicentric and multiple lesions and lesions with pathological epithelial dysplasia are prone to develop cancer [44, 45]. Furthermore, it is considered that lesions with higher degree of epithelial dysplasia develop cancers in shorter period [43].

1.6 Multiple Cancers and Double Cancers

Recently the number of multiple and double cancers is increasing. The causes include super-aging of patients, improvement of a cure rate in oral cancer, and exposure to a variety of carcinogens from diet and environmental factors. Favorite sites and frequency of double cancer in patients with head and neck cancer including oral cancer are explained in this section.

Plurally developed cancers are referred to as multiple primary cancers or multicentric cancers. Meanwhile, a number of cancers that occurred in the same organ are referred to as multiple cancers, and a number of cancers that occurred in

Table 1.5 Clinical features of multiple primary cancer

Case no.	Age	Gender	Drinking	Smoking	Site 1st	2nd	3rd	4th	5th	6th	7th	Carcinogenesis time	Observation period (month)	Outcome
1	63	M	No	No	T	T	–	–	–	–	–	Heterochronous	15	Alive
2	70	M	Yes	Yes	T	OF	–	–	–	–	–	Heterochronous	20	Alive
3	54	F	No	No	T	ManG	–	–	–	–	–	Heterochronous	30	Alive
4	55	F	No	No	MaxG	ManG	–	–	–	–	–	Heterochronous	33	Alive
5	73	M	No	No	MaxG	ManG	–	–	–	–	–	Heterochronous	79	Death
6	67	F	No	No	MaxG	ManG	–	–	–	–	–	Heterochronous	76	Death
7	82	F	No	No	MaxG	ManG	–	–	–	–	–	Heterochronous	25	Unknown
8	61	M	Yes	Yes	ManG	T	–	–	–	–	–	Heterochronous	33	Unknown
9	82	F	Yes	Yes	ManG	T	–	–	–	–	–	Heterochronous	54	Unknown
10	66	F	No	No	ManG	T	–	–	–	–	–	Heterochronous	108	Alive
11	74	M	Yes	No	ManG	T	–	–	–	–	–	Heterochronous	77	Alive
12	67	M	Yes	Yes	ManG	ManG	–	–	–	–	–	Heterochronous	52	Alive
13	67	M	No	Yes	ManG	ManG	–	–	–	–	–	Heterochronous	43	Alive
14	70	F	Yes	No	BM	T	–	–	–	–	–	Heterochronous	17	Alive
15	15	M	Yes	Yes	P	T	–	–	–	–	–	Heterochronous	25	Death
16	71	M	Yes	No	L	MaxG	ManG	–	–	–	–	Heterochronous	42	Alive
17	59	F	No	No	MaxG	L	BM	T	–	–	–	Heterochronous	137	Alive
18	70	F	No	No	ManG	MaxG	T	MaxG	–	–	–	Heterochronous	78	Death
19	84	F	Yes	No	L	ManG	T	ManG	–	–	–	Synchronous	0	Alive
20	59	F	No	No	MaxG	MaxG	MaxG	L	ManG	P	–	Synchronous	34	Death
21	78	F	Yes	No	OF	T	–	–	–	–	–	Heterochronous	16	Alive
22	58	F	Yes	No	ManG	ManG	–	–	–	–	–	Heterochronous	55	Alive
23	71	F	Yes	No	MaxG	BM	T	MaxG	MaxG	BM	BM	Heterochronous	43	Alive
24	72	M	Yes	No	T	T	–	–	–	–	–	Synchronous	0	Alive
25	74	F	Yes	No	ManG	BM	–	–	–	–	–	Heterochronous	42	Alive
26	68	F	Yes	No	BM	BM	–	–	–	–	–	Synchronous	5	Alive

T tongue, *ManG* mandibular gingiva, *MaxG* maxillary gingiva, *OF* oral floor, *BM* buccal mucosa, *P* palate, *L* lip

different organs are referred to as double cancers. These are divided into synchronous type and metachronous type according to the timing of development [46–48].

It is considered that most of cancers that redundantly occurred with oral cancer are upper digestive tract cancer and lung cancer, and frequency of double cancers is 11.0–16.2 % [49].

Results of our clinical study on multiple cancers and double cancers treated by authors are shown here. Multiple cancer subjects included 696 patients with oral squamous cell cancer who visited Department of Dental Surgery, Tokyo Dental College during a period of over 26 years from 1982 to 2008, and double cancer subjects included 497 patients during a period of over 16 years since the introduction of endoscopic examination from 1992 to 2008. As a result (Tables 1.5 and 1.6), multiple cancers occurred in 26 of 696 patients (3.7 %). Primary site of the multiple cancers was the lip in most cases (18.2 %), and the highest number of multiple cancers was the 7th cancer. On the other hand, double cancers occurred in 43 of 497 patients (8.7 %). Most of double cancers occurred as esophageal cancer (58.1 %). Most of double oral cancers occurred in the oral floor (32.6 %). The outcome of double cancers included 12 survivals (48.8 %), 16 deaths (37.2 %) (including 8 deaths due to the original disease, 3 deaths due to esophageal cancer, 2 deaths due to stomach cancer, and 3 deaths due to other diseases), and 6 unknown cases (20.0 %). Five-year survival rate of oral cancers alone was 77.8 %, and 10-year survival rate was 73.2 % with Kaplan–Meier analysis. Meanwhile, for double cancers, 5-year survival rate of oral cancer alone was 64.7 %, and 10-year survival rate was 49.3 % and low. Significant difference in survival rate was observed between double cancers and oral cancers alone with log-rank test ($P<0.01$) (Fig. 1.15). The outcome of multiple cancers included 18 survivals (69.2 %), 5 deaths (19.2 %) (including 4 deaths due to the original disease and 1 death due to other disease), and 3 unknown cases (11.5 %).

Characteristics of double cancers in patients with head and neck cancer including oral cancer include that the occurrence frequency is rapidly increasing for the last 20 years, that most of second cancers occur in the surrounding areas, that the second cancer often occurred after treatment for head and neck cancer, and that 60–70 % of double cancers occurred in the upper digestive tract or lung [50].

An explanation for that the double cancer often occurs with the upper digestive tract includes the concept of field

Table 1.6 Clinical features of double cancer

Case no.	Age	Gender	Drinking	Smoking	Primary site	Carcinogenesis time	Observation period (month)	Outcome
1	43	M	Yes	Yes	ManG	Synchronous	0	Unknown
2	68	M	Yes	Yes	T	Synchronous	6	Death
3	62	M	Yes	Yes	T	Synchronous	68	Alive
4	46	F	Yes	No	ManG	Synchronous	104	Alive
5	58	M	Yes	Yes	BM	Heterochronous	71	Alive
6	64	M	Yes	Yes	P	Synchronous	110	Alive
7	52	M	Yes	Yes	T	Synchronous	24	Death
8	73	M	Yes	Yes	MaxG	Heterochronous	12	Death
9	49	M	Yes	Yes	OF	Synchronous	81	Alive
10	69	M	Yes	Yes	ManG	Heterochronous	30	Death
11	54	M	Yes	Yes	OF	Synchronous	24	Death
12	51	M	Yes	Yes	T	Synchronous	0	Unknown
13	60	M	Yes	Yes	OF	Synchronous	36	Death
14	67	M	Yes	Yes	T	Synchronous	107	Alive
15	75	M	Yes	Yes	OF	Synchronous	36	Death
16	72	M	Yes	Yes	T	Synchronous	41	Alive
17	58	M	Yes	Yes	OF	Heterochronous	33	Alive
18	66	M	Yes	Yes	MaxG	Heterochronous	94	Alive
19	61	M	Yes	Yes	BM	Synchronous	0	Unknown
20	73	M	Yes	Yes	T	Synchronous	38	Alive
21	63	M	Yes	Yes	MaxG	Synchronous	0	Unknown
22	70	M	Yes	Yes	T	Heterochronous	58	Alive
23	83	M	Yes	Yes	MaxG	Synchronous	0	Unknown
24	63	M	Yes	Yes	T	Synchronous	6	Death
25	55	M	Yes	Yes	MaxG	Synchronous	0	Unknown
26	60	M	Yes	Yes	OF	Heterochronous	120	Death
27	62	M	Yes	Yes	OF	Heterochronous	46	Alive
28	62	M	Yes	Yes	OF	Synchronous	62	Alive
29	67	M	Yes	Yes	P	Heterochronous	87	Death
30	64	M	Yes	Yes	OF	Synchronous	30	Alive
31	72	M	Yes	Yes	ManG	Synchronous	51	Alive
32	69	M	Yes	Yes	T	Synchronous	6	Death
33	52	F	Yes	Yes	T	Heterochronous	120	Death
34	68	M	Yes	Yes	ManG	Synchronous	72	Death
35	63	F	Yes	Yes	BM	Synchronous	6	Death
36	53	M	Yes	Yes	T	Synchronous	17	Alive
37	67	M	Yes	Yes	OF	Synchronous	31	Death
38	55	F	Yes	No	ManG	Synchronous	33	Alive
39	62	F	No	No	OF	Synchronous	45	Alive
40	64	F	No	No	OF	Synchronous	103	Alive
41	70	F	Yes	Yes	OF	Synchronous	17	Death
42	57	M	Yes	Yes	OF	Synchronous	115	Alive
43	63	M	Yes	Yes	ManG	Synchronous	24	Alive

T tongue, *ManG* mandibular gingiva, *MaxG* maxillary gingiva, *OF* oral floor, *BM* buccal mucosa, *P* palate

cancerization because the oral cavity, pharynx, esophagus, and stomach are under the same carcinogenic environment [51]. Furthermore, background factors of double cancers of oral cancer include sex, lifestyle habits, and excessive smoking and drinking [52–55].

Complication of precancerous lesion such as oral leukoplakia [40, 56] and the existence of double cancers have influences on therapeutic choice and treatment results for oral cancer [57, 58]. Therefore, examination of the upper digestive tract and lungs is required before and after the treatment [59–61].

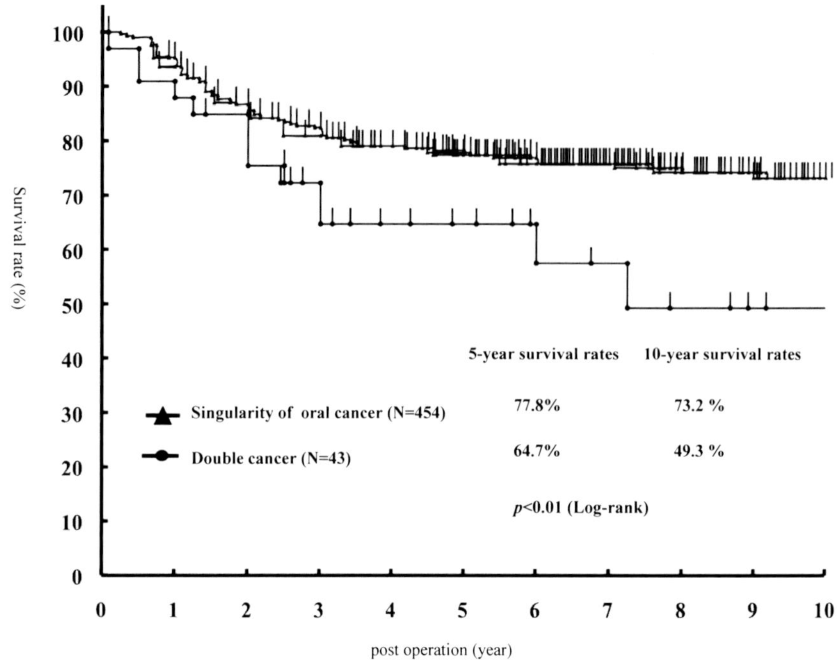

Fig. 1.15 Relations with double cancer and prognosis. Significant difference in survival rate was observed between double cancers and oral cancers alone ($P<0.01$)

1.7 Oral Cancer Screening

1. Oral cancer screening in Japan

Mass screening for gastric cancer, uterine cancer, breast cancer, lung cancer, and colorectal cancer has already been implemented in Japan, and it is known that prognosis of cancers detected with such mass screening is extremely good as compared to that of non-screened population [62–67]. Early detection and early treatment are most important to improve the cure rate of oral cancer and cancer in other organs. Oral cancer screening conducted in Japan is shown in Fig. 1.16. Oral cancer screening has been reported since around 1985. Most of the screenings are conducted in collaboration among dental associations in cities and towns, dental surgery departments of dental schools and dental oral surgery departments of medical schools, and dental oral surgery departments of major hospitals [68–73]. Currently oral cancer screenings conducted by dentists are divided into screening at mass level (mass screening) and at individual level (individual screening).

Most of mass screenings are regularly conducted in collaboration with the government, dentists, and dental oral surgery departments of university hospitals and national, prefectural, municipal, and other public hospitals. In addition, oral mucosal diseases are incorporated into examination items for dental checkup conducted in business places in some cases.

For individual screenings, on the other hand, dental examination and oral cancer screening are often conducted in dentistry of hospitals as optional screening for complete medical checkups. In addition, oral cancer screening is also conducted in dental clinics focusing on prevention. Furthermore, an endeavor to implement oral cancer screening in general private dental clinics is recently attempted in cooperation with dentists and dental oral surgery departments and clinical laboratory of major hospitals, and their performances are reported [74].

Authors have been conducting oral cancer screening and educational activities about oral health every year in cooperation with dental associations since 1992. Here, we would like to introduce current oral cancer screening conducted in our department and future perspective.

2. Flow and method of mass screening of oral cancer (Fig. 1.17)

Subjects of screening are recruited through city bulletin, posters, newspapers, or TV in advance and accept reservation for all subjects to avoid confusion on the day of screening. Subjects are males and females of 40 years or older in consideration of a cancer-prone age. First, subjects are asked to fill out a questionnaire. Mainly history talking, visual inspection, and palpation are performed based on this questionnaire. Members of dental associations conduct preliminary examination, and then dental surgery specialists, who are mainly engaged in the diagnosis and treatment of oral cancer in our department, conduct direct medical examination. The subjects are referred to a secondary medical facility when some kind of abnormity was found and determined that close examination is required. We also positively provide consultation and direction for oral diseases other than cancers.

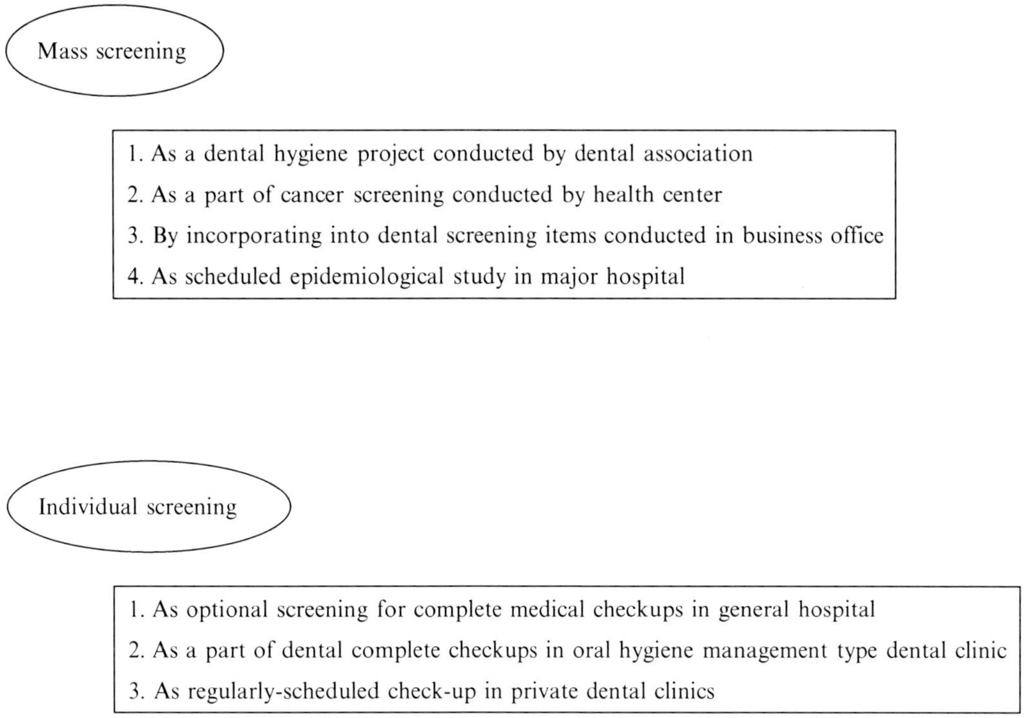

Fig. 1.16 Oral cancer screening currently conducted in Japan

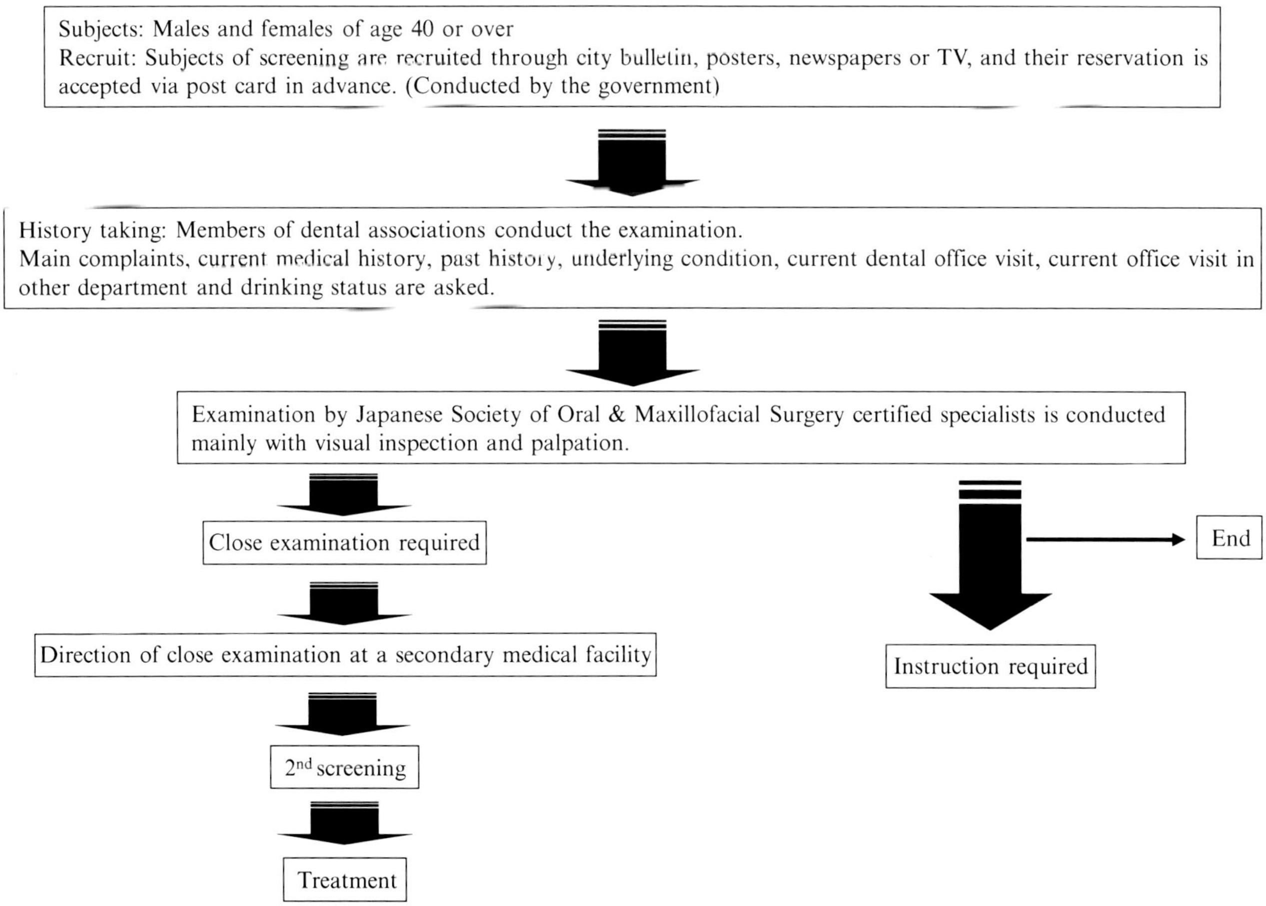

Fig. 1.17 Flow and method of mass screening for oral cancer

Table 1.7 Result of mass screening

Discovery rate of oral cancer (%)	0.01
Rate of patients requiring close examination (%)	7.10
Rate of cancer in the patients required close examination (%)	1.27
Discovery rate of precancerous lesion (%)	0.52

	Oral cancer[a]	Stomach cancer	Lung cancer	Colorectal cancer	Uterine cancer	Breast cancer
Total patients who received cancer screening (*n*)	9,934	4,262,048	7,506,113	7,176,312	3,538,132	1,892,834
Patients who required close examination (*n*)	706	427,949	211,154	521,695	40,023	161,971
Patients with discovered cancer (*n*)	9	6,551	3,516	12,284	1,921	5,193
Percentage of the patients who received cancer screening (%)	0.01	0.15	0.05	0.17	0.05	0.27
Percentage of the patients who required close examination (%)	1.27	1.53	1.67	2.35	4.80	3.21

Data for stomach cancer, lung cancer, colorectal cancer, uterine cancer, and breast cancer are excerpts from the project report of healthcare of the aged (2007) by Health, Labour and Welfare Ministry

[a]Data for oral cancers are obtained in authors' department (for 20 years from 1992 to 2011)

3. Results of mass screening of oral cancer (Table 1.7)
   People in their 50's and 60's, called cancer-prone ages, accounted for most of patients who underwent the mass screening of oral cancer. The number of patients who underwent the screening was 9,934 (males, 2,480; females, 7,454) for two decades from 1992 to 2011. The number of female patients was 3 times higher than male patients, which indicated that females have a higher level of interest in the screening than males.

   The motive for visiting the office for the screening included request for close examination although having no particular subjective symptoms (38 %), which was the highest, followed by chief complaints (swelling, bleeding, pain) about gingiva (35 %), chief complaints (pain or uncomfortable sensation of the tongue) about tongue (19 %), and chief complaints about oral mucosa (18 %).

   The most common diagnosis was gingivitis and periodontitis (11 %), followed by glossodynia and stomatitis (10 %) and benign tumor (3 %); and leukoplakia, lichen planus, xerostomia, and ptyalolithiasis were also observed and varied. Three cases of oral cancers were found in the past screening, and the discovery rate of oral cancer was 0.14 % in the screening participants for 20 years. The rate of oral cancer occurrence is estimated to be 1 in 100,000 patients; therefore, it may be said that this discovery rate is high.
4. Eight items for early detection of oral cancer (Fig. 1.18)
   It is very important how to find early cancers efficiently by extracting high-risk group of people with drinking and smoking habits for screening through oral cancer examination. Therefore, we distribute a pamphlet for general readers entitled "Eight items for early detection of oral cancer—Have no fear but oral cancer with early discovery," which explains subjective and objective symptoms to look out for oral mucosal lesion in an easily understood manner.
5. Significance of implementation of oral cancer screening
   Oral cancer tends to develop in the sites where it is relatively easy to detect at an early stage with visual inspection and palpation; however, early detection is not adequately realized in the present circumstances. Taking the increase in the prevalence of oral cancer together, early detection should be realized more than now. Mass screening is one of the important measures.

   Ohno et al. [75] described conditions for conducting a cancer screening as follows: (1) the prevalence and mortality of the cancer are high; (2) the method is collectively applicable; (3) the method has high diagnostic accuracy; (4) early detection and early treatment have a therapeutic effect on the cancer; (5) the cost efficiency is balanced; (6) it is efficient and effective; and (7) the method is safe. There was a significance of implementation of oral cancer screening as compared with our results, 0.14 % of discovery rate of oral cancer in our mass screening for 20 years.
6. Current status of oral cancer screening overseas
   Most of cancer screenings currently conducted in Japan included local screenings implemented by the administrative authorities based on the Health and Medical Services Act for the Aged and occupational field screenings. In addition, some cancer screenings are conducted aiming at studying to evaluate accuracy of the screening method and efficacy of the screening in certain model areas. Such efforts are implemented in the USA and in other parts of the world.

   A preventive campaign against oral cancer in the USA has been conducted mainly by the American Dental Association (hereinafter referred to as ADA), which plays a central role. Investigation of the campaign has been started from 1996, and then a full-scale campaign was started from the fall of 2003. The main framework of the campaign was established and implemented in accordance with a national policy for laryngeal and oral cancer prevention proposed by the US government.

1. Wart-like white bulge, which often found in the gingiva or buccal mucosa, and have almost no symptoms.

2. White spot slightly raised from the surrounding normal mucosa with ruggedness and irregularity on the surface or partial red parts.

3. A mucosal wound caused by stimulus with edging or spring of denture or sharp edge of a tooth, and does not cure even after 2 weeks or more.

4. When there is no obvious wound on the surface of the mucosa but there is a hard lump with unclear border and without pain under the mucosa, and it gradually becomes bigger.

5. A mucosal wound of unknown cause, and does not cure even after 2 weeks or more.

6. When a wound after dental extraction is hard to heal, and red and easily-bleeding bulging spots of flesh when touching is appearing from the wound site.

7. Certain area of the mucosal surface became red and broke out in sores, and hard to heal.
8. When you have a pain of unknown cause, and this pain gradually changes to numbness.

Meanwhile, if you have cancer patients among parents and brothers and sisters, you are prone to develop cancer by constitution. Please keep your eye on these symptoms.
In addition, smoking and high concentration of alcoholic drinks become carcinogenic stimulation. You had better abstain from them if possible.

Fig. 1.18 Eight items for early discovery of oral cancer

In brief, the campaign is dealt with by state governments state by state, and the state governments establish a system for screening in collaboration with universities, dental associations, and health service-related organizations. At the same time, education for dentists as well as staff who engage in the operation is conducted. This is mainly conducted within a postgraduate education program in dental school of universities. Furthermore, it is proposed that it is important to ensure budget and monetary resources for prosecution of the program and to incorporate the oral cancer screening into private insurance program to continue this effort. The final goal of this screening is to enlighten the nation about oral cancer prevention including risk factors of oral cancer such as smoking and drinking.

7. Future perspectives and the latest navigation system for oral cancer screening
It is a future subject how to promote screening of males aged 40 or over with drinking and/or smoking habits, who have especially high risk of oral cancer in the general population. However, current approach cannot narrow down a target to this high-risk group. Accordingly, for example, it is considered that the examination rate of the high-risk group may increase if oral cancer screening can be incorporated into dental checkups conducted in companies and health insurance associations. In addition, we believe that diagnostic techniques for oral mucosal disease and oral cancer can be disseminated by conducting existing oral cancer screening in cooperation with local dentists.

Moreover, the "navigation system for oral cancer screening [76]" started from 2012 is a system that author's department answers questions from general dental clinics about individual examination, as a control center. The system is characterized by support for necessary close examination and referral to higher-level medical facilities, and provision of opinion of specialists at chairside. Popularization of this system all over the country and construction of standardized oral cancer screening are expected in the future.

References

1. Cancer Information Service, Center for Cancer Control and Information Services, National Cancer Center, Japan. Summary of the latest statistics for cancer in Japan. ganjoho.jp
2. Tominaga S, Oshima A, Ishiguro T et al (eds) (1999) White paper on cancer statistics: affection, death, prognosis. Shinoharashinsha Publisher Inc, Tokyo, pp 159–170
3. Foundation for Promotion of Cancer Research (2009) Cancer statistics 2008. Foundation for Promotion of Cancer Research, Tokyo, pp 26–29
4. Sobue T (2005) Update on cancer prevention and screening. Curr Treat Cancer 12:5–34
5. Tanaka S, Sobue T (2005) Comparison of oral and pharyngeal cancer mortality in five countries: France, Italy, Japan, UK and USA from WHO mortality database (1960–2000). Jpn J Clin Oncol 35:488–491
6. Japan Society for Oral Tumors and Japanese Society of Oral and Maxillofacial Surgeons Co-Edition (2013) Evidence based guidelines for oral cancer care, 2013th edn. Kanehara, Tokyo
7. Japan Society for Oral Tumors Edition (2010) Handling stipulations for oral cancer, 1st edn. Kanehara, Tokyo

8. Japan Society for Head and Neck Cancer Edition (2012) Handling stipulations for head and neck cancer, 5th edn. Kanehara, Tokyo
9. Hermanek P (ed) (1997) UICC international union against cancer. TNM atlas, 4th edn. Springer, New York
10. Krolls SO, Hoffman S (1976) Squamous cell of the oral soft tissues: a statistic analysis of 14,253 cases by age, sex, and race of patients. JADA 92:571–574
11. Kirida T, Zheng Y, Kurumaya N et al (1997) Epidemiological study of oral cancer in Japan: changes and future prospects. Jpn J Oral Maxillofac Surg 43:140–147
12. Uchida Y (1988) Epidemiological study of based on national statistics of dental surgery for oral cancer: 1497 cases in 1986. J Jpn Assoc Dental Sci 7:16–26
13. Clinical Staging System on TNM Classification (1989) Material for study on TNM classification for head and neck area (Trends in TNM classification and primary treatment of cases in 1986). Head and neck area subcommittee edition
14. Ariyoshi Y, Shimabara M, Omura K et al (2006) Epidemiological research 2002 on malignant tumor of stomatognathic area visited Japanese society of oral and maxillofacial surgery designated training facilities designated. Jpn J Oral Maxillofac Surg 52:401–410
15. Bolt WJ, McLaughlin JK, Winn DM et al (1988) Smoking and drinking in relation to oral and pharyngeal cancer. Cancer Res 48:3282–3287
16. Gupta PC, Mehta FS, Daftary DK et al (1980) Incidence rates of oral cancer and natural history of oral precancerous lesions in a 10-year follow-up study of Indian villagers. Community Dent Oral Epidemiol 8:283–333
17. Petti S, Scully C (2005) Oral cancer: the association between nation-based alcohol-drinking profiles and oral cancer mortality. Oral Oncol 41:828–834
18. Sankaranarayanan R, Ramadas K, Thomas G et al (2005) Effect of screening on oral cancer mortality in Kerala, India: a cluster-randomised controlled trial. Lancet 365:1972–1933
19. Khanna JN, Andrade NN (1995) Oral submucous fibrosis: a new concept in management, report of 100 cases. Int J Oral Maxillofac Surg 24:433–439
20. Shibahara T, Noma H, Kakizawa T et al (2002) Oral cancer research with an emphasis on genomic analysis. Bull Tokyo Dent Coll 43:209–222
21. Wynder EL, Bross IJ, Feldman RM (1957) A study of the etiological factors in cancer of the mouth. Cancer 10:1300–1323
22. Kamiyama I, Ikuno T, Narita M et al (2005) A study of drinking smoking as carcinogens in the oral cancer. Shikwa Gakuho 105:446–452
23. The Ministry of Health and Welfare (1995) Smoking and health, 2nd edn. Hokendojinsha Inc, Tokyo
24. Takeshi N, Chihaya T, Tomohiro Y et al (2003) A clinical study of double cancers in patients with oral squamous cell carcinoma. J Korean Assoc Oral Maxillofac Surg 29:278
25. International Agency for Research on Cancer (1988) Alcohol drinking. In: IARC monographs on the evaluation of the carcinogenic risks to humans, vol 44. IARC, Lyon
26. Homann N, Tillonen J, Rintamäki H et al (2001) Poor dental status increases acetaldehyde production from ethanol in saliva: a possible link to increased oral cancer risk among heavy drinkers. Oral Oncol 37:153–158
27. Takeshi N, Hiroyasu N, Takahiko S et al (2000) Aldehyde dehydrogenase 2 and glutathione S-transferase M1 polymorphisms in relation to the risk for oral cancer in Japanese drinkers. Oral Oncol 36:42–46
28. Stefania B, Mia H, Paola G et al (2009) Aldehyde dehydrogenase 2 and head and neck cancer: a meta-analysis implementing a mendelian randomization approach. Cancer Epidemiol Biomarkers Prev 18:248–254
29. Yeudall WA (1993) Human papilloma viruses and oral neoplasia. Oral Oncol Eur J Cancer Res 53:4811–4816
30. Myers JN, Elkins T, Roberts D et al (2000) Squamous cell carcinoma of the tongue in young adults: increasing incidence and factors that predict treatment outcomes. Otolaryngol Head Neck Surg 122:44–51
31. Stimson PS, Guo-Pci Y (2002) Head and neck cancer incidence trends in young Americans, 1973–1997, with special analysis for tongue cancer. Arch Otolaryngol 128:268–274
32. Maruoka Y, Ando T, Ogiuchi Y et al (2005) Squamous cell carcinoma of the tongue in patients less than forty. Jpn J Oral Diag 18:214–218
33. Saito Y, Takahara M, Knazawa H et al (1996) Clinico-statistical analysis of oral carcinoma in young patients. Jpn J Oral Maxillofac Surg 42:503–505
34. Takahara T, Fujitani T, Inoue K et al (1988) Cancer of the oral cavity and oropharynx in patients less than 40 years of age: clinical appearance and treatment results. J Otolaryngol Jpn 91:204–209
35. Garavello W, Spreafico R, Gaini RM et al (2007) Oral tongue cancer in young patients: a matched analysis. Oral Oncol 43:894–897
36. Hasegawa H, Matsuura H, Ito Y et al (1995) Squamous cell carcinoma of the tongue in patients under 40 years of age. Head Neck Cancer 21:93–98
37. Pindborg JJ, Reichart PA, Smith CJ et al (1997) Histological typing of cancer and precancer of the oral mucosa, 2nd edn. Springer, Berlin
38. Waldron CA, Shafer WG (1975) Leukoplakia revisited. A clinicopathologic study of 3,256 oral leukoplakias. Cancer 36:1386–1392
39. Silverman S, Bhargava K, Smith LW et al (1976) Malignant transformation and natural history of oral leukoplakia in 57,518 industrial workers of Gujarat, India. Cancer 38:1790–1795
40. Silverman S Jr, Gorsky M, Francina L et al (1984) Oral leukoplakia and malignant transformation. A follow-up study of 257 patients. Cancer 53:563–568
41. Washizu K, Ono I, Ebihara T et al (1981) Clinical study of oral precancerous stage. Jpn J Cancer Clin 27:942–947
42. Kurokawa H, Yamasaki K, Yamashita Y et al (1998) Clinicopathological study on oral leukoplakia. J Jpn Stomatol Soc 47:61–67
43. Amagasa T, Yamashiro M, Ishikawa H et al (2006) Oral leukoplakia related to malignant transformation. Oral Sci Int 3:45–55
44. Washizu K (1981) Study of early diagnosis and establishment of criterion for treatment in tongue cancer. Reports of studies funded by grant-in-aid for cancer research from The Ministry of Health and Welfare1980. National Cancer Center, Japan, pp 462–470
45. Ohta K, Katsumoto A, Misumi S et al (2003) Clinicopathological study of oral leukoplakia. Jpn J Oral Maxillofac Surg 49:439–445
46. Warren S, Gates O (1932) Multiple primary malignant tumors, a surgery of the literature and a statistical study. Am J Cancer 16:1358–1414
47. Moertel CG, Dockerty MB, Baggenstoss AH et al (1961) Multiple primary malignant neoplasms. I. Introduction and presentation of data. Cancer 14:221–230
48. Tanaka A, Tsuchikawa K, Tsuchimochi M et al (1994) Clinical study of multiple primary cancers, highlighting on the oral and maxillofacial region. Head Neck Cancer 20:57–62
49. Miyahara H (2004) Introduction to head and neck tumor. Igakusha, Tokyo, pp 61–68
50. Horiuchi M (2001) Double cancer in head and neck cancer cases. Illustrated new otorhinolaryngology, head-neck surgery course, head and neck tumor, vol 5. Medical View Co. Ltd, Tokyo, pp 8–9
51. Thomson PJ (2002) Field change and oral cancer: new evidence for widespread carcinogenesis? Int J Oral Maxillofac Surg 31:262–266
52. Kawakami M, Ikemura K (2004) Multiple primary malignant tumors in patients with squamous cell carcinoma of the oral cavity: influence on the 5-year survival rate. J Jpn Stomatol Soc 53:9–13
53. Nakamizo M, Kamata N, Kawabata K et al (1993) Double cancer and history of smoking and drinking in head and neck cancer: analysis based on person-year method. J Otolaryngol Jpn 96: 1501–1509

54. Yambe M, Tohnai I, Ueda M et al (1996) A case-control study of oral cancer part 1. Relation to smoking, drinking and dietary habits. Jpn J Oral Maxillofac Surg 42:42–50
55. Blot WJ, McLaughlin JK, Winn DM et al (1988) Smoking and drinking in relation to oral and pharyngeal cancer. Cancer Res 48:3282–3287
56. Shibuya H, Amagasa T, Seto K et al (1986) Leukoplakia-associated multiple carcinomas in patients with tongue carcinoma. Cancer 57:843–846
57. Kawabe R, Omura S, Saito T et al (1999) Risk factors for multiple primary squamous cell carcinomas of the oral cavity. Jpn J Oral Maxillofac Surg 45:421–426
58. Shibuya H, Hisamitsu S, Shioiri S et al (1987) Multiple primary cancer risk in patients with squamous cell carcinoma of the oral cavity. Cancer 60:3083–3086
59. Saikawa M, Ebihara S, Yoshizumi T et al (1991) Multiple primary cancers in patients with squamous cell carcinoma of the oral cavity. Jpn J Cancer Res 82:40–45
60. Yamamoto T, Katayama K, Ueda E et al (2004) A clinical investigation on oral carcinoma patients with ectopic second primary carcinomas: especially on the importance of second primary carcinomas. J Jpn Stomatol Soc 53:161–166
61. McGuirt WF (1982) Panendoscopy as a screening examination for simultaneous primary tumors in head and neck cancer: a prospective sequential study and review of the literature. Laryngoscope 92:569–576
62. Yamada T, Ikeda S, Iwasaki M et al (1999) Summary of national survey of digestive system mass screening 1996, I. Summary of national survey of gastric mass screening, II. Summary of national survey of colorectal mass screening, III. Summary of national survey of esophageal and liver mass screenings. Jpn Soc Gastroenterol Mass Surv 37:212–230
63. Shigematsu T (1992) Group medical examination and screening. its concept and requirements. J Jpn Med Assoc 107:517–521
64. Yanagawa H, Sakata K, Tsukuda A (1992) Current circumstances and issues of cancer mass screening. J Jpn Med Assoc 107:522–526
65. Oshima A (1992) Basics of evaluation techniques for cancer mass screening. J Jpn Med Assoc 107:527–530
66. Koinuma N (1992) Cancer mass screening as viewed from the economic perspective. J Jpn Med Assoc 107:531–535
67. Watanabe S (1992) 5. Mass screening in cancer countermeasures. J Jpn Med Assoc 107:536–541
68. Ikeda N, Ishii T, Iida S et al (1988) A study of mass screening for oral mucosal diseases of adults. Jpn J Oral Maxillofac Surg 34:2394–2402
69. Yamamoto N, Nomura T, Takeda E et al (2005) The present conditions and the future prospects of oral cancer examination running in our department: the oral cancer examination cooperated with dental society. Shikwa Gakuho 105:96–102
70. Ohno K, Yamamoto N, Nomura T et al (2009) Mass examination for oral cancer with Narashino city dental association: clinical data from past 10 years. Shikwa Gakuho 109:270–275
71. Nomura T, Kasahara K, Takagi R et al (2009) Future prospects for screening for oral cancer: 11-year clinical study by Tokyo dental college and Sakura-region dental association. Shikwa Gakuho 109:362–368
72. Sugahara K, Takahashi M, Kawachi H et al (2010) Government mass screening examination of oral cancer in Ichihara city. J J Gerodont 25:340–346
73. Shibahara T, Nomura T, Yamauchi T et al (2011) Effectiveness of mass screening for oral cancer: cooperated with Chiba city dental association duration 20 years. Head Neck Cancer 37:381–385
74. Tanaka Y (2012) Detecting early-stage oral cancer, close teamwork with general hospital and dental office and role of pathology. Shikwa Gakuho 112:22–31
75. Ohno Y, Yanagawa H (1986) Adult health manual (III-3 cancer prevention and countermeasures). Nanzando, Tokyo, pp 136–153
76. Bessho H, Shibahara T (2013) Oral cancer screening navigation system for general practitioner. Quintessence 32:79–87

2 Surgical Pathology of Oral Cancer

Toshiyuki Izumo

Abstract

This chapter reviews the surgical pathologic findings that provided the framework for the General Rules for Clinical and Pathological Studies on Oral Cancer (first edition), which currently serves as the common foundation for the diagnosis, treatment, and study of oral cancer in Japan. Although oral cancer varies from case to case, the clinical findings to which attention should be paid were determined for different cancer types after investigating the factors that can be used to accurately predict clinical manifestations and prognosis. It took approximately 10 years to accumulate a sufficient number of cases and perform data analysis, the findings of which were amassed in the general rules, thereby providing the current notions on oral cancer. We also review the pathologic and prognostic factors, such as clinical type, tumor depth, and invasion route; oral intraepithelial neoplasia/carcinoma in situ; and the histopathological factors associated with malignancy, such as mode of invasion and mode of mandibular invasion.

Keywords

Bone infiltration pattern • Intraepithelial neoplasia • Oral cancer • Prognostic factor • Surgical pathology

2.1 Introduction

For medical professionals in different disciplines to have common knowledge for the diagnosis, treatment, and study of oral cancer, it is necessary to establish criteria and general rules for the management of oral cancer, as exists for other cancers, in Japan. Proper oral cancer general rules will enable the same standards to be used to search imaging, surgical, and pathological findings of oral cancers and to understand the intricate pathology. Useful information should also be accumulated on actual clinical cases across institutions. All of the above will contribute to advancing the diagnostic, treatment, and research approaches for different cancers.

The Japan Society for Oral Tumors (JSOT) focuses on the issues and cases associated with oral cancer. After 10 years of review by 19 oral surgeons, oral radiologists, and oral pathologists, the society published the first edition of General Rules for Clinical and Pathological Studies on Oral Cancer in 2010 [1, 2]. In this chapter, we introduce some of the current notions about oral cancer by reviewing the surgical pathologic findings that served as the foundation for the general rules.

In principle, these general rules conform to the classification recommended by the International Union against Cancer (UICC) [3] and the World Health Organization (WHO) [4]. However, some general rule items were thought to require some modification from these international classifications, and these modifications were proposed in the official journal [5–8] and website of the JSOT.

In this chapter, oral cancer is defined as primary, not secondary, mucosal carcinoma originating at 6 locations in the oral cavity, as defined in the UICC classification: (1) tongue

T. Izumo, D.D.S., Ph.D. (✉)
Section of Diagnostic Oral Pathology, Tokyo Medical and Dental University, Tokyo, Japan
e-mail: izumo.dlab@tmd.ac.jp

T. Kirita and K. Omura (eds.), *Oral Cancer: Diagnosis and Therapy*, DOI 10.1007/978-4-431-54938-3_2, © Springer Japan 2015

cancer, (2) upper gingival and alveolar cancer, (3) lower gingival and alveolar cancer, (4) buccal mucosal cancer, (5) floor of mouth (FOM) cancer, and (6) hard palate cancer.

2.2 Primary Lesion

The oral cavity is lined with stratified squamous epithelium and is anatomically adjacent to the oropharynx, extending from the upper and lower lips to the terminal sulcus of tongue—the palatoglossal arch—to the posterior margin of the hard palate. The upper and lower teeth and gingiva separate the oral cavity into the oral vestibule and the oral cavity proper. The oral cavity is also the opening to the digestive tract and plays a role in respiration and articulation.

2.2.1 Anatomical Sites and Subsites

Tongue (TON-0, 1, 2)
Upper gingiva and alveolus (UG)
Lower gingiva and alveolus (LG)
Buccal mucosa (BM-0, 1, 2, 3, 4)
Floor of mouth (FOM)
Hard palate (HP)

(1) Tongue: The lingual mucosa encompasses the dorsal surface of the tongue anterior to the circumvallate papillae (anterior 2/3) and the lateral borders (anterior 2/3) and inferior surface of the tongue.
(2) Gingival and alveolar mucosa (maxillary or mandibular): There are two types of gingiva: free gingiva and attached gingiva. The latter is contiguous with the alveolar mucosa and occupies the area surrounded by a transition region to the lips and cheeks on the buccolabial side, the borderline between the horizontal region and the transverse ridges or the vertical region of the upper palate, and the borderline between the horizontal and vertical regions of the soft palate on the labiomandibular side. Although there is no anatomical name for the gingiva of edentulous alveolar ridges because the study of anatomy involves only normal body structures, "alveolar ridge mucosa" may most appropriately explain the gingiva of edentulous alveolar ridges. Gingival cancers include cancers originating from alveolar and alveolar ridge mucosae (Fig. 2.1).
(3) Buccal mucosa: According to the UICC classification, the mucosal layer of the cheeks, mucosa of the upper and lower alveolobuccal sulci (oral vestibule), mucosa in the retromolar areas, and labial mucosa of the upper and lower lips are collectively termed the buccal mucosa.
    (a) Mucosal layer of the cheeks: Area between the upper and lower buccal sulci.
    (b) Upper and lower alveolobuccal sulci (oral vestibule): Area extending from the distal surface of the canine anteriorly to the palatoglossal arch posteriorly. This square-shaped area is surrounded by the mucogingival junction and the junction on the buccal mucosa 1 cm from the deepest point in the buccal sulcus.
    (c) Retromolar areas: The area posterior to the gingiva, forming the margin of the tonsillar fossa.
    (d) Labial mucosa of the upper and lower lips: A square region bordered by the line connecting the corner of the mouth and the distal surface of the canine on the maxilla or mandible, the mucocutaneous junction, and the line 1 cm from the deepest part of the labial groove toward the mucocutaneous junction.
(4) Floor of mouth: The mucosa of the FOM is bordered by the mucogingival junction on the lingual side of the mandible and the tongue–FOM junction.

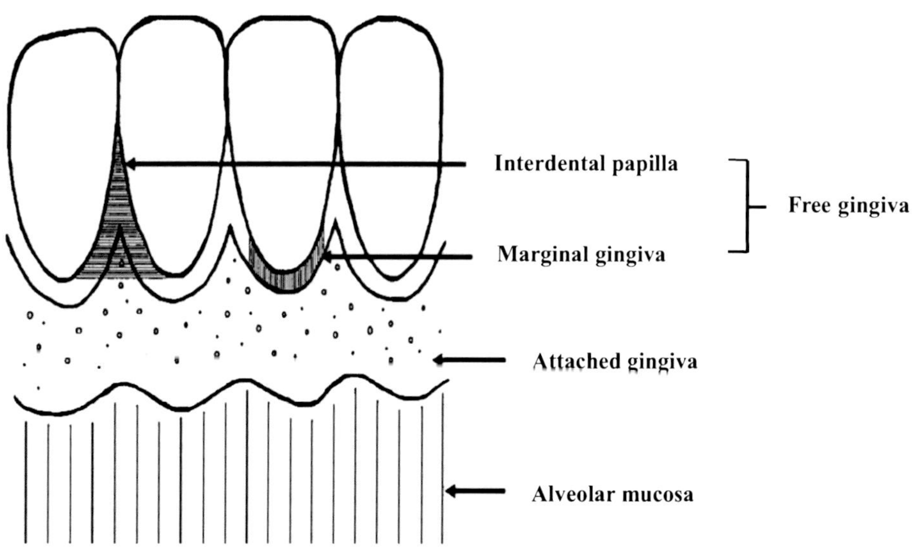

Fig. 2.1 Anatomical structure of the mandibular gingiva

Tongue (TON)
- **Dorsal surface (TON-0)**
- **Lateral boader (TON 1)**
- **Inferior surface (TON 2)**

Upper alveolus and gingiva (UG)
Lower alveolus and gingiva (LG)
Buccal mucosa (BM)
- **Buccal mucosa (BM-0)**
- **Upper bucco-alveolar sulci (BM-1U)**
- **Lower bucco-alveolar sulci (BN-1L)**
- **Retromolar areas (BM-2)**
- **Mucosa of upper lip (BM-3)**
- **Mucosa of lower lip (BM-4)**

Floor of mouth (FOM)
Hard palate (HP)

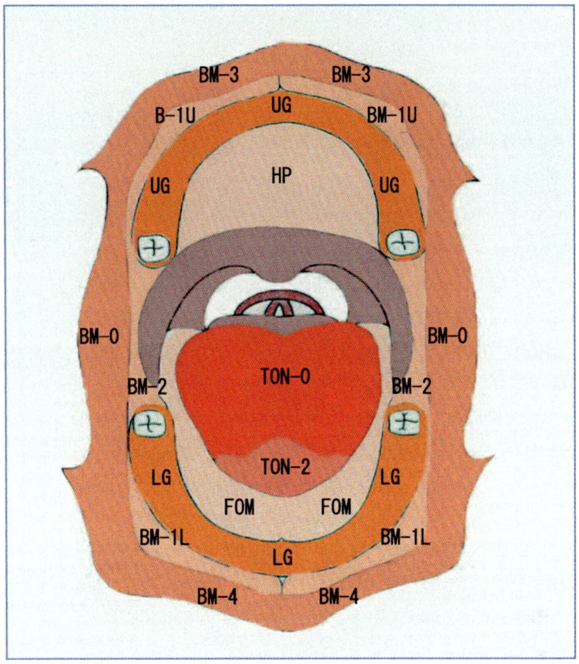

Fig. 2.2 Anatomical sites and subsites

(5) Hard palate: The mucosa of the hard palate is the triangular region encompassed within the borderline between the horizontal and vertical regions of the palate, the midline of the palate, and the borderline with the soft palate which lacks bone.

2.2.2 Locations of the Lesions (Fig. 2.2)

Tongue (TON-0, 1, 2)—dorsal surface (0)/lateral borders (1)/ventral surface (2)
Upper gingival and alveolus (UG)
- Dentulous jaw (teeth: 8/7/6/5/4/3/2/1/1/2/3/4/5/6/7/8)
- Edentulous jaw (Molar/Premolar/Canine/Incisor/I/C/P/M)

Lower gingiva and alveolus (LG)
- Dentulous jaw (teeth: 8/7/6/5/4/3/2/1/1/2/3/4/5/6/7/8)
- Edentulous jaw (Molar/Premolar/Canine/Incisor/I/C/P/M)

Buccal mucosa (BM-0, 1, 2, 3, 4)
- Buccal mucosa (0)/upper buccoalveolar sulcus (oral vestibule) (1U)/lower buccoalveolar sulcus (oral vestibule) (1 L)/retromolar area(2)/upper labial mucosa (3)/lower labial mucosa (4)
- Anterior type (a)/posterior type (b)

Floor of mouth (FOM)—median type (a)/lateral type (b)
Hard palate (HP)

(1) According to the UICC classification, the tongue is divided into three subsites: the dorsum of the tongue anterior to the circumvallate papillae (anterior 2/3 of the tongue) (TON-0), the lateral boaders of the tongue (TON-1), and the inferior (or ventral) surface of the tongue (TON-2).
(2) The location of lesions in the upper and lower gingival cancer is determined in relation to the teeth on the dentulous jaw or the corresponding teeth on the edentulous jaw. In the latter case, the location of lesion may be specified as an anterior teeth region (A), premolar region (P), or molar region (M). Because the presence and absence of teeth is thought to affect the progress of gingival cancer, the presence of impacted teeth should be recorded.
(3) Similarly, the location of buccal mucosal cancers is determined by dividing the buccal mucosa into five subsites: the mucosa of the cheeks (BM-0), the upper and lower alveolobuccal sulcus (oral vestibule) (BM-1), the retromolar area (BM-2), the labial mucosa of the upper lip (BM-3), and the labial mucosa of the lower lip (BM-4). In addition, because the tissue structure deep inside the oral mucosa varies depending on the anatomical locations, buccal mucosal cancers are further classified into the anterior or posterior type. Anterior type (the mucosa of the cheeks, most of the oral vestibule, and the upper and lower labial mucosae): muscles and fat tissue are present beneath the mucosa, and the outermost layer is the skin. Posterior type (primarily retromolar area): due to the presence of the masseter muscle just adjacent to the buccinator muscle, the medial pterygoid muscle on the side of the pharynx, and the mandible, tumors readily extend into the space between the muscles of mastication (hereinafter masticator space), which is among the poor prognostic factors for oral cancer. Consequently, it is useful to subclassify buccal mucosal

cancers into the anterior or posterior type with respect to the anterior margin of the masseter muscle.

(4) FOM cancers are subclassified into the medial and lateral types. Medial FOM cancers are located in the anterior region of the FOM mesial to the junction of the canine and the first premolar on the mandible. Any cancers located in the posterior region of the FOM distal to the region defined above are considered the lateral type. Medial-type FOM cancers, which account for the majority of FOM cancers, often expand into the opening of the salivary gland, sublingual caruncle, and eventually into the contralateral side of the FOM. This type of FOM cancer may also extend to the Wharton tube, sublingual gland, genioglossus muscle, geniohyoid muscle, and the lower anterior tooth area. The submandibular lymph nodes are a frequent site of cervical lymph node metastasis, but metastasis to the submental lymph nodes is rare. Lateral-type FOM cancers often originate from the lateral margin or the root of the tongue, and the determination of tumor range is sometimes difficult in advanced cases. There are two routes for lateral FOM cancers to invade adjacent tissues. First, along the mandibular periosteum, they may invade the mylohyoid muscle and submandibular space from the sublingual gland. These cancers may also invade internally the genioglossus muscle, geniohyoid muscle, styloglossus, and then the hyoglossus and posteriorly the medial pterygoid muscle (masticator space). Cervical lymph node metastasis often involves the submandibular and upper jugular lymph nodes.

2.2.3 Size

(long diameter) × (short diameter) × (thickness) cm
(mesiodistal diameter) × (buccolingual diameter) × (thickness) cm

2.2.4 Clinical Types

Superficial type: tumors primarily showing superficial growth
Exophytic type: those primarily showing exophytic growth
Endophytic type: those primarily showing endophytic growth
Unclassified type: those not belonging to any of the above types

Oral cancers are classified into superficial (Fig. 2.3a), exophytic (Fig. 2.3b), and endophytic (Fig. 2.3c) types based on the clinical manifestations. In general, early (T1, T2) tongue cancers are diagnosed by visual inspection and palpation; however, it is preferable to perform ultrasonographic (US) imaging to confirm the diagnosis. Although visual inspection and palpation are performed to determine tumor invasion depth in or under the mucosal layer, because of individual variations in palpation skills among clinicians, diagnostic accuracy may have a margin of error of ±0.5 cm. Nonetheless, for the diagnosis of T1-2 cancers in soft tissue, palpation can provide fairly accurate supplementary findings to visual inspection. With continued advances in and dissemination of probe-based US examination, it may be possible in the near future to determine the invasion depth of tumors in millimeter increments. At that point, it will be necessary to reestablish a next-generation classification method for invasion patterns of tumors including those in gastric cancer.

A previous study investigating the efficacy of clinical classification in 2,224 patients with T1-2 tongue cancer [5] revealed that this clinical type can be used as a prognostic factor for local recurrence, lymph node metastasis, distant metastasis, and 5-year survival rate (Fig. 2.4a, b). Although such classification has some utility in buccal mucosa and FOM cancers, utility is affected by the site of the tumor. Consequently, we decided to subclassify buccal mucosa and FOM cancers into anterior/posterior type and medial/lateral type [6]. However, the utility of clinical classification based on growth patterns is not clear for cancers with a risk of bone invasion, such as gingival and hard palate cancers [7, 8], necessitating further investigation. As we describe later, the classification of lower gingival cancer by mandibular resorption type [9], which reflects mandibular invasion pattern [10], has proven useful [7, 10–13]. After incorporating diagnostic imaging that shows the pathological features at the apical end of cancer invasion, this classification method may be considered to fulfill all the requirements of a next-generation method. However, we decided to record the invasion of adjacent tissues in advanced oral cancers in detail without performing clinical classification, due to unproven utility.

The clinical types of oral cancer, which are the superficial, exophytic, and endophytic types, correspond to the macroscopic classification of digestive tract cancers (e.g., esophageal, gastric, and colon cancers [14–16]), namely, type 0, type 1, and type 2–4, respectively. A small number of endophytic oral cancers are reported to be highly malignant, corresponding to type 4 oral cancer. Preliminary investigation of clinical cases at Saitama Cancer Center showed that 5 % of all T1-2 tongue cancers were the scirrhous type exhibiting the characteristic macroscopic features of a small ulcer with broad expansion into the deep tissue layer and with broad hard induration (Fig. 2.5a). In addition to these invasion patterns, such as broad invasion at depth and submucosal lateral infiltration (Fig. 2.5b Left, c), these cancers also exhibited histopathological features corresponding to a Yamamoto-Kohama's (YK) Mode of Invasion [17] (Fig. 2.5b Right) of YK-4D and a scirrhous pattern, and they were also identified as a subtype with particularly poor prognosis, even among endophytic oral cancers (Fig. 2.5d). To improve the treatment of tongue cancer, further retrospective studies are being conducted to elucidate the pathological features associated with poor prognosis.

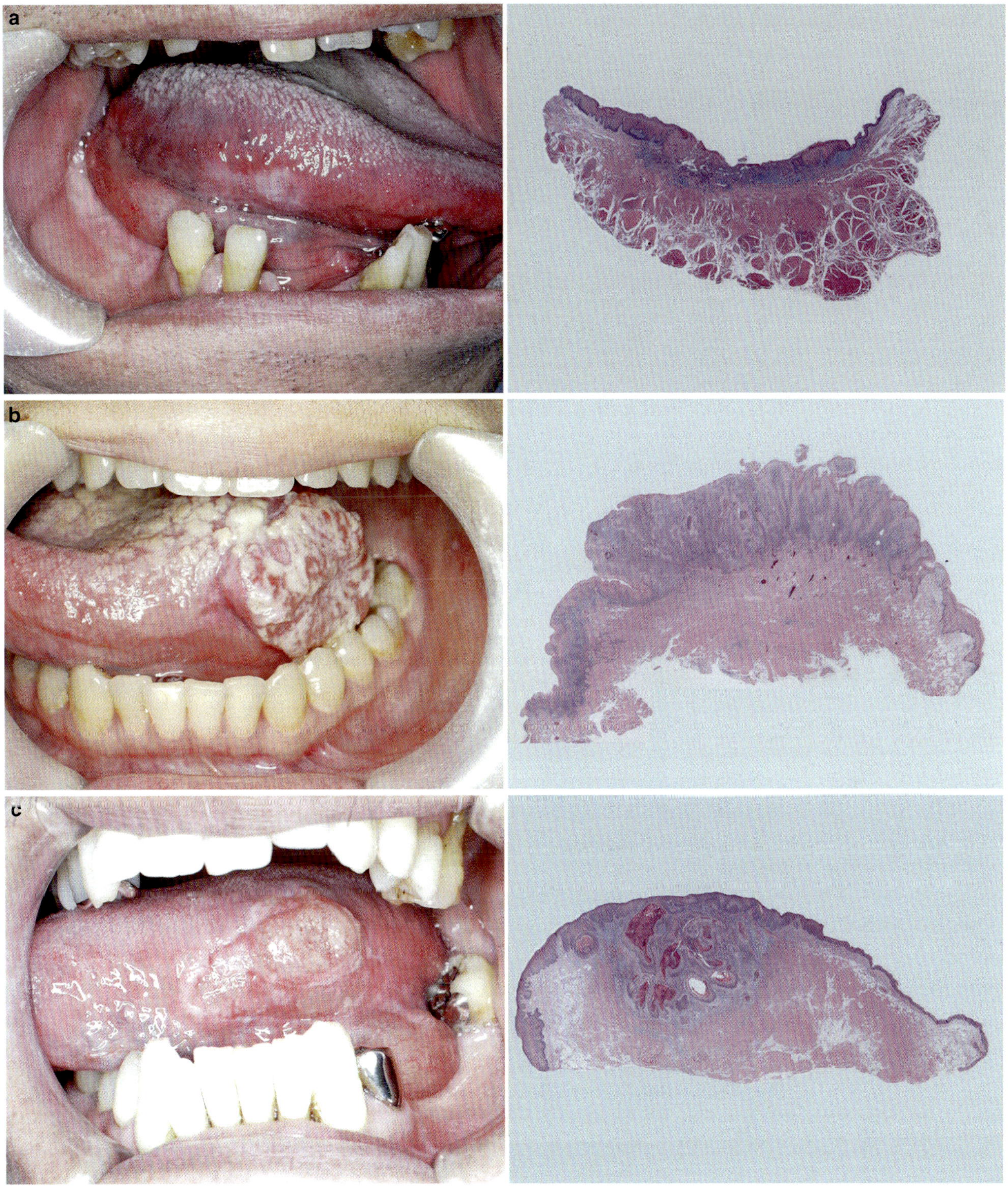

Fig. 2.3 Clinical types. (**a**) Superficial type. (**b**) Exophytic type. (**c**) Endophytic type

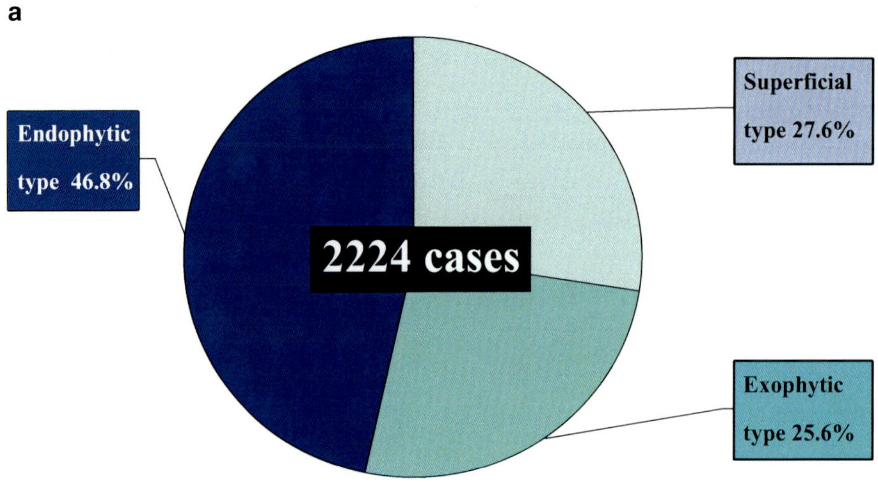

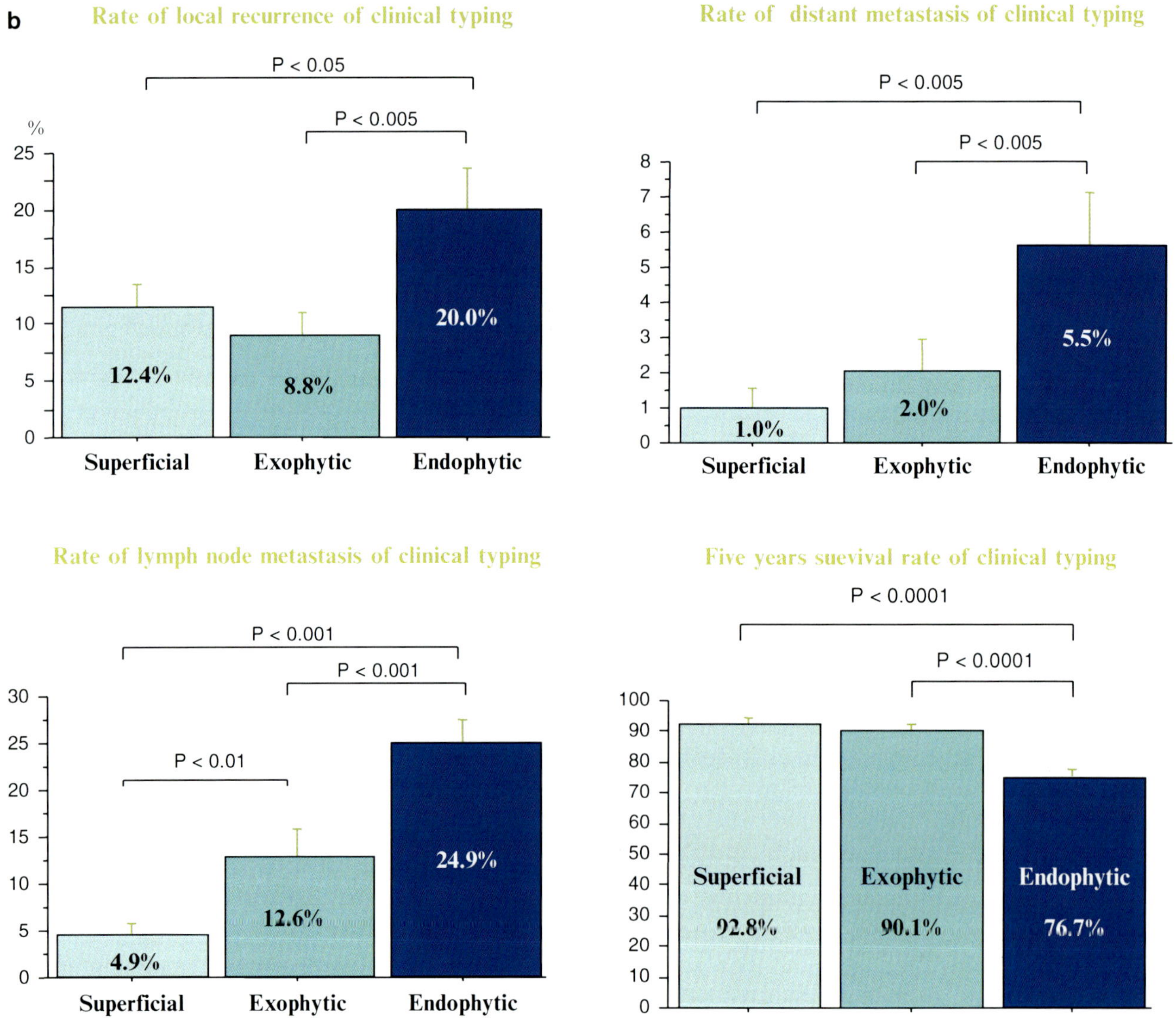

Fig. 2.4 (**a**) Frequency of clinical types in lingual carcinoma. (**b**) Prognostic factors of clinical types

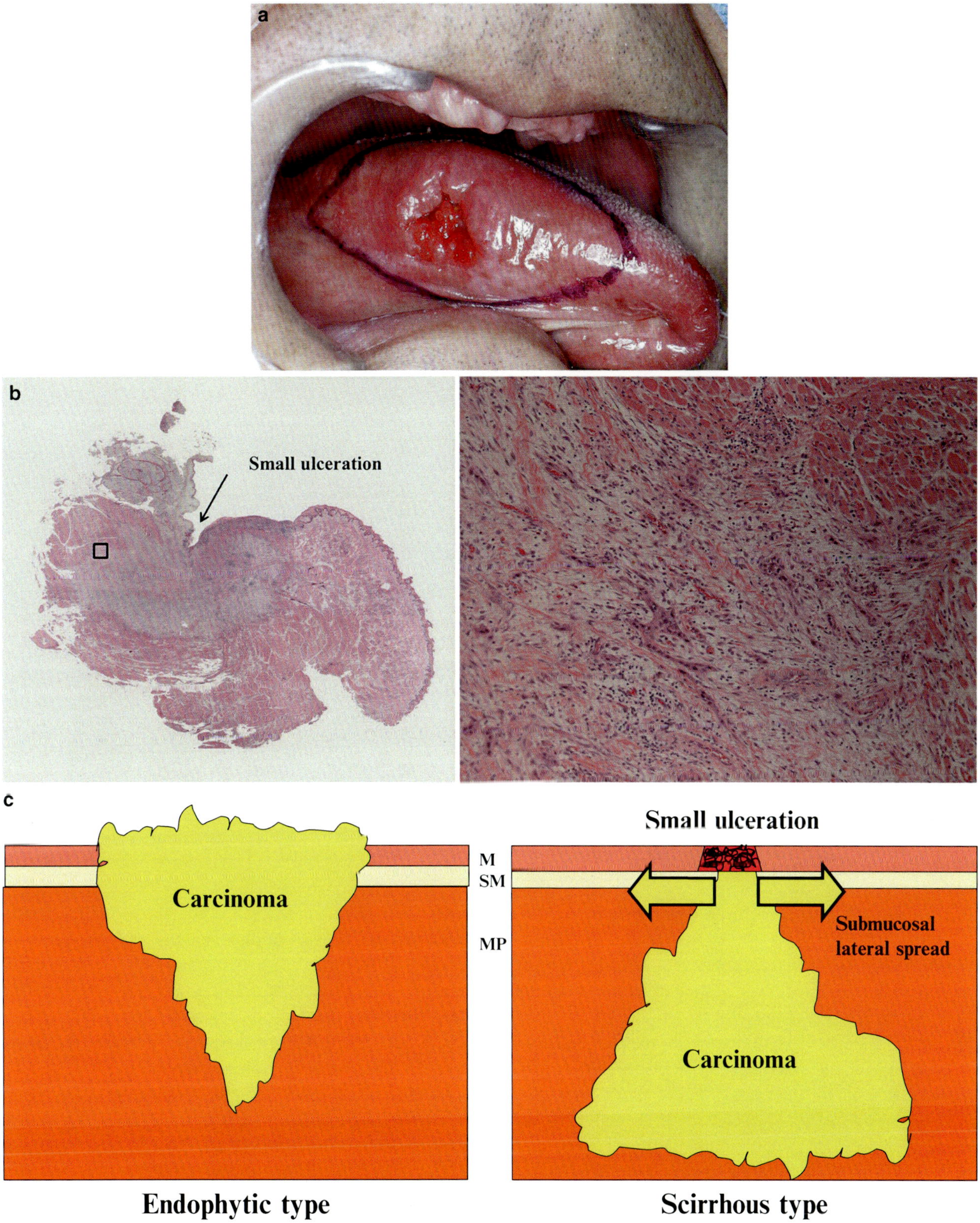

Fig. 2.5 (**a**) Macroscopic presentation of the scirrhous type of lingual carcinoma. Palpation of a small ulcer with broad expansion into the deep tissue layer and extensive induration (*outlined in ink*). (**b**) Histologic presentation of the scirrhous type of lingual carcinoma. *Left panel*: low-magnification image showing a small ulcer on the surface with broad expansion into the deep tissue layer. *Right panel*: high-magnification image of the opening showing diffuse invasion (YK-4D) of small nests or single cells. (**c**) Spread pattern of endophytic and scirrhous types of lingual carcinoma. *Left panel*: broad endophytic ulcer with tapering depth. *Right panel*: small ulcer with broad expansion in the deep tissue layer and lateral expansion in the submucosal layer. (**d**) Prognostic factors of the endophytic and scirrhous types of lingual carcinoma

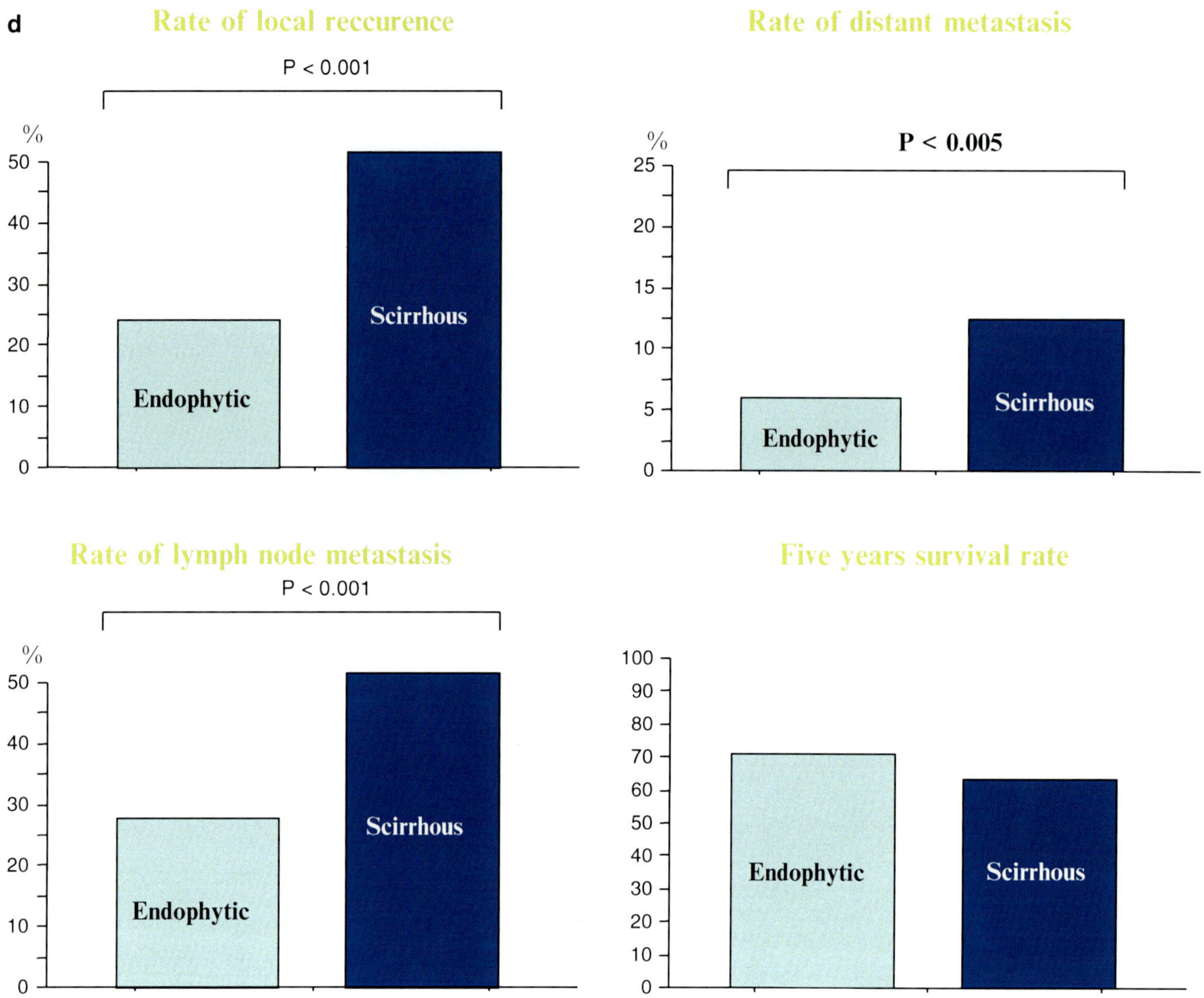

Fig. 2.5 (continued)

2.2.5 Depth and Deepness of Invasion

Depth: Tissue name of the deepest part of cancer invasion. (See tissue names below according to subsite. Underlined tissue names refer to *adjacent tissues*.)

Deepness: Distance from the surface of the assumed normal mucosa to the deepest part of cancer invasion, which is different from the thickness of tumor.

T factors in the UICC classification of oral cancers are determined based on greatest tumor diameter. However, the prognosis of primary tumors correlates with tumor invasion depth much more strongly than with tumor diameter. For this reason, we plan to define the invasion depth of a tumor as the T factor in future studies. Determination of invasion depth is relatively easy in esophageal and gastric cancers because of the six clear layers of the wall: the mucosa (M), muscularis mucosae (MM), submucosa (SM), muscularis propria (MP), subserosa (SS), and serosa (S).

However, in oral cancers, it is not possible to standardize tumor depth because of the complex three-dimensional structure of the oral cavity, which has different deep tissue structures at different anatomical locations. Accordingly, albeit somewhat cumbersome, invasion depth of the vertical structures is recorded in detail from the mucosa to the deeper layers by anatomical site and subsite.

In the present rules, original evaluation criteria were developed for the invasion of adjacent tissues (T4a) by considering evaluation of the depth.

(1) Invasion depth of tongue cancer

Tongue (TON): mucosa (M)/submucosa (SM)/shallow part of the proper muscle layer of the tongue (MP1)/deep part of the proper muscle layer of the tongue (MP2)/extrinsic muscles of the tongue (HG)

Scanning of a healthy tongue with the most widely used US [18–20] device shows three layers of different US intensities and features at the lateral boarder of the

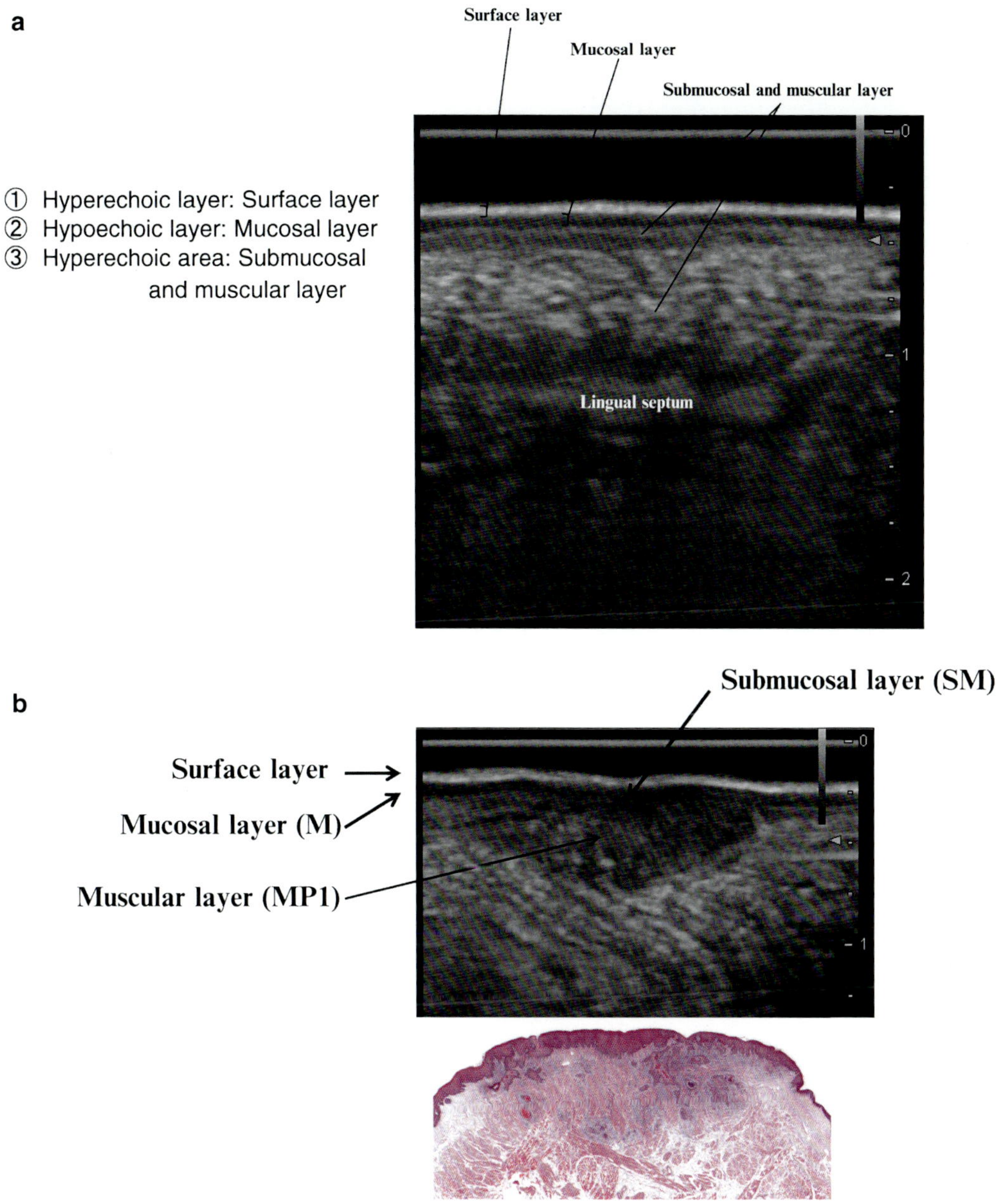

Fig. 2.6 (**a**) Ultrasonographic findings of normal lingual tissue. (**b**) Assessment of tumor invasion in the muscular layer and comparison between ultrasonographic and histological images. (**c**) Assessment of tumor depth

tongue, which is the most frequent site of the cancer. These are the outermost, second, and innermost layers of heterogenous hyperechoic or hypoechoic signal intensity (Fig. 2.6a). The outermost hyperechoic layer is thought to represent signal reflection at the mucosal surface, the second hypoechoic layer likely represents mucosa (M), and the innermost layer therefore represents submucosa (SM) and muscularis propria (MP). Because of the hyperechoic signal in the muscularis propria, cancer invading this layer is displayed as an area of hypoechoic intensity (Fig. 2.6b).

Given the extroverted growth of the tumor and the formation of a depression due to ulcer, it is important to measure the deepness of tumor from the assumed normal mucosal surface, instead of measuring the actual thickness of tumor (Fig. 2.6c). It is also important to record the method of measurement (palpation or US), the extent of tumor invasion in the existing structure, and the depth of invasion in centimeters if palpated or millimeters if scanned by US.

(2) Invasion depth of upper gingival cancer

Upper gingival and alveolus (UG): mucosa (M)/ submucosa (SM)/periosteum (PER)/ cortical bone (CB)/

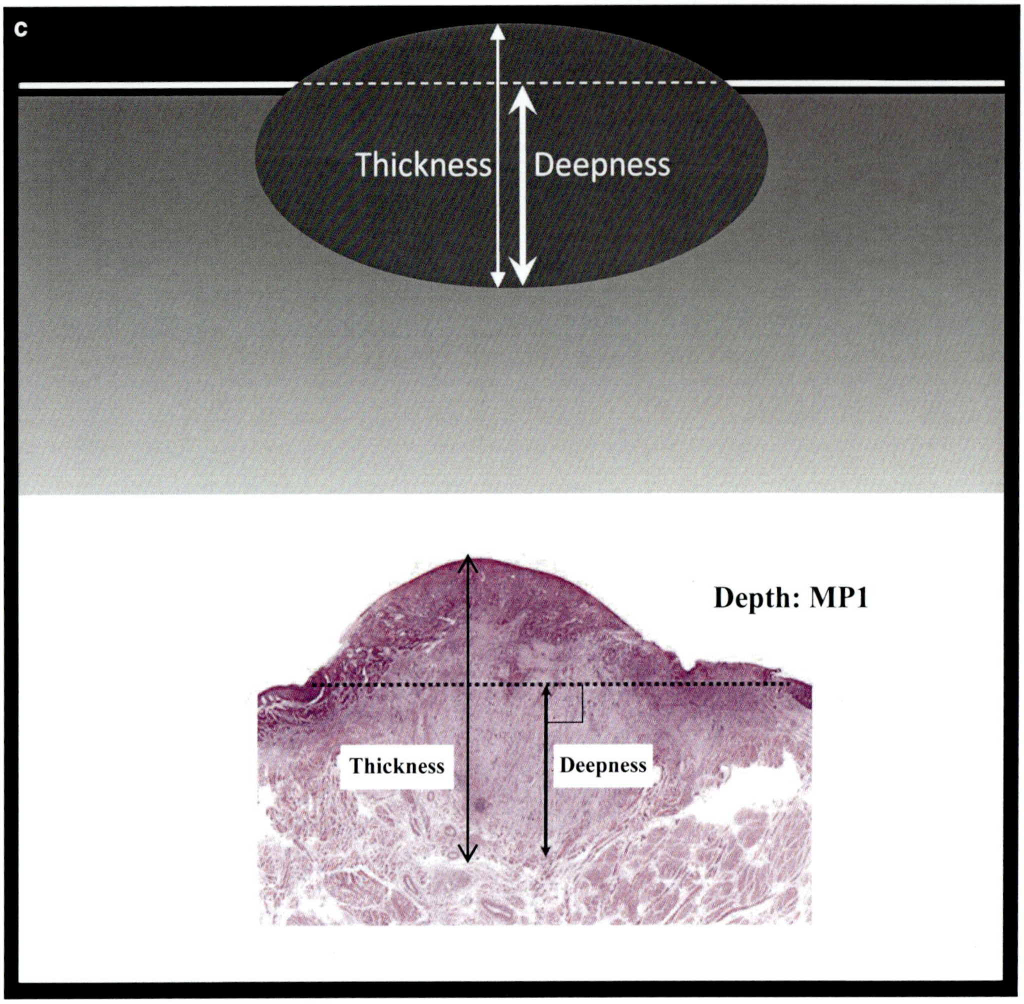

Fig. 2.6 (continued)

bone marrow (CAN)/maxillary sinus (MS) and nasal cavity (NC)

At present, we tentatively use the sinus and nasal floor (SNF) criteria [21, 22] which classify tumor invasion in the maxillary sinus and nasal cavity as T4a.

(3) Invasion depth of lower gingival cancer

Lower gingiva and alveolus (LG): mucosa (M)/submucosa (SM)/periosteum (PER)/cortical bone (CB)/upper part of the mandibular canal in bone marrow (CAN1)/*lower part of the mandibular canal in bone marrow (CAN2)*

According to the UICC classification, superficial erosion alone of the bone/tooth socket by gingival primary carcinoma is not sufficient to classify a tumor as T4a, and consequently, the diagnosis of any mandibular infiltration beyond this point is crucial. By classifying mandibular infiltration patterns as shown in Fig. 2.7, the JSOT demonstrated the appropriateness of mandibular canal classification that defines CAN2 as T4a in a multicenter study of 1,187 cases of mandibular gingival cancer [23]. The present general rules define CAN2 in mandibular bone invasion as T4a.

The mandibular invasion of lower gingival cancer is an important indication for surgery. The invasion depth of squamous cell carcinoma (SSC) in the mandible shows a fair correlation with the degree of mandibular resorption on X-ray absorptiometry [9, 12]. By also assessing the pattern of bone resorption, it is possible to determine which resection method is appropriate for the mandible [9, 11–13, 23]. Consequently, in addition to the invasion depth from the gingival mucosa, the images of mandibular resorption by lower gingival cancer should be examined carefully for the following points.

Note: Images of mandibular resorption

In the evaluation of the depth of lower gingival cancer, additional comments concerning the following findings on X-ray studies are attached.

(a) Type of images examined
(b) Degree of mandibular resorption: none/alveolar process of bone marrow/upper mandibular canal of bone marrow/lower mandibular canal of bone marrow

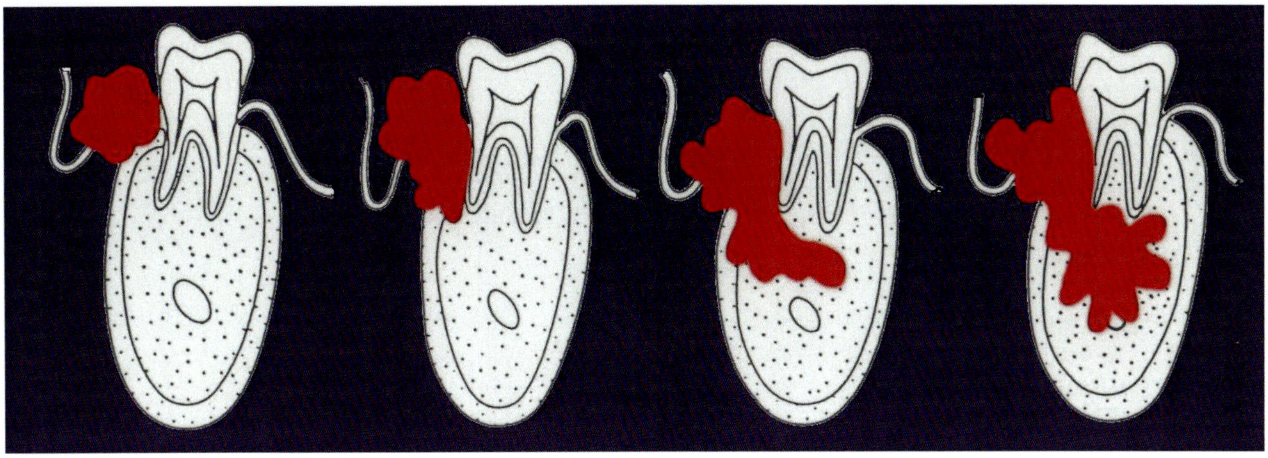

Fig. 2.7 Invasion depth of lower gingival carcinoma

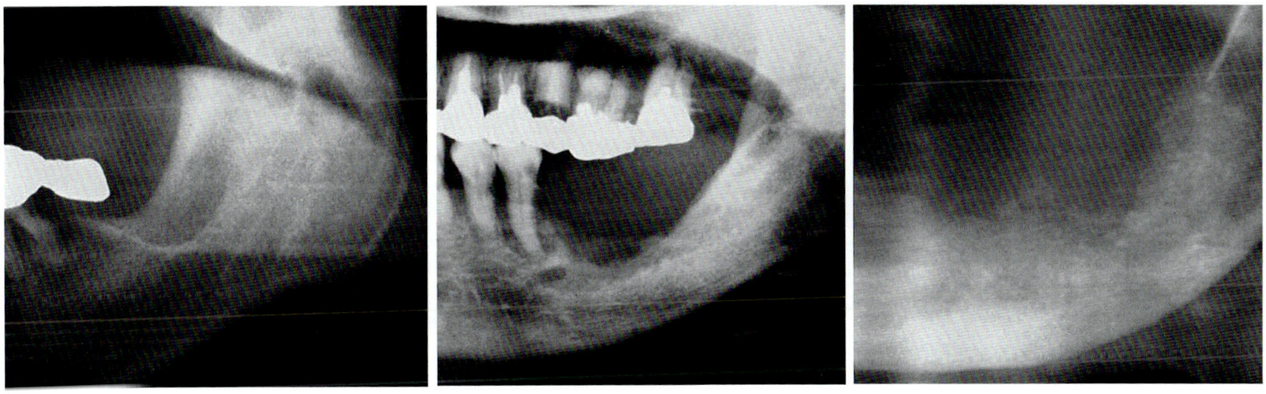

Fig. 2.8 Patterns of bone resorption in lower gingival carcinoma

(c) Deepest part of mandibular bone resorption:
Dentulous jaw (Retromolar/8/7/6/5/4/3/2/1/2/3/4/5/6/7/8/R)
Edentulous jaw (Retromolar/ Molar/Premolar/Canine/Incisor/I/C/P/M/R)

(d) Mandibular resorption type: pressure type/mixed type/moth-eaten type
The patterns of bone resorption on radiograms are grouped into the pressure type, moth-eaten type, and mixed type in accordance with the Swearingen classification [9] (Fig. 2.8). It is common to observe all bone resorption patterns distributed continuously on the same radiogram of upper or lower gingival cancer.
(1) Pressure type: The margins of bone resorption are clear and smooth with no displaced bone fragments.
(2) Mixed type: Despite somewhat unclear and irregular margins of bone resorption, no displaced bone fragments are observed.
(3) Moth-eaten type: The margins are unclear and irregular, and bone fragments are observed.
In the initial examination of bone resorption, panoramic radiograms may be useful for differential diagnosis of the pressure and moth-eaten types. However, computed tomography (CT) or other imaging modality is necessary to obtain higher detailed imaging findings [24–26].

(4) Invasion depth of buccal mucosal cancer
Buccal mucosa (BM): mucosa (M)/submucosa (SM)/buccinator muscle (oral orbicular muscle) (BM, OOM)/buccal sulcus (BS)/buccal fat (BF)/muscles of

facial expression and superficial musculoaponeurotic system (SMAS) (FM)/subcutaneous fat (SCF)

Anterior type: buccal space→muscles of facial expression and superficial musculoaponeurotic system (SMAS) (FM)/subcutaneous fat (SCF)

Posterior type: buccal space→masticator muscle space (MS)

Because of the small number of cases and the complex deep tissue structure, a search of the literature does not produce sufficient information on the clinical and pathological features of buccal mucosal cancer. In the general rules, buccal mucosal cancers are subclassified into the anterior and posterior type on the basis of deep tissue structure. It is important to carefully examine diagnostic images and histopathological samples to accumulate sufficient information on tumor depth in the mucosa, submucosal tissues, buccinator muscle, buccal space, buccal fat pad, muscles of facial expression interlinked via the superficial musculoaponeurotic system (SMAS) [27, 28], subcutaneous fat, skin, masticator space, maxilla, and mandible, as well as information on the invasion of the surrounding tissues.

(5) Invasion depth of FOM cancer

Floor of mouth (FOM): mucosa (M)/submucosa (SM)/sublingual space (SLS)/mylohyoid muscle (MH)/submandibular space (SMS)

Median type: sublingual space→genioglossus muscle (GG)/geniohyoid muscle (GH)/ mylohyoid muscle (MH)/submandibular space (SMS)

Lateral type: sublingual space→mylohyoid muscle (MH)/submandibular space (SMS)

Median-type FOM cancers infiltrate into the tissues surrounding the Wharton duct immediately below the mucosa and sublingual gland in the relatively early stages; these cancers infiltrate into the genioglossus (extrinsic tongue muscle) and may further advance into the geniohyoideus and mylohyoideus muscles and the submental space. Lateral-type FOM cancers infiltrate into the mylohyoid and submandibular space vertically via the tissues surrounding the Wharton duct and sublingual gland. In addition, it is important to pay clinical attention to the invasion of the intrinsic muscles of the tongue, the outer periosteum on the mandibular lingual side, and the masticator space.

(6) Invasion depth of hard palate cancer

Hard palate (HP): mucosa (M)/submucosa (SM)/periosteum (PER)/cortical bone (CB)/bone marrow (CAN)/maxillary sinus (MS) and nasal cavity (NC)

In general, hard palate cancers located in the posterior region have poor prognosis and a high risk of lymph node metastasis. Prognosis for hard palate cancers invading the nasal cavity and maxillary sinus is thought to be even worse; however, hard palate cancers have not been studied in great detail due to the extremely small number of cases. To reveal their clinical manifestations, it is necessary to carefully investigate their invasion depth into surrounding tissues, including the nasal cavity and maxillary sinus. At present, we tentatively use the SNF criteria [21, 22], which classify tumor invasion in the maxillary sinus and nasal cavity as T4a.

2.2.6 Invasion into Adjacent Structures

In principle, the UICC TNM classification of malignant tumors [3] is used to assess the infiltration of primary lesions, except T4a lesions, into surrounding tissues. For T4a lesions, we propose our own classification criteria specific to the site of invasion, as described below. In the following section, we review the association between T factors and the UICC classification.

(1) Invasion into adjacent tissues by tongue cancer

None/FOM/sublingual space/mylohyoid muscle/extrinsic muscles of the tongue/root of the tongue/gingiva/mandibular cortex/mandibular bone marrow

The tongue consists of four extrinsic muscles (genioglossus, hyoglossus, styloglossus, and palatoglossus) and four intrinsic muscles (superior longitudinal, inferior longitudinal, verticalis, and transversus muscles). Infiltration into the intrinsic muscles is used as an indication of deep tissue invasion in T4a tumors. Infiltration into individual intrinsic muscles is not regarded as an indication of T4a tumors. The intrinsic muscles move the tongue, whereas the extrinsic muscles change its shape during swallowing and speech. For example, the genioglossus muscle moves the tongue anteriorly or toward the mentum, whereas the hyoglossus pulls the root of the tongue posteriorly. In addition, the styloglossus pulls the tongue toward the upper posterior direction, and the palatoglossus plays a role in narrowing the faucial area by elevating the root of tongue and lowering the palate. The lingual and hypoglossal nerves serve to regulate the tongue's sensory and motor functions, respectively. The extent of invasion is diagnosed while taking account of the function of individual muscles and nerves as well as the current symptoms. With regard to bone metastasis, infiltration into bone marrow is clearly an indication of T4a. In addition, as in the other oral cancers, the diagnosis of T4a is made when the submandibular space is infiltrated via the mylohyoid muscle. Invasion into the skin, which also appears in the UICC classification criteria, occurs only through the mandible or submandibular space and therefore is excluded from the criteria for T4a lesions in these general rules. T4b is also diagnosed upon tumor invasion into the posteriorly located masticator space. The UICC T4b criteria are

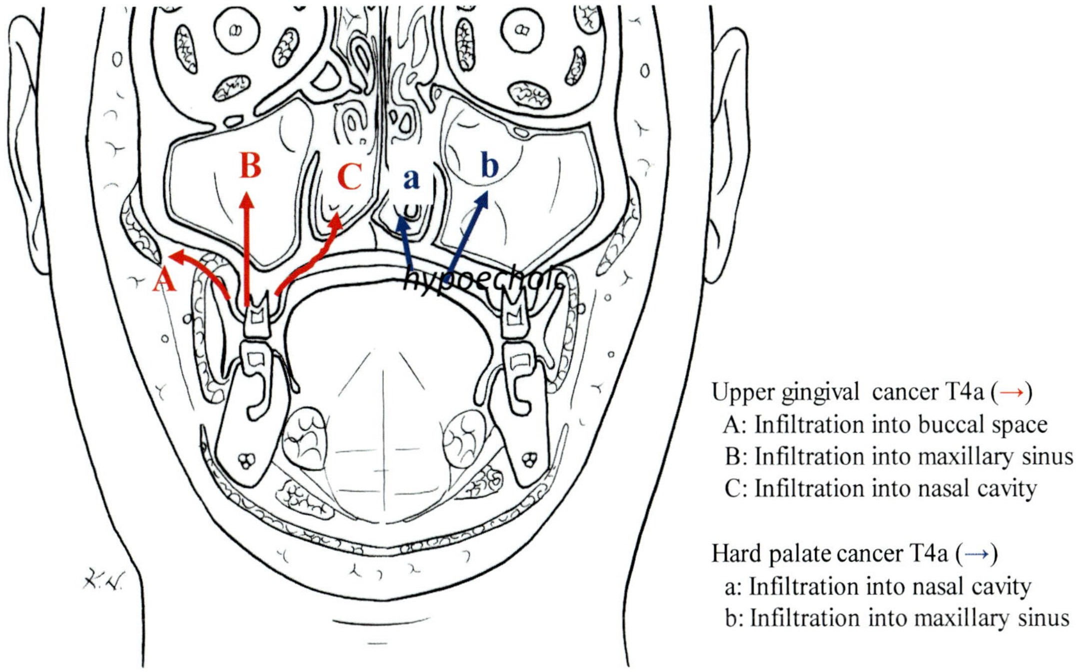

Fig. 2.9 Invasion routes of upper gingival and hard palate carcinomas on a coronal section

used for infiltration into the internal carotid artery and pterygoid process, both of which rarely occur without the invasion of the masticator space.

(2) Invasion of adjacent tissues by upper gingival cancer
None/maxillary sinus/nasal cavity/buccinator muscles/buccal space/muscles of facial expression/masticator space/pterygoid plate/skull base/internal carotid artery/subcutaneous fat/skin

Figure 2.9 shows the potential infiltration routes of upper gingival and hard palate cancers into the surrounding tissues in the coronal section. In these general rules, infiltration into surrounding tissues beyond the buccinator muscle is classed as T4a in upper and in lower gingival cancer. Because the orbicularis oris muscle and buccinator muscles are adjacent to each other, any tumor invasion beyond the orbicularis oris muscle is diagnosed as T4a as well. In contrast to the UICC classification for lower gingival cancer, which defines T4a by bone marrow infiltration, we define tumor invasion reaching the mandibular canal as T4a. However, compared with the mandible, the bone cortex of the maxilla is thin and thus readily allows tumor invasion into the bone marrow. Accordingly, the invasion of the nasal cavity or maxillary sinus, but not the bone marrow, is also defined as T4a for upper gingival cancers in accordance with the SNF criteria (Fig. 2.10). Infiltration into the skin, which is described in the UICC classification, occurs only through the buccinator muscle and therefore is excluded from the T4a criteria in these general rules. As described earlier, anterior and posterior infiltration into the buccal space and subcutaneous fat is considered to be T4a. However, as described in the section on buccal mucosal cancer, none of the infiltration routes in the horizontal direction (Fig. 2.11) are considered T4b (the routes in Figs. 2.9a and 2.11a). The most important factor that affects prognosis is tumor invasion in a posterior direction. Because infiltration into the medial and lateral pterygoid muscles, masseter muscle, and temporal muscle is invasion of the muscles of mastication (the routes in Fig. 2.11c–e) and because of the potential invasion of the pterygoid process (the route in Fig. 2.11b), infiltration into these muscles is defined as T4b in accordance with the UICC classification.

(3) Invasion of adjacent tissues by lower gingival cancer
None/FOM/sublingual space/tongue/buccal mucosa/buccinator muscles/buccal space/ masticator space/muscles of facial expression/subcutaneous fat/skin

The progression of lower gingival cancer toward the buccal mucosa may lead to tumor infiltration into the buccinator muscle, buccal space, and even the skin (Fig. 2.12a). In the direction of the FOM, lower gingival cancer may infiltrate superficially into the lingual gingiva, FOM mucosa, and even the tongue (Fig. 2.12b) and infiltrate deeply into the sublingual gland, Wharton duct, lingual nerve, and as far as the submandibular space via the mylohyoid muscle (Fig. 2.12c). The progression of lower gingival cancer toward the retromolar areas may cause invasion of the submandibular space via the posterior edge of the mylohyoid muscle medially (Fig. 2.12d), invasion of the masseter muscle via the buccinator

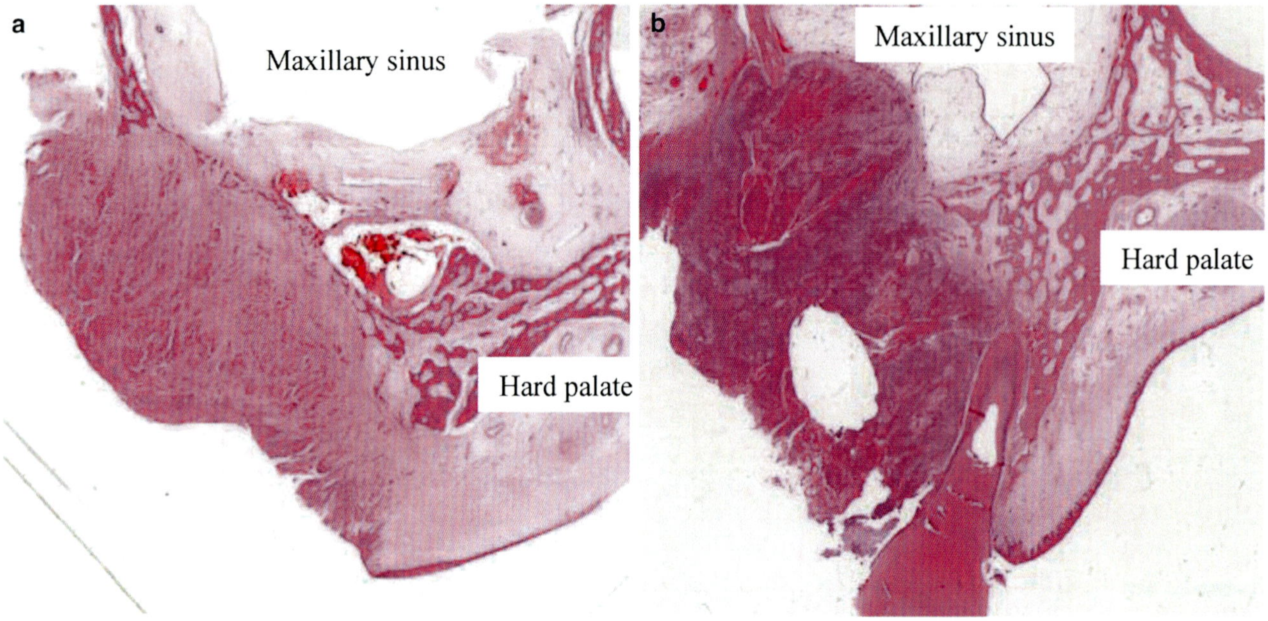

Fig. 2.10 Maxillary invasion of upper gingival carcinoma according to the sinus and nasal floor criteria. (**a**) The carcinoma advancing through and expansively absorbing the bone marrow on the buccal side is not classified as T4a because of no infiltration into the maxillary sinus. (**b**) The carcinoma infiltrating the maxillary sinus through the bone is classified as T4a

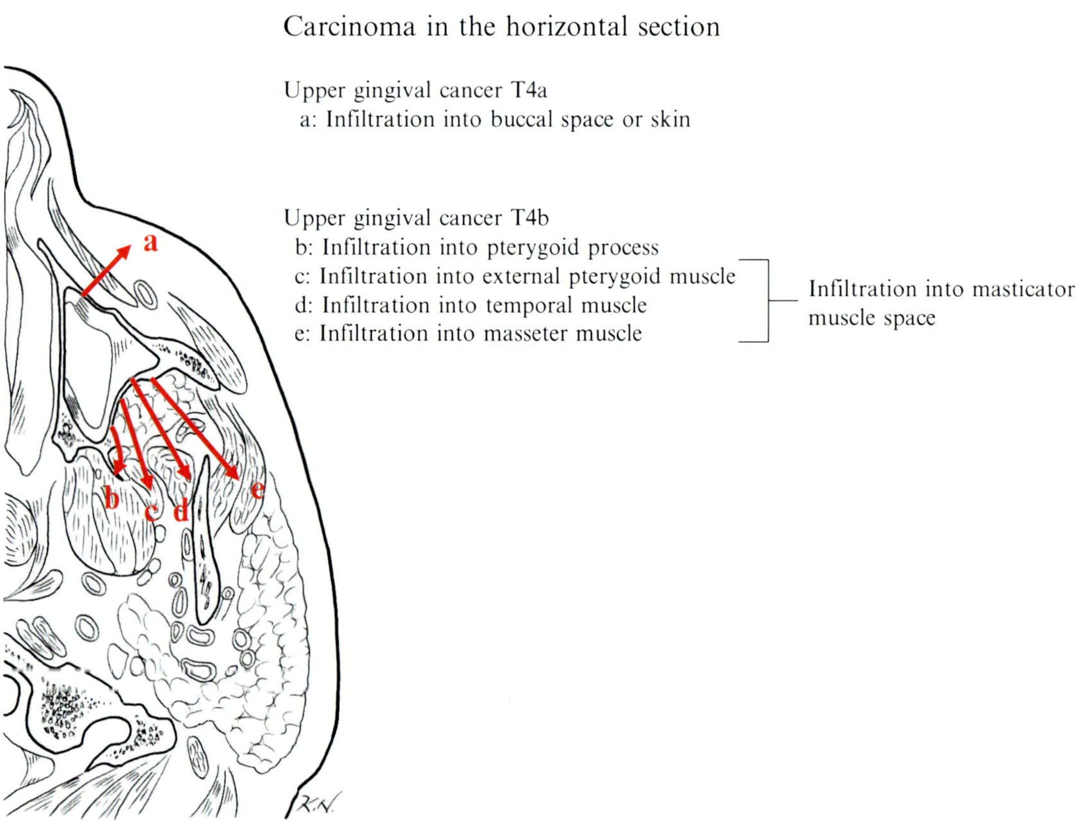

Fig. 2.11 Invasion routes of upper gingival carcinoma in the horizontal section

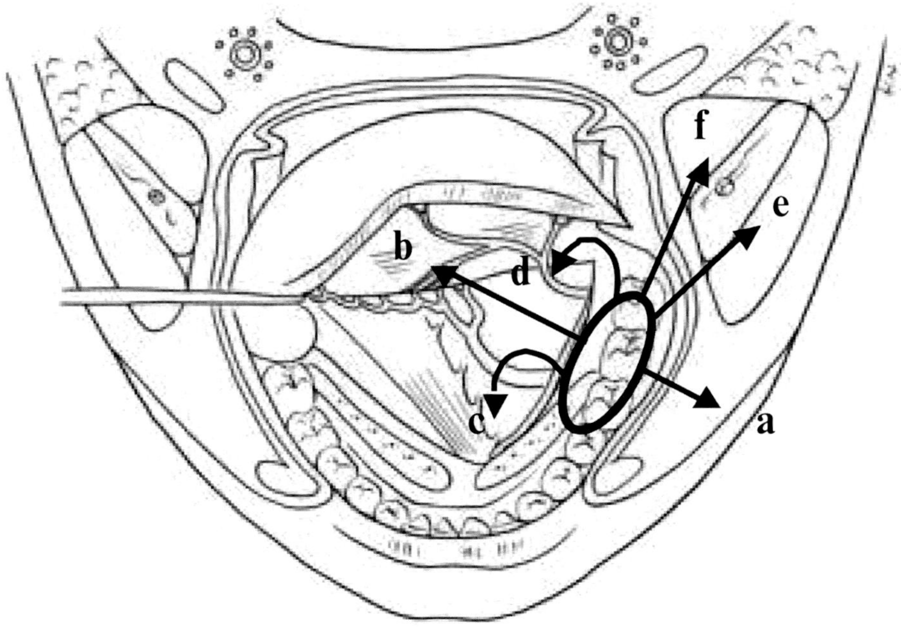

a. Infiltration into skin
b. Infiltration into tongue
c. Infiltration into submandibular space beyond the mylohyoid muscle
d. Infiltration into submandibular space from the posterior margin of the mylohyoid muscle
e. Infiltration into the masseter muscle
f. Infiltration into pterygomandiular space

Fig. 2.12 Invasion routes of lower gingival carcinoma

muscle laterally (Fig. 2.12e), and invasion of the base of the skull and the parapharyngeal space via the pterygomandibular space posteriorly (Fig. 2.12f). In the JSOT general rules, tumor infiltration reaching the mandibular canal via the deep interior region of the mandible is defined as T4a. Invasion of the adjacent tissues that are defined as T4a includes the extrinsic muscles of the tongue on the FOM side, the submandibular space, and the skin, buccal space, and even subcutaneous fat on the buccal mucosal side. The problem associated with the UICC criteria of T4b for lower gingival cancers is the invasion of the masticator space because lower gingival cancers originating from the retromolar areas readily invade the masticator space (Fig. 2.13).

(4) Invasion of adjacent tissues by buccal mucosal cancer
None/masticator space/lower gingiva/mandibular cortex/mandibular bone marrow/FOM/upper gingiva/maxillary cortex/maxillary bone marrow/ oropharynx/lips/subcutaneous fat/skin

The major invasion routes of FOM cancers into the adjacent tissues and the relationship between the routes and fascial spaces are shown in Fig. 2.14. In the upper and lower gingival cancer section of the JSOP general rules, the invasion of buccal space or subcutaneous fat is defined as T4a. However, it can be problematic to apply this definition as is because buccal mucosal cancers easily invade the buccal space. Figure 2.15 therefore shows the different degrees of invasion of buccal mucosal cancers in the coronal plane. The buccal space is present between the buccinator muscle and the SMAS muscles for facial expression and contains the buccal fat pad with a distinctive coating. Although invasion into the skin is defined as T4a in the UICC classification, the JSOT general rules define invasion of the subcutaneous fat via the buccal space or via the orbicularis oris muscle which lacks the buccal space as T4a. On the other hand, the invasion of the maxilla and mandible (Fig. 2.15f1, f2) is defined as T4a only when accompanied by bone marrow invasion, in accordance with the UICC classification. The posterior type of buccal mucosal cancer may bypass the buccal space and posteriorly invade the masseter muscle, i.e., the masticator space (the route in Fig. 2.14b). In this case, the invasion is defined as T4b in accordance with the UICC classification.

(5) Invasion of adjacent tissues by FOM cancer
None/mylohyoid muscle/tongue/extrinsic muscles of the tongue /gingiva/mandibular cortex/mandibular bone marrow/submandibular space/masticator space/oropharynx

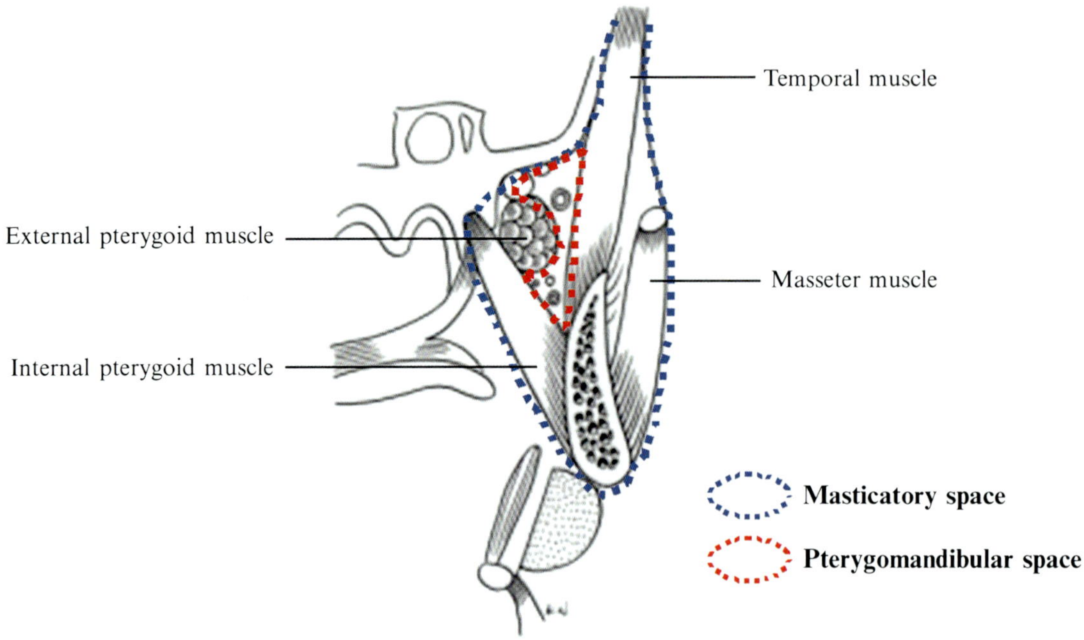

Fig. 2.13 Masticatory space and pterygomandibular space

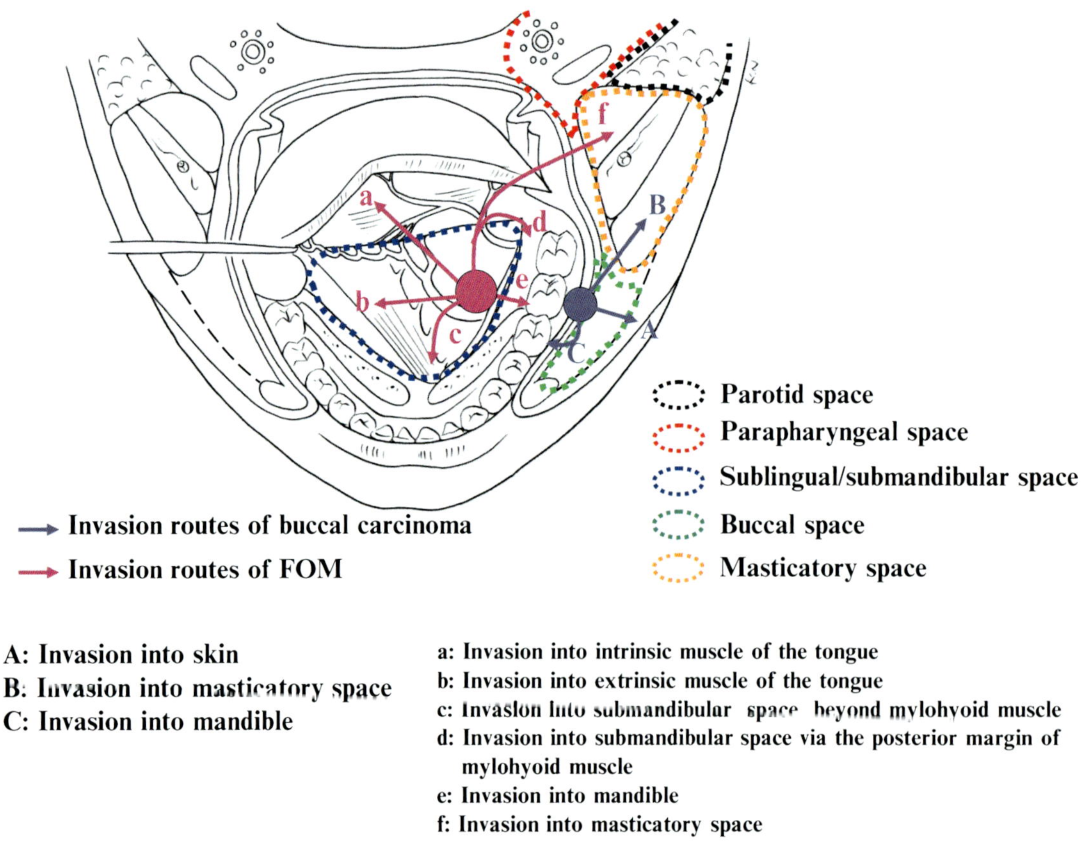

Fig. 2.14 Invasion routes of buccal mucosal and floor of mouth (*FOM*) carcinoma and fascial spaces

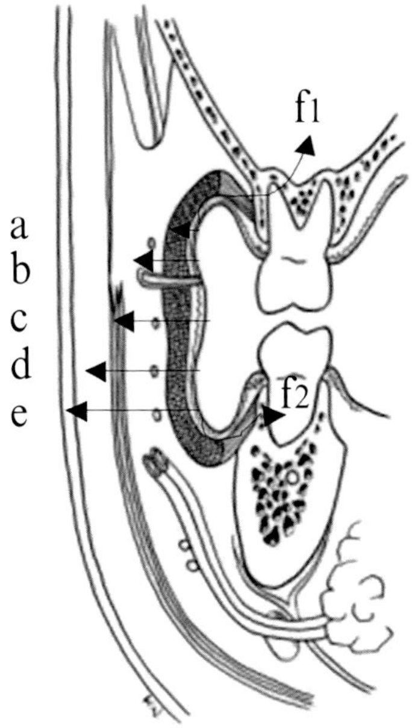

Fig. 2.15 Depth of buccal carcinoma on a coronal section

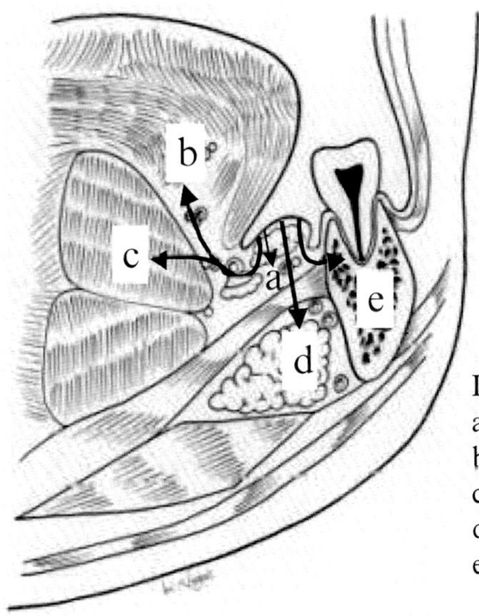

Fig. 2.16 Invasion routes of FOM carcinoma on a coronal section

The invasion routes of FOM cancers in the coronal plane may involve the sublingual gland (a), intrinsic tongue muscles (b), extrinsic tongue muscles (c), mylohyoid muscle (d), and mandible (e), as shown in Fig. 2.16. Non-superficial lesions generally involve tumor invasion into the sublingual gland and rarely infiltration into the mandible or the submandibular space beyond the mylohyoid muscle. However, with regard to the progression of lateral FOM cancers in the posterior direction, attention must be paid to the invasion of the submandibular space via the posterior margin of the mylohyoid muscle and the invasion of the medial pterygoid muscle. The T4a definitions of FOM cancers conform to the corresponding UICC criteria, and accordingly, FOM cancers are defined as T4a when accompanied by the invasion of the extrinsic tongue muscles and mandibular bone marrow and the invasion of the submandibular space by coming around the posterior margin of the mylohyoid muscle (the route in Fig. 2.14d) or by passing over the mylohyoid muscle (the route in Fig. 2.14c). Invasion into the skin is excluded from the UICC T4a criteria because it is possible only via the mandible or submandibular space. Invasion of the medial pterygoid muscle is defined as T4b in accordance with the UICC classification because the invasion is equivalent to the invasion of the masticator space (the route in Fig. 2.14f).

(6) Invasion of adjacent tissues by hard palate cancer
None/maxillary sinus/nasal cavity/gingiva/soft palate/masticator space/ pterygoid plate/skull base/internal carotid artery

The potential invasion routes of upper gingival and hard palate cancers in the coronal plane are shown in Fig. 2.9. Although hard palate cancers may invade posteriorly into the soft palate, pterygoid process, and medial pterygoid muscle (masticator space), invasion of the soft palate is not included in the UICC T4 criteria. On the other hand, despite the contiguous mucosal structure, invasion of soft palate cancer (oropharyngeal cancer) into the hard palate is considered to be T4a according to the UICC criteria. To ensure consistency among the criteria, it may be necessary to define the invasion of hard palate cancer into the soft palate as T4a. However, define such simple invasion of contiguous anatomical regions as T4a independently of the depth is questionable. We will therefore continue to investigate the prognosis of soft palate cancer accompanied by invasion of the hard palate.

Note: Description of the superficial muscular aponeurotic system (SMAS)

In 1976, Mitz et al. reported the presence of the SMAS [27], which is connected to the platysma muscle, muscles of facial expression, temporoparietal fascia, and galea aponeurotica [28]. The SMAS is an important anatomical structure in cosmetic surgery, especially rhytidectomy, because the system stabilizes facial expression and transmits contraction signals to the facial skin. Compared with the adipose tissue medial to the SMAS, the adipose tissue lateral to it (i.e., toward the skin) contains small adipocytes partitioned by fibrous tissues that transmit muscular movement to the skin. The SMAS is wide at the para-parotid gland area but becomes thinner and discontinuous anteriorly. As indicated by the arrow in the coronal section of the masseter muscle stained with hematoxylin and eosin of Fig. 2.17, the SMAS is contiguous to the platysma muscle and forms a thin layer of muscle or a layer of connective tissue outside the masseter muscle.

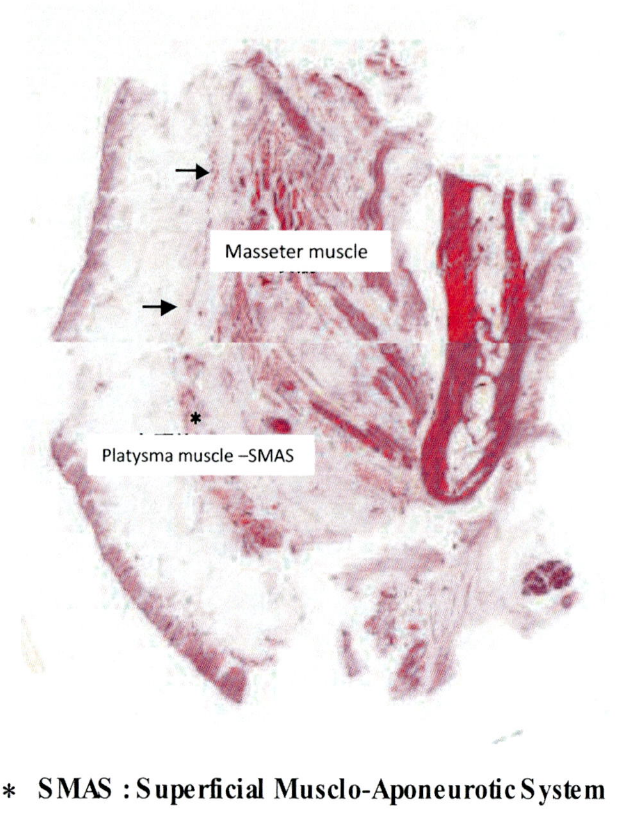

Fig. 2.17 Histologic figure at the masseter muscle on a coronal section

2.2.7 *T* Score

The assessment of *T* score in primary tumors, except T4a tumors, is performed in accordance with the UICC TNM malignant tumor criteria [3].

TX: Primary tumor cannot be assessed
T0: No evidence of primary tumor
Tis: Carcinoma in situ (squamous intraepithelial neoplasia)
T1: Maximum diameter $\leq$2 cm
T2: Maximum diameter >2 and $\leq$4 cm
T3: Maximum diameter >4 cm
T4: Invasion into adjacent structures

However, as stated earlier, the criteria for T4a lesions were developed by invasion sites, and therefore we summarize the differences between our general rules and the UICC classification below.

In addition, tumors 2–3 and 3–4 cm in the greatest diameter are occasionally called early T2 and late (or advanced) T2, respectively. This appears to be an effective subclassification for:

<Comparative relations to the UICC T4a criteria>

(1) Tongue cancer:
T4a: Invasion into the mandibular bone marrow, invasion into the submandibular space, and invasion into the extrinsic tongue muscles
T4b: Invasion into the masticator space, invasion into the pterygoid plate, invasion into the skull base, and invasion circumferentially surrounding the internal carotid artery

- Addition of "invasion into the submandibular space"
- Omission of "invasion into the skin" in the UICC classification because it does not occur without the invasion of the mandible or submandibular space
- Deletion of "invasion into the maxillary sinus" in the UICC classification

- Retention of "invasion into the mandibular bone marrow" and "invasion into the extrinsic tongue muscles" in the UICC classification

(2) Upper gingival cancer:
T4a: Invasion into the maxillary sinus and nasal cavity and invasion into the buccal space or subcutaneous fat
T4b: Invasion into the masticator space, invasion into the pterygoid plate, invasion into the skull base, and invasion circumferentially surrounding the internal carotid artery
Note 1: If the tumor is confined to the alveolar bone, the tumor is classified as T1-3 according to its size.
Note 2: Tumors invading the maxillary sinus are judged to be T4a regardless of their size.

- Omission of "invasion of the bone marrow" and change of "invasion of the maxillary sinus" in the UICC classification to "invasion of the maxillary sinus and nasal cavity"
- Change of "invasion of the skin" in the UICC classification to "invasion of the buccal space or subcutaneous fat"
- Omission of "invasion of the extrinsic tongue muscles" in the UICC classification

(3) Lower gingival cancer:
T4a: Invasion reaching the mandibular canal, invasion into the buccal space or subcutaneous fat, invasion into the submandibular space, and invasion into the extrinsic tongue muscles
T4b: Invasion into the masticator space, invasion into the pterygoid plate, invasion into the skull base, and invasion circumferentially surrounding the internal carotid artery
Note 1: If the tumor is confined to the upper part of the mandibular canal in the bone marrow, the tumor is classified as T1-3 according to its size.
Note 2: Tumors invading the mandibular canal are judged to be T4a regardless of their size.

- Addition of "invasion of the submandibular space"
- Change of "invasion of the skin" in the UICC classification to "invasion of the buccal space or subcutaneous fat"
- Change of "invasion of the bone marrow" in the UICC classification to "invasion reaching the mandibular canal"
- Omission of "invasion of the maxillary sinus" in the UICC classification
- Retention of "invasion of the extrinsic tongue muscles" in the UICC classification"

(4) Buccal mucosal cancer:
T4a: Invasion into the subcutaneous fat, invasion into the maxillary and mandibular bone marrow, and invasion into the maxillary sinus
T4b: Invasion into the masticator space, invasion into the pterygoid plate, invasion into the skull base, and invasion circumferentially surrounding the internal carotid artery

- Change of "invasion of the skin" in the UICC classification to "invasion of the subcutaneous fat"
- Retention of "invasion of the mandibular bone marrow" and "invasion of the maxillary sinus" in the UICC classification
- Omission of "invasion of the extrinsic tongue muscles" in the UICC classification

(5) FOM cancer:
T4a: Invasion into the mandibular bone marrow, invasion into the submandibular space, and invasion into the extrinsic tongue muscles
T4b: Invasion into the masticator space, invasion into the pterygoid plate, invasion into the skull base, and invasion circumferentially surrounding the internal carotid artery

- Addition of "invasion of the submandibular space"
- Omission of "invasion of the skin" in the UICC classification because it does not occur without the invasion of the mandible or submandibular space
- Omission of "invasion of the maxillary sinus" in the UICC classification
- Retention of "invasion of the mandibular bone marrow" and "invasion of the extrinsic muscles of the tongue" in the UICC classification

(6) Hard palate cancer:
T4a: Invasion into the maxillary sinus and nasal cavity
T4b: Invasion into the masticatory muscle space, invasion into the pterygoid process, invasion into the base of the skull, and invasion circumferentially surrounding the internal carotid artery

- Addition of "nasal cavity" into "invasion of the maxillary sinus" in the UICC classification while omitting "invasion of the mandibular bone marrow"
- Change of "invasion of the skin" in the UICC classification to "invasion of the buccal space or subcutaneous fat"
- Omission of "invasion of the extrinsic tongue muscles" in the UICC classification

2.2.8 Histological Classification

2.2.8.1 Tis Cancer: Oral Intraepithelial Neoplasia (OIN)/Carcinoma In Situ

(1) Basaloid type
(2) Differentiated type

The histological classification of early oral SCC has been performed universally in accordance with WHO's classification of "dysplasia" [29–31], which grades the severity of dysplasia as mild, moderate, or severe and defines carcinoma in situ (CIS) as a precursor to oral SCC. The definition of CIS as the presence of atypical cells in all layers of the epithelium has remained unchanged since the first edition (1971). However, this diagnostic criterion is controversial because the criterion was established by emulating the pathological concept of dysplasia in cervical cancer [32–34] and because differentiated precancerous lesions and CIS are typically present in the mucosa of the oral cavity, pharynx, and larynx [35–41]. Against this background, when the classification of squamous intraepithelial neoplasia (SIN) [39–42] and the Ljubljana classification of laryngeal lesions [43–54] were proposed, WHO included these classifications alongside the criteria for dysplasia in head and neck tumors (2005) [31]. Nevertheless, in the WHO classification, the pathologic concept of dysplasia and SIN includes both neoplastic lesion and atypical reactive lesion. This concept is not only incomplete for pathological classification but also useless as a diagnostic indicator for deciding the treatment strategy. Furthermore, it remains a descriptive diagnosis and cannot be used to qualitatively diagnose tumor malignancy.

Although the WHO classification has been conventionally used in Japan, recent developments in oral oncology have promoted certain modifications in the diagnosis of early cancerous lesions in the oral cavity. After conducting its own investigation of precancerous lesions, in 2005 the Working Group of the JSOT proposed the differentiated type of CIS [5, 35]. In 2007, the other group of the Japan Society for Oral Pathology published an Oral CIS Catalog which contained histopathological variations including a histological image of differentiated CIS [36, 37]. These studies revealed the existence of an oral type of Tis SCC derived from atypical squamous epithelial lesions distinct from "full thickness or almost full thickness architectural abnormalities," one of the diagnostic criteria for CIS in the WHO classification. Differentiated type is a type of CIS that becomes cancerous while maintaining the maturation and differentiation of stratified squamous epithelium and accounts for the majority of oral CIS [1, 35–37]. Therefore, the dysplasia-carcinoma sequence theory, which was established for cervical cancer and classifies atypical cells into mild, moderate, and severe dysplasia based on the involvement of 3 epithelial layers before turning into CIS, should not be used to define precancerous lesions in oral cancer. Because of the difficulty in diagnosing cellular atypia in the stratum corneum or superficial layer using this criterion based on three layers, it is highly possible to underdiagnose moderate dysplasia [31, 55, 56]. For diagnosing CIS in oral mucosa, cytologic atypia is more important than the classification based on layers. It is important to remember that in histological examination, many CIS in the oral mucosa are highly differentiated, unlike cervical and esophageal cancers. Against this background, the first edition of the General Rules for Clinical and

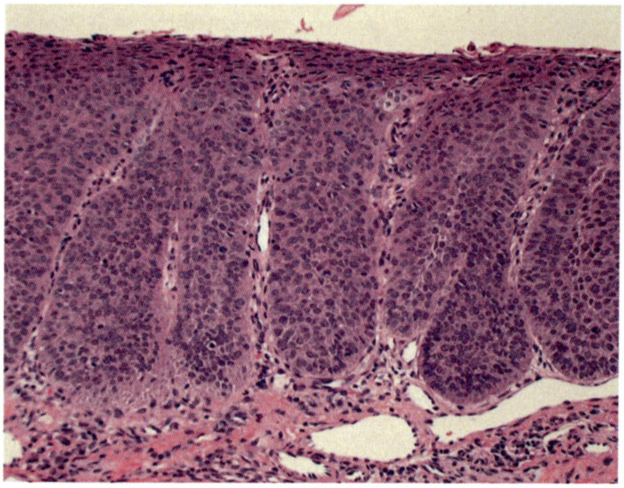

Fig. 2.18 Basaloid type of oral intraepithelial neoplasia/carcinoma in situ (OIN/CIS)

Pathological Studies on Oral Cancer published in 2010 [1, 2] clearly states the concept of oral intraepithelial neoplasia (OIN), which takes the place of CIS. OIN was used to avoid confusion with CIS in WHO's diagnostic criteria and to define a pathological feature specific to oral cancer. Although histological examination shows the basaloid type and differentiated type, OIN often reveals a transition between the two.

(1) The basaloid type of OIN/CIS corresponds to CIS in the WHO classification, and the histological images of OIN show basal-like cells in all or almost all layers (Fig. 2.18). Although in reality it is rare to observe this type of OIN in the oral cavity, when present, macroscopic observation reveals an erosive erythroid lesion, which rapidly progresses to invasive carcinoma within 6 months.
(2) The differentiated type of OIN/CIS is specific to the oral type of intraepithelial neoplasia and shows highly atypical cells in the basal layer, but not in the stratum corneum or stratum spinosum. It is histopathologically important to pay attention to atypical cells in the first layer of the stratum basale and to examine for irregularities in the size and shape of the nucleus, the ratio of the nucleus to the cytoplasm, prominent nucleolus, mitotic features, and the disturbance and loss of polarity (Fig. 2.19). Because oncogenic transformation occurs while maintaining the maturation and differentiation characteristics of the stratified squamous epithelium, it is often difficult to recognize structural atypia in this type of OIN. However, the diagnosis of intraepithelial neoplasia can be made based on the specific pathological features of CIS, including the formation of a tumor front between the lesion and adjacent mucosal epithelium and the establishment of other aspects of CIS, after multilayer formation and lateral expansion of atypical cells. Most OIN in the oral cavity are the differentiated type or

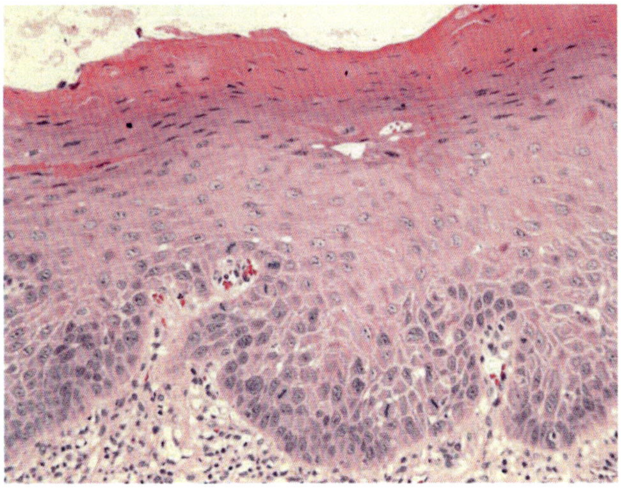

Fig. 2.19 Differentiated type of OIN/CIS

the mixed type of CIS. These OIN have white lesions and progress to invasive carcinoma within 5 years.

(a) Molecular markers

Although it is difficult to differentiate OIN, especially the differentiated type of OIN, from oral epithelial dysplasia (see below) and reactive atypical epithelium, many studies have reported the utility of morphological diagnostic criteria and immunostaining with Ki-67, cytokeratin 13, and cytokeratin 17 [1, 35, 37, 57–73]. However, immunostaining findings should be supplementary to histopathological findings because the gene expression mechanism of cytokeratin with a molecular weight different from that of the common type of cytokeratin has not been elucidated. Here, we introduce several useful immunostaining findings.

(1) Ki-67/MIB1 (Fig. 2.20)

Cell-cycle cells are immunoreactive for Ki-67/MIB1. In healthy oral mucosa, cells positive for Ki-67/MIB1 are scattered in the second basal layer.

Ki-67/MIB1 immunoreactive cells with a large nucleus and prominent nucleolus are observed in the stratum basale of OIN.

Multilayer Ki-67/MIB1 immunoreactive cells are observed throughout the parabasal and spinous layers of OIN.

(2) Cytokeratins 13 and 17 (Fig. 2.21)

In the oral cavity, healthy mucosal cells are negative, while OIN are positive for CK13 immunoreactivity.

OIN, but not healthy mucosal cells, is immunoreactive for CK17.

The above changes are sometimes observed in reactive atypical lesions.

A number of gene expression and immunohistochemical studies indicate that transglutaminase 3, a squamous differentiated marker, is useful for the diagnosis of OIN [71, 72, 74], although further examination is required to substantiate these findings. It is anticipated that an increase in the number of useful molecular markers available will improve the objectivity of diagnosis. The justification for diagnosis on which the OIN classification as well as the other classifications relies is based on findings from retrospective studies, and there have been only a few prospective studies that have examined the description of oncogenesis at the molecular level. It is well known that genomic instability due to telomere shortening plays an important role in carcinoma development. Telomere shortening is the initial phenomenon in cancerization, and genomic instability is accelerated by the chromosomal instability that results from such shortening [75, 76]. It has been reported that mean telomere length was significantly shorter in OIN cases diagnosed histopathologically than in normal mucosal epithelium [77].

(b) Relations with other classification methods

Table 2.1 shows the comparative relations among different classification methods [35]. Although a one-to-one comparison is not made here because the methods used different diagnostic criteria, this table shows their comparative relationships conceptually. It has long been known that some cases of mild to moderate dysplasia diagnosed according to the WHO classification develop into invasive cancer later on. We believe such cases actually involve superficial and differentiated intraepithelial neoplasia.

Note: Oral epithelial dysplasia (OED)

Atypical epithelium is divided into two pathological entities, one with progression to cancer (true preinvasive SCC, OIN/CIS) and the other without (reactive atypical epithelium). However, as it is difficult in practice to distinguish between these clearly at present, the term "OED" is used to denote a borderline lesion that is difficult to differentiate from reactive atypical epithelium, although OIN/CIS may be suspected. These cases require 5 years or more of long-term follow-up [1]. Although dysplasia in the esophagus is defined as an intraepithelial neoplastic lesion [78], in the oral mucosa located in front of Waldeyer's tonsillar ring, the differential diagnosis of neoplastic lesion and reactive atypical epithelium is frequently difficult to make. Therefore, practically speaking, the application of this boundary classification to the oral mucosa is useful [1].

Note: Lugol (iodine) staining

It is very difficult to detect OIN/CIS on macroscopic examination. Generally, OIN/CIS is composed of flat or slight elevated white or erosive red lesions, or an admixture of focal white and red ones. It can be detected as an

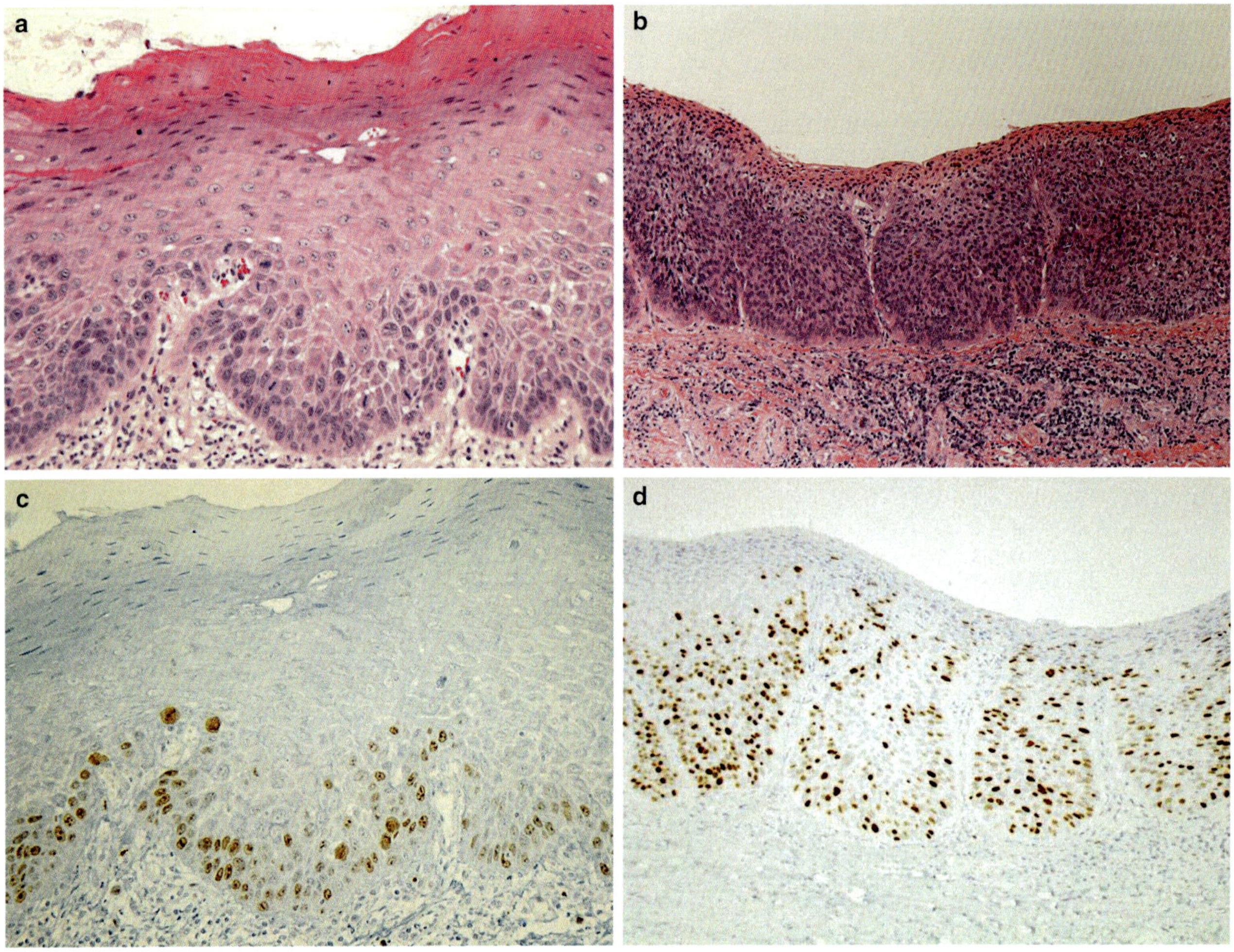

Fig. 2.20 Immunohistochemistry for Ki-67/MIB1 of OIN. (**a**) OIN, differentiated type. (**b**) OIN, basaloid type. (**c**) Large immunoreactive atypical cells in the first basal layer. (**d**) Immunoreactive cells across several layers

unstained area by Lugol's (iodine) staining [1, 79–81] (Fig. 2.22). Since superficial layers of the normal squamous mucosa are rich in glycogen, any lesions with a loss of superficial glycogen, such as reactive atypical epithelium, oral epithelial dysplasia, oral intraepithelial neoplasia, or early invasive squamous cell carcinoma (Fig. 2.23), can be recognized as unstained areas [1, 5–8]. However, in hyperkeratinized mucosa, especially in the gingiva and palate, Lugol may not show a clear unstained area or may instead show a lightly stained area [1]. Although further classification of any iodine-free areas is necessary, in principle it is desirable to resect an iodine-free area in the vicinity of cancer as much as possible.

2.2.8.2 Squamous Cell Carcinoma, Common Type

(1) Histological Grade (WHO) (Fig. 2.24):
 Grade 1: Well-differentiated type
 Grade 2: Moderately differentiated type
 Grade 3: Poorly differentiated type

Histological grading is a useful indicator for the degree of malignancy in SCC. The WHO grading system [29, 30], which was derived from the Broders' classification for lip cancer (1920) [82] and classifies oral SCC into well-, moderately, and poorly differentiated tumors based on the degree of cell differentiation, has been the most widely used method worldwide. The method is still used routinely at many institutions because of its moderate correlation with prognosis and lymph node metastasis reported by a large-population study.

However, the WHO grading system is not particularly useful for determining treatment options in individual cases, and consequently various malignancy grading systems have been proposed including the Jakobsson classification (1973) [83], Willen classification [84], and Anneroth classification [85, 86]. These grading systems evaluate factors related to tumor–host interactions as well as tumor-related factors to diagnose the degree of malignancy, by scoring 6–8 factors at the tumor–host junction

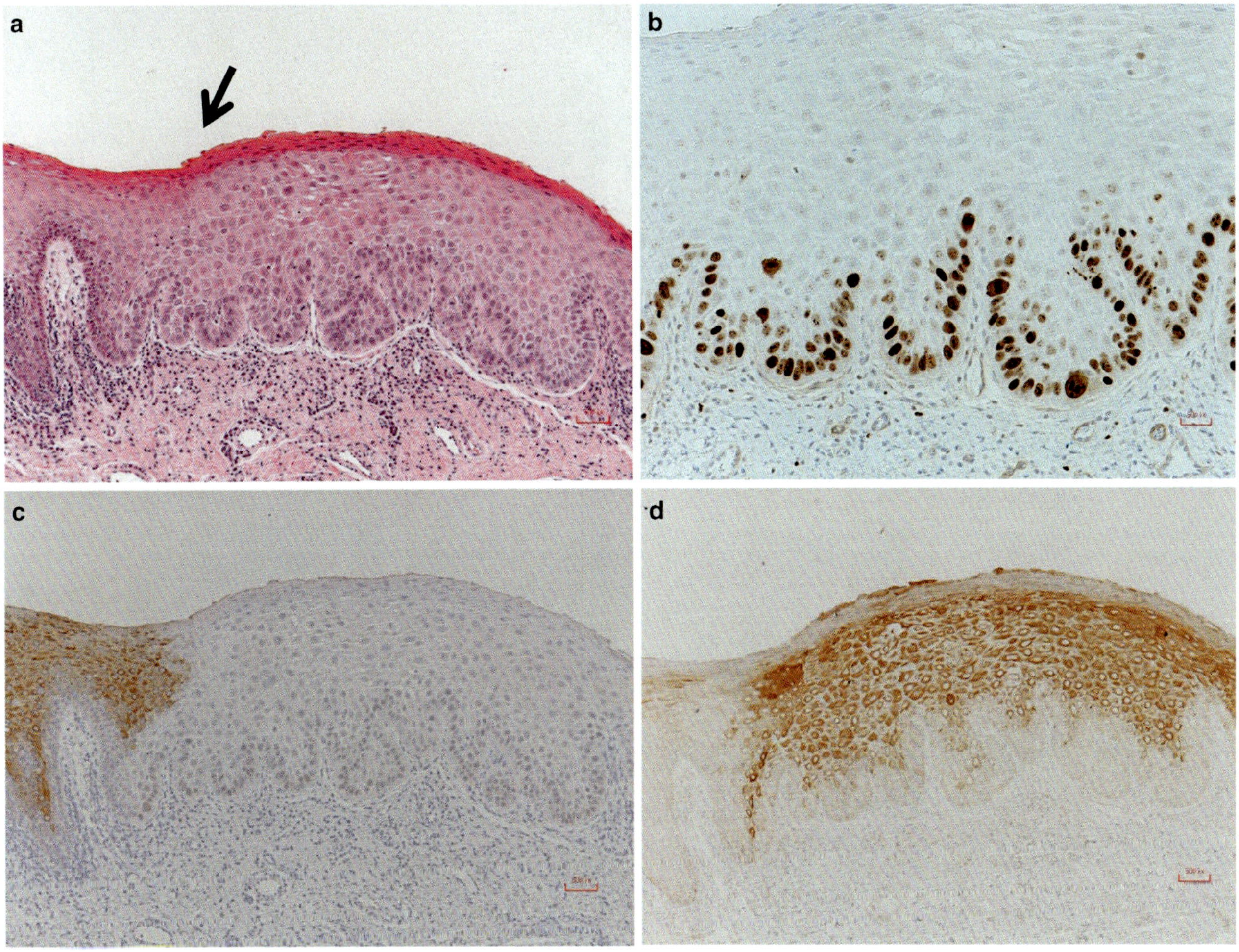

Fig. 2.21 Immunohistochemistry for cytokeratin 13 and 17 of OIN. (**a**) OIN, *arrow* shows the front line. (**b**, **c**) Immunohistochemistry for ki-67/MIB1 (**b**), cytokeratin 13 (**c**), and cytokeratin 17 (**d**)

Table 2.1 Schemas for histologically categorizing precursor CIS and related lesions

WHO	SIN	SIL*	OIN/CIS system	
		Hyperplasia/keratosis	Reactive atypical epithelium	
Mild dysplasia	SIN1			
		SIL I	OED →	Follow up
Moderate dysplasia	SIN2	(Low grade)		
Severe dysplasia	SIN3	SIL II (high grade)	OIN/CIS →	Mucosal resection
CIS				

WHO World Health Organization, *SIN* squamous intraepithelial neoplasia, *SIL* modified binary system of SIN, *OIN/CIS* oral intraepithelial neoplasia/carcinoma in situ, *OED* oral epithelial dysplasia

and calculating the total score. Despite their proven efficacy in many studies, these systems are not widely used because of their complexity.

In Japan, Imai conducted a study on tumor growth by focusing on tumor–host interactions and compared SCC in the oral cavity, larynx, and uterine cervix with adenocarcinoma in the stomach and breast (1954) [87]. The author classified tumors into elongation, hypertrophic, and budding growth types based on the morphology of the tumor margin and reported that the budding-type tumors had the worst prognosis. The author defines budding-type tumors as small tumor nests containing approximately 2–3 tumor cells on average or free tumors growing individually.

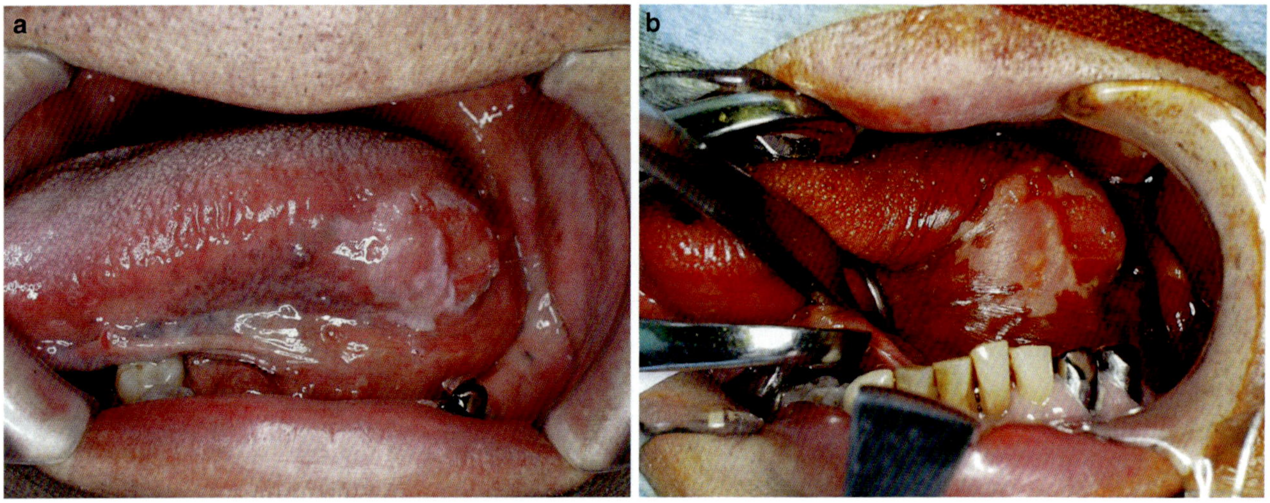

Fig. 2.22 Lugol's (iodine) staining of OIN. (**a**) Macroscopic presentation of early invasive cancer located posterior to OIN and appearing *white*. (**b**) Lugol's (iodine) staining showing lightly stained early invasive cancer located posterior to the OIN and appearing as an unstained area

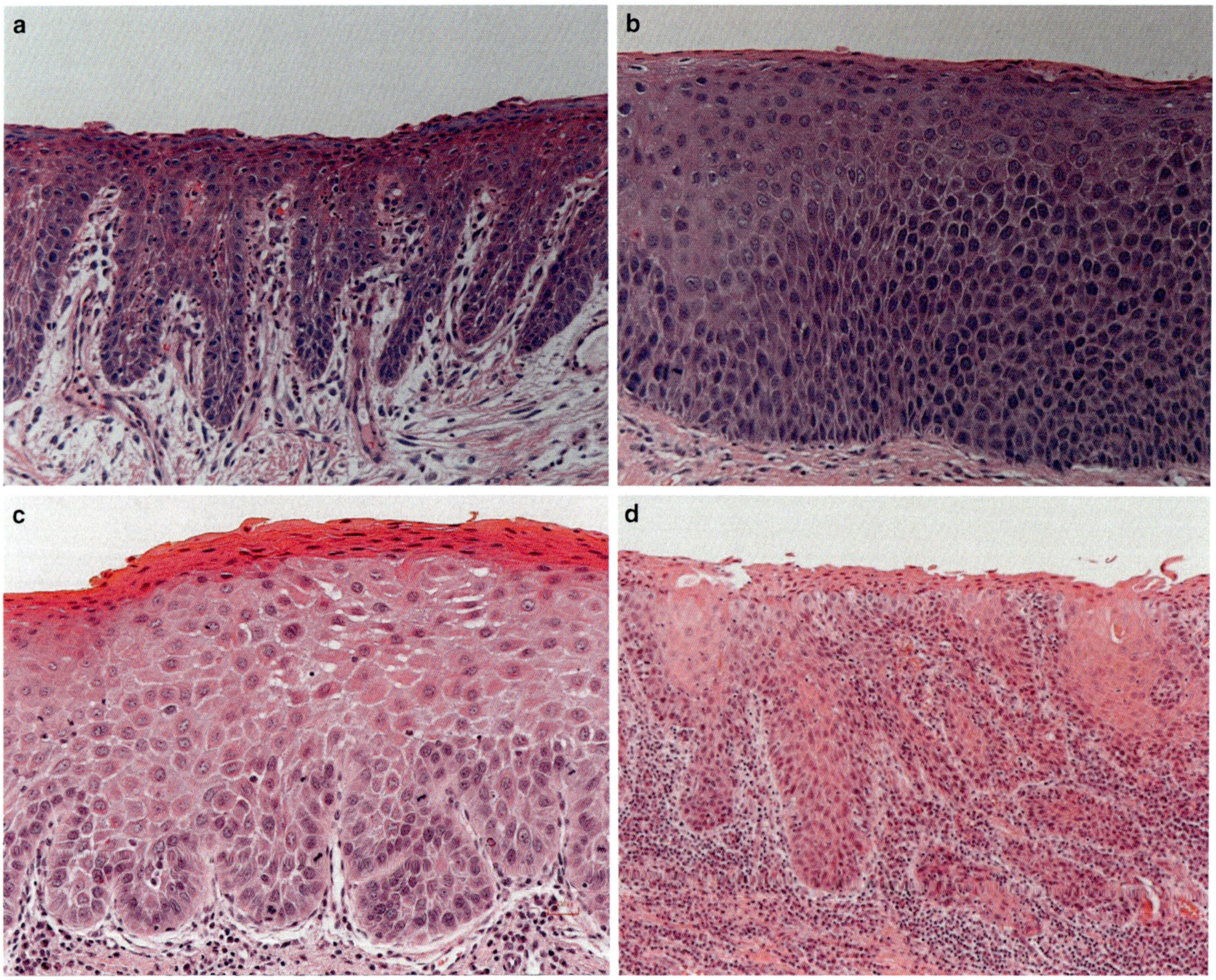

Fig. 2.23 Histological varieties of Lugol-free oral mucosa. (**a**) Reactive atypical epithelium. (**b**) Oral epithelial dysplasia. (**c**) Oral intraepithelial neoplasia. (**d**) Early invasive squamous cell carcinoma

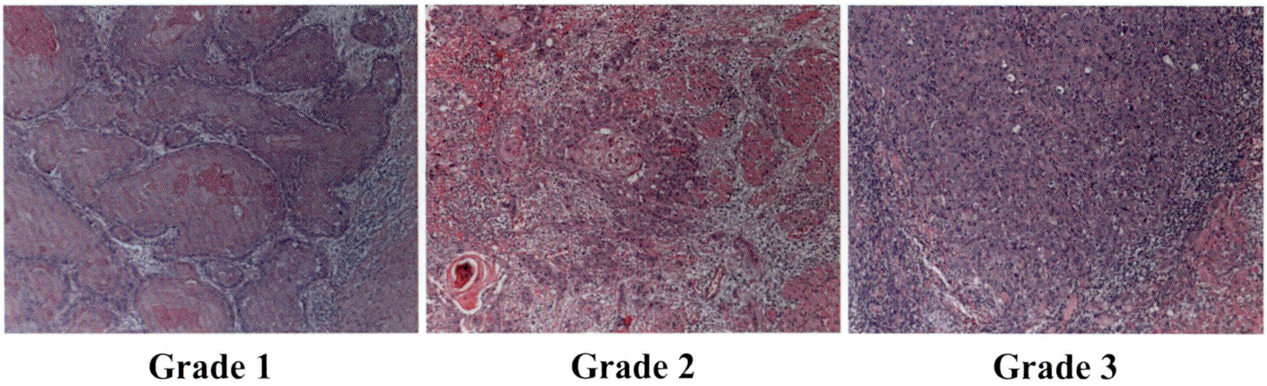

Fig. 2.24 World Health Organization histological grade of SCC

(2) Mode of Invasion/YK classification (Fig. 2.25):
YK-1: Well-defined borderline
YK-2: Cords, less-marked borderline
YK-3: Groups of cells, no distinct borderline
YK-4C: Diffuse invasion, cord-like type invasion
YK-4D: Diffuse invasion, diffuse-type invasion

After reporting that invasion characteristics are the most important indicator of malignancy among the histopathological factors used in the Jakobsson classification [83], Yamamoto systematically continued his study for many years before eventually elucidating their biological property [17, 88]. In Japan, a relatively large number of oral surgery clinics use tumor classification based on the patterns of tumor invasion, namely the YK Mode of Invasion that focuses on invasion patterns at tumor–host junctions and correlates highly with lymph node metastasis [89] and prognosis compared with the WHO grading system. The YK Mode of Invasion is also compatible with infiltrative growth patterns (INF: INFa, INFb, and INFc) observed in gastrointestinal cancer (esophageal, gastric, and colorectal cancers) [14–16], showing that YK-1, YK-2, YK-3, and YK-4C/4D correspond to oral cancer-specific well-differentiated SCC, INFa, INFb, and INFc, respectively. Although rare, YK-4D is highly malignant and possesses a specific biological property accompanied by desmoplastic reaction [89].

(3) Mode of mandibular invasion (Figs. 2.26, 2.27, 2.28, and 2.29):
Expansive type/invasive type
The malignancy of mandibular gingival cancer may be graded using the patterns of mandibular invasion [10, 12]. According to the mode of mandibular invasion, lower gingival carcinomas are histologically classified into two groups: invasive type and expansive type. The invasive type has a diffuse irregular margin, while the expansive type has a well-defined borderline. The pathological changes during bone resorption are comparable in both types of carcinoma. Histologically, in the invasive type, a large number of Howship's lacunae are observed in the resorption phase. In the expansive type, Howship's lacunae are relatively marked by reversal lines in the formation phase. Scanning electron microscopy of the invasive type has shown marked destruction of the bone surface with Howship's lacunae in the resorption phase, whereas scanning electron microscopy in the expansive type of carcinoma has shown a smooth bone surface with Howship's lacunae in the formation phase.

The utility of mandibular invasion patterns in determining tumor malignancy was investigated in a previous study examining 102 cases (1975–1990) [10, 12] and our multi-institutional study of 524 cases (1992–2005) [7] (Fig. 2.30). In both studies, a significant difference was observed in prognosis, but not lymph node metastasis, between the expansive and invasive types, indicating that the use of mandibular invasion patterns is an effective grading system that reflects the activity of local invasion. Furthermore, because of the correlation with imaging findings of bone resorption, this grading system may be regarded as a clinical classification method, as in the classification based on invasion patterns.

Note: Correlation between mode of mandibular invasion and image classification of bone resorption

Because radiographic findings of bone resorption simply reflect bone resorption caused by tumor invasion, they may not necessarily reflect the front line of bone invasion histopathologically. Yet, there is a certain correlation between the types of bone resorption and the patterns of bone invasion in SCC. A previous study comparing imaging findings of a surgical specimen using soft X-ray with histopathological findings revealed that the radiographic images of SCC of the mandibular gingiva show two types of bone resorption which reflect tumor invasion patterns. The two types of bone resorption correspond to the pressure and moth-eaten types in the conventional Swearingen classification [9], where

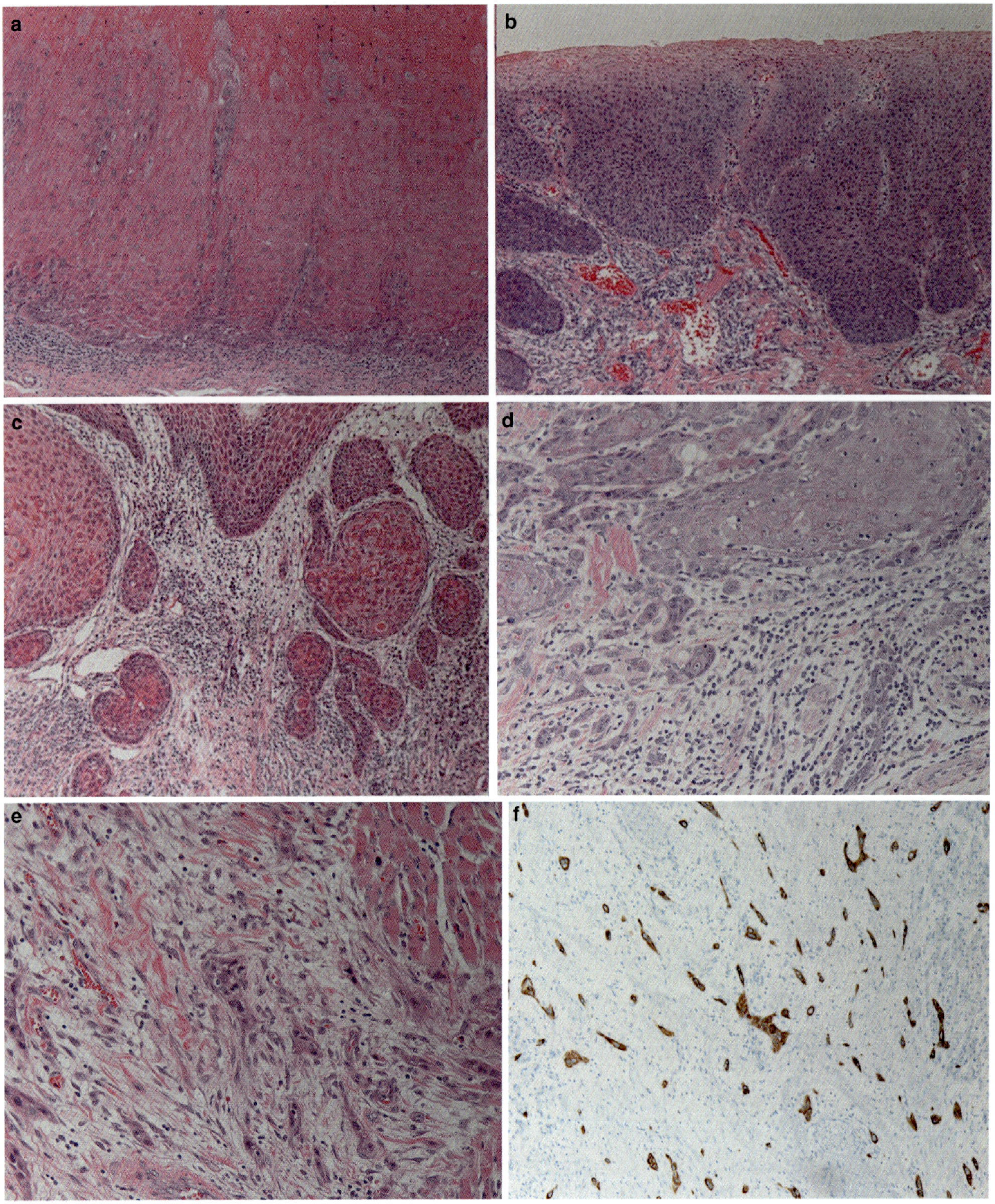

Fig. 2.25 YK-classification histologic figures. (**a**) YK-1, (**b**) YK-2, (**c**) YK-3, (**d**) YK-4C, (**e**) YK-4D, (**f**) YK-4D, immunohistochemistry for cytokeratin

the lesions with relatively uniform X-ray transmission and with clear and smooth bone resorption margins are defined as the pressure type and where lesions with uneven transmission due to diffused moth-eaten patterns are defined as the moth-eaten type (Fig. 2.31). The pressure and moth-eaten types correspond to the expansive and invasive types described in the previous section, with a significant correlation between the patterns of mandibular invasion and bone resorption and with a diagnostic accuracy of 76 % [10]. However, it is often difficult to classify actual clinical images into either type; consequently, the mixed type was introduced into

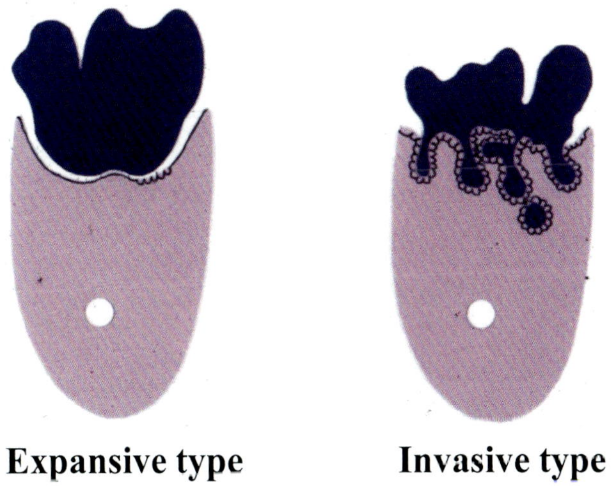

Fig. 2.26 Schemas for mode of mandibular invasion. *Left panel*: the expansive type of carcinoma has a well-defined borderline. *Right panel*: the invasive type of carcinoma has a diffuse irregular margin

the present general rules as the third bone resorption pattern. The clinical approach of this mixed type is similar to that of the moth-eaten type.

The diagnostic accuracy of bone resorption is affected by images used for the assessment, as shown by a study comparing the histological patterns of bone invasion with the patterns of bone resorption on panoramic X-ray images and CT images. Both types of image were statistically significantly correlated with bone invasion patterns; however, the correlation differed by pattern, and a greater correlation was observed between prognosis and bone resorption diagnosed by CT. Moreover, because a simple radiographic image compresses an entire visual plane, there is a chance of misdiagnosing the type of bone resorption, as an area of bone resorption could overlap with healthy trabecular bone located outside of the zone of tumor invasion. It is therefore necessary to incorporate the most advanced imaging technology to make clinically a significant diagnosis of bone resorption.

(4) Route of intramandibular development:
Development through the periodontal membrane (+/-)
Development in the mandibular canal (+/-)

It should be noted that tumor invasion in the mandibular soft tissue is not displayed as bone resorption on radiographic images. When assessing the range of tumor invasion, potential tumor invasion routes to consider are the periodontal ligament space and mandibular canal. Regardless of bone invasion patterns, the periodontal ligament space is the invasion route for early-stage cancers in the dentulous mandible (Fig. 2.32a). In contrast, tumor progression to the mandibular canal is observed only in the invasive type of pT4 cancers (Fig. 2.32b).

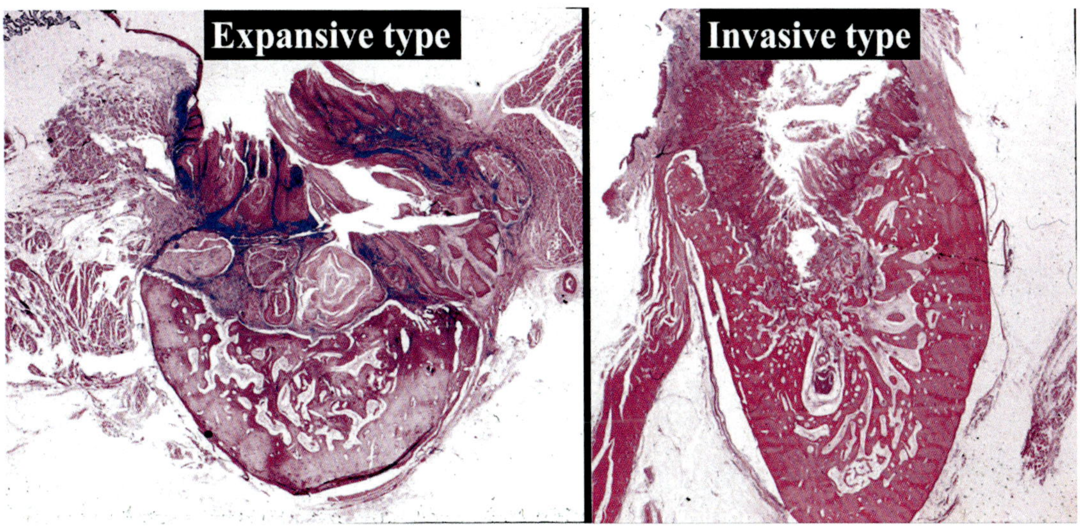

Fig. 2.27 Mode of mandibular invasion showing an image obtained using a magnifying glass. *Left panel*: expansive type of lower gingival carcinoma infiltrating the mandibular canal. *Right panel*: invasive type of lower gingival carcinoma infiltrating the mandibular canal

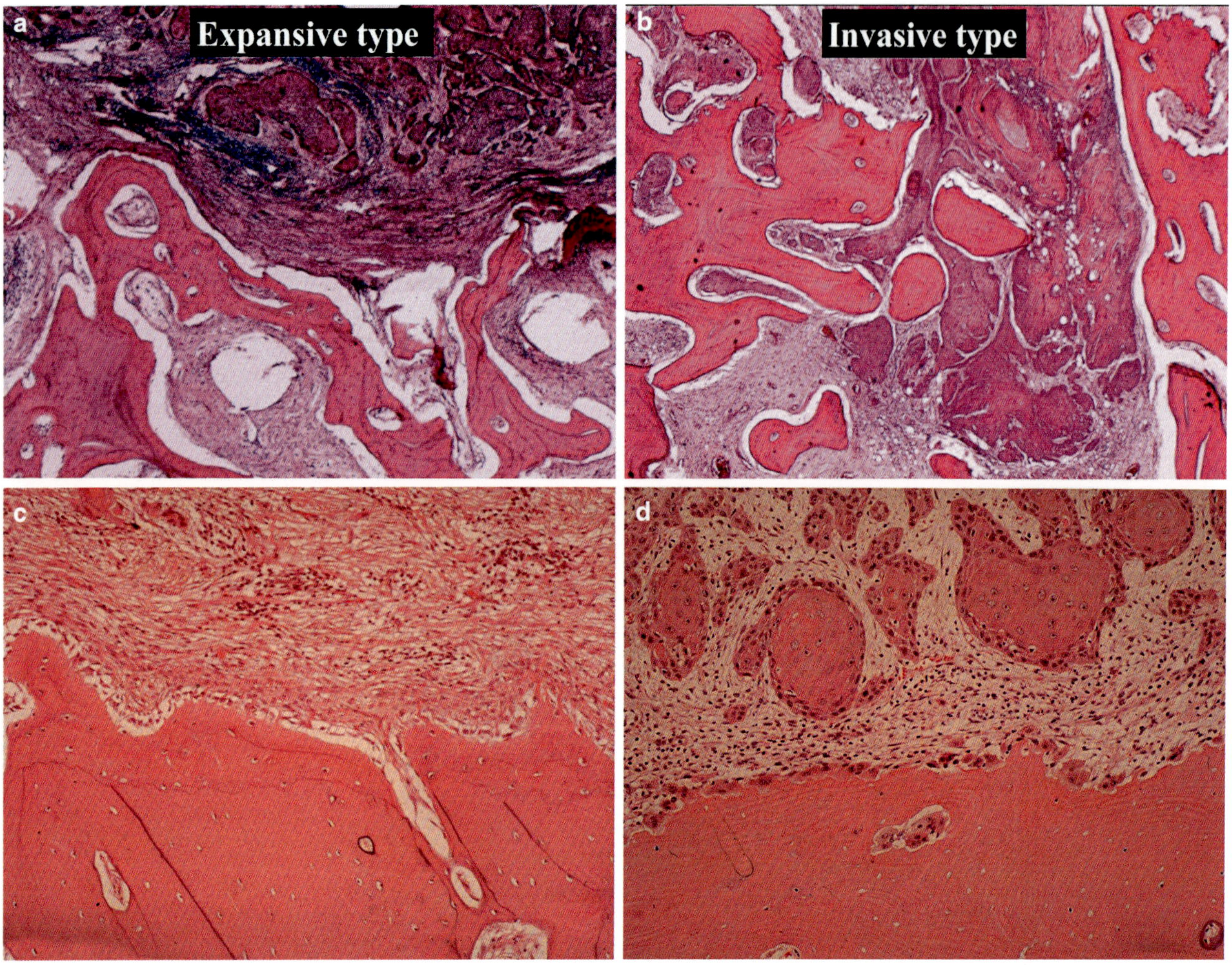

Fig. 2.28 Mode of mandibular invasion showing histologic presentation. (**a**) Expansive type carcinoma having a well-defined margin. (**b**) Invasive type carcinoma having diffuse irregular margins. (**c**) Reversal line seen on the bone surface, indicating that the bone is in the remodeling phase. (**d**) Howship's lacunae accompanied by a large number of osteoclasts, indicating that the bone is in the resorption phase

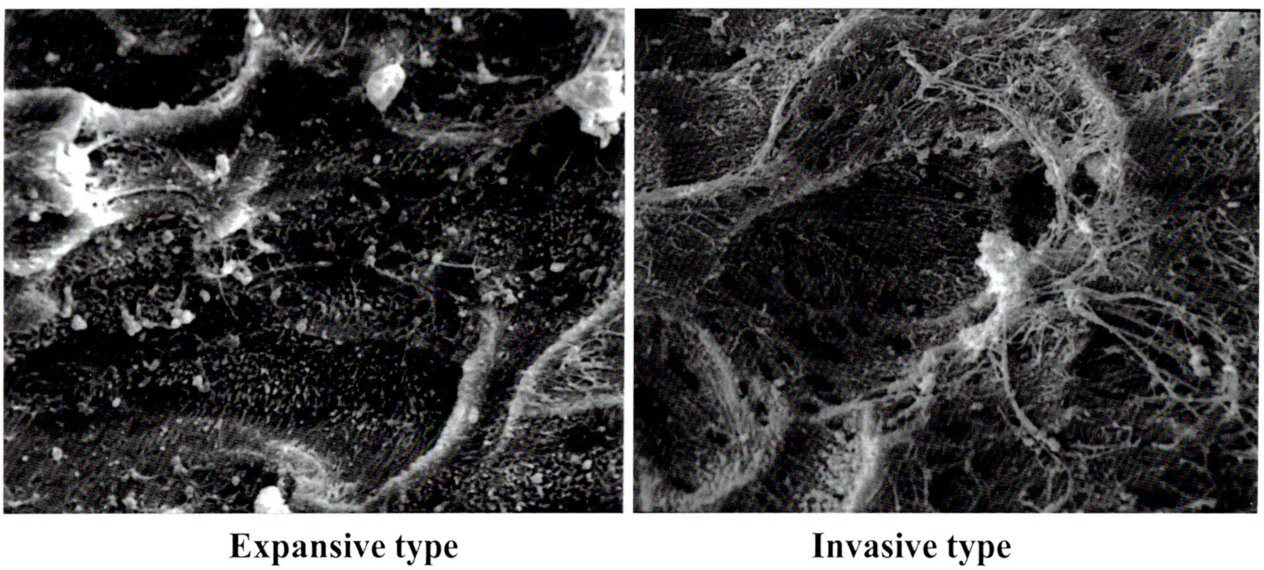

Fig. 2.29 Mode of mandibular invasion on scanning electron microscopy. *Left panel*: shallow Howship's lacunae accompanied by remineralization. *Right panel*: deep Howship's lacunae with many bone canaliculi at the *bottom*

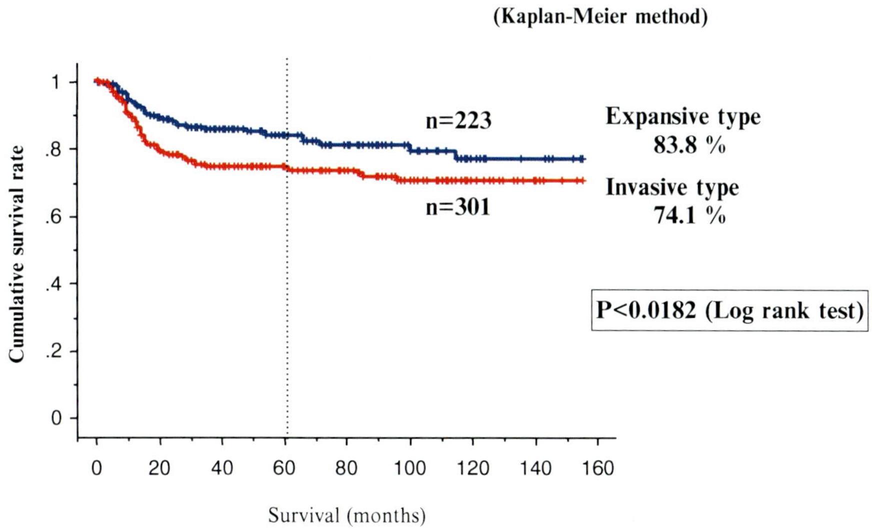

Fig. 2.30 Mode of mandibular invasion and prognosis

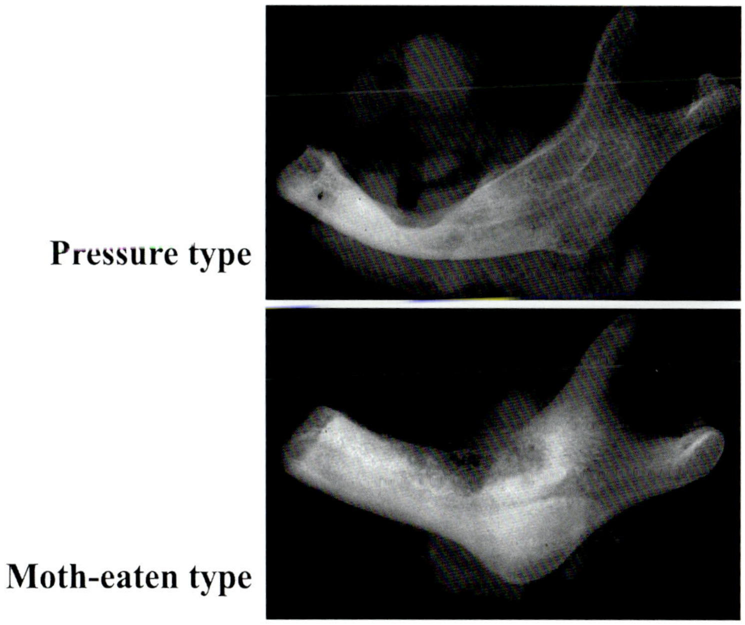

Fig. 2.31 Soft X-ray image of a surgical specimen of mandibular gingival squamous cell carcinoma. *Upper panel*: expansive type of lower gingival carcinoma. *Lower panel*: invasive type of lower gingival carcinoma

2.2.8.3 Squamous Cell Carcinoma, Variants

(1) Verrucous carcinoma (Fig. 2.33a)

This is a high-grade carcinoma that exhibits prominent exophytic growth of well-differentiated keratinized stratified squamous epithelium and locally destructive expansive subepithelial growth. It is difficult to diagnose this carcinoma when biopsy findings lack clear images of expansive growth into the subepithelial tissues. Although metastasis is an extremely rare clinical occurrence, attention must be paid to the fact that approximately 20 % of verrucous carcinoma cases are accompanied by typical SCC.

(2) Basaloid squamous cell carcinoma (Fig. 2.33b)

This is a highly malignant carcinoma that resembles the basal cells and is accompanied in part by clearly differentiated SCC. Basaloid SCC cells are either solid or arranged in cords, and a palisade arrangement of tumor cells is often observed in the vicinity of tumor nests, while coagulative necrosis of tumor nests and an expanding cystic cavity are observed in the central area.

(3) Adenoid squamous cell carcinoma (Fig. 2.33c)

This SCC presents with histological findings of adenosquamous carcinoma due to false spaces and ducts on diagnostic images caused by the liquefactive necrosis

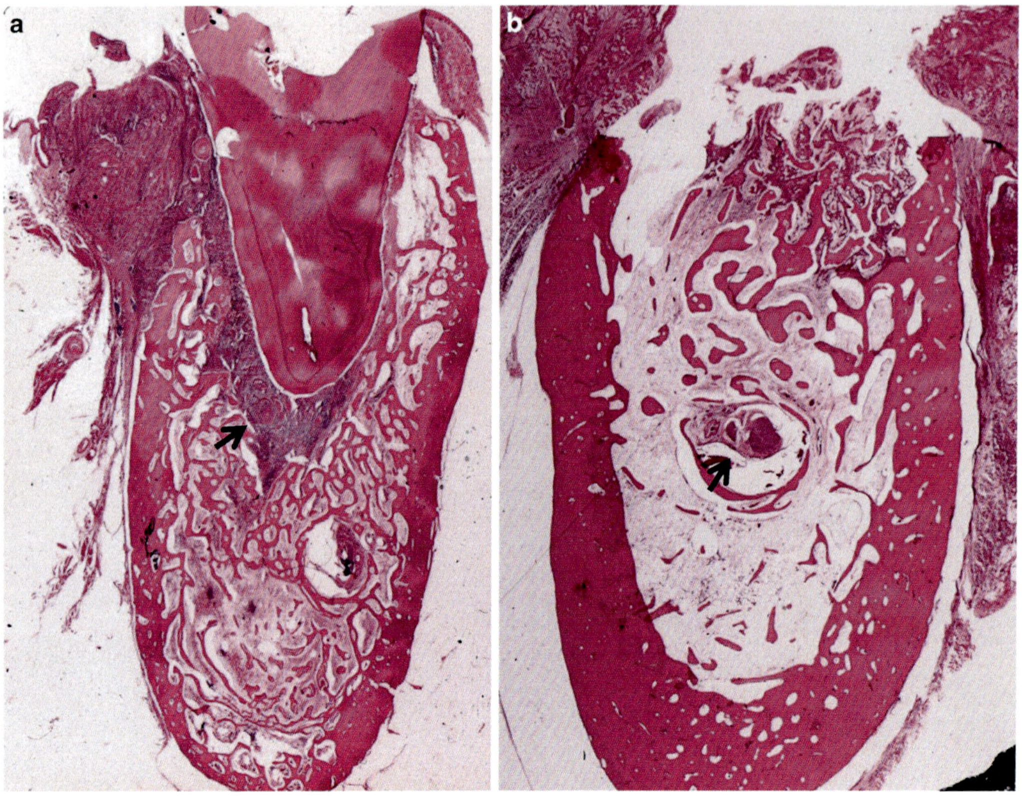

Fig. 2.32 Routes of intramandibular spread. (**a**) Developmental route through the periodontal membrane. (**b**) Developmental route in the mandibular canal

of the nests. No epithelial mucus is present. Although currently unclear, the clinicopathological malignancy of this SCC is thought to be similar to typical SCC. The classification of this SSC is currently under debate.

(4) Spindle cell carcinoma (Fig. 2.33d)
This is a highly malignant carcinoma that presents with sarcoma-like histological findings due to the proliferation of mostly spindle cells and other polygonal cells. It is occasionally accompanied by CIS or SCC. These cells are positive for vimentin and some cytokeratins. It is important to perform complete resection of spindle cell carcinoma in the early stages when it presents with pedunculated or sessile exophytic growth.

(5) Adenosquamous carcinoma (Fig. 2.33e)
This is a highly malignant carcinoma with histological findings of SCC and adenocarcinoma, with a ductal structure and mucus. The pathological features of invasion rather resemble those of adenocarcinoma, and attention must be paid to tumor progression through the trabecular bone so that bone destruction does not occur.

(6) Papillary squamous cell carcinoma (Fig. 2.33f)
This invasive SCC presents with exophytic papillary growth as well as expansive growth similar to verrucous carcinoma at the tumor–host margin, with clear cellular atypia. For definitive diagnosis, it is important to examine for invasive characteristics.

2.2.9 Invasion to Lymphatic Vessels, Veins, and Nerves

(1) Lymphatic vessel invasion
ly0: No lymphatic vessel invasion
ly1: Mild lymphatic vessel invasion
ly2: Marked lymphatic vessel invasion
Note: If immunostaining has been used for the evaluation of lymphatic vessel invasion, it must be recorded.

(2) Venous invasion
v0: No venous invasion
v1: Mild venous invasion
v2: Marked venous invasion
Note: If elastic fiber staining has been used for the evaluation of venous invasion, it must be recorded.

(3) Neural invasion
neu0: No neural invasion
neu1: Mild neural invasion
neu2: Marked neural invasion
Note: If immunostaining has been used for the evaluation of neural invasion, it must be recorded.

When examining the invasion of vessels, it is important to separate the invasion of lymph vessels (ly) and veins (v). When they are indistinguishable on a hematoxylin–eosin-stained specimen, elastic fiber staining such as Elastica van Gieson staining and

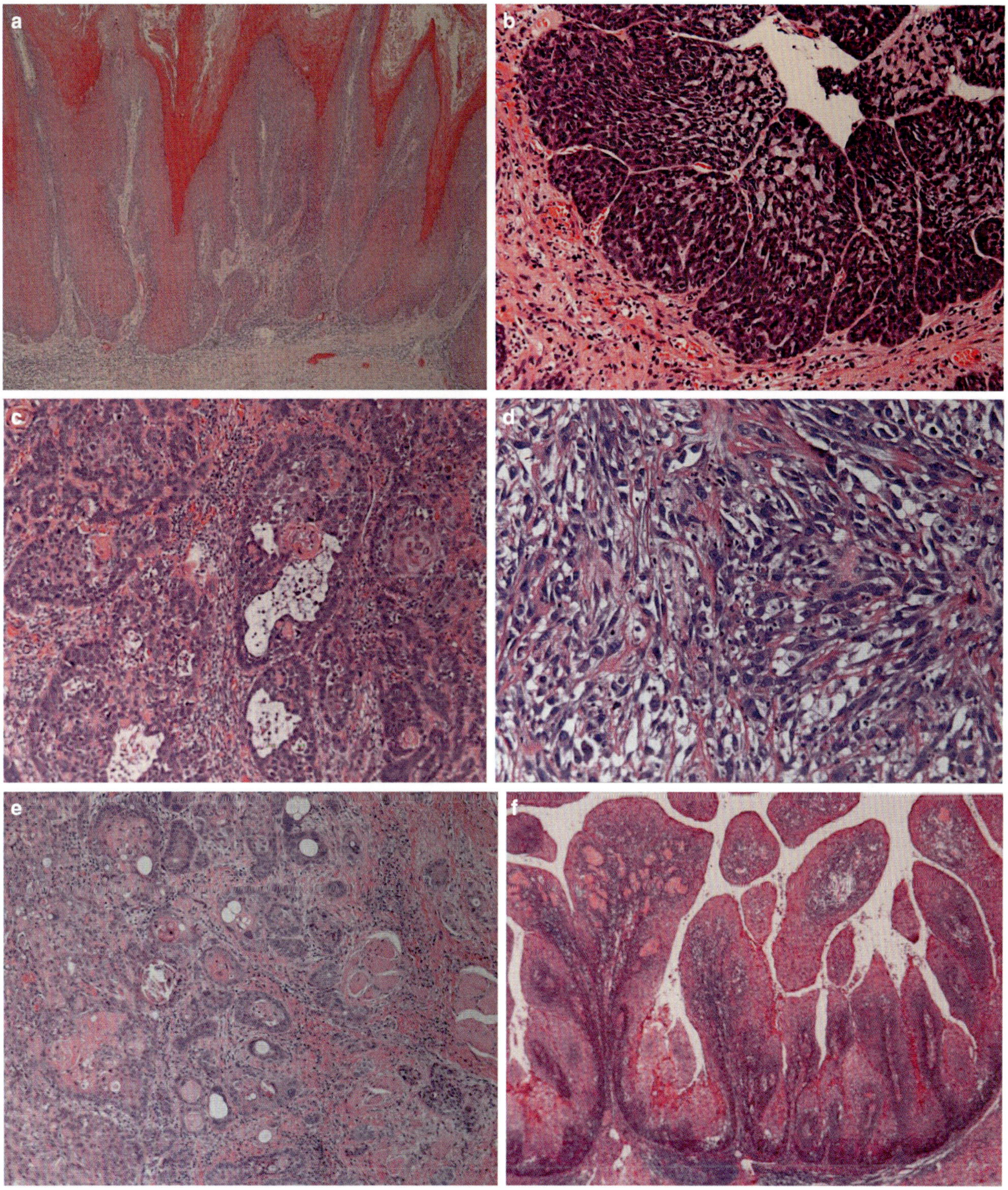

Fig. 2.33 Histological variants of squamous cell carcinoma. (**a**) Verrucous carcinoma, (**b**) basaloid squamous cell carcinoma, (**c**) adenoid squamous cell carcinoma, (**d**) spindle cell carcinoma, (**e**) adenosquamous carcinoma, (**f**) papillary squamous cell carcinoma

immunostaining with monoclonal antibody D2-40 are used to confirm v and ly, respectively.

Among oral cavity cancers, perineural infiltration by adenoid cystic carcinoma is well known to affect prognosis. In SCC, it is rare for perineural infiltration to extend very far from the primary lesion site. However, it is important to pay attention to neural invasion near the resection margin or neural invasion into the mandibular canal.

2.2.10 Evaluation of the Resection Margin

(1) Horizontal margin (HM), distance from margin ( ) mm
 pHMX Impossible to evaluate the resection margin
 pHM0 Margin (-)
 pHM1 Margin (+)
 Note: Also record presence or absence of OED at the mucosal stump.
(2) Vertical margin (VM), distance from margin ( ) mm
 pVMX Impossible to evaluate the resection margin
 pVM0 Margin (-)
 pVM1 Margin (+)
 Note: Also record the results of evaluation of the bone stump in patients after osteotomy and stump of the inferior alveolar nerve in patients after mandibular/mandibular canal resection.

The most important point to remember during the histopathological examination of the resected specimen in oral cavity cancer is to determine the presence of cancer cells. For this reason, the pathologist should be provided with clinical information about where to conduct detailed examination. It is a good idea to mark (e.g., using a thread) the region of tissue suggestive of Ca(+) or (+/-) based on the preoperative findings of tumor margin, intraoperative palpation, and postoperative visual inspection of the specimen. It is also important to explain whether the resection margin in the mucosal surface was set in the area stained by iodine.

2.3 Regional Lymph Node Metastasis

The classification and range of cervical lymph nodes are the same as described in the Rules Regarding Lymph Nodes by the Japan Society of Clinical Oncology (JSCO) (Fig. 2.34), and lymph node metastasis was evaluated according to the UICC classification. Internationally, the level classification (Fig. 2.35) system by ACHNSO based on the area of neck dissection is widely used, and the American Academy of Otolaryngology-Head and Neck Surgery (AAO-HNS) classification, a fragmented version of the ACHNSO classification, has also been proposed.

(1) Site
 Regional lymph node groups (JSCO), level classification (AAO-HNS)

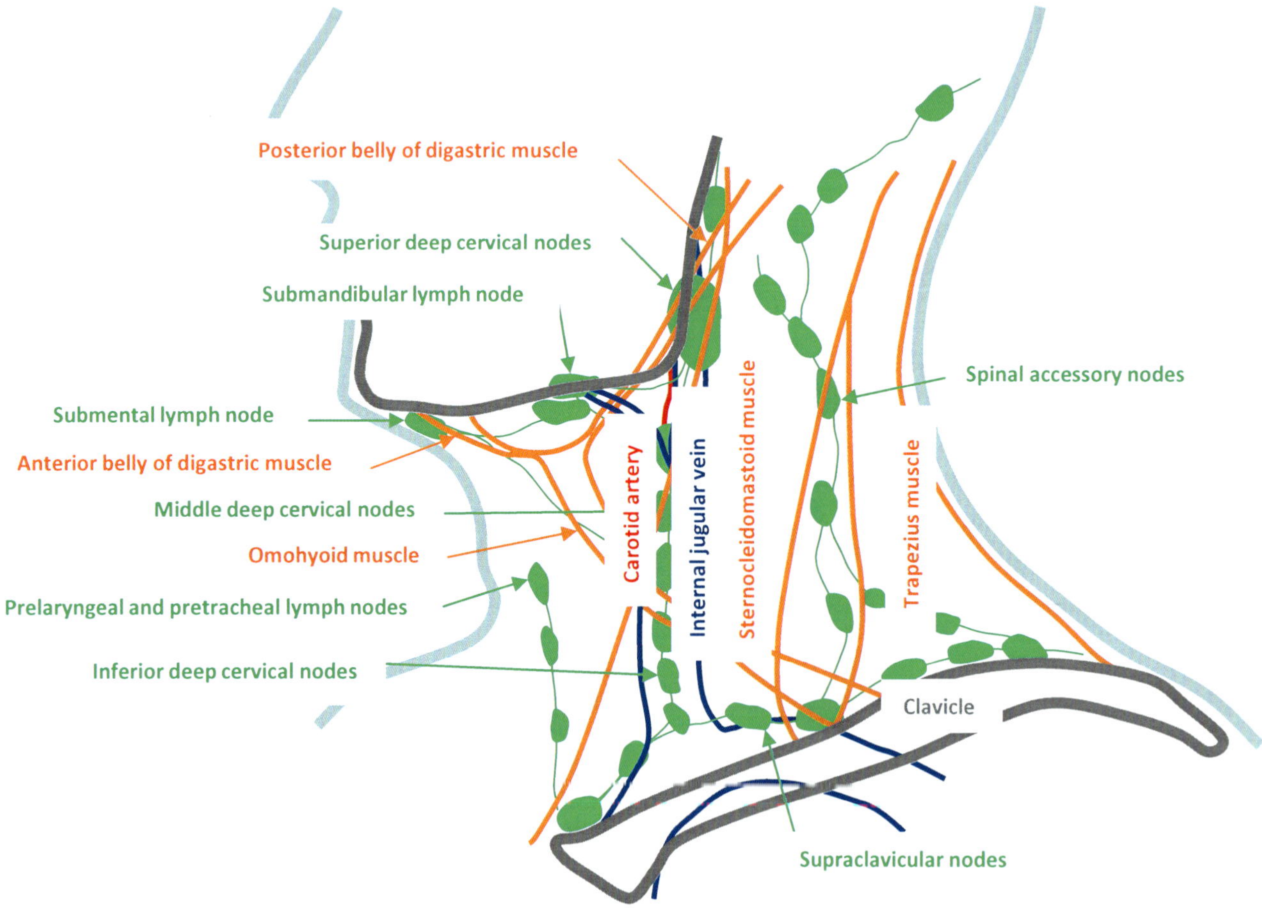

Fig. 2.34 Classification of cervical lymph nodes according to the classification of regional lymph nodes published by the Japan society of clinical oncology

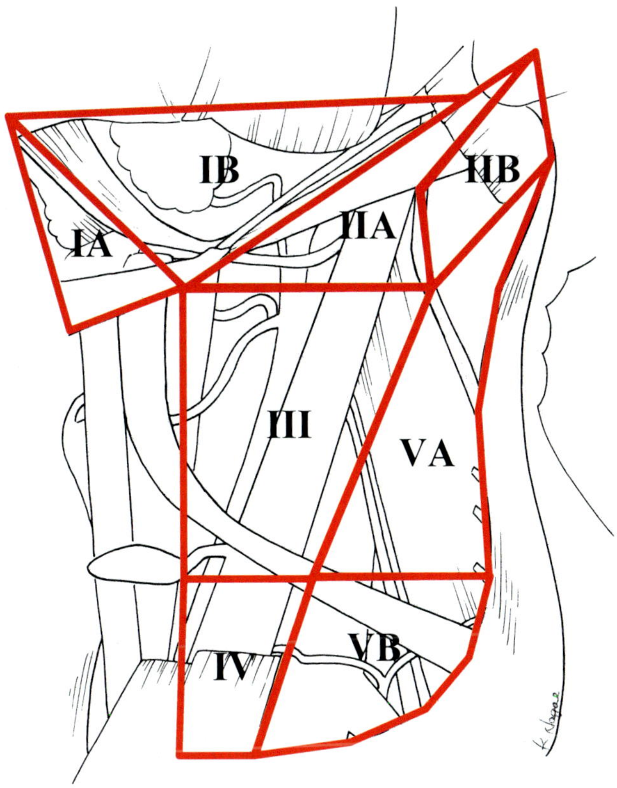

Fig. 2.35 Classification of cervical lymph node levels

(2) Number of metastasis
Number of metastatic lymph nodes/number of resected lymph nodes
(3) Size (<3<6<) cm
(4) Adhesiveness (–/+), extranodal invasion (–/+)
(5) N factor
NX: Regional lymph nodes cannot be assessed
N0: No regional lymph node metastasis
N1: Metastasis in a single ipsilateral lymph node, ≤3 cm in greatest dimension
N2a: Metastasis in a single ipsilateral lymph node, >3 cm but ≤6 cm in greatest dimension
N2b: Metastasis in multiple ipsilateral lymph nodes, none >6 cm in greatest dimension
N2c: Metastasis in bilateral or contralateral lymph nodes, none >6 cm in greatest dimension
N3: Metastasis in a lymph node, >6 cm in greatest dimension
Note 1: Lymph nodes of the median region are ipsilateral lymph nodes.
Note 2: Direct invasion of the primary tumor to lymph nodes is classified as lymph node metastasis.
Note 3: Tumors ≥ 3 mm at sites corresponding to lymph nodes are classified as regional lymph node metastases even without a histological lymph node remnant.
Note 4: If the size is within the evaluation criteria of the pN classification, the size of the metastatic focus rather than the entire lymph node is measured.
Level classification (Fig. 2.35)
Level IA: Submental lymph nodes
Level IB: Submandibular lymph nodes
Level IIA: Superior deep cervical lymph nodes (jugulodigastric nodes) (anterior)
Level IIB: Superior deep cervical lymph nodes (jugulodigastric nodes) (posterior)
Level III: Middle deep cervical lymph nodes (juguloomohyoid nodes)
Level IV: Inferior deep cervical lymph nodes
Level VA: Spinal accessory lymph nodes
Level VB: Supraclavicular lymph nodes

Note: Examination of sentinel lymph node

Sentinel nodes (SNs) are the first lymph nodes to receive lymph flowing from a tumor. The SN theory states that the tumor metastasizes further after invading an SN. If this theory is correct, cases without SN metastasis are thought to be free of lymph node metastasis and therefore require no neck dissection. Consequently, by using SNs as an indicator of metastasis and performing detailed examination of SNs, it is possible to perform highly sensitive and effective diagnosis of micrometastasis. In recent years, the SN-based diagnosis of metastasis has produced good clinical outcomes in many fields.

In oral cancers, the site and frequency of SN metastasis vary due to individual variations in lymph drainage and to differences in tumor sites and tissue types. However, it is possible to determine the area of lymph node dissection required individually based on the severity of SN metastasis. Clinical application of SN biopsy in treating oral cavity cancer is expected to become widespread in the future; however, further studies are needed to improve the accuracy of intraoperative diagnosis of micrometastasis.

2.4 *M* Score

MX: Presence of distant metastasis cannot be assessed
M0: No distant metastasis
M1: Distant metastasis

The category M1 may be further specified according to the following notation:

Pulmonary (PUL), hepatic (HEP), osseous (OSS), lymph nodes (LYM), adrenal gland (ADR), brain (BRA), skin (SKI), and other (OTH)

2.5 Staging

The stage is determined according to the UICC classification. The *T*, *N*, and *M* scores and stage are recorded (Table 2.2).

2.6 Multiple, Double, and Multiple Primary Cancers

(1) Multiple oral cancers: The occurrence of 2 or more primary cancers fulfilling the following conditions:
  (a) Cancers located at different sites according to the UICC classification.
  (b) Cancers located at corresponding contralateral sites.
  (c) Cancers located at ipsilateral sites, but not continuous and are clinically separated by ≥1.5 cm.
  (d) Each lesion is histopathologically confirmed to be a carcinoma.

(2) Double cancer: The concurrence of primary oral cancer with primary malignant tumors of other organs. If both multiple and double cancers are observed, they are expressed as multiple-double cancers.

(3) Multiple primary cancers: The term multiple primary cancers is used to comprehensively express multiple and double cancers.

(4) Synchronous and heterochronous cancers
  (a) Cancers diagnosed within a period of <1 year are defined as synchronous cancers.
  (b) Cancers diagnosed at an interval of ≥1 year are defined as heterochronous cancers.
  (c) If there are both synchronous and heterochronous cancers, they are called synchronous/heterochronous cancers.

  Note 1: The organs affected by double cancers are indicated.

  Note 2: Whether the cancers are synchronous or heterochronous is indicated.

2.7 Histological Evaluation of Therapeutic Effect

If radiation therapy or chemotherapy has been used to treat oral cancer, conditions of treatment including the dose and method of irradiation, the kind, dose, and administration method of the drugs used, and the time from last treatment to resection of the lesion should be recorded.

In examining patients after preoperative treatment, specimens of the grossly estimated lesion must be prepared as thoroughly as possible, and the state of the remaining tumor must be evaluated histologically.

Table 2.2 Staging

	N0	N1	N2	N3	M1
Tis	0				
T1	I	III	IVA	IVB	IVC
T2	II	III	IVA	IVB	IVC
T3	III	III	IVA	IVB	IVC
T4a	IVA	IVA	IVA	IVB	IVC
T4b	IVB	IVB	IVB	IVB	IVC

Grade 0: Ineffective

No therapeutic effect is noted in cancer tissue or cancer cells.

Grade 1: Slightly effective

Some degenerative change is noted in cancer tissue/cells, but cancer cells considered capable of proliferation (those showing eosinophilic cytoplasm with vacuolation and enlargement of the nucleus are also included) occupy ≥1/3 of the cancer in a tissue section.

Grade 1a: Very slightly effective

Cancer cells considered "capable of proliferation" occupy ≥2/3 of the cancer.

Grade 1b: Mildly effective

Cancer cells considered "capable of proliferation" occupy between 1/3 and 2/3 of the cancer.

Grade 2: Moderately effective

Cancer cells considered "capable of proliferation" occupy <1/3 of the cancer, and those showing a tendency toward nuclear disintegration are dominant.

Grade 3: Markedly effective

No cancer cells considered "capable of proliferation" are observed, and all cancer cells show a tendency toward nuclear disintegration, or only a trace of cancer is noted.

Note: If a section clearly judged to be a focus of reproliferation is noted in a treated cancer focus, the entry "evidence of reproliferation (+)" should be made after the judgment.

(1) Study methods

  To histologically assess the treatment outcome, it is necessary to examine all specimens for morphological changes in cancer cells, cell nests, and cytoplasm with the emphasis on changes in cancer cell morphology and the degree of destruction in cell nests. The ratio of areas showing any of the changes stated above is calculated by setting the entire section containing the cancerous tissue as 1. It is also important to record treatment conditions and preoperative duration because these factors influence tissue morphology.

(2) Histological changes observed in cancer cells and cell nests (Fig. 2.36)
  (a) Changes in cancer cells
    (1) Increase in abnormal mitotic figures
    (2) Enlarged nucleus, prominent nucleolus, chromatin condensation on the nuclear membrane, and appearance of multinucleated giant cell

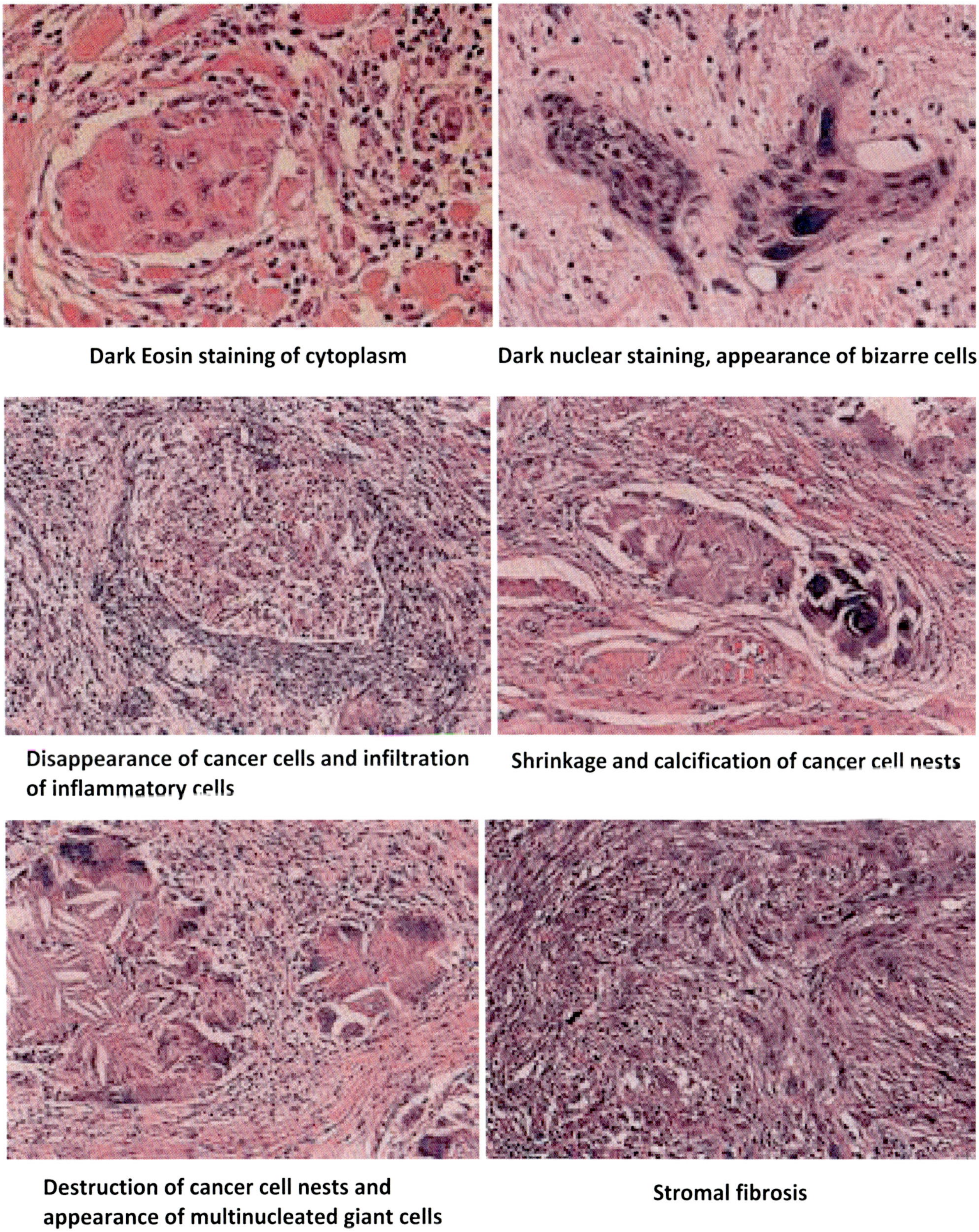

Fig. 2.36 Histologic findings showing the effect of radiotherapy and chemotherapy

(3) Lysis of cancer cells and nuclei, dark staining of cytoplasm with eosin, dark staining of the nucleus, and appearance of bizarre cells

(b) Changes in cancer cell nests
   (1) Lymphocyte infiltration around cancer cell nests
   (2) Lysis of cancer cells and inflammatory cell infiltration
   (3) Moth-eaten-like changes to cell nests and shrinkage and disappearance of cell nests
   (4) Foreign-body granuloma and xanthomatous granuloma

(c) "Nonviable cells"
   (1) Greatly eosinophilic cytoplasm
   (2) Pyknosis or karyolysis
   (3) Karyorrhexis
   (4) Cell membrane lysis
   (5) Cellular infiltration of leukocytes

(d) "Viable cells"
   Active cells without the features of "nonviable cell"

2.8 Biopsy

When obtaining a biopsy specimen prior to treatment, it is common to perform wedge biopsy, where a wedge-shaped specimen contains both the tumor and non-tumorous mucosa. The purpose of biopsy is not only to verify the presence of cancerous lesions but also to obtain detailed clinical information, including histological grade, invasion features, vascular invasion, and prediction of lymph node metastasis. At biopsy, a tissue specimen greater than 5 mm in diameter that contains invasion front tissue is collected. However, if vital iodine staining reveals a wide iodine-free area in the vicinity of the tumor, it is important to obtain a wedge-shape tissue specimen containing both the stained and non-stained areas with the aim to determine tumor resection margin.

Mucosal resection including the iodine-free area is recommended when the diagnosis of a small, early cancer (up to early T2) is made after careful assessment of tumor depth by palpation and diagnostic imaging.

2.9 Handling of Surgical Materials

2.9.1 Sectioning Method

It is a principle of surgical pathological studies of mucosal cancer to prepare cross sections perpendicular to the mucosal surface.

(1) Sampling of soft tissues of the tongue, buccal mucosa, and FOM
   In cancers of the tongue, buccal mucosa, and FOM, examination of coronal sections is preferable. Sections are obtained at intervals of 5–7 mm by step sectioning, and tumoral and ulcerative lesions in each section are photographed as magnified images. Large samples containing skin, muscle, or bone tissue are sectioned at intervals of 1–2 cm and photographed after checking the spread of the tumor on the mucosal surface and depth. Subsequently, a tissue block 4–5 mm thick is sectioned from a representative cross section to prepare specimens (Figs. 2.37, 2.38, 2.39, and 2.40).

(2) Sampling of maxillary or mandibular gingival cancer
   (a) Surgical sample consisting of only soft tissues
   After checking the extent of the lesion (particularly, the anteroposterior dimension, lateral margins, and gingival margin at the dental neck adjacent to the next tooth), the sample is sectioned coronally or sagittally by referring to image information such as CT and MRI. First, the resection margin is sectioned and then the center of the primary lesion, and serial sections are obtained at intervals of 4–5 mm.
   (b) Surgical samples containing hard tissues
      (1) Method to examine the sample without separating hard and soft tissues
      The basic method to section samples of upper or lower gingival cancer containing tooth or bone tissue is to section them perpendicularly to the dental arch, centering around the deepest part of the primary tumor. If the tumor is located in the incisor region, the dental arch is markedly curved, so the sample should be sectioned radially. Because the lateral and molar regions are also arched gently, sections should be made by checking the direction of the teeth. Sections containing hard tissue are cut out at intervals of 7–8 mm using a diamond cutter and decalcified after photographing the cross sections (Fig. 2.39).
      (2) Method to examine the sample by separating soft tissue and bone
      Since the stainability of soft tissue is expected to be reduced by the decalcification of bone, specimens may also be prepared after separating hard and soft tissues. When this method is employed, accurate diagnosis is impossible unless the spatial relationship between bone and soft tissue is clear. Their locations must be determined on photographs or through other such techniques, and the spatial relationships of invasion sites and the resection margin should be clarified before their separation. In mandibular gingival cancer, because tumor cells are more numerous in the margin of soft tissue than in bone, judgment

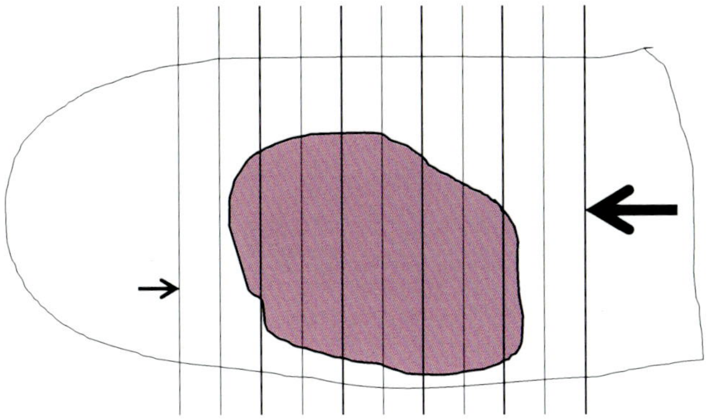

Fig. 2.37 How to resect tongue cancer

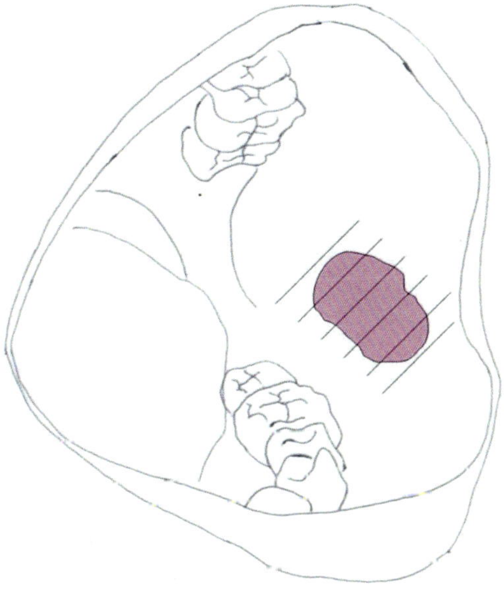

Fig. 2.38 How to resect buccal mucosal cancer

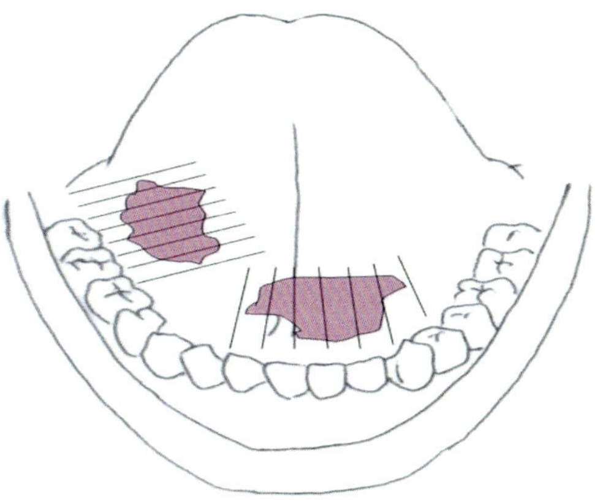

Fig. 2.39 How to resect floor of mouth cancer

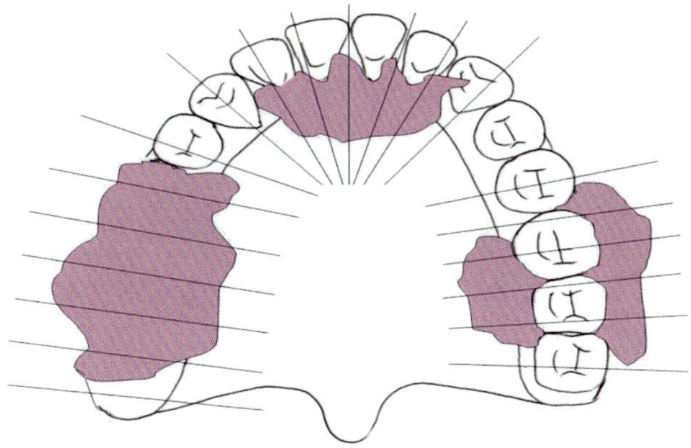

Fig. 2.40 How to resect upper gingival cancer

using high-quality specimens is meaningful. Particularly in patients who have undergone preoperative treatments such as chemotherapy, the judgment of the therapeutic effect using decalcified soft tissue specimens is often difficult.

2.9.2 Decalcification Methods

Tissue sections 7–8 mm thick containing hard tissue are placed in a decalcification solution after washing under running water, without washing, or after defatting in a mixture of equal volumes of methanol and chloroform for 1 day as a pretreatment. Plank-Rychlo's rapid decalcification solution is typically used. Stainability after decalcification is preserved by performing low-temperature decalcification in a refrigerator (low temperature decalcification). A sufficient amount of decalcification solution for the sample (several tens of times) should be prepared and changed during the decalcification process when considered appropriate. Decalcification is accelerated by shaking the decalcification solution. EDTA decalcification solution must be used if a process such as immunostaining is anticipated.

Acknowledgments Development of the first edition of General Rules for Clinical and Pathological Studies on Oral Cancer was made possible by the efforts of many oral surgeons, oral radiologists, and oral pathologists. We thank Eiichiro Ariji, Satoru Ozeki, Norihiko Okada, Sadao Okabe, Yuichiro Okazaki, Ken Omura, Tadaaki Kirita, Mikio Kusama, Toru Sato, Masanori Shinohara, Kazuo Shimozato, Satoru Shintani, Yoichi Tanaka, Eiji Nakayama, Takahumi Hayashi, Akihiro Miyazaki, HisaoYagishita, and Masayuki Yamane for their contribution to many parts of this chapter.

References

1. Japan Society for Oral Tumors (2010) General rules for clinical and pathological studies on oral cancer (in Japanese), 1st edn. Kanehara, Tokyo
2. Izumo T, Kirita T, Ajiri E et al (2012) General rules for clinical and pathological studies on oral cancer: a synopsis. Jpn J Clin Oncol 42:1099–1109
3. Sobin LH, Gospodarowicz MK, Wittekind C (eds) (2009) TNM classification of malignant tumours, 7th edn. UK Wiley-Blackwell, Chichester
4. Barnes L, Everson JW, Reichart P et al (eds) (2005) World Health Organization classification on tumours: pathology and genetics of head and neck tumours. IARC Press, Lyon
5. Working Group 1, Scientific Committee, Japan Society for Oral Tumors (2005) General rules for the clinical and pathological studies on oral carcinoma: 1, carcinoma of the tongue (in Japanese). J Jpn Soc Oral Tumor 17:13–86
6. Working Group 1, Scientific Committee, Japan Society for Oral Tumors (2008) General rules for the clinical and pathological studies on oral carcinoma: 3, carcinoma of the buccal mucosa and floor of mouth (in Japanese). J Jpn Soc Oral Tumor 20:25–117
7. Working Group 1, Scientific Committee, Japan Society for Oral Tumors (2007) General rules for the clinical and pathological studies on oral carcinoma: 2, Carcinoma of the lower gingiva (in Japanese). J Jpn Soc Oral Tumor 19:37–124
8. Working Group 1, Scientific Committee, Japan Society for Oral Tumors (2009) General rules for the clinical and pathological studies on oral carcinoma: 3, carcinoma of the upper gingiva and palate (in Japanese). J Jpn Soc Oral Tumor 20:25–117
9. Swearingen AG, McGraw JP, Palumbo VD (1966) Roentgenographic pathologic correlation of carcinoma of the gingiva involving the mandible. Am J Roentgenol Radium Ther Nucl Med 96:15–18
10. Izumo T (1986) Bone resorption by invasive squamous cell carcinoma of mandibular gingiva (in Japanese). J Stomatol Soc Jpn 53:343–356
11. Totsuka Y, Usui T, Tei K et al (1991) Mandibular involvement by squamous cell carcinoma of the lower alveolus: analysis and comparative study of histologic and radiologic features. Head Neck 13:40–50
12. Izumo T (2001) Surgical pathology of squamous cell carcinoma in the mandibular gingiva: mode of mandibular invasion (in Japanese). J Jpn Soc Oral Tumor 13:223–228
13. Tei K, Totsuka Y, Iizuka T et al (2004) Marginal resection for carcinoma of the mandibular alveolus and gingiva where radiologically detected bone defects do not extend beyond the mandibular canal. J Oral Maxillofac Surg 62:834–839
14. Japanese Society for Esophageal Diseases (2008) Japanese classification of esophageal cancer. Kanehara, Tokyo
15. Japanese Gastric Cancer Association (2011) Japanese classification of gastric carcinoma: 3rd edition. Gastric Cancer 14:101–112
16. Japanese Society for Cancer of the Colon and Rectum (2009) Japanese classification of colorectal carcinoma. Kanehara, Tokyo
17. Yamamoto E, Kohama G, Sunakawa H et al (1983) Mode of invasion, bleomycin sensitivity, and clinical course in squamous cell carcinoma of the oral cavity. Cancer 51:2175–2180
18. Hayashi T, Ito J, Taira S et al (2001) The relationship of primary tumor thickness in carcinoma of the tongue to subsequent lymph node metastasis. Dentomaxillofac Radiol 30:242–245
19. Shintani S, Yoshihama Y, Ueyama Y et al (2001) The usefulness of intraoral ultrasonography in the evaluation of oral cancer. Int J Oral Maxillofac Surg 30:139–143
20. Kimura Y, Ariji Y, Gotoh M et al (2001) Doppler sonography of the deep lingual artery. Acta Radiol 42:306–311
21. Sasaki T, Fujibayashi T, Imai Y et al (1999) A study on T-classifications of carcinomas of upper alveolus and gingiva and carcinoma of hard palate: a proposal of "sinus and nasal floor (SNF) criteria" (in Japanese). J Jpn Soc Oral Tumor 11:98–105
22. Sasaki T, Imai Y, Fujibayashi T (2004) New proposal for T classification of gingival carcinomas arising in the maxilla. Int J Oral Maxillofac Surg 33:349–352
23. Fujibayashi T (2004) Level of mandibular canal (LMC) criteria of lower gingival carcinomas and mode of mandibulectomy according to LMC criteria and bone invasion pattern (in Japanese). J Jpn Soc Oral Tumor 16:35–48
24. Nakayama E, Yoshiura K, Ozeki S et al (2003) The correlation of histologic features with a panoramic radiography pattern and a computed tomography pattern of bone destruction in carcinoma of the mandibular gingiva. Oral Surg Oral Med Oral Pathol Oral Radiol Endod 96:774–782
25. Nakayama E, Yoshiura K, Yuasa K et al (2000) A study of the association between the prognosis of carcinoma of the mandibular gingiva and the pattern of bone destruction on computed tomography. Dentomaxillofac Radiol 29:163–169
26. Kimura Y, Sumi M, Sumi T et al (2002) Deep extension from carcinoma arising from the gingiva: CT and MR imaging features. AJNR Am J Neuroradiol 23:468–472
27. Mitz V, Peyronie M (1976) The superficial musculo-aponeurotic system (SMAS) in the parotid and cheek area. Plast Reconstr Surg 58:80–88
28. Janfaza P, Fabian RL (2011) Fasciae and fascial spaces of the head and neck. In: Janfaza P, Nadol JB, Galla R et al (eds) Surgical anatomy of the head and neck. Harvard University Press, Cambridge, pp 685–703
29. Wahi PN, Cohen B, Luthra UK et al (1971) Histological typing of oral and oropharyngeal tumours, vol 4, International histological classification of tumours. World Health Organization, Geneva
30. Pindborg JJ, Reichart P, Smith CJ et al (1997) World Health Organization: histological typing of cancer and precancer of the oral mucosa, 2nd edn. Springer, Berlin
31. Gale N, Westra W, Pilch BZ et al (2005) Epithelial precursor lesions. In: Barnes L, Everson JW, Reichart P et al (eds) World Health Organization classification on tumours: pathology and genetics of head and neck tumours. IARC Press, Lyon, pp 177–179
32. International Committee on Histological Definition (1962) An international agreement on histological terminology for the lesions of the uterine cervix. Acta Cytol 6:235–236
33. Reagan JW, Hamonic MJ (1956) Dysplasia of the uterine cervix. Ann N Y Acad Sci 63:1236–1244
34. Poulsen HE, Taylor CW, Sobin LH (1975) Histological typing of female genital tract tumours, vol 13, International histological classification of tumours. World Health Organization, Geneva
35. Izumo T (2011) Oral premalignant lesions: from the pathological view-point. Int J Clin Oncol 16:15–26
36. Working Committee of New Histopathological Criteria for Borderline Malignancies of the Oral Mucosa, Japanese Society for Oral Pathology (JSOP) (2007) JSOP Oral CIS Catalog: histopathological variations. Sunashobo Publishing, Tokyo
37. Working Committee of New Histopathological Criteria for Borderline Malignancies of the Oral Mucosa, Japanese Society for Oral Pathology (JSOP) (2014) Carcinoma in-situ of the oral mucosa: its pathological diagnostic concept based on the recognition of histological varieties proposed in the JSOP Oral CIS Catalog. J Oral Maxillofacial Surg Med Pathol 26:397–406. doi:10.1016/j.ajoms.2013.11.003
38. Shafer WG (1975) Oral carcinoma in situ. Oral Surg 39:227–238
39. Crissman JD, Zarbo RJ (1989) Dysplasia, in situ carcinoma, and progression to invasive squamous cell carcinoma of the upper aerodigestive tract. Am J Surg Pathol 13:5–16

40. Crissman JD, Sakr WA (2001) Squamous intraepithelial neoplasia of upper aerodigestive tract. In: Diagnostic surgical pathology of the head and neck. Saunders, Philadelphia, pp 1–17
41. Sakr WA, Gale N, Gnepp DR et al (2009) Squamous intraepithelial neoplasia of the upper aerodigestive tract. In: Diagnostic surgical pathology of the head and neck, 2nd edn. Saunders, Philadelphia, pp 1–44
42. Kuffer R, Lombardi T (2002) Premalignant lesions of the oral mucosa. A discussion about the place of oral intraepithelial neoplasia (OIN). Oral Oncol 38:125–130
43. Crissman JD, Zarbo RJ, Drozdowicz S et al (1988) Carcinoma in situ and microinvasive squamous carcinoma of the laryngeal glottis. Arch Otolaryngol Head Neck Surg 114:299–307
44. Sllamniku B, Bauer W, Painter C et al (1989) The transformation of laryngeal keratosis into invasive carcinoma. Am J Otolaryngol 10:42–54
45. Crissman JD, Visscher DW, Sarkar FH (1993) Premalignant lesion of the upper aerodigestive tract: biomakers of genetic alterations, proliferation, and differentiation. J Cell Biochem Suppl 17F:192–198
46. Blackwell KE, Fu YS, Calcaterra TC (1995) Laryngeal dysplasia. A clinico-pathologic study. Cancer 75:457–463
47. Kambic V (1997) Epithelial hyperplastic lesions-a challenging topic in laryngology. Acta Otolaryngol Suppl 527:7–11
48. Michaels L (1997) The Kambic-Gale method of assessment of epithelial hyperplastic lesions of the larynx in comparison with the dysplasia grade method. Acta Otolaryngol 527:17–20
49. Hellquist H, Cardesa A, Gale N et al (1999) Criteria for grading in Ljubljana classification of epithelial hyperplastic laryngeal lesions. A study by members of the working group on epithelial hyperplastic laryngeal lesions of the European Society of Pathology Histopathology 34:226–233
50. Gale N, Kambic V, Michaels L et al (2000) The Ljubljana classification: a practical strategy for the diagnosis of laryngeal precancerous lesions. Adv Anat Pathol 7:240–251
51. Gale N, Zidar N, Fischinger J et al (2000) Clinical applicability of the Ljubljana classification of epithelial hyperplastic laryngeal lesions. Clin Otolaryngol 25:227–232
52. Warnakulasuriya S (2001) Histological grading of oral epithelial dysplasia: revisited. J Pathol 194:294–297
53. Koren R, Kristt D, Shvero J et al (2002) The spectrum of laryngeal neoplasia: the pathologist's view. Pathol Res Pract 198:709–715
54. Gale N, Michaels L, Luzar B et al (2009) Current review on squamous intraepithelial lesions of the larynx. Histopathology 54:639–656
55. Robinson RA (2010) Upper airway squamous dysplasia, early invasive squamous carcinoma, and squamous carcinoma variant. In: Head and neck pathology: atlas for histologic and cytologic diagnosis. Lippincott Williams & Wilkins, Philadelphia
56. Richardson MS, Barns L, Carison DL et al (2012) Protocol for the examination of specimens from patients with carcinoma of the lip and oral cavity, 7th edn. College of American Pathologists. http://www.cap.org/apps/docs/committees/cancer/cancer_protocols/2012/LipOralCav_12protocol.pdf. Accessed 1 July 2012
57. Mikata T, Cheng J, Maruyama S et al (2011) Emergence of keratin 17 vs. loss of keratin 13: their reciprocal immunohistochemical profiles in oral carcinoma in situ. Oral Oncol 47:497–503
58. Pitiyage G, Tilakaratne WM, Tavhvash M et al (2009) Molecular markers in oral epithelial dysplasia: review. J Oral Pathol Med 38:737–752
59. Hunter K, Thurlow JK, Fleming J et al (2006) Divergent routes to oral cancer. Cancer Res 66:7405–7413
60. Braakhuis BJM, Leemans CR, Brakenhoff RH (2004) A genetic progression model of oral cancer: current evidence and clinical implications. J Oral Pathol Med 33:317–322
61. Tabor MP, Braakhuis BJM, van der Wal JE et al (2003) Comparative molecular and histological grading of epithelial dysplasia of oral cavity and the oropharynx. J Pathol 199:354–360
62. Brieger J, Jacob R, Riazimand HS et al (2003) Chromosomal aberrations in premalignant and malignant squamous epithelium. Cancer Genet Cytogenet 144:148–155
63. Ha PK, Pilkington TA, Westra WH et al (2002) Progression of microsatellite instability from premalignant lesion to tumors of head and neck. Int J Cancer 102:615–617
64. Gelb AB, Kamel OW, LeBrun DP et al (1992) Estimation of tumor growth fractions in archival formalin-fixed, paraffin-embedded tissues using two anti-PCNA/cyclin monoclonal antibodies: factors affecting reactivity. Am J Pathol 141:1453–1458
65. Scott RE, Wilke MS, Wille JJ et al (1988) Human squamous carcinoma cells express complex defects in the control of proliferation and differentiation. Am J Pathol 133:374–380
66. Lindberg K, Rheinwald JG (1989) Suprabasal 40 kd keratin (K19) expression as an immunohistologic marker of premalignancy in oral epithelium. Am J Pathol 134:89–98
67. Klijanienko J, Micheau C, Carluc-Caillaud JM (1989) Significance of keratin 13 and 6 expression in normal, dysplastic and malignant squamous epithelium of pyriform fossa. Virchows Arch A Pathol Anat Histopathol 416:121–124
68. Coltrera MD, Zarbo RJ, Sakr WA et al (1992) Markers for dysplasia of the upper aerodigestive tract. Suprabasal expression of PCNA, p53, CK19 in alcohol-fixed, embedded tissue. Am J Pathol 141:817–825
69. Ogden GR, Chisholm DM, Adi M et al (1993) Cytokeratin expression in oral cancer and its relationship to tumor differentiation. J Oral Pathol Med 22:82–86
70. Kobayashi T, Ida H, Cheng J et al (2005) Histopathological evaluation of borderline malignancies of the oral mucosa by the aid of immunohistochemistry for keratin species and Ki-67. Oral Med Pathol 10:45
71. Kondoh N, Ohkura S, Arai M et al (2007) Gene expression signature that can discriminate oral leukoplakia subtypes and squamous cell carcinoma. Oral Oncol 43:455–462
72. Ohkura S, Kondoh N, Arai M et al (2005) Differential expression on the keratin-4, -13, -14, -17 and transglutaminase 3 genes during the development of oral squamous cell carcinoma from leukoplakia. Oral Oncol 41:607–613
73. Whipple ME, Mendez E, Farwell DG et al (2004) A genomic predictor of oral squamous cell carcinoma. Laryngoscope 114:1364–1354
74. Izumo T (2009) Squamous intraepithelial neoplasia (SIN) of the oral mucosa (in Japanese). J Jpn Soc Oral Tumors 22:15–24
75. Londono-Vallejo JA (2008) Telomere instability and cancer. Biochimie 90:73–82
76. Luzar B, Poljak M, Marin IJ et al (2003) Telomerase reaction is an early event in laryngeal carcinogenesis. Mod Pathol 16:841–848
77. Aida J, Izumo T, Shimomura N et al (2010) Telomere lengths in the oral epithelia with and without carcinoma. Eur J Cancer 46:430–439
78. Hamilton SR, Aaltonen LA (2000) World Health Organization classification of tumours: pathology and genetics of tumours of the digestive system. IARC, Lyon, pp 9–19
79. Epstein JB, Scully C, Spinelli JJ (1992) Toluidine blue and Lugol's iodine application in the assessment of oral malignant disease and lesions at risk of malignancy. J Oral Patho Med 21:160–163
80. Kurita H, Kurashina K (1996) Vital staining with iodine solution in delineating the border of oral dysplastic lesions. Oral Surg Oral Med Oral Pathol 81:275–280
81. Shibahara T, Tanaka Y (2000) New method for detecting early oral cancer: a study of image uptake analysis with magnifying endoscopy (in Japanese). Oral Tumors 22:2–9
82. Broders AC (1920) Squamous-cell epithelioma of the lip. LAMA 74:656–664
83. Jakobsson PA, Eneroth CM, Killander D et al (1973) Histological classification and grading of malignancy in carcinoma of larynx. Acta Radiol 12:1–7

84. Willen R, Nathanson A, Moberger G et al (1975) Squamous cell carcinoma of the gingiva. Histological classification and grading of malignancy. Acta Otolaryngol 79:146–154
85. Anneroth G, Hansen LS (1984) A methodologic study of histologic classification and grading of malignancy in oral squamous cell carcinoma. Scand J Dent Res 92:448–468
86. Anneroth G, Batsakis J, Luna M (1987) Review of the literature and a recommended system of malignant grading in oral squamous cell carcinoma. Scand J Dent Res 95:229–249
87. Imai K (1954) Jintai ganshu hatsuiku joukyo no keitaigakuteki kousatsu. (in Japanese). Fukuoka Acta Medica 45:72–102
88. Yamamoto E, Kawajiri H, Katou K, Yoshizawa K, Noguchi N, Kitahara H (2009) Biological characteristics of the most invasive squamous cell carcinoma (Grade 4D) of the oral cavity (in Japanese). J Jpn Soc Oral Tumor 21:131–169
89. Yamamoto E, Miyakawa A, Kohama G (1984) Mode of invasion and lymph node metastasis in squamous cell carcinoma of the oral cavity. Head Neck Surg 6:938–947

3 Molecular Biology of the Oral Cancer

Tomonori Sasahira and Hiroki Kuniyasu

Abstract

Head and neck cancer, including oral squamous cell carcinoma (OSCC) and salivary gland cancer, is the sixth most common cancer in the world. OSCC has a high potential for local invasion and nodal metastasis, and the overall 5-year survival rate has not significantly improved during the past three decades. The need to understand the detailed molecular mechanisms of OSCC is urgent. Recent studies have clarified the molecular mechanisms of carcinogenesis, tumor progression, and metastasis of head and neck cancer. Although pathology is based on morphological findings, knowledge of molecular pathology is essential for the current pathology and oncology fields. In this chapter, we describe the molecular biological findings related to OSCC, such as the genetic events leading to OSCC development, human papillomavirus (HPV)-related OSCC, hallmarks of cancer, epithelial-mesenchymal transition (EMT), and microRNA. We also discuss the novel molecular pathological findings obtained by our laboratory related to OSCC, salivary gland adenoid cystic carcinoma (ACC), and mucoepidermoid carcinoma (MEC).

Keywords

Hallmarks of cancer • Molecular biology • Oral cancer • Salivary gland cancer

3.1 General

Head and neck cancer, including oral squamous cell carcinoma (OSCC) and salivary gland cancer, is the sixth most common cancer worldwide [1] and the leading cause of cancer death in Southern Asia [2]. The incidence of OSCC is estimated to be 263,900 cases and 128,000 deaths annually [3]; it is predicted that 7,850 patients will die from this disease in the United States in 2012 [4]. Furthermore, mortality from OSCC is 3.7 per 100,000 in Japan [5]. OSCC has a high potential for local invasion and lymph node metastasis. Over 80 % of early stage OSCC can be cured by treatment, whereas more than 70 % of the advanced stage cases cannot be rescued. Moreover, the overall 5-year survival rate of OSCC, less than 50 %, has not significantly improved during the past three decades [6, 7]. Therefore, it is urgently necessary to detect oral cancer early and to clarify its detailed molecular mechanism. In this chapter, we outline the latest molecular biological findings concerning oral cancer. Furthermore, we briefly describe salivary gland cancer, which is widespread in Japan, adenoid cystic carcinoma (ACC), and mucoepidermoid carcinoma (MEC).

3.2 Genetic Alterations Leading to OSCC Development

It is generally accepted that OSCC arises from multiple genetic alterations caused by chronic exposure to carcinogens such as alcohol, smoking, viral infections, and inflammation. These genetic alterations, which include deletions, point mutations, promoter methylation, and gene amplification of

T. Sasahira (✉) • H. Kuniyasu
Department of Molecular Pathology, Nara Medical University, Kashihara, Nara 634-8521, Japan
e-mail: sasa@naramed-u.ac.jp

T. Kirita and K. Omura (eds.), *Oral Cancer: Diagnosis and Therapy*, DOI 10.1007/978-4-431-54938-3_3, © Springer Japan 2015

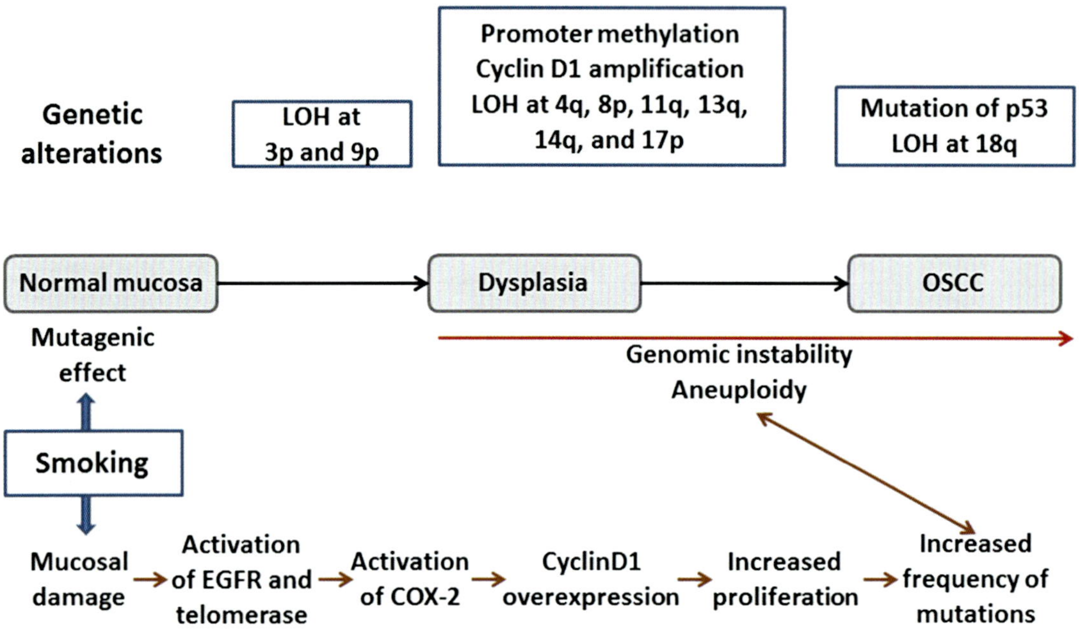

Fig. 3.1 Hypothetical molecular progression model for oral carcinogenesis. This figure was modified from previous reports [9–12]. OSCC is caused by multiple genetic and epigenetic alterations

oncogenes, inactivate tumor suppressor genes. Leukoplakia and erythroplakia are the most famous precancerous lesions of OSCC. In the presence of moderate to severe dysplasia, they are regarded as oral intraepithelial neoplasia (OIN)/carcinoma in situ (CIS), according to the latest Japanese guidelines on oral cancer [8]. Figure 3.1 shows a hypothetical genetic multistep model for OSCC [9–12]. The loss of chromosomal region 9p21 is found in 70–80 % of oral dysplasia, and this loss appears to be an early event in oral carcinogenesis [9–12]. Chromosomal region 9p21 is the gene locus of cyclin-dependent kinase inhibitor 2A (CDKN2A), and it encodes the tumor suppressors p16 and p14^{ARF}, G_1 cell cycle regulators. p16 is frequently inactivated by promoter hypermethylation [11–13]. Loss of chromosomal region 3p is another common early genetic event in oral carcinogenesis; loss of heterozygosity (LOH) of 3p is found in 60–70 % of OSCC [14]. The tumor suppressor genes fragile histidine triad (FHIT) and Ras association (RalGDS/AF-6) domain family member 1 (RASSF1) map to 3p14 and 3p21; exonic deletion of FHIT and hypermethylation of RASSF1 are observed in 50–80 % of OSCC [11, 12]. LOH of 17p (50–70 %) and p53 mutation (50 %) occur in the late stage of progression from dysplasia to invasive OSCC [11, 12]. Shahnavaz et al. reported that mutation of p53 occurs in 8 % of dysplasia and 75 % of invasive OSCC [15]. Boyle et al. also identified the p53 mutation in 19 % of dysplasia and CIS cases [16]. The amplification of 11q13 and the activation of cyclin D1 are seen in 30–60 % of OSCC [11]. Cyclin D1 is a cell cycle regulator from G1 to S phase, and its overexpression is associated with poor prognosis [17]. The activation of cyclooxygenase-2 (COX-2) and the phosphorylation of epidermal growth factor receptor (EGFR) are also crucial events in oral carcinogenesis [10]. The evaluation of the ploidy of oral leukoplakia is a useful tool to predict the risk of malignancy [18, 19]. Only 3 % of diploids develop invasive OSCC, whereas 84 % of aneuploid cases develop invasive lesions [18]. Patients with aneuploid leukoplakia had a 96 % rate of primary OSCC, an 81 % rate of recurrent or second primary oral cancer, and a 78 % rate of death from disease even in the case of pathologically negative surgical margins [19]. Thus, ploidy and chromosomal status may be risk factors for OSCC from precancerous lesions.

3.3 Human Papillomavirus in OSCC

Human papillomavirus (HPV) is strongly correlated with cervical carcinoma. HPV DNA has been identified in approximately 24 % of OSCC, with HPV-16 and HPV-18, the most common types, accounting for almost 70 % and 8 % of HPV-positive OSCC, respectively [20–22]. High-risk oncogenic HPV-16 and HPV-18 contain two oncogenes, E6 and E7, which induce cell transformation and cause cell cycle dysregulation [11]. E7 induces the proteolytic degradation of phosphorylated retinoblastoma (pRb), and E6 inhibits p53 activation by facilitating its ubiquitin-mediated proteolysis [11, 23]. Typical HPV-positive head and neck cancer is associated with poorly differentiated, nonkeratinizing, basaloid morphology, wild-type p53, overexpression of p16, and inactivation of cyclin D1 and Rb [11, 24]. Table 3.1 summarizes the different characteristics of HPV-negative and HPV-positive OSCC [25].

Table 3.1 Differential features of HPV-positive and HPV-negative OSCC

Characteristics	HPV-positive OSCC	HPV-negative OSCC
Risk factor	Oral sex	Smoking, alcohol abuse
Age	Under 60 years	Above 60 years
Field carcinogenesis	Yes or no	Yes
Mutation of p53	Infrequently	Frequently
Susceptible site	Oropharynx	Various sites
Outcome	Good	Bad

3.4 Hallmarks of Cancer

Hanahan and Weinberg proposed six hallmarks of the cancer cell model: sustained proliferative signals, evasion of growth suppressors, resistance to cell death, replicative immortality, induction of angiogenesis, and activation of invasion and metastasis [26]. Recently, they added two emerging hallmarks, avoidance of immune destruction and deregulation of cellular energetics, and two enabling characteristics, genome instability and mutation and tumor-promoting inflammation (Fig. 3.2) [27]. Below, we describe OSCC-associated signals according to their recent model.

3.4.1 Sustained Proliferative Signals

Normal cells regulate growth signals through soluble and membrane-bound growth factors, but cancer cells are characterized by autonomous, chaotic growth because of the deregulation of growth signals.

3.4.1.1 EGFR

EGFR belongs to the membrane-bound receptor tyrosine kinase family comprising ErbB1 or human epidermal growth factor receptor 1 (HER1), ErbB2 or HER2, ErbB3 or HER3, and ErbB4 or HER4 [28]. The binding of EGFR and EGF or transforming growth factor-α (TGFα) enhances Ras/Raf/mitogen-activated kinase protein (MAPK), phosphatidylinositol-3-kinase (PI3K)/protein kinase B (AKT), mammalian target of rapamycin (mTOR), Janus tyrosine kinase (JAK), signal transducers and activators of transcription (STAT), and protein kinase C (PKC) signaling pathways [12]. Overexpression of EGFR is observed in almost all patients with head and neck cancer and is correlated with advanced clinical stage and poor survival [29]. Additionally, overexpression of HER2 in head and neck squamous cell carcinoma (SCC) is correlated with nodal metastasis and poor outcome [30]. Cetuximab is an EGFR monoclonal antibody, and gefitinib and erlotinib are small-molecule EGFR tyrosine kinase inhibitors [12]. Molecular therapy targeting EGFR may be useful for OSCC.

3.4.1.2 Ras

The Ras family comprises H-Ras, K-Ras, and N-Ras in humans [31]. Approximately 30 % of all malignancies show mutations of Ras [32]. In advanced OSCC, a high frequency of H-Ras mutation is detected in Asian populations associated with betel nut chewing [33, 34]. On the other hand, mutations of H-Ras are not frequent (less than 6 %) in Western countries [35].

3.4.1.3 HGF/c-Met

Hepatocyte growth factor (HGF) regulates cell growth, cell motility, and morphogenesis by activating tyrosine kinase signaling after binding to its receptor, c-Met[36]. In OSCC, HGF/c-Met promotes invasion and metastasis through the destruction of E-cadherin[37]. The expression rates of HGF in oral dysplasia and OSCC are higher than in non-tumor oral mucosa [38]. Through effects on matrix metalloproteinase (MMP)-1, MMP-2, and MMP-9 expression, overexpression of c-Met is correlated with nodal metastasis and poor outcome caused by enhanced migration and invasion [39]. Furthermore, c-Met induces lymphangiogenesis via potentiation of vascular endothelial growth factor (VEGF)-C [38].

3.4.1.4 NFκB

Nuclear factor-kappa B (NFκB) is a ubiquitous nuclear transcription factor implicated in inflammation and the immune response [12, 32]. In its inactive state, NFκB is located in the cytoplasm bound to members of the NFκB inhibitor (IκB) family. After the phosphorylation, ubiquitination, and degradation of IκB, activated NFκB translocates to the nucleus and regulates the expression of target genes [40]. In OSCC, NFκB promotes lymphatic metastasis, invasion, and angiogenesis[41–43]. Moreover, the expression of NFκB has been shown to be related to resistance to chemoradiation therapy in OSCC [44].

3.4.1.5 PI3K-AKT

PI3K/AKT is a downstream target of EGFR that promotes the cell growth and proliferation of cancer cells [45]. PI3K is a heterodimeric kinase consisting of p85 and p110α (PI3KCA). Activation of PI3KCA and inactivation of phosphatase and tensin homolog (PTEN) have been found in approximately 10 % of head and neck SCC [25, 46]. In OSCC, EGFR-independent activation of PI3K/AKT is frequently observed and strongly related to radiation resistance [45]. Furthermore, in their review article, Leemans et al. reported that the PI3K-PTEN-AKT pathway is one of the important signaling events in head and neck cancers, including OSCC [25].

3.4.1.6 Cyclin D1

Cyclin D1 is a cell cycle regulator from G1 to S phase. It interacts with calcium-dependent kinase 4 (CDK4) [17].

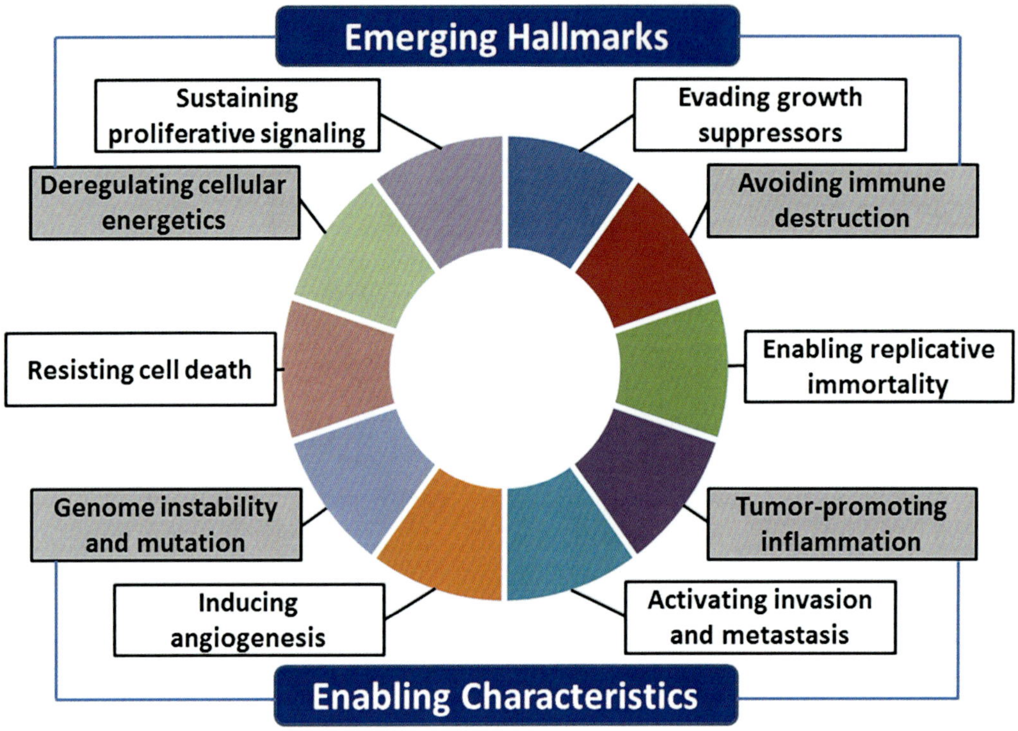

Fig. 3.2 The hallmarks of cancer. The new hallmarks of cancer were proposed by Hanahan et al. in 2011 [27]. This schema shows the ten hallmark capabilities including sustaining proliferative signals, evading growth suppressors, resisting cell death, enabling replicative immortality, inducing angiogenesis, activating invasion and metastasis and two emerging hallmarks, avoiding immune destruction, and deregulating cellular energetics and two enabling characteristics, genome instability and mutation and tumor-promoting inflammation

Overexpression of cyclin D1, found in 25–70 % of OSCC, is a nodal metastatic and poor prognostic factor [47, 48]. In signaling analysis using OSCC cells, the enhancement of extracellular signal-regulated kinase (ERK1/2) induces cyclin D1 expression [48]. Moreover, cyclin D1 is involved in cisplatin resistance through the repression of apoptosis and the activation of NFκB[49]. In HPV-related oral cancer, cyclin D1 activity is inhibited after the downregulation of p53 and pRb by E6 and E7, respectively [32].

3.4.1.7 STAT

Members of the STAT family are cytoplasmic transcription factors [12, 32]. STAT3 is activated by JAK or interleukin-6 (IL-6), EGF, platelet-derived growth factor (PDGF), VEGF, and others in several malignancies [50]. A recent study indicates that inactivation of STAT3 decreases hypoxia-inducible factor 1α (HIF-1α) expression, inhibits cell growth, and augments the radiosensitivity of OSCC cells [51]. In immunohistochemical analysis using human OSCC specimens, pSTAT3 expression is correlated with poor prognosis and is observed in premalignant lesions [52]. Co-expression of STAT3 and c-Met is involved in OSCC progression [53].

3.4.2 Evasion of Growth Suppressors

Many tumor suppressor genes related to anti-growth signals are downregulated by mutation, deletion, and methylation in cancer cells. In the next sections, we review the functions of p53, p16, p21, and PTEN in OSCC.

3.4.2.1 p53

The p53 gene is located on chromosome 17p13.1. p53 plays a pivotal role in the regulation of cell cycle, cellular differentiation, DNA repair, and apoptosis [12]. It is generally accepted that p53 is a gatekeeper of the genome [12]. Hypoxia, oncogenic stimulation by $p14^{ARF}$ activation, and DNA double-strand breaks increase p53 expression [54, 55]. Somatic mutations in p53 are detected in 60–80 % of head and neck cancers, including OSCC [25], and in 13 % of oral dysplasia [56]. Aside from mutations, the inactivation of $p14^{ARF}$ and the overexpression of mouse double minute 2 (MDM2) can also inhibit the tumor-suppressive function of p53 [12, 28]. Another mechanism for the deactivation of wild-type p53 is through high-risk HPV infection, such as HPV-16 and HPV-18. In HPV-positive OSCC, the inactivation of p53 occurs through the interaction with E6, which increases the ubiquitination and proteolysis of p53 [12, 57].

3.4.2.2 p16^{INK4A}

The p16 tumor suppressor gene is located on chromosome 9p21-22. p16 disrupts the phosphorylation of Rb and induces the separation of E2F via binding with CDK4 and CDK6 [58]. Thus, p16 regulates the cell cycle from G1 to S phase [59]. Loss of p16 activation by methylation is frequently observed in OSCC, and p16 alteration is one of the initial events in oral carcinogenesis [60–62]. In contrast, Mendenhall et al. reported that high-risk HPV-related OSCC is associated with the overexpression of p16 [63].

3.4.2.3 p21^{WAF1}

The cyclin-dependent kinase inhibitor p21 plays an essential role in regulating the G1-S transition of the cell cycle, cellular growth suppressors, and apoptosis [12, 32]. p21 is located downstream of p53, and wild-type p53 induces p21 expression in response to DNA damage [64, 65]. The expression of p21 is observed not only in OSCC but also in the dysplastic lesions of the oral cavity; thus, activation of p21 is thought to be an early step in the malignant transformation of oral cancer [66]. Reduction of p21 levels is associated with poor outcome in OSCC [67]. However, other studies have shown that overexpression of p21 is correlated with poor prognosis [68]. In HPV-positive OSCC cases, p21 expression is a significant predictor of a favorable outcome [69]. Thus, the function of p21 in OSCC is controversial.

3.4.2.4 PTEN

The PTEN gene is located on chromosome 10q23.3 [70]. PTEN acts as a tumor suppressor through negative feedback of the PI3K/AKT pathway [71]. Deletion or somatic mutation of the PTEN gene has been detected in various carcinomas [70–74]. More recently, it was reported that reduction of PTEN is associated with poor prognosis. Therefore, the expression of PTEN may be a useful marker for radiotherapy in OSCC [75]. Kurasawa et al. reported that PTEN expression is downregulated in OSCC compared to the expression in normal oral mucosa [76]. They also observed restoration of PTEN mRNA in human OSCC-derived HSC3, HSC4, Ho-1-N-1, and SCC4 cells after treatment with 5-aza-2′-deoxycytidine (5-Aza-dc), a demethylation reagent. These results indicate that PTEN inactivation in OSCC may be due to gene methylation.

3.4.3 Resistance to Cell Death

Apoptosis, a programmed form of cell death, plays an important role in cellular homeostasis [12]. Apoptosis can occur through both extrinsic (receptor-initiated death) and intrinsic (mitochondrial) pathways. The extrinsic pathway is initiated by the binding of tumor necrosis factor-α (TNFα) or Fas to TNF-related apoptosis-inducing ligand (TRAIL) or Fas ligand (FasL), leading to the activation of caspases 8 and 3. The intrinsic pathway is induced by the activation of BH3-containing proteins through various stimuli, prompting the release of cytochrome C and enhancement of caspases 9 and 3. Some important factors in apoptosis are the antiapoptotic proteins B-cell CLL/lymphoma 2 (Bcl-2) and Bcl-X_L and the proapoptotic proteins Bax and Bak[12, 27, 32]. Figure 3.3 shows the process of apoptosis.

3.4.3.1 Bcl-2, Bcl-XL, Bax, and Bak

Previous reports suggested that the overexpression of Bcl-2 is a useful predictive marker of poor prognosis in OSCC [77]. Other reports linked the upregulation of Bcl-XL and wild-type p53 with cisplatin resistance in head and neck SCC cells [78]. Although Bax and Bak are proapoptotic proteins, previous studies demonstrated that their high expression is associated with poor prognosis in OSCC [79, 80]. However, another report showed that low expression of Bax is associated with poor prognosis [81]. Furthermore, decreased levels of Bax and Bak are found in hypoxia-induced apoptosis in OSCC [82].

3.4.4 Replicative Immortality

Telomeres are tandem repeats of the DNA sequence TTAGGG present at the linear ends of chromosomes. They become shortened in somatic cells [83]. The enzyme telomerase maintains telomere length. Its activity is regulated by the expression of human telomerase reverse transcriptase (hTERT), the catalytic subunit of telomerase [12]. Activation of hTERT enables a cancer cell to maintain its telomeric length [32]. Recently, it was reported that hTERT stimulates epithelial-mesenchymal transition (EMT) via the Wnt/β-catenin pathway and induces the stemness of cancer cells [84]. Telomerase or hTERT activity is found in 80 % of head and neck cancer, including OSCC [9]. Chen et al. reported that the activation of hTERT may be an early event of oral carcinogenesis, with high expression levels of hTERT related with poor outcome [85]. Furthermore, a recent report indicated that telomere dysfunction is a useful predictor of radioresistance in OSCC [86].

3.4.5 Induction of Angiogenesis

Angiogenesis and lymphangiogenesis are pivotal events in tumor progression and metastasis. The major angiogenic and lymphangiogenic factors are VEGF-A-VEGF receptor-1/2 (VEGFR-1/2) and the VEGF-C/D-VEGFR-3 system, respectively [87]. We recently showed that high microvessel density (MVD) and lymphovessel density (LVD) are strongly

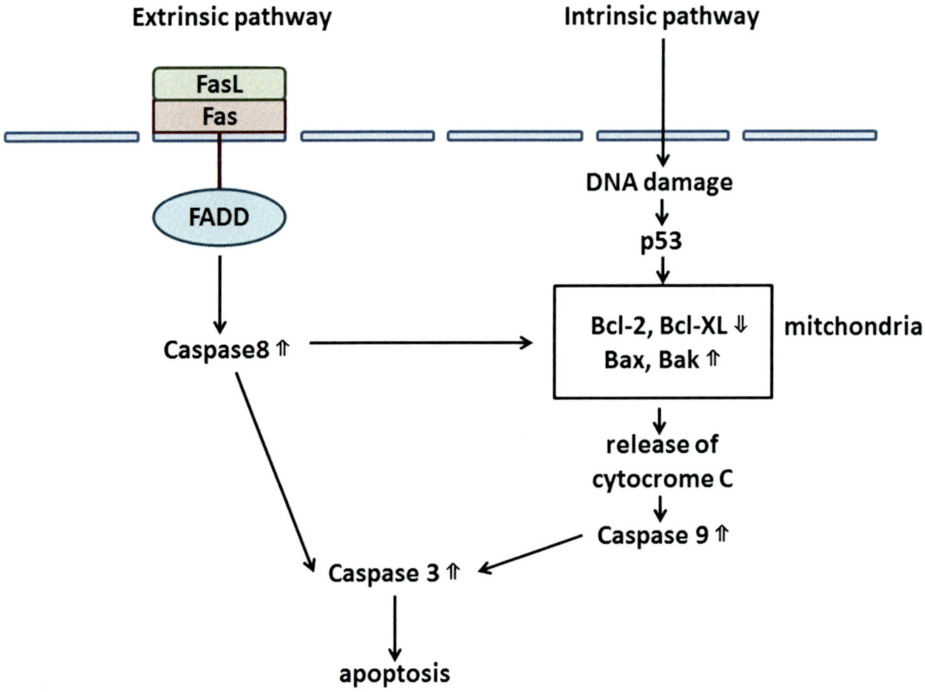

Fig. 3.3 Apoptotic pathways. There are two major programs of apoptosis: extrinsic and intrinsic pathways

associated with T grade, clinical stage, nodal metastasis, local recurrence, and poor outcome in OSCC [88]. Other important factors for angiogenesis and lymphangiogenesis include basic fibroblast growth factor (bFGF) [89], interleukin (IL)-8 [90], platelet-derived growth factor beta polypeptide (PDGFB) [89], angiopoietin2 [91], FoxC2 [92], Prox1 [93], and neuropilin2 [94].

3.4.5.1 VEGF Family

The VEGF family includes VEGF-A, VEGF-B, placenta growth factor (PlGF), VEGF-C, VEGF-D, and VEGF-E and plays a key role in developmental vasculogenesis and inflammatory angiogenesis[87]. We performed immunohistochemistry of VEGF family using OSCC samples and found that VEGF-A expression was related to tumor progression, lymph node metastasis, disease recurrence, and poor prognosis; the expression of VEGF-C and VEGF-D was only linked to nodal metastasis. Furthermore, VEGF-D was induced only in lymphangiogenesis, whereas VEGF-A and VEGF were induced in both angiogenesis and lymphangiogenesis in OSCC [88]. The recently developed drug bevacizumab is an anti-VEGF-A agent, and it may be useful for the treatment of OSCC [95].

3.4.6 Activation of Invasion and Metastasis

The following steps are necessary for cancer cell invasion and metastasis: destruction of the basal membrane, decreased adhesion and isolation of cancer cells, acquisition of cancer cell migration and stromal infiltration, vascular invasion, intravascular migration, and cancer cell growth in the metastatic organ. Here, we review E-cadherin, MMPs, and integrins.

3.4.6.1 E-Cadherin

E-cadherin, a calcium-dependent intracellular adhesion molecule, plays an important role in maintaining cell-to-cell connections in normal epithelial cells [96]. In OSCC, reduction of E-cadherin is associated with invasion [97], nodal metastasis [96], and poor prognosis [98]. Inactivation of E-cadherin can be induced by methylation [99]. Its transcriptional inhibition results from the activation of Snail, Slug, zinc finger E-box binding homeobox 2 (ZEB2), and Twist [100]. Thus, E-cadherin plays a pivotal role in EMT.

3.4.6.2 MMPs

MMPs are extracellular proteases involved in extracellular matrix modulation [12, 32]. Many studies have described the relationship between MMPs and OSCC. MMP-2 is a good predictive marker of invasion and metastasis in OSCC [101]. The high expression of MMP-7 has been linked to invasion and poor prognosis [102]. MMP-3, MMP-9, MMP-10, and MMP-11 may also take part in the progression of OSCC [103–106]. Tissue inhibitors of metalloproteinase (TIMP), antagonists of MMPs, are associated with the progression of OSCC [105, 107]. However, the relationship between TIMP/MMPs and clinical features is controversial.

3.4.6.3 Integrins

Integrins are heterodimeric cellular transmembrane proteins that mediate cell-to-cell and cell-to-extracellular matrix interactions [32]. In OSCC, integrins $\alpha_3\beta_1$ and $\alpha6A\beta_1$ are related to invasion, metastasis, and poor prognosis [108]. The interaction of integrin α_5 and hypoxia-inducible factor-1 (HIF-1α) promotes the invasion of OSCC cells under hypoxic conditions [109]. Recently, Li et al. revealed that the overexpression of integrin $\alpha_v\beta_6$ is related to unfavorable clinical prognostic factors and decreased survival [110]. The upregulation of integrin $\alpha_v\beta_6$ is also found in oral dysplasia [111]. However, the role of integrins in cancer is complicated, and further studies are needed.

3.4.7 Avoidance of Immune Destruction

The function of immune cell cancer is an emerging hallmark of cancer [27]. The marked infiltration of $CD8^+$ cytotoxic T lymphocytes (CTLs) and natural killer (NK) cells is related to a favorable outcome in colon and ovarian cancers [27, 112, 113]. A previous report suggested that TGFα secreted by cancer cells confuses infiltrating CTLs and NK cells [114], whose activation is also attenuated by tumor-infiltrating myeloid cells [115]. Toll-like receptors (TLRs) are single transmembrane cell-surface receptors with tumor immune escape and resistance to apoptosis properties [116]. In OSCC, TLR3, 4, 7, and 9 are correlated with invasion, apoptosis, necrosis, and cell proliferation [117–120].

3.4.8 Tumor-Promoting Inflammation

Inflammation can change the tumor microenvironment by inducing growth factors and modifying the extracellular matrix, thus facilitating angiogenesis, invasion, and metastasis [27]. Furthermore, chronic inflammation increases cancer risk because activated inflammatory cells release reactive oxygen species (ROS) and reactive nitrogen intermediates (RNI) and induce DNA damage and genomic instability [121]. Therefore, it is now believed that chronic inflammation promotes tumor progression.

3.4.8.1 COX-2

COX-2 is a proinflammatory enzyme that converts arachidonic acid to prostaglandins. Despite the lack of COX-2 expression in normal epithelium, increased expression is found in OSCC and is related to apoptosis inhibition [28, 32]. Overexpression of COX-2 is found in higher grades of oral epithelial dysplasia and in invasion and nodal metastasis of OSCC [122–124]. Additionally, COX-2 inhibition suppresses proliferation, migration, and invasion in OSCC cells [125].

3.4.9 Genome Instability and Mutation

Epigenetic mechanisms, such as DNA methylation and histone deacetylation, play pivotal roles in silencing tumor suppressor genes. One of the famous methylated genes in OSCC is CDKN2A, which controls the cell cycle [126, 127]. Loss of E-cadherin (*CDH1* gene) is observed in 64 % of primary OSCC, 67 % of nodal metastases, and 71 % of recurrent tumors [128]. Furthermore, the DNA repair genes O^6-methylguanine-DNA-methyltransferase (MGMT) and death-associated protein kinase (DAPK) were methylated in 52 % and 68 % of OSCCs, respectively [129]. Retinoic acid receptor-β2 (RAR-β2) is a member of the thyroid-steroid hormone receptor superfamily of nuclear transcriptional regulators. Youssef and colleagues reported that RAR-β2 methylation is found in 66 % of head and neck SCC, including OSCC, and 53 % of oral leukoplakia [130].

3.4.10 Deregulation of Cellular Energetics

Under aerobic conditions, normal cells produce adenosine triphosphate (ATP) from glucose through the tricarboxylic acid (TCA) cycle in the mitochondria and oxidative phosphorylation in the electron transfer system. In addition, ATP is also produced through the anaerobic glycolytic pathway, which breaks down glucose in the cytoplasm and generates lactic acid under anaerobic conditions. However, cancer cells can produce ATP through aerobic glycolysis even in the presence of oxygen. This phenomenon is called the Warburg effect[27]. In clinical settings, glucose metabolism in tumors is assessed by positron emission tomography (PET) using ^{18}F-fluorodeoxyglucose (FDG).

3.4.10.1 GLUT-1

Glucose transporter 1 (GLUT-1) is a 12-pass transmembrane protein that transports glucose and belongs to the sugar porter family. In OSCC, a significant association was found between the expression of GLUT-1 and resistance to radiation or poor prognosis [131–133].

3.4.10.2 HIF-1

HIF-1 is composed of HIF-1α, which modulates the transactivation of target genes under hypoxic conditions by binding to hypoxia-responsive elements, and HIF-1β, a key regulator of oxygen homeostasis [82, 134]. HIF-1α plays an important role in angiogenesis by activating VEGF-A and inhibiting apoptosis; it is associated with poor prognosis in OSCC [82, 135–137]. Moreover, HIF-1α promotes nodal metastasis by the induction of lymphangiogenesis via VEGF-C [138].

3.5 EMT

EMT, characterized by the loss of epithelial differentiation and the acquisition of a mesenchymal phenotype, plays a key role in cancer metastasis [139]. The important factors for EMT are TGFβ, Wnt, Notch, interleukin-like EMT inducer (ILEI), HGF, EGF, and PDGF. TGFβ acts as tumor suppressor by inhibiting cell growth and facilitating apoptosis, but it has tumor-promoting effects by inducing EMT in advanced cancers [140]. Cancer cells with induced EMT display a loss of epithelial cell-to-cell contacts, with suppression of E-cadherin, ZO-1, and claudin-1/-7, among others, and expression of mesenchymal markers such as α-smooth muscle actin (SMA), vimentin, N-cadherin, and desmin [140, 141]. In cancer cells, the upregulation of transcription factors such as Snail, Slug, Twist, ZEB1/2, and/or E47 is necessary for the maintenance of EMT [141]. The induction of EMT is also critical for the progression of OSCC [139, 142, 143].

3.6 MicroRNA

MicroRNAs (miRNAs) are noncoding small RNAs of approximately 18–25 nucleotides that regulate gene expression by binding to the 3′-untranslated region (UTR) of target mRNAs [144]. Mature miRNAs derive from primary miRNAs (pri-miRNAs), which are processed in the nucleus into precursor miRNAs (pre-miRNAs) by the RNase Drosha and its cofactor DiGeorge syndrome critical region gene 8 (DCRG8). The pre-miRNAs are exported to the cytoplasm by exportin-5 and processed into mature miRNAs by the RNase Dicer. Once integrated into the RNA-induced silencing complex (RISC), the mature miRNAs mediate target gene mRNA expression (Fig. 3.4) [145–148]. Here, we summarize the role of several miRNAs in OSCC [146, 147].

3.6.1 Upregulation of miRNAs in OSCC

Overexpression of miR-21, which targets tropomyosin 1 (TPM1) and PTEN, is related to the reduction of apoptosis [146, 147, 149]. Similarly, upregulation of miR-24 reduces apoptosis by inhibiting RNA-binding protein dead end 1 (DND1) and promotes proliferation through the downregulation of cyclin-dependent kinase inhibitor 1B (CDKN1B), a downstream target of DND1 [146, 147, 150]. Elevated expression of miR-222 inhibits cell invasion by directly regulating MMP-1 and indirectly reducing manganese superoxide dismutase 2 (SOD2) expression [146, 147, 151]. Another report showed that high expression of miR-211 is correlated with nodal metastasis, vascular invasion, and poor prognosis and that the increment of miR-211 expression results in the attenuation of α-galactosidase and the LacZ operon [146, 147, 152]. The upregulation of miR-31 directly represses factor-inhibiting hypoxia-inducible factor (FIH) expression. The plasma level of miR-31 in patients with OSCC is higher than that in controls [146, 147, 153, 154]. Moreover, overexpression of miR-23a and miR-98 suppresses the expression of topoisomerase IIβ (TOP2B) that is an inhibitor of TOP2 and high-mobility group box A2 (HMGA2) that is an enhancer of cisplatin and doxorubicin resistance, respectively [146, 147, 155, 156].

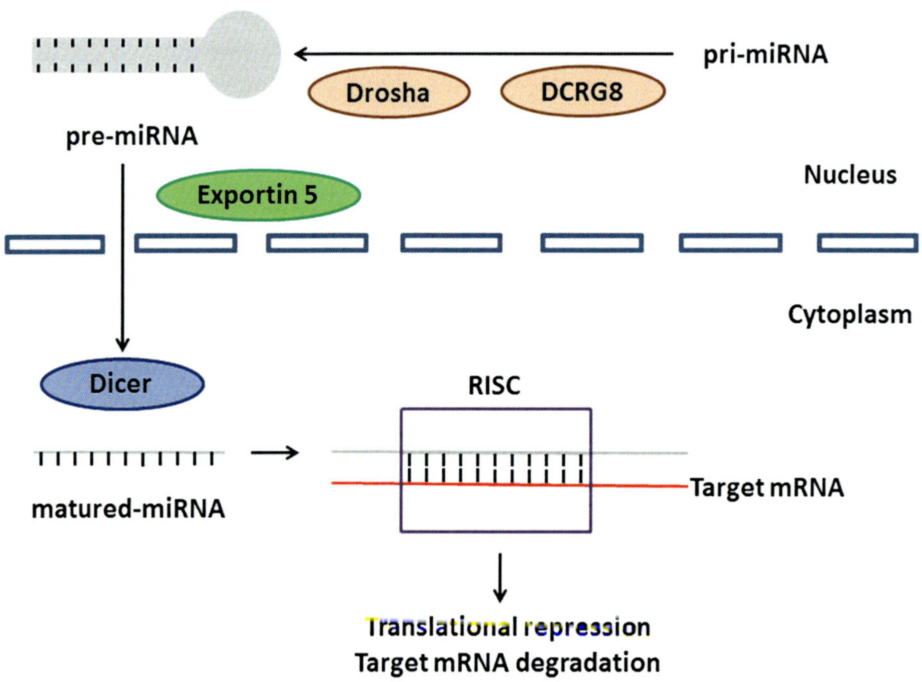

Fig. 3.4 The cascade of miRNA in humans. This schema was modified from previous findings [147, 148]. The pri-miRNAs are processed in the nucleus into pre-miRNAs with the help of Drosha and its cofactor DCRG8. The pre-miRNAs are exported to the cytoplasm by exportin-5 and processed into mature miRNAs by another Dicer. The mature miRNAs are integrated into the RISC and regulate target gene mRNA expression

3.6.2 Downregulation of miRNAs in OSCC

Underexpression of miR-133a elevates the expression of pyruvate kinase type M2 (PKM2) and glutathione-S-transferase P1 (GSTP1) and is associated with promotion of cell proliferation and inhibition of apoptosis [146, 147, 157, 158]. Liu et al. revealed that low miR-138 expression affects metastasis by directly targeting Rho-related GTP-binding protein C (RhoC) and Rho-associated, coiled-coil-containing protein kinase 2 (ROCK2) [146, 147]. miR-15a is also downregulated in OSCC, resulting in regulation of PKCα and cyclin E expression, which in turn affects DNA synthesis [146, 147, 158]. Furthermore, diminished expression of miR-7 and miR-124, which target insulin-like growth factor 1 (IGF1) and integrin beta-1 (ITGB1), respectively, is observed in OSCC [147, 159, 160].

3.7 The Novel OSCC-Related Molecular Markers

3.7.1 RAGE-HMGB1 Signal

Receptor for advanced glycation end products (RAGE) is a multi-ligand receptor that belongs to the immunoglobulin superfamily [161]. High-mobility group box 1 (HMGB1), AGE, S100 protein, and β amyloid are major ligands of RAGE, whose associated intracellular signaling pathways involve GTPases, Rac1/Cdc42, MAPK, ERK1/2, c-Jun N-terminal kinase (JNK), and NFκB[162]. HMGB1 is a nuclear chromatin protein and cytokine that participates in inflammation and cancer progression [163]. Extracellular HMGB1 is associated with endotoxin-induced tissue injury, macrophage infiltration, and tumor advancement [163, 164] We previously reported that the RAGE-HMGB1 system is deeply correlated with tumor progression, metastasis, prognosis of gastrointestinal cancer [161–163], prostate cancer [165], and malignant transformation of colorectal adenoma [166].

The RAGE-HMGB1 system also plays an important role in OSCC. Increased expression of RAGE was linked to invasion depth and poor prognosis, and multivariate analysis demonstrated a significant relationship between RAGE expression levels and disease-free survival [167]. Furthermore, RAGE-HMGB1 signaling induces angiogenesis by activation of VEGF-A [168], and it is responsible for migration, invasion, and MMP-9 production in OSCC cells [169]. Moreover, RAGE is involved in rat tongue carcinogenesis induced by 4-nitroquinoline 1-oxide (4-NQO) [170]. Interestingly, a selective COX-2 inhibitor, etodolac, significantly reduced the expression of RAGE in dysplasia and OSCC. Our findings suggest that the RAGE-HMGB1 system might be a good marker for malignancy potential in OSCC and a useful target for the diagnosis and treatment of OSCC.

3.7.2 MIA Gene Family

The melanoma inhibitory activity (MIA) gene family contains MIA, MIA2, MIA3, and otoraplin (OTOR), which share 47–59 % cDNA sequence and 34–45 % amino acid homology [171]. Previous reports indicated that MIA promotes the progression and metastasis of malignant melanoma and other malignancies [172, 173]. MIA accelerates the cell detachment, migration, invasion, apoptosis resistance, and infiltration of lymphokine-activated killer cells [174]. MIA inhibits cell-to-stromal interaction by binding to fibronectin via SH3 domain-like structures [174, 175]. Bauer et al. also revealed that MIA is a ligand for selected integrins by demonstrating its ability to bind integrins $\alpha_4\beta_1$ and $\alpha_5\beta_1$ [176]. Recently, we elucidated the functional role of MIA in OSCC [177, 88]. The interplay between intracellular HMGB1 and NFκB p65 facilitated MIA expression. MIA also regulated the phosphorylation of ERK1/2 and MAPK p38, the induction of angiogenesis and lymphangiogenesis, and the activation of VEGF-A/-C/-D in OSCC cells. Analysis of OSCC specimens revealed that MIA expression was strongly related with nodal metastasis, poor prognosis, MVD, LVD, and high expression levels of HMGB1 and VEGF family members. Figure 3.5 summarizes the roles of MIA in OSCC.

The activation of MIA2 is transcriptionally regulated by the hepatocyte nuclear factor (HNF)-1 binding site [178]. Although MIA2 expression is increased chronic hepatitis and liver cirrhosis [179], MIA2 inhibits the growth and invasion of hepatocellular carcinoma (HCC) [180]. In OSCC, MIA2 expression was strongly correlated with tumor progression and nodal metastasis and was negatively associated with cytotoxic T lymphocyte infiltration [181]. In in vitro

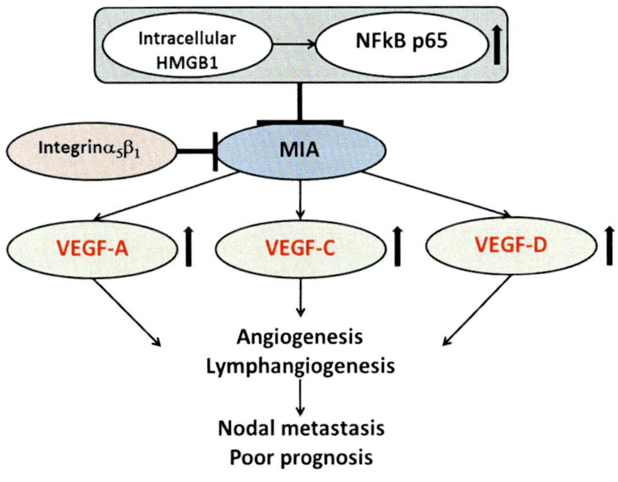

Fig. 3.5 The schema of the roles of MIA in OSCC. MIA acts as oncogene by induction of angiogenesis and lymphangiogenesis via activation of VEGF family and is associated with nodal metastasis and poor prognosis in OSCC

examinations using OSCC cells, modulation of cancer cell invasion, antiapoptotic effect, VEGF family expression, and host anticancer immunity were found to be related to MIA2. Moreover, MIA2 regulated the phosphorylation of MAPK p38 and JNK by binding to integrins α_4 and α_5.

MIA3 acts as tumor suppressor in melanoma, colorectal cancer, and HCC [182, 183]. We also showed that it induces angiogenesis and lymphangiogenesis in OSCC (unpublished data). OTOR expression is highly restricted in healthy eyes, cochlea, and cartilage [184], and its involvement in cancer has not been reported yet. Our results suggest that the MIA gene family might be important for tumor progression in OSCC.

3.7.3 Trk

Tropomyosin receptor kinases (Trk) have a high affinity for neurotrophins. Nerve growth factor (NGF), brain-derived neurotrophic factor (BDNF) or neurotrophin 4/5 (NT4/5), and NT3 are the ligands for TrkA, TrkB, and TrkC, respectively [185]. Trks regulate neuronal survival and differentiation [186]. Trks also act as oncogenes in many tumors, and the overexpression of TrkA is found in thyroid and ovarian cancer [187, 188]. Overexpression of TrkB has been found in hepatocellular carcinoma [189], pancreatic cancer [190], and neuroblastoma [191]; it is correlated with more aggressive tumor behavior. TrkB and TrkC also inhibit apoptosis in ovarian cancer and neuroblastoma cells, respectively, by activating PI3K signaling [192, 193]. Furthermore, we showed that TrkB and TrkC have a tumor progression function in colorectal cancer [194]. However, it has been reported that TrkB is downregulated in prostate cancer [195]. In neuroblastoma, patients with high expression of TrkA or TrkC have a better prognosis [196, 197], and TrkC plays a favorable role in medulloblastoma, leading to a good clinical outcome [198]. Therefore, the detailed functional roles of Trks in malignancies are not clearly understood.

We recently reported the functional roles of Trks in OSCC [199]. Although all Trks inhibited apoptosis by activating caspase 3, regulation of cell growth by TrkB- and MMP-2/-9-mediated enhancement of invasive ability by TrkC was observed. The gene expression of Trks was modulated by methylation of runt-related transcription factor 3 (RUNX3). VEGF family-dependent and VEGF family-independent angiogenesis and lymphangiogenesis were induced by TrkB and TrkC, respectively. In immunohistochemical analysis using OSCC specimens, the expression of TrkB was significantly associated with MVD, LVD, and poor outcome, whereas the immunoreactivity of TrkC was strongly correlated with clinical stage, nodal metastasis, MVD, LVD, and poor prognosis. These results indicate that Trks might be a useful diagnostic and therapeutic tool for OSCC. The functional roles of Trks in OSCC are summarized in Fig. 3.6.

3.7.4 miR-126

miR-126 is an endothelial-specific miRNA that is located within intron 7 of epidermal growth factor-like domain 7 (EGFL7). Its overexpression in endothelial cells enhances VEGF-A activity and promotes vessel formation by repressing the expression of sprouty-related protein-1 (Spred-1) in developmental angiogenesis and vasculogenesis in wound healing [200, 201]. Low expression of miR-126 is found in pancreatic cancer, where it is associated with the activation of K-Ras[202], and it is significantly associated with short survival in non-small cell lung carcinoma (NSCLC) and renal cell carcinoma [203, 204]. Downregulation of miR-126 and EGFL7 by DNA hypermethylation has been reported in

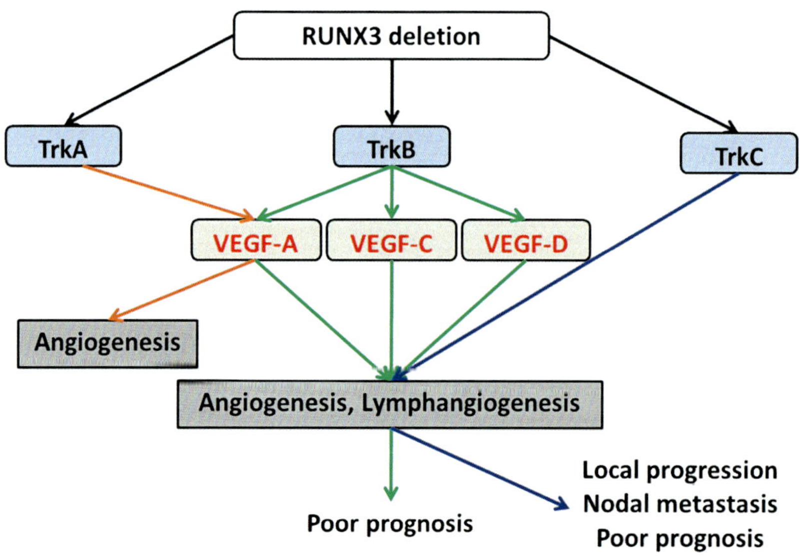

Fig. 3.6 The schema of the function of Trk in OSCC. Trks are regulator of angiogenesis and lymphangiogenesis and promote tumor progression, nodal metastasis, and poor outcome of OSCC

urologic cancer and NSCLC [205, 206]. However, miR-126 promotes gastric carcinogenesis and metastasis in prostatic adenocarcinoma [207, 208]. Thus, the functional role of miR-126 in cancer is still unknown. We clarified that miR-126 negatively regulates VEGF-A activation and promotes cell proliferation. Demethylation upon 5-Aza-dc treatment increased the expression of miR-126 and EGFL7 in OSCC cells [209]. A significant relationship was also found between decreased expression of miR-126 and tumor progression, nodal metastasis, induction of angiogenesis/lymphangiogenesis, and poor prognosis in 118 OSCC cases. Moreover, low expression of miR-126 was a prognostic factor for disease-free survival according to multivariate analysis. Our results imply that the restoration of miR-126 expression could be a useful therapeutic target for human OSCC.

3.8 Salivary Gland Cancer

Salivary gland cancer is a rare tumor whose estimated annual incidence in Japan is approximately 400 cases [210]. The expression of HER2 [211] and the downregulation of E-cadherin[212] and p27 [213] have been reported to promote tumor progression in ACC. Cyclic adenosine monophosphate response element binding protein (CREB)-regulated transcription coactivator 1-mastermind-like gene family (CRTC1-MAML2) fusion oncogene is a good marker for MEC [214]. However, the useful molecular markers associated with tumor progression of ACC and MEC remain controversial. Below, we describe our findings concerning ACC and MEC, the representative salivary gland cancers in Japan.

3.8.1 Reg IV

Regenerating islet-derived family member 4 (Reg IV), a member of the Reg gene family, belongs to the calcium-dependent superfamily. Its expression is confined to the gastrointestinal tract and pancreas in normal tissue, and it was detected in Crohn's disease, ulcerative colitis, and the intestinal metaplasia of gastric mucosa [215]. In malignancies, upregulation of Reg IV is found in gastric, colorectal, pancreatic, and prostate cancer [216–219]. We recently reported that Reg IV accelerates peritoneal metastasis and is detected in lavage fluids in patients with gastric adenocarcinoma [220]. We also revealed that 41 % of ACC expresses Reg IV and that overexpression of Reg IV is strongly associated with tumor recurrence and poor prognosis [221]. Furthermore, we reported that Reg IV induces EGFR phosphorylation and promotes cell growth in ACC. Reg IV has been observed in intestinal-type gastric cancer cells that express the intestinal mucin marker MUC2 [216]; however, no relationship was found between Reg IV and MUC2 expression in ACC. Thus, Reg IV might not be related to the specific differentiation of salivary gland epithelial cells. Our results suggest that Reg IV will be a good marker for poor prognosis in salivary gland ACC.

3.8.2 RUNX3

RUNX3 is a transcription factor that belongs to the TGFβ superfamily [222]. RUNX3 possesses tumor-suppressive functions, and its expression is decreased or abolished by CpG island hypermethylation in its promoter region in several tumors [223]. Additionally, cytoplasmic mislocalization of RUNX3 is associated with inactive tumor suppressor function [224]. We described the expression and methylation status of RUNX3 in salivary gland ACC and MEC [225]. Using immunohistochemical analysis, we showed that RUNX3 was mislocalized, decreased, or absent in all cases examined and that the decrease or deletion of RUNX3 was significantly correlated with tumor progression and short disease-free periods in ACC and MEC. Furthermore, by methylation-specific PCR and bisulfite genomic sequencing using microdissected cDNA, low mRNA expression and enhanced DNA hypermethylation of RUNX3 were found in ACC and MEC, when compared to benign salivary gland tumor and normal salivary gland. These results indicate that restoring the tumor-suppressive ability of RUNX3 may be a useful therapeutic target in salivary gland ACC and MEC.

3.9 Conclusions

The molecular mechanisms of carcinogenesis, tumor progression, and metastasis of head and neck cancer have been elucidated by recent advances in molecular biology. However, many unsolved questions remain. Current understanding of pathology is based on morphological findings. However, the molecular pathological approach is becoming mainstream in current pathological research because pathologists are increasingly required to master molecular biological knowledge. Our future efforts will focus on the elucidation of the morphology and molecular pathology of oral cancer.

References

1. Argiris A, Karamouzis MV, Raben D, Ferris RL (2008) Head and neck cancer. Lancet 371(9625):1695–1709. doi:10.1016/s0140-6736(08)60728-x
2. Paterson IC, Eveson JW, Prime SS (1996) Molecular changes in oral cancer may reflect aetiology and ethnic origin. Eur J Cancer Pt B Oral Oncol 32B(3):150–153
3. Jemal A, Bray F, Center MM, Ferlay J, Ward E, Forman D (2011) Global cancer statistics. CA Cancer J Clin 61(2):69–90. doi:10.3322/caac.20107

4. Siegel R, Naishadham D, Jemal A (2012) Cancer statistics, 2012. CA Cancer J Clin 62(1):10–29. doi:10.3322/caac.20138
5. Tanaka S, Sobue T (2005) Comparison of oral and pharyngeal cancer mortality in five countries: France, Italy, Japan, UK and USA from the WHO Mortality Database (1960–2000). Jpn J Clin Oncol 35(8):488–491. doi:10.1093/jjco/hyi133
6. Alvi A, Johnson JT (1997) Development of distant metastasis after treatment of advanced-stage head and neck cancer. Head Neck 19(6):500–505
7. Marsh D, Suchak K, Moutasim KA, Vallath S, Hopper C, Jerjes W, Upile T, Kalavrezos N, Violette SM, Weinreb PH, Chester KA, Chana JS, Marshall JF, Hart IR, Hackshaw AK, Piper K, Thomas GJ (2011) Stromal features are predictive of disease mortality in oral cancer patients. J Pathol 223(4):470–481. doi:10.1002/path.2830
8. Izumo T, Kirita T, Ariji E, Ozeki S, Okada N, Okabe S, Okazaki Y, Omura K, Kusama M, Sato T, Shinohara M, Shimozato K, Shintani S, Tanaka Y, Nakayama E, Hayashi T, Miyazaki A, Yagishita H, Yamane M, Working Group 1 on the Guidelines for C, Pathological Studies of Oral Cancer SCJSfOT (2012) General rules for clinical and pathological studies on oral cancer: a synopsis. Jpn J Clin Oncol 42(11):1099–1109. doi:10.1093/jjco/hys141
9. Califano J, van der Riet P, Westra W, Nawroz H, Clayman G, Piantadosi S, Corio R, Lee D, Greenberg B, Koch W, Sidransky D (1996) Genetic progression model for head and neck cancer: implications for field cancerization. Cancer Res 56(11): 2488–2492
10. Lippman SM, Sudbo J, Hong WK (2005) Oral cancer prevention and the evolution of molecular-targeted drug development. J Clin Oncol 23(2):346–356. doi:10.1200/jco.2005.09.128
11. Perez-Ordonez B, Beauchemin M, Jordan RC (2006) Molecular biology of squamous cell carcinoma of the head and neck. J Clin Pathol 59(5):445–453. doi:10.1136/jcp.2003.007641
12. Choi S, Myers JN (2008) Molecular pathogenesis of oral squamous cell carcinoma: implications for therapy. J Dental Res 87(1):14–32
13. Reed AL, Califano J, Cairns P, Westra WH, Jones RM, Koch W, Ahrendt S, Eby Y, Sewell D, Nawroz H, Bartek J, Sidransky D (1996) High frequency of p16 (CDKN2/MTS-1/INK4A) inactivation in head and neck squamous cell carcinoma. Cancer Res 56(16):3630–3633
14. Garnis C, Baldwin C, Zhang L, Rosin MP, Lam WL (2003) Use of complete coverage array comparative genomic hybridization to define copy number alterations on chromosome 3p in oral squamous cell carcinomas. Cancer Res 63(24):8582–8585
15. Shahnavaz SA, Regezi JA, Bradley G, Dube ID, Jordan RC (2000) p53 gene mutations in sequential oral epithelial dysplasias and squamous cell carcinomas. J Pathol 190(4):417–422. doi:10.1002/(sici)1096-9896(200003)190:4<417::aid-path544>3.0.co;2-g
16. Boyle JO, Hakim J, Koch W, van der Riet P, Hruban RH, Roa RA, Correo R, Eby YJ, Ruppert JM, Sidransky D (1993) The incidence of p53 mutations increases with progression of head and neck cancer. Cancer Res 53(19):4477–4480
17. Yu Z, Weinberger PM, Haffty BG, Sasaki C, Zerillo C, Joe J, Kowalski D, Dziura J, Camp RL, Rimm DL, Psyrri A (2005) Cyclin d1 is a valuable prognostic marker in oropharyngeal squamous cell carcinoma. Clin Cancer Res 11(3):1160–1166
18. Sudbo J, Kildal W, Risberg B, Koppang HS, Danielsen HE, Reith A (2001) DNA content as a prognostic marker in patients with oral leukoplakia. New Engl J Med 344(17):1270–1278. doi:10.1056/nejm200104263441702
19. Sudbo J, Lippman SM, Lee JJ, Mao L, Kildal W, Sudbo A, Sagen S, Bryne M, El-Naggar A, Risberg B, Evensen JF, Reith A (2004) The influence of resection and aneuploidy on mortality in oral leukoplakia. New Engl J Med 350(14):1405–1413. doi:10.1056/NEJMoa033374
20. Kreimer AR, Clifford GM, Boyle P, Franceschi S (2005) Human papillomavirus types in head and neck squamous cell carcinomas worldwide: a systematic review. Cancer Epidemiol Biomarkers Prev 14(2):467–475. doi:10.1158/1055-9965.epi-04-0551
21. Adelstein DJ, Ridge JA, Gillison ML, Chaturvedi AK, D'Souza G, Gravitt PE, Westra W, Psyrri A, Kast WM, Koutsky LA, Giuliano A, Krosnick S, Trotti A, Schuller DE, Forastiere A, Ullmann CD (2009) Head and neck squamous cell cancer and the human papillomavirus: summary of a National Cancer Institute State of the science meeting, November 9–10, 2008, Washington, DC. Head Neck 31(11):1393–1422. doi:10.1002/hed.21269
22. Syrjanen S, Lodi G, von Bultzingslowen I, Aliko A, Arduino P, Campisi G, Challacombe S, Ficarra G, Flaitz C, Zhou HM, Maeda H, Miller C, Jontell M (2011) Human papillomaviruses in oral carcinoma and oral potentially malignant disorders: a systematic review. Oral Dis 17(Suppl 1):58–72. doi:10.1111/j.1601-0825.2011.01792.x
23. Munger K, Howley PM (2002) Human papillomavirus immortalization and transformation functions. Virus Res 89(2):213–228
24. Li W, Thompson CH, Cossart YE, O'Brien CJ, McNeil EB, Scolyer RA, Rose BR (2004) The expression of key cell cycle markers and presence of human papillomavirus in squamous cell carcinoma of the tonsil. Head Neck 26(1):1–9. doi:10.1002/hed.10335
25. Leemans CR, Braakhuis BJ, Brakenhoff RH (2011) The molecular biology of head and neck cancer. Nat Rev Cancer 11(1):9–22. doi:10.1038/nrc2982
26. Hanahan D, Weinberg RA (2000) The hallmarks of cancer. Cell 100(1):57–70
27. Hanahan D, Weinberg RA (2011) Hallmarks of cancer: the next generation. Cell 144(5):646–674. doi:10.1016/j.cell.2011.02.013
28. Pitiyage G, Tilakaratne WM, Tavassoli M, Warnakulasuriya S (2009) Molecular markers in oral epithelial dysplasia: review. J Oral PatholMed38(10):737–752.doi:10.1111/j.1600-0714.2009.00804.x
29. Reuter CW, Morgan MA, Eckardt A (2007) Targeting EGF-receptor-signalling in squamous cell carcinomas of the head and neck. Br J Cancer 96(3):408–416. doi:10.1038/sj.bjc.6603566
30. Cavalot A, Martone T, Roggero N, Brondino G, Pagano M, Cortesina G (2007) Prognostic impact of HER-2/neu expression on squamous head and neck carcinomas. Head Neck 29(7):655–664. doi:10.1002/hed.20574
31. Cox AD, Der CJ (2003) The dark side of Ras: regulation of apoptosis. Oncogene 22(56):8999–9006. doi:10.1038/sj.onc.1207111
32. Grimminger CM, Danenberg PV (2011) Update of prognostic and predictive biomarkers in oropharyngeal squamous cell carcinoma: a review. Eur Arch Oto-Rhino-Laryngol 268(1):5–16. doi:10.1007/s00405-010-1369-x
33. Das N, Majumder J, DasGupta UB (2000) Ras gene mutations in oral cancer in eastern India. Oral Oncol 36(1):76–80
34. Murugan AK, Hong NT, Cuc TT, Hung NC, Munirajan AK, Ikeda MA, Tsuchida N (2009) Detection of two novel mutations and relatively high incidence of H-RAS mutations in Vietnamese oral cancer. Oral Oncol 45(10):e161–166. doi:10.1016/j.oraloncology.2009.05.638
35. Weber A, Langhanki L, Sommerer F, Markwarth A, Wittekind C, Tannapfel A (2003) Mutations of the BRAF gene in squamous cell carcinoma of the head and neck. Oncogene 22(30):4757–4759. doi:10.1038/sj.onc.1206705
36. Shojaei F, Lee JH, Simmons BH, Wong A, Esparza CO, Plumlee PA, Feng J, Stewart AE, Hu-Lowe DD, Christensen JG (2010) HGF/c-Met acts as an alternative angiogenic pathway in sunitinib-resistant tumors. Cancer Res 70(24):10090–10100. doi:10.1158/0008-5472.can-10-0489
37. Murai M, Shen X, Huang L, Carpenter WM, Lin CS, Silverman S, Regezi J, Kramer RH (2004) Overexpression of c-met in oral SCC promotes hepatocyte growth factor-induced disruption of cadherin junctions and invasion. Int J Oncol 25(4):831–840

38. Chen YS, Wang JT, Chang YF, Liu BY, Wang YP, Sun A, Chiang CP (2004) Expression of hepatocyte growth factor and c-met protein is significantly associated with the progression of oral squamous cell carcinoma in Taiwan. J Oral Pathol Med 33(4):209–217. doi:10.1111/j.0904-2512.2004.00118.x
39. Lim YC, Han JH, Kang HJ, Kim YS, Lee BH, Choi EC, Kim CH (2012) Overexpression of c-Met promotes invasion and metastasis of small oral tongue carcinoma. Oral Oncol 48(11):1114–1119. doi:10.1016/j.oraloncology.2012.05.013
40. Sun XF, Zhang H (2007) NFKB and NFKBI polymorphisms in relation to susceptibility of tumour and other diseases. Histol Histopathol 22(12):1387–1398
41. Yan M, Xu Q, Zhang P, Zhou XJ, Zhang ZY, Chen WT (2010) Correlation of NF-kappaB signal pathway with tumor metastasis of human head and neck squamous cell carcinoma. BMC Cancer 10:437. doi:10.1186/1471-2407-10-437
42. Furuta H, Osawa K, Shin M, Ishikawa A, Matsuo K, Khan M, Aoki K, Ohya K, Okamoto M, Tominaga K, Takahashi T, Nakanishi O, Jimi E (2012) Selective inhibition of NF-kappaB suppresses bone invasion by oral squamous cell carcinoma in vivo. Int J Cancer 131(5):E625–635. doi:10.1002/ijc.27435
43. Watari K, Nakamura M, Fukunaga Y, Furuno A, Shibata T, Kawahara A, Hosoi F, Kuwano T, Kuwano M, Ono M (2012) The antitumor effect of a novel angiogenesis inhibitor (an octahydronaphthalene derivative) targeting both VEGF receptor and NF-kappaB pathway. Int J Cancer 131(2):310–321. doi:10.1002/ijc.26356
44. Tamatani T, Azuma M, Ashida Y, Motegi K, Takashima R, Harada K, Kawaguchi S, Sato M (2004) Enhanced radiosensitization and chemosensitization in NF-kappaB-suppressed human oral cancer cells via the inhibition of gamma-irradiation- and 5-FU-induced production of IL-6 and IL-8. Int J Cancer 108(6):912–921. doi:10.1002/ijc.11640
45. Bussink J, van der Kogel AJ, Kaanders JH (2008) Activation of the PI3-K/AKT pathway and implications for radioresistance mechanisms in head and neck cancer. Lancet Oncol 9(3):288–296. doi:10.1016/s1470-2045(08)70073-1
46. Murugan AK, Hong NT, Fukui Y, Munirajan AK, Tsuchida N (2008) Oncogenic mutations of the PIK3CA gene in head and neck squamous cell carcinomas. Int J Oncol 32(1):101–111
47. Miyamoto R, Uzawa N, Nagaoka S, Hirata Y, Amagasa T (2003) Prognostic significance of cyclin D1 amplification and overexpression in oral squamous cell carcinomas. Oral Oncol 39(6):610–618
48. Wang L, Liu T, Nishioka M, Aguirre RL, Win SS, Okada N (2006) Activation of ERK1/2 and cyclin D1 expression in oral tongue squamous cell carcinomas: relationship between clinicopathological appearances and cell proliferation. Oral Oncol 42(6):625–631. doi:10.1016/j.oraloncology.2005.11.002
49. Zhou X, Zhang Z, Yang X, Chen W, Zhang P (2009) Inhibition of cyclin D1 expression by cyclin D1 shRNAs in human oral squamous cell carcinoma cells is associated with increased cisplatin chemosensitivity. Int J Cancer 124(2):483–489. doi:10.1002/ijc.23964
50. Yu H, Pardoll D, Jove R (2009) STATs in cancer inflammation and immunity: a leading role for STAT3. Nat Rev Cancer 9(11):798–809. doi:10.1038/nrc2734
51. Adachi M, Cui C, Dodge CT, Bhayani MK, Lai SY (2012) Targeting STAT3 inhibits growth and enhances radiosensitivity in head and neck squamous cell carcinoma. Oral Oncol 48(12):1220–1226. doi:10.1016/j.oraloncology.2012.06.006
52. Macha MA, Matta A, Kaur J, Chauhan SS, Thakar A, Shukla NK, Gupta SD, Ralhan R (2011) Prognostic significance of nuclear pSTAT3 in oral cancer. Head Neck 33(4):482–489. doi:10.1002/hed.21468
53. Klosek SK, Nakashiro K, Hara S, Li C, Shintani S, Hamakawa H (2004) Constitutive activation of Stat3 correlates with increased expression of the c-Met/HGF receptor in oral squamous cell carcinoma. Oncol Rep 12(2):293–296
54. Vogelstein B, Lane D, Levine AJ (2000) Surfing the p53 network. Nature 408(6810):307–310. doi:10.1038/35042675
55. Shiraishi K, Kato S, Han SY, Liu W, Otsuka K, Sakayori M, Ishida T, Takeda M, Kanamaru R, Ohuchi N, Ishioka C (2004) Isolation of temperature-sensitive p53 mutations from a comprehensive missense mutation library. J Biol Chem 279(1):348–355. doi:10.1074/jbc.M310815200
56. Ries JC, Schreiner D, Steininger H, Girod SC (1998) p53 mutation and detection of p53 protein expression in oral leukoplakia and oral squamous cell carcinoma. Anticancer Res 18(3B):2031–2036
57. Nagpal JK, Patnaik S, Das BR (2002) Prevalence of high-risk human papilloma virus types and its association with P53 codon 72 polymorphism in tobacco addicted oral squamous cell carcinoma (OSCC) patients of Eastern India. Int J Cancer 97(5):649–653
58. Sun P, Nallar SC, Raha A, Kalakonda S, Velalar CN, Reddy SP, Kalvakolanu DV (2010) GRIM-19 and p16(INK4a) synergistically regulate cell cycle progression and E2F1-responsive gene expression. J Biol Chem 285(36):27545–27552. doi:10.1074/jbc.M110.105767
59. Schlosshauer PW, Deligdisch L, Penault-Llorca F, Fatemi D, Qiao R, Yao S, Pearl M, Yang Z, Sheng T, Dong J (2011) Loss of p16INK4A expression in low-grade ovarian serous carcinomas. Int J Gynecol Pathol 30(1):22–29. doi:10.1097/PGP.0b013e3181ed89b3
60. Viswanathan M, Tsuchida N, Shanmugam G (2003) Promoter hypermethylation profile of tumor-associated genes p16, p15, hMLH1, MGMT and E-cadherin in oral squamous cell carcinoma. Int J Cancer 105(1):41–46. doi:10.1002/ijc.11028
61. Ruesga MT, Acha-Sagredo A, Rodriguez MJ, Aguirregaviria JI, Videgain J, Rodriguez C, de Pancorbo Mde L, Aguirre JM (2007) p16(INK4a) promoter hypermethylation in oral scrapings of oral squamous cell carcinoma risk patients. Cancer Lett 250(1):140–145. doi:10.1016/j.canlet.2006.10.001
62. Su PF, Huang WL, Wu HT, Wu CH, Liu TY, Kao SY (2010) p16(INK4A) promoter hypermethylation is associated with invasiveness and prognosis of oral squamous cell carcinoma in an age-dependent manner. Oral Oncol 46(10):734–739. doi:10.1016/j.oraloncology.2010.07.002
63. Mendenhall WM, Logan HL (2009) Human papillomavirus and head and neck cancer. Am J Clin Oncol 32(5):535–539. doi:10.1097/COC.0b013e31818b8fee
64. el-Deiry WS, Tokino T, Velculescu VE, Levy DB, Parsons R, Trent JM, Lin D, Mercer WE, Kinzler KW, Vogelstein B (1993) WAF1, a potential mediator of p53 tumor suppression. Cell 75(4):817–825
65. el-Deiry WS, Tokino T, Waldman T, Oliner JD, Velculescu VE, Burrell M, Hill DE, Healy E, Rees JL, Hamilton SR et al (1995) Topological control of p21WAF1/CIP1 expression in normal and neoplastic tissues. Cancer Res 55(13):2910–2919
66. Agarwal S, Mathur M, Shukla NK, Ralhan R (1998) Expression of cyclin dependent kinase inhibitor p21waf1/cip1 in premalignant and malignant oral lesions: relationship with p53 status. Oral Oncol 34(5):353–360
67. Kudo Y, Takata T, Ogawa I, Sato S, Nikai H (1999) Expression of p53 and p21CIP1/WAF1 proteins in oral epithelial dysplasias and squamous cell carcinomas. Oncol Rep 6(3):539–545
68. Nemes JA, Nemes Z, Marton IJ (2005) p21WAF1/CIP1 expression is a marker of poor prognosis in oral squamous cell carcinoma. J Oral Pathol Med 34(5):274–279. doi:10.1111/j.1600-0714.2005.00310.x
69. Hafkamp HC, Mooren JJ, Claessen SM, Klingenberg B, Voogd AC, Bot FJ, Klussmann JP, Hopman AH, Manni JJ, Kremer B, Ramaekers FC, Speel EJ (2009) P21 Cip1/WAF1 expression is strongly associated with HPV-positive tonsillar carcinoma and a favorable prognosis. Modern Pathol 22(5):686–698. doi:10.1038/modpathol.2009.23

70. Li J, Yen C, Liaw D, Podsypanina K, Bose S, Wang SI, Puc J, Miliaresis C, Rodgers L, McCombie R, Bigner SH, Giovanella BC, Ittmann M, Tycko B, Hibshoosh H, Wigler MH, Parsons R (1997) PTEN, a putative protein tyrosine phosphatase gene mutated in human brain, breast, and prostate cancer. Science 275(5308):1943–1947
71. Kim S, Domon-Dell C, Wang Q, Chung DH, Di Cristofano A, Pandolfi PP, Freund JN, Evers BM (2002) PTEN and TNF-alpha regulation of the intestinal-specific Cdx-2 homeobox gene through a PI3K, PKB/Akt, and NF-kappaB-dependent pathway. Gastroenterology 123(4):1163–1178
72. Guldberg P, thor Straten P, Birck A, Ahrenkiel V, Kirkin AF, Zeuthen J (1997) Disruption of the MMAC1/PTEN gene by deletion or mutation is a frequent event in malignant melanoma. Cancer Res 57(17):3660–3663
73. Yokomizo A, Tindall DJ, Drabkin H, Gemmill R, Franklin W, Yang P, Sugio K, Smith DI, Liu W (1998) PTEN/MMAC1 mutations identified in small cell, but not in non-small cell lung cancers. Oncogene 17(4):475–479. doi:10.1038/sj.onc.1201956
74. Kinross KM, Brown DV, Kleinschmidt M, Jackson S, Christensen J, Cullinane C, Hicks RJ, Johnstone RW, McArthur GA (2011) In vivo activity of combined PI3K/mTOR and MEK inhibition in a Kras(G12D); Pten deletion mouse model of ovarian cancer. Mol Cancer Therap 10(8):1440–1449. doi:10.1158/1535-7163.mct-11-0240
75. Snietura M, Jaworska M, Mlynarczyk-Liszka J, Goraj-Zajac A, Piglowski W, Lange D, Wozniak G, Nowara E, Suwinski R (2012) PTEN as a prognostic and predictive marker in postoperative radiotherapy for squamous cell cancer of the head and neck. PLoS One 7(3):e33396. doi:10.1371/journal.pone.0033396
76. Kurasawa Y, Shiiba M, Nakamura M, Fushimi K, Ishigami T, Bukawa H, Yokoe H, Uzawa K, Tanzawa H (2008) PTEN expression and methylation status in oral squamous cell carcinoma. Oncol Rep 19(6):1429–1434
77. Kato K, Kawashiri S, Yoshizawa K, Kitahara H, Yamamoto E (2008) Apoptosis-associated markers and clinical outcome in human oral squamous cell carcinomas. J Oral Pathol Med 37(6):364–371. doi:10.1111/j.1600-0714.2008.00642.x
78. Bauer JA, Trask DK, Kumar B, Los G, Castro J, Lee JS, Chen J, Wang S, Bradford CR, Carey TE (2005) Reversal of cisplatin resistance with a BH3 mimetic, (-)-gossypol, in head and neck cancer cells: role of wild-type p53 and Bcl-xL. Mol Cancer Therap 4(7):1096–1104. doi:10.1158/1535-7163.mct-05-0081
79. Staibano S, Mignogna MD, Lo Muzio L, Di Alberti L, Di Natale E, Lucariello A, Mezza E, Bucci E, DeRosa G (1998) Overexpression of cyclin-D1, bcl-2, and bax proteins, proliferating cell nuclear antigen (PCNA), and DNA-ploidy in squamous cell carcinoma of the oral cavity. Hum Pathol 29(11):1189–1194
80. Xie X, Clausen OP, Boysen M (2003) Prognostic value of Bak expression in oral tongue squamous cell carcinomas. Oncol Rep 10(2):369–374
81. Camisasca DR, Honorato J, Bernardo V, da Silva LE, da Fonseca EC, de Faria PA, Dias FL, Lourenco Sde Q (2009) Expression of Bcl-2 family proteins and associated clinicopathologic factors predict survival outcome in patients with oral squamous cell carcinoma. Oral Oncol 45(3):225–233. doi:10.1016/j.oraloncology.2008.05.021
82. Sasabe E, Tatemoto Y, Li D, Yamamoto T, Osaki T (2005) Mechanism of HIF-1alpha-dependent suppression of hypoxia-induced apoptosis in squamous cell carcinoma cells. Cancer Sci 96(7):394–402. doi:10.1111/j.1349-7006.2005.00065.x
83. McCaul JA, Gordon KE, Clark LJ, Parkinson EK (2002) Telomerase inhibition and the future management of head-and-neck cancer. Lancet Oncol 3(5):280–288
84. Liu Z, Li Q, Li K, Chen L, Li W, Hou M, Liu T, Yang J, Lindvall C, Bjorkholm M, Jia J, Xu D (2012) Telomerase reverse transcriptase promotes epithelial-mesenchymal transition and stem cell-like traits in cancer cells. Oncogene. doi:10.1038/onc.2012.441
85. Chen HH, Yu CH, Wang JT, Liu BY, Wang YP, Sun A, Tsai TC, Chiang CP (2007) Expression of human telomerase reverse transcriptase (hTERT) protein is significantly associated with the progression, recurrence and prognosis of oral squamous cell carcinoma in Taiwan. Oral Oncol 43(2):122–129. doi:10.1016/j.oraloncology.2006.01.011
86. McCaul JA, Gordon KE, Minty F, Fleming J, Parkinson EK (2008) Telomere dysfunction is related to the intrinsic radio-resistance of human oral cancer cells. Oral Oncol 44(3):261–269. doi:10.1016/j.oraloncology.2007.02.010
87. Lohela M, Bry M, Tammela T, Alitalo K (2009) VEGFs and receptors involved in angiogenesis versus lymphangiogenesis. Curr Opin Cell Biol 21(2):154–165. doi:10.1016/j.ceb.2008.12.012
88. Sasahira T, Kirita T, Kurihara M, Yamamoto K, Bhawal UK, Bosserhoff AK, Kuniyasu H (2010) MIA-dependent angiogenesis and lymphangiogenesis are closely associated with progression, nodal metastasis and poor prognosis in tongue squamous cell carcinoma. Eur J Cancer 46(12):2285–2294. doi:10.1016/j.ejca.2010.04.027
89. Li C, Shintani S, Terakado N, Klosek SK, Ishikawa T, Nakashiro K, Hamakawa H (2005) Microvessel density and expression of vascular endothelial growth factor, basic fibroblast growth factor, and platelet-derived endothelial growth factor in oral squamous cell carcinomas. Int J Oral Maxillofac Surg 34(5):559–565. doi:10.1016/j.ijom.2004.10.016
90. Watanabe H, Iwase M, Ohashi M, Nagumo M (2002) Role of interleukin-8 secreted from human oral squamous cell carcinoma cell lines. Oral Oncol 38(7):670–679
91. Fagiani E, Lorentz P, Kopfstein L, Christofori G (2011) Angiopoietin-1 and -2 exert antagonistic functions in tumor angiogenesis, yet both induce lymphangiogenesis. Cancer Res 71(17):5717–5727. doi:10.1158/0008-5472.can-10-4635
92. Dagenais SL, Hartsough RL, Erickson RP, Witte MH, Butler MG, Glover TW (2004) Foxc2 is expressed in developing lymphatic vessels and other tissues associated with lymphedema-distichiasis syndrome. Gene Expr Patterns 4(6):611–619. doi:10.1016/j.modgep.2004.07.004
93. Van den Eynden GG, Van der Auwera I, Van Laere SJ, Trinh XB, Colpaert CG, van Dam P, Dirix LY, Vermeulen PB, Van Marck EA (2007) Comparison of molecular determinants of angiogenesis and lymphangiogenesis in lymph node metastases and in primary tumours of patients with breast cancer. J Pathol 213(1):56–64. doi:10.1002/path.2211
94. Kim WH, Lee SH, Jung MH, Seo JH, Kim J, Kim MA, Lee YM (2009) Neuropilin2 expressed in gastric cancer endothelial cells increases the proliferation and migration of endothelial cells in response to VEGF. Exp Cell Res 315(13):2154–2164. doi:10.1016/j.yexcr.2009.04.018
95. Jayson GC, Hicklin DJ, Ellis LM (2012) Antiangiogenic therapy: evolving view based on clinical trial results. Nat Rev Clin Oncol 9(5):297–303. doi:10.1038/nrclinonc.2012.8
96. Huber GF, Zullig L, Soltermann A, Roessle M, Graf N, Haerle SK, Studer G, Jochum W, Moch H, Stoeckli SJ (2011) Down regulation of E-Cadherin (ECAD): a predictor for occult metastatic disease in sentinel node biopsy of early squamous cell carcinomas of the oral cavity and oropharynx. BMC Cancer 11(217):211–218. doi:10.1186/1471-2407-11-217
97. Wang X, Zhang J, Fan M, Zhou Q, Deng H, Aisharif MJ, Chen X (2009) The expression of E-cadherin at the invasive tumor front of oral squamous cell carcinoma: immunohistochemical and RT-PCR analysis with clinicopathological correlation. Oral Surg Oral Med Oral Pathol Oral Radiol Endod 107(4):547–554. doi:10.1016/j.tripleo.2008.11.021
98. Diniz-Freitas M, Garcia-Caballero T, Antunez-Lopez J, Gandara-Rey JM, Garcia-Garcia A (2006) Reduced E-cadherin expression is an indicator of unfavourable prognosis in oral squamous cell carcinoma. Oral Oncol 42(2):190–200. doi:10.1016/j.oraloncology.2005.07.010

99. Kudo Y, Kitajima S, Ogawa I, Hiraoka M, Sargolzaei S, Keikhaee MR, Sato S, Miyauchi M, Takata T (2004) Invasion and metastasis of oral cancer cells require methylation of E-cadherin and/or degradation of membranous beta-catenin. Clin Cancer Res 10(16):5455–5463. doi:10.1158/1078-0432.ccr-04-0372
100. Larue L, Bellacosa A (2005) Epithelial-mesenchymal transition in development and cancer: role of phosphatidylinositol 3′ kinase/AKT pathways. Oncogene 24(50):7443–7454. doi:10.1038/sj.onc.1209091
101. Gao ZB, Duan YQ, Zhang L, Chen DW, Ding PT (2005) Expression of matrix metalloproteinase 2 and its tissue inhibitor in oral squamous cell carcinoma. Int J Mol Med 16(4):599–603
102. de Vicente JC, Lequerica-Fernandez P, Santamaria J, Fresno MF (2007) Expression of MMP-7 and MT1-MMP in oral squamous cell carcinoma as predictive indicator for tumor invasion and prognosis. J Oral Pathol Med 36(7):415–424. doi:10.1111/j.1600-0714.2007.00546.x
103. Liu SY, Liu YC, Huang WT, Huang GC, Su HJ, Lin MH (2007) Requirement of MMP-3 in anchorage-independent growth of oral squamous cell carcinomas. J Oral Pathol Med 36(7):430–435. doi:10.1111/j.1600-0714.2007.00524.x
104. Yorioka CW, Coletta RD, Alves F, Nishimoto IN, Kowalski LP, Graner E (2002) Matrix metalloproteinase-2 and -9 activities correlate with the disease-free survival of oral squamous cell carcinoma patients. Int J Oncol 20(1):189–194
105. Mashhadiabbas F, Mahjour F, Mahjour SB, Fereidooni F, Hosseini FS (2012) The immunohistochemical characterization of MMP-2, MMP-10, TIMP-1, TIMP-2, and podoplanin in oral squamous cell carcinoma. Oral Surg Oral Med Oral Pathol Oral Radiol 114(2):240–250. doi:10.1016/j.oooo.2012.04.009
106. Arora S, Kaur J, Sharma C, Mathur M, Bahadur S, Shukla NK, Deo SV, Ralhan R (2005) Stromelysin 3, Ets-1, and vascular endothelial growth factor expression in oral precancerous and cancerous lesions: correlation with microvessel density, progression, and prognosis. Clin Cancer Res 11(6):2272–2284. doi:10.1158/1078-0432.ccr-04-0572
107. Perez-Sayans Garcia M, Suarez-Penaranda JM, Gayoso-Diz P, Barros-Angueira F, Gandara-Rey JM, Garcia-Garcia A (2012) Tissue inhibitor of metalloproteinases in oral squamous cell carcinomas: a therapeutic target? Cancer Lett 323(1):11–19. doi:10.1016/j.canlet.2012.03.040
108. Ohara T, Kawashiri S, Tanaka A, Noguchi N, Kitahara H, Okamune A, Kato K, Hase T, Nakaya H, Yoshizawa K (2009) Integrin expression levels correlate with invasion, metastasis and prognosis of oral squamous cell carcinoma. Pathol Oncol Res 15(3):429–436. doi:10.1007/s12253-008-9142-9
109. Ryu MH, Park HM, Chung J, Lee CH, Park HR (2010) Hypoxia-inducible factor-1alpha mediates oral squamous cell carcinoma invasion via upregulation of alpha5 integrin and fibronectin. Biochem Biophys Res Commun 393(1):11–15. doi:10.1016/j.bbrc.2010.01.060
110. Li HX, Zheng JH, Fan HX, Li HP, Gao ZX, Chen D (2013) Expression of alphavbeta6 integrin and collagen fibre in oral squamous cell carcinoma: association with clinical outcomes and prognostic implications. J Oral Pathol Med. doi:10.1111/jop.12044
111. Hamidi S, Salo T, Kainulainen T, Epstein J, Lerner K, Larjava H (2000) Expression of alpha(v)beta6 integrin in oral leukoplakia. Br J Cancer 82(8):1433–1440. doi:10.1054/bjoc.1999.1130
112. Nelson BH (2008) The impact of T-cell immunity on ovarian cancer outcomes. Immunol Rev 222:101–116. doi:10.1111/j.1600-065X.2008.00614.x
113. Pages F, Galon J, Dieu-Nosjean MC, Tartour E, Sautes-Fridman C, Fridman WH (2010) Immune infiltration in human tumors: a prognostic factor that should not be ignored. Oncogene 29(8):1093–1102. doi:10.1038/onc.2009.416
114. Yang L, Pang Y, Moses HL (2010) TGF-beta and immune cells: an important regulatory axis in the tumor microenvironment and progression. Trends Immunol 31(6):220–227. doi:10.1016/j.it.2010.04.002
115. Ostrand-Rosenberg S, Sinha P (2009) Myeloid-derived suppressor cells: linking inflammation and cancer. J Immunol 182(8):4499–4506. doi:10.4049/jimmunol.0802740
116. Paulos CM, Kaiser A, Wrzesinski C, Hinrichs CS, Cassard L, Boni A, Muranski P, Sanchez-Perez L, Palmer DC, Yu Z, Antony PA, Gattinoni L, Rosenberg SA, Restifo NP (2007) Toll-like receptors in tumor immunotherapy. Clin Cancer Res 13(18 Pt 1):5280–5289. doi:10.1158/1078-0432.ccr-07-1378
117. Chuang HC, Huang CC, Chien CY, Chuang JH (2012) Toll-like receptor 3-mediated tumor invasion in head and neck cancer. Oral Oncol 48(3):226–232. doi:10.1016/j.oraloncology.2011.10.008
118. Sun Z, Luo Q, Ye D, Chen W, Chen F (2012) Role of toll-like receptor 4 on the immune escape of human oral squamous cell carcinoma and resistance of cisplatin-induced apoptosis. Mol Cancer 11:33. doi:10.1186/1476-4598-11-33
119. Ahn MY, Kwon SM, Cheong HH, Park JH, Lee J, Min SK, Ahn SG, Yoon JH (2012) Toll-like receptor 7 agonist, imiquimod, inhibits oral squamous carcinoma cells through apoptosis and necrosis. J Oral Pathol Med 41(7):540–546. doi:10.1111/j.1600-0714.2012.01158.x
120. Min R, Zun Z, Siyi L, Wenjun Y, Lizheng W, Chenping Z (2011) Increased expression of Toll-like receptor-9 has close relation with tumour cell proliferation in oral squamous cell carcinoma. Arch Oral Biol 56(9):877–884. doi:10.1016/j.archoralbio.2011.01.010
121. Grivennikov SI, Greten FR, Karin M (2010) Immunity, inflammation, and cancer. Cell 140(6):883–899. doi:10.1016/j.cell.2010.01.025
122. Shibata M, Kodani I, Osaki M, Araki K, Adachi H, Ryoke K, Ito H (2005) Cyclo-oxygenase-1 and -2 expression in human oral mucosa, dysplasias and squamous cell carcinomas and their pathological significance. Oral Oncol 41(3):304–312. doi:10.1016/j.oraloncology.2004.09.009
123. Kurihara Y, Hatori M, Ando Y, Ito D, Toyoshima T, Tanaka M, Shintani S (2009) Inhibition of cyclooxygenase-2 suppresses the invasiveness of oral squamous cell carcinoma cell lines via down-regulation of matrix metalloproteinase-2 production and activation. Clin Exp Metastasis 26(5):425–432. doi:10.1007/s10585-009-9241-3
124. Morita Y, Hata K, Nakanishi M, Nishisho T, Yura Y, Yoneda T (2012) Cyclooxygenase-2 promotes tumor lymphangiogenesis and lymph node metastasis in oral squamous cell carcinoma. Int J Oncol 41(3):885–892. doi:10.3892/ijo.2012.1529
125. Kwak YE, Jeon NK, Kim J, Lee EJ (2007) The cyclooxygenase-2 selective inhibitor celecoxib suppresses proliferation and invasiveness in the human oral squamous carcinoma. Ann NY Acad Sci 1095:99–112. doi:10.1196/annals.1397.014
126. Nakahara Y, Shintani S, Mihara M, Ueyama Y, Matsumura T (2001) High frequency of homozygous deletion and methylation of p16(INK4A) gene in oral squamous cell carcinomas. Cancer Lett 163(2):221–228
127. Ha PK, Califano JA (2006) Promoter methylation and inactivation of tumour-suppressor genes in oral squamous-cell carcinoma. Lancet Oncol 7(1):77–82. doi:10.1016/s1470-2045(05)70540-4
128. Chang HW, Chow V, Lam KY, Wei WI, Yuen A (2002) Loss of E-cadherin expression resulting from promoter hypermethylation in oral tongue carcinoma and its prognostic significance. Cancer 94(2):386–392. doi:10.1002/cncr.10211
129. Kulkarni V, Saranath D (2004) Concurrent hypermethylation of multiple regulatory genes in chewing tobacco associated oral squamous cell carcinomas and adjacent normal tissues. Oral Oncol 40(2):145–153
130. Youssef EM, Lotan D, Issa JP, Wakasa K, Fan YH, Mao L, Hassan K, Feng L, Lee JJ, Lippman SM, Hong WK, Lotan R (2004)

Hypermethylation of the retinoic acid receptor-beta(2) gene in head and neck carcinogenesis. Clin Cancer Res 10(5):1733–1742
131. Kunkel M, Reichert TE, Benz P, Lehr HA, Jeong JH, Wieand S, Bartenstein P, Wagner W, Whiteside TL (2003) Overexpression of Glut-1 and increased glucose metabolism in tumors are associated with a poor prognosis in patients with oral squamous cell carcinoma. Cancer 97(4):1015–1024. doi:10.1002/cncr.11159
132. Kunkel M, Moergel M, Stockinger M, Jeong JH, Fritz G, Lehr HA, Whiteside TL (2007) Overexpression of GLUT-1 is associated with resistance to radiotherapy and adverse prognosis in squamous cell carcinoma of the oral cavity. Oral Oncol 43(8):796–803. doi:10.1016/j.oraloncology.2006.10.009
133. Eckert AW, Lautner MH, Taubert H, Schubert J, Bilkenroth U (2008) Expression of Glut-1 is a prognostic marker for oral squamous cell carcinoma patients. Oncol Rep 20(6):1381–1385
134. Zhu GQ, Tang YL, Li L, Zheng M, Jiang J, Li XY, Chen SX, Liang XH (2010) Hypoxia inducible factor 1alpha and hypoxia inducible factor 2alpha play distinct and functionally overlapping roles in oral squamous cell carcinoma. Clin Cancer Res 16(19):4732–4741. doi:10.1158/1078-0432.ccr-10-1408
135. Brennan PA, Mackenzie N, Quintero M (2005) Hypoxia-inducible factor 1alpha in oral cancer. J Oral Pathol Med 34(7):385–389. doi:10.1111/j.1600-0714.2005.00335.x
136. Eckert AW, Lautner MH, Schutze A, Taubert H, Schubert J, Bilkenroth U (2011) Coexpression of hypoxia-inducible factor-1alpha and glucose transporter-1 is associated with poor prognosis in oral squamous cell carcinoma patients. Histopathology 58(7):1136–1147. doi:10.1111/j.1365-2559.2011.03806.x
137. Naruse T, Kawasaki G, Yanamoto S, Mizuno A, Umeda M (2011) Immunohistochemical study of VEGF expression in oral squamous cell carcinomas: correlation with the mTOR-HIF-1alpha pathway. Anticancer Res 31(12):4429–4437
138. Liang X, Yang D, Hu J, Hao X, Gao J, Mao Z (2008) Hypoxia inducible factor-alpha expression correlates with vascular endothelial growth factor-C expression and lymphangiogenesis/angiogenesis in oral squamous cell carcinoma. Anticancer Res 28(3A):1659–1666
139. Chaw SY, Majeed AA, Dalley AJ, Chan A, Stein S, Farah CS (2012) Epithelial to mesenchymal transition (EMT) biomarkers–E-cadherin, beta-catenin, APC and Vimentin–in oral squamous cell carcinogenesis and transformation. Oral Oncol 48(10):997–1006. doi:10.1016/j.oraloncology.2012.05.011
140. Heldin CH, Vanlandewijck M, Moustakas A (2012) Regulation of EMT by TGFbeta in cancer. FEBS Lett 586(14):1959–1970. doi:10.1016/j.febslet.2012.02.037
141. Shirkoohi R (2013) Epithelial mesenchymal transition from a natural gestational orchestration to a bizarre cancer disturbance. Cancer Sci 104(1):28–35. doi:10.1111/cas.12074
142. Qiao B, Johnson NW, Gao J (2010) Epithelial-mesenchymal transition in oral squamous cell carcinoma triggered by transforming growth factor-beta1 is Snail family-dependent and correlates with matrix metalloproteinase-2 and -9 expressions. Int J Oncol 37(3):663–668
143. Zhao D, Tang XF, Yang K, Liu JY, Ma XR (2012) Over-expression of integrin-linked kinase correlates with aberrant expression of Snail, E-cadherin and N-cadherin in oral squamous cell carcinoma: implications in tumor progression and metastasis. Clin Exp Metastasis 29(8):957–969. doi:10.1007/s10585-012-9485-1
144. Melo SA, Kalluri R (2012) Molecular pathways: microRNAs as cancer therapeutics. Clin Cancer Res 18(16):4234–4239. doi:10.1158/1078-0432.ccr-11-2010
145. Chen CZ (2005) MicroRNAs as oncogenes and tumor suppressors. New Engl J Med 353(17):1768–1771. doi:10.1056/NEJMp058190
146. Wu BH, Xiong XP, Jia J, Zhang WF (2011) MicroRNAs: new actors in the oral cancer scene. Oral Oncol 47(5):314–319. doi:10.1016/j.oraloncology.2011.03.019
147. Perez-Sayans M, Pilar GD, Barros-Angueira F, Suarez-Penaranda JM, Fernandez AC, Gandara-Rey JM, Garcia-Garcia A (2012) Current trends in miRNAs and their relationship with oral squamous cell carcinoma. J Oral Pathol Med 41(6):433–443. doi:10.1111/j.1600-0714.2011.01121.x
148. Merritt WM, Lin YG, Han LY, Kamat AA, Spannuth WA, Schmandt R, Urbauer D, Pennacchio LA, Cheng JF, Nick AM, Deavers MT, Mourad-Zeidan A, Wang H, Mueller P, Lenburg ME, Gray JW, Mok S, Birrer MJ, Lopez-Berestein G, Coleman RL, Bar-Eli M, Sood AK (2008) Dicer, Drosha, and outcomes in patients with ovarian cancer. New Engl J Med 359(25):2641–2650. doi:10.1056/NEJMoa0803785
149. Li J, Huang H, Sun L, Yang M, Pan C, Chen W, Wu D, Lin Z, Zeng C, Yao Y, Zhang P, Song E (2009) MiR-21 indicates poor prognosis in tongue squamous cell carcinomas as an apoptosis inhibitor. Clin Cancer Res 15(12):3998–4008. doi:10.1158/1078-0432.ccr-08-3053
150. Liu X, Wang A, Heidbreder CE, Jiang L, Yu J, Kolokythas A, Huang L, Dai Y, Zhou X (2010) MicroRNA-24 targeting RNA-binding protein DND1 in tongue squamous cell carcinoma. FEBS Lett 584(18):4115–4120. doi:10.1016/j.febslet.2010.08.040
151. Liu X, Yu J, Jiang L, Wang A, Shi F, Ye H, Zhou X (2009) MicroRNA-222 regulates cell invasion by targeting matrix metalloproteinase 1 (MMP1) and manganese superoxide dismutase 2 (SOD2) in tongue squamous cell carcinoma cell lines. Cancer Genomics Proteomics 6(3):131–139
152. Chang KW, Liu CJ, Chu TH, Cheng HW, Hung PS, Hu WY, Lin SC (2008) Association between high miR-211 microRNA expression and the poor prognosis of oral carcinoma. J Dental Res 87(11):1063–1068
153. Liu CJ, Tsai MM, Hung PS, Kao SY, Liu TY, Wu KJ, Chiou SH, Lin SC, Chang KW (2010) miR-31 ablates expression of the HIF regulatory factor FIH to activate the HIF pathway in head and neck carcinoma. Cancer Res 70(4):1635–1644. doi:10.1158/0008-5472.can-09-2291
154. Liu CJ, Kao SY, Tu HF, Tsai MM, Chang KW, Lin SC (2010) Increase of microRNA miR-31 level in plasma could be a potential marker of oral cancer. Oral Dis 16(4):360–364. doi:10.1111/j.1601-0825.2009.01646.x
155. Yu ZW, Zhong LP, Ji T, Zhang P, Chen WT, Zhang CP (2010) MicroRNAs contribute to the chemoresistance of cisplatin in tongue squamous cell carcinoma lines. Oral Oncol 46(4):317–322. doi:10.1016/j.oraloncology.2010.02.002
156. Hebert C, Norris K, Scheper MA, Nikitakis N, Sauk JJ (2007) High mobility group A2 is a target for miRNA-98 in head and neck squamous cell carcinoma. Mol Cancer 6:5. doi:10.1186/1476-4598-6-5
157. Wong TS, Liu XB, Chung-Wai Ho A, Po-Wing Yuen A, Wai-Man Ng R, Ignace Wei W (2008) Identification of pyruvate kinase type M2 as potential oncoprotein in squamous cell carcinoma of tongue through microRNA profiling. Int J Cancer 123(2):251–257. doi:10.1002/ijc.23583
158. Mutallip M, Nohata N, Hanazawa T, Kikkawa N, Horiguchi S, Fujimura L, Kawakami K, Chiyomaru T, Enokida H, Nakagawa M, Okamoto Y, Seki N (2011) Glutathione S-transferase P1 (GSTP1) suppresses cell apoptosis and its regulation by miR-133alpha in head and neck squamous cell carcinoma (HNSCC). Int J Mol Med 27(3):345–352. doi:10.3892/ijmm.2010.589
159. Jiang L, Liu X, Chen Z, Jin Y, Heidbreder CE, Kolokythas A, Wang A, Dai Y, Zhou X (2010) MicroRNA-7 targets IGF1R (insulin-like growth factor 1 receptor) in tongue squamous cell carcinoma cells. Biochem J 432(1):199–205. doi:10.1042/bj20100859
160. Hunt S, Jones AV, Hinsley EE, Whawell SA, Lambert DW (2011) MicroRNA-124 suppresses oral squamous cell carcinoma motility by targeting ITGB1. FEBS Lett 585(1):187–192. doi:10.1016/j.febslet.2010.11.038

161. Kuniyasu H, Oue N, Wakikawa A, Shigeishi H, Matsutani N, Kuraoka K, Ito R, Yokozaki H, Yasui W (2002) Expression of receptors for advanced glycation end-products (RAGE) is closely associated with the invasive and metastatic activity of gastric cancer. J Pathol 196(2):163–170. doi:10.1002/path.1031
162. Kuniyasu H, Chihara Y, Kondo H (2003) Differential effects between amphoterin and advanced glycation end products on colon cancer cells. Int J Cancer 104(6):722–727. doi:10.1002/ijc.11016
163. Kuniyasu H, Yano S, Sasaki T, Sasahira T, Sone S, Ohmori H (2005) Colon cancer cell-derived high mobility group 1/amphoterin induces growth inhibition and apoptosis in macrophages. Am J Pathol 166(3):751–760. doi:10.1016/s0002-9440(10)62296-1
164. Tang D, Shi Y, Jang L, Wang K, Xiao W, Xiao X (2005) Heat shock response inhibits release of high mobility group box 1 protein induced by endotoxin in murine macrophages. Shock 23(5):434–440
165. Kuniyasu H, Chihara Y, Kondo H, Ohmori H, Ukai R (2003) Amphoterin induction in prostatic stromal cells by androgen deprivation is associated with metastatic prostate cancer. Oncol Rep 10(6):1863–1868
166. Sasahira T, Akama Y, Fujii K, Kuniyasu H (2005) Expression of receptor for advanced glycation end products and HMGB1/amphoterin in colorectal adenomas. Virchows Arch 446(4):411–415. doi:10.1007/s00428-005-1210-x
167. Sasahira T, Kirita T, Bhawal UK, Yamamoto K, Ohmori H, Fujii K, Kuniyasu H (2007) Receptor for advanced glycation end products (RAGE) is important in the prediction of recurrence in human oral squamous cell carcinoma. Histopathology 51(2):166–172. doi:10.1111/j.1365-2559.2007.02739.x
168. Sasahira T, Kirita T, Bhawal UK, Ikeda M, Nagasawa A, Yamamoto K, Kuniyasu H (2007) The expression of receptor for advanced glycation end products is associated with angiogenesis in human oral squamous cell carcinoma. Virchows Arch 450(3):287–295. doi:10.1007/s00428-006-0359-2
169. Bhawal UK, Ozaki Y, Nishimura M, Sugiyama M, Sasahira T, Nomura Y, Sato F, Fujimoto K, Sasaki N, Ikeda MA, Tsuji K, Kuniyasu H, Kato Y (2005) Association of expression of receptor for advanced glycation end products and invasive activity of oral squamous cell carcinoma. Oncology 69(3):246–255. doi:10.1159/000087910
170. Yamamoto K, Kitayama W, Denda A, Sasahira T, Kuniyasu H, Kirita T (2006) Expression of receptor for advanced glycation end products during rat tongue carcinogenesis by 4-nitroquinoline 1-oxide and effect of a selective cyclooxygenase-2 inhibitor, etodolac. Pathobiology 73(6):317–324. doi:10.1159/000099127
171. Bosserhoff AK, Moser M, Buettner R (2004) Characterization and expression pattern of the novel MIA homolog TANGO. Gene Expr Patterns 4(4):473–479. doi:10.1016/j.modgep.2003.12.002
172. Bosserhoff AK, Moser M, Hein R, Landthaler M, Buettner R (1999) In situ expression patterns of melanoma-inhibiting activity (MIA) in melanomas and breast cancers. J Pathol 187(4):446–454. doi:10.1002/(sici)1096-9896(199903)187:4<446::aid-path267>3.0.co;2-y
173. Perez RP, Zhang P, Bosserhoff AK, Buettner R, Abu-Hadid M (2000) Expression of melanoma inhibitory activity in melanoma and nonmelanoma tissue specimens. Hum Pathol 31(11):1381–1388
174. Jachimczak P, Apfel R, Bosserhoff AK, Fabel K, Hau P, Tschertner I, Wise P, Schlingensiepen KH, Schuler-Thurner B, Bogdahn U (2005) Inhibition of immunosuppressive effects of melanoma-inhibiting activity (MIA) by antisense techniques. Int J Cancer 113(1):88–92. doi:10.1002/ijc.20549
175. Bosserhoff AK, Stoll R, Sleeman JP, Bataille F, Buettner R, Holak TA (2003) Active detachment involves inhibition of cell-matrix contacts of malignant melanoma cells by secretion of melanoma inhibitory activity. Lab Invest 83(11):1583–1594
176. Bauer R, Humphries M, Fassler R, Winklmeier A, Craig SE, Bosserhoff AK (2006) Regulation of integrin activity by MIA. J Biol Chem 281(17):11669–11677. doi:10.1074/jbc.M511367200
177. Sasahira T, Kirita T, Oue N, Bhawal UK, Yamamoto K, Fujii K, Ohmori H, Luo Y, Yasui W, Bosserhoff AK, Kuniyasu H (2008) High mobility group box-1-inducible melanoma inhibitory activity is associated with nodal metastasis and lymphangiogenesis in oral squamous cell carcinoma. Cancer Sci 99(9):1806–1812. doi:10.1111/j.1349-7006.2008.00894.x
178. Hellerbrand C, Bataille F, Schlegel J, Hartmann A, Muhlbauer M, Scholmerich J, Buttner R, Hofstadter F, Bosserhoff AK (2005) In situ expression patterns of melanoma inhibitory activity 2 in healthy and diseased livers. Liver Int 25(2):357–366. doi:10.1111/j.1478-3231.2005.01099.x
179. Bosserhoff AK, Moser M, Scholmerich J, Buettner R, Hellerbrand C (2003) Specific expression and regulation of the new melanoma inhibitory activity-related gene MIA2 in hepatocytes. J Biol Chem 278(17):15225–15231. doi:10.1074/jbc.M212639200
180. Hellerbrand C, Amann T, Schlegel J, Wild P, Bataille F, Spruss T, Hartmann A, Bosserhoff AK (2008) The novel gene MIA2 acts as a tumour suppressor in hepatocellular carcinoma. Gut 57(2):243–251. doi:10.1136/gut.2007.129544
181. Kurihara M, Kirita T, Sasahira T, Ohmori H, Matsushima S, Yamamoto K, Bosserhoff AK, Kuniyasu H (2013) Protumoral roles of melanoma inhibitory activity 2 in oral squamous cell carcinoma. Br J Cancer 108(7):1460–1469. doi:10.1038/bjc.2013.27
182. Arndt S, Bosserhoff AK (2006) TANGO is a tumor suppressor of malignant melanoma. Int J Cancer 119(12):2812–2820. doi:10.1002/ijc.22242
183. Arndt S, Bosserhoff AK (2007) Reduced expression of TANGO in colon and hepatocellular carcinomas. Oncol Rep 18(4):885–891
184. Bosserhoff AK, Buettner R (2002) Expression, function and clinical relevance of MIA (melanoma inhibitory activity). Histol Histopathol 17(1):289–300
185. Thiele CJ, Li Z, McKee AE (2009) On Trk–the TrkB signal transduction pathway is an increasingly important target in cancer biology. Clin Cancer Res 15(19):5962–5967. doi:10.1158/1078-0432.ccr-08-0651
186. Laramore C, Maymind E, Shifman MI (2011) Expression of neurotrophin and its tropomyosin-related kinase receptors (Trks) during axonal regeneration following spinal cord injury in larval lamprey. Neuroscience 183:265–277. doi:10.1016/j.neuroscience.2011.03.024
187. Bounacer A, Schlumberger M, Wicker R, Du-Villard JA, Caillou B, Sarasin A, Suarez HG (2000) Search for NTRK1 proto-oncogene rearrangements in human thyroid tumours originated after therapeutic radiation. Br J Cancer 82(2):308–314. doi:10.1054/bjoc.1999.0920
188. Davidson B, Reich R, Lazarovici P, Nesland JM, Skrede M, Risberg B, Trope CG, Florenes VA (2003) Expression and activation of the nerve growth factor receptor TrkA in serous ovarian carcinoma. Clin Cancer Res 9(6):2248–2259
189. Yang ZF, Ho DW, Lam CT, Luk JM, Lum CT, Yu WC, Poon RT, Fan ST (2005) Identification of brain-derived neurotrophic factor as a novel functional protein in hepatocellular carcinoma. Cancer Res 65(1):219–225
190. Sclabas GM, Fujioka S, Schmidt C, Li Z, Frederick WA, Yang W, Yokoi K, Evans DB, Abbruzzese JL, Hess KR, Zhang W, Fidler IJ, Chiao PJ (2005) Overexpression of tropomyosin-related kinase B in metastatic human pancreatic cancer cells. Clin Cancer Res 11 (2 Pt 1):440–449
191. Nakagawara A, Azar CG, Scavarda NJ, Brodeur GM (1994) Expression and function of TRK-B and BDNF in human neuroblastomas. Mol Cell Biol 14(1):759–767
192. Yu X, Liu L, Cai B, He Y, Wan X (2008) Suppression of anoikis by the neurotrophic receptor TrkB in human ovarian cancer. Cancer Sci 99(3):543–552. doi:10.1111/j.1349-7006.2007.00722.x

193. Bouzas-Rodriguez J, Cabrera JR, Delloye-Bourgeois C, Ichim G, Delcros JG, Raquin MA, Rousseau R, Combaret V, Benard J, Tauszig-Delamasure S, Mehlen P (2010) Neurotrophin-3 production promotes human neuroblastoma cell survival by inhibiting TrkC-induced apoptosis. J Clin Invest 120(3):850–858. doi:10.1172/jci41013
194. Sasahira T, Ueda N, Kurihara M, Matsushima S, Ohmori H, Fujii K, Bhawal UK, Yamamoto K, Kirita T, Kuniyasu H (2013) Tropomyosin receptor kinases B and C are tumor progressive and metastatic marker in colorectal carcinoma. Hum Pathol. doi:10.1016/j.humpath.2012.09.016
195. Satoh F, Mimata H, Nomura T, Fujita Y, Shin T, Sakamoto S, Hamada Y, Nomura Y (2001) Autocrine expression of neurotrophins and their receptors in prostate cancer. Int J Urol 8(7):S28–34
196. Nakagawara A, Arima-Nakagawara M, Scavarda NJ, Azar CG, Cantor AB, Brodeur GM (1993) Association between high levels of expression of the TRK gene and favorable outcome in human neuroblastoma. New Engl J Med 328(12):847–854. doi:10.1056/nejm199303253281205
197. Yamashiro DJ, Liu XG, Lee CP, Nakagawara A, Ikegaki N, McGregor LM, Baylin SB, Brodeur GM (1997) Expression and function of Trk-C in favourable human neuroblastomas. Eur J Cancer 33(12):2054–2057
198. Segal RA, Goumnerova LC, Kwon YK, Stiles CD, Pomeroy SL (1994) Expression of the neurotrophin receptor TrkC is linked to a favorable outcome in medulloblastoma. Proc Natl Acad Sci USA 91(26):12867–12871
199. Sasahira T, Ueda N, Yamamoto K, Bhawal UK, Kurihara M, Kirita T, Kuniyasu H (2013) Trks are novel oncogenes involved in the induction of neovascularization, tumor progression, and nodal metastasis in oral squamous cell carcinoma. Clin Exp Metastasis 30(2):165–176. doi:10.1007/s10585-012-9525-x
200. Fish JE, Santoro MM, Morton SU, Yu S, Yeh RF, Wythe JD, Ivey KN, Bruneau BG, Stainier DY, Srivastava D (2008) miR-126 regulates angiogenic signaling and vascular integrity. Dev Cell 15(2):272–284. doi:10.1016/j.devcel.2008.07.008
201. Wang S, Aurora AB, Johnson BA, Qi X, McAnally J, Hill JA, Richardson JA, Bassel-Duby R, Olson EN (2008) The endothelial-specific microRNA miR-126 governs vascular integrity and angiogenesis. Dev Cell 15(2):261–271. doi:10.1016/j.devcel.2008.07.002
202. Jiao LR, Frampton AE, Jacob J, Pellegrino L, Krell J, Giamas G, Tsim N, Vlavianos P, Cohen P, Ahmad R, Keller A, Habib NA, Stebbing J, Castellano L (2012) MicroRNAs targeting oncogenes are down-regulated in pancreatic malignant transformation from benign tumors. PLoS One 7(2):e32068. doi:10.1371/journal.pone.0032068
203. Donnem T, Fenton CG, Lonvik K, Berg T, Eklo K, Andersen S, Stenvold H, Al-Shibli K, Al-Saad S, Bremnes RM, Busund LT (2012) MicroRNA signatures in tumor tissue related to angiogenesis in non-small cell lung cancer. PLoS One 7(1):e29671. doi:10.1371/journal.pone.0029671
204. Slaby O, Redova M, Poprach A, Nekvindova J, Iliev R, Radova L, Lakomy R, Svoboda M, Vyzula R (2012) Identification of MicroRNAs associated with early relapse after nephrectomy in renal cell carcinoma patients. Genes Chromosomes Cancer 51(7):707–716. doi:10.1002/gcc.21957
205. Saito Y, Friedman JM, Chihara Y, Egger G, Chuang JC, Liang G (2009) Epigenetic therapy upregulates the tumor suppressor microRNA-126 and its host gene EGFL7 in human cancer cells. Biochem Biophys Res Commun 379(3):726–731. doi:10.1016/j.bbrc.2008.12.098
206. Watanabe K, Emoto N, Hamano E, Sunohara M, Kawakami M, Kage H, Kitano K, Nakajima J, Goto A, Fukayama M, Nagase T, Yatomi Y, Ohishi N, Takai D (2012) Genome structure-based screening identified epigenetically silenced microRNA associated with invasiveness in non-small-cell lung cancer. Int J Cancer 130(11):2580–2590. doi:10.1002/ijc.26254
207. Otsubo T, Akiyama Y, Hashimoto Y, Shimada S, Goto K, Yuasa Y (2011) MicroRNA-126 inhibits SOX2 expression and contributes to gastric carcinogenesis. PLoS One 6(1):e16617. doi:10.1371/journal.pone.0016617
208. Watahiki A, Wang Y, Morris J, Dennis K, O'Dwyer HM, Gleave M, Gout PW, Wang Y (2011) MicroRNAs associated with metastatic prostate cancer. PLoS One 6(9):e24950. doi:10.1371/journal.pone.0024950
209. Sasahira T, Kurihara M, Bhawal UK, Ueda N, Shimomoto T, Yamamoto K, Kirita T, Kuniyasu H (2012) Downregulation of miR-126 induces angiogenesis and lymphangiogenesis by activation of VEGF-A in oral cancer. Br J Cancer 107(4):700–706. doi:10.1038/bjc.2012.330
210. Uchida D, Kuribayashi N, Kinouchi M, Ohe G, Tamatani T, Nagai H, Miyamoto Y (2013) Expression and function of CXCR4 in human salivary gland cancers. Clin Exp Metastasis 30(2):133–142. doi:10.1007/s10585-012-9518-9
211. Shintani S, Funayama T, Yoshihama Y, Alcalde RE, Ootsuki K, Terakado N, Matsumura T (1995) Expression of c-erbB family gene products in adenoid cystic carcinoma of salivary glands: an immunohistochemical study. Anticancer Res 15(6B):2623–2626
212. Franchi A, Gallo O, Bocciolini C, Franchi L, Paglierani M, Santucci M (1999) Reduced E-cadherin expression correlates with unfavorable prognosis in adenoid cystic carcinoma of salivary glands of the oral cavity. Am J Clin Pathol 111(1):43–50
213. Takata T, Kudo Y, Zhao M, Ogawa I, Miyauchi M, Sato S, Cheng J, Nikai H (1999) Reduced expression of p27(Kip1) protein in relation to salivary adenoid cystic carcinoma metastasis. Cancer 86(6):928–935
214. Anzick SL, Chen WD, Park Y, Meltzer P, Bell D, El-Naggar AK, Kaye FJ (2010) Unfavorable prognosis of CRTC1-MAML2 positive mucoepidermoid tumors with CDKN2A deletions. Genes Chromosomes Cancer 49(1):59–69. doi:10.1002/gcc.20719
215. Kamarainen M, Heiskala K, Knuutila S, Heiskala M, Winqvist O, Andersson LC (2003) RELP, a novel human REG-like protein with up-regulated expression in inflammatory and metaplastic gastrointestinal mucosa. Am J Pathol 163(1):11–20. doi:10.1016/s0002-9440(10)63625-5
216. Oue N, Mitani Y, Aung PP, Sakakura C, Takeshima Y, Kaneko M, Noguchi T, Nakayama H, Yasui W (2005) Expression and localization of Reg IV in human neoplastic and non-neoplastic tissues: Reg IV expression is associated with intestinal and neuroendocrine differentiation in gastric adenocarcinoma. J Pathol 207(2):185–198. doi:10.1002/path.1827
217. Oue N, Kuniyasu H, Noguchi T, Sentani K, Ito M, Tanaka S, Setoyama T, Sakakura C, Natsugoe S, Yasui W (2007) Serum concentration of Reg IV in patients with colorectal cancer: overexpression and high serum levels of Reg IV are associated with liver metastasis. Oncology 72(5–6):371–380. doi:10.1159/000113147
218. Takehara A, Eguchi H, Ohigashi H, Ishikawa O, Kasugai T, Hosokawa M, Katagiri T, Nakamura Y, Nakagawa H (2006) Novel tumor marker REG4 detected in serum of patients with resectable pancreatic cancer and feasibility for antibody therapy targeting REG4. Cancer Sci 97(11):1191–1197. doi:10.1111/j.1349-7006.2006.00297.x
219. Ohara S, Oue N, Matsubara A, Mita K, Hasegawa Y, Hayashi T, Usui T, Amatya VJ, Takeshima Y, Kuniyasu H, Yasui W (2008) Reg IV is an independent prognostic factor for relapse in patients with clinically localized prostate cancer. Cancer Sci 99(8):1570–1577. doi:10.1111/j.1349-7006.2008.00846.x
220. Kuniyasu H, Oue N, Sasahira T, Yi L, Moriwaka Y, Shimomoto T, Fujii K, Ohmori H, Yasui W (2009) Reg IV enhances peritoneal metastasis in gastric carcinomas. Cell Prolif 42(1):110–121. doi:10.1111/j.1365-2184.2008.00577.x

221. Sasahira T, Oue N, Kirita T, Luo Y, Bhawal UK, Fujii K, Yasui W, Kuniyasu H (2008) Reg IV expression is associated with cell growth and prognosis of adenoid cystic carcinoma in the salivary gland. Histopathology 53(6):667–675. doi:10.1111/j.1365-2559.2008.03188.x
222. Lee CW, Ito K, Ito Y (2010) Role of RUNX3 in bone morphogenetic protein signaling in colorectal cancer. Cancer Res 70(10):4243–4252. doi:10.1158/0008-5472.can-09-3805
223. Chuang LS, Ito Y (2010) RUNX3 is multifunctional in carcinogenesis of multiple solid tumors. Oncogene 29(18):2605–2615. doi:10.1038/onc.2010.88
224. Ito K, Liu Q, Salto-Tellez M, Yano T, Tada K, Ida H, Huang C, Shah N, Inoue M, Rajnakova A, Hiong KC, Peh BK, Han HC, Ito T, Teh M, Yeoh KG, Ito Y (2005) RUNX3, a novel tumor suppressor, is frequently inactivated in gastric cancer by protein mislocalization. Cancer Res 65(17):7743–7750. doi:10.1158/0008-5472.can-05-0743
225. Sasahira T, Kurihara M, Yamamoto K, Bhawal UK, Kirita T, Kuniyasu H (2011) Downregulation of runt-related transcription factor 3 associated with poor prognosis of adenoid cystic and mucoepidermoid carcinomas of the salivary gland. Cancer Sci 102(2):492–497. doi:10.1111/j.1349-7006.2010.01787.x

Oral Potentially Malignant Disorders

4

Teruo Amagasa

Abstract

At a World Health Organization workshop held in 2005, the term "oral potentially malignant disorders" (OPMDs) was recommended instead of "premalignant lesions and conditions." This chapter describes two OPMDs, namely, oral leukoplakia and erythroplakia. Oral leukoplakia is a newly defined entity of white plaques of questionable risk after excluding (other) known diseases or disorders carrying no increased risk for cancer. The clinical findings of patients with leukoplakia may depend on the oral habits of tobacco chewing and smoking. The risk factors for the development of oral squamous cell carcinoma (OSCC) in patients with leukoplakia are female sex, age >50 years, large lesions, tongue or floor of mouth, the buccal mucosa in association with tobacco habits, non-homogeneous and epithelial dysplasia. Surgery has been recommended for leukoplakia by some researchers, though some reviewers have voiced their concerns over a lack of evidence for surgery. The author proposes that oral leukoplakia should be surgically removed with sufficient margin using iodine staining and that patients having leukoplakias with or without epithelial dysplasia should be followed up at regular intervals with or without surgery in order to detect recurrent or new lesions in the initial stage. Erythroplakia is a rare OPMD in which the soft palate, floor of mouth, and buccal mucosa are commonly affected, but the tongue and any other site of the oral cavity can also be affected. As erythroplakia has the highest malignant potential of the OPMDs, surgery is recommended for its treatment, and regular follow-up is important for decreasing the development of OSCC from erythroplakia.

Keywords

Epithelial dysplasia • Erythroplakia • Leukoplakia • Malignant transformation • Oral potentially malignant disorders • Premalignant lesion

4.1 Introduction

A working group of the World Health Organization (WHO) held in 1973 later proposed in 1978 that clinical presentations of the oral cavity recognized as precancerous should be classified into two broad groups: precancerous lesions and precancerous conditions [1, 2]. A precancerous lesion is defined as "morphologically altered tissue in which oral cancer is more likely to occur than in its apparently normal counterpart" and includes leukoplakia, erythroplakia, and palatal lesions in reverse smokers. A precancerous condition is defined as "a generalized state associated with a significantly increased risk of cancer."

In 1984, the first international conference on oral leukoplakia was held in Malmo, Sweden [3], and in 1994, an international symposium on oral leukoplakia was held in Uppsala, Sweden [4, 5]. The wording of the definitions of leukoplakia

T. Amagasa (✉)
Tokyo Medical and Dental University, Tokyo, Japan

Department of Dentistry and Oral Surgery, Hidaka Hospital, Takasaki, Japan
e-mail: tamagasa@mopera.net

T. Kirita and K. Omura (eds.), *Oral Cancer: Diagnosis and Therapy*, DOI 10.1007/978-4-431-54938-3_4, and erythroplakia was slightly changed, but the terms "precancerous lesion" and "precancerous condition" remained unchanged at these meetings. In the past three decades, many studies have been conducted on premalignant lesions and conditions.

At a WHO workshop held in 2005, the terminology, definitions, and classification of oral lesions with a predisposition for malignant transformation were discussed [6], and the term "potentially malignant" was preferred over "premalignant" or "precancerous." Furthermore, it was recommended to abandon the traditional distinction between potentially malignant lesions and potentially malignant conditions and instead to use the term "potentially malignant disorders" (PMDs) [6].

In this chapter, the term PMDs is discussed, and the clinical and histopathological findings and malignant transformation of PMDs are described with a focus on leukoplakia and erythroplakia.

4.2 Terminology and Concept of Potentially Malignant Disorders

At the WHO workshop held in 2005, the working group discussed the concept of "precancerous" based on the following findings [6]:

1. In longitudinal studies, areas of tissue with certain alterations in clinical appearance identified at the first assessment as "precancerous" were found during follow-up to have undergone malignant transformation.
2. Some of these alterations, particularly red and white patches, were observed to coexist at the margins of overt oral squamous cell carcinoma (OSCC).
3. A proportion of these lesions may share the morphological and cytological changes observed in epithelial malignancies, but without frank invasion.
4. Some of the chromosomal, genomic, and molecular alterations found in clearly invasive oral cancers were detected in these presumptive "precancerous" or "premalignant" phases.

When the terms "precancerous lesion" and "precancerous condition" were used at first, the origin of an oral malignancy in a patient with a precancerous lesion was considered to correspond the site of the lesion. On the other hand, in precancerous conditions, cancer may arise in any anatomical site of the mouth or pharynx (Table 4.1) [2]. It is now known

Table 4.1 Classification of precancerous lesions and conditions [1]

Precancerous lesions	Precancerous conditions
Leukoplakia	Submucous fibrosis
Erythroplakia	Actinic keratosis
Palatal lesions in reverse smokers	Lichen planus
	Discoid lupus erythematosus

Table 4.2 Potentially malignant disorders revised from the literatures [6, 9]

Potentially malignant disorders	
Leukoplakia	Oral submucous fibrosis
Erythroplakia	Lichen planus
Palatal lesions in reverse smokers	Actinic keratosis
	Discoid lupus erythematosus
	Hereditary or some disorders with increased risk[a]

[a]Including xeroderma pigmentosum, epidermolysis bullosa, etc.

even in cases where the mucosa has a clinically "normal" appearance in a patient with a precancerous lesion that dysplasia may exist at the contralateral anatomic site [7] or that molecular aberrations may be present in other oral mucosal sites, suggestive of a pathway to malignant transformation, and that cancer could subsequently arise in apparently normal tissue [8]. The current working group, therefore, did not favor subdividing "precancerous" into lesions and conditions, and the consensus was to refer to all clinical presentations carrying a risk of cancer as PMDs to reflect their widespread anatomical distribution [6]. The PMDs adopted by the working group are listed in Table 4.2 [6, 9].

4.3 Leukoplakia

4.3.1 Criteria and Diagnosis

4.3.1.1 Definition

In the 1978 report on the meeting for establishing the histological definition of precancerous lesions, oral leukoplakia was defined as "a white patch or plaque that cannot be characterized clinically or pathologically as any other disease" [2]. In 1984, the first international conference on oral leukoplakia was held in Malmo Sweden [3], where leukoplakia was defined as "a white patch or plaque that cannot be characterized clinically or pathologically as any other disease and is not associated with any physical or chemical causative agent except the use of tobacco" [3]. In 1994, an international symposium was held in Uppsala, Sweden, and leukoplakia was defined as "a predominantly white lesion of the oral mucosa that cannot be characterized as any other definable diseases (lesions)" [4, 5]. At a WHO workshop held in 2005, it was decided to use the term "leukoplakia" for "white plaques of questionable risk after excluding (other) known diseases or disorders carrying no increased risk for cancer" [6].

4.3.1.2 Diagnosis

The current working group recommended the use of a three-step flowchart for the diagnosis of oral leukoplakia (Fig. 4.1) [6]. According to the flowchart, in the presence of possible etiological factors, including tobacco habits, the patient

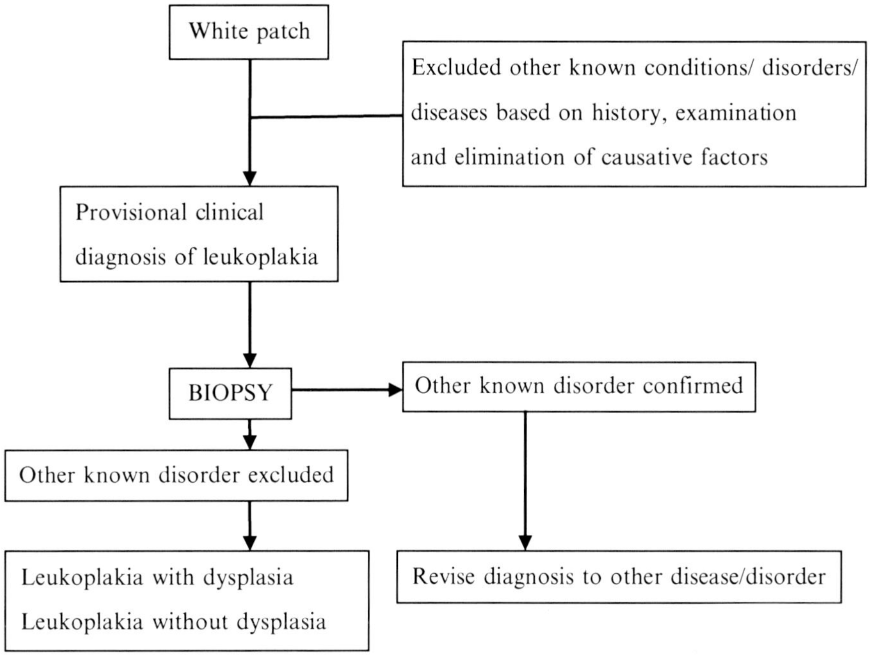

Fig. 4.1 Schematic representation of the steps in diagnosis of oral leukoplakia [6]

should be observed after not more than a somewhat arbitrarily chosen 2–4 weeks, which seems an acceptable period for observing possible regression after eliminating such factors. However, most leukoplakic lesions do not usually regress in such a short period, especially in smokers. Examples of white or predominantly white diseases of the oral mucosa carrying no increased risk for cancer development are listed in Table 4.3 [9].

van der Waal [9] proposed that the term leukoplakia can be used at different levels of certainty (C-factor) as a clinical term (C1, diagnosed from a single visit, or C2, diagnosed by a negative results of elimination of etiologic factors) or a clinicopathological term (C3, confirmed pathologically on incisional biopsy, or C4, confirmed pathologically in a resected specimen) [9]. Amagasa et al. recommended biopsy for the accurate diagnosis of leukoplakia, especially for investigating the malignant transformation of leukoplakia, which is in agreement with other studies on the malignant transformation of leukoplakia [10].

4.3.2 Clinical Aspects

4.3.2.1 Sex

With regard to the sex of patients with leukoplakia, many studies have reported a predominance of oral leukoplakia in men [11–24], with an extreme predominance in men in India and other countries where tobacco chewing and/or smoking habits are prevalent [19, 25–27]. On the contrary, some studies have reported an equal male-to-female ratio or a slight female predominance in the United States, other Western countries, and Japan [28–31].

4.3.2.2 Age

With regard to the age of patients with leukoplakia, a majority of patients in developed countries (United States, Europe, and Japan) were in their 40s–60s [10, 12, 27, 29, 32], whereas patients in India and other Asian countries with tobacco habits were younger [19, 25, 26, 33].

4.3.2.3 Site

With regard to the site of oral leukoplakia, many studies have reported the buccal mucosa as a common site [12, 13, 16, 24, 25, 30]. In India and other countries with tobacco chewing and/or smoking habits, the vast majority of leukoplakia cases were located on the buccal mucosa and labial commissure, with a few on the tongue or floor of mouth [20, 26, 27]. In Japan, however, the lower gum/alveolar ridge and the tongue were the most frequent sites followed by the buccal mucosa and upper gum/alveolar ridge [10], which is partially in agreement with other studies conducted in Japan [31, 34]. In the Netherlands, the tongue and floor of mouth were reported as the most frequently affected sites [29]. The sites commonly affected by oral leukoplakia may be the result of oral habits, especially tobacco smoking and/or various unknown causes.

4.3.2.4 Clinical Features and Types

Pindborg et al. [35] described in 1963 that speckled leukoplakia is often associated with epithelial dysplasia and carcinoma, and other researchers have reported their clinical types of oral leukoplakia with epithelial dysplasia and malignant transformation [12, 20, 29, 36]. In 1978, leukoplakia was divided into two main types: homogeneous and nonhomogeneous [2]. Homogeneous leukoplakia was subclassified into flat, corrugated, wrinkled, and pumice-like, while

Table 4.3 The most common white or predominantly white benign diseases of the oral mucosa and their main diagnostic criteria [9]

Lesion	Main diagnostic criteria
Aspirin burn	History of local application of aspirin tablets
Candidiasis, pseudomembranous	Clinical aspect (pseudomembranes, often of symmetrical pattern)
Candidiasis, hyperplastica[a]	
Frictional lesion	Presence of mechanical irritation (e.g., habit of vigorous toothbrushing)
Hairy leukoplakia	Clinical aspect (incl. bilateral localization on the tongue); histopathology (incl. EBV)
Leukoedema	Clinical aspect (incl. symmetrical pattern)
Linea alba	Clinical aspect (incl. location on the line of occlusion in the cheek mucosa)
Lupus erythematosus	History of skin lesions; clinical appearance (incl. bilateral pattern); histopathology
Morsicatio (habitual chewing or biting of the cheek, tongue, lips)	History of habitual chewing or biting; clinical aspects
Papilloma and allied lesions	Clinical aspect; histopathology
Syphilis, secondary ("mucous patches")	Clinical aspect: histopathology
	T. pallidum; serology
Tobacco-induced lesions[b]	
Smoker's palate (nicotinic stomatitis)	Clinical aspect; history of smoking
Snuff induced lesion	Clinical aspect; site were snuff is placed
White sponge nevus	Family history; clinical aspect (often symmetrical pattern)

[a]There is no consensus in the literature as whether to recognize a hyperplastic subtype of oral candidiasis: some prefer to these lesions as *Candida-associated* leukoplakia

[b]Palatal lesions in reverse smokers are considered potential malignant disorders

Table 4.4 Classification of oral leukoplakia [5]

Homogeneous	Nonhomogeneous
Flat	Verrucous
Corrugated	Nodular
Wrinkled	Ulcerated
Pumice-like	Erythroleukoplakia

non-homogeneous leukoplakia was subclassified into verrucous, nodular, ulcerated, and erythroleukoplakia (Table 4.4); these classifications were recognized by the WHO in 1994 [4, 5].

At a WHO workshop held in 2005, the working group noted that nonhomogeneous varieties include speckled, nodular, and verrucous types; however, the working group consensus was that broadly dividing leukoplakia into homogeneous or non-homogeneous categories was imprecise and of limited value. Nevertheless, patients with mixed white and red plaques should be recognized as having a higher risk status, and such cases should be denoted as "erythroleukoplakia" [6]. Proliferative verrucous leukoplakia (PVL), which was reported in 1984 by Hansen et al. [37], was also recognized at the workshop. This form of leukoplakia is characterized by multiple, simultaneous leukoplakias as the disease is visibly multifocal and frequently presents across a wide area of the oral mucosa with most patients developing OSCC over long follow-up periods [37, 38]. Unfortunately, this type of leukoplakia cannot be determined in the initial stage and is diagnosed during or after its course.

4.3.3 Histopathological Aspects

4.3.3.1 Epithelial Dysplasia

It is largely accepted worldwide that a general disturbance of the epithelium is designated as "dysplasia" and that the potential for developing invasive carcinoma increases with the severity of dysplasia [5, 39]. Epithelial dysplasia is conventionally classified into mild, moderate, and severe including carcinoma in situ (CIS). Many reports have attempted to show a typical sample for each degree of epithelial dysplasia [5, 39, 40]. However, the degree of epithelial dysplasia is difficult to diagnose and several studies have reported great interexaminer and intraexaminer variability when assessing the presence or absence, as well as the grade, of oral epithelial dysplasia [41–43]. To increase the likelihood of agreement between oral pathologists by reducing the number of choices, a two-tier classification system (no/questionable/mild denoting low risk and moderate/severe denoting high risk) was considered at the 2005 Oral Cancer and Precancer Workshop coordinated by the WHO, with samples of each of the three grades of epithelial dysplasia [44].

The book *World Health Organization Classification of Tumours* (2005) recommended using the new concept of "epithelial precursor lesions," which were previously termed "premalignant lesions," and the terms "squamous intraepithelial neoplasia" and "squamous intraepithelial lesions" according to the Ljubljana Classification instead of "epithelial dysplasia" [45]. Although this classification was reported to be useful for predicting the malignant transformation of

Table 4.5 Clinical classification of oral leukoplakia [10]

Type I	Flat, white patch/plaque without red components
Type II	Flat, white patch/plaque with erosion or red components
Type III	Slightly raised or elevated white patch/plaque
Type IV	Markedly raised or elevated white patch/plaque

the hypopharynx and larynx [45–49], the WHO consensus group did not favor its use for oral mucosal lesions [44]. In addition, the current working group [6] did not actively accept the term "epithelial precursor lesions", but adopted the new term "potentially malignant disorders."

CIS of the oral mucosa is defined in the WHO classification as histologic changes involving the full thickness or almost the full thickness of squamous epithelium showing cellular features of carcinoma without stromal invasion [5, 39, 40, 50] and is in agreement with the definition proposed by the current working group [44]. Typically, most CIS of the upper aero digestive tract are nonkeratinizing, although keratinizing CIS can be encountered in the vocal cords or oral cavity [51]. Lesions with similar histological figures in the esophagus are considered to be squamous cell CIS (noninvasive squamous cell carcinoma) by Japanese pathologists and high-grade intraepithelial neoplasia by Western pathologists [52]. Izumo [53] in his review article noted that CIS of the oral mucosa show superficial maturation and differentiation. Some recent clinicopathological examinations in Japan have also revealed several variations of CIS of the oral mucosa [54] that are not included in the WHO classification [44, 45]. In the future, the suitability of the CIS criteria proposed by Japanese oral pathologists will be evaluated.

In relation between the clinical classification and epithelial dysplasia, Sugár and Bánóczy [55] reported in their three-tiered clinical classification in 1969 that leukoplakia erosiva and leukoplakia verrucosa were more often associated than leukoplakia simplex with epithelial dysplasia. In 1977, Amagasa et al. [56] developed a clinical classification system for oral leukoplakia based on lesions with or without elevation and with or without red components that was further developed in 2006 [10]. In this system, oral leukoplakia was classified into four clinical types: type I, a flat white patch or plaque without red components; type II, a flat white patch or plaque with red components; type III, a slightly raised or elevated white plaque; and type IV, a markedly raised or elevated white plaque (Table 4.5, Fig. 4.2a–d). With regard to epithelial dysplasia (Fig. 4.3a–c) in our classification system, type II leukoplakia was found to be significantly associated with epithelial dysplasia (Table 4.6) [10].

4.3.3.2 Diagnosis of Epithelial Dysplasia with a Colorimeter and Iodine Staining

Biopsy or a surgical procedure should always be performed for the diagnosis of epithelial dysplasia. However, diagnosis of this disease by a noninvasive procedure is desirable. The efficacy of vital iodine staining for the diagnosis of cancer or dysplasia has been reported in some papers [57–60]. In particular, Maeda et al. attempted to use a colorimeter after iodine staining to clarify the relationship between lesion color (i.e., the color of the unstained lesion) and histopathological findings after staining (Fig. 4.4a, b) [61] and found a significant color difference between lesions with moderate to severe dysplasia and those with mild to no epithelial dysplasia. Colorimetry with iodine staining for premalignant lesions may be useful for distinguishing moderate to severe dysplasia from mild to no dysplasia before biopsy. However, this combination method for PMD lesions is only suitable in the two-tier pathological classification system proposed by the working group.

Maeda et al. also measured the deviation of the macroscopic and histopathological boundary of oral leukoplakia after iodine staining. The histopathological boundary of the lesions with epithelial dysplasia was at most 4.36 mm beyond the macroscopic boundary, suggesting that PMDs should be surgically removed with a safety margin >5 mm after iodine staining [62].

4.3.4 Prognosis and Development of Oral Squamous Cell Carcinoma

4.3.4.1 Prognosis

Development of OSCC in patients with oral leukoplakia is a serious problem; however, knowing the natural history of oral leukoplakia is also important for both aggressive and conservative treatment of oral leukoplakia (Fig. 4.5a–e). Mehta et al. reported that 42.5 % of untreated leukoplakias disappeared within 5 years and 45.3 % within 10 years in persons who chewed tobacco, whereas 41.5 % of untreated lesions remained unchanged in 5 years and 31.6 % in 10 years in smokers in India [20]. During follow-up of patients in India, approximately 30–40 % of oral leukoplakias had decreased in size or disappeared, 30–60 % remained unchanged, and 11 % had increased in size [18–20], and regression was more frequently observed in tobacco chewers and pipe smokers than in those who smoked cigarettes [63].

On the other hand, during follow-up periods of 1–10 years for 248 patients with leukoplakia in Denmark, lesions disappeared in 43 (20.1 %), decreased in size in 38 (17.8 %), and increased in size in 7 (3.3 %) [36]. Silverman reported that lesions in patients in the United States decreased or disappeared in 49 of 133 current smokers (37 %), in 22 of 50 past smokers (44 %), and in only 2 of 74 nonsmokers (3 %) [28]. Including the above reports, approximately 20–37 % of lesions completely disappeared after eliminating the causative factors, including a reduction in tobacco consumption or abstinence; 20–50 % or more decreased in size; and only 10 % or less increased in size in developed countries [28, 64, 65]. However, similar decreases in the number or size of oral leukoplakias were not observed in Japan during follow-up [10, 11].

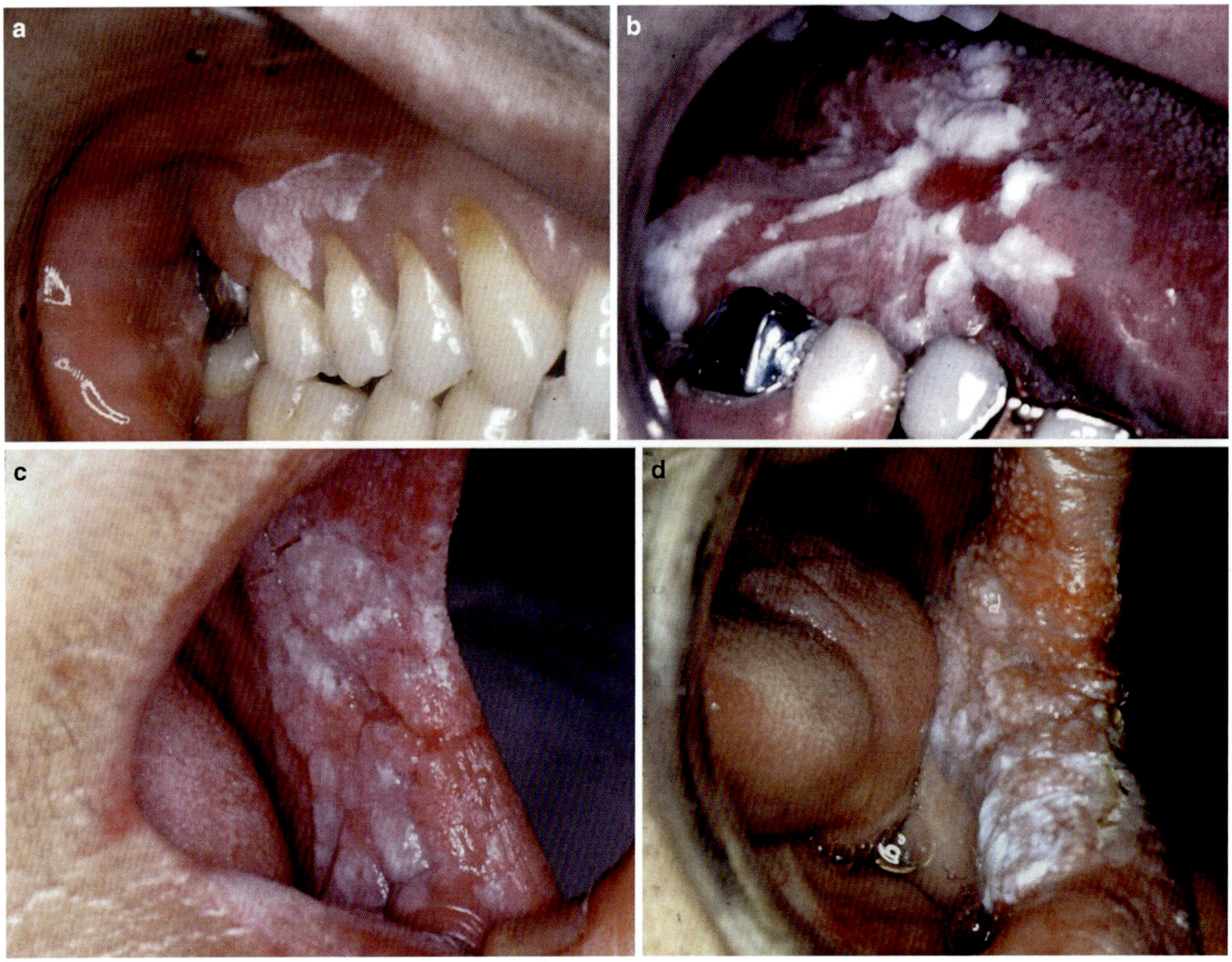

Fig. 4.2 Clinical features of leukoplakia can be classified into four types: type I (**a**) flat white patch on the of the maxillary gingival, type II (**b**) white patch and plaque with erosion on the tongue, type III (**c**) slightly elevated white plaque on the buccal mucosa, and type IV (**d**) markedly elevated white plaque with partly granular appearance on the buccal mucosa [10]

4.3.4.2 Development of Oral Squamous Cell Carcinoma

Malignant Transformation Rate and Cumulative Malignant Transformation Rate

Many studies have reported so-called malignant transformation rates of oral leukoplakia ranging from 0.13 to 17.5 % (Table 4.7) [10, 12, 18–22, 28, 29, 32, 36, 66–68]. Among these reports, a community-based survey in India revealed a malignant transformation rate of oral leukoplakia of 0.13–2.2 %. However, the rate of oral leukoplakia derived from studies of hospital-based samples was 3.6–17.5 %, showing a higher incidence of malignant transformation than in India. The rate of malignant transformation may increase when patients are followed over a longer term and may decrease when patients are lost early to follow up. The resulting rate of malignant transformation may therefore be unreliable. To eliminate this bias, calculation of the cumulative survival rate is necessary to determine the cumulative malignant transformation rate. The cumulative transformation rates reported by some researchers are shown in Table 4.8; the 5-year cumulative malignant transformation rate ranged from 1.2 to 14.5 % [29, 31, 32, 34, 69, 70].

4.3.4.3 Sex and Malignant Transformation

With regard to the relationship between sex and malignant transformation, of 331 patients with leukoplakia in Denmark, 5.8 % of women developed OSCC in contrast to 2.1 % of men (2.8-fold higher in women) [66]. In the United States, an equal sex ratio was found for leukoplakia (125 men vs. 132 women) with slightly more women having cancer (26 women vs. 19 men). Therefore, the rate of malignant change in women was 1.3-fold higher than in men [28]. In Japan, of 444 patients with oral leukoplakia, 17 of 275 men (6.2 %) and 18 of 169 women (10.7 %) developed OSSC (1.7-fold higher in women) [10]. Reports on the malignant transformation of oral leukoplakia in developed countries showed relatively more frequent development of OSCC from leukoplakia in women than in men [18, 66].

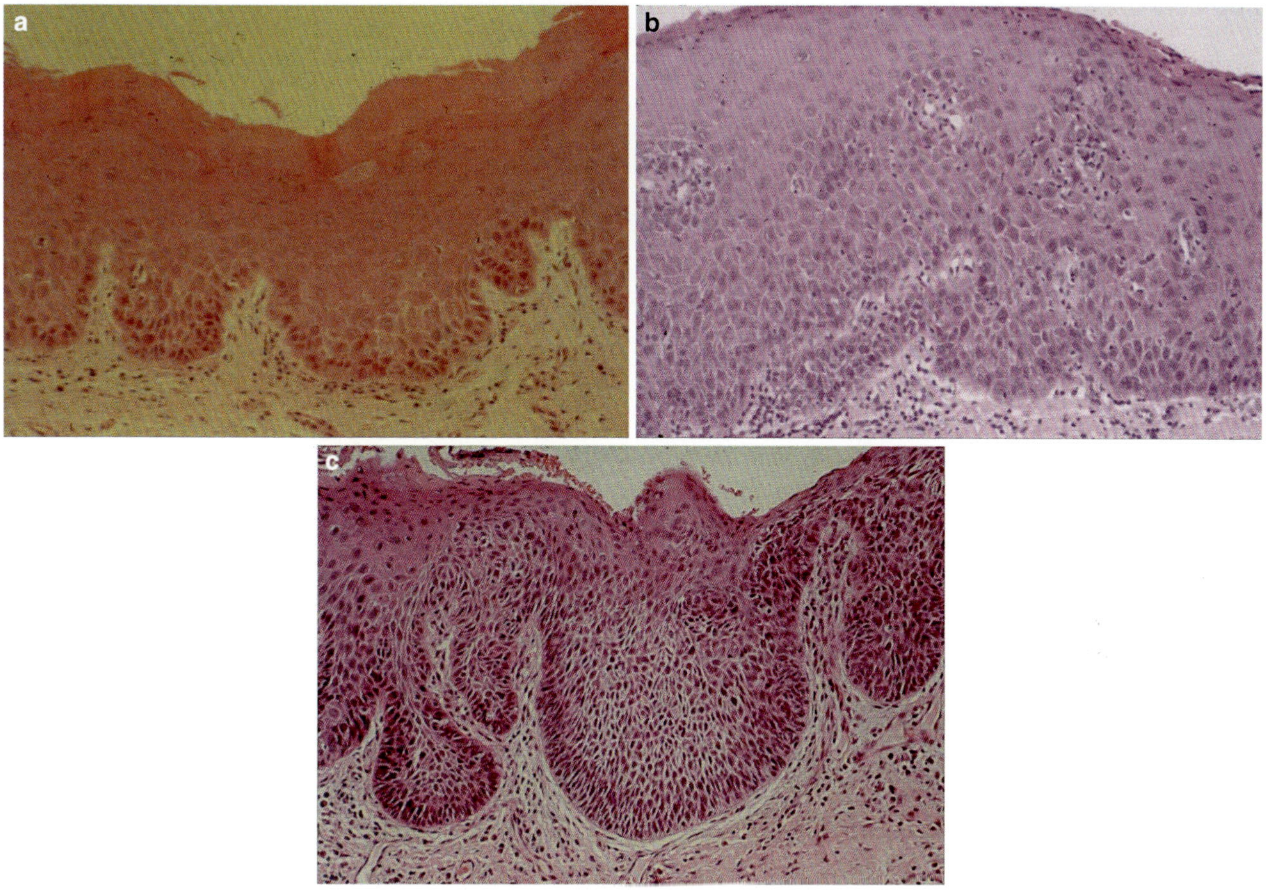

Fig. 4.3 Histopathological features of leukoplakia (**a**) Mild dysplasia: slightly irregular epithelial architecture limited to the lower third of the epithelium. Basal–parabasal cells show hyperchromatic large nuclei and loss of polarity. (**b**) Moderate dysplasia: hyperplastic epithelium with increased number of polymorphic cells extends up to two-thirds of the epithelium, and cellular atypia is more pronounced with nuclear pleomorphism. (**c**) Severe dysplasia: the atypical basal-like and spinous-like cells occupy almost all epithelial layers. Squamous epithelium is of variable thickness with drop-shaped rete ridges and prominent cytologic atypia [10]

Table 4.6 Incidence of epithelial dysplasia in each clinical type of oral leukoplakia [10]

Type	Cases	No dysplasia	Dysplasia			Total number of dysplasia (%)
			Mild	Moderate	Severe	
I	328	203	86	30	9	125 (38.1)*
II	71	13	31	16	11	58 (81.7)*
III	24	11	10	2	1	13 (54.2)*
IV	21	7	11	1	2	14 (66.7)*
Total (%)	444	234 (52.7)	138 (31.1)	49 (11.0)	23 (5.2)	210 (47.3)

*Statistically difference ($p<0.01$) between type II and type I, $p<0.05$ between type I and types II, III, and IV

Lind [68] reported that women were more likely to undergo malignant transformation than men and that epithelial dysplasia was more prevalent in women. This was further supported by the findings of other authors [12, 21, 31, 36]. The following risk factors for malignant transformation were listed by Schepman et al. [29]: female sex, absence of smoking habits in women ($p<0.05$), and nonhomogeneous clinical aspects ($p<0.01$).

However, other studies revealed greater malignant transformation potential in men in India, particularly in association with tobacco chewing and smoking [18–20]. These differences in the common site for developing OSCC may be the result of causative agents or oral habits, especially tobacco chewing and/or smoking.

4.3.4.4 Age and Malignant Transformation

Over a 30-year research period, Bánóczy [12] in Hungary identified a higher prevalence of leukoplakia in 50- to 60-year-old subjects, but found the highest risk of malignant transformation in 60- to 70-year-old subjects. Some studies

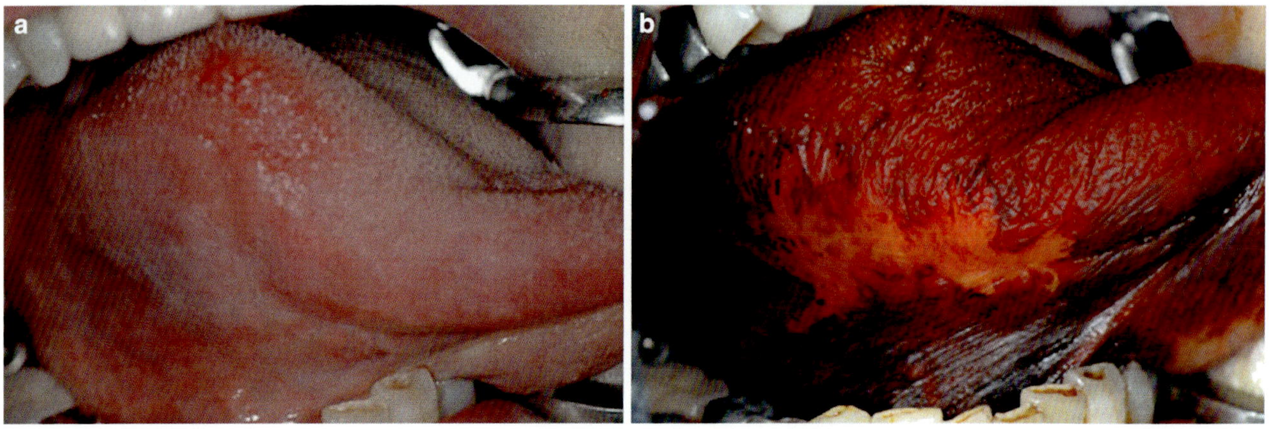

Fig. 4.4 Leukoplakia on the lateral border of tongue, showing dull border before 3 % iodine staining (**a**) and showing a clear border after staining (**b**) [87]

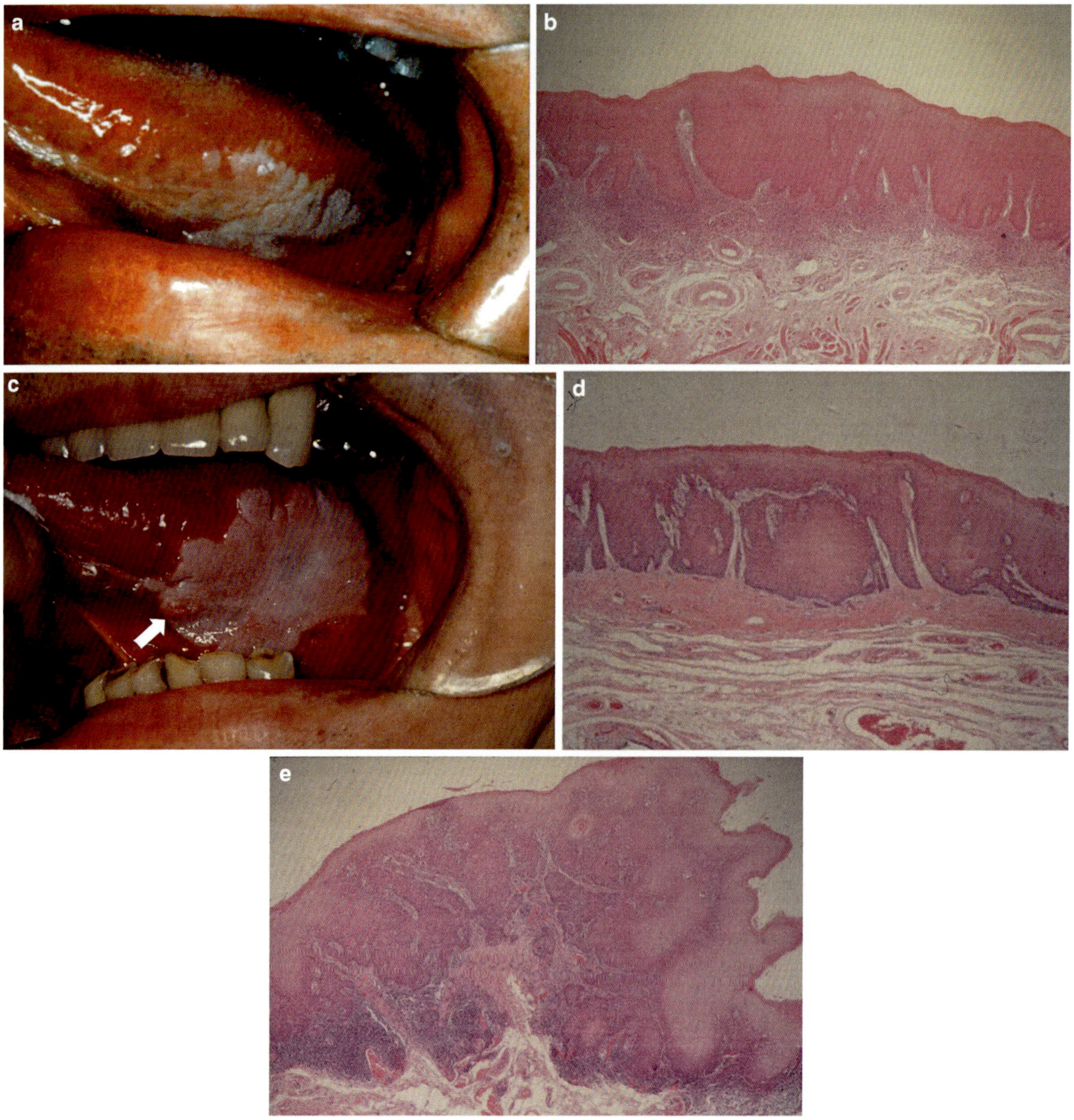

Fig. 4.5 Leukoplakia on the tongue showing a flat white plaque (**a**) and a biopsy specimen of the leukoplakia showing hyperplasia with moderate epithelial dysplasia (**b**). Seven years later without any treatment, a small-red-exophytic growth developed at the white plaque (↑) (**c**), a resected material specimen showing sever epithelial dysplasia (**d**) with early invasive squamous carcinoma (**e**) [87]

Table 4.7 Malignant transformation rates of oral leukoplakia [10]

Authors [references]	Country	Year	Number of patients	Malignant transformation (%)	Observation periods (mean) years
Silverman et al. [18]	India	1976	4,762	0.13	2
Gupta et al. [19]	India	1980	360	0.3	1–10 (7)
Mehta et al. [20]	India	1972	117	0.8	10
Gupta et al. [19]	India	1980	410	2.2	1–10 (8)
Roed-Peterson et al. [66]	Denmark	1971	331	3.6	1≦(4.3)
Einhorn et al. [32]	Sweden	1967	782	4.0	1–20
Pindborg et al. [36]	Denmark	1968	248	4.4	1–9
Kramer et al. [67]	England	1969	187	4.8	1–16
Silverman et al. [21]	USA	1968	117	6.0	1–11
Banocy et al. [12]	Hungary	1977	670	6.0	1–30
Amagasa et al. [10]	Japan	2006	444	7.9	1–29
Lind [68]	Norway	1987	157	8.9	6≦
Gangadharan et al. [22]	India	1971	626	10.0	1–19
Schepman et al. [29]	Holland	1998	166	12.0	6 months–17 (2.7)
Silverman et al. [28]	USA	1984	257	17.5	6 months–39 (7.2)

Table 4.8 Cummulative malignant transformation rates of oral leukoplakia [10]

Authors (year)	Country	Number of patients	5-year (%)	10-year (%)	Follow-up period (mean)
Einhorn et al. [32]	USA	782	1.6	2.4	1–20 years
Amagasa et al. [69]	Japan	169	12.0	21.0	1–20 years
Inoue et al. [70]	Japan	75	4.5	9.7	7 months–26 years (12 years 8 months)
Kirita et al. [31]	Japan	102	1.2	6.6	7 months–12 years 1 months (6 years 2 months)
Schepman et al. [29]	Netherlands	166	14.5	29.0	6 months–16 years 9 months [6 years 2 months]
Kawabe et al. [34]	Japan	237	4.7	11.1	(56.5 ± 43.4 months) [median]

have reported that older patients have a higher malignant transformation rate of leukoplakia than younger patients [29, 32, 64]. Furthermore, a study in Japan revealed a statistically significant difference in the malignant transformation rate between ≥50-year-old subjects and <50-year-old subjects (Table 4.9) [10], supporting the findings of Chiesa et al. [71] with statistical significance. The relationship between the higher malignant transformation rate and older patients may suggest that patients with longer exposure to oral leukoplakia are more prone to malignant transformation [10].

4.3.4.5 Site and Malignant Transformation

Knowing the common site of leukoplakia with developing OSSC is important for investigating the causes and selecting an appropriate therapy. Some authors reported that leukoplakia of the tongue and floor of mouth has a high risk of malignant transformation [66, 72, 73]. In Japan, the malignant transformation rate of oral leukoplakia of the tongue has been reported to be significantly higher than that of the buccal mucosa and other sites [10]. These results are supported by other studies conducted in Japan and in some European countries [12, 31, 34, 66, 70] and are in contrast to those in other reports which identified the buccal mucosa and labial commissure as the areas with the highest malignant transformation rate, particularly in tobacco chewers and smokers in rural India [18–20, 25]. On the other hand, some reports have shown that no oral subsites are associated with a high risk of malignant transformation [29, 74]. These differences might be related to the presence or absence of various oral habits in certain groups or populations.

4.3.4.6 Clinical Type and Malignant Transformation

Pinborg et al. [35] reported that speckled leukoplakia is often associated with epithelial dysplasia and carcinoma, and many reports on the correlation between the clinical type of oral leukoplakia and malignant transformation have since been published [20, 29, 36, 66, 75, 76]. Sugár and Bánóczy [17] reported that leukoplakia erosiva has a higher potential than simplex leukoplakia for malignant transformation. Lind et al. [68] reported that 157 leukoplakias in Norwegians were divided into four groups: homogeneous ($n=60$), verrucous ($n=41$), erosive ($n=28$), and nodular ($n=28$). OSCC developed in only one subject (1.7 %) with homogeneous leukoplakia, in two (4.9 %) with verrucous leukoplakia, in three (10.7 %) with erosive leukoplakia, and in eight (28.6 %) with nodular leukoplakia during the follow-up periods. Nodular leukoplakia had the highest malignant potential

Table 4.9 The incidence of malignant transformation of oral leukoplakia according to sex and age [10]

Age	Male	Female	Total (%)
18–19	0/2	0/0	0/2 (0.0)*
20–29	0/12	1/7	1/19 (5.3)*
30–39	1/24	1/14	2/38 (5.3)*
40–49	1/52	1/34	2/86 (2.3)*
50–59	6/90	6/58	12/148 (8.1)*
60–69	7/62	7/31	14/93 (15.1)*
70–79	1/29	1/23	2/52 (5.8)*
80	1/4	1/2	2/6 (33.0)*
Total (%)	17/275 (6.2)	18/169 (11.2)	35/444 (7.9)

*Statistically significant difference in the malignant transformation rate between ≥50-year-old subjects and <50-year-old subjects ($p<0.05$)

Table 4.10 The incidence of malignant transformation of oral leukoplakias according to epithelial dysplasia [10]

Epithelial dysplasia	Number of cases	Number of malignant transformation (%)
None	234	7 (3.0)*
Mild	138	18 (13.0)*
Moderate	49	7 (14.3)*
Severe	23	3 (13.0)*
Total	444	35 (7.9)

*Statistically significant difference in the malignant transformation rate between with and without epithelial dysplasia ($p<0.05$)

followed by the erosive and the verrucous types. Holmstrup et al. [74] examined 236 patients with leukoplakia and showed via logistic regression analysis a sevenfold increase in the risk of malignant transformation (odds ratio, 7.0) in non-homogeneous leukoplakia compared with homogeneous leukoplakia. Amagasa et al. [10] reported that the malignant transformation rate was the highest in type II lesions (21.4 %), followed by type III (6.9 %) and type IV (6.7 %), and lowest in type I (2.8 %). Statistical differences were noted between type I and type II ($p<0.01$) and between type I and types II, III, and IV (i.e., all non-homogeneous leukoplakias) ($p<0.05$). Despite the fact that various criteria are used to evaluate the clinical types of oral leukoplakia, we concur that leukoplakia with red components and the so-called non-homogeneous leukoplakia, including the verrucous and raised type, carry a high risk of malignant transformation.

4.3.4.7 Epithelial Dysplasia and Malignant Transformation

It is largely accepted that lesions with epithelial dysplasia have higher malignant potential to develop into OSCC than those without. Among the 444 patients with oral leukoplakia reported in Japan, 28 of 210 (13.3 %) with leukoplakia and epithelial dysplasia underwent malignant transformation, while only 7 of 234 (3.0 %) with leukoplakia and no epithelial dysplasia had malignant transformation. A significant difference was observed between the malignant transformation rate of oral leukoplakia with epithelial dysplasia and that without. However, no correlation was evident between the malignant transformation rate and the degree of epithelial dysplasia (Table 4.10) [10] because many leukoplakias with moderate or severe dysplasia were selectively excised. The malignant transformation rates of oral leukoplakia with and without dysplasia reported by several authors are listed in Table 4.11 [10, 16, 28, 77–80]. The malignant transformation rates of oral leukoplakia with epithelia dysplasia were 6.6–36.4 %, whereas those without epithelial dysplasia were 1.0–9.8 %. Several studies have shown that the malignant transformation rate of oral leukoplakia with epithelial dysplasia was significantly higher than that of oral leukoplakia without epithelial dysplasia [28, 80]. Kawabe et al. [34] reported using the Cox proportional hazard model that only the presence of epithelial dysplasia and a past history of oral cancer are significant predictors for the malignant transformation of leukoplakia.

On the contrary, Holmstrup et al. [74] reported that the presence of epithelial dysplasia in oral leukoplakia was not a significant factor for malignant transformation based on logistic regression analysis. They mentioned that this factor may, however, vary in the level of significance due to the subjectivity in diagnosing epithelial dysplasia [41, 42].

4.3.4.8 Epithelial Dysplasia and the Period to Developing Oral Squamous Cell Carcinoma

Some studies have reported patients developing OSCC within 5 years of being diagnosed as having oral leukoplakia [36, 63]. On the other hand, some patients were reported to develop OSCC after 5 years [28, 68]. These reports made no mention of lesions with or without epithelial dysplasia. In our previous study [11], 17 of 35 (48 %) cases developed OSCC >5 years after the initial biopsy of oral leukoplakia, and all of those cases without epithelial dysplasia developed OSCC >5 years after the initial biopsy. The shortest malignant transformation periods (≦ 5 years) were observed for oral leukoplakia with severe epithelia dysplasia, followed by moderate dysplasia, mild dysplasia, and no dysplasia from 5 to 25 years and 6 months (Table 4.12) [10]. These findings suggest a relationship between the severity of epithelial dysplasia and the period of malignant transformation from oral leukoplakia to cancer.

4.3.4.9 Size and Malignant Transformation

Few studies have been conducted on the relationship between the size of leukoplakia lesions and malignant transformation. Among 331 cases of leukoplakia in Denmark followed for more than 1 year, eight of nine leukoplakias that developed into OSCC were larger than the mean size of 5.5 cm^2 [66], similar to the findings of another study [71]. Logistic regression analysis of 236 patients with leukoplakia by Holmstrup et al. [74] revealed that lesions >200 mm^2 showed a 5.4-fold

Table 4.11 Malignant transformation rates of oral leukoplakia with dysplasia [10]

	Number of leukoplakia with epithelial dysplasia		Number of leukoplakia without epithelial dysplasia		Follow-up
References	Number of Cases	Number of malignant transformation (%)	Number of cases	Number of malignant transformation (%)	Period (year)
Mincer et al. [77]	45	5 (11.1)			Up to 8
Banoczy and Csiba [16]	68	9 (13.2)			1–20 (mean 6.3)
Pindborg et al. [78]	61	4 (6.6)			Up to 7
Silverman et al. [28]	22	8 (36.4)	235	23 (9.8)	Mean 8.1
Lumerman et al. [79]	44	7 (16.0)			Up to 6.5
Amagasa et al. [10]	210	28 (13.3)	234	7 (3.0)	1–29
Cowan et al. [80]	165	25 (15.0)	1,182	12 (1.0)	More than 20
Total	615	86 (13.9)	1,647	42 (2.6)	

Table 4.12 Malignant transformation periods of 35 oral leukoplakias according to epithelial dysplasia [10]

Epithelial dysplasia	Period (years) ≦2	≦5	≦7	≦10	10<	Total
None	0	0	1	5	1	7
Mild	4	6	3	2	3	18
Moderate	1	4	2	0	0	7
Severe	1	2	0	0	0	3
Total (%)	6 (17.2)	12 (34.3)	6 (17.1)	7 (20.0)	4 (11.4)	35 (100.0)

Table 4.13 Reported risk factors of statistical significance for malignant transformation of leukoplakia [9]

Female gender
Long duration of leukoplakia
Leukoplakia in nonsmokers (idiopathic leukoplakia)
Leukoplakia on the tongue and/or floor of the mouth
Size ≧200 mm^2
Nonhomogeneous type
Presence of *Candida albicans*
Presence of epithelial dysplasia

increase in the risk of malignant transformation compared with those <200 mm^2. Napier et al. [81] using multivariate survival analysis reported that in 50 patients with leukoplakia from Northern Ireland, neither duration nor clinical appearance was associated with the development of OSCC. The risk of malignant progression was noted to be approximately sixfold higher in patients with large confluent leukoplakia and approximately fourfold higher in patients with leukoplakia affecting a single anatomical site than in those with multiple lesions.

4.3.4.10 Treatment and Malignant Transformation

It is a very important to select an appropriate therapy as not all treatments will reduce the progression of OSCC in patients with oral leukoplakia. To date, the risk of developing cancer from oral leukoplakia has not been significantly reduced by surgical intervention [74, 82, 83]. Moreover, some reviewers have stated that it is unclear whether removal of the lesion decreases malignant transformation of oral leukoplakia because of the lack of randomized controlled trials comparing different treatment modalities [84, 85].

Nevertheless, research conducted by Amagasa et al. [86] showed that the malignant transformation rate of leukoplakia treated by surgery was significantly lower than that without any treatment or without surgery. Therefore, we believe that surgical excision with an adequate safety margin coupled with well-timed follow-up evaluation of oral leukoplakia is effective for preventing the malignant transformation of these lesions [87]. These findings are supported by those of other reports [88, 89]. van der Waal noted in his review article [9] that although no scientific evidence shows that treatment truly prevents future development of OSCC [84], it seems a safe practice to actively treat leukoplakias irrespective of the absence or presence of epithelial dysplasia [90].

Some studies have reported that laser treatment for oral leukoplakia is a useful modality because of the low recurrence and no or rare progression to OSCC [91, 92]. However, a cohort study of 100 patients presenting with new, single oral dysplastic PMD lesions showed that in patients followed for up to 10 years after laser treatment [93], 17 had the same site of recurrence, 14 developed further PMDs at new sites, 5 underwent malignant transformation at the same sites, and 2 developed OSCC at new oral sites. These findings are consistent with those of other studies [71].

Cancer development from oral leukoplakia rarely or occasionally occurs in patients with leukoplakia treated by surgery [74]. We propose that this observation may be associated with the following courses of cancer development after surgery [87]:

Course A: OSCC develops in a short period after surgery because of insufficient surgical margin.

Course B: OSCC develops in a short or relatively long period, even after sufficient surgery for one or more lesions because of obscure or small remaining lesions in cases of multiple leukoplakias.

Course C: OSCC develops from a new lesion over a long period even after sufficient surgery and develops because of the unchanged causative environment of the oral cavity.

With regard to Course A, van der Waal et al. [94] reported that the difficulties in determining a sufficient surgical margin provide a possible explanation for the comparatively high recurrence rate after surgery [71, 81, 95]. Course B has been reported by a number of groups [96, 97].

We would like to propose that the recurrence rate and malignant transformation rate of oral leukoplakia will be reduced if iodine staining of leukoplakia is conducted and if the unstained lesions are removed with adequate safety margins [87]. On the other hand, several comparative studies (excluding surgical treatment) have found no treatment procedures that can effectively prevent malignant transformation of oral leukoplakia [84, 98, 99]. Although vitamin A and other retinoids [100], as well as topical bleomycin [101], are used for the treatment of leukoplakia, they are reported to have only a limited effect in controlling oral leukoplakia and preventing malignant transformation.

4.3.4.11 Etiological Factors of Oral Leukoplakia

Many studies on the pathogenesis of oral leukoplakia have shown that malignant transformation of oral leukoplakia is likely associated with oral habits, in particular, tobacco chewing and smoking [18–20, 26, 63, 75, 76]. A case–control study performed in Taiwan showed adjusted odds ratios for betel nut chewing and smoking with respect to the occurrence of leukoplakia of 17.43 [95 % confidence interval (CI), 1.94–156.27] and 3.22 (95 % CI, 1.06–9.78), respectively [102]. Quitting smoking is expected to reduce the cases of leukoplakia by 36 %, whereas eliminating betel nuts is estimated to decrease the cases of leukoplakia by 62 % and malignant transformation to oral carcinoma by 26 % in the underlying population [102]. Yen et al. [103] reported that among individuals chewing betel quid and smoking, the risk of developing oral cancer after 20 years was 42.2 % for leukoplakia and 95.0 % for erythroleukoplakia.

However, an association between smoking and the malignant transformation of oral leukoplakia has not always been found. Silverman et al. [28] showed that the clinical presence of erythroplasia (erythroleukoplakia) and a clinical verrucous-papillary hyperkeratotic pattern was a high risk for malignant transformation and that nonsmokers were also at risk. Moreover, Schepman et al. [29] reported that the parameters associated with an increased risk of malignant transformation were female sex ($p<0.025$), absence of smoking habits in women ($p<0.05$), and nonhomogeneous clinical aspects ($p<0.01$).

Recently, many reports have suggested that human papillomavirus (HPV) may be the cause of oral leukoplakia and its malignant transformation [104–109]. Miller and Johnstone [106] reported an increased frequency of HPV in oral dysplastic and carcinomatous epithelium compared with a normal mucosa. Specifically, HPV was detected in 36 % (13/36) of patients with oral tongue cancer compared with 4 % (1/25) of controls. In the HPV-positive group of patients with oral tongue cancer, HPV-13 was detected in 55 % (6/11). Moreover, the HPV-16-positive group showed shallower stromal invasion than the HPV-16-negative group ($p=0.045$). Thus, HPV-16 may be one of the causative factors of early OSCC of the tongue [109]. In contrast, Campisi et al. remarked in their review that HPV was identified to play a controversial role in oral oncogenesis and in premalignant and malignant lesions [110].

It is important to note that conflicting data have been reported [111, 112]. Accordingly, further investigations are needed to determine the nature of the association between HPV and malignant transformation.

4.4 Erythroplakia

Oral erythroplakia has been considered to have the greatest potential for malignant transformation in the mouth [1–5, 113, 114]. However, there were a small number of reports on erythroplakia. Therefore, the clinical and pathological findings remain unclear.

4.4.1 Historical Aspects

In 1911, Queyrat described a sharply defined, bright-red, glistening, velvety precancerous lesion of the glans penis, which was termed "erythroplasie" in French. Blau and Hyman [115] noted that erythroplasia of Queyrat clinically involved the mucosal and mucocutaneous areas of the genitalia with similar histologic features to those of Bowen's disease of the skin. Graham and Helwig [116], however, showed that erythroplasia of Queyrat is a distinct clinicopathologic entity from Bowen's disease. Moreover, Shear [117] pointed out that "erythroplasie" in French should be translated to "erythroplakia" in English since "leukoplakia" in English corresponds with "leucoplasie" in French.

4.4.2 Criteria and Clinicopathological Findings

Erythroplakia is defined as "a fiery bright-red patch that cannot be characterized clinically or pathologically as any other definable lesion" [2–6]. However, the author proposed in a review that the term "erythroplakia" should be used analogously to leukoplakia to designate lesions of the oral mucosa presenting as "a predominantly red lesion of the oral mucosa that cannot be characterized as any other definable lesion" (Fig. 4.6a–d) [118].

The typical clinical appearance of erythroplakia is a flat, fiery, bright-red lesion with a well-defined margin adjacent to the normal mucosa that is seldom dull red or granular on

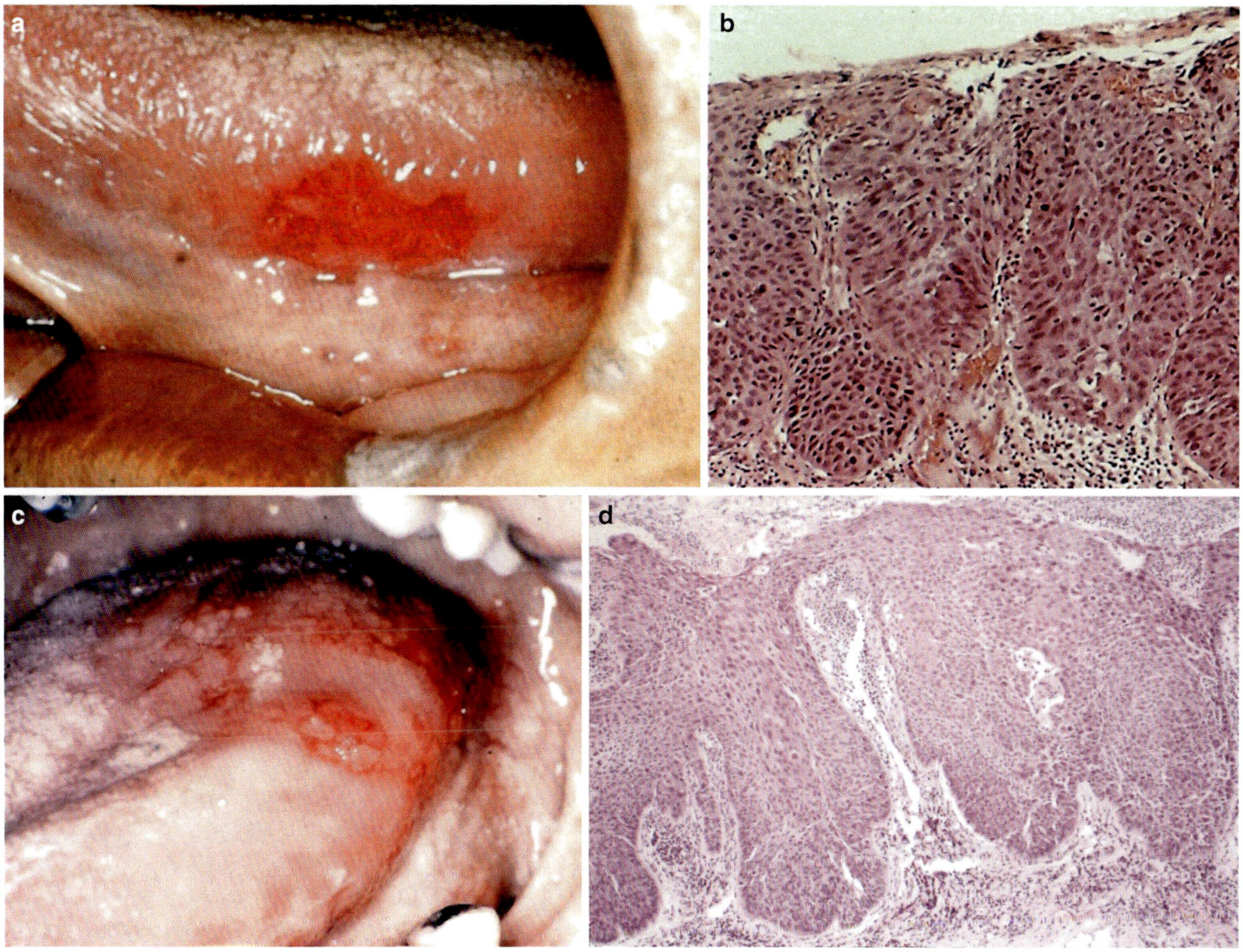

Fig. 4.6 A erythroplakia on the tongue showing a fiery bright-red patch with well-defined margin (**a**), its histology showing CIS (**b**), and a erythroplakia on the tongue showing a wide and red patch (**c**) with CIS (**d**)

the surface [117, 119]. In the case of a mixture of red and white changes, such lesions are usually categorized as nonhomogeneous leukoplakia (erythroleukoplakia) [4–6, 114].

Reichart et al. [114] stated in a review that erythroplakia occurs mainly in middle-aged and elderly individuals [119–123]. Moreover, no distinct sex preference is evident [119–121]. The soft palate, the floor of the mouth, and the buccal mucosa are the most common sites; however, any sites in the mouth are affected [5, 114, 120]. Erythroplakia lesions are typically <1.5 cm in diameter [114], but lesions >4 cm have been reported [124] and a rare case with widespread in the mouth was reported in Japan [119]. A study on the etiology of erythroplakia revealed a strong association between tobacco use and alcohol consumption [114, 121, 123, 125, 126]; however, half of the patients were women and half were nonsmokers and nondrinkers [119]. Tobacco chewing/smoking and alcohol drinking are important etiologic factors for some patients with erythroplakia but the other unknown factor might be.

As for the pathology of erythroplakia, most cases have moderate to severe epithelial dysplasia including CIS [113, 114, 116–120]. Shafer and Waldron [120] reported in 58 patients with histologically documented oral erythroplakia of the homogeneous type (typical erythroplakia) that 51 % showed invasive carcinoma, 40 % CIS, and 9 % mild or moderate dysplasia. However, the authors would like to strongly recommend the exclusion of the 51 % with invasive carcinoma from the erythroplakia group.

4.4.3 Treatment and Development of Oral Squamous Cell Carcinoma

Our previous studies showed that in seven patients with erythroplakia except early invasive SCC followed between 1 year and 4 months and 7 years and 6 months, three patients treated by surgery did not develop OSCC but three of four patients by radiation and /or chemotherapy developed OSCC [118]. In our opinion, surgery remains the appropriate treatment choice as sufficient data on laser excision are not available in the literature [114]. Taken together, the malignant transformation rates of oral erythroplakia (14–59 %) [114, 124] including a few lesions without erythroplakia were notable higher than those of oral leukoplakia (0.1–17.5 %) [10], and appropriate surgical treatment coupled with a suitable follow-up period is important for preventing the development of OSCC from oral erythroplakia.

References

1. World Health Organization (1973) Report of a meeting of investigators on the histological definition of precancerous lesions. World Health Organization, Geneva
2. World Health Organization Collaborating Centre for Oral Precancerous lesions (1978) Definition of leukoplakia and related lesions: an aid to studies on oral precancer. Oral Surg Oral Med Oral Pathol 46:518–539
3. Axéll T, Holmstrup P, Kramer IRH, Pindborg JJ, Shear M (1984) International seminar on oral leukoplakia and associated lesions related to tobacco habits. Community Dent Oral Epidemiol 12:145–154
4. Axéll T, Pindborg JJ, Smith CJ, Van der Waal I, An International Collaborative Group on Oral White Lesions (1996) Oral white lesions with special reference to precancerous and tobacco-related lesions: conclusions of an international symposium held in Uppsala, Sweden, May 18–21, 1994. J Oral Pathol Med 25:49–54
5. Pindborg JJ, Reichart PA, Smith CJ, van der Waal I, in Collaboration with Sobin LH and Pathologists in 9 Countries, WHO International Histological Classification of Tumours (1997) Histological typing of cancer and precancer of the oral mucosa, 2nd edn. Springer, Berlin
6. Warnakulasuriya S, Johnson NW, van der Waal I (2007) Nomenclature and classification of potentially malignant disorders of the oral mucosa. J Oral Pathol Med 36:575–580
7. Thompson PJ (2002) Field change and oral cancer: new evidence for widespread carcinogenesis? Int J Oral Maxillofac Surg 31:262–266
8. Bremmer JF, Braakhuis BJM, Ruijter-Schippers HJ et al (2005) A non invasive genetic screening test to detect oral preneoplastic lesions. Lab Invest 85:1481–1488
9. van der Waal I (2009) Potentially malignant disorders of the oral mucosa and oropharyngeal mucosa; terminology, classification and present concepts of management. Oral Oncol 45:317–323
10. Amagasa T, Yamashiro M, Ishikawa H (2006) Oral leukoplakia related malignant transformation. Oral Sci Int 3:45–55
11. Amagasa T, Fujii E, Suzuki T, Yamashiro M, Ogura I, Miyakura T, Negishi A, Uzawa N, Iwaki H (1999) Clinical characteristics of precancerous lesions and early squamous cell carcinoma in the oral cavity. J Jpn Soc Oral Tum 11:357–363 (In Japanese)
12. Banoczy J (1977) Follow-up studies in oral leukoplakia. J Maxillofac Surg 5:69–75
13. Banoczy J, Rigo O (1991) Prevalence study of oral precancerous lesions within a complex screening system in Hungary. Community Dent Oral Epidemiol 19:265–267
14. Reichart PA (2000) Oral mucosal lesions in a representative cross-sectional study of aging Germans. Community Dent Oral Epidemiol 28:390–398
15. Shafer WG, Waldron CA (1961) A clinical and histopathologic study of oral leukoplakia. Surg Gynec Obstet 112:411–420
16. Bánóczy J, Csiba Á (1976) Occurrence of epithelial dysplasia in oral leukoplakia: analysis and follow-up study of 120 cases. Oral Surg Oral Med Oral Pathol 42:766–774
17. Sugár L, Bánóczy J (1969) Follow-up studies in oral leukoplakia. Bull WHO 41:289–293
18. Silverman S Jr, Bhargava K, Smith LW, Malaowalla AM (1976) Malignant transformation and natural history of oral leukoplakia in 57,518 industrial workers of Gujarat, India. Cancer 8: 1790–1795
19. Gupta PC, Mehta FS, Daftary DK et al (1980) Incidence rates of oral cancer and natural history of oral precancerous lesions in a 10 year follow-up study of Indian villagers. Community Dent Oral Epidemiol 8:287–333
20. Mehta FS, Shroff BC, Gupta PC, Daftary DK (1972) Oral leukoplakia in relation to tobacco habits. A ten-year follow-up study of Bombay policemen. Oral Surg Oral Med Oral Pathol 34:426–433
21. Silverman S Jr, Rozen RD (1968) Observations on the clinical characteristics and natural history of oral leukoplakia. J Am Dent Assoc 76:772–777
22. Gangadharan P, Paymaster JC (1971) Leukoplakia. An epidemiologic study of 1504 cases observed at the Tata Memorial Hospital, Bombay, India. Br J Cancer 25:657
23. Pindborg JJ, Reibel J, Roed-Peterson B, Mehta FS (1980) Tobacco-induced changes in oral leukoplakic epithelium. Cancer 45:2330–2336
24. Waldron CA, Shafer WG (1975) Leukoplakia revisited, a clinicopathologic study 3256 oral leukoplakias. Cancer 36:1386–1392
25. Bhargava K, Smith LW, Mani NJ, Silverman S, Malaowalla AM, Billimoria KF (1975) A follow-up study of oral cancer and precancerous lesions in 57518 industrial workers in Gujarat, India. Indian J Cancer 12:124–129
26. Mehta FS, Pindborg JJ, Gupta PC, Daftary DK (1969) Epidemiologic and histologic study of oral cancer and leukoplakia among 50,915 villagers in India. Cancer 24:832–849
27. Axéll T (1987) Occurrence of leukoplakia and some other oral white lesions among 20333 adult Swedish people. Community Dent Oral Epidemiol 15:46–51
28. Silverman S Jr, Gorsky M, Lozada F (1984) Oral leukoplakia and malignant transformation: a follow-up study of 257 patients. Cancer 53:563–568
29. Schepman KP, van der Meij EH, Smeele LE, van der Waal I (1998) Malignant transformation of oral leukoplakia: a follow- up study of a hospital-based population of 166 patients with oral leukoplakia from The Netherlands. Oral Oncol 34:270–275
30. Bouquot JE, Gorlin RJ (1986) Leukoplakia, lichen planus, and other oral keratoses in 23,616 white Americans over the age of 35 years. Oral Surg Oral Med Oral Pathol 61:373–381
31. Kirita T, Horiuchi K, Tsuyuki M, Ohgi K, Okamoto M et al (1995) Clinico-pathological study on oral leukoplakia- evaluation of potential for malignant transformation. Jpn J Oral Maxillofac Surg 41:26–35
32. Einhorn J, Wersall J (1967) Incidence of oral carcinoma in patients with leukoplakia of the oral cavity. Cancer 20:2189–2193
33. Yen AMF, Chen SC, Chen THH (2007) Dose–response relationships of oral habits associated with the risk of oral premalignant lesions among men who chew betel quid. Oral Oncol 43:634–638
34. Kawabe R, Fujita K (2001) Survival analysis: application to evaluation of risk factors for cancer development in oral leukoplakia. Jpn J Oral Mucosa 7:45–58 (in Japanese)
35. Pindborg JJ, Renstrup G, Poulsen HE, Silverman S Jr (1963) Studies on oral leukoplakias. V. Clinical and histologic signs of malignancy. Acta Odont Scand 21:407–414
36. Pindborg JJ, Jølst O, Renstrup G, Roed-Petersen B (1968) Studies in oral leukoplakia: a preliminary report on the period prevalence of malignant transformation in leukoplakia based on a follow-up study of 248 patients. J Am Dent Assoc 76:767–771
37. Hansen LS, Olson JA, Silverman S Jr (1985) Proliferative verrucous leukoplakia. A long-term study of thirty patients. Oral Surg Oral Med Oral Pathol 60:285–298
38. Silverman S Jr, Gorsky M (1997) Proliferative verrucous leukoplakia: a follow-up study of 54 cases. Oral Surg Oral Med Oral Pathol Oral Radiol Endod 84:154–157

39. Kramer IRH, Lucas RB, Pindborg JJ et al (1978) Definition of leukoplakia and related lesions: an aid to studies on oral precancer. Oral Surg Oral Med Oral Pathol 46:518–539
40. Pindborg JJ (1980) Oral cancer and precancer. John Wright & Sons Ltd, Bristol
41. Pindborg JJ, Reibel J, Holmstrup P (1985) Subjectivity in evaluating oral epithelial dysplasia, carcinoma in situ and initial carcinoma. J Oral Pathol 14:698–708
42. Abbey L, Kaugars GE, Gunsolley JC et al (1995) Intraexaminer and interexaminer reliability in the diagnosis of oral epithelial dysplasia. Oral Surg Oral Med Oral Pathol 80:188–191
43. Karabulut A, Reibel J, Therkildsen MH et al (1995) Observer variability in the histologic assessment of oral premalignant lesions. J Oral Pathol Med 24:198–200
44. Warnakulasuriya S, Reibel J, Bouquot J et al (2008) Oral epithelial dysplasia classification systems: predictive value, utility, weaknesses and scope for improvement. J Oral Pathol Med 37:127–133
45. World Health Organization (2005) World health organization classification of tumours. In: Barnes L, Eveson JW, Reichart P, Sidransky D (eds) Pathology and genetics. Head and neck tumours. International Agency for Research on Cancer (IARC), IARC, Lyon
46. Gale N, Kambic V, Michaels L et al (2000) The Ljubljana classification: a practical strategy for the diagnosis of laryngeal precancerous lesions. Adv Anat Pathol 7:240–251
47. Hellquist H, Cardesa A, Gale N et al (1999) Criteria for grading in the Ljubljana classification of epithelial hyperplastic laryngeal lesions. A study by members of the Working Group on Epithelial Hyperplastic Laryngeal Lesions of the European Society of Pathology. Histopathology 34:226–233
48. Hellquist H, Lundgren J, Olofsson J (1982) Hyperplasia, keratosis, dysplasia and carcinoma in situ of the vocal cords a follow-up study. Clin Otolaryngol 7:11–27
49. Kambic V, Gale N (1995) Epithelial hyperplastic lesions of the larynx. Elsevier, Amsterdam
50. Amagasa T, Yokoo E, Sato K et al (1985) A study of the clinical characteristics and treatment of oral carcinoma in situ. Oral Surg Oral Med Oral Pathol 60:50–55
51. Sakr WA, Gale N, Gnepp DR et al (2009) Squamous intraepithelial neoplasia of the upper aerodigestive tract. In: Gnepp DR (ed) Diagnostic surgical pathology of the head and neck, 2nd edn. Saunders, Philadelphia
52. Shimizu M, Nagata K, Yamaguchi H et al (2009) Squamous intraepithelial neoplasia of the esophagus: past, present, and future. J Gastroenterol 44:103–112
53. Izumo T (2011) Oral premalignant lesions: from the pathological viewpoint. Int J Clin Oncol 16:15–26
54. The Working Committee of New Histopathological Criteria for Borderline Malignancies of the Oral Mucosa, Japanese Society for Oral Pathology (2007) Oral CIS (JSOP) catalog: histopathological variations. Sunashobo Publishing Co Ltd, Tokyo
55. Sugar L, Banoczy J (1969) Follow-up studies in oral leukoplakia. Bull WHO 41:289–293
56. Amagasa T, Michi K, Saito K et al (1977) Clinical classification of oral leukoplakia. Jpn J Oral Maxillofac Surg 23:89–96 (in Japanese)
57. Dawsey SM, Fleischer DE, Wang GQ et al (1998) Mucosal iodine staining improves endoscopic visualization of squamous dysplasia and squamous cell carcinoma of the esophagus in Linxian, China. Cancer 83:220–231
58. Freitag CP, Barros SG, Kruel CD et al (1999) Esophageal dysplasias are detected by endoscopy with Lugol in patients at risk for squamous cell carcinoma in southern Brazil. Dis Esophagus 12:191–195
59. Nakanishi Y, Ochiai A, Yoshimura K (1998) The clinicopathologic significance of small areas unstained by Lugol's iodine in the mucosa surrounding resected esophageal carcinoma. Cancer 82:1454–1459
60. Shimizu Y, Tsukagoshi H, Fujita M et al (2001) Endoscopic screening for early esophageal cancer by iodine staining in patients with other current or prior primary cancers. Gastrointest Endosc 53:1–5
61. Maeda K, Suzuki T, Ohyama Y, Nakakuki K, Yamashiro M, Okada N, Amagasa T (2009) Colorimetric analysis of unstained lesions surrounding oral squamous cell carcinomas and oral potentially malignant disorders using iodine. Int J Oral Maxillofac Surg 39:486–492
62. Maeda K, Yamashiro M, Michi Y, Suzuki T, Ohyama Y, Okada N, Amagasa T (2009) Effective staining method with iodine for leukoplakia and lesions surrounding squamous cell carcinoma of the tongue assessed by colorimetric analysis. J Med Dent Sci 56: 123–130
63. Napier SS, Speight PM (2008) Natural history of potentially malignant oral lesions and conditions: an overview of the literature. J Oral Pathol Med 37:1–10
64. Bánóczy J, Sugár L (1972) Longitudinal studies in oral leukoplakias. J Oral Pathol 1:265–272
65. Pindborg JJ, Roed-Petersen B, Renstrup G (1972) Role of smoking in floor of the mouth leukoplakias. J Oral Pathol 1:22–29
66. Roed-Petersen B (1971) Cancer development in oral leukoplakia follow-up of 331 patients. J Dent Res 50:711 (abstract)
67. Kramer IRH (1969) Precancerous conditions of oral mucosa: a computer aided study. Ann R Coll Surg Eng 45:340–356
68. Lind PO (1987) Malignant transformation in oral leukoplakia. Scand J Dent Res 95:449–455
69. Amagasa T (1982) Precancerous lesions; its diagnosis and treatment plan. Shika-Rinshou-Kouza, Ishiyaku Shuppan Inc., Tokyo, pp 509–516 (in Japanese)
70. Inoue A, Sakamoto A, Uchida M, Kamata S (1985) Malignant progression of oral leukoplakia. J Jpn Soc Cancer Ther 20:18–24
71. Chiesa F, Boracchi P, Tradati N, Rossi N, Costal L, Giardini R, Marazza M, Zurrida S (1993) Risk of preneoplastic and neoplastic events in operated oral leukoplakias. Eur J Cancer B Oral Oncol 29B:23–28
72. Kramer IRH, El-Labban N, Lee KW (1978) The clinical features and risk of malignant transformation in sublingual keratosis. Br Dent J 144:171–180
73. Pogrel MA (1979) Sublingual keratosis and malignant transformation. J Oral Pathol 8:176–178
74. Holmstrup P, Vedtofte P, Reibel J, Stolze K (2006) Long-term treatment outcome of oral premalignant lesions. Oral Oncol 42:461–474
75. Mehta FS, Gupta PC et al (1981) Chewing and smoking habits in relation to precancer and oral cancer. J Cancer Res Clin Oncol 99:35–39
76. Gupta PC, Bhonsle RB, Murti PR, Daftary DK, Mehta FS, Pindborg JJ (1989) An epidemiologic assessment of cancer risk in oral precancerous lesions in India with special reference to nodular leukoplakia. Cancer 63:2247–2252
77. Mincer HH, Coleman SA, Hopkins KP (1972) Observations on the clinical characteristics of oral lesions showing histologic epithelial dysplasia. Oral Surg Oral Med Oral Pathol 33: 389–399
78. Pindborg JJ, Daftary DK, Mehta FS (1977) A follow-up study of sixty-one oral dysplastic precancerous lesions in Indian villagers. Oral Surg Oral Med Oral Pathol 43:383–390
79. Lumerman H, Freedman P, Kerpel S (1995) Oral epithelial dysplasia and the development of invasive squamous carcinoma. Oral Surg Oral Med Oral Pathol 79:321–329

80. Cowan CG, Gregg TA et al (2001) Potentially malignant oral lesions in northern Ireland: a 20-year population-based perspective of malignant transformation. Oral Dis 7:18–24
81. Napier SS, Cowan CG, Gregg TA, Stevenson M, Lamey P-J, Toner PG (2003) Potentially malignant lesions in Northern Ireland: size (extent) matters. Oral Dis 9:129–137
82. Vedtofte P, Holmstrup P, Hjorting-Hansen E et al (1987) Surgical treatment of premalignant lesions of the oral mucosa. Int J Oral Maxillofac Surg 16:656–664
83. Schoelch ML, Sekandari N, Regezi JA et al (1999) Laser management of oral leukoplakias: a follow-up study of 70 patients. Laryngoscope 109:949–953
84. Lodi G, Sardella A, Bez C et al. (2006) Interventions for treating oral leukoplakia. Cochrane Database Syst Rev (4):CD001829
85. Lodi G, Porter S (2008) Management of potentially malignant disorders: evidence and critique. J Oral Pathol Med 37(2):63–69
86. Amagasa T, Fujii E, Hasegawa K, Shioda S (1989) Clinicopathology of oral cancer and precancerous lesions. In: International congress of oral cancer, New Delhli, India, 14 Nov 1989
87. Amagasa T, Yamashiro M, Uzawa N (2011) Oral premalignant lesions: from a clinical perspective. Int J Clin Oncol 16:5–14
88. Saito T, Sugiura C, Hirai A et al (2001) Development of squamous cell carcinoma from pre-existent oral leukoplakia: with respect to treatment modality. Int J Oral Maxillofac Surg 30:49–53
89. Zhang L, Poh CF, Lam WL et al (2001) Impact of localized treatment in reducing risk of progression of low-grade oral dysplasia: molecular evidence of incomplete resection. Oral Oncol 37:505–512
90. Tradati N, Grigolat R, Calabrese L et al (1997) Oral leukoplakias: to treat or not? Oral Oncol 33:317–321
91. Roodenburg JL, Panders AK, Vermey A (1991) Carbon dioxide laser surgery of oral leukoplakia. Oral Surg Oral Med Oral Pathol 71:670–674
92. Ishii J, Fujita K, Munemoto S et al (2004) Management of oral leukoplakia by laser surgery: relation between recurrence and malignant transformation and clinicopathological features. J Clin Laser Med Surg 22:27–33
93. Diajil A, Robinson CM, Sloan P, Thomson PJ (2013) Clinical outcome following oral potentially malignant disorder treatment: a 100 patient cohort study. Int J Dent. doi:10.1155/2013/809248
94. van der Waal I, Schepman KP, van der Meiji EH et al (1997) Oral leukoplakia: a clinicopathological review. Oral Oncol 33:291–301
95. Browne RM, Potts AJC (1986) Dysplasia in salivary gland ducts in sublingual leukoplakia and erythroplakia. Oral Oncol 62:44–49
96. Hays GL, Lippman SM, Flaitz CM et al (1995) Co-carcinogenesis and field cancerization: oral lesions offer first signs. J Am Dent Assoc 126:47–51
97. Scholes AG, Woolgar JA, Boyle MA et al (1998) Synchronous oral carcinomas: independent or common clonal origin? Cancer Res 58:2003–2006
98. Lele S (2005) Although leukoplakia responds to some treatments relapses and adverse effects are common. Evid Based Dent 6:15–16
99. Lodi G, Sardella A, Bez C et al (2002) Systematic review of randomized trials for the treatment of oral leukoplakia. J Dent Educ 66:896–902
100. Epstein JB, Gorsky M (1999) Topical application of vitamin A to oral leukoplakia: a clinical case series. Cancer 86:921–927
101. Epstein JB, Gorsky M, Wong FLW et al (1998) Topical bleomycin for the treatment of dysplastic oral leukoplakia. Cancer 83:629–634
102. Shiu MN, Chen THH, Chang SH et al (2000) Risk factors for leukoplakia and malignant transformation to oral carcinoma: a leukoplakia cohort in Taiwan. Br J Cancer 82:1871–1874
103. Yen AM, Chen SC, Chang SH et al (2008) The effect of betel quid and cigarette on multistate progression of oral premalignancy. J Oral Pathol Med 37(7):417–422
104. Palefsky JM, Silverman S Jr, Abdel-Salaam M et al (1995) Association between proliferative verrucous leukoplakia and infection with human papillomavirus type 16. J Oral Pathol Med 24:193–197
105. Bouda M, Gorgoulis VG, Kastrinakis NG et al (2000) High risk HPV types are frequently detected in potentially malignant and malignant oral lesions, but not in normal mucosa. Mod Pathol 13:644–653
106. Miller CS, Johnstone BM (2001) Human papillomavirus as a risk factor for oral squamous cell carcinoma: a meta-analysis, 1982–1997. Oral Surg Oral Med Oral Pathol Oral Radiol Endod 91:622–635
107. Chang KC, Su IJ, Tsai ST et al (2002) Pathological features of betel quid-related oral epithelial lesions in Taiwan with special emphasis on the tumor progression and human papillomavirus association. Oncology 63:362–369
108. Szarka K, Tar I, Feher E et al (2009) Progressive increase of human papillomavirus carriage rates in potentially malignant and malignant oral disorders with increasing malignant potential. Oral Microbiol Immunol 24(4):314–318
109. Lee SY, Cho NH, Choi EC et al (2010) Relevance of human papillomavirus (HPV) infection to carcinogenesis of oral tongue cancer. Int J Oral Maxillofac Surg 39:678–683
110. Campisi G, Panzarella V, Giuliani M et al (2007) human papillomavirus: its identikit and controversial role in oral oncogenesis, premalignant and malignant lesions. Int J Oncol 30:813–823
111. Yang SW, Lee YS et al (2009) Human papillomavirus in oral leukoplakia is no prognostic indicator of malignant transformation. Cancer Epidemiol 33(2):118–122
112. Acay R, Rezende N et al (2008) Human papillomavirus as a risk factor in oral carcinogenesis: a study using in situ hybridization with signal amplification. Oral Microbiol Immunol 23(4): 271–274
113. Scully C, Sudbø J, Speight PM (2003) Progress in determining the malignant potential of oral lesions. J Oral Pathol Med 32:251–256
114. Reichart PA, Philipsen HP (2005) Oral erythroplakia—a review. Oral Oncol 41:551–561
115. Blau S, Hyman AB (1955) Erythroplasia of Queyrat. Acta Dermatol Venerol 35:341–378
116. Graham JH, Helwig EB (1973) Erythroplakia of Queyrat. A clinicopathologic and histochemical study. Cancer 32:1396–1414
117. Shear M (1972) Erythroplakia of the mouth. Int Dent J 22: 460–473
118. Amagasa T (2011) Oral premalignant lesions. Int J Clin Oncol 16:1–4
119. Amagasa T, Masuo K, Takagi M, Michi K, Saito K (1979) Clinicopathological study of erythroplasia of the oral mucosa. Jpn J Oral Surg 25:514–522
120. Shafer WG, Waldron CA (1975) Erythroplakia of the oral cavity. Cancer 36:1021–1028
121. Hashibe M, Mathew B, Kuruvilla B, Thomas G, Sankaranarayanan B, Parkin DM et al (2000) Chewing tobacco, alcohol and the risk of erythroplakia. Cancer Epidemiol Biomarkers Prev 9: 639–645
122. Feller L, Altini M, Slabbert H (1991) Pre-malignant lesions of the oral mucosa in a South Africa sample—a clinicopathological study. J Dent Assoc S Af 46:262–265
123. Hashibe M, Jacob BJ, Thomas G, Ramadas K, Mathew B, Sankaranarayanan R et al (2003) Socioeconomic status, life- style factors and oral premalignant lesions. Oral Oncol 39:664–671
124. Bouquot JE, Ephros H (1995) Erythroplakia: the dangerous red mucosa. Pract Periodontics Aesthet Dent 7:59–67
125. Thomas G, Hashibe M, Jacob BJ, Ramadas K, Mathew B, Sankaranarayanan R et al (2003) Risk factors for multiple oral premalignant lesions. Int J Cancer 107:285–291
126. Jacob BJ, Straif K, Thomas G, Kunnambathu R, Mathew B, Zhang ZF et al (2004) Betel quid without tobacco as a risk factor for oral precancers. Oral Oncol 40:697–704

Imaging and Classification of Staging

5

Takafumi Hayashi

Abstract

A detailed and accurate pretherapeutic evaluation of stage plays a crucial role in the prognosis as well as the choice and extent of the therapeutic procedure required for patients with oral cancer. For this purpose, various modern diagnostic imaging modalities are routinely used. In this section, the potential roles of conventional X-rays, computed tomography (CT), magnetic resonance imaging (MRI), ultrasonography (US), and positron emission tomography (PET)/CT in the staging of oral cancer are addressed.

Keywords

Diagnostic imaging • Magnetic resonance imaging • Ultrasonography • X-ray computed tomography

5.1 Imaging Techniques

5.1.1 Conventional X-Ray in Oral Cancer

A conventional X-ray is commonly used for surveillance of oral cancer. Because of the limited viewing direction, its role in staging of oral cancer is limited. This technique renders a three-dimensional volume onto a two-dimensional plane. As a consequence, overlying and underlying tissues and structures are superimposed, which generally results in reduced conspicuity as well as subject contrast.

5.1.1.1 Dental X-Ray

The detailed shape of the margins of bone absorption in gingival carcinoma can be assessed with a dental X-ray. Small fragments of the destroyed bone can also be detected. The exact extent of the tumor involvement can hardly be evaluated because of the superimposition of adjacent structures.

5.1.1.2 Orthopantomography (Panoramic X-Ray)

Orthopantomography is a two-dimensional half-circle view of the upper and lower jaws from ear to ear obtained by panoramic X-ray scanning. Its intrinsic value is screening for malignancy in routine dental practice. Marked maxillary or mandibular bone absorption caused by gingival, floor of mouth, and tongue carcinomas can be detected by orthopantomography. However, the diagnostic sensitivity for the extent of tumor involvement is insufficient compared with modern sectional imaging modalities such as computed tomography (CT) and magnetic resonance imaging (MRI), because of the limited viewing direction. From the viewpoint of treatment outcome, the Japan Society for Oral Tumors (JSOT) proposed a classification regarding the shape of the absorbed bone involved in gingival carcinoma [1]. The characteristic shape of the absorbed bone margin was classified into three types: pressure type; moth-eaten type; and intermediate type (Fig. 5.72). Moth-eaten type, which commonly shows a poorer outcome, is applied if an ill-defined permeated margin and small bone fragments within the lesion are observed.

T. Hayashi, D.D.S., Ph.D. (✉)
Division of Oral and Maxillofacial Radiology, Niigata University Graduate School of Medical and Dental Sciences, 2-5274 Gakkocho-dori, Chuo-ku, Niigata 951-8514, Japan
e-mail: hayashi@dent.niigata-u.ac.jp

T. Kirita and K. Omura (eds.), *Oral Cancer: Diagnosis and Therapy*, DOI 10.1007/978-4-431-54938-3_5, © Springer Japan 2015

5.1.1.3 Other Conventional X-Ray

Posteroanterior projection and Waters projection X-rays can occasionally reveal bone destruction at the lateral portion of the maxilla and mandibular bone structure, which might be overlooked by orthopantomography.

5.1.2 CT in Oral Cancer

5.1.2.1 Plain CT and CECT

CT is a fundamental cross-sectional imaging modality for evaluating oral cancer and is superior for detecting cortical bone destruction and intratumoral calcification compared with other imaging modalities [2]. As modern CT equipment can deal with isotropic voxel data, three-dimensional evaluation using multiplanar reformatted images is routinely used to define the extent of tumor involvement. Contrast-enhanced CT (CECT) using iodine contrast materials is an excellent modality for oral cancer staging, i.e., determining the tumor extent (especially depth of invasion) and size, identifying lymph node metastases, assessing response to therapy, and evaluating recurrent disease.

On CT, tumors appear as homogeneous or heterogeneous soft-tissue-attenuated lesions that are variably enhanced after intravenous administration of iodine contrast materials [3]. Commonly, the tumor is intensely enhanced compared with adjacent normal structures because of the tumor neoangiogenesis, and a central necrotic portion is frequently identified as a non-enhanced or barely enhanced hypodense area within the tumor mass. There may be early or prominent enhancement of the tumor margins, because of the higher vascularity of the tumor periphery.

Tumors located around the occlusal plane level are frequently obscured with metallic artifacts caused by dental prostheses. A CT image is also degraded by motion artifacts, but is less affected by breathing and swallowing artifacts than MRI. Good-quality imaging obtained with CT is readily reproducible. A soft-tissue window setting image with a soft-tissue algorithm at a level of 40–50 with a window width of 250–350 is recommended for discrimination of enhanced tumor tissue. In addition, a bone window setting with a bone algorithm should be used for osseous involvement of the tumor (thin slice images of less than 1 mm are preferable). For routine examination in oral cancer, contiguous scanning from the level of the nasopharynx to the level of the supraclavicular fossa is recommended.

5.1.2.2 CT Perfusion

CT Perfusion (CTP) is a technique that measures the parameters of tissue perfusion through dynamic acquisition of images after contrast material administration (Fig. 5.130) [2]. The physiologic basis of contrast enhancement on CT closely mimics the physiologic effects of tumor angiogenesis. Angiogenesis is a key factor for tumor growth and metastasis and is a complex process that includes endothelial cell breakdown, proliferation, and migration stimulated by angiogenic factors. CTP can be routinely performed on all modern CT equipment and is potentially useful to distinguish neoplasms from normal structures and posttreatment changes. The major drawback of CTP is an excessive radiation exposure dose, and therefore lower tube voltages and mAs are recommended.

5.1.3 CBCT in Oral Cancer

As a modern cone-beam CT (CBCT) system has relatively higher spatial resolution compared with a CT system, the significance of CBCT in the evaluation of osseous involvement is almost equal or superior to the bone-algorithm CT. The major disadvantage of CBCT is poor soft-tissue contrast because of the limited radiation exposure. The tumor mass is hardly visualized clearly with CBCT, and therefore neoplastic processes are frequently overlooked. The limited field of view is another drawback of CBCT in the evaluation of tumor extent. Therefore, the role of CBCT in oral cancer staging is limited.

5.1.4 MRI in Oral Cancer

5.1.4.1 Plain MRI and Contrast-Enhanced MRI

MRI uses the magnetic properties of hydrogen and its interactions with both a large external magnetic field and radio waves to produce highly detailed images of the human body.

MRI has superior soft-tissue contrast compared with CT and may provide better delineation of soft-tissue invasion of the carcinoma [3]. The lack of ionizing radiation makes it the preferred technique in patients with iodine allergy. There is also the advantage of reduced metallic artifacts from metallic dental prostheses. However, the images are often degraded by magnetic metallic materials and unexpected oral motion. The major drawbacks of MRI are the relatively high cost and claustrophobia.

On conventional T1-weighted images obtained without fat saturation, a squamous cell carcinoma (SCC) has intermediate signal intensity and is generally isointense to muscle. On T2-weighted images, an SCC is typically heterogeneous and hyperintense to normal muscle, making it more conspicuous. However, the tumor size might be overestimated on T2-weighted images because the tumor cannot be distinguished from surrounding inflammation and edema. On gadolinium-enhanced T1-weighted images, the tumor has variable enhancement and conspicuity. Fat-saturated images are helpful in distinguishing tumors from normal surrounding structures. Axial and coronal contrast-enhanced T1-weighted images with fat saturation are superior to CT for defining the soft-tissue extent. One of the disadvantages of fat saturation is increased susceptibility to artifacts, particularly in locations near the bone or air.

MRI is the optimal modality for detection of perineural tumor spreading [3]. Direct signs of perineural tumor spreading are enlargement, irregularity, and abnormal enhancement of the major cranial nerves and their branches. Replacement of high-intensity fat-containing spaces adjacent to the major skull foramina, such as the pterygopalatine fossa, by tumor tissue is also a valuable clue to the presence of perineural tumor spreading. Although CT is generally considered superior for detection of cortical erosion, MRI is more sensitive for identification of early bone marrow invasion. Findings suggestive of marrow invasion are replacement of normal high-intensity marrow fat by tumor tissue. Dynamic contrast-enhanced MRI provides better delineation of the tumor margin.

5.1.4.2 Diffusion-Weighted MRI

Diffusion reflects the random motion of molecules, and diffusion-weighted imaging (DWI) is an MRI technique wherein images are weighted with the local characteristics of water diffusion [2]. The apparent diffusion coefficient (ADC) is a measure of the magnitude of freedom of water diffusion. Higher ADC values indicate greater magnitude of water diffusion, while lower ADC values indicate lesser magnitude of water diffusion and restricted motion. The DWI signal intensity is dependent on the magnitude of water motion. Highly cellular tissues exhibit lower ADC values than acellular or hypocellular tissues. Generally, the ADC of malignant lesions is lower than that of benign lesions (Figs. 5.54, 5.80 and 5.103). Malignant lymph nodes tend to have lower ADC values than nonmalignant lymph nodes.

5.1.5 Ultrasonography (US) in Oral Cancer

US is based on the pulse-echo principle, in which a short burst of ultrasound is emitted from a transducer and directed into a tissue, and echoes are produced as a result of the interactions of the ultrasound with the tissue, traveling back to the transducer. By timing the period that elapses between the emission of the pulse and the reception of the echo, the distance between the transducer and the echo-producing structure can be calculated. US is a real-time, multiplanar, dynamic assessment technique for oral, maxillofacial, and neck structures. The high spatial resolution of modern US equipment is superior to CT and MRI. US has limited beam penetration, with the depth inversely proportional to the frequency. Power or color Doppler sonography is useful for detection of blood flow. Elastosonography has a potential role in differentiating benign tissue from malignant tissue (Figs. 5.123 and 5.129).

5.1.5.1 Intraoral US

A small carcinoma (T1, T2) of the mobile tongue and buccal mucosa may be visualized by intraoral US (Figs. 5.60 and 5.68) [1]. Intraoral US is performed by direct contact with the surface of the carcinoma, and therefore a small intraoperative transducer is preferable. If a thin polymer gel pad is placed as an acoustic coupling device between the probe surface and the tumor surface, three layers are clearly distinguished: (a) surface layer (hyperechoic line); (b) mucosal layer (hypoechoic line); and (c) submucosal and muscular layer (heterogeneous internal echo). Commonly, an SCC arising from the mucous membrane appears as a focal hypoechoic area continuous with the surrounding normal mucosal layer and the depth of invasion can be measured accurately (Figs. 5.60 and 5.68). Evaluation of the invasion depth of a tongue carcinoma may be useful for prediction of subsequent lymph node metastasis. In addition, Doppler US demonstrates prominent vascularity around the deep margins, arising from neoangiogenesis at the tumor invasion front. Intraoral US has a superior ability to evaluate the depth of invasion of a tumor compared with other imaging modalities.

5.1.5.2 Face and Neck US

Nodal involvement is the most important prognostic factor for oral cancer. US is the most accurate method currently available for detecting neck lymph node metastasis. Retropharyngeal and mediastinal nodes are inaccessible by US and require evaluation by CT or MRI. The US features of metastatic nodes are round shape, heterogeneity, loss of normal hilum, internal necrosis, and peripheral vascularity (Figs. 5.122 and 5.128). An ill-defined border in a metastatic node suggests extracapsular spread. With regard to internal necrosis, marked cystic degeneration is interpreted as a hypoechoic or non-echoic area with an irregular margin, whereas keratinization is demonstrated as an ill-defined hyperechoic area within a node [1]. However, diffuse-spreading tumor tissue that lacks obvious necrosis may be overlooked on a routine B-mode image only.

5.1.6 PET/CT in Oral Cancer

Positron emission tomography (PET)/CT, reflecting PET combined with CT, is the best modality for staging, monitoring, and surveillance of advanced oral cancer (Fig. 5.125) [2]. The utility of PET/CT in staging depends on the size of the primary tumor, and therefore PET/CT is not useful for a very small tumor. PET/CT is useful for identifying unsuspected additional primary tumors and/or distant metastases at the time of staging of a known primary tumor. 18F-fluorodeoxyglucose (FDG) is transported into cells like glucose by transmembrane transporters and becomes trapped, thereby accumulating in cells with high glucose metabolism. The standardized uptake value (SUV) is the quantified measure of FDG uptake. However, the SUV is highly dependent on the machine used and the patient characteristics. A small tumor size limits the detection of FDG uptake and the minimal size limit is about 5 mm. Normal physiologic uptake should be encountered. Normal salivary glands exhibit low-level FDG uptake, while lymphoid tissue uptake is highly variable, especially at the tonsils and tongue base.

5.2 Sectional Anatomy of the Oral Cavity (Figs. 5.1, 5.2, 5.3, 5.4, 5.5, 5.6, 5.7, 5.8, 5.9, 5.10, 5.11, 5.12, 5.13, 5.14, 5.15, 5.16, 5.17, 5.18, 5.19, 5.20, 5.21, 5.22, 5.23, 5.24, 5.25, 5.26, 5.27, 5.28, 5.29, 5.30, 5.31, 5.32, 5.33, 5.34, 5.35, 5.36, 5.37, 5.38, 5.39, 5.40, 5.41, 5.42, 5.43, 5.44, 5.45, 5.46 and 5.47)

5.3 Oral Cancer Staging

5.3.1 TNM (UICC Staging)

(Mainly cited from: 2010 American Joint Committee on Cancer Definitions of TNM for the Lip and Oral avity [4])

5.3.2 Primary Tumor (T)

T factor

TX Primary tumor cannot be assessed
T0 No evidence of primary tumor
Tis Carcinoma in situ

T1 Tumor 2 cm or less in greatest dimension
T2 Tumor more than 2 cm but not more than 4 cm in greatest dimension

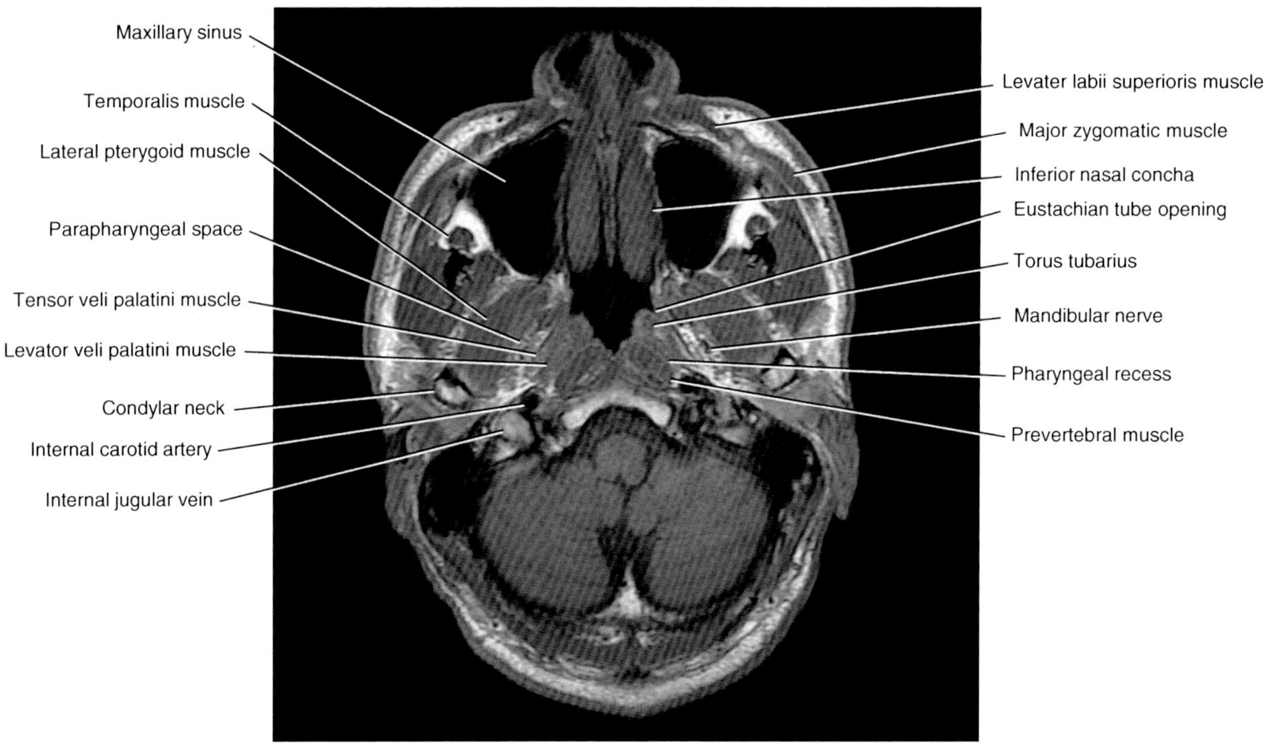

Fig. 5.1 Axial T1-weighted MRI

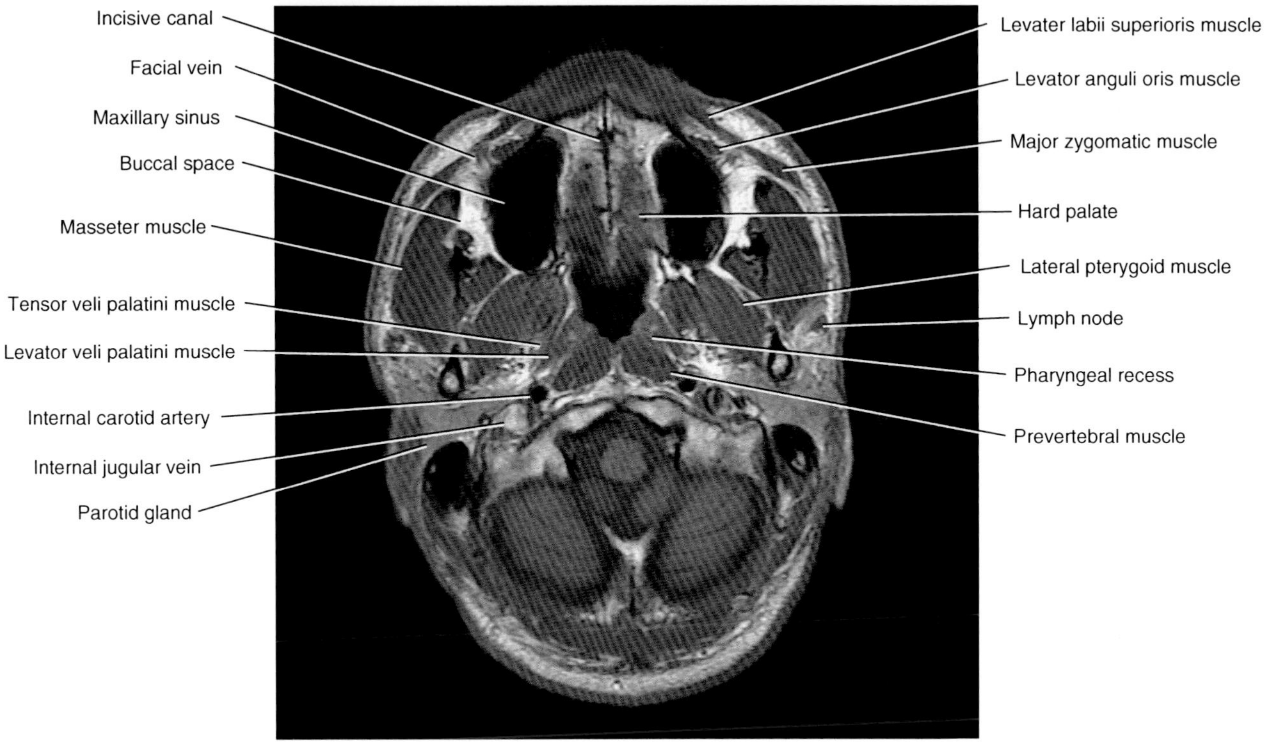

Fig. 5.2 Axial T1-weighted MRI

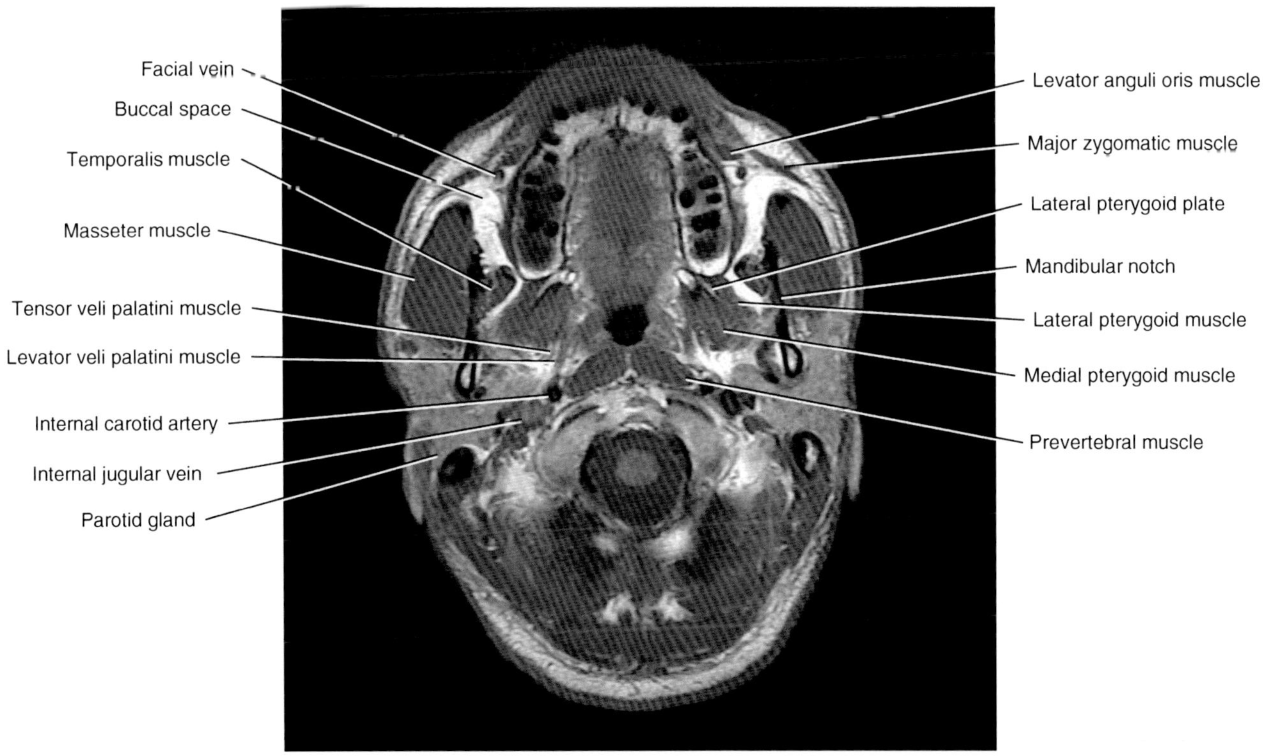

Fig. 5.3 Axial T1-weighted MRI

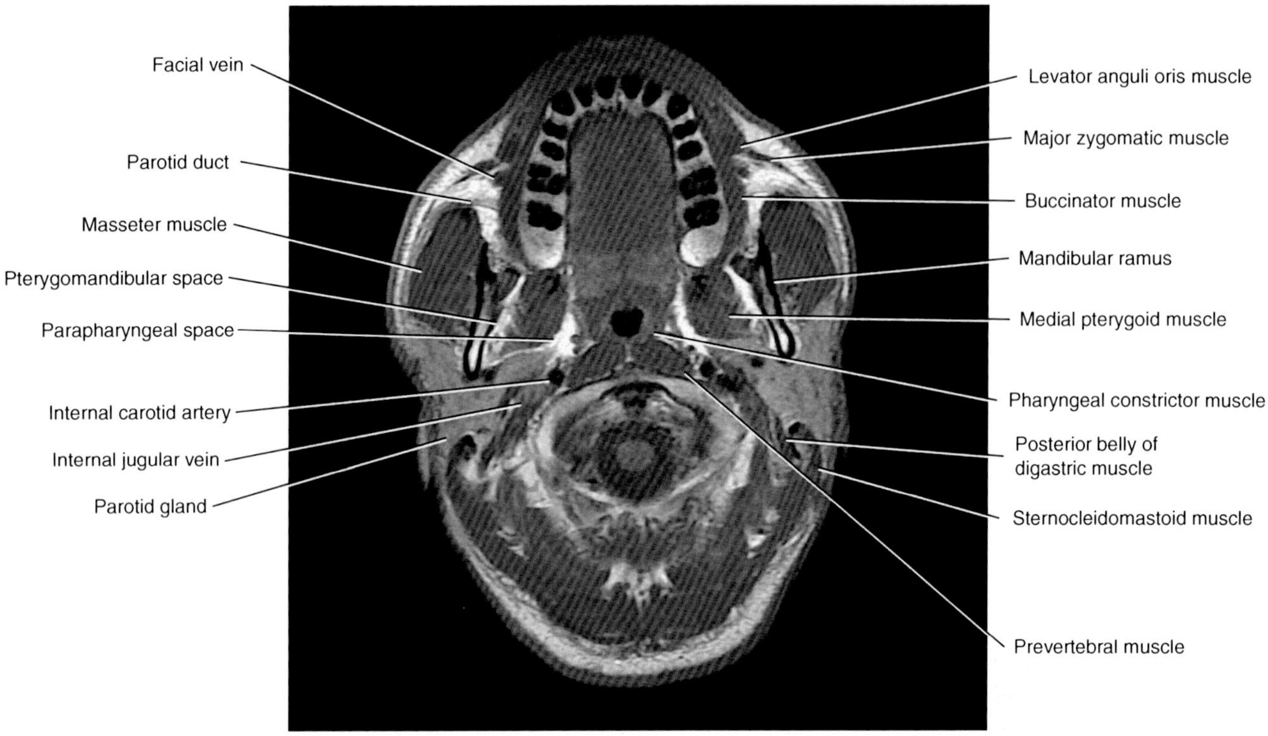

Fig. 5.4 Axial T1-weighted MRI

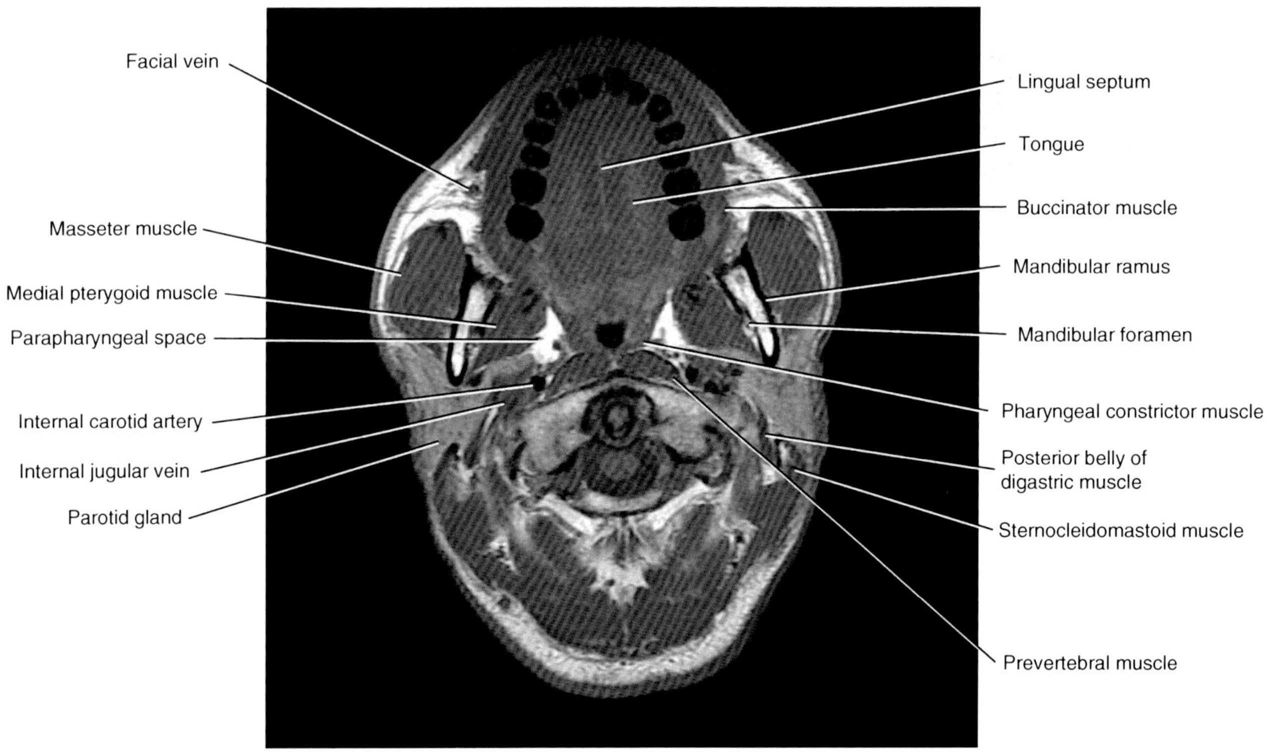

Fig. 5.5 Axial T1-weighted MRI

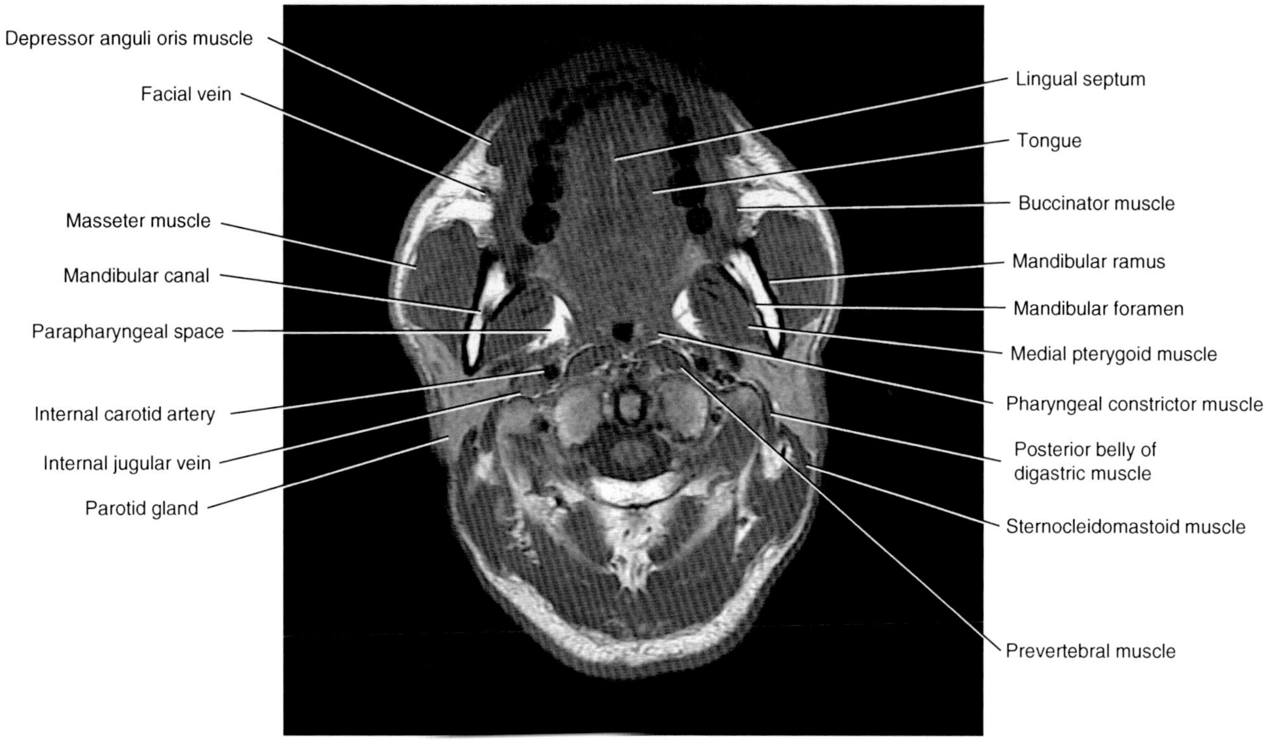

Fig. 5.6 Axial T1-weighted MRI

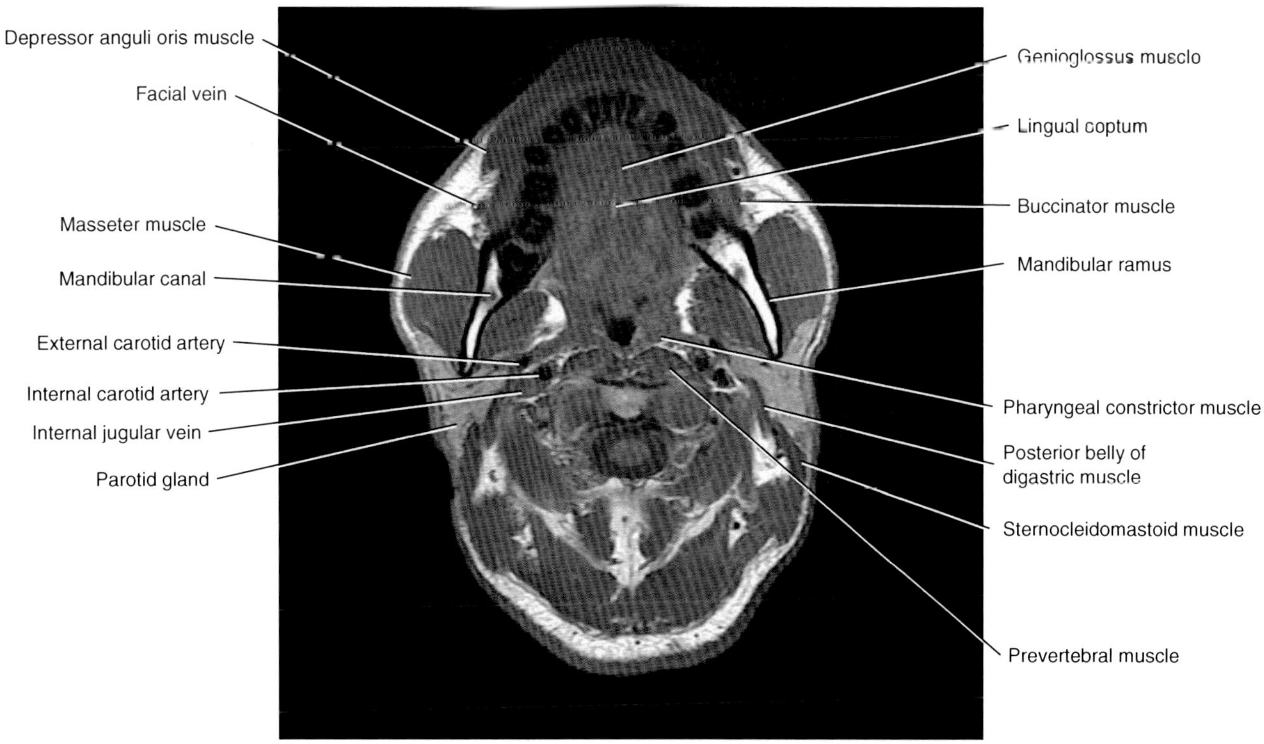

Fig. 5.7 Axial T1-weighted MRI

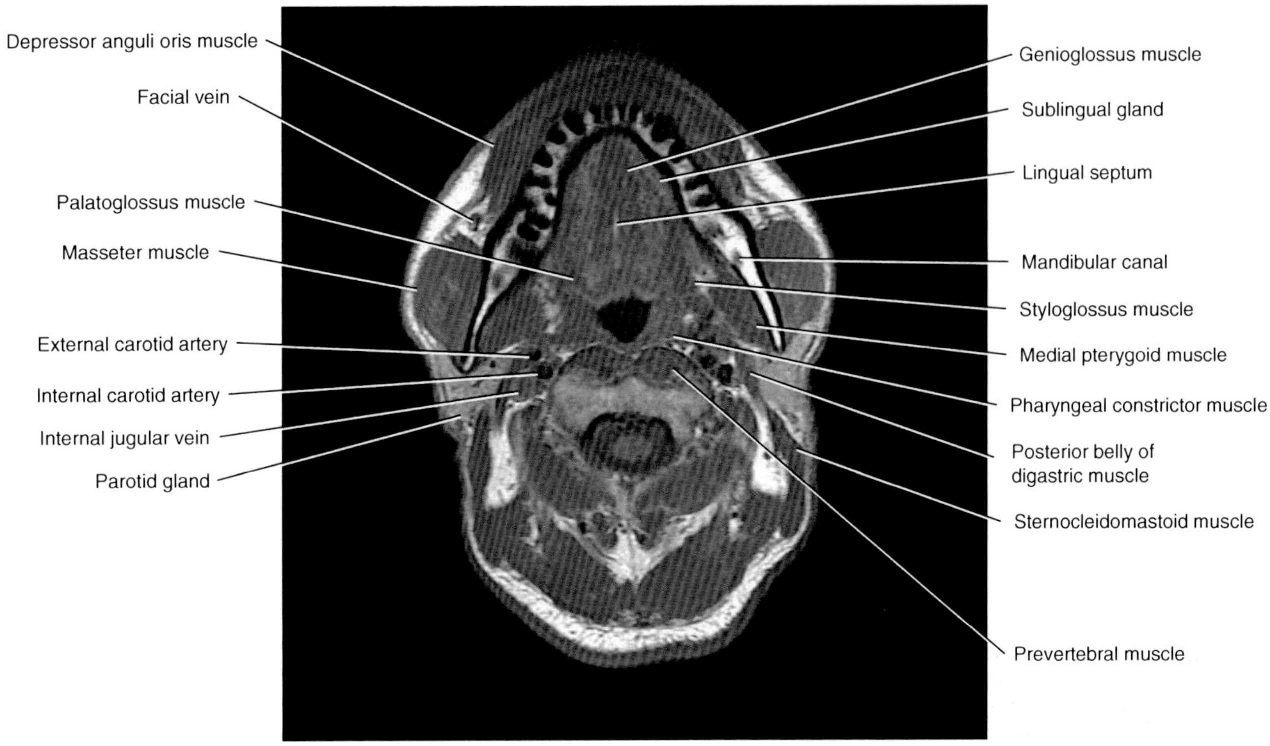

Fig. 5.8 Axial T1-weighted MRI

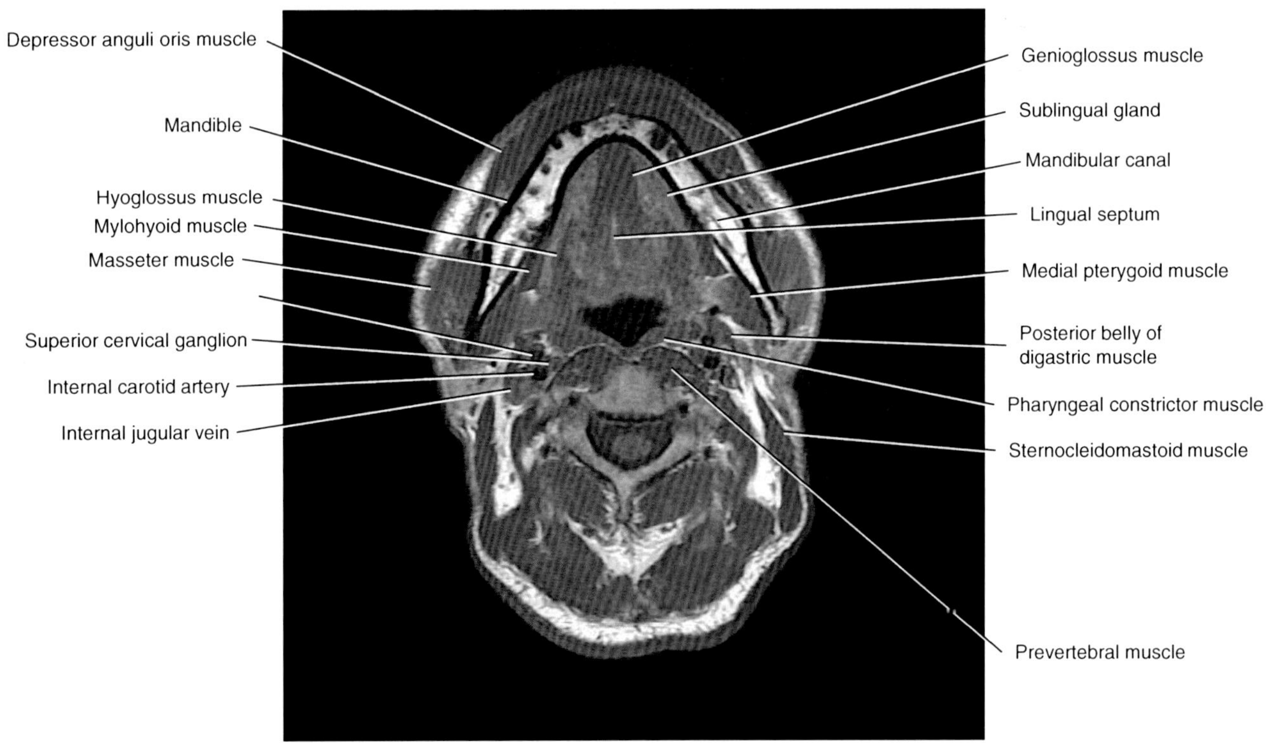

Fig. 5.9 Axial T1-weighted MRI

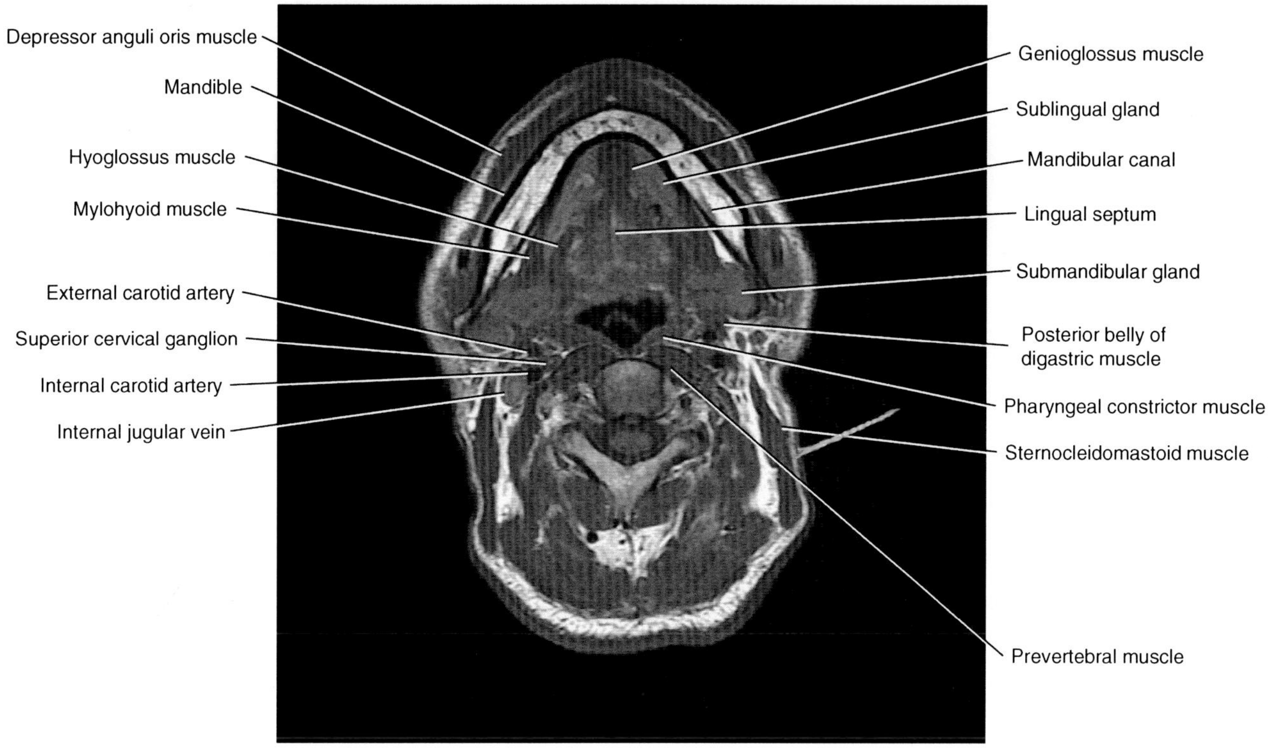

Fig. 5.10 Axial T1-weighted MRI

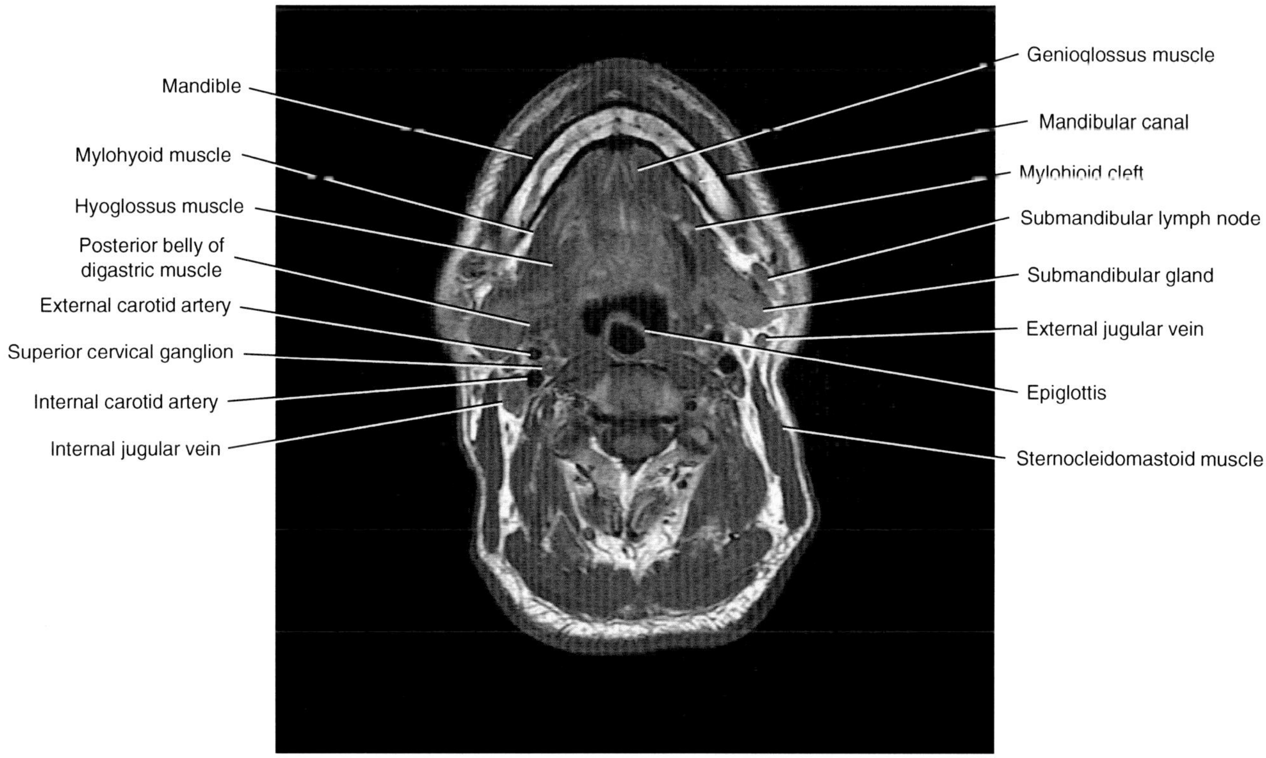

Fig. 5.11 Axial T1-weighted MRI

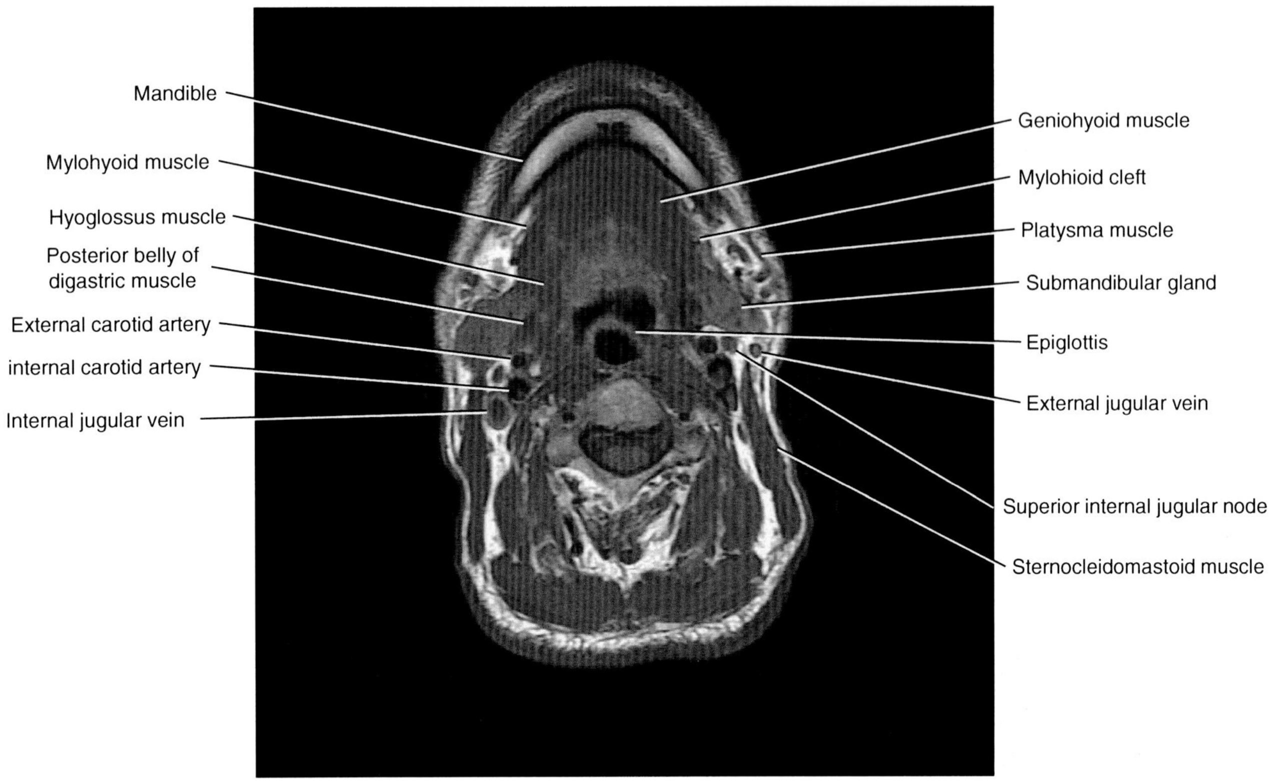

Fig. 5.12 Axial T1-weighted MRI

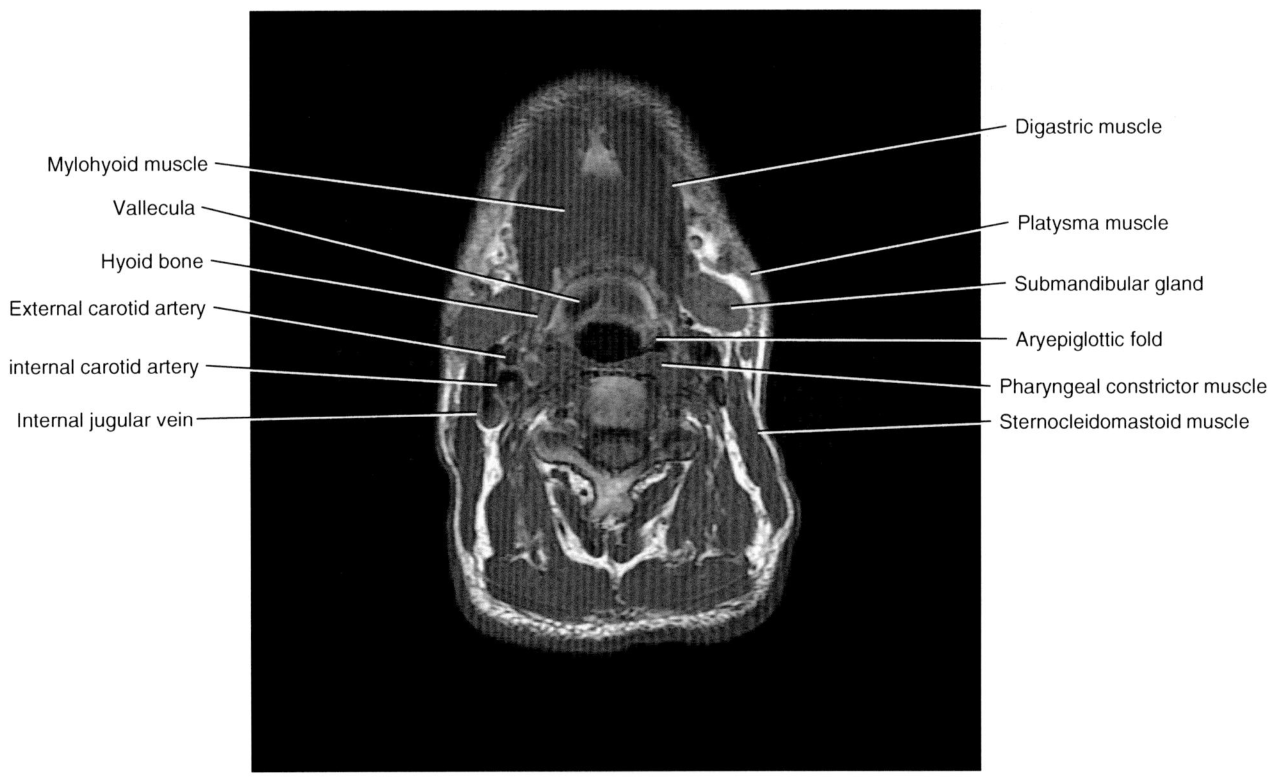

Fig. 5.13 Axial T1-weighted MRI

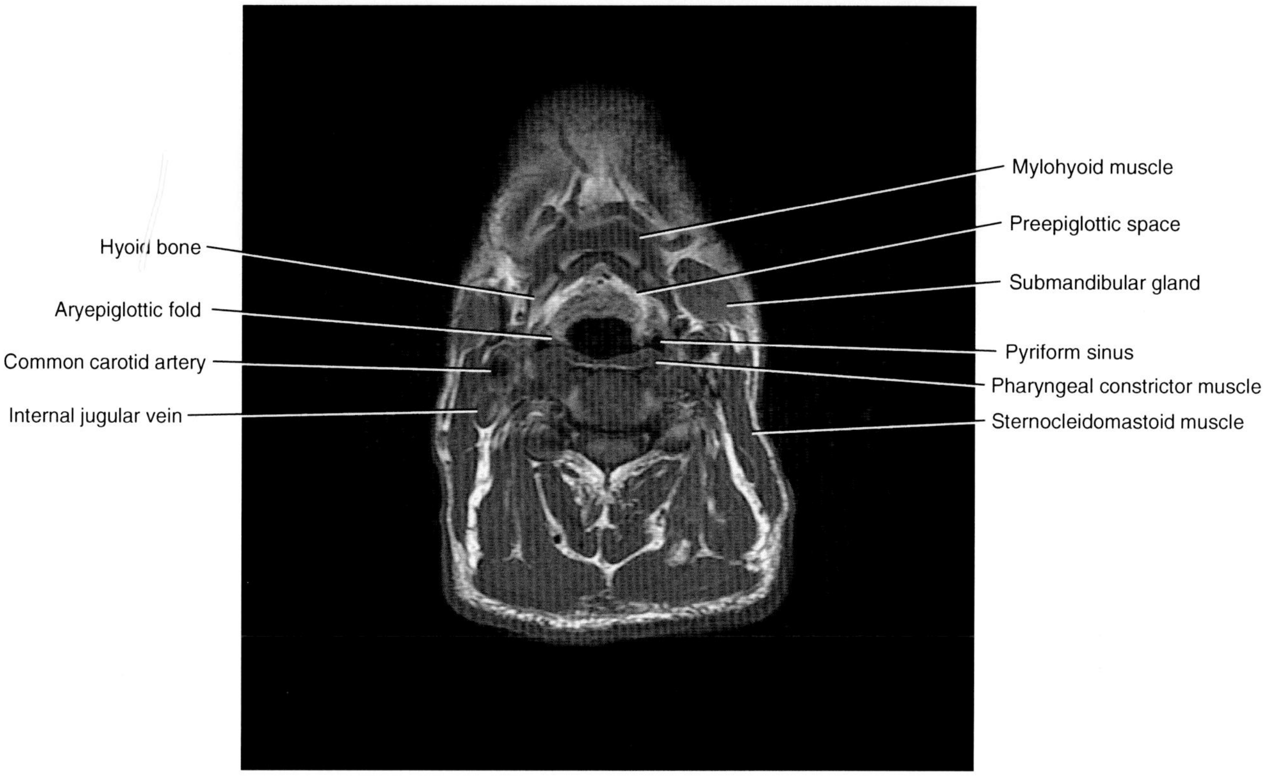

Fig. 5.14 Axial T1-weighted MRI

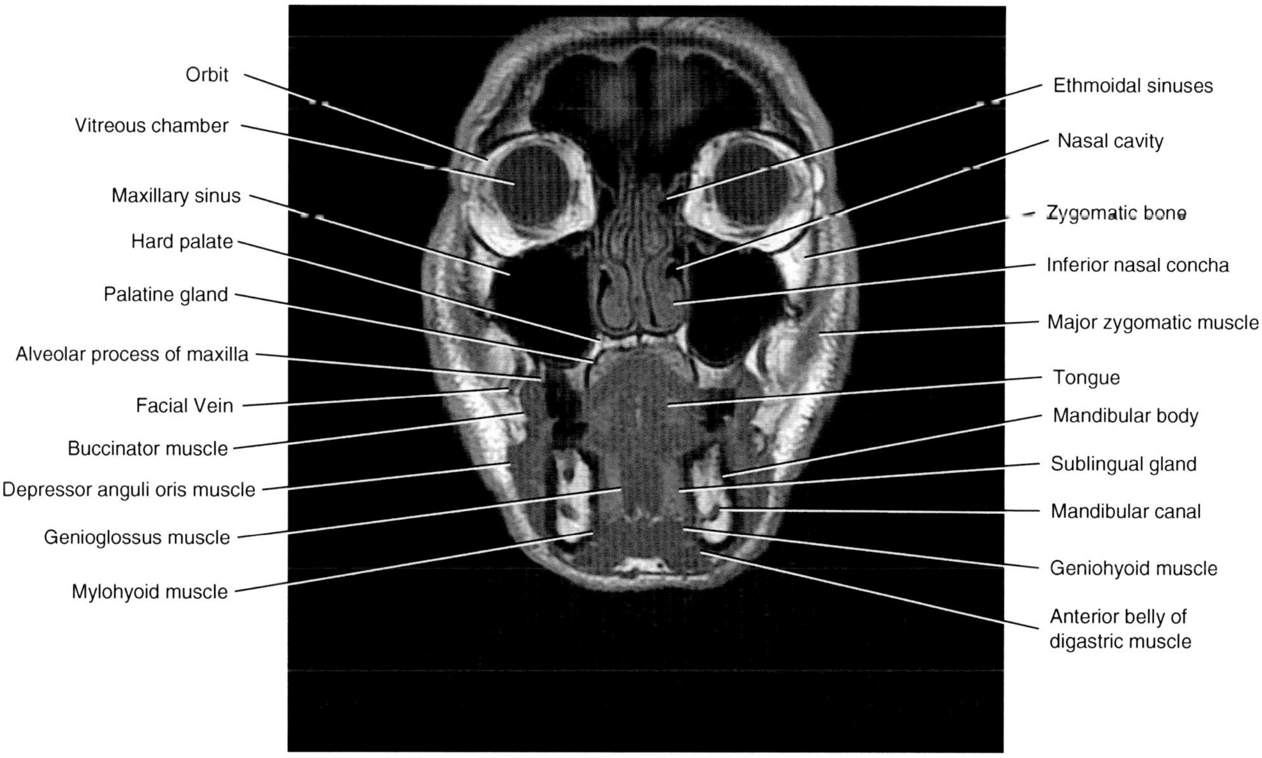

Fig. 5.15 Coronal T1-weighted MRI

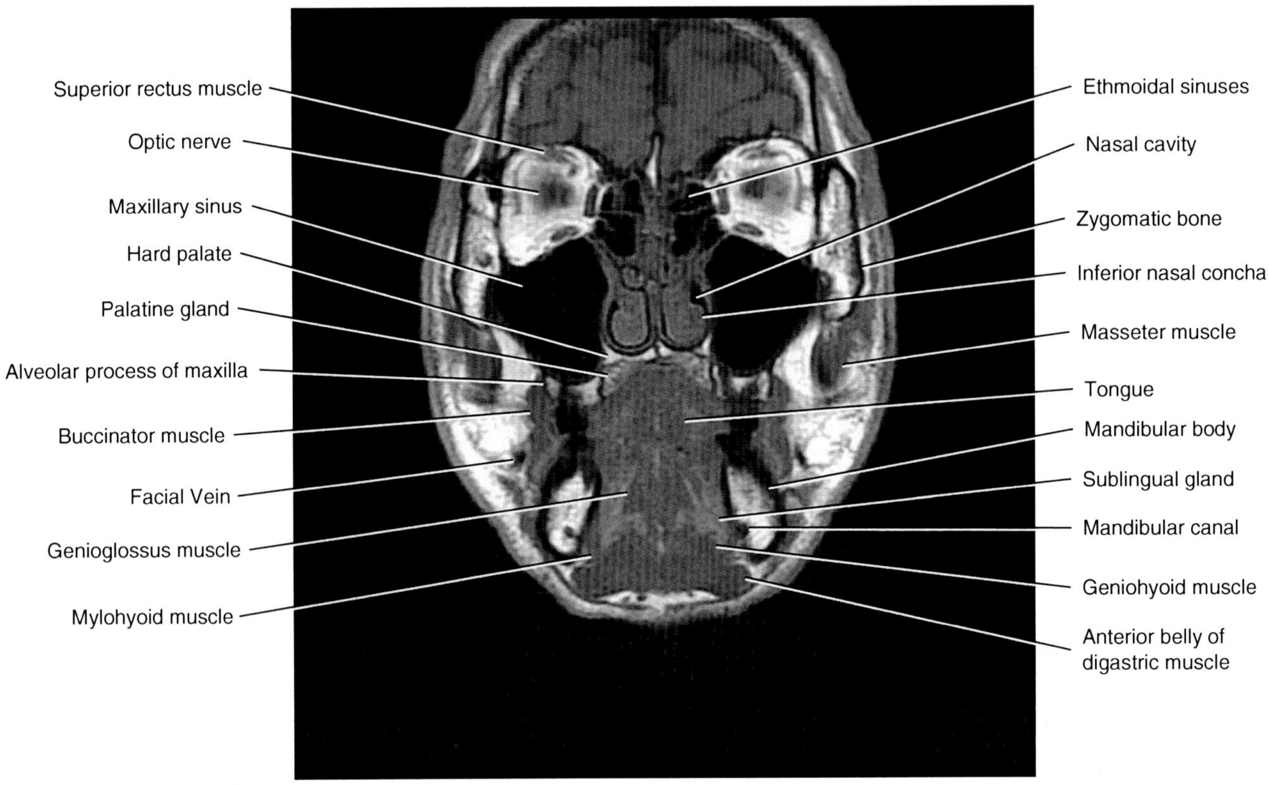

Fig. 5.16 Coronal T1-weighted MRI

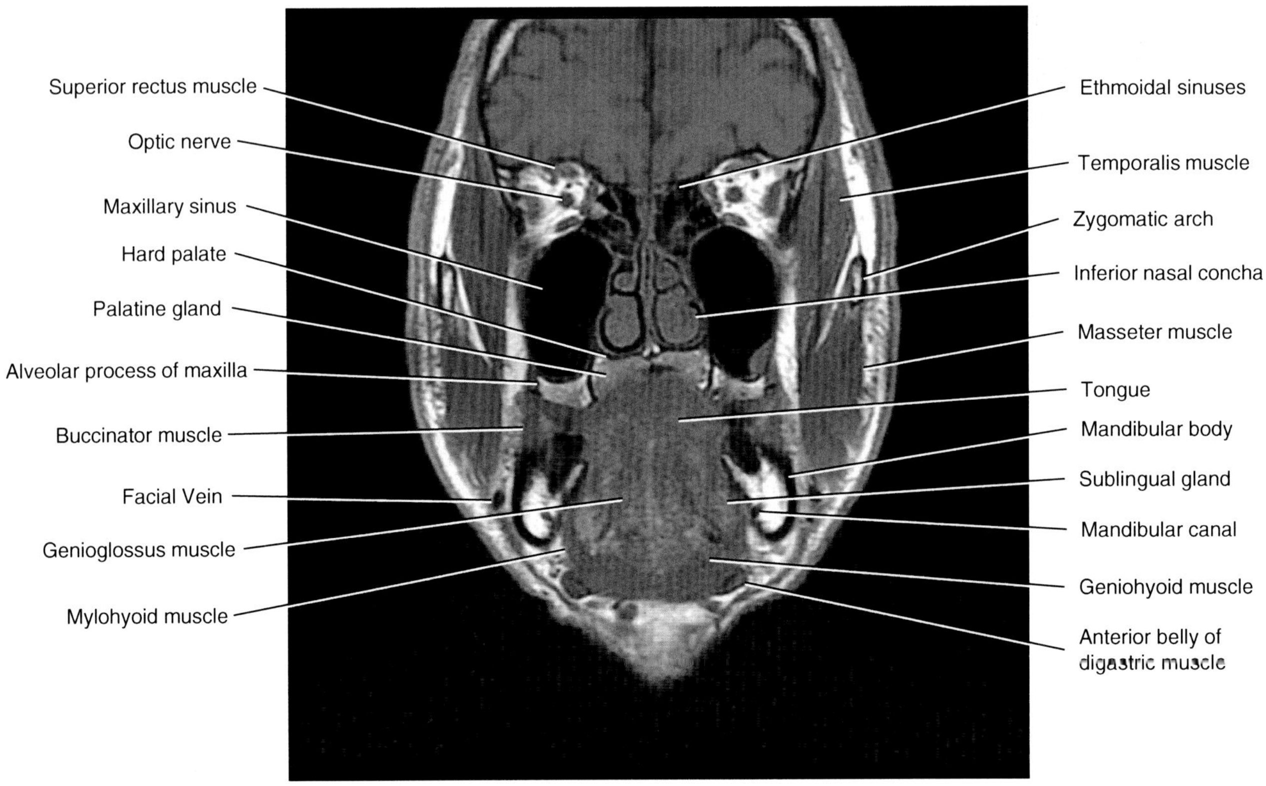

Fig. 5.17 Coronal T1-weighted MRI

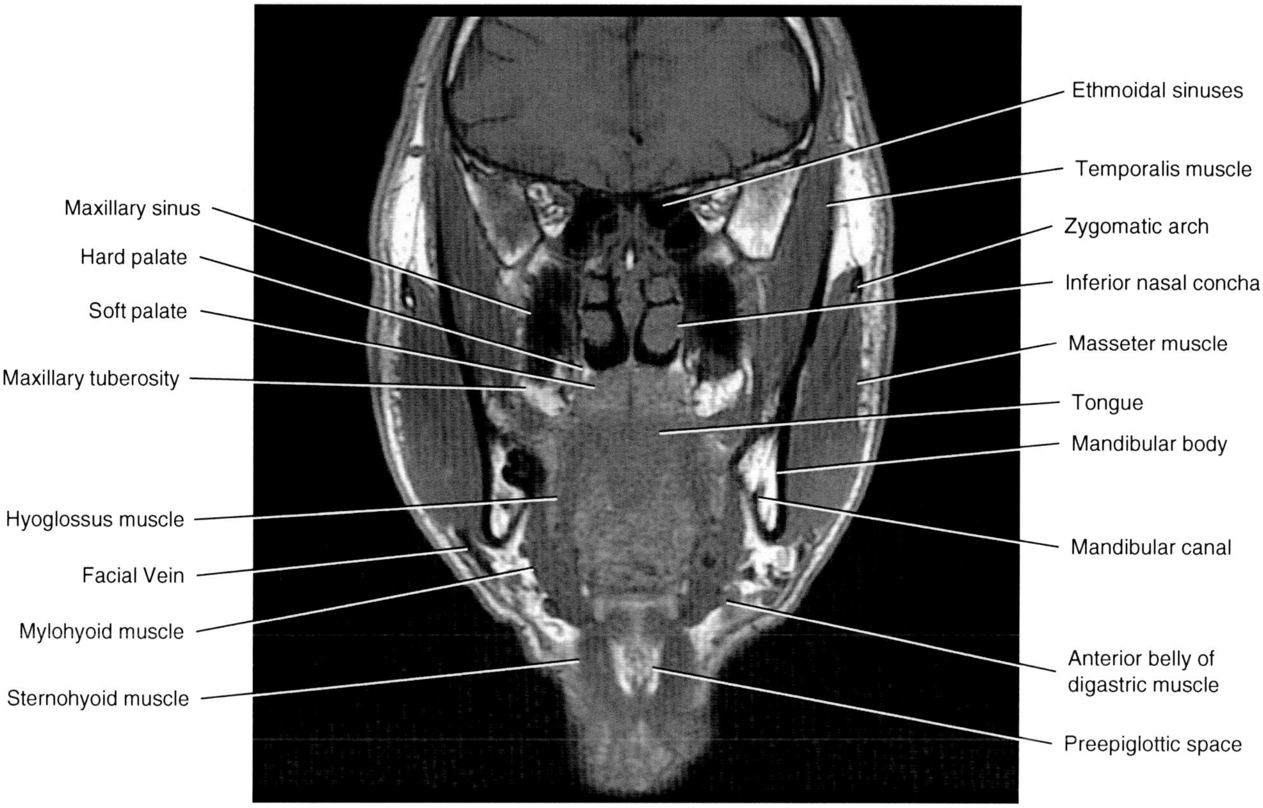

Fig. 5.18 Coronal T1-weighted MRI

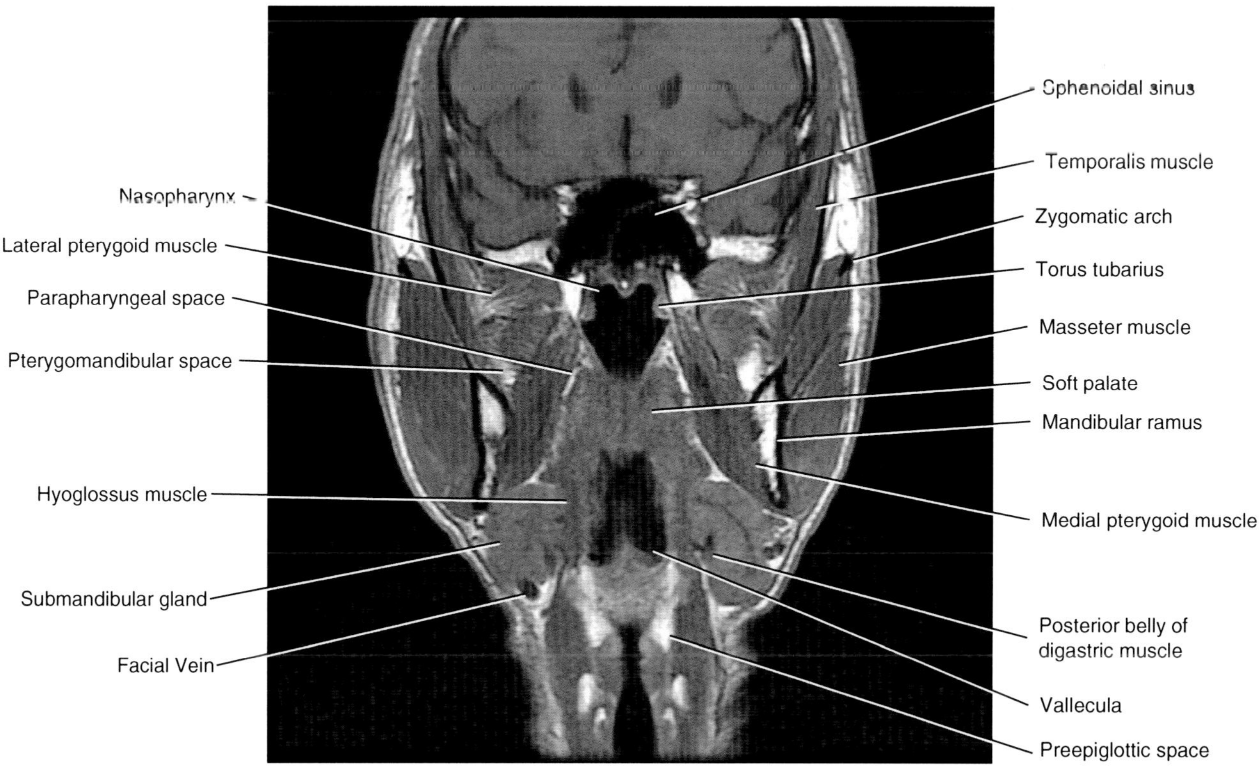

Fig. 5.19 Coronal T1-weighted MRI

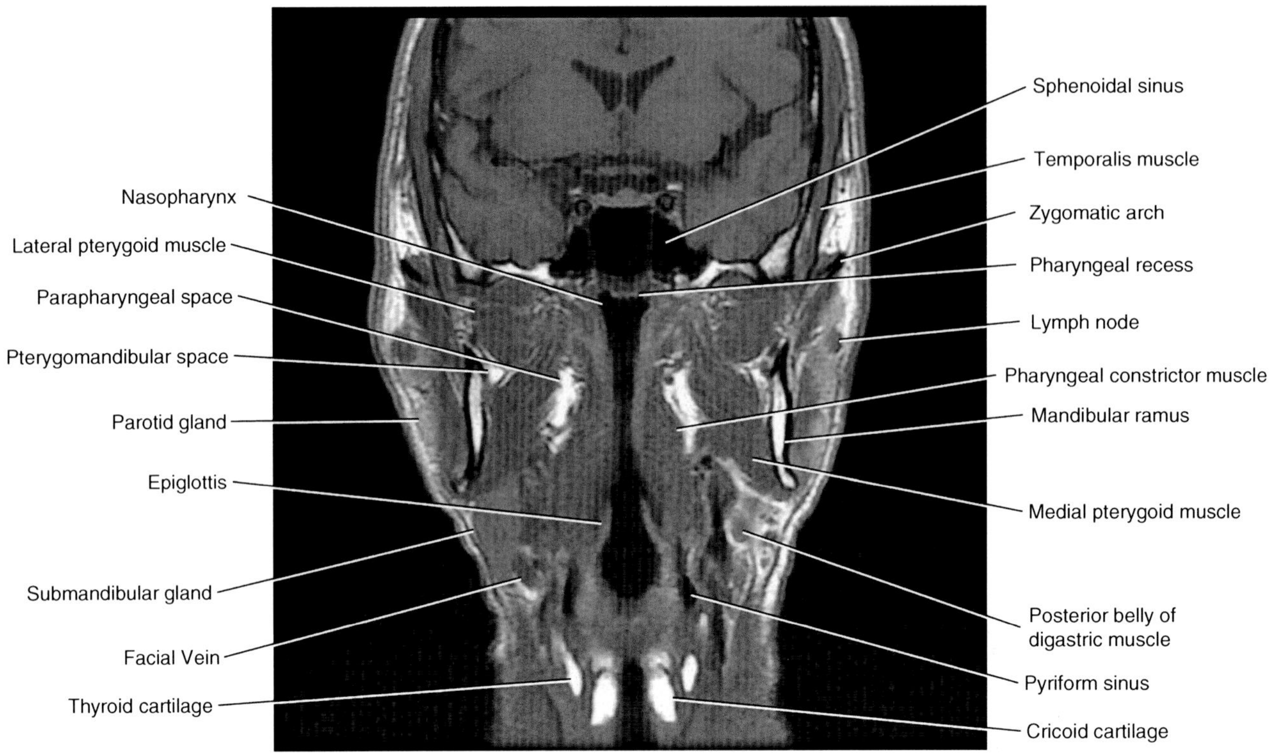

Fig. 5.20 Coronal T1-weighted MRI

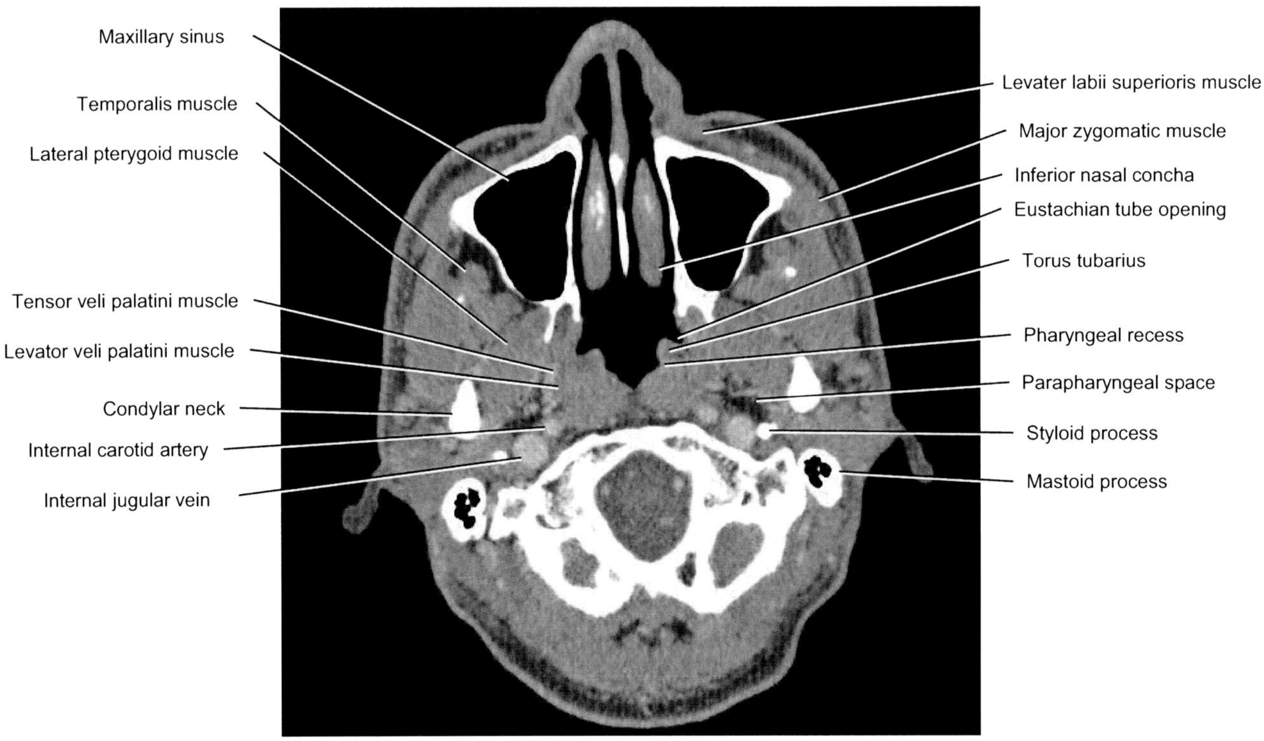

Fig. 5.21 Axial CECT

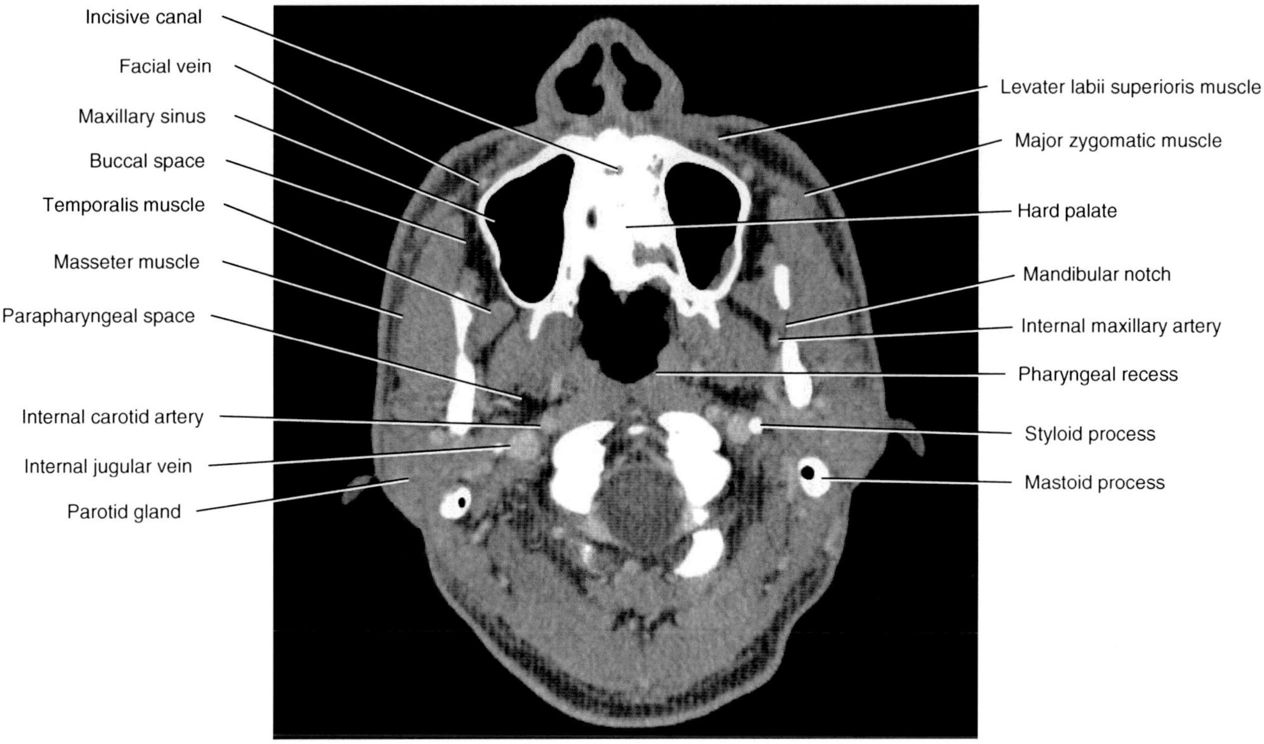

Fig. 5.22 Axial CECT

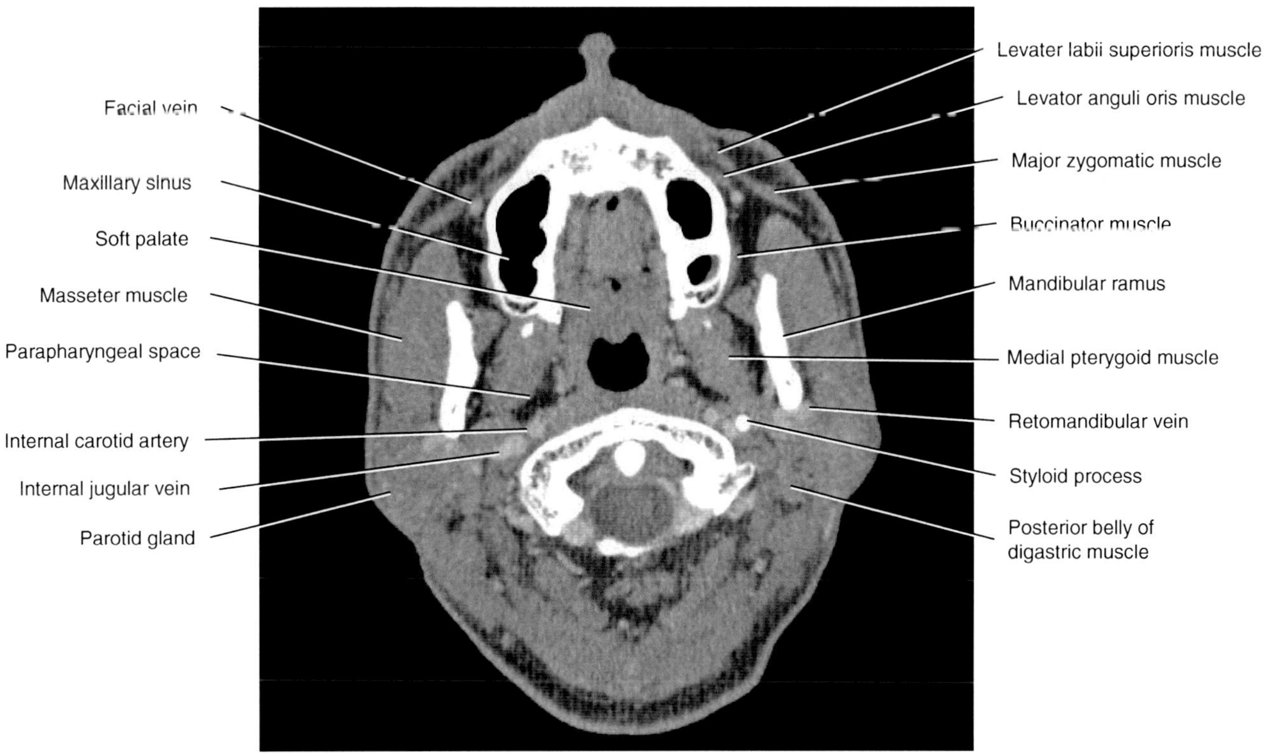

Fig. 5.23 Axial CECT

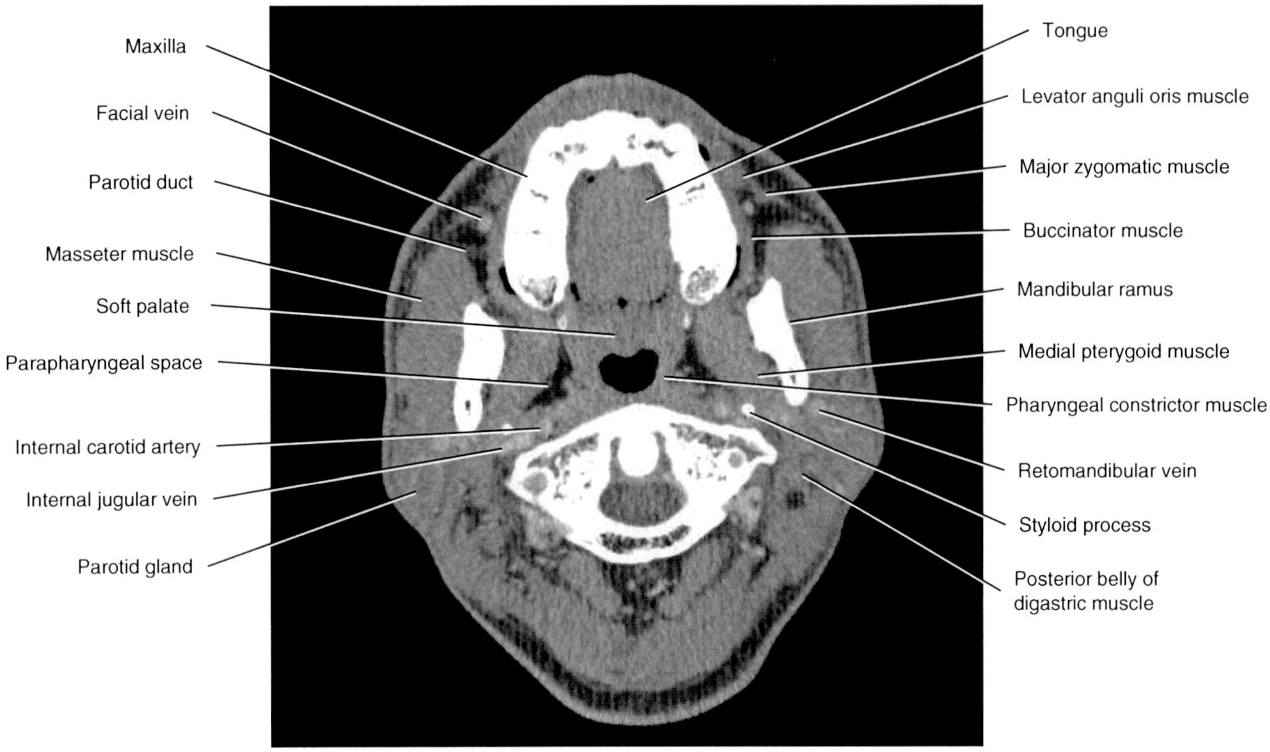

Fig. 5.24 Axial CECT

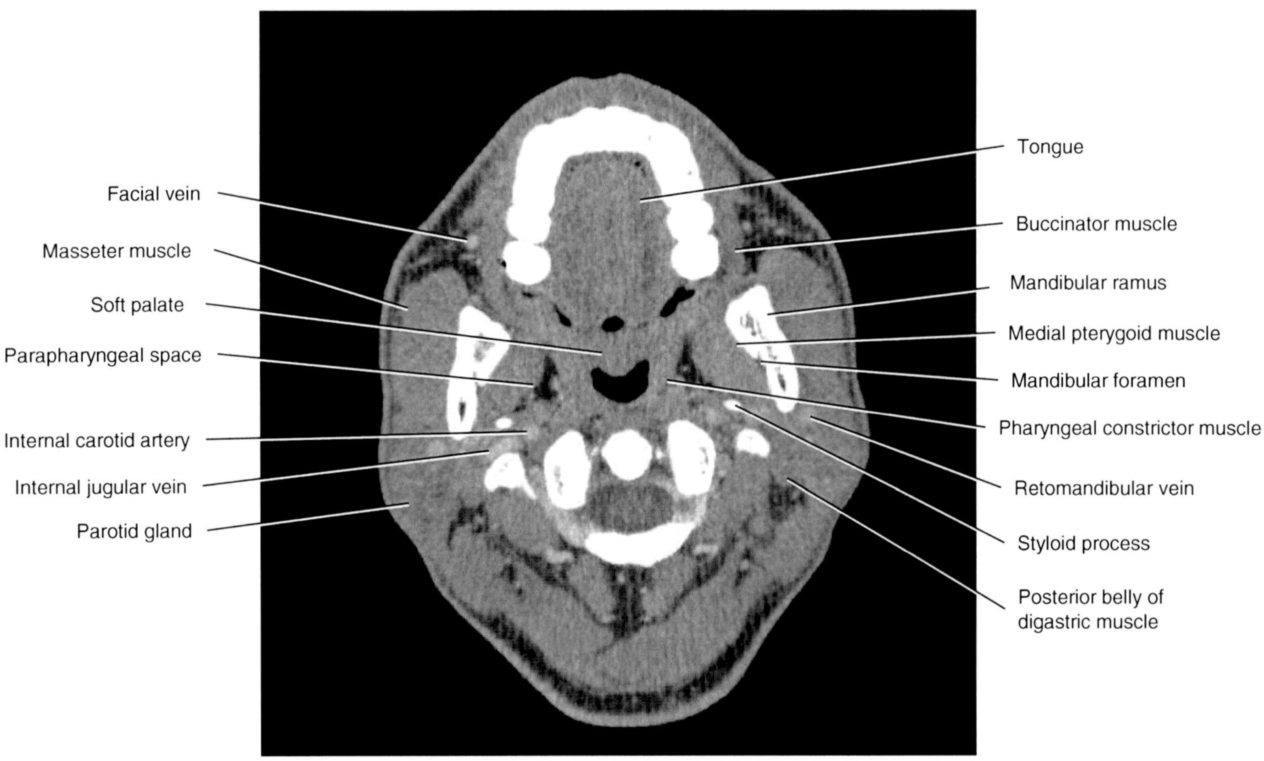

Fig. 5.25 Axial CECT

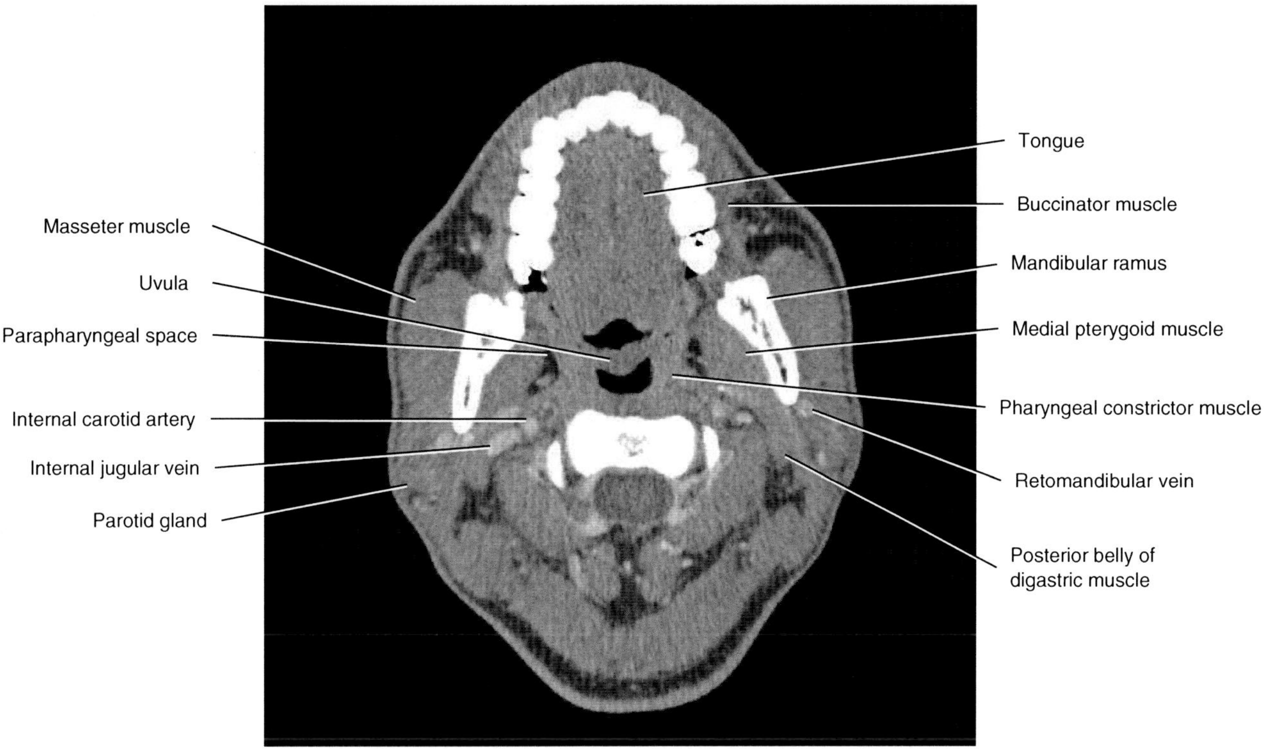

Fig. 5.26 Axial CECT

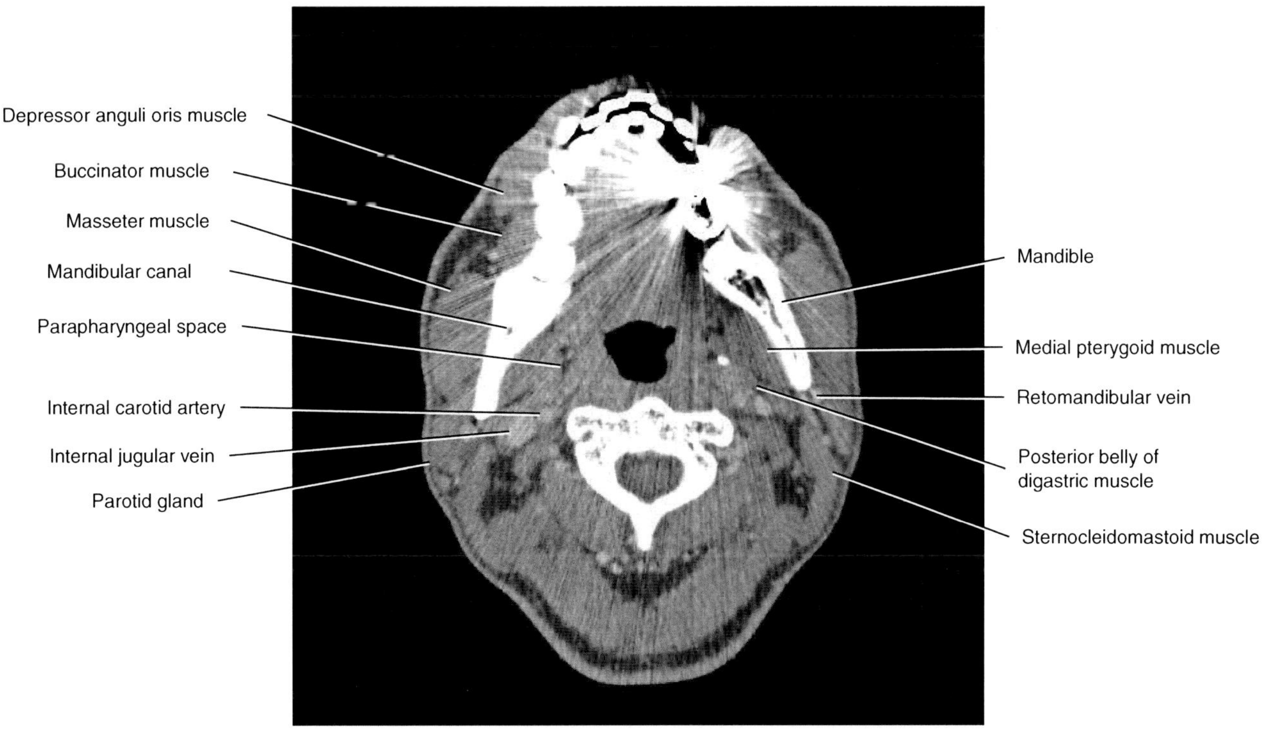

Fig. 5.27 Axial CECT

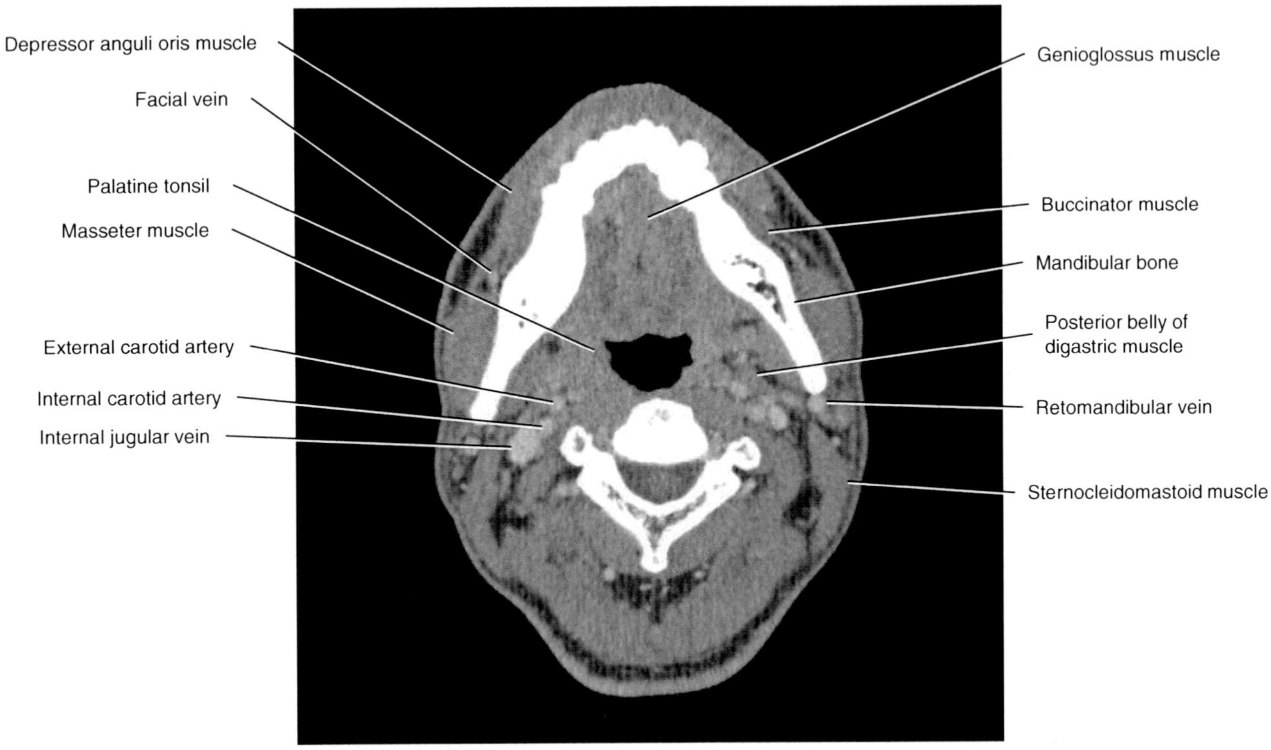

Fig. 5.28 Axial CECT

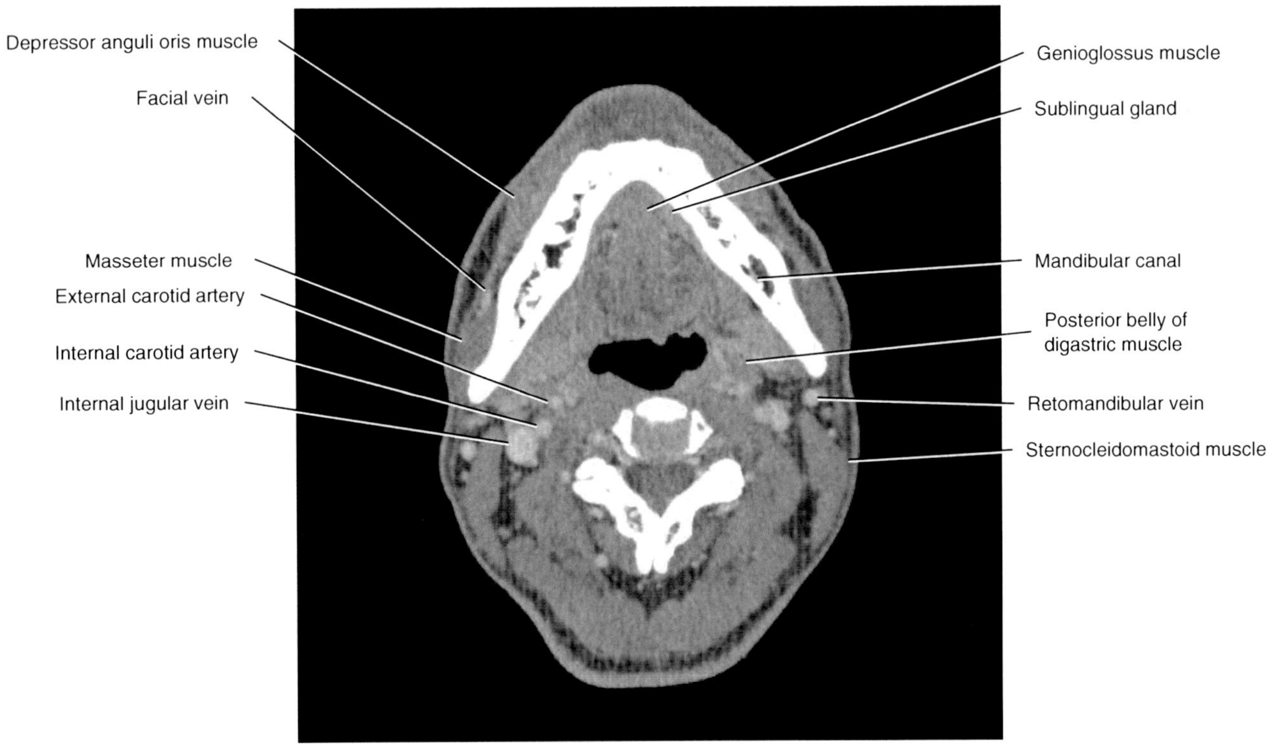

Fig. 5.29 Axial CECT

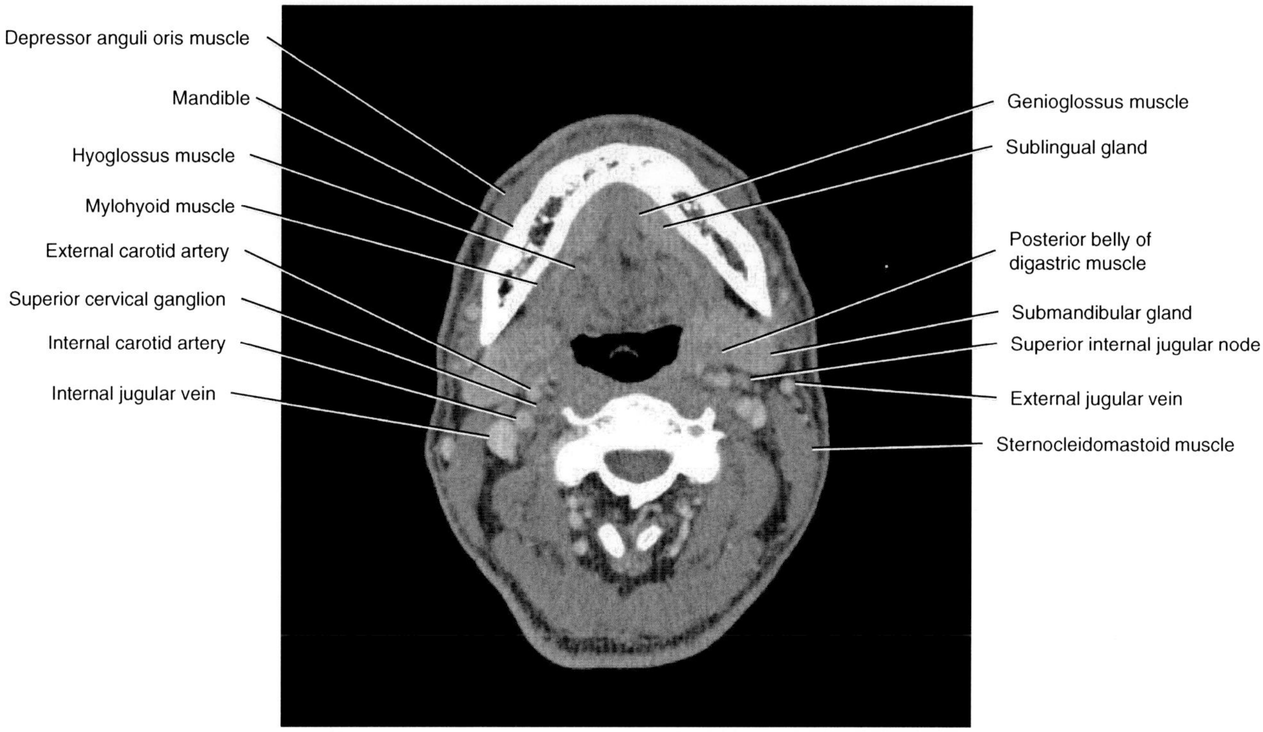

Fig. 5.30 Axial CECT

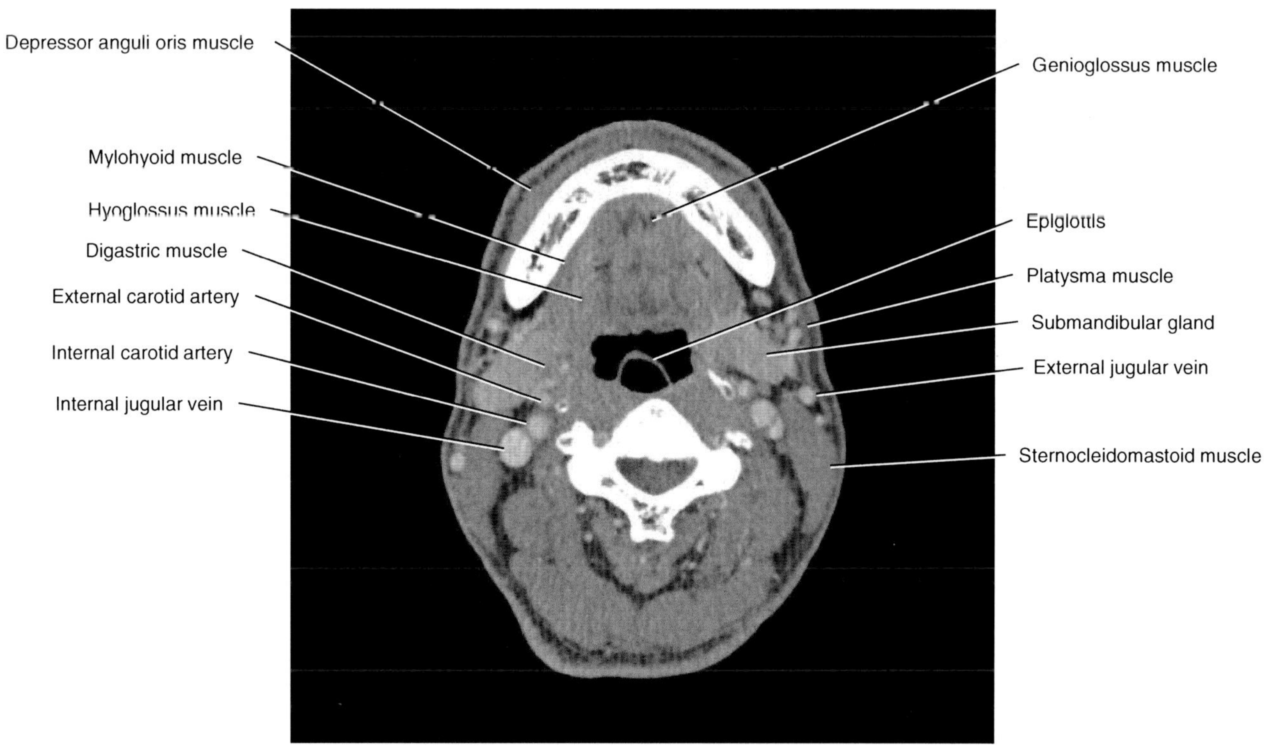

Fig. 5.31 Axial CECT

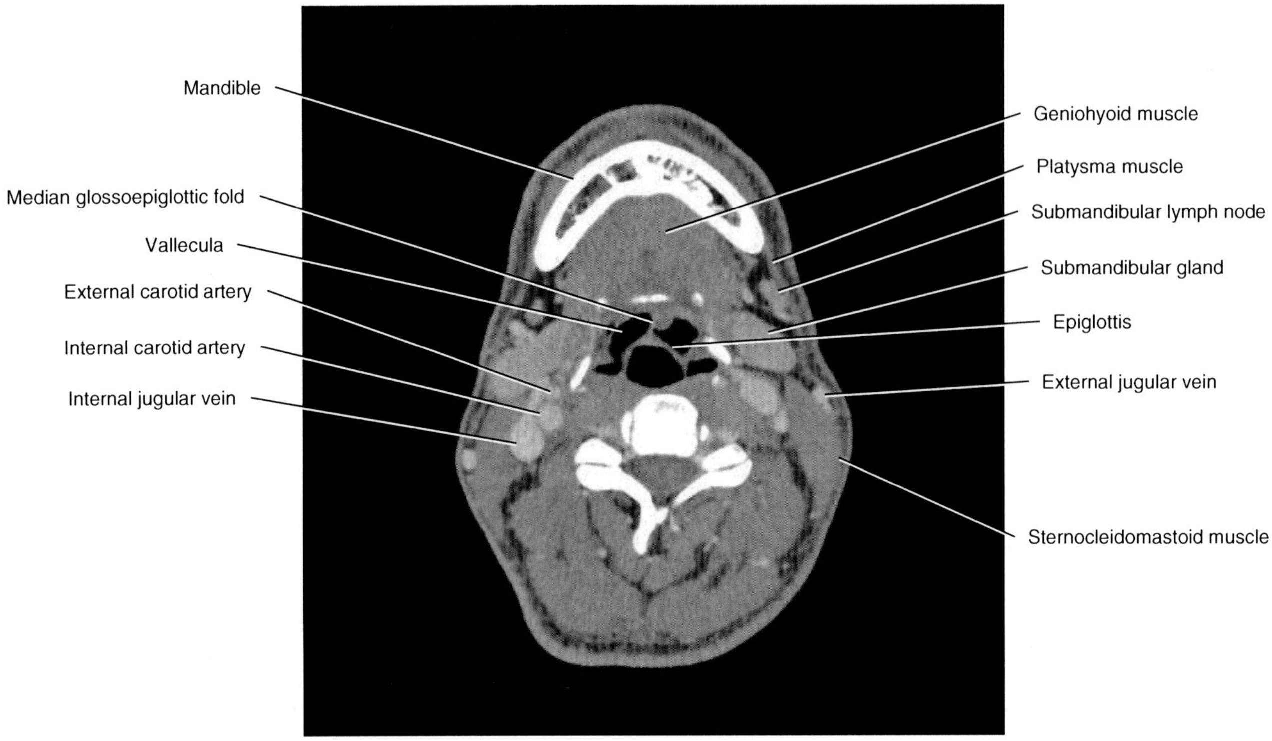

Fig. 5.32 Axial CECT

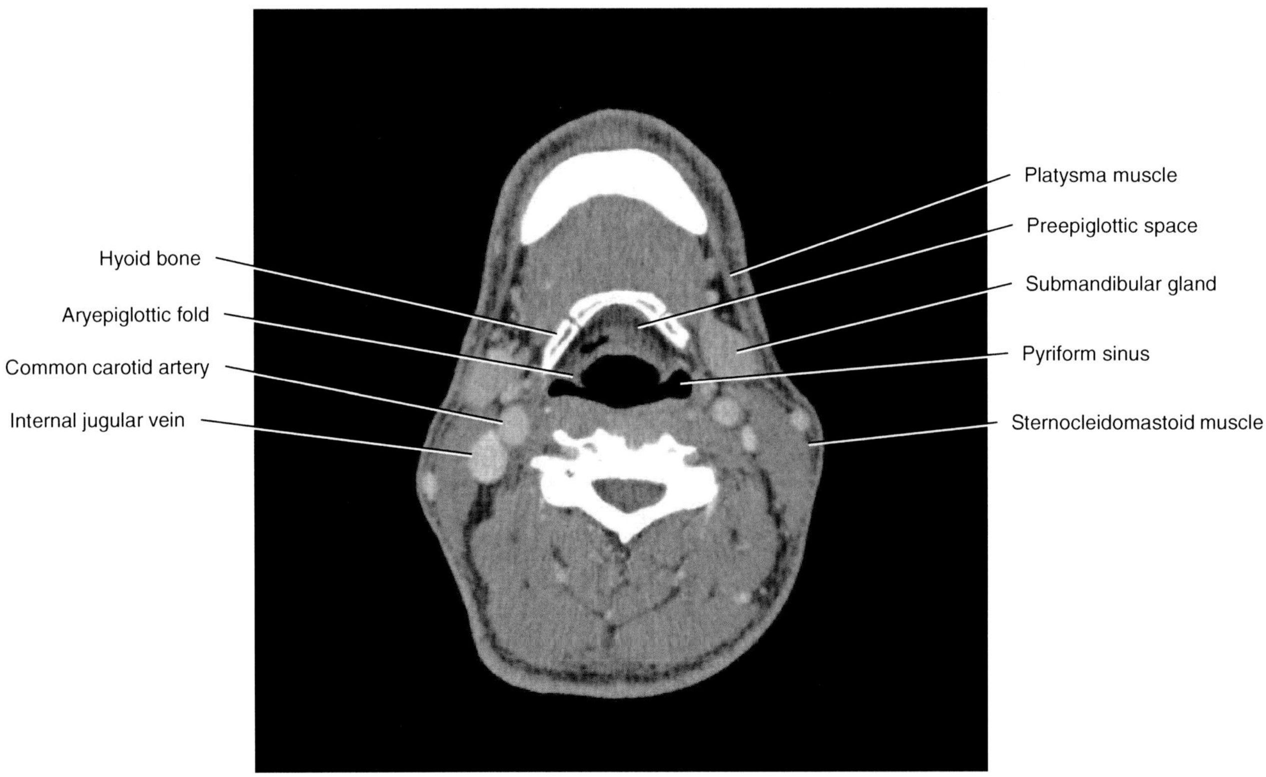

Fig. 5.33 Axial CECT

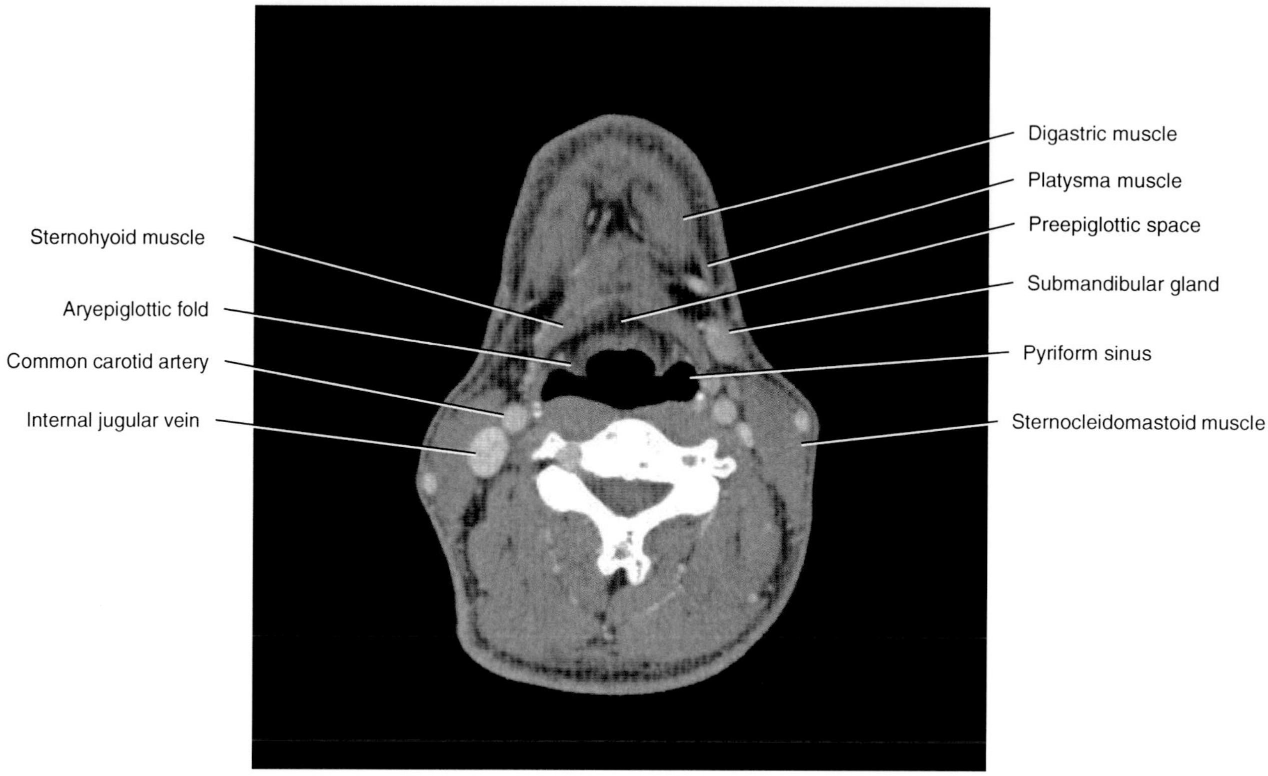

Fig. 5.34 Axial CECT

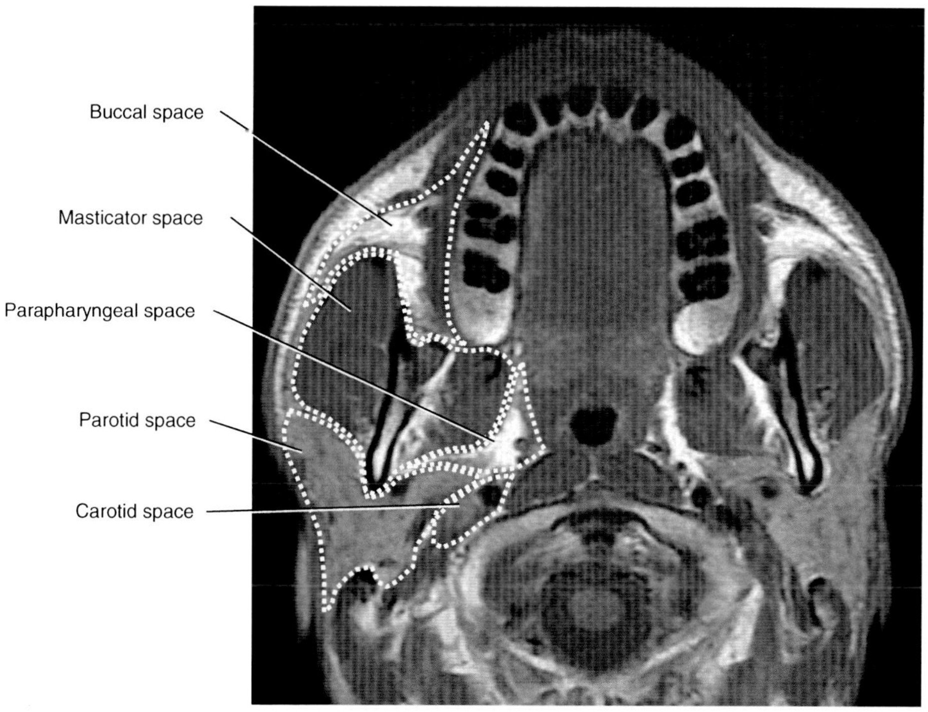

Fig. 5.35 Axial T1-weighted MRI at the level of the maxillary alveolar process

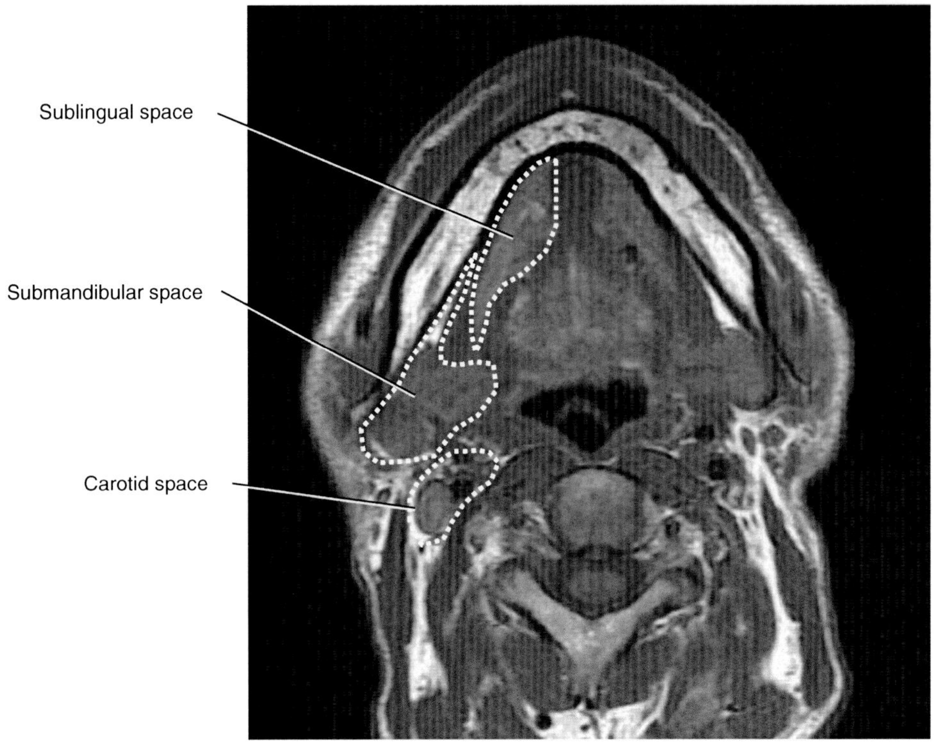

Fig. 5.36 Axial T1-weighted MRI at the level of the mental foramen

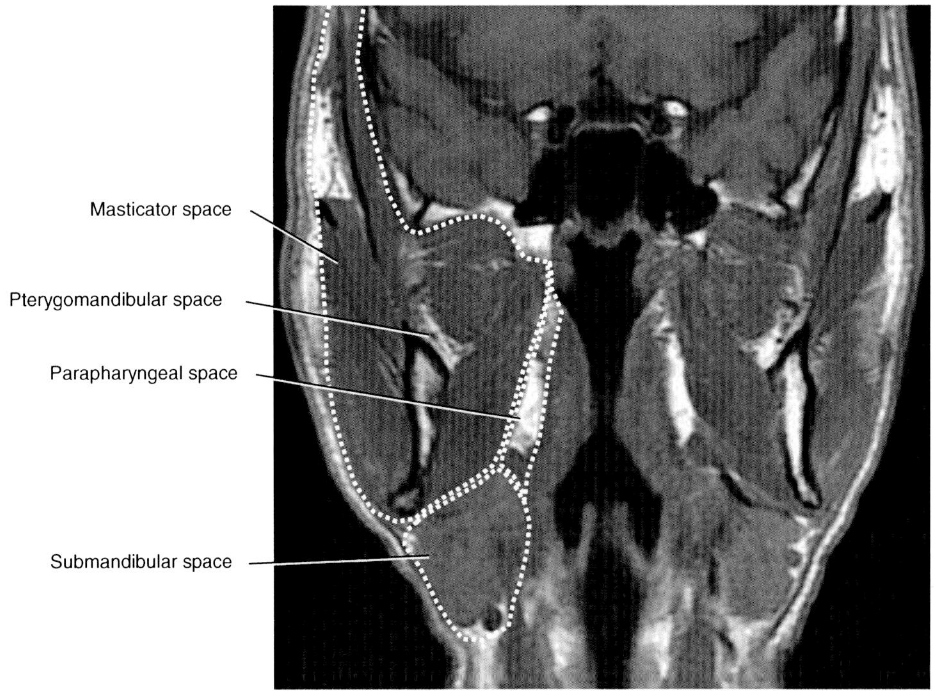

Fig. 5.37 Coronal T1-weighted MRI of the pharyngeal airway

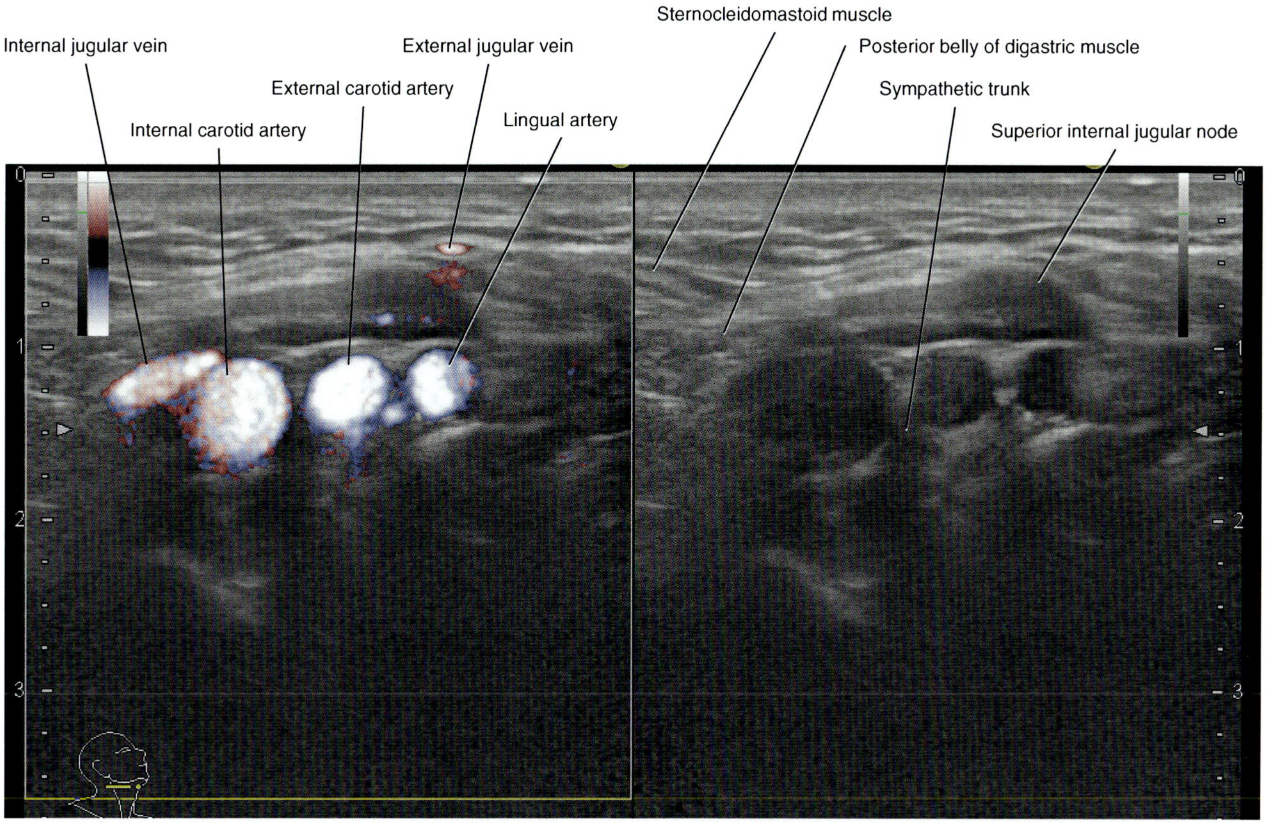

Fig. 5.38 Transverse neck US, right superior internal jugular node (left, fine flow Doppler; right, B-mode)

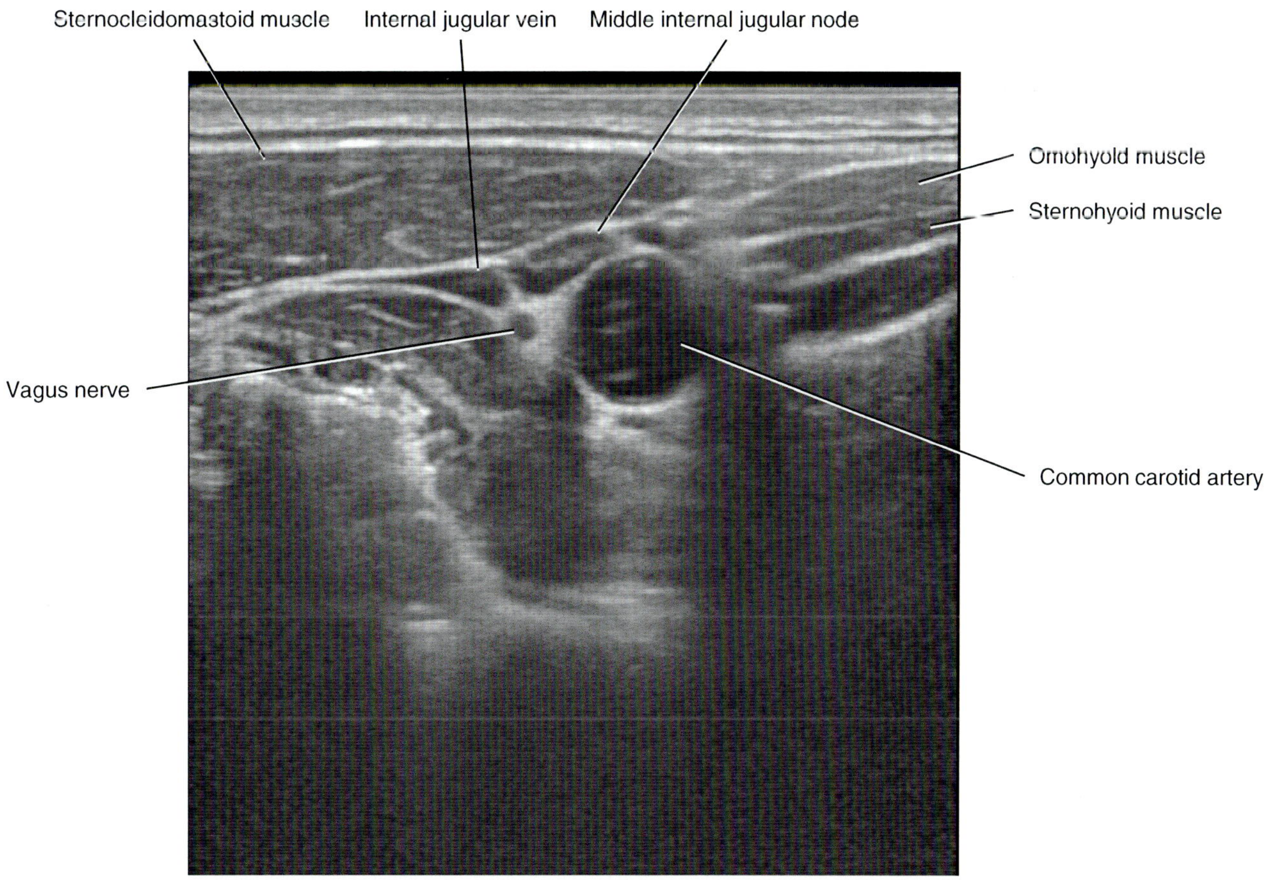

Fig. 5.39 Transverse neck US, right middle internal jugular node

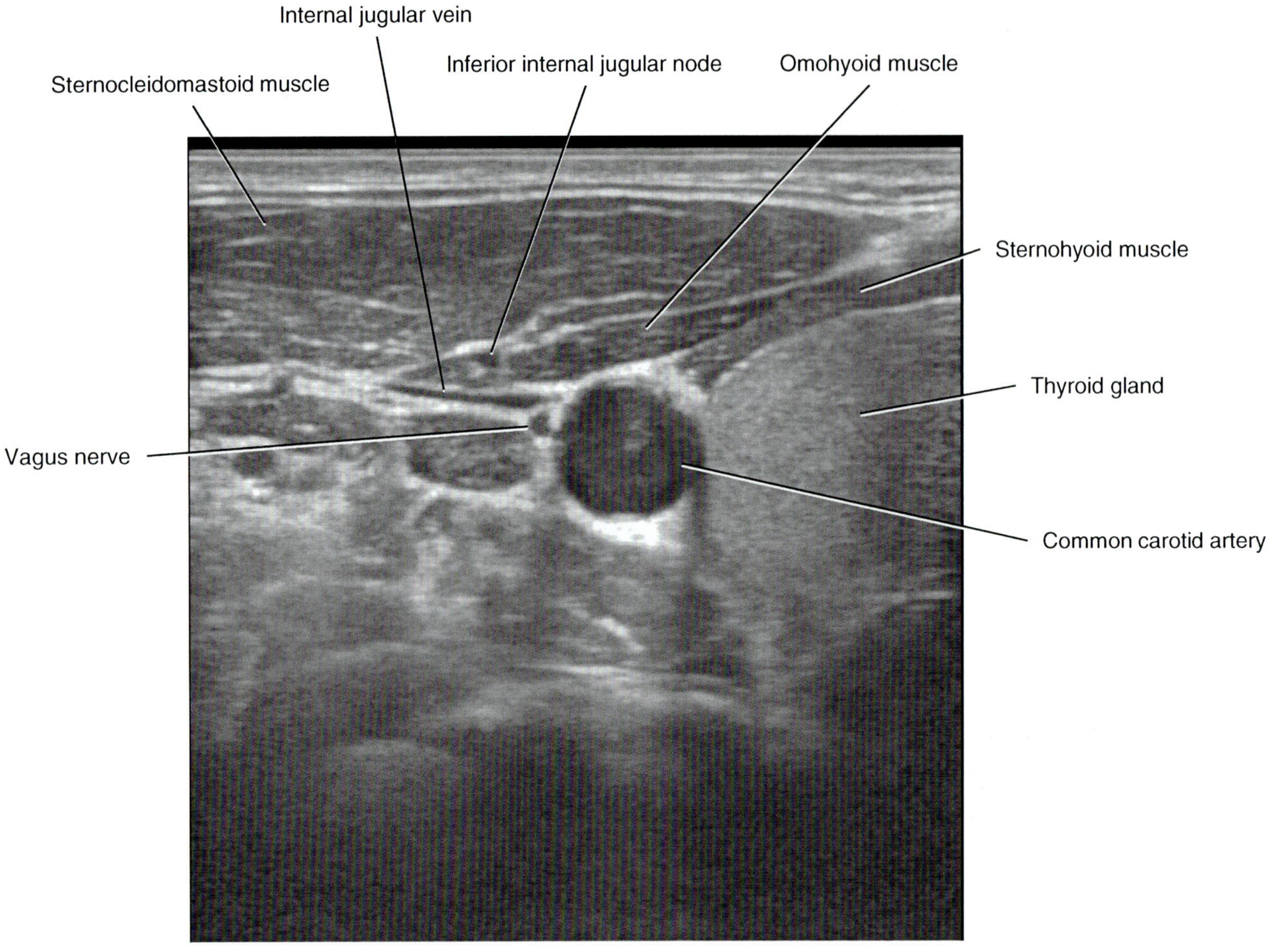

Fig. 5.40 Transverse neck US, right inferior internal jugular node

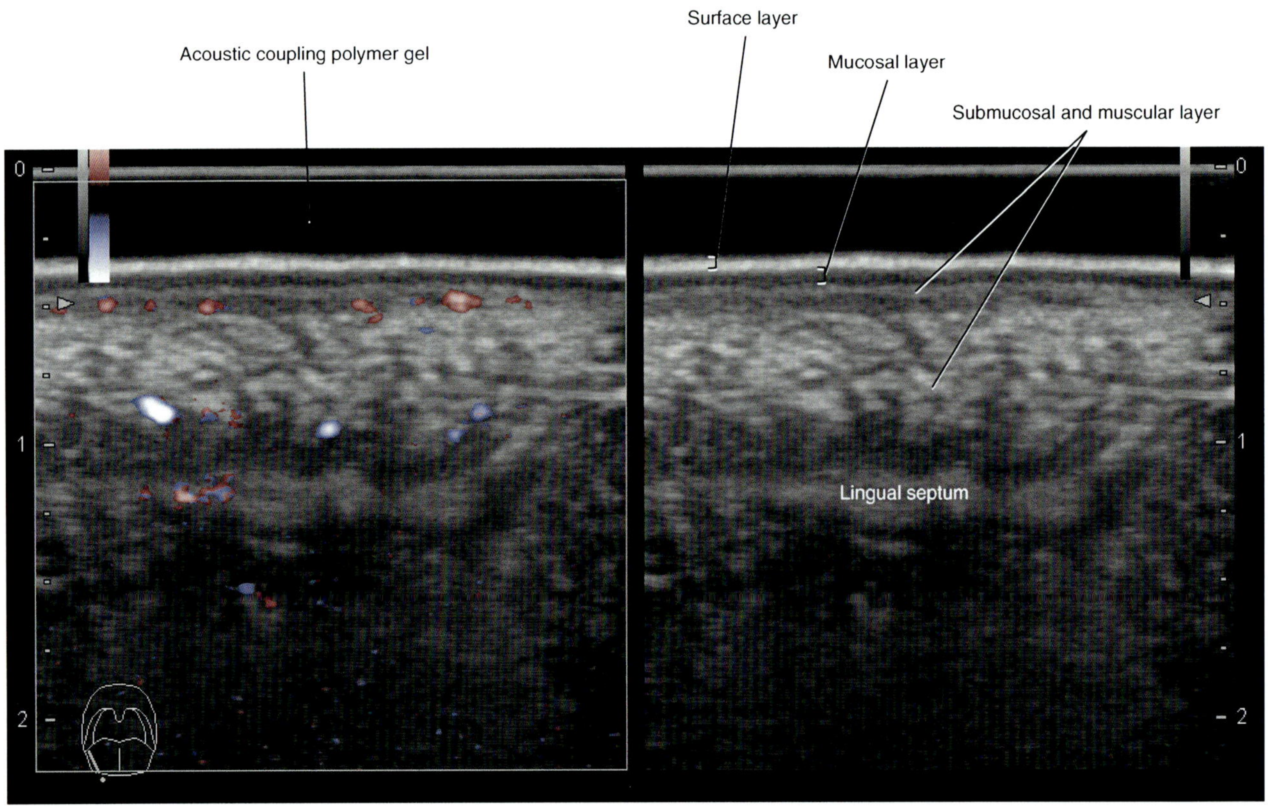

Fig. 5.41 Transverse intraoral US, right lateral margin of the tongue (left, fine flow Doppler; right, B-mode)

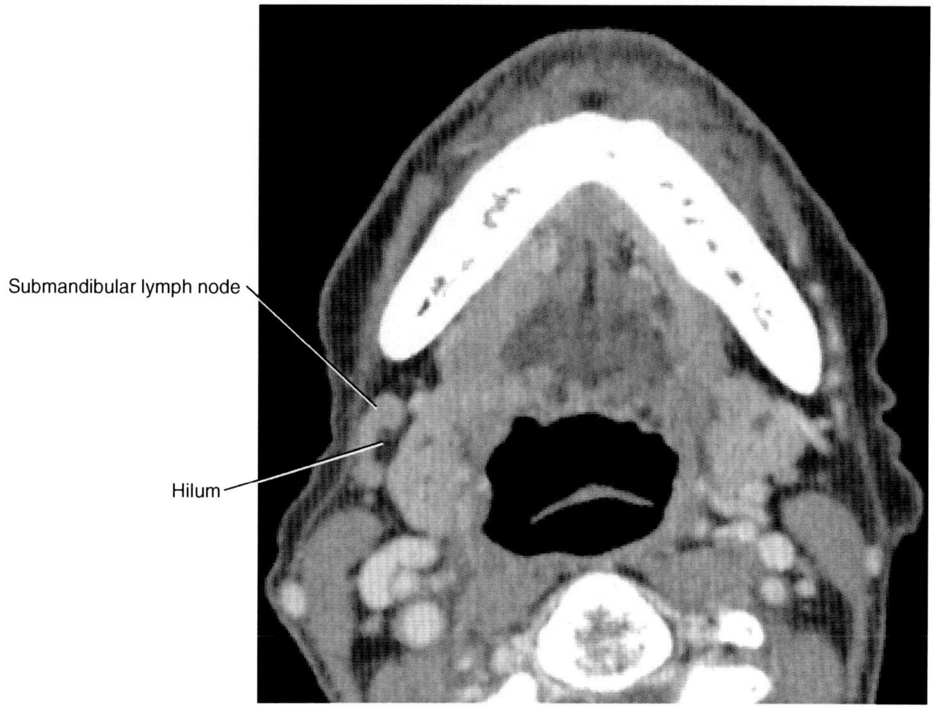

Fig. 5.42 Axial CECT of the right normal submandibular lymph node

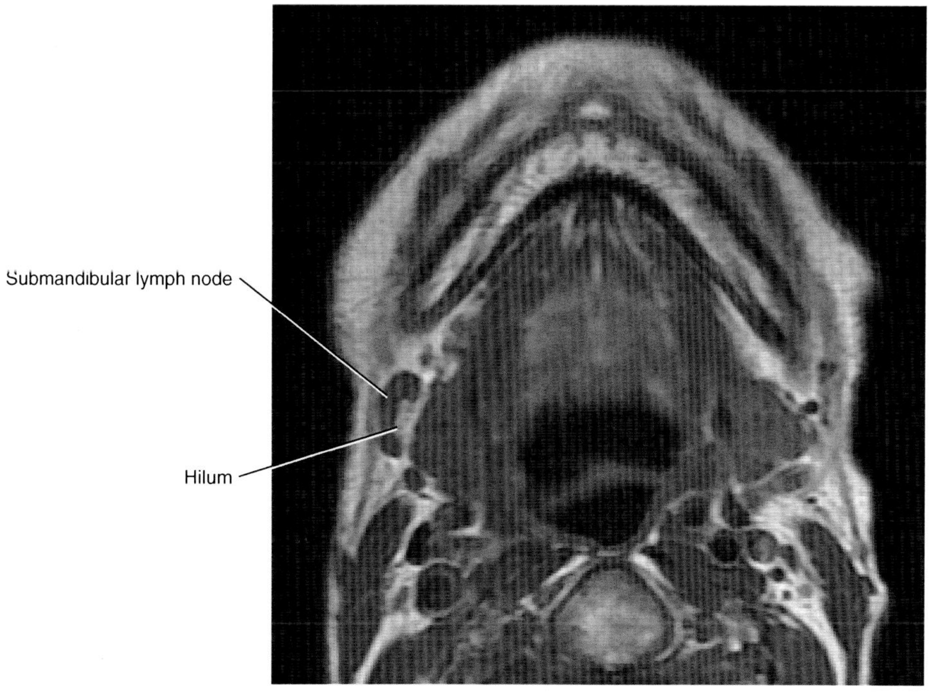

Fig. 5.43 Axial T1-weighted MRI of the right normal submandibular lymph node

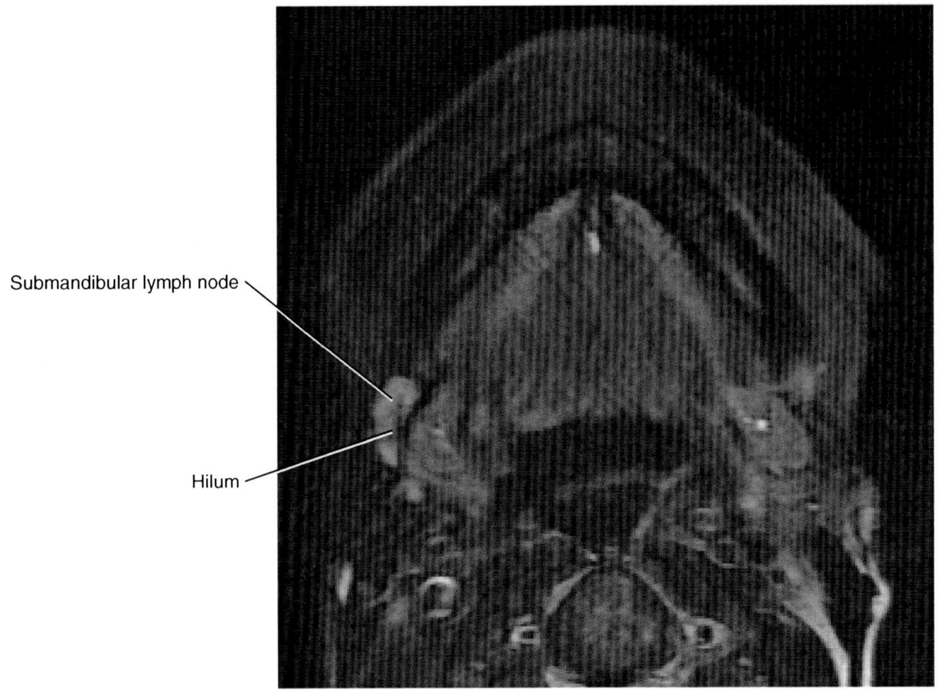

Fig. 5.44 Axial fat-saturated T2-weighted MRI of the right normal submandibular lymph node

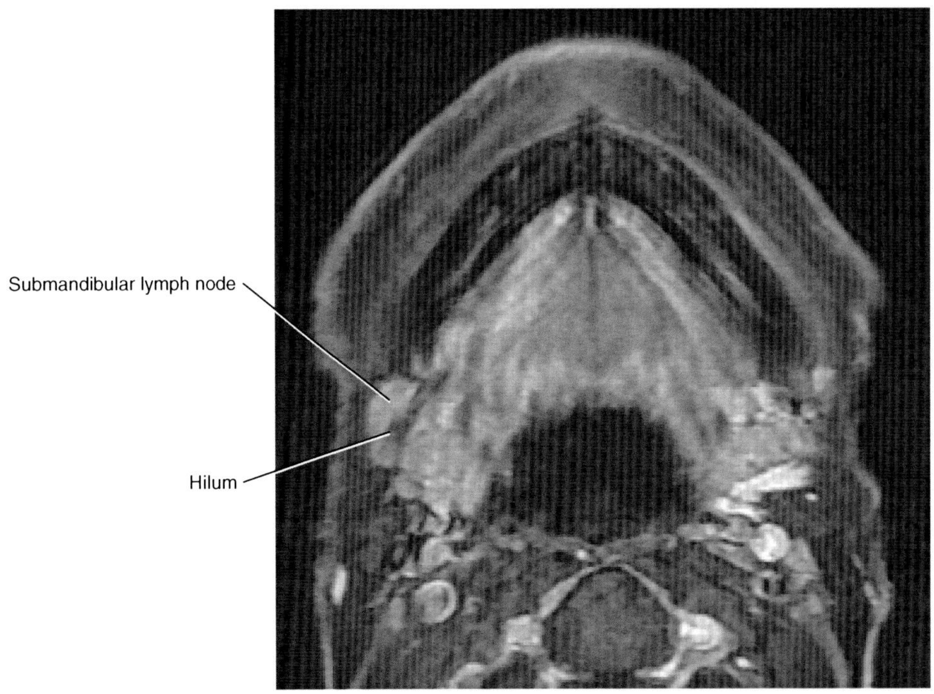

Fig. 5.45 Axial post-contrast fat-saturated T1-weighted MRI of the right normal submandibular lymph node

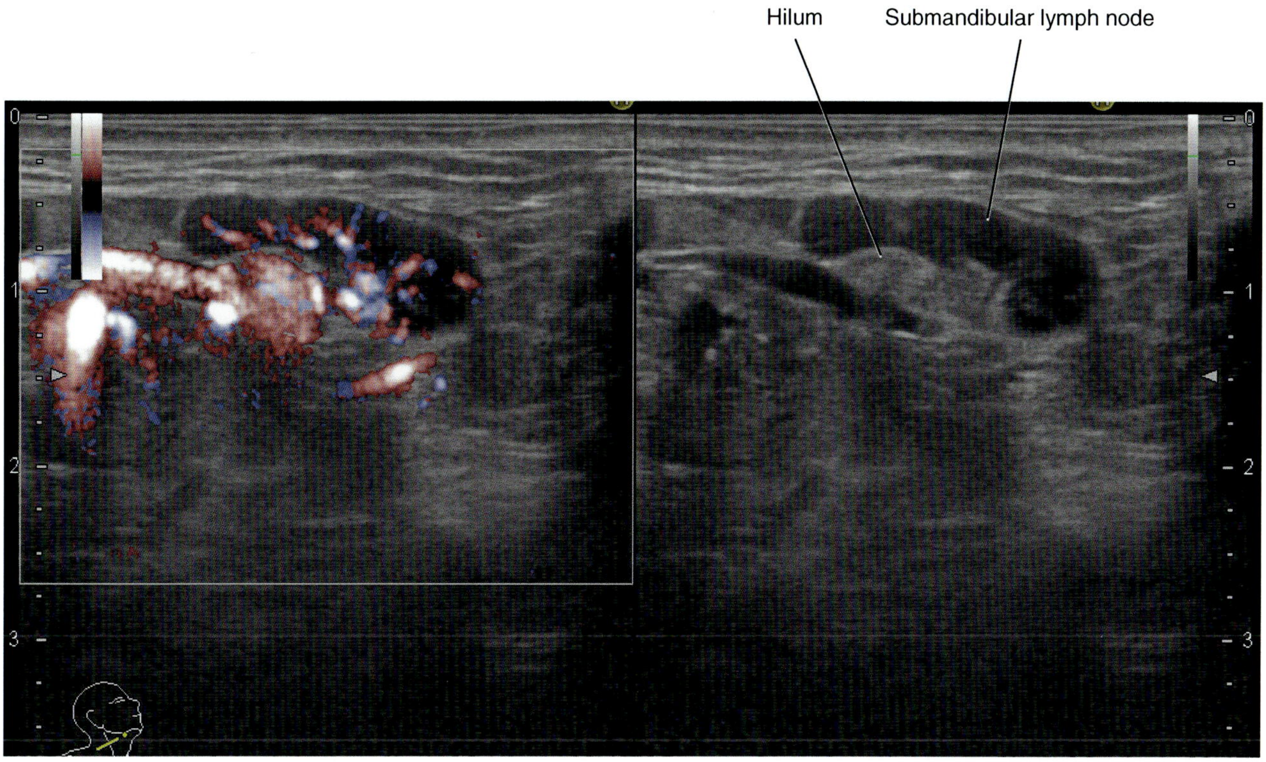

Fig. 5.46 Sagittal ultrasonography of the right normal submandibular lymph node (left, fine flow Doppler; right, B-mode)

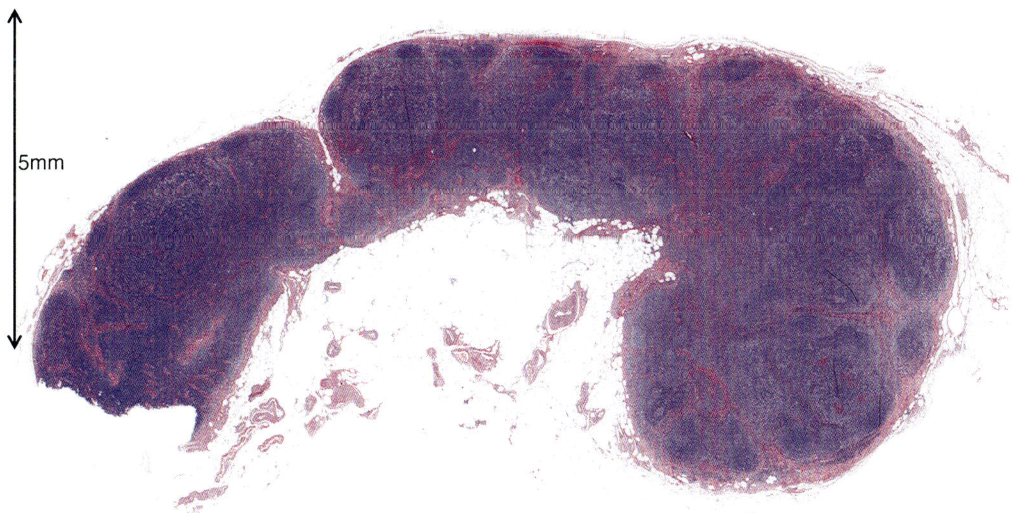

Fig. 5.47 Photomicrograph of histopathological specimen of the right normal submandibular lymph node (hematoxylin-eosin stain)

T3 Tumor more than 4 cm in greatest dimension

T4a Moderately advanced local disease; tumor invades adjacent structures

(according to the 2012 General Rules for Clinical and Pathological Studies on Oral Cancer by the Scientific Committee of Japan Society for Oral Tumors [5]):

1. Tongue: invasion into the mandibular bone marrow, invasion into the submandibular space, and invasion into the extrinsic muscles of the tongue
2. Upper gingiva: invasion into the maxillary sinus and nasal cavity and invasion into the buccal space or subcutaneous fat
3. Lower gingiva: invasion reaching the mandibular canal, invasion into the buccal space or subcutaneous fat, invasion into the submandibular space, and invasion into the extrinsic muscles of the tongue
4. Buccal mucosa: invasion into the subcutaneous fat, invasion into the maxillary and mandibular bone marrow, and invasion into the maxillary sinus
5. Floor of the mouth: invasion into the mandibular bone marrow, invasion into the submandibular space, and invasion into the extrinsic muscles of the tongue
6. Hard palate: invasion into the maxillary sinus and nasal cavity

T4b Very advanced local disease; tumor invasion into the masticator space, invasion into the pterygoid plate, invasion into the skull base, and invasion circumferentially surrounding the internal carotid artery

5.3.3 Regional Lymph Nodes (N)

The classification and range of cervical lymph nodes are the same as described in the Rules Regarding Lymph Nodes by the Japan Society of Clinical Oncology (JSCO), and lymph node metastasis is evaluated according to the UICC classification. Internationally, the level classification system by the Academy's Committee for Head and Neck Surgery and Oncology (ACHNSO) based on the area of neck dissection is widely used, and the AAO-HNS classification, a fragmented version of the ACHNSO classification, has also been proposed [5].

N factor

NX Regional lymph nodes cannot be assessed

N0 No regional lymph node metastasis

N1 Metastasis in a single ipsilateral lymph node, 3 cm or less in greatest diameter

N2 Metastasis in a single ipsilateral lymph node, more than 3 cm but not more than 6 cm in greatest dimension; or in multiple ipsilateral lymph nodes, none more than 6 cm in greatest dimension; or in bilateral or contralateral lymph nodes, none more than 6 cm in greatest dimension

N2a Metastasis in a single ipsilateral lymph node, more than 3 cm but not more than 6 cm in greatest dimension

N2b Metastasis in multiple ipsilateral lymph nodes, none more than 6 cm in greatest dimension

N2c Metastasis in bilateral or contralateral lymph nodes, none more than 6 cm in greatest dimension

N3 Metastasis in a lymph node, more than 6 cm in greatest dimension

5.3.4 Distant Metastasis (M)

M Factor

M0 No distant metastasis

M1 Distant metastasis present

Staging

0 Tis, N0, M0

I T1, N0, M0

II T2, N0, M0

III T3, N0, M0
T1, T2 or T3, N1, M0

IVA T4a, N0 or N1, M0
T1, T2, T3 or T4a, N2, M0

IVB Any T, N3, M0
T4a and any N, M0

IVC Any T and any N M1

Level Classification (Fig. 5.48)

Level IA Submental lymph nodes; they lie between medial margins of the anterior bellies of the digastric muscles.

Level IB Submandibular lymph nodes; on each side, they lie lateral to the level IA nodes and anterior to the back of each submandibular gland.

Level IIA Superior internal jugular lymph nodes, superior deep cervical lymph nodes (jugulodigastric nodes, anterior); they lie either anterior, medial, lateral, or posterior to the internal jugular vein. If posterior to the vein, the node is inseparable from the vein.

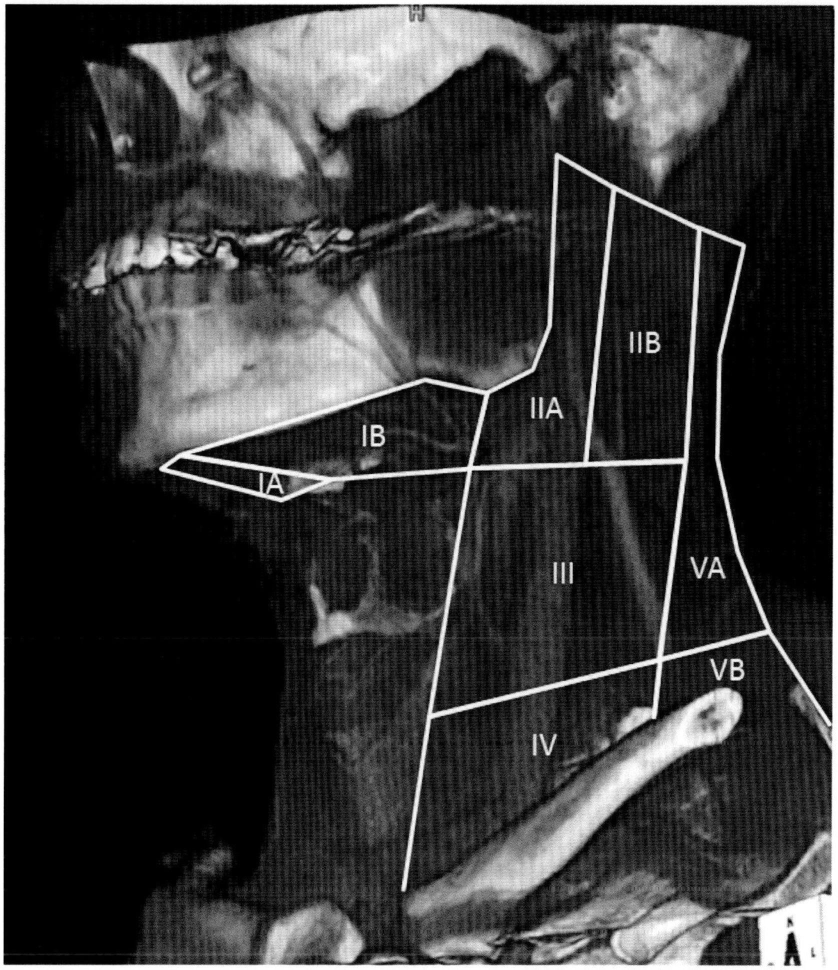

Fig. 5.48 Level classification

Level IIB	Superior internal jugular lymph nodes, superior deep cervical lymph nodes (jugulodigastric nodes, posterior); they lie posterior to the internal jugular vein and have a fat plane separating it from the vein.
Level III	Middle internal jugular lymph nodes, middle deep cervical lymph nodes (jugulo-omohyoid nodes); they extend from the level of the bottom of the body of the hyoid bone to the level of the bottom of the cricoid arch. They lie anterior to the back of the sternocleidomastoid muscle.
Level IV	Inferior internal jugular lymph nodes, inferior deep cervical lymph nodes; they extend from the level of the bottom of the cricoid arch to the level of the clavicle.
Level VA	Spinal accessory lymph nodes; they extend from the skull base to the level of the bottom of the cricoid arch.
Level VB	Supraclavicular lymph nodes; they extend from the level of the bottom of the cricoid arch to the level of the clavicle.

5.4 Oral Cavity Malignancies

5.4.1 Tongue Carcinoma [Squamous Cell Carcinoma (SCC)]

5.4.1.1 Case 1: 82-Year-Old Female, Left-Tongue SCC T4aN0 (Figs. 5.49, 5.50, 5.51, 5.52, 5.53, 5.54, 5.55, 5.56, 5.57, 5.58 and 5.59)

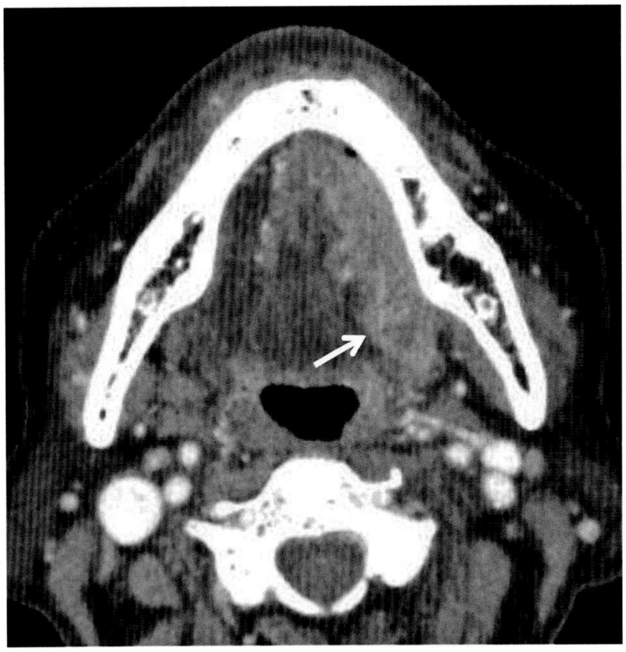

Fig. 5.49 Axial CECT. Tumor is demonstrated as an ill-defined enhancing mass at the left lateral margin of the tongue involving the floor of the mouth (*arrow*)

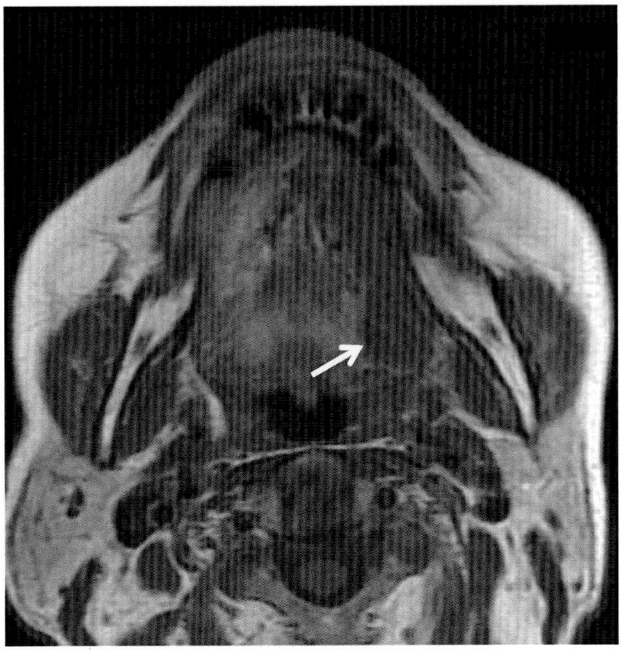

Fig. 5.51 Axial T1-weighted MRI. Tumor is demonstrated as an intermediate signal intensity area with an ill-defined margin (*arrow*)

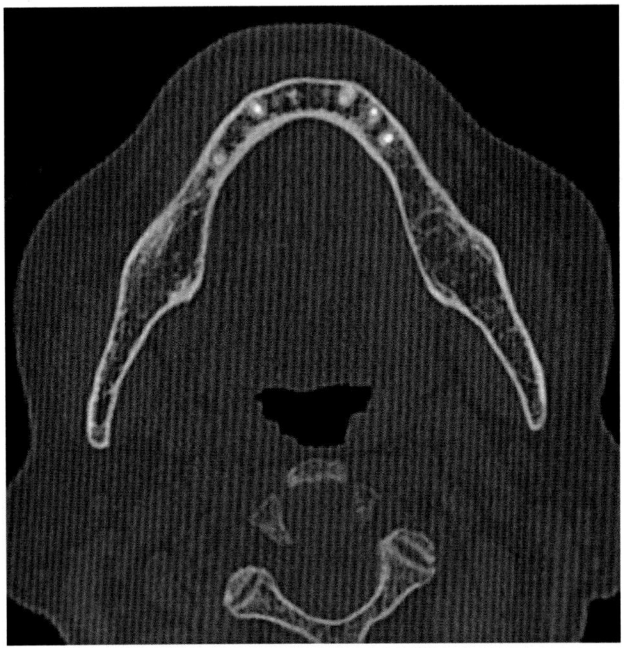

Fig. 5.50 Axial plain CT with bone window. No apparent destruction of adjacent bone cortex of the mandible is seen

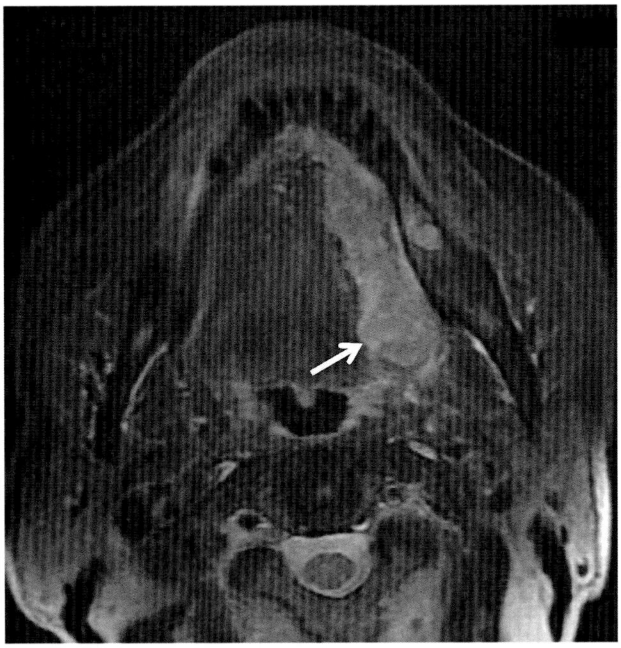

Fig. 5.52 Axial fat-saturated T2-weighted MRI. Tumor is demonstrated as relatively high heterogeneous intensity area with an ill-defined margin (*arrow*)

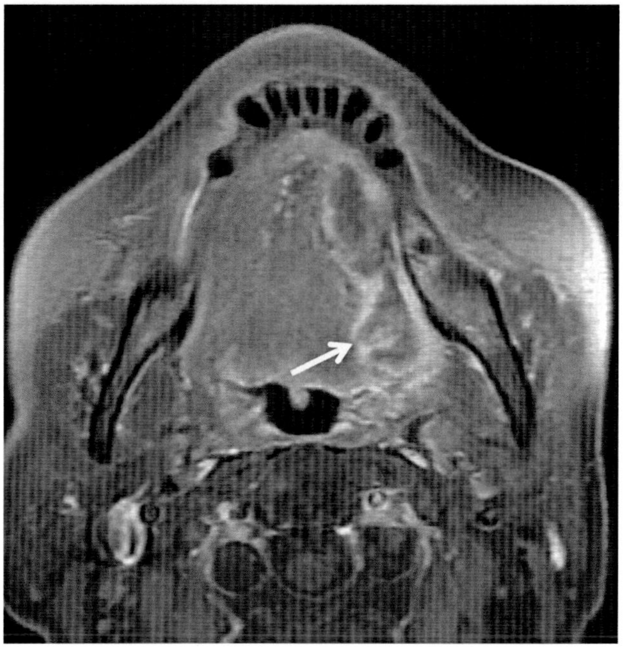

Fig. 5.53 Axial fat-saturated post-contrast T1-weighted MRI. Tumor enhances heterogeneously (*arrow*) and the peripheral portion of the tumor enhances prominently

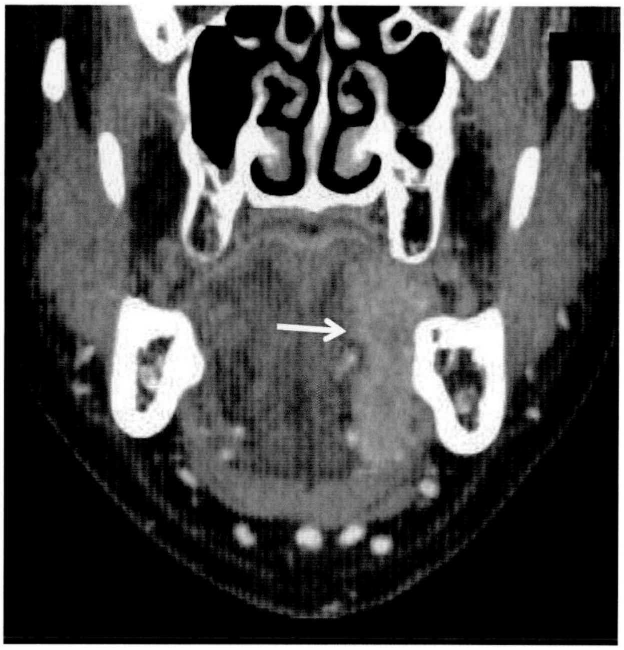

Fig. 5.55 Coronal CECT. Tumor (*arrow*) involves the left sublingual space and the hyoglossus muscle

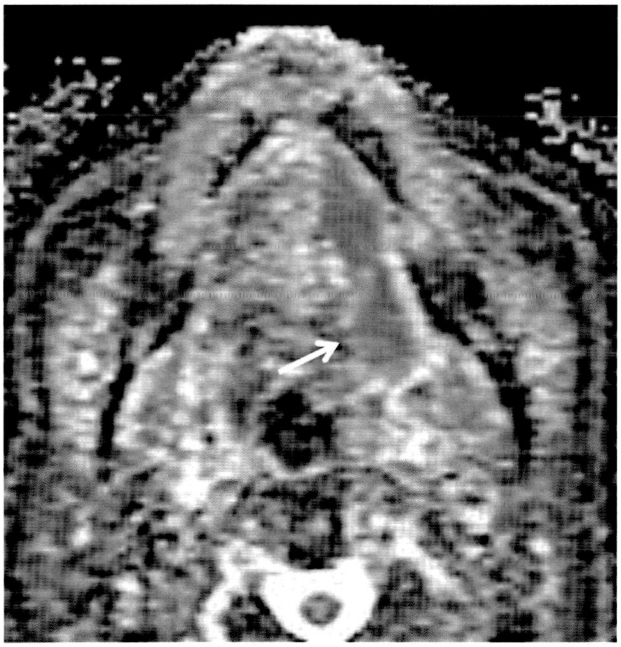

Fig. 5.54 Axial ADC map MRI. Tumor is demonstrated as a restricted diffusion area (*arrow*)

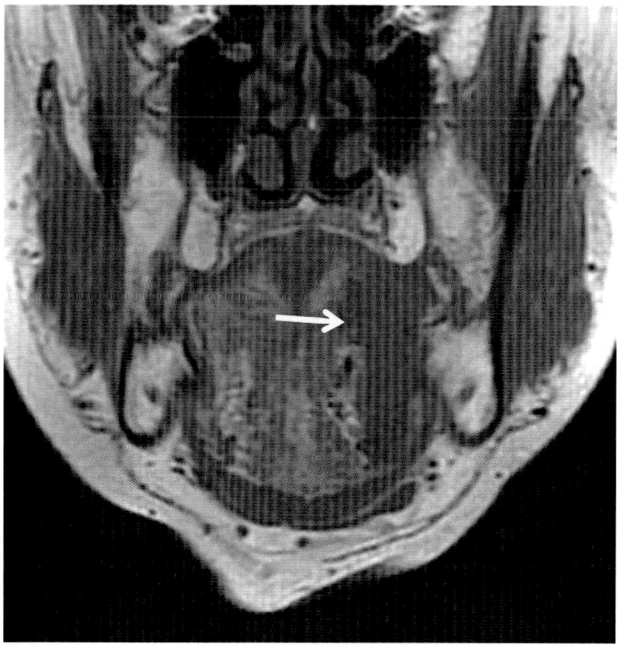

Fig. 5.56 Coronal T1-weighted MRI. Tumor is demonstrated as intermediate signal intensity (*arrow*)

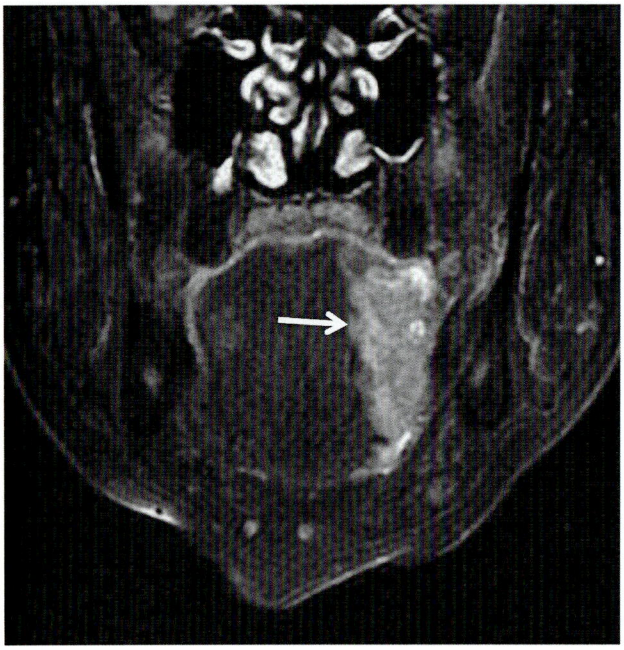

Fig. 5.57 Coronal fat-saturated T2-weighted MRI. Tumor is demonstrated as relatively high heterogeneous intensity (*arrow*)

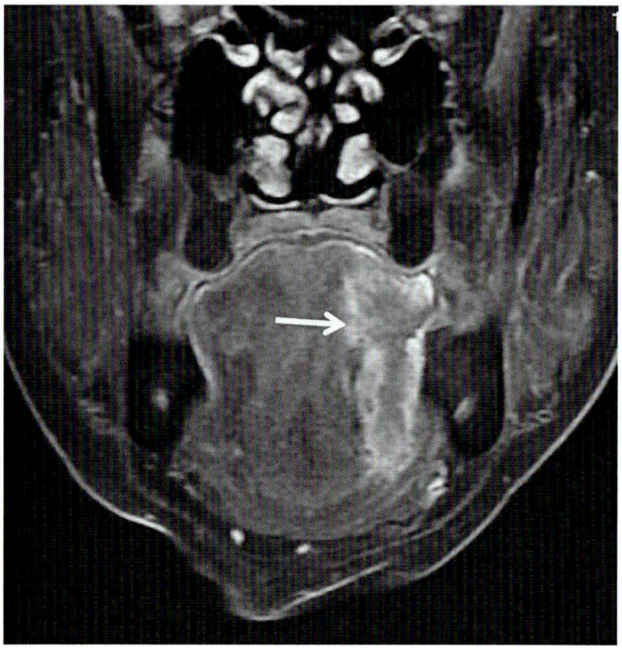

Fig. 5.58 Coronal fat-saturated post-contrast T1-weighted MRI. Tumor (*arrow*) enhances heterogeneously and involves the hyoglossus muscle

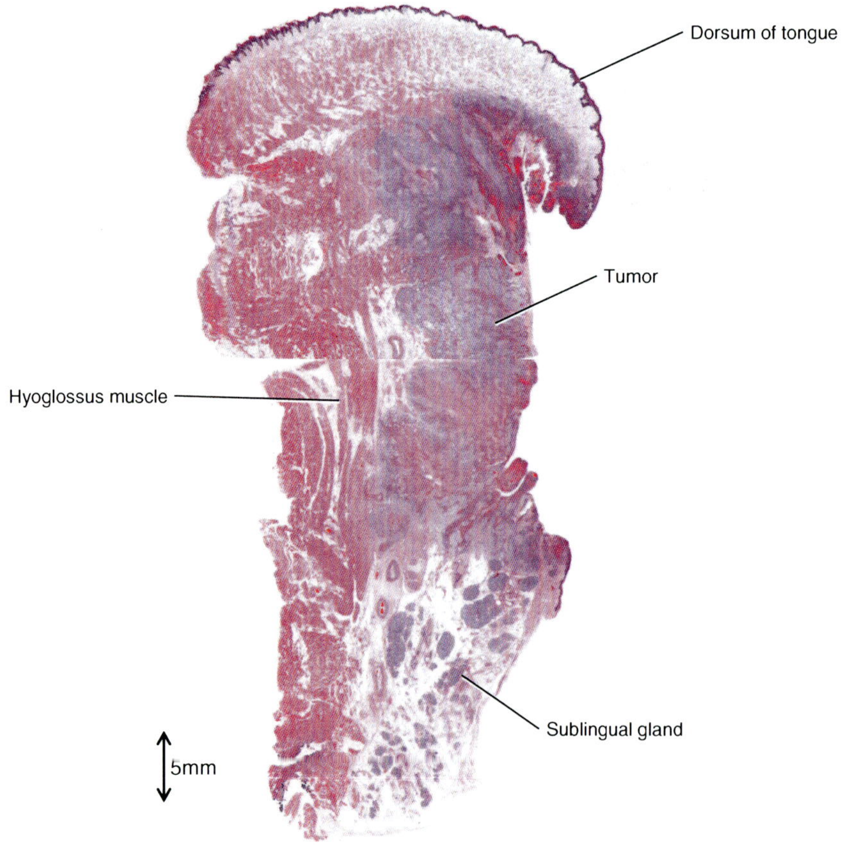

Fig. 5.59 Photomicrograph of histopathological specimen, coronal section (hematoxylin-eosin stain)

5.4.1.2 Case 2: 60-Year-Old Female, Left-Tongue SCC T4aN0 (Figs. 5.60, 5.61, 5.62, 5.63, 5.64, 5.65, 5.66 and 5.67)

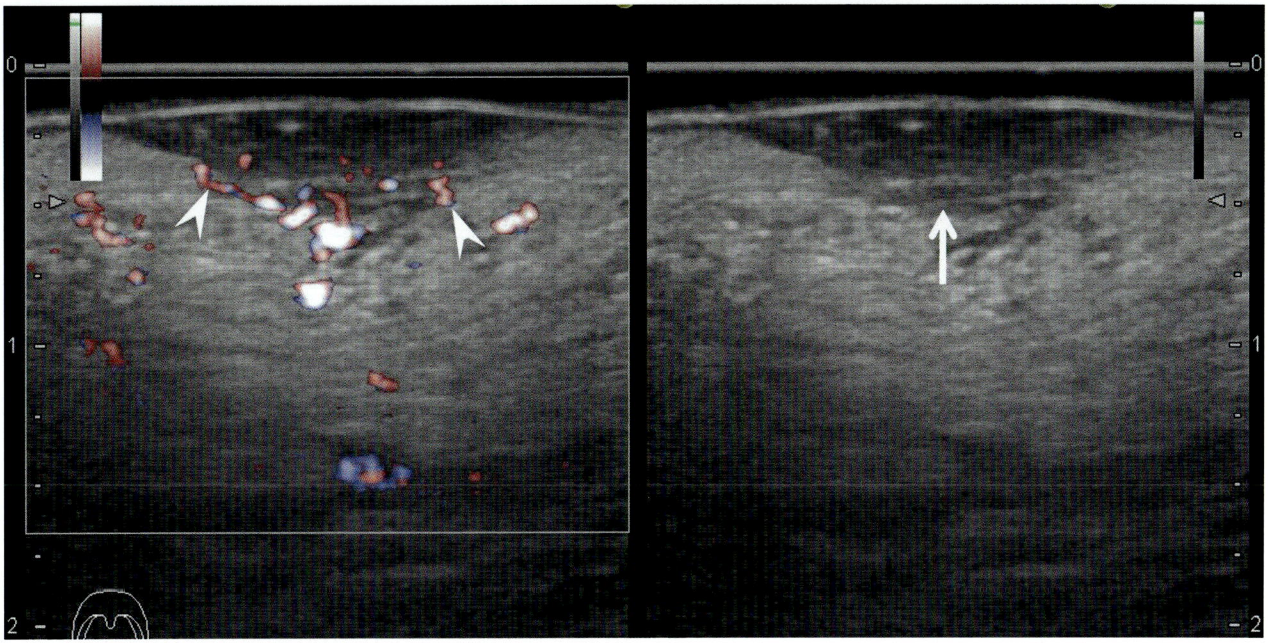

Fig. 5.60 Intraoral ultrasonography with the acoustic coupling device between the probe surface and the tumor surface (left, fine flow Doppler; right, B-mode). Tumor is demonstrated as an ill-defined hypoechoic area (*arrow*) continuous with the surrounding normal mucosal layer. Note the vascularity around the deep margins arising from neoangiogenesis at the tumor invasion front (*arrowheads*)

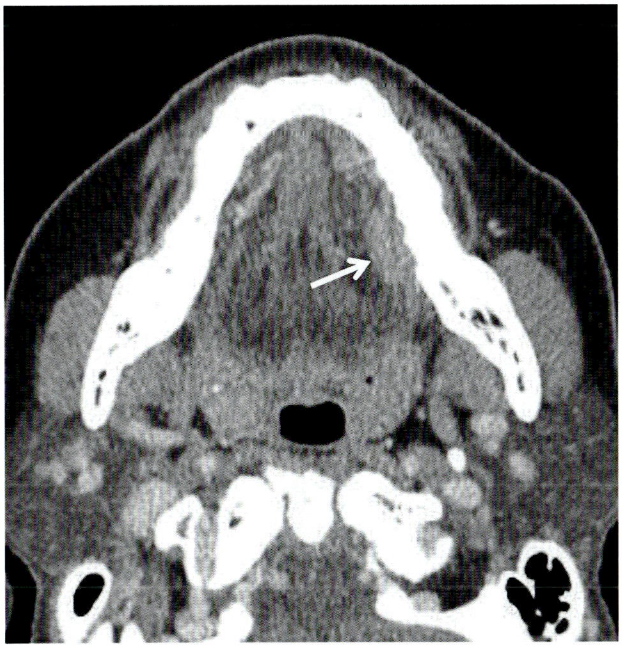

Fig. 5.61 Axial CECT. Tumor is demonstrated as an ill-defined enhancing mass at the left lateral margin of the tongue (*arrow*)

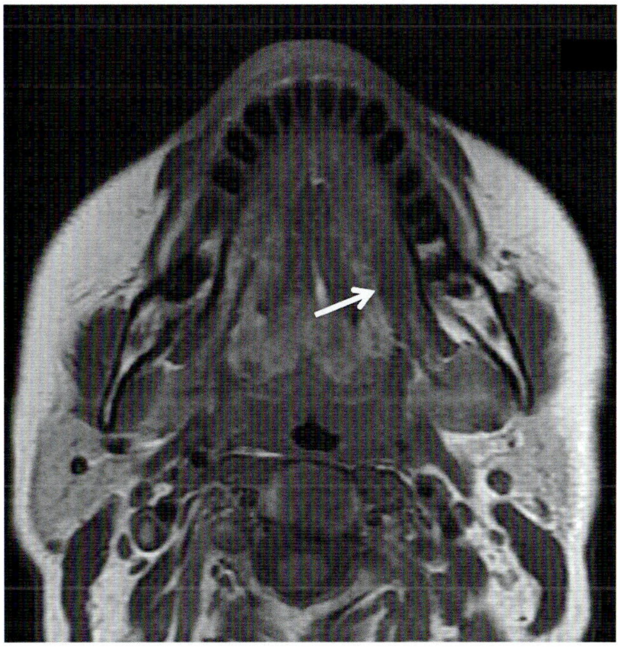

Fig. 5.62 Axial T1-weighted MRI. Tumor (*arrow*) is demonstrated as an intermediate signal intensity area with an ill-defined margin involving the left hyoglossus muscle

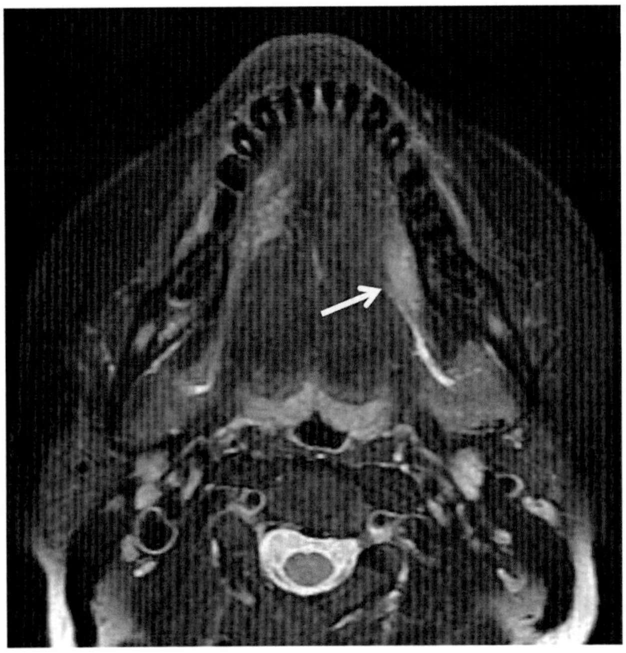

Fig. 5.63 Axial fat-saturated T2-weighted MRI. Tumor is demonstrated as relatively high heterogeneous intensity area with an ill-defined margin (*arrow*)

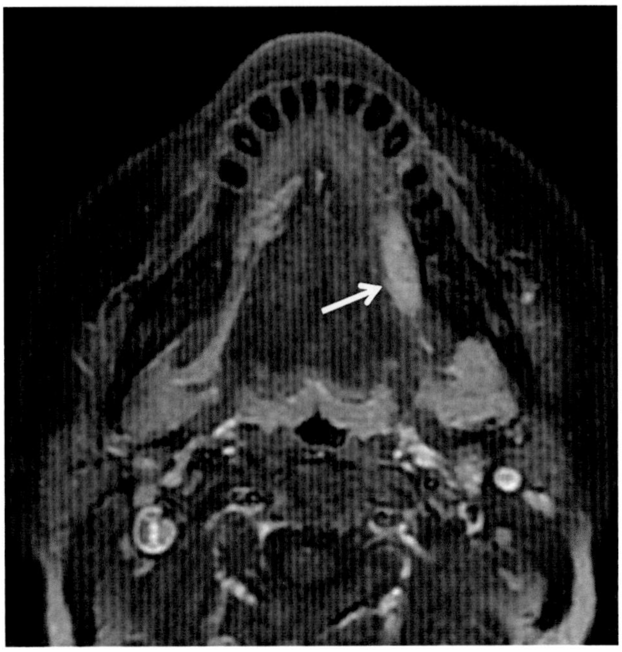

Fig. 5.64 Axial dynamic MRI. Tumor enhances homogeneously (*arrow*)

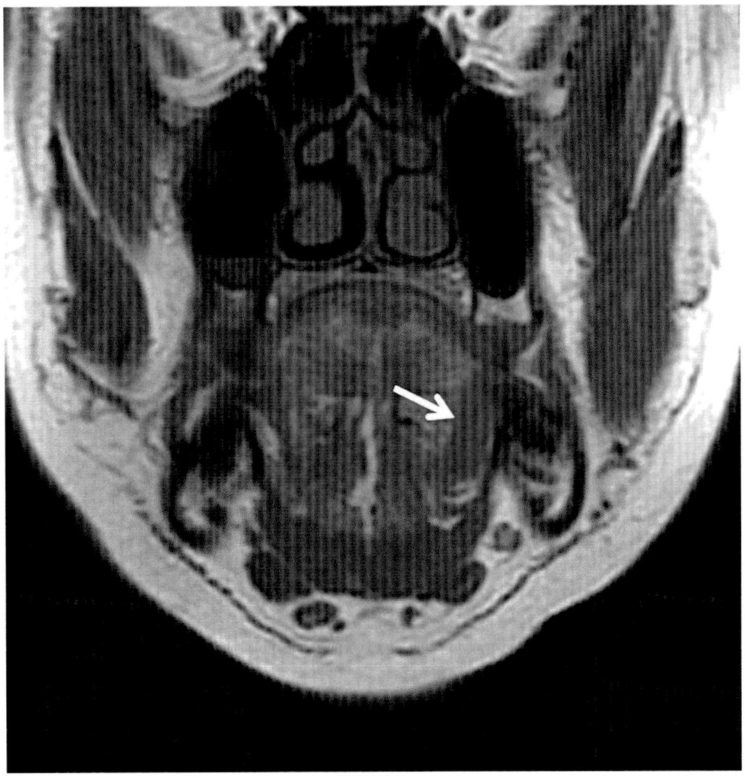

Fig. 5.65 Coronal T1-weighted MRI. Tumor is demonstrated as intermediate signal intensity (*arrow*)

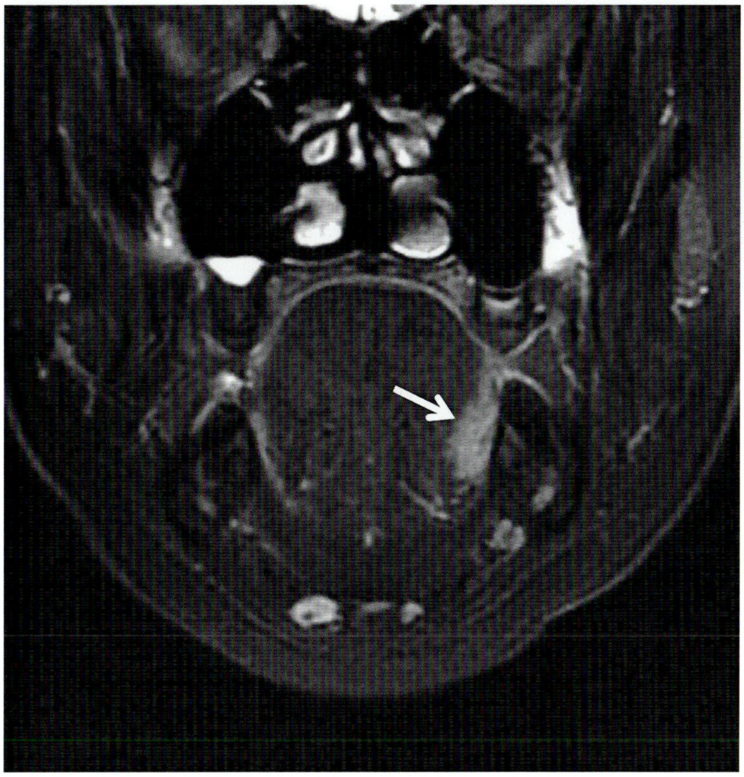

Fig. 5.66 Coronal fat-saturated T2-weighted MRI. Tumor is demonstrated as relatively high heterogeneous intensity (*arrow*)

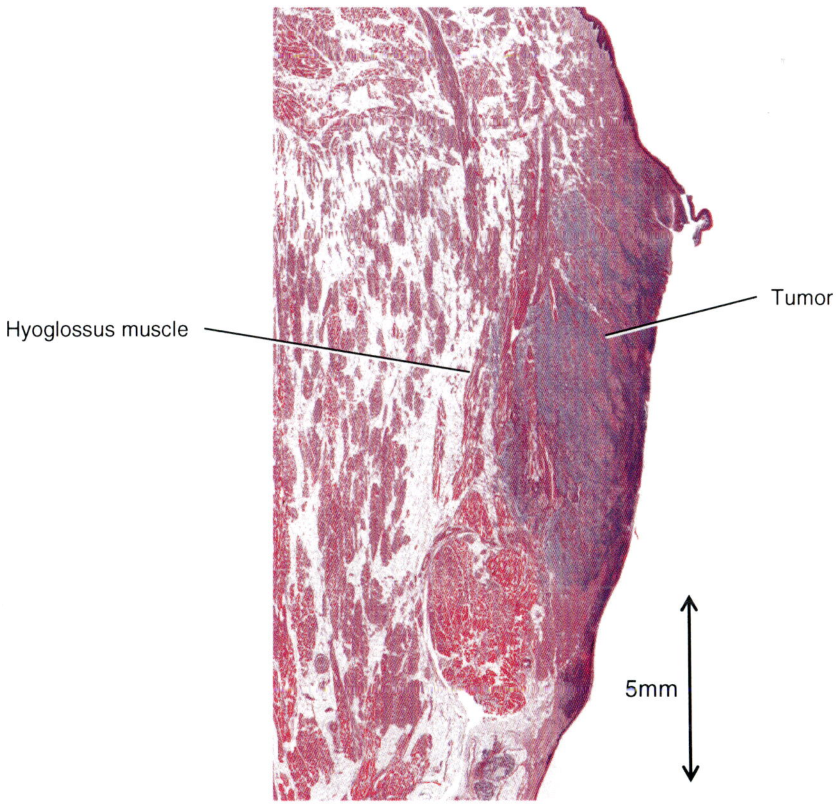

Fig. 5.67 Photomicrograph of histopathological specimen, coronal section (hematoxylin-eosin stain)

5.4.1.3 Case 3: 60-Year-Old Female, Right-Tongue SCC T2N0 (Figs. 5.68, 5.69, 5.70 and 5.71)

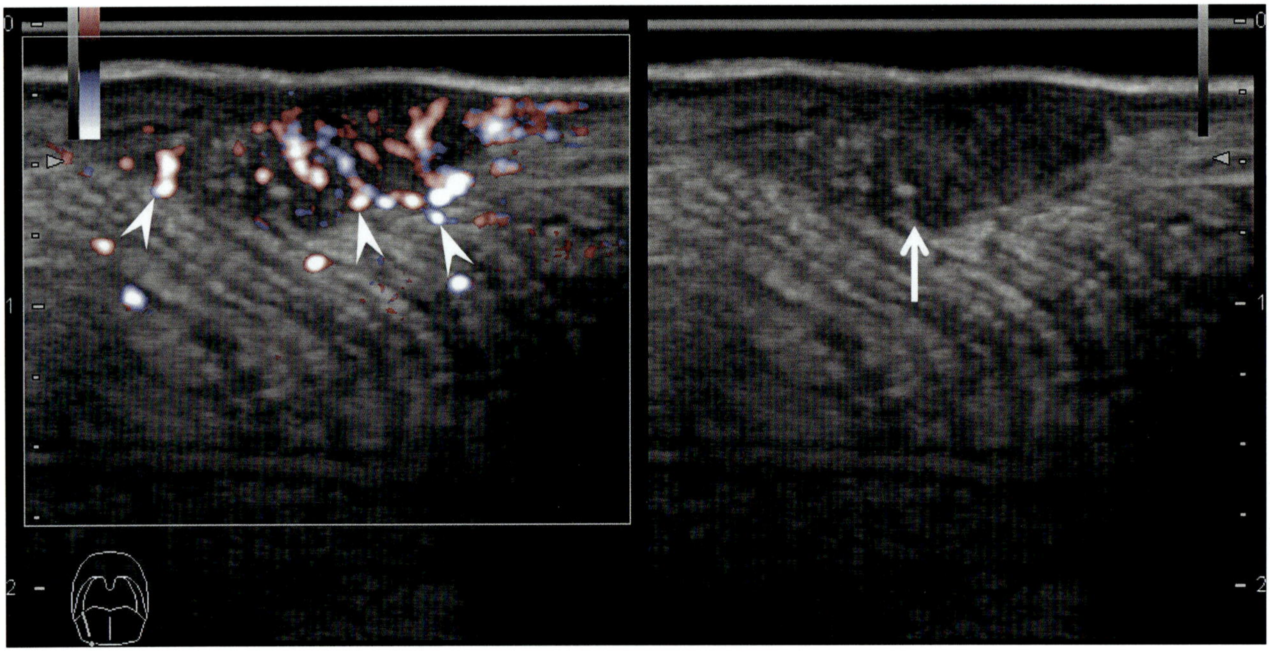

Fig. 5.68 Intraoral ultrasonography with the acoustic coupling device between the probe surface and the tumor surface (left, fine flow Doppler; right, B-mode). Tumor is demonstrated clearly as an ill-defined hypoechoic area (*arrow*) continuous with the surrounding normal mucosal layer. Note the prominent vascularity around the deep margins arising from neoangiogenesis at the tumor invasion front (*arrowheads*)

Fig. 5.69 Axial CECT. Tumor is markedly obscured by severe metal artifact of dental prosthesis

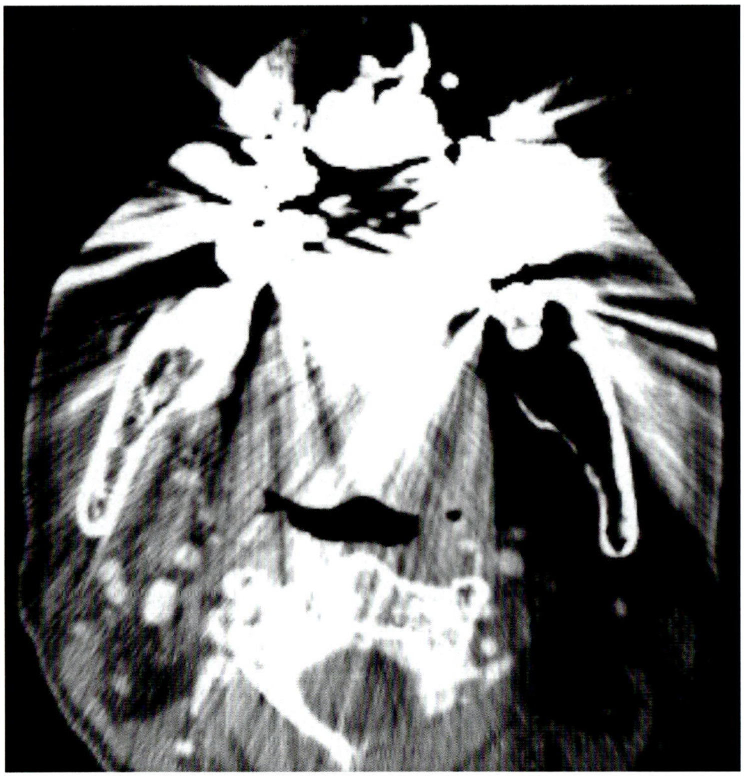

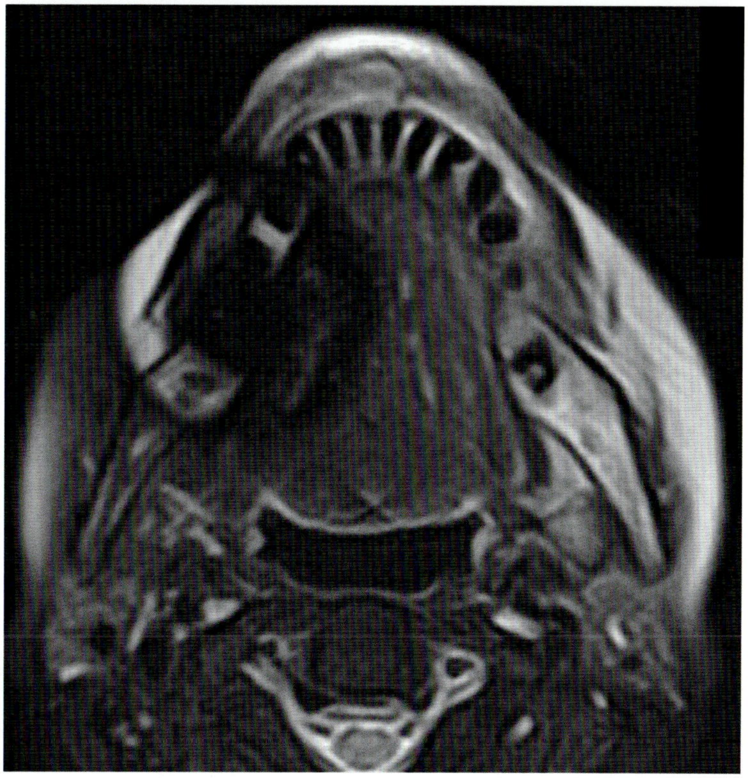

Fig. 5.70 Axial post-contrast T1-weighted MRI. Tumor is also obscured by susceptibility artifact of dental prosthesis

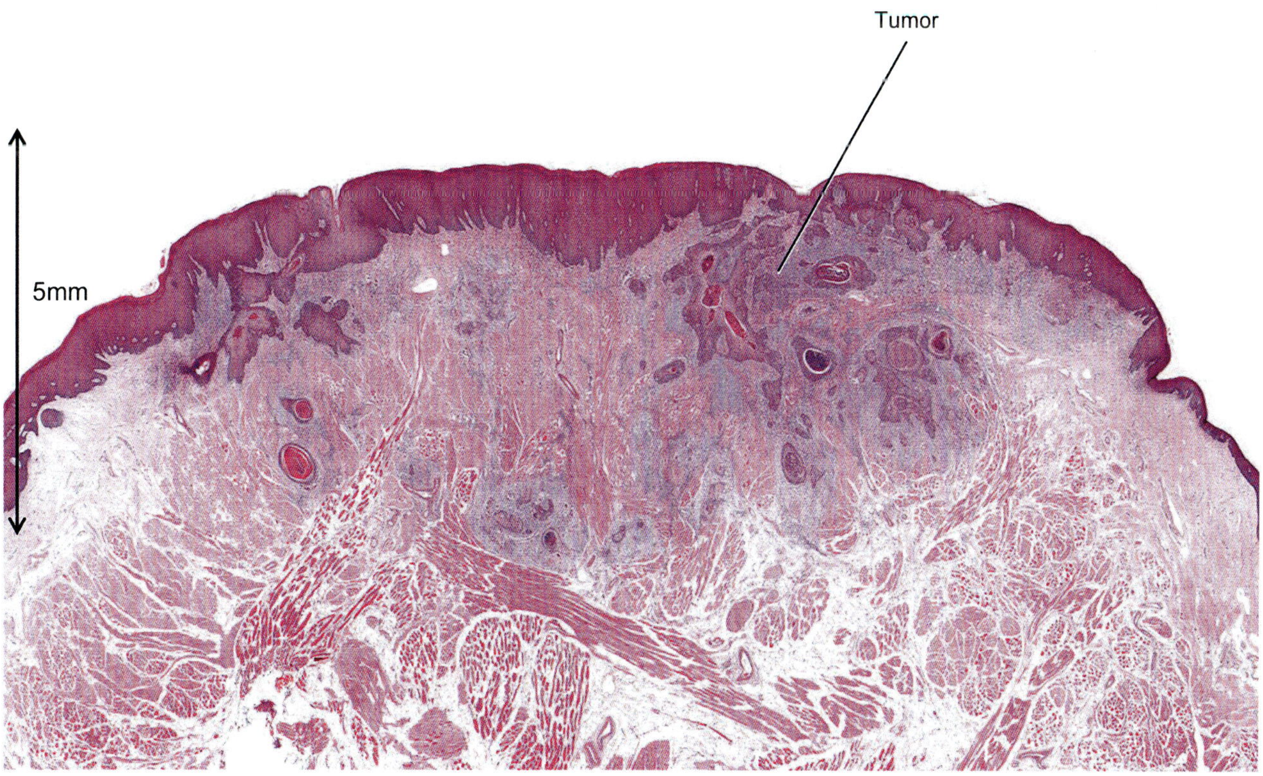

Fig. 5.71 Photomicrograph of histopathological specimen, coronal section (hematoxylin-eosin stain)

5.4.2 Gingival Carcinoma

5.4.2.1 Case 3: 62-Year-Old Male, Left-Mandibular Gingival SCC T4aN0 (Figs. 5.72, 5.73, 5.74, 5.75, 5.76, 5.77, 5.78, 5.79, 5.80, 5.81, 5.82, 5.83 and 5.84)

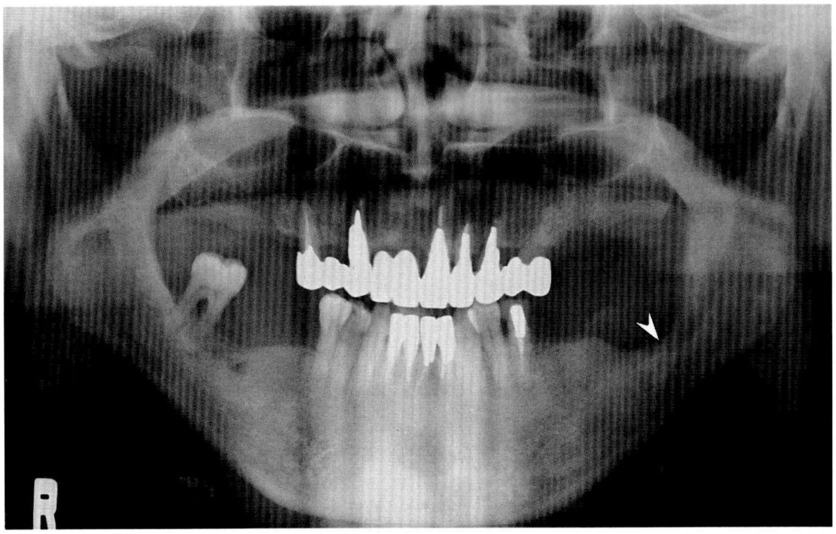

Fig. 5.72 Orthopantomography. An ill-defined bone destruction possibly caused by gingival SCC is demonstrated as an intermediate-type absorption at the left lower molar region possibly involving the mandibular canal (*arrowhead*)

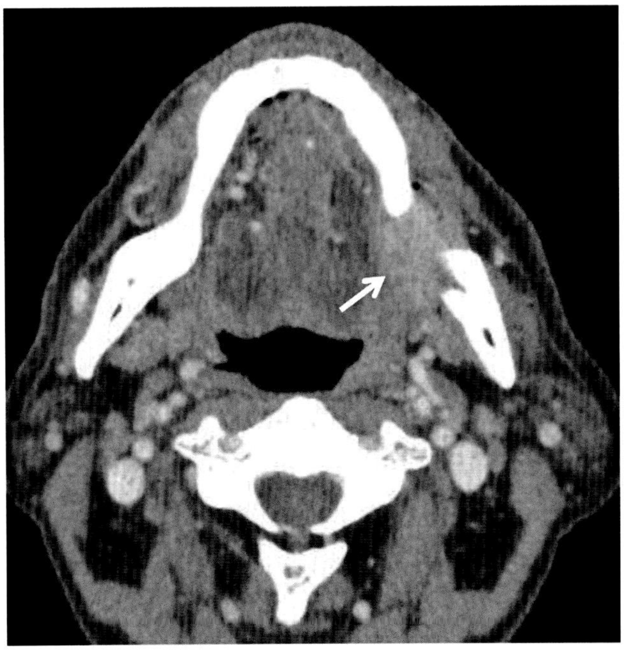

Fig. 5.73 Axial CECT. Tumor is demonstrated as an ill-defined enhancing mass involving the floor of the mouth (*arrow*)

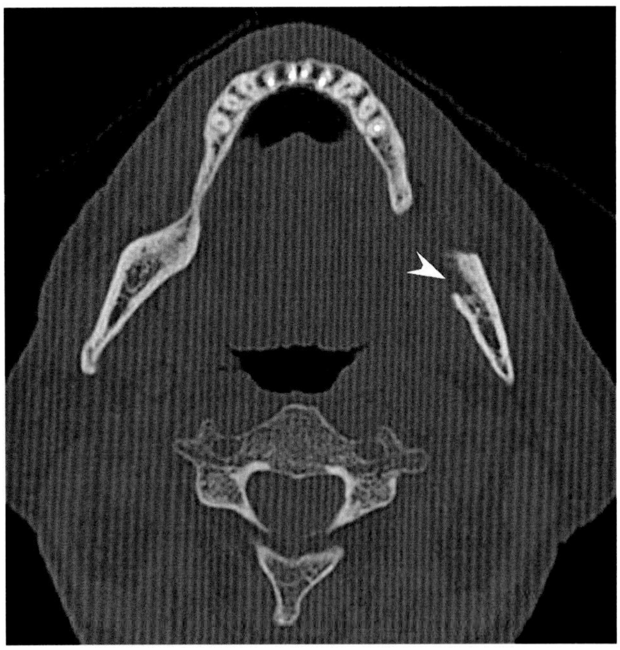

Fig. 5.74 Axial plain CT with bone window

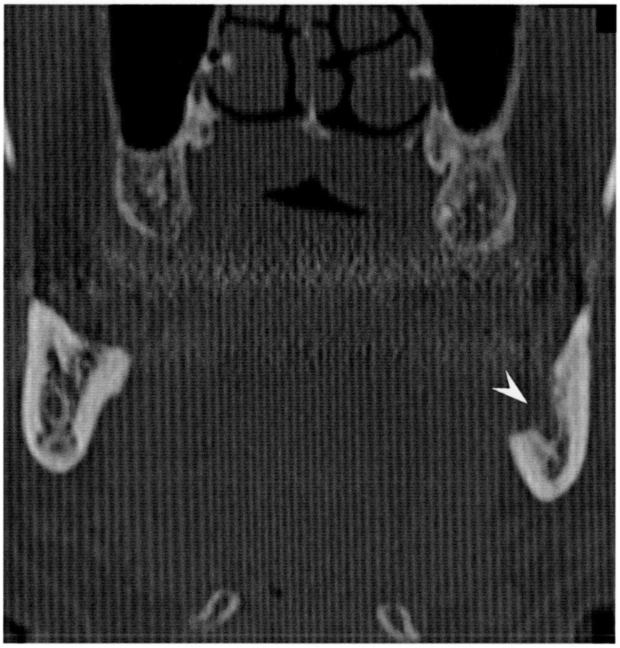

Fig. 5.75 Coronal plain CT with bone window

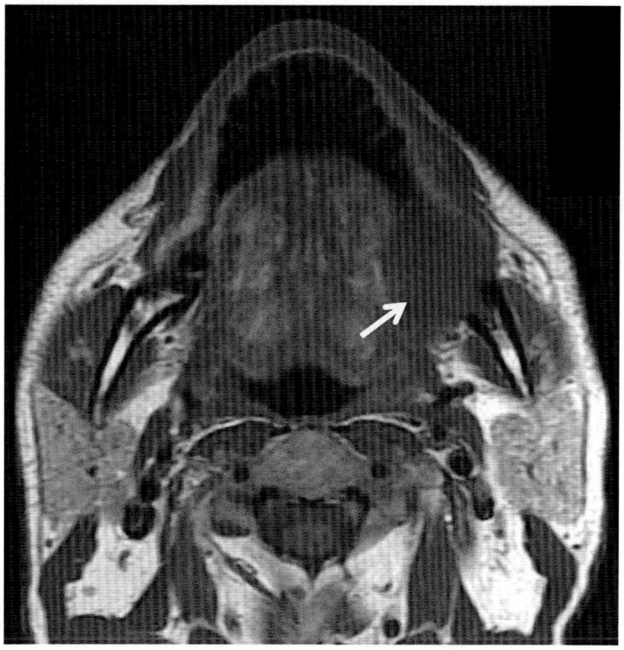

Fig. 5.77 Axial T1-weighted MRI. Tumor is demonstrated as an intermediate signal intensity area (*arrow*) with an ill-defined margin

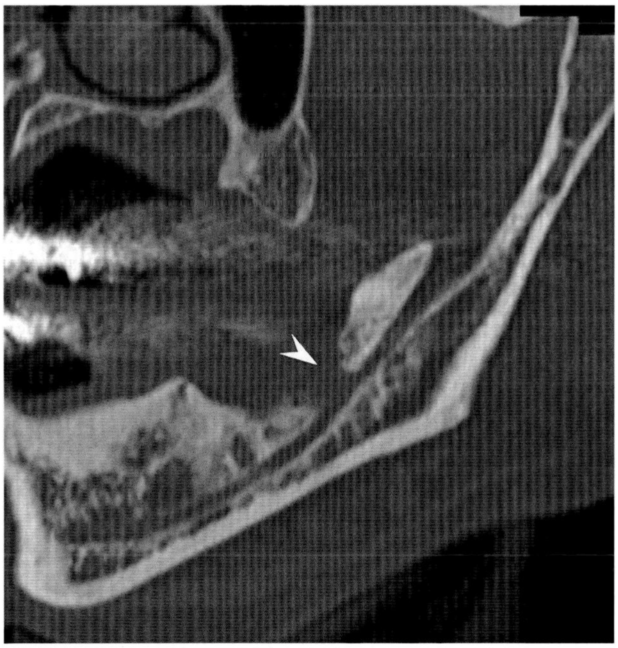

Fig. 5.76 Parasagittal plain CT with bone window. Destruction of the lower alveolar bone with an irregular margin possibly involving the mandibular canal wall is demonstrated (*arrowhead*)

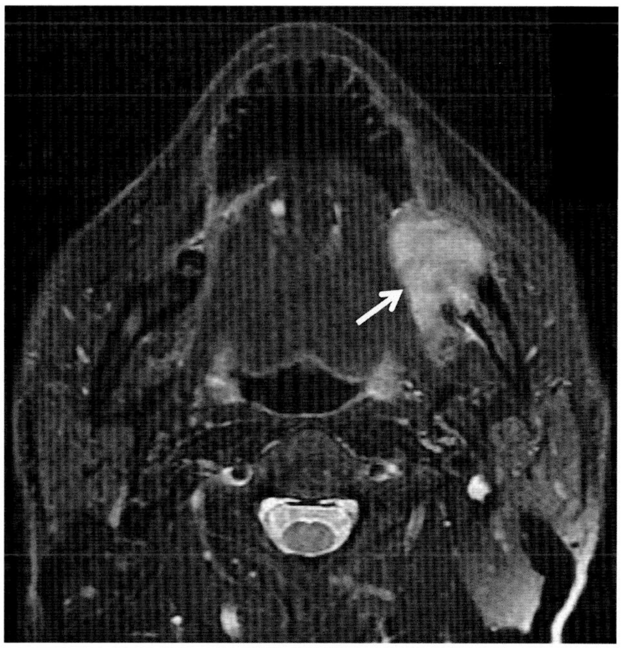

Fig. 5.78 Axial fat-saturated T2-weighted MRI. Tumor is demonstrated as relatively high heterogeneous intensity area (*arrow*) with bone marrow involvement

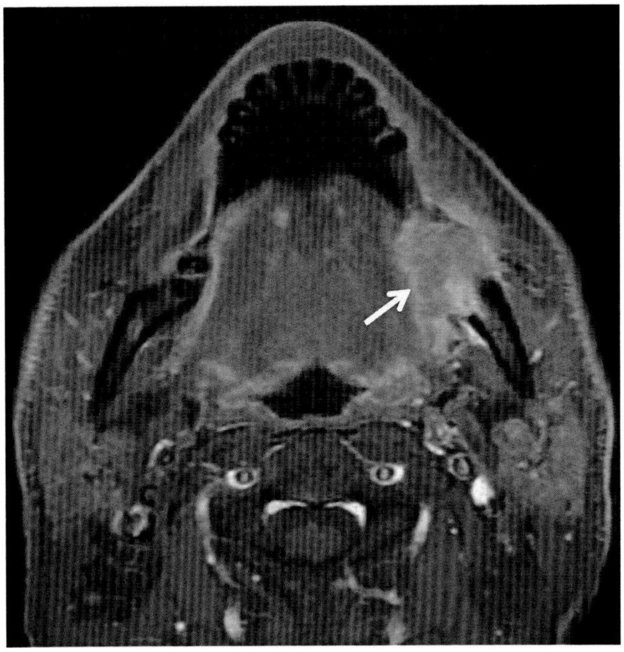

Fig. 5.79 Axial fat-saturated post-contrast T1-weighted MRI. Tumor enhances heterogeneously (*arrow*) and the peripheral portion of the tumor enhances prominently

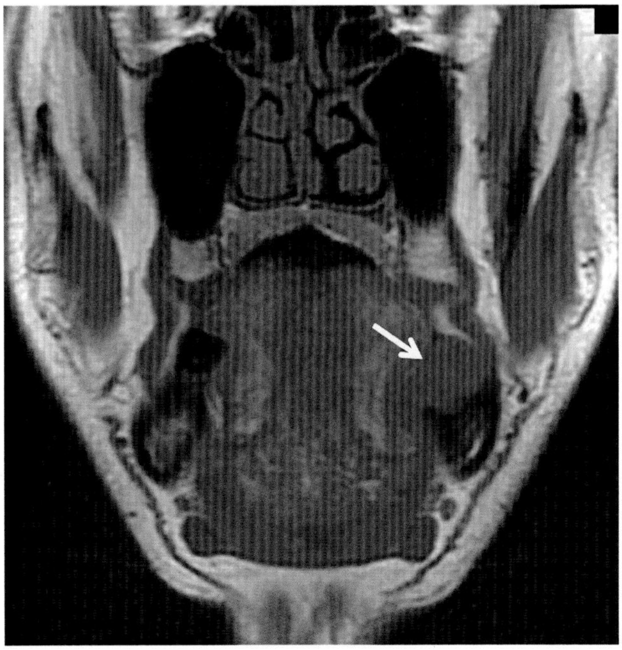

Fig. 5.81 Coronal T1-weighted MRI. Tumor is demonstrated as an intermediate signal intensity area involving the left mylohyoid muscle

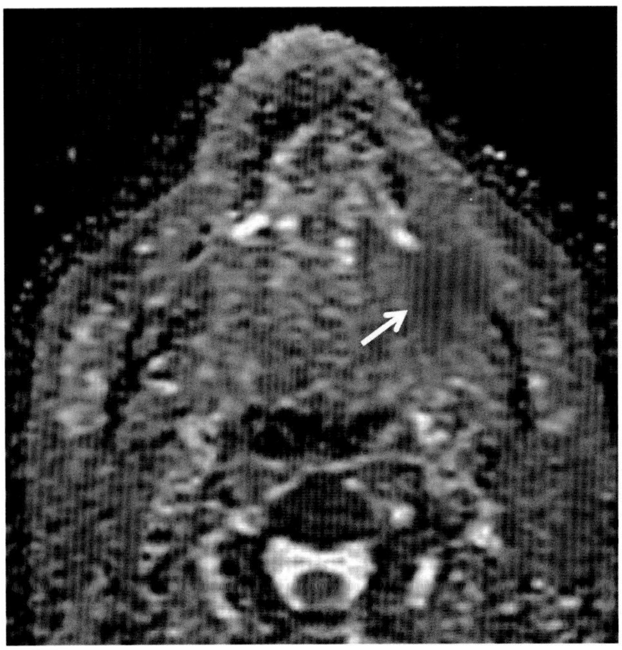

Fig. 5.80 Axial ADC map MRI. Tumor is demonstrated as a restricted diffusion area (*arrow*)

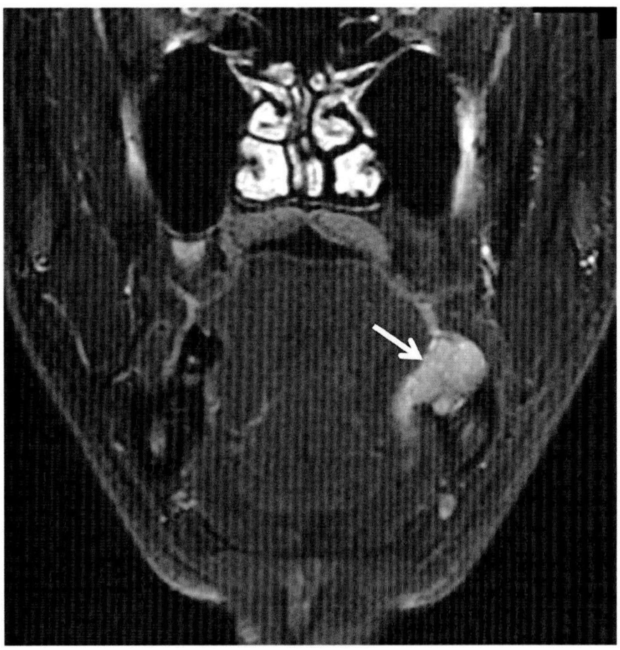

Fig. 5.82 Coronal fat-saturated T2-weighted MRI. Tumor is demonstrated as relatively high heterogeneous intensity (*arrow*)

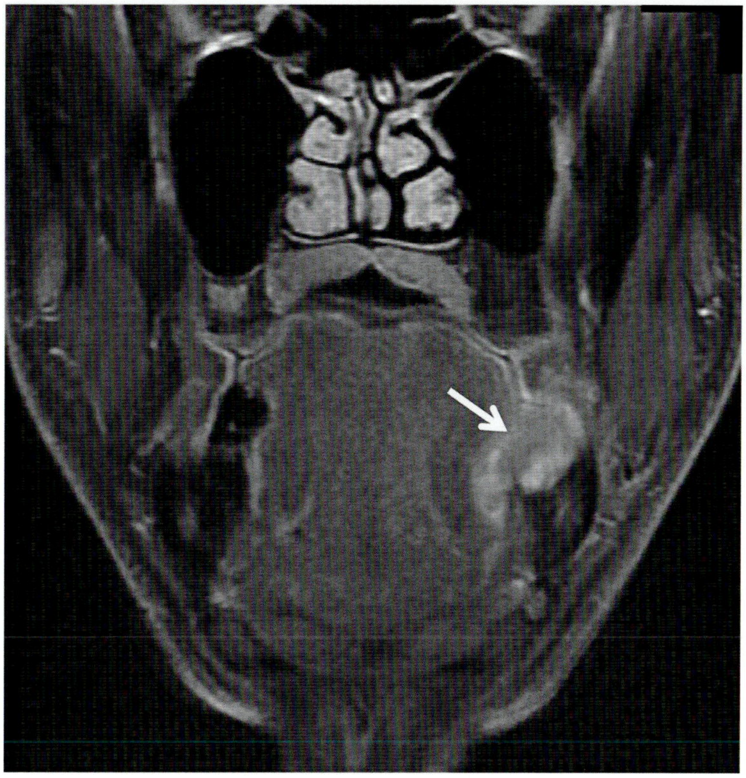

Fig. 5.83 Coronal fat-saturated post-contrast T1-weighted MRI. Tumor (*arrow*) enhances heterogeneously

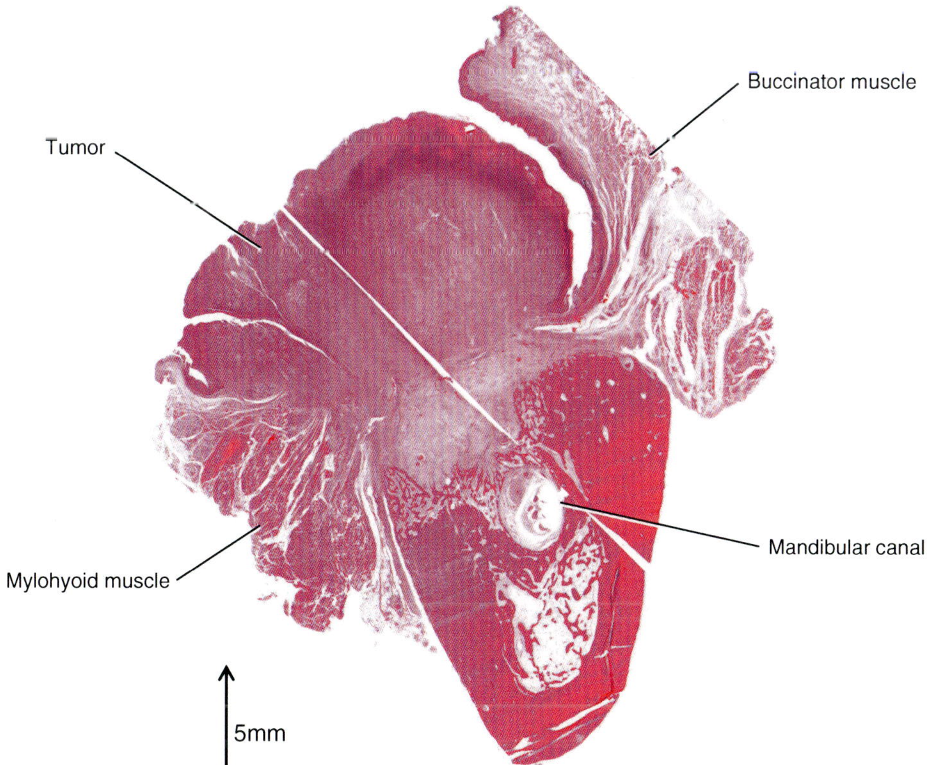

Fig. 5.84 Photomicrograph of histopathological specimen, coronal section (hematoxylin-eosin stain)

5.4.2.2 Case 4: 85-Year-Old Male, Right-Maxillary Gingival SCC, T4aN0 (Figs. 5.85, 5.86, 5.87, 5.88, 5.89, 5.90, 5.91, 5.92, 5.93, 5.94, 5.95 and 5.96)

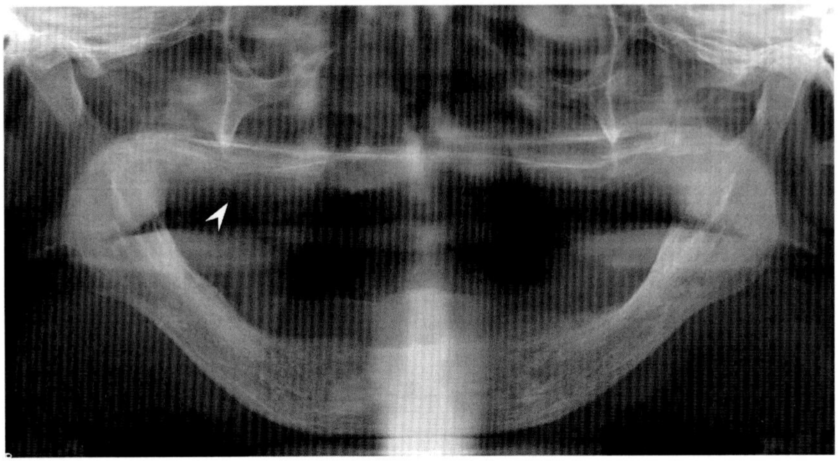

Fig. 5.85 Orthopantomography. An ill-defined bone destruction possibly caused by gingival SCC is demonstrated at the right upper molar region possibly involving the maxillary sinus (*arrowhead*)

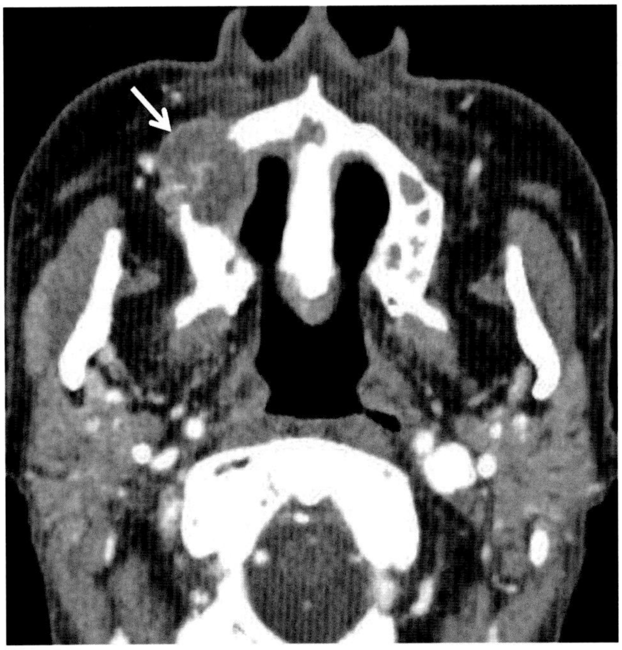

Fig. 5.86 Axial CECT. Tumor is demonstrated as an ill-defined heterogeneously enhancing mass (*arrow*) and the periphery and central portions of the tumor enhance prominently

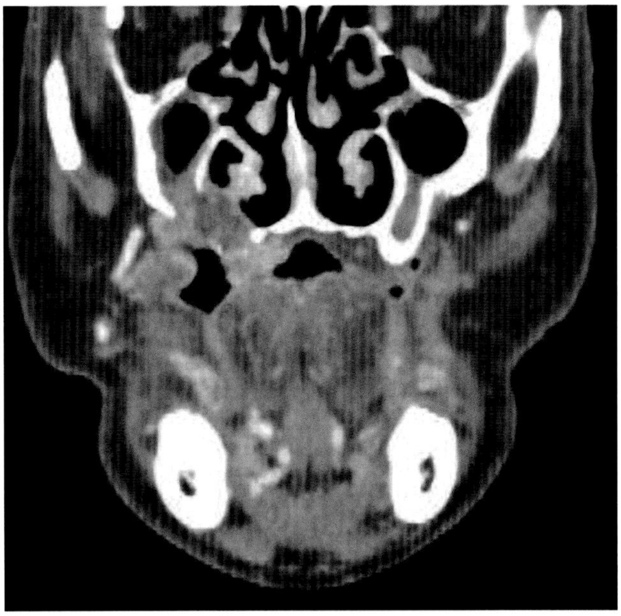

Fig. 5.87 Coronal CECT. Tumor (*arrow*) involves the buccinators muscle, the maxillary sinus, the nasal cavity, and the hard palate

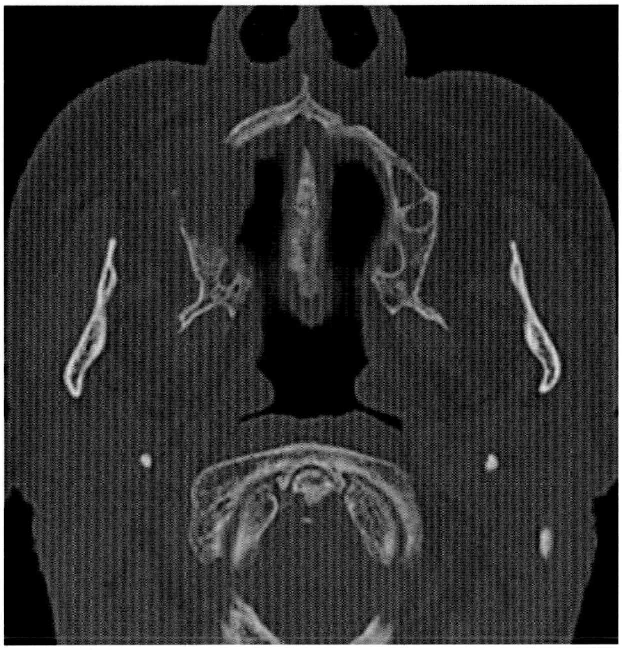

Fig. 5.88 Axial plain CT with bone window

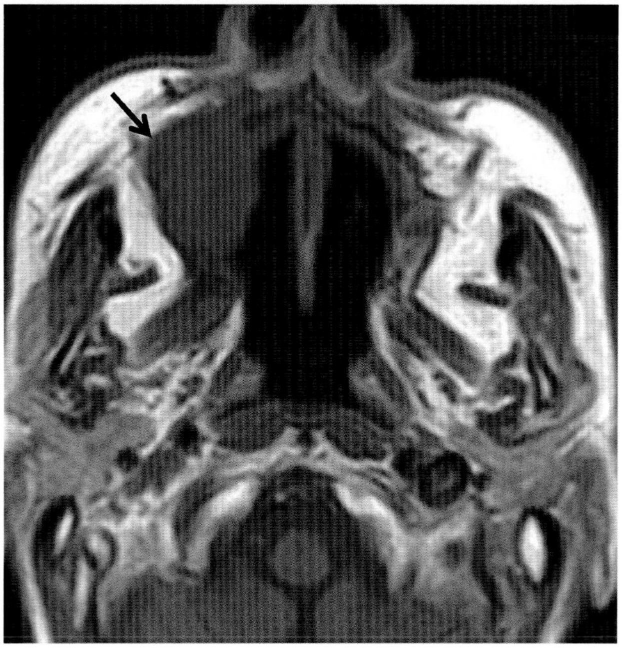

Fig. 5.90 Axial T1-weighted MRI. Tumor is demonstrated as an intermediate signal intensity area (*arrow*) with an ill-defined margin

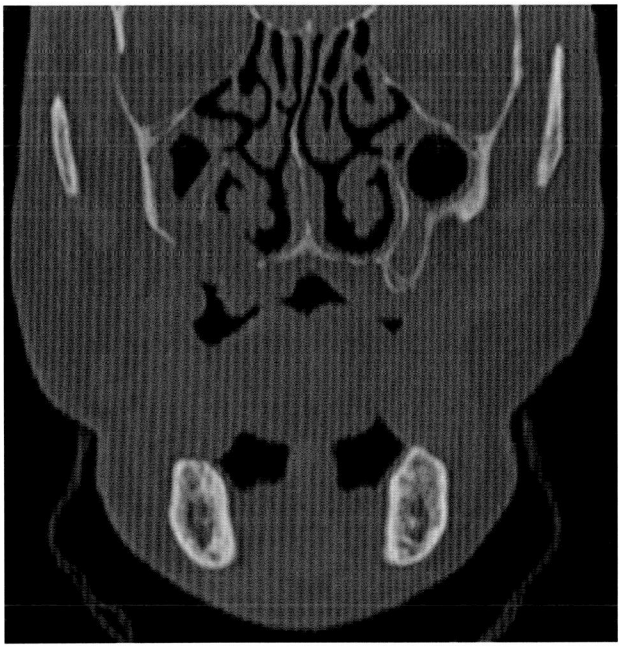

Fig. 5.89 Coronal plain CT with bone window. Destruction of the upper alveolar process, floor of the maxillary sinus, lateral wall of the nasal cavity, and the hard palate are demonstrated

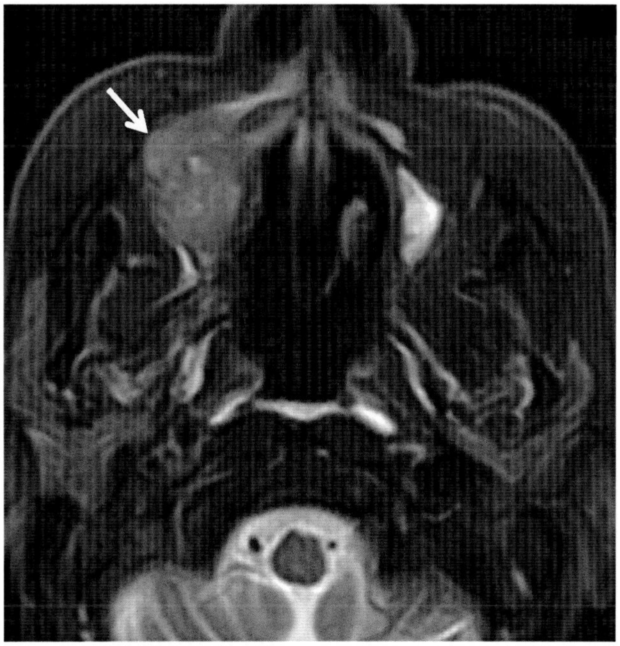

Fig. 5.91 Axial fat-saturated T2-weighted MRI. Tumor is demonstrated as relatively high heterogeneous intensity area (*arrow*)

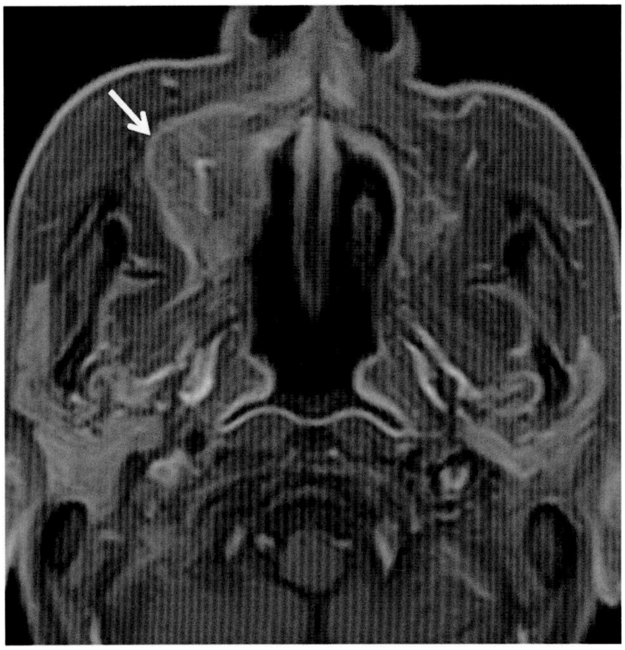

Fig. 5.92 Axial fat-saturated post-contrast T1-weighted MRI. Tumor enhances heterogeneously with an ill-defined margin (*arrow*) and the periphery and central portions of the tumor enhance prominently

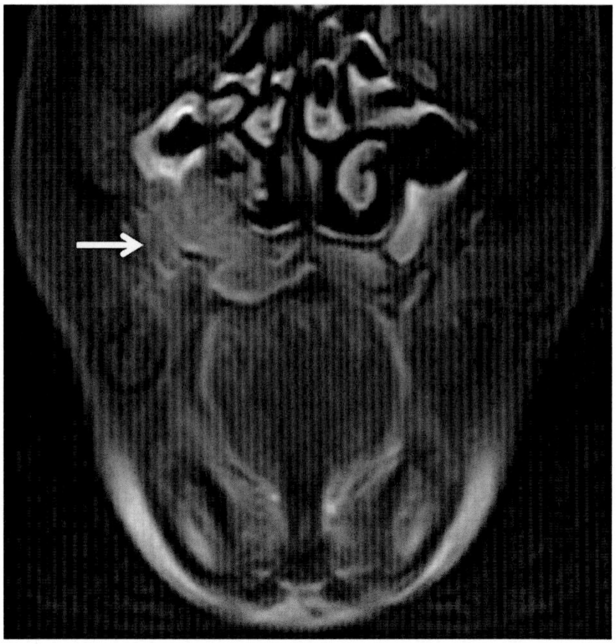

Fig. 5.94 Coronal fat-saturated T2-weighted MRI. Tumor is demonstrated as relatively high heterogeneous intensity (*arrow*). The signal intensity of the tumor is lower than that of thickened mucous membrane locating just above the tumor

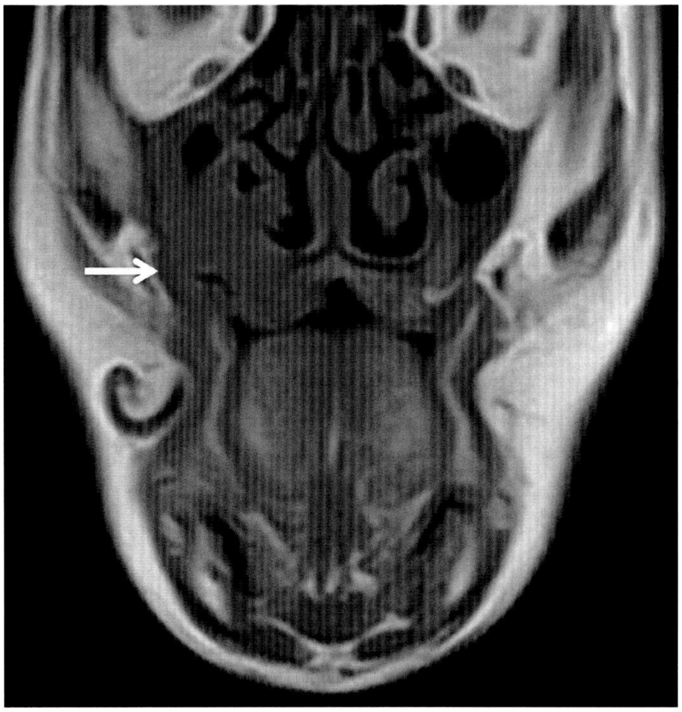

Fig. 5.93 Coronal T1-weighted MRI. Tumor is demonstrated as an intermediate signal intensity area (*arrow*)

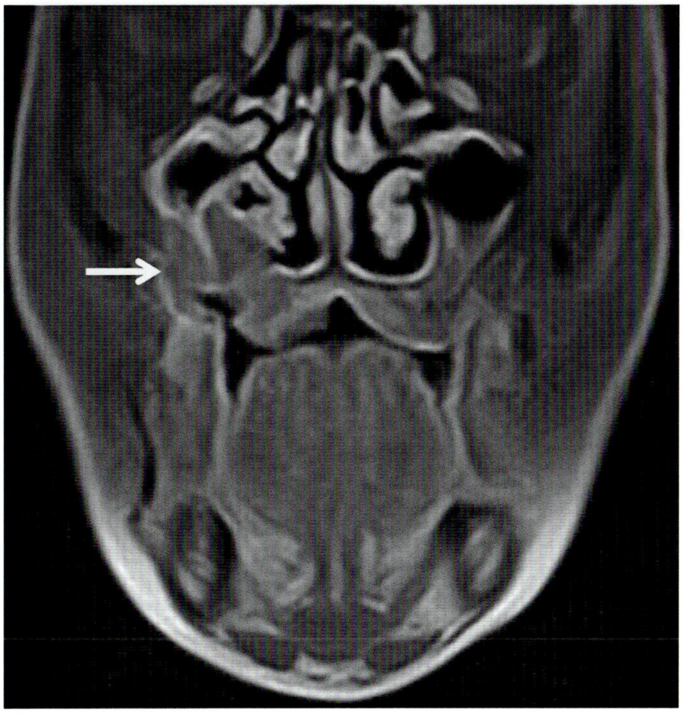

Fig. 5.95 Coronal fat-saturated post-contrast T1-weighted MRI. Tumor enhances heterogeneously and the signal intensity of the enhanced tumor is lower than that of thickened mucous membrane

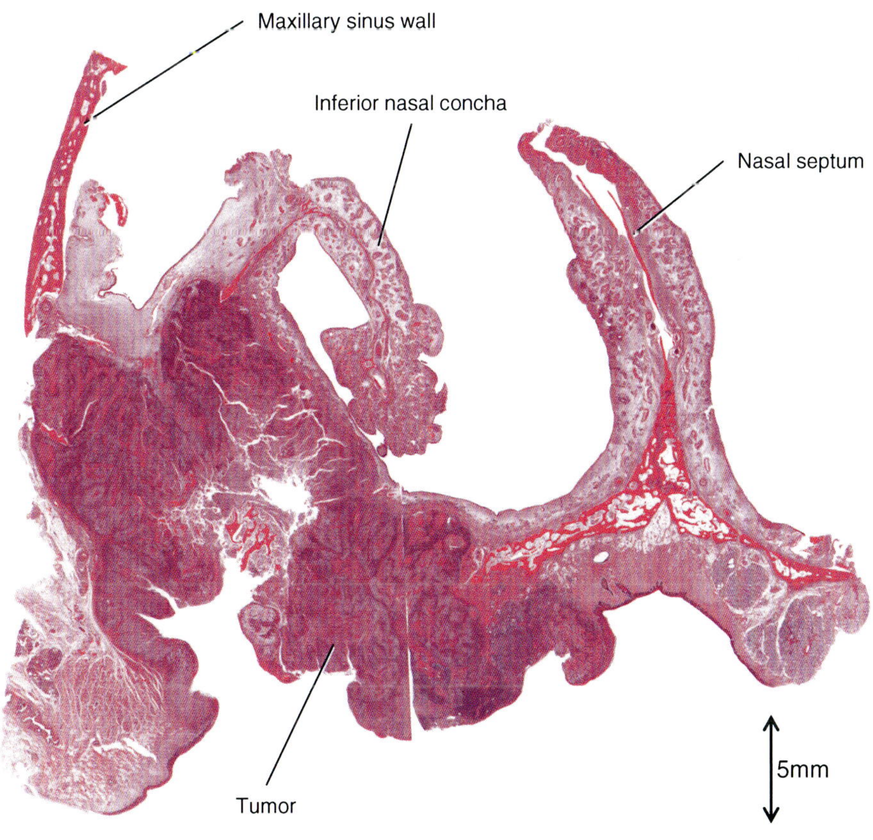

Fig. 5.96 Photomicrograph of histopathological specimen, coronal section (hematoxylin-eosin stain)

5.4.3 Floor of the Mouth Carcinoma

5.4.3.1 Case 5: 64-Year-Old Male, Floor of the Mouth SCC T4aN2c (Figs. 5.97, 5.98, 5.99, 5.100, 5.101, 5.102, 5.103, 5.104 and 5.105)

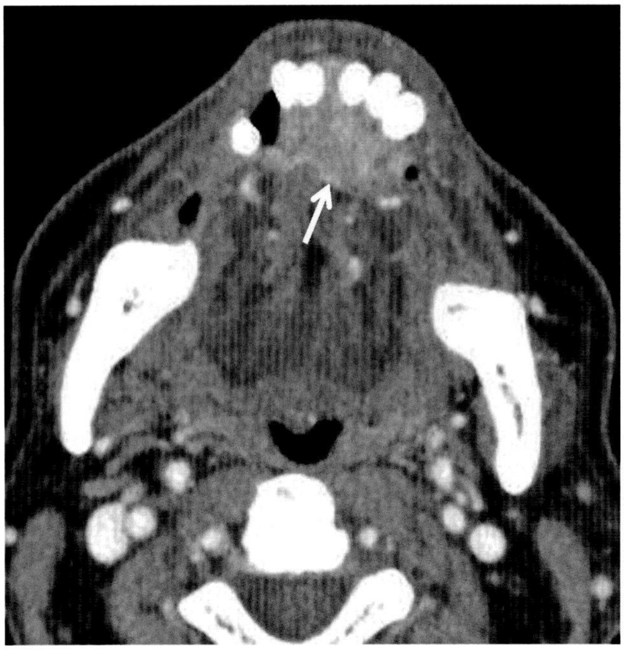

Fig. 5.97 Axial CECT. Tumor is demonstrated as an ill-defined heterogeneously enhancing mass (*arrow*) involving the bilateral sublingual space

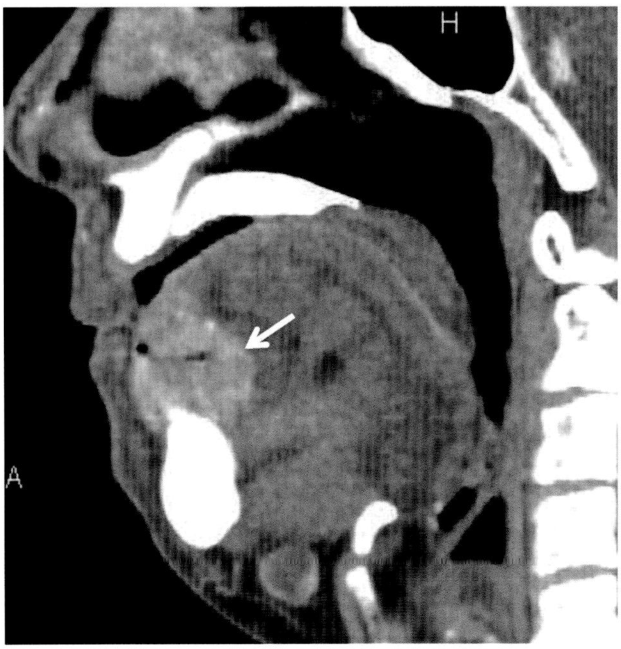

Fig. 5.98 Sagittal CECT. Tumor (*arrow*) involves the gingival mucosa and the genioglossus muscle

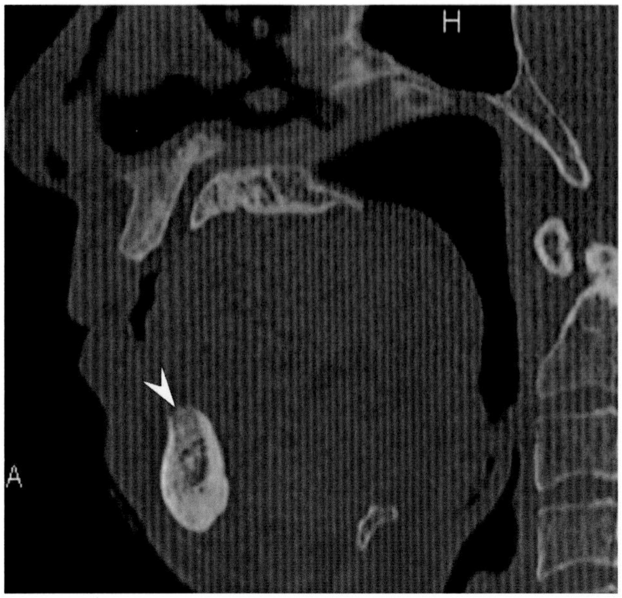

Fig. 5.99 Sagittal plain CT with bone window. Erosion of the cortex of the lower alveolar ridge is demonstrated (*arrowheads*)

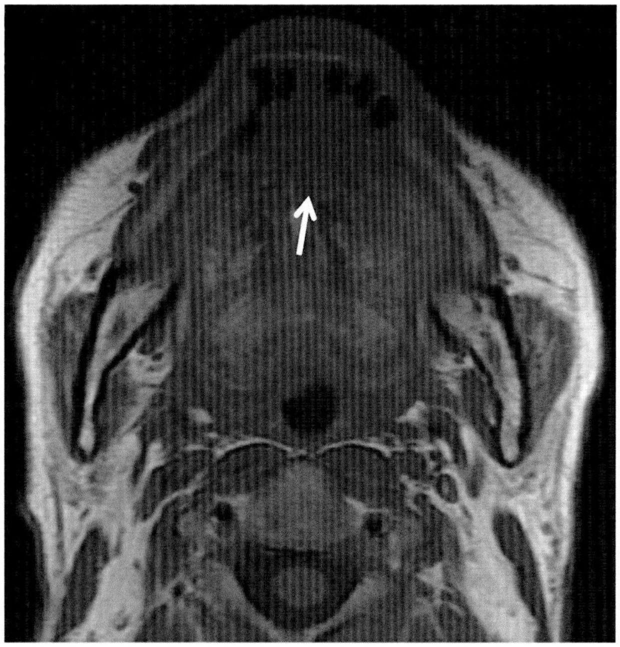

Fig. 5.100 Axial T1-weighted MRI. Tumor is demonstrated as an intermediate signal intensity area (*arrow*) with an ill-defined margin. Tumor (*arrow*) involves the genioglossus muscle

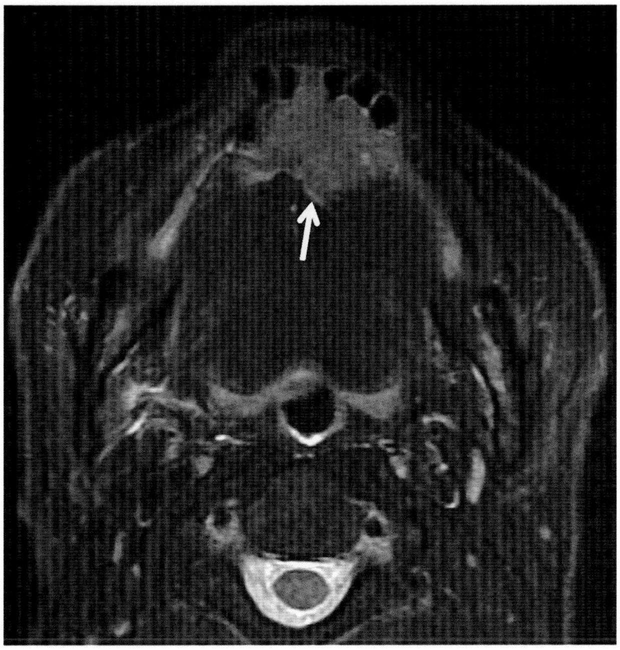

Fig. 5.101 Axial fat-saturated T2-weighted MRI. Tumor is demonstrated as relatively high heterogeneous intensity area (*arrow*)

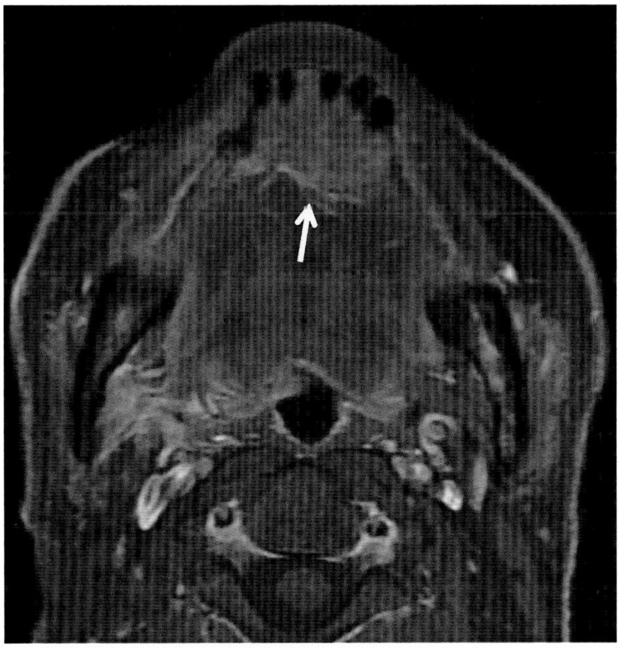

Fig. 5.102 Axial fat-saturated post-contrast T1-weighted MRI. Tumor enhances heterogeneously with an ill-defined margin (*arrow*)

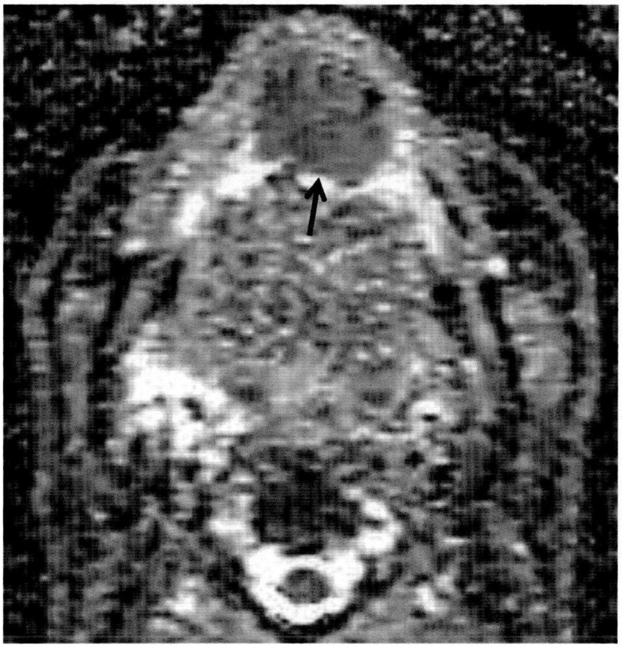

Fig. 5.103 Axial ADC map MRI. Tumor is demonstrated as a restricted diffusion area (*arrow*)

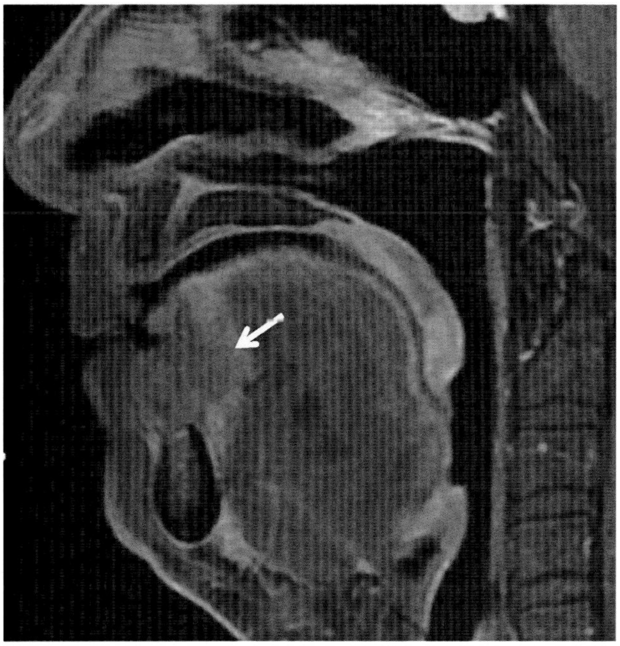

Fig. 5.104 Sagittal fat-saturated post-contrast T1-weighted MRI. Tumor enhances heterogeneously with an ill-defined margin (*arrow*)

5.4.4 Buccal Mucosa Carcinoma

5.4.4.1 Case 6: 78-Year-Old Male, Buccal Mucosa SCC T2N0 (Figs. 5.106, 5.107, 5.108, 5.109, 5.110, 5.111, 5.112, 5.113, 5.114 and 5.115)

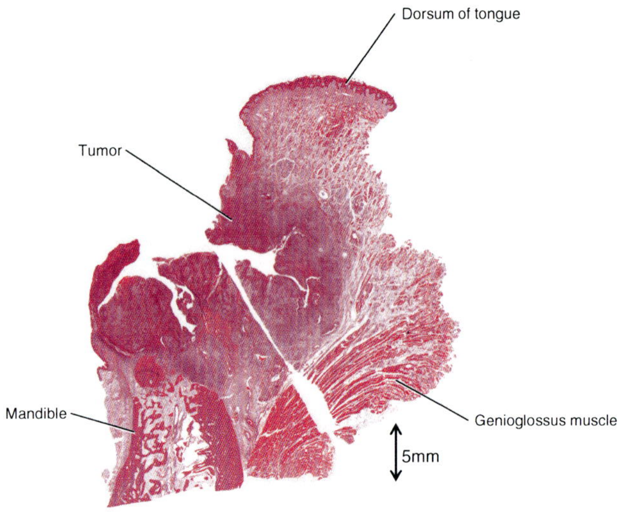

Fig. 5.105 Photomicrograph of histopathological specimen, sagittal section (hematoxylin-eosin stain)

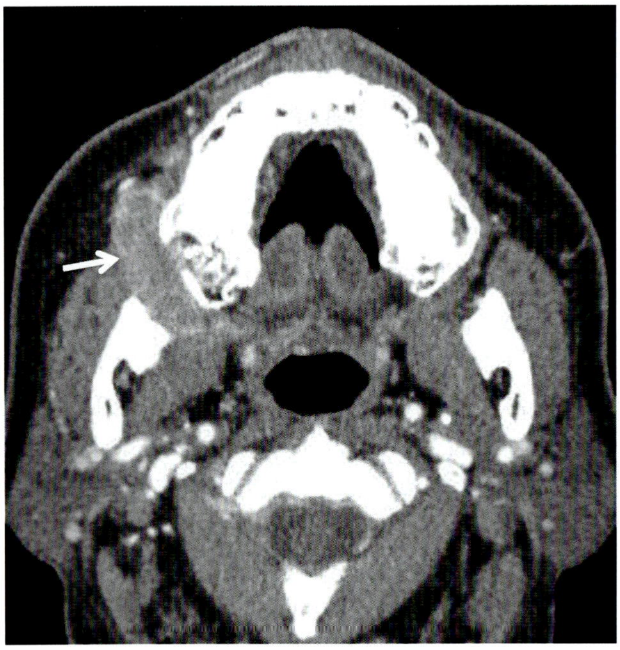

Fig. 5.106 Axial CECT. Tumor is demonstrated as an ill-defined heterogeneously enhancing mass (*arrow*) involving the buccinator muscle

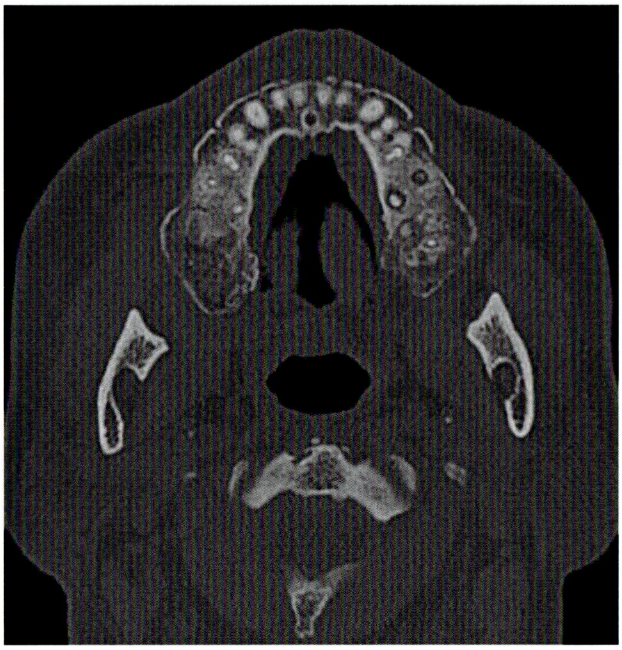

Fig. 5.107 Axial plain CT with bone window. No apparent destruction of adjacent bone cortex of the maxilla is observed

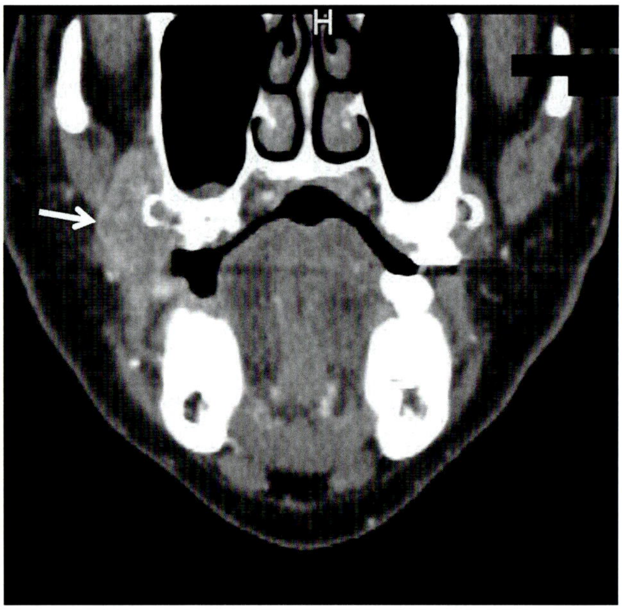

Fig. 5.108 Coronal CECT. Tumor (*arrow*) involves the buccal space

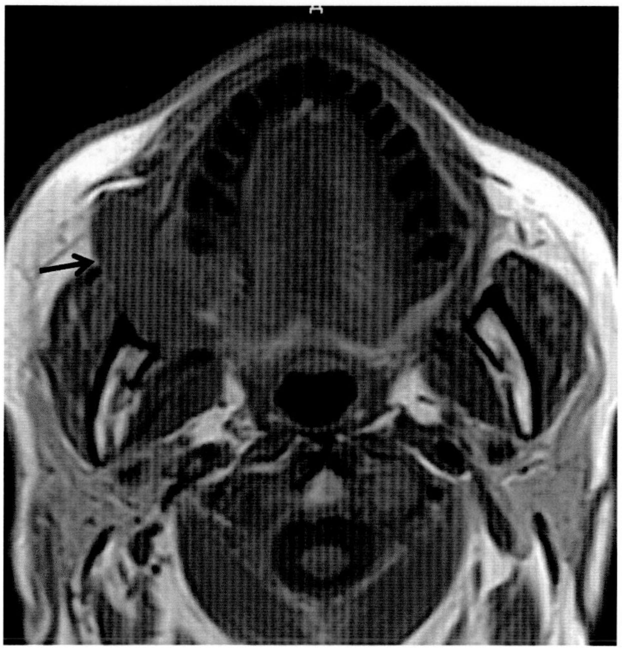

Fig. 5.109 Axial T1-weighted MRI. Tumor is demonstrated as an intermediate signal intensity area (*arrow*) with an ill-defined margin

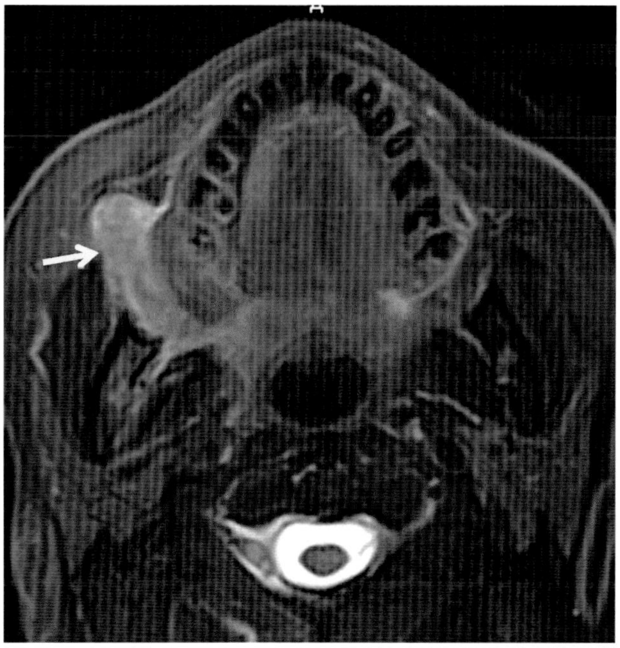

Fig. 5.110 Axial fat-saturated T2-weighted MRI. Tumor is demonstrated as relatively high heterogeneous intensity area (*arrow*)

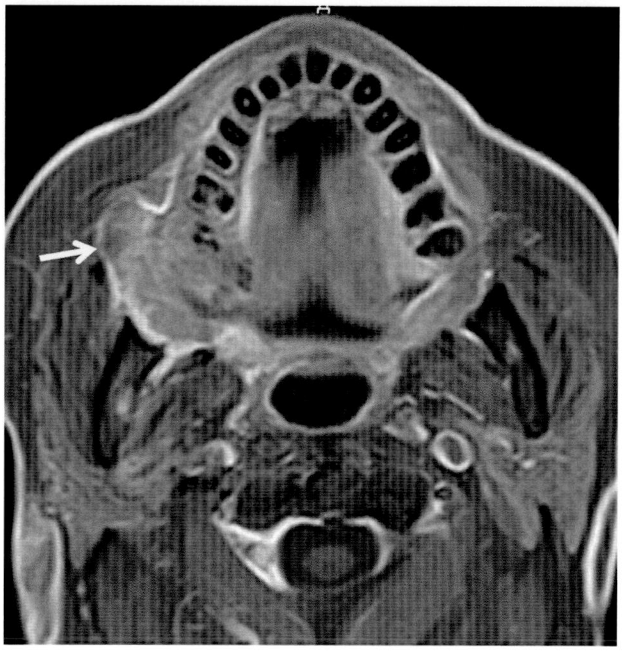

Fig. 5.111 Axial fat-saturated post-contrast T1-weighted MRI. Tumor enhances heterogeneously with an ill-defined margin (*arrow*)

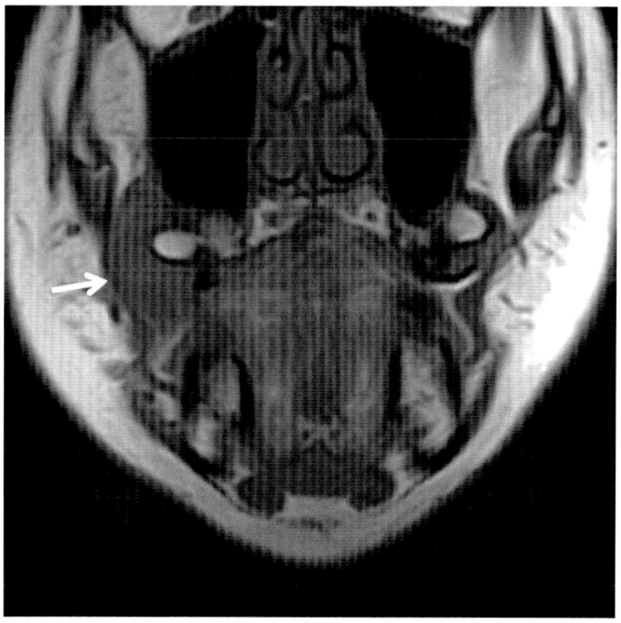

Fig. 5.112 Coronal T1-weighted MRI. Tumor is demonstrated as an intermediate signal intensity area (*arrow*)

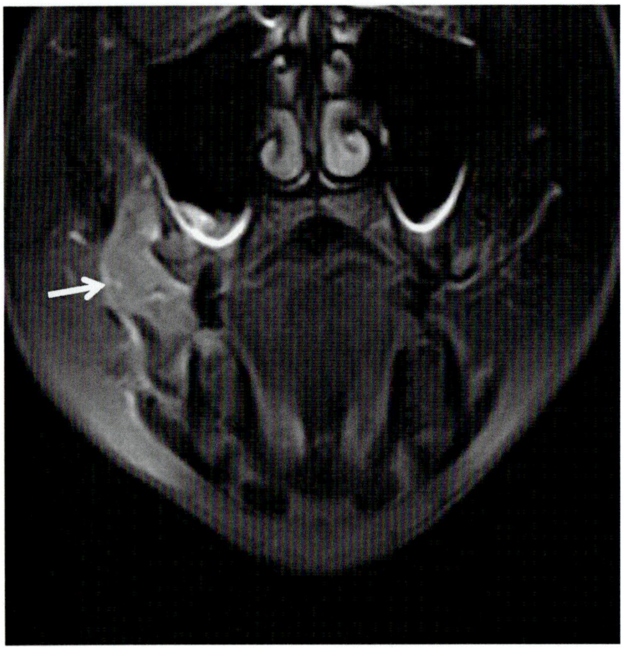

Fig. 5.113 Coronal fat-saturated T2-weighted MRI. Tumor is demonstrated as relatively high heterogeneous intensity (*arrow*). The signal intensity of the tumor is lower than that of thickened mucous membrane at the floor of the maxillary sinus

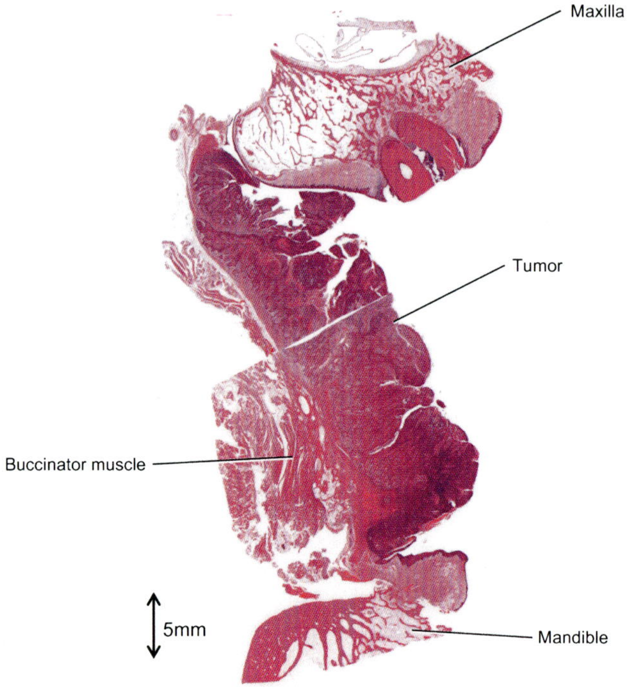

Fig. 5.115 Photomicrograph of histopathological specimen, coronal section (hematoxylin-eosin stain)

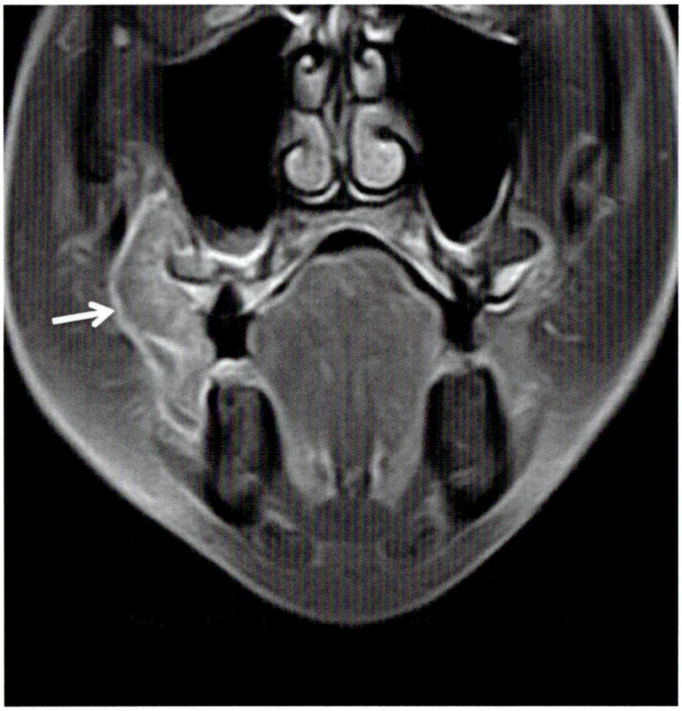

Fig. 5.114 Coronal fat-saturated post-contrast T1-weighted MRI. Tumor enhances heterogeneously (*arrow*) and the peripheral portion of the tumor enhances prominently

5.4.5 Lymph Node Metastasis

5.4.5.1 Case 7: 64-Year-Old Male, Floor of the Mouth SCC T4aN2c (Figs. 5.116, 5.117, 5.118, 5.119, 5.120, 5.121, 5.122, 5.123, 5.124, 5.125 and 5.126)

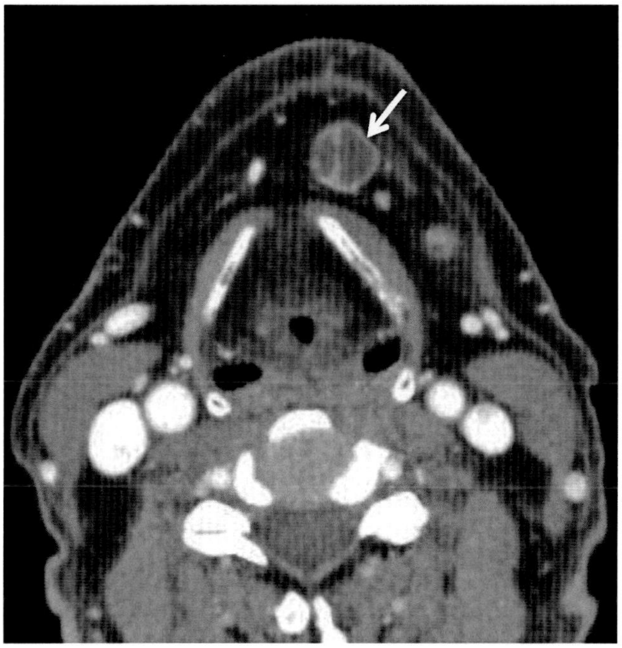

Fig. 5.116 Axial CECT. The metastatic left submental lymph node (*arrow*) is demonstrated as an oval-shaped nodule without distinct fatty hilum. Note the enhancing margin (rim enhancement) and central low-density area caused by central necrosis

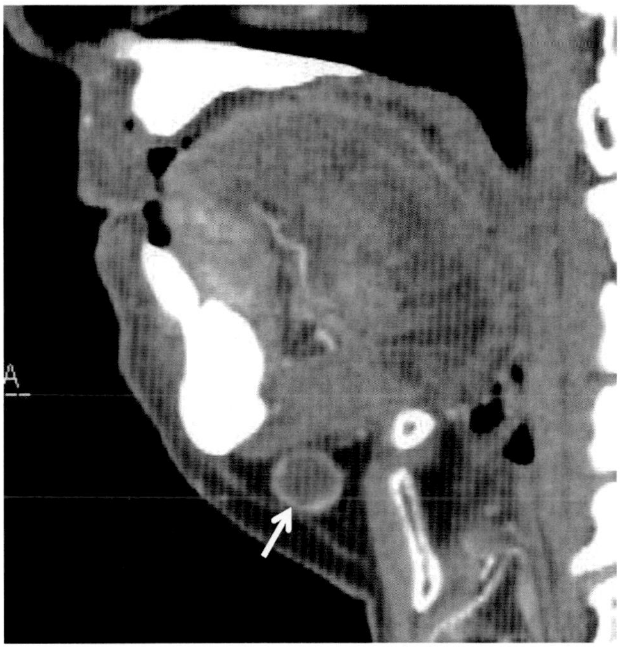

Fig. 5.117 Sagittal CECT. The left submental lymph node with rim enhancement is demonstrated (*arrow*)

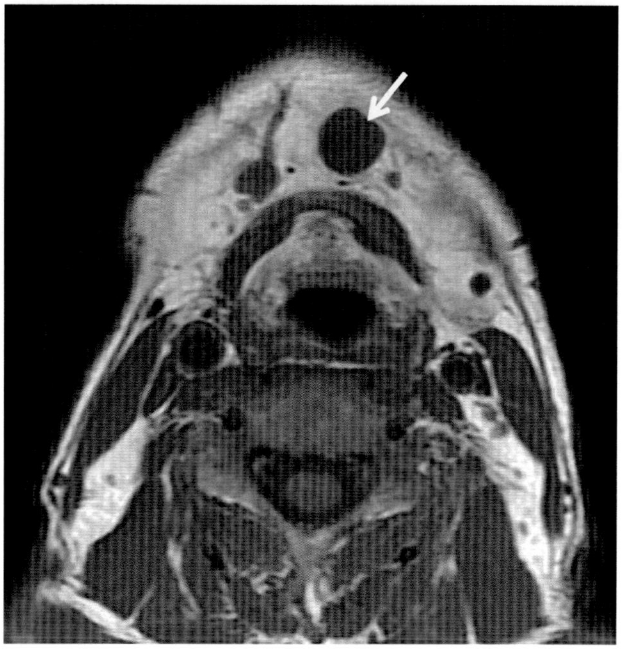

Fig. 5.118 Axial T1-weighted MRI. The left submental lymph node shows intermediate signal intensity

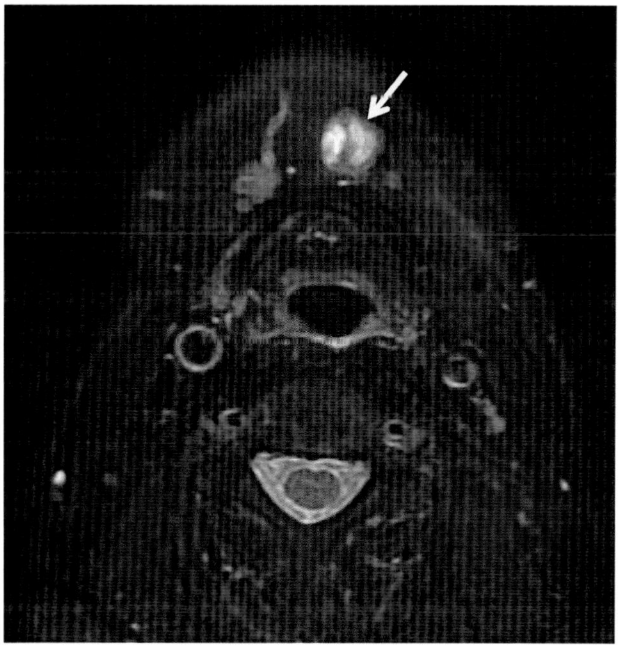

Fig. 5.119 Axial fat-saturated T2-weighted MRI. The left submental lymph node (*arrow*) shows heterogeneous intensity. Marginal portion of the node shows intermediate intensity and central portion shows high intensity

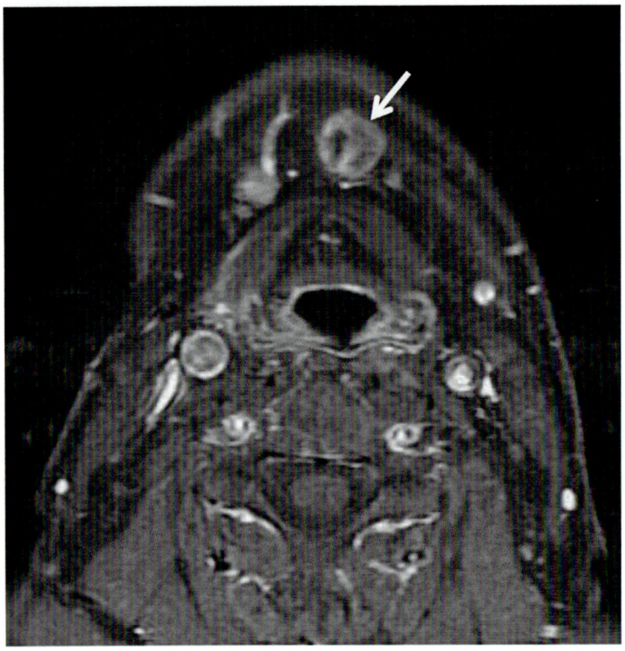

Fig. 5.120 Axial fat-saturated post-contrast T1-weighted MRI. Marginal portion of the left submental lymph node enhances and central portion remains unenhanced

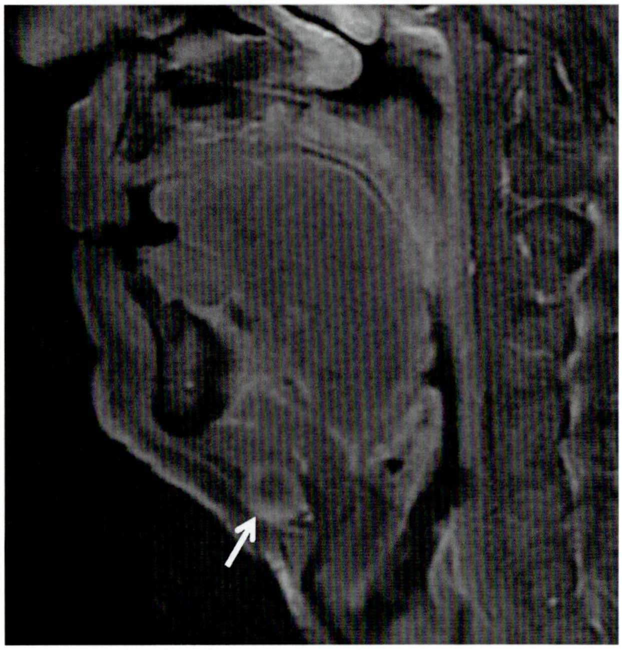

Fig. 5.121 Sagittal fat-saturated post-contrast T1-weighted MRI. The left submental lymph node with rim enhancement is demonstrated (*arrow*)

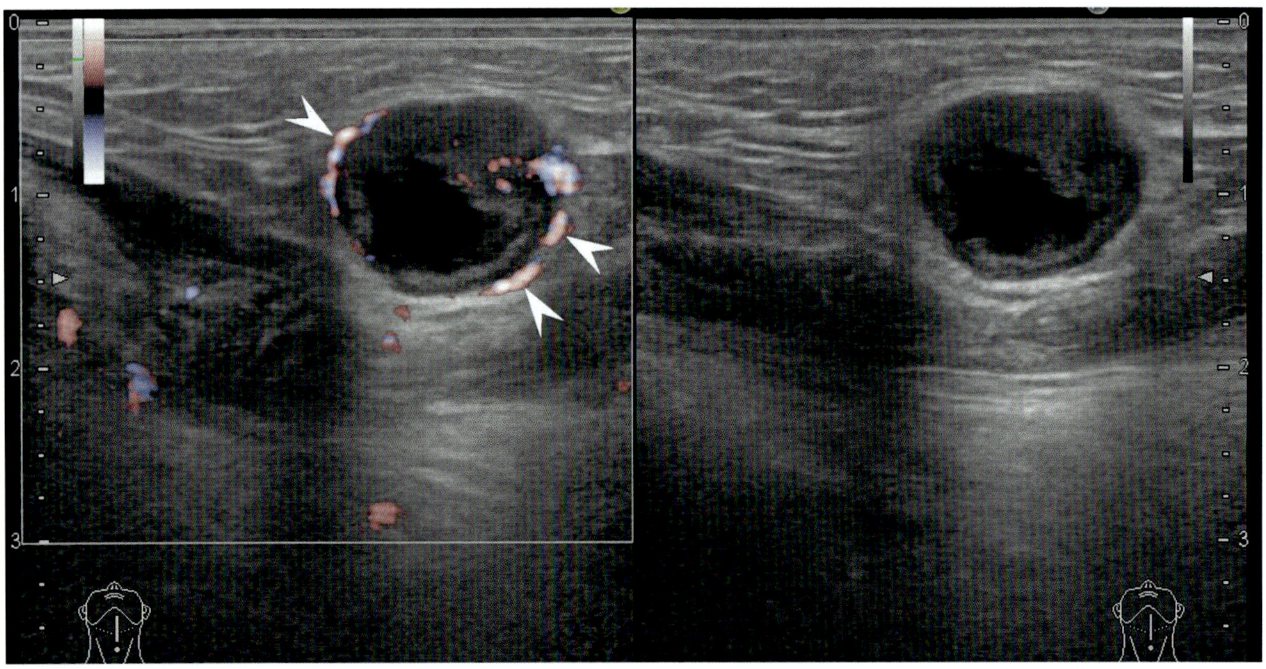

Fig. 5.122 Sagittal ultrasonography of the submental region (left, fine flow Doppler; right, B-mode). The left submental lymph node with anechoic area caused by central necrosis is demonstrated. Note the characteristic peripheral vascularity (*arrowheads*)

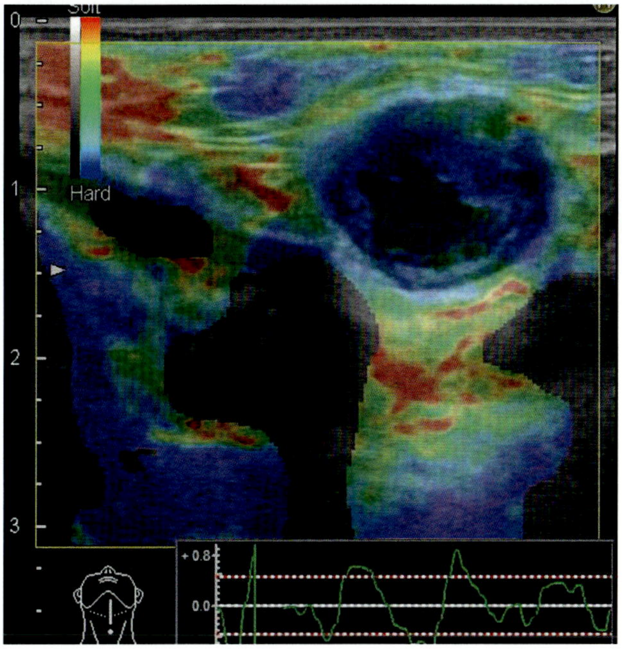

Fig. 5.123 Sagittal elastosonography of the left submental lymph node. Almost the whole node is occupied with a blue, hard area suggesting malignancy

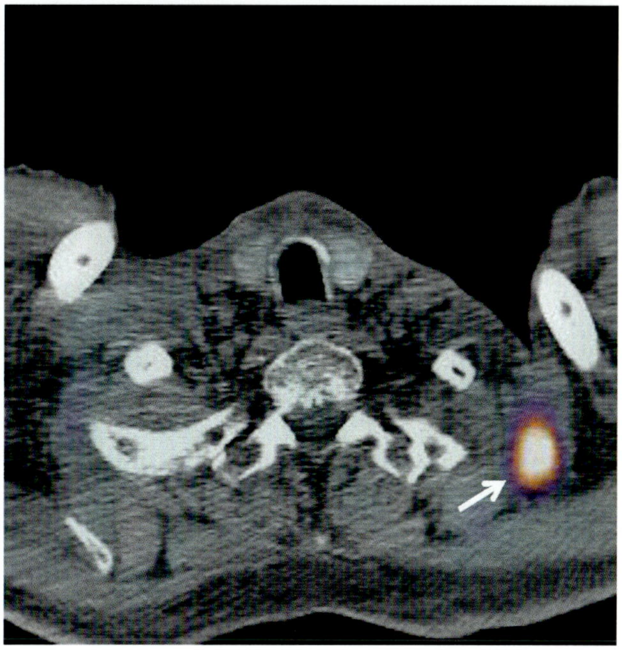

Fig. 5.125 Axial PET/CT. Recurrent tumor locating at the left supraclavicular fossa is disclosed after initial treatment (*arrow*)

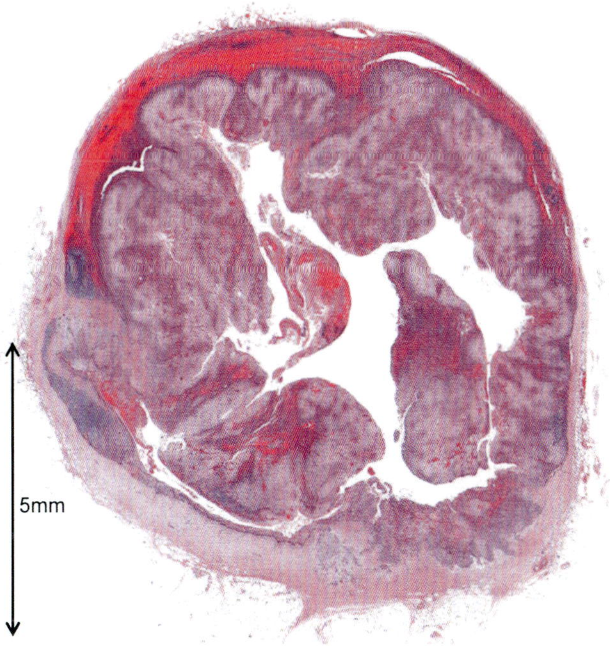

Fig. 5.124 Photomicrograph of histopathological specimen of the left submental lymph node (hematoxylin-eosin stain)

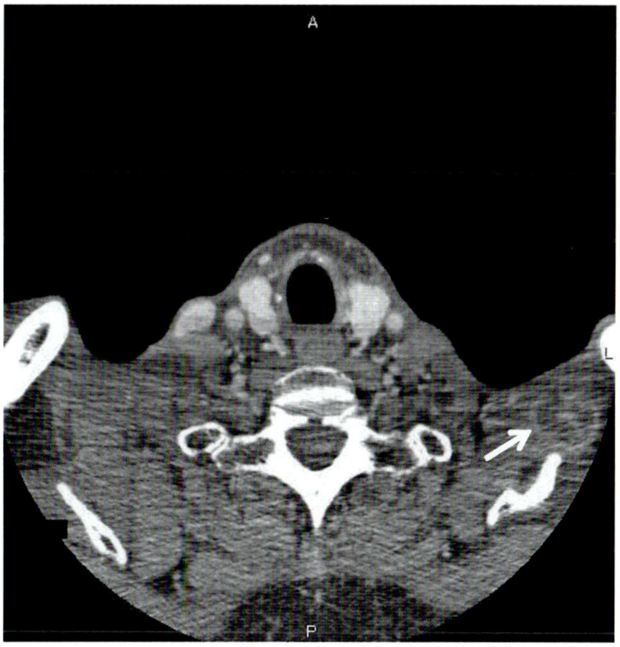

Fig. 5.126 Axial CECT. Recurrent tumor locating at the left supraclavicular fossa (*arrow*)

5.4.5.2 Case 8: 61-Year-Old Male, Left-Maxillary Gingival SCC T1N2b (Figs. 5.127, 5.128, 5.129, 5.130 and 5.131)

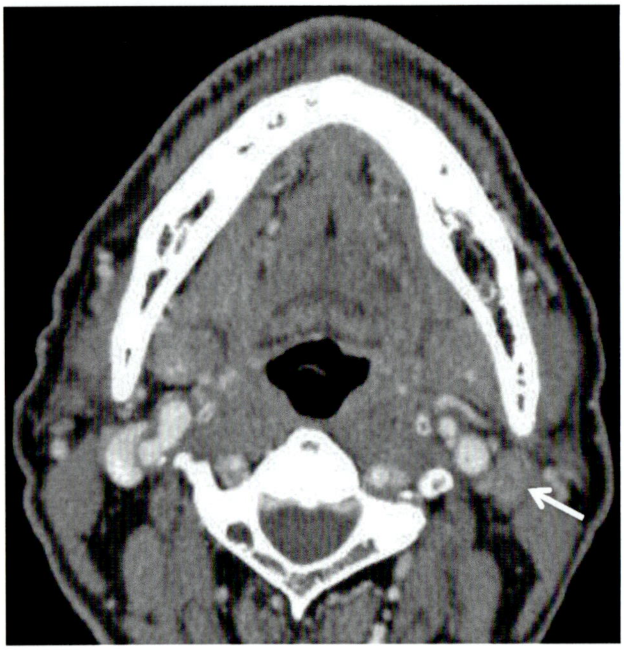

Fig. 5.127 Axial CECT. An enlarged homogenously enhancing superior internal jugular node is demonstrated (*arrow*). No apparent necrosis is observed

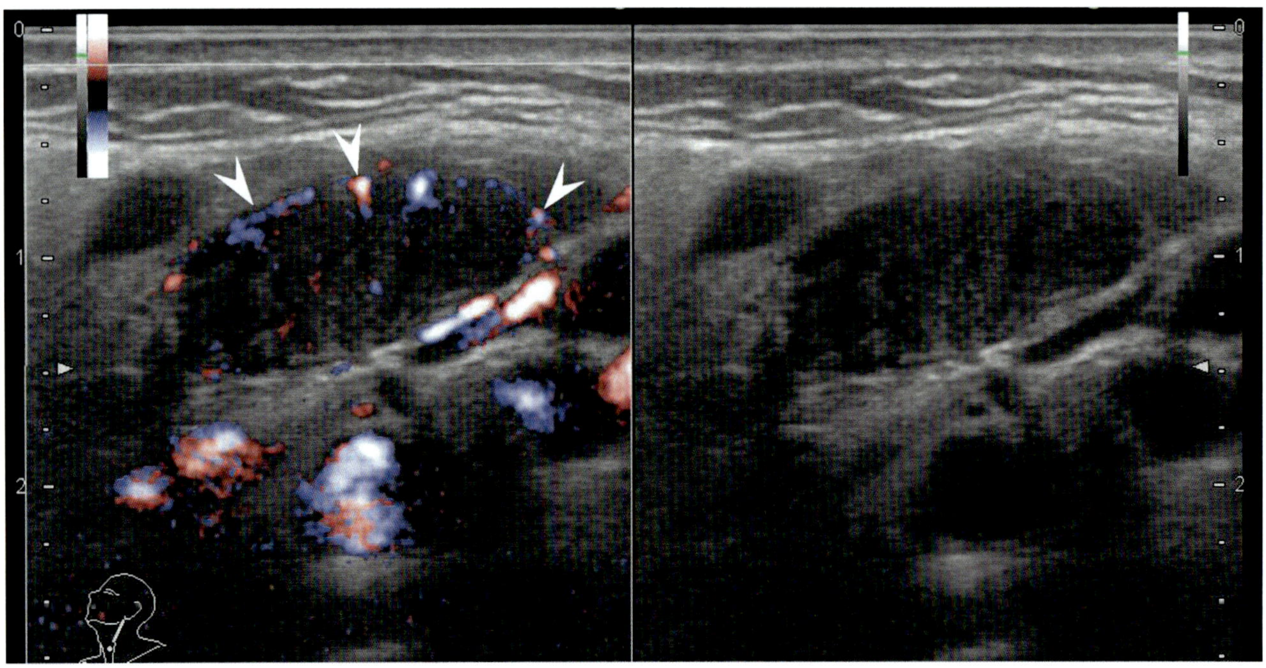

Fig. 5.128 Transverse ultrasonography at the upper neck level (left, fine flow Doppler; right, B-mode). An enlarged superior internal jugular node with an ill-defined margin is demonstrated. Note the characteristic peripheral vascularity (*arrowheads*)

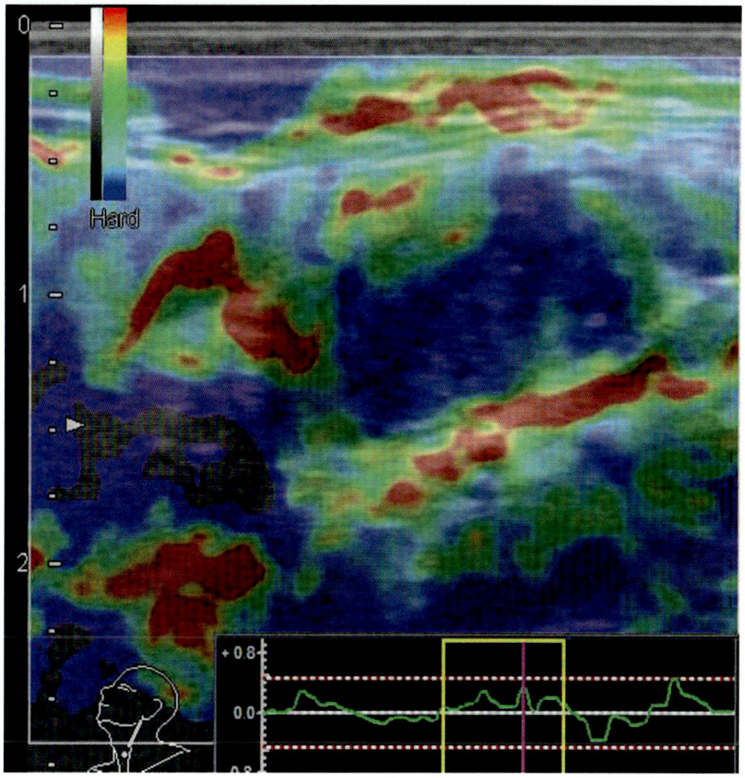

Fig. 5.129 Transverse elastosonography of the superior internal jugular node. The most part of the node is occupied with a blue, hard area suggesting malignancy

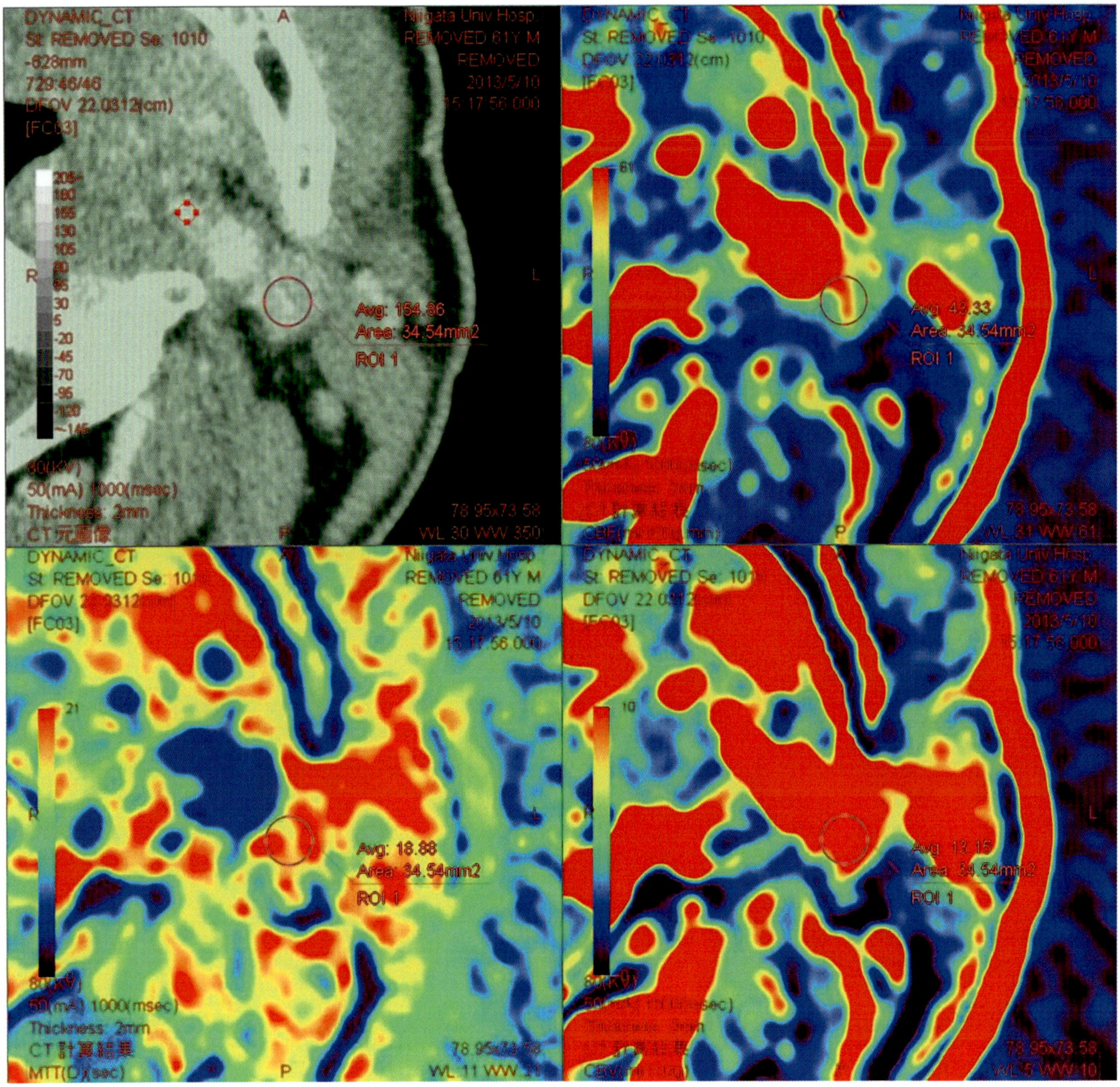

Fig. 5.130 CTP at the level of the superior internal jugular node. According to the CTP analysis, blood flow and mean transit time of the superior internal jugular node present significantly different values compared with normal contralateral node

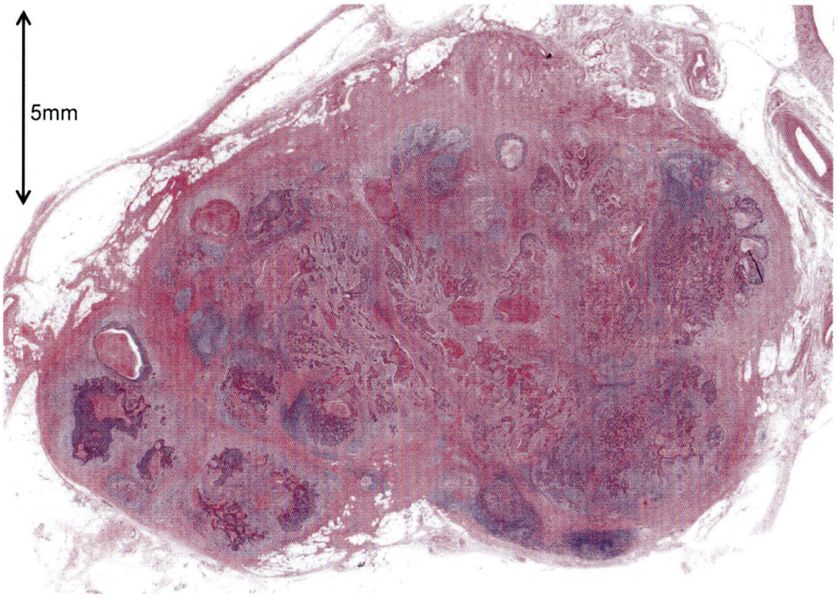

Fig. 5.131 Photomicrograph of histopathological specimen of the superior internal jugular node (hematoxylin-eosin stain)

References

1. Izumo T, Ariji E, Ozeki S, Okada N, Okabe S, Okazaki Y, Omura K, Kirita T, Kusama M, Sato T, Shinohara M, Shimozato K, Shintani S, Tanaka Y, Nakayama E, Hayashi T, Miyazaki A, Yagishita H, Yamane M, Working Group 1 on the 'Guidelines for Clinical and Pathological Studies of Oral Cancer', Scientific Committee, Japan Society for Oral Tumors (2010) General rules for clinical and pathological studies on oral cancer, 1st edn. Kaneharashuppan, Tokyo
2. Glastonbury CM, Harnsberger HR, Michel MA, Branstetter BF, Hudgins PA, Shatzkes D (eds) (2012) Specialty imaging: head and neck cancer: state of the art diagnosis, staging, and surveillance. Amirsys Publishing, Inc., Salt Lake City
3. Som PM, Curtin HD (2011) Head and neck imaging, 5th edn. Elsevier Mosby Inc., St. Louis
4. Edge SB, Byrd DR, Compton CC et al (eds) (2010) AJCC cancer staging manual, 7th edn. Springer, New York
5. Izumo T, Kirita T, Ariji E, Ozeki S, Okada N, Okabe S, Okazaki Y, Omura K, Kusama M, Sato T, Shinohara M, Shimozato K, Shintani S, Tanaka Y, Nakayama E, Hayashi T, Miyazaki A, Yagishita H, Yamane M, Working Group 1 on the "Guidelines for Clinical and Pathological Studies of Oral Cancer", Scientific Committee, Japan Society for Oral Tumors (2012) General rules for clinical and pathological studies on oral cancer: a synopsis. Jpn J Clin Oncol 42:1099–1109. doi:10.1093/jjco/hys141

Clinical Evaluation and Differential Diagnosis

6

Seiji Nakamura

Abstract

In this chapter, the focus is on the clinical characteristics of oral cancers. The general characteristics regarding site distribution, observational findings, symptoms, examinations to diagnose, and evaluate, and site-specific clinical characteristics are described. Second, other oral lesions with clinical similarities to oral cancers, precancerous lesions and conditions with early malignant changes, and other malignancies in the oral cavity, which occasionally involve the oral cavity and should be carefully differentiated from oral cancers, are listed and their clinical characteristics are described.

Keywords

Clinical evaluation • Differential diagnosis • Oral cancer • Precancerous lesion • Squamous cell carcinoma

6.1 Clinical Evaluation and Differential Diagnosis

6.1.1 Clinical Evaluation of Oral Cancers

6.1.1.1 General Clinical Characteristics of Oral Cancers

Oral cancers generally refer to squamous cell carcinomas originating in the covering mucosa in the oral cavity, although carcinomas occasionally arise in the salivary gland. According to the UICC classification [1], the oral mucosa is divided into six sites—buccal mucosa, upper alveolus and gingiva, lower alveolus and gingiva, hard palate, tongue, and floor of mouth—and among these, carcinoma of the tongue is the most commonly occurring. The clinical diagnosis of oral cancers presents few diagnostic difficulties, and provided that the dentist or oral surgeon carries out a systematic examination of the oral cavity, there is little chance of oral cancers being overlooked. Difficulty can arise only if the lesion is exceptionally small or if it lies in an anatomically inaccessible area.

Oral cancers usually develop as an erosive, ulcerative, verrucous, nodular, or granular lesion with white patch or erythema and thereafter show various findings including ulcer, induration, and tumor formation in progression. Lesions are always painless in the early stages, although general symptoms vary according to the site of the lesion. Pain and tenderness only develop when an ulcerative lesion becomes secondarily infected or if the lesion involves a sensory nerve. In the late stages, symptoms of the lesion include pain due to secondary infection or involvement of the sensory nerves in the region, excessive salivation, difficulty with speech, mastication and swallowing, and hemorrhage that usually manifests as blood-contaminated saliva.

A number of clinical classification methods based on observational findings have been proposed so far [2–10]. One of the conventional methods proposed by Ueno classified oral cancer into five types: indurative, ulcerative, granular, leukoplakic, and papillary [10]. Clinical characteristics of each type are as follows: (1) The indurative type is a bulged lesion with elevated mucosal surface and extensive deep induration caused by submucosal and deep invasion of

S. Nakamura, D.D.S., Ph.D. (✉)
Section of Oral and Maxillofacial Oncology, Division of Maxillofacial Diagnostic and Surgical Sciences, Faculty of Dental Science, Kyushu University, Fukuoka, Japan
e-mail: seiji@dent.kyushu-u.ac.jp

T. Kirita and K. Omura (eds.), *Oral Cancer: Diagnosis and Therapy*, DOI 10.1007/978-4-431-54938-3_6, © Springer Japan 2015

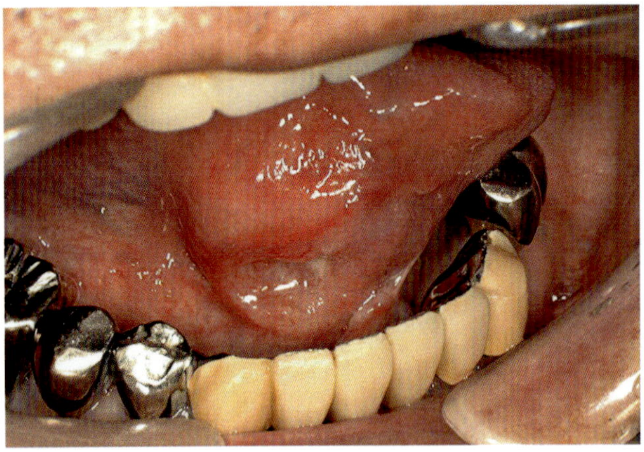

Fig. 6.1 A squamous cell carcinoma of the tongue showing the indurative type of observational findings and the endophytic type of clinical growth pattern

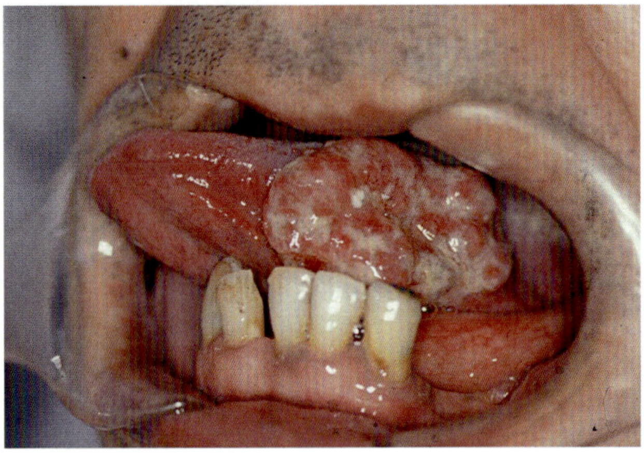

Fig. 6.3 A squamous cell carcinoma of the tongue showing the granular type of observational findings and the exophytic type of clinical growth pattern

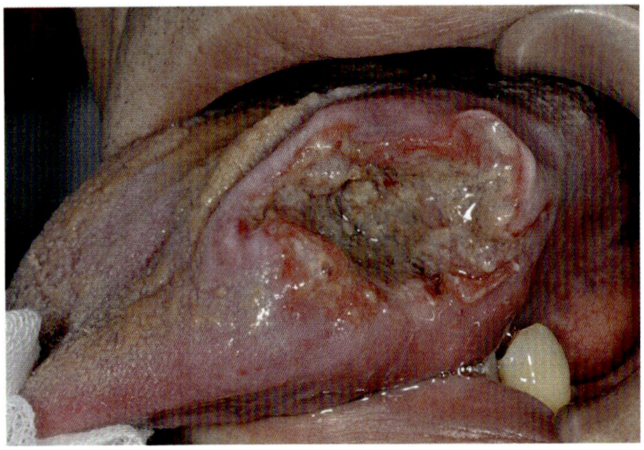

Fig. 6.2 A squamous cell carcinoma of the tongue showing the ulcerative type of observational findings and the endophytic type of clinical growth pattern

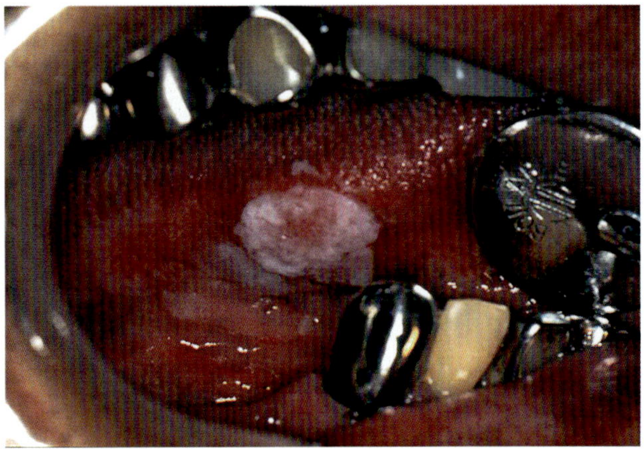

Fig. 6.4 A squamous cell carcinoma of the tongue showing the leukoplakic type of observational findings and the superficial type of clinical growth pattern

tumor cells (Fig. 6.1). (2) The ulcerative type is a poorly defined erosive or ulcerative lesion with raised or rolled edges and extensive deep induration (Fig. 6.2). (3) The granular type is a granulomatous lesion with a granular surface caused by exposure of tumor cells and with moderately deep induration (Fig. 6.3). (4) The leukoplakic type is a white, patchy, and slightly thick lesion lacking deep induration and with partial erosions and ulcerations (Fig. 6.4). (5) The papillary type is a whitish and hard lesion with moderately deep induration, which takes on a verrucous, fissuring, fungating, nodular, or papillomatous form (Fig. 6.5).

Recently, a more universal and reproducible classification based on clinical growth patterns judged by close inspection and digital palpation has been proposed, which divides oral cancer into three types: superficial, exophytic, and endophytic [11]. These superficial, exophytic, and endophytic types are leukoplakic or erythroplakic lesions lacking deep indurations (Fig. 6.4), granular or papillary lesions with moderately deep indurations (Figs. 6.3 and 6.5), and indurative or ulcerative lesions with extensive deep indurations (Figs. 6.1 and 6.2), respectively. Especially in carcinoma of the tongue, the endophytic type is more closely associated with poor prognosis in comparison with the other types. This classification

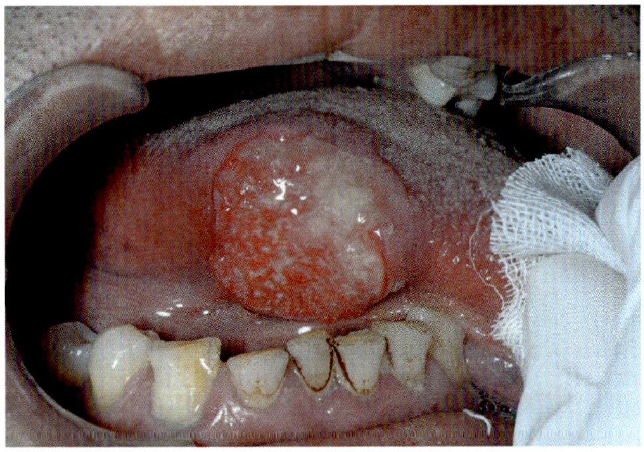

Fig. 6.5 A squamous cell carcinoma of the tongue showing the papillary type of observational findings and the exophytic type of clinical growth pattern

thus provides clinically useful information as a prognostic factor for recurrence, metastasis, and survival rate.

In addition to macroscopic inspection and digital palpation, pathological examination is indispensable for definite and accurate evaluation of lesions. Cancer tissue together with adjacent noncancerous mucosa is generally sampled using wedge resections as biopsy specimens. The objective of a biopsy is not only to make a definitive diagnosis of cancer but also to obtain detailed information concerning the degree of histological malignancy, mode of invasion, stage of invasion, vascular invasion, cellular response, and probability of lymph node metastasis.

Furthermore, oral cancers should be evaluated using imaging with X-ray examinations including pantomography, CT, MR, ultrasonography, and PET. X-ray examinations, CT and MR, are extremely supportive to identify the invasion of adjacent tissues by attaching importance to the evaluation of depth. Furthermore, bone resorption patterns identified using imaging provide clinically useful information to evaluate malignancy of oral cancers. The patterns are usually classified into two types: pressure and moth-eaten types [11]. The pressure type shows flat, saucer-shaped, or U-shaped margin and is observed in association with slowly growing and non-invasive lesions (Fig. 6.6). In contrast, the moth-eaten type is irregular with an indistinct margin and is closely associated with rapidly growing and highly invasive lesions (Fig. 6.7).

Cervical lymph node metastasis should be evaluated using CT and ultrasonography, as well as careful digital

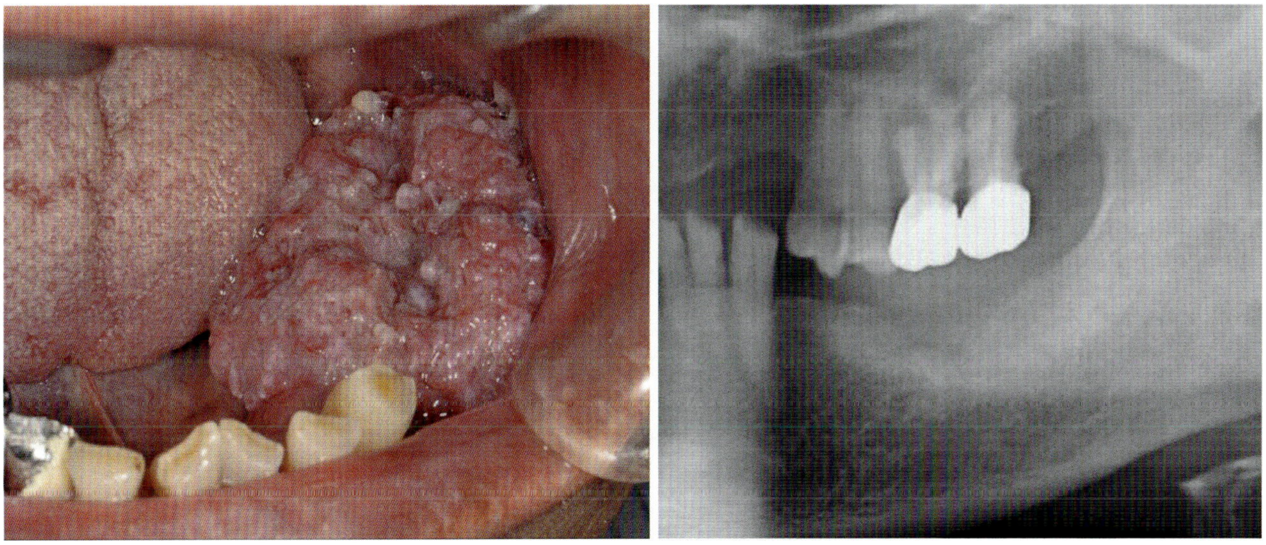

Fig. 6.6 A squamous cell carcinoma of the lower gingiva showing the granular type of observational findings, the exophytic type of clinical growth pattern, and the pressure type of bone resorption

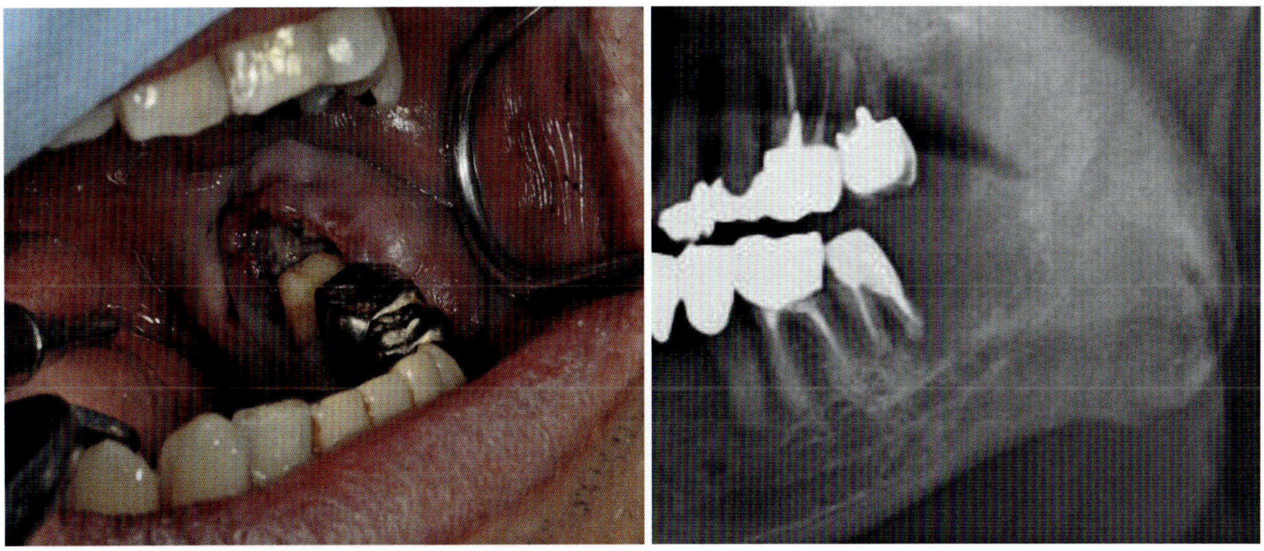

Fig. 6.7 A squamous cell carcinoma of the lower gingiva showing the indurative type of observational findings, the endophytic type of clinical growth pattern, and the moth-eaten type of bone resorption

palpation, since approximately 30 % of oral cancers metastasize to the regional lymph node(s) in the ipsilateral and/or contralateral neck. MR and PET are occasionally supportive. Distant metastasis is identified only in approximately 1 % of oral cancers, but should be routinely evaluated using chest X-ray examination, as lung is one of the most frequent distant organs to which oral cancers metastasize. ^{67}Ga and bone scintigraphies, and recently PET, are useful to identify distant metastasis to other organs.

6.1.1.2 Site-Specific Clinical Characteristics of Oral Cancers

Buccal Mucosa

In the Indian subcontinent, oral cancers account for more than one third of all malignancies, and buccal mucosa is the most common site for them. This is probably related to the widespread habit of betel- and tobacco-chewing. Carcinomas of the buccal mucosa account for approximately 10 % of oral cancers. The tumors usually involve the mucosa opposite the lower third molar tooth and retromolar pad and are predominantly well and moderately differentiated squamous cell carcinomas.

The early lesion is painless and may form a white or speckled patch or an indurated nodule or ulcer. As the tumor enlarges exophytically, it usually becomes ulcerated or papillary and then invades into the surrounding muscle and bones (Figs. 6.8 and 6.9). Nodal involvement, usually in the jugulodigastric, submandibular or upper deep cervical lymph nodes, is seen in 35–50 % of patients.

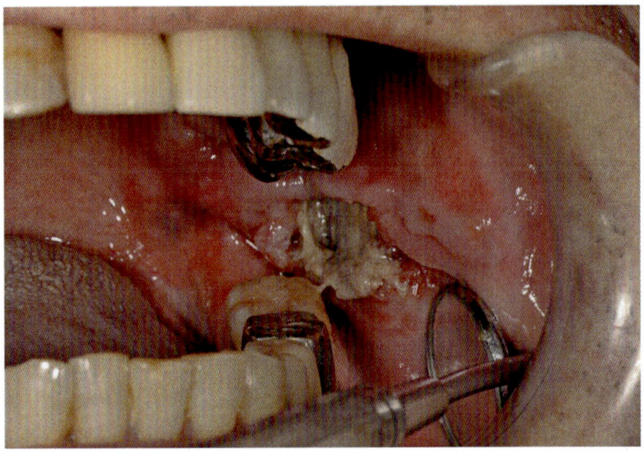

Fig. 6.8 A squamous cell carcinoma of the buccal mucosa showing the ulcerative type of observational findings and the endophytic type of clinical growth pattern

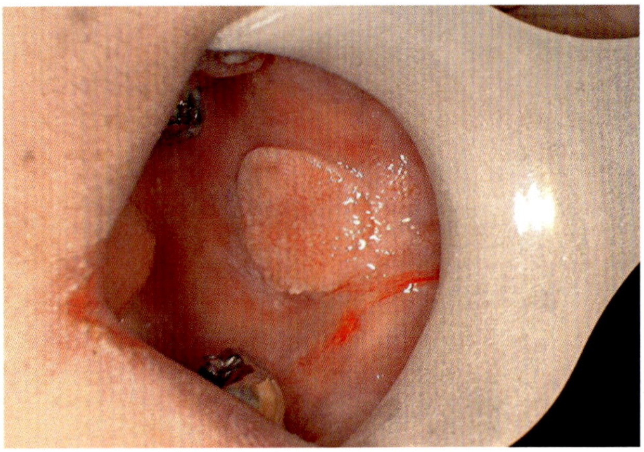

Fig. 6.9 A squamous cell carcinoma of the buccal mucosa showing the papillary type of observational findings and the exophytic type of clinical growth pattern

Upper Alveolus and Gingiva

Carcinomas of the upper alveolus and gingiva account for approximately 10 % of oral cancers, and the incidence is apparently lower than that of carcinomas of the lower alveolus and gingiva. These carcinomas are commonly well and moderately differentiated squamous cell carcinomas.

The tumor may present as a lump or as a more obvious vegetating mass and tends to involve the bone at a relatively early stage. Bone resorption patterns classified into either pressure or moth-eaten type provide clinically useful information to evaluate the malignancy of the tumor. The speckled appearance of the granular and exophytic mass is most frequently seen and the ulcerated mass is also seen (Fig. 6.10). If teeth are present in relation to the tumor, they may become loose, painful, and periostitic. Carcinomas of the maxillary sinus and malignant lymphomas invade the alveolus and/or palate to present in a similar manner. The submandibular and upper deep cervical lymph nodes are the most frequent sites of secondary spread and nodal involvement is evident in 20–30 % of patients.

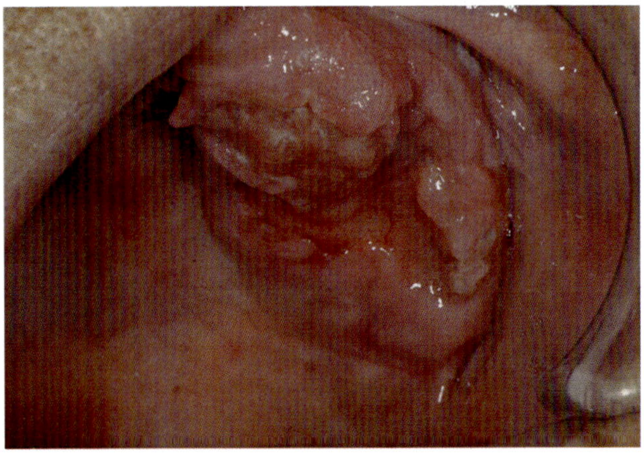

Fig. 6.10 A squamous cell carcinoma of the upper alveolus showing the granular type of observational findings and the exophytic type of clinical growth pattern

Lower Alveolus and Gingiva

Carcinomas of the lower alveolus and gingiva account for as many as 20 % of oral cancers, and the incidence is two times higher than that of carcinomas of the upper alveolus and gingiva. The carcinomas are pathologically squamous cell carcinomas with high or moderate differentiation.

The tumor is most commonly granular and exophytic and may be indurative, ulcerative, or papillary, while the leukoplakic type is less commonly presented (Figs. 6.6, 6.7, and

6.11). As carcinomas of the upper alveolus and gingiva, the tumor frequently involves the bone at a relatively early stage, and bone resorption patterns, either pressure or moth-eaten type, provide clinically useful information to evaluate the malignancy of the tumor. If teeth are present in relation to the tumor, they may become loose, painful, and periostitic. Once the tumor invades into a mandibular canal, anesthesia of the lower lip is quite commonly detected, which may be accompanied by a pathologic fracture of the mandible. Metastasis of the tumor to regional lymph nodes, particularly submandibular and submental lymph nodes, is more frequently evident than that of carcinomas of the upper alveolus and gingiva, and the incidence is 30–40 % of patients.

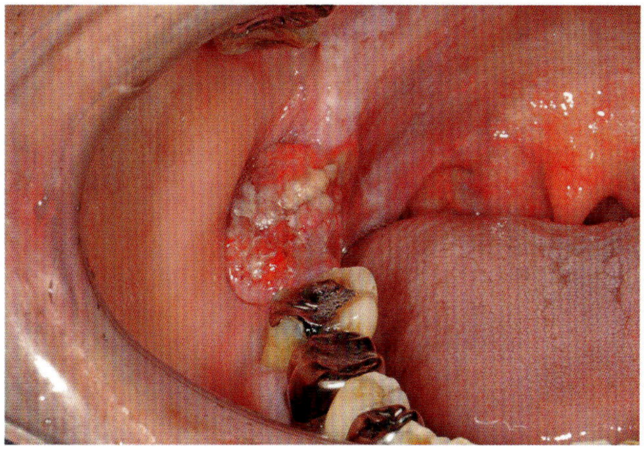

Fig. 6.11 A squamous cell carcinoma of the lower alveolus showing the ulcerative type of observational findings and the endophytic type of clinical growth pattern

Hard Palate

Carcinomas of the palate are rare and account for approximately 3 % of oral cancers, but are fairly common in countries where reverse cigarette smoking is practiced. Most of them are highly differentiated squamous cell carcinomas. It should be noted that the most common site of intraoral salivary gland tumors is also the palate. The incidence of carcinomas of the palate is almost the same as that of salivary gland malignancies in the palate. Furthermore, it is occasionally difficult to distinguish it from a carcinoma of the maxillary sinus that has spread to the palate.

The tumor is often ulcerative or papillary and usually spreads extensively before it affects the bone (Fig. 6.12). The incidence and mode of lymphatic metastasis is almost the same as that of carcinomas of the upper alveolus and gingiva, but lymphatic spread rarely occurs to the retropharyngeal group of nodes.

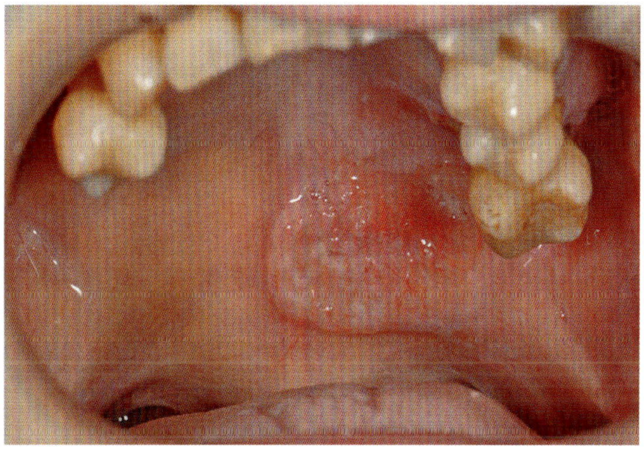

Fig. 6.12 A squamous cell carcinoma of the hard palate showing the ulcerative type of observational findings and the superficial type of clinical growth pattern

Tongue

The tongue is the most common site of oral cancers, and carcinomas of the tongue account for almost a half of all oral cancers. Tobacco use, heavy drinking of alcohol, mucosal atrophy caused by Plummer-Vinson syndrome or vitamin deficiency, and infections such as tertiary syphilis and chronic candidiasis are predisposing factors. Most tumors are on the lateral border extending on to the ventrum of the tongue, while tumors on the dorsum and tip are rare. Carcinomas of the tongue are pathologically squamous cell carcinomas with high or moderate differentiation.

The earliest symptom is a painless swelling; an inconspicuous white, red, or speckled patch; an ulcer; or a small nodule or fissure. Once the ulcer is established, pain is continuous and severe and may radiate to the ear and beyond. It is accompanied by excessive salivation and there is marked halitosis, hemorrhage, and finally immobility of the tongue as it becomes fixed to the floor of the mouth. Dysarthria and dysphagia may also occur. Almost any type of tumor may develop, but ulcerative, indurative, or leukoplakic types are common (Figs. 6.1, 6.2, 6.3, 6.4, and 6.5). The spread to regional lymph nodes depends on the location of the tumor and it may be bilateral. Tumors at the tip of the tongue tend to spread to the submental and jugulo-omohyoid lymph nodes, whereas more distal tumors spread to the submandibular and jugulodigastric lymph nodes and extend down the deep cervical chain. The tumor tends to metastasize early, and 30–40 % of patients have one or more enlarged lymph nodes on initial examination.

Floor of the Mouth

Carcinomas of the floor of the mouth account for approximately 10 % of oral cancers and affect males more frequently than females with stronger sexual predilection than that of other oral cancers. The central part of the floor of the mouth is the most common site. The carcinomas are pathologically squamous cell carcinomas with high or moderate differentiation.

Early carcinoma of the floor of the mouth may be asymptomatic, but tumors at this site tend to invade adjacent structures extensively, such as the alveolar and tongue, and many patients present with advanced disease. Ankyloglossia and dysarthria may be the initial symptoms. The tumor may form an exophytic mass but more commonly presents as a typical malignant ulcer (Fig. 6.13). The submandibular and jugulodigastric lymph nodes are the most frequent sites of secondary spread and more than half the patients have evidence of lymphatic metastasis when initially examined. The bilateral lymph nodes are frequently metastatic and the incidence of lymphatic metastasis is highest in oral cancers.

6.1.2 Differential Diagnosis of Oral Cancers

6.1.2.1 Other Oral Nonmalignant Lesions with Similarities to Oral Cancer

Chronic inflammation, such as marginal and apical periodontitis, pyogenic granuloma, epulis, denture fibroma or granuloma, and incomplete healing after tooth extraction, may present as a suspicious swollen or granular mass (Figs. 6.14, 6.15, 6.16, and 6.17) and must be distinguished from the indurative or granular types of oral cancers. In these chronic inflammatory lesions, the induration, as in oral cancers, is not usually palpable, or the mass is sharply demarcated or pedunculated.

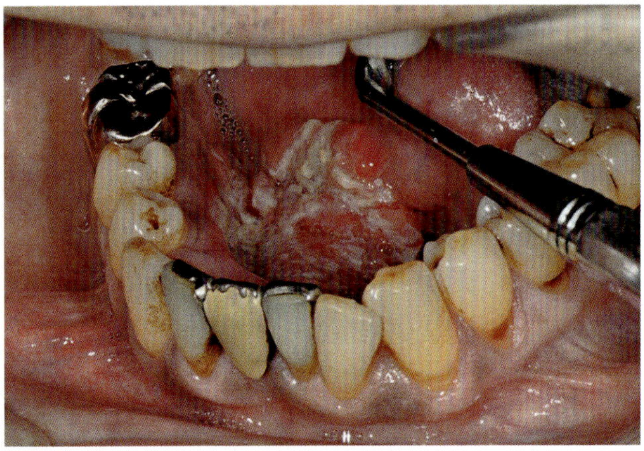

Fig. 6.13 A squamous cell carcinoma of the floor of the mouth showing the ulcerative type of observational findings and the endophytic type of clinical growth pattern

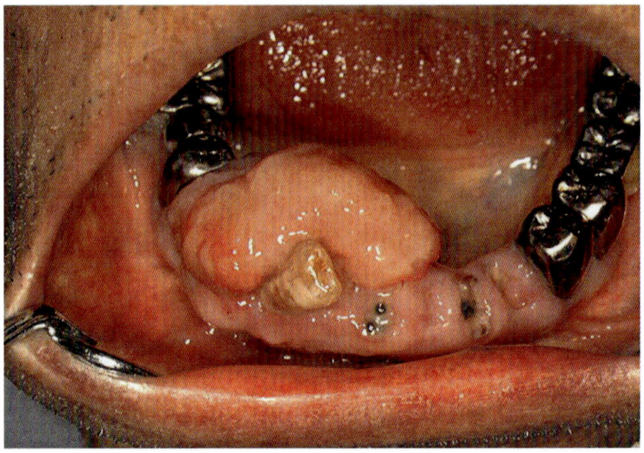

Fig. 6.15 An epulis of the lower gingiva

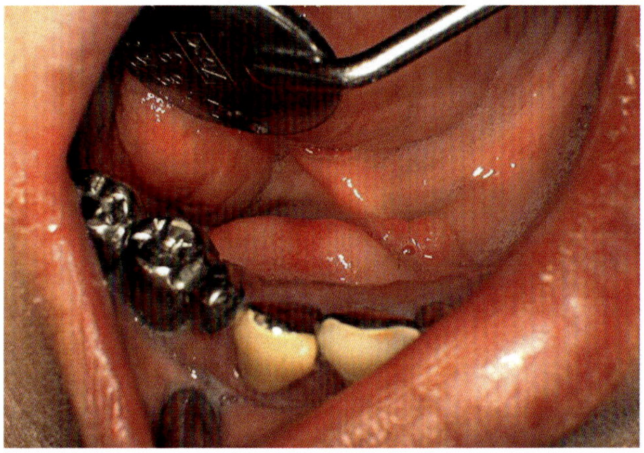

Fig. 6.16 A denture fibroma of the lower gingiva caused by the lingual bar of partial denture

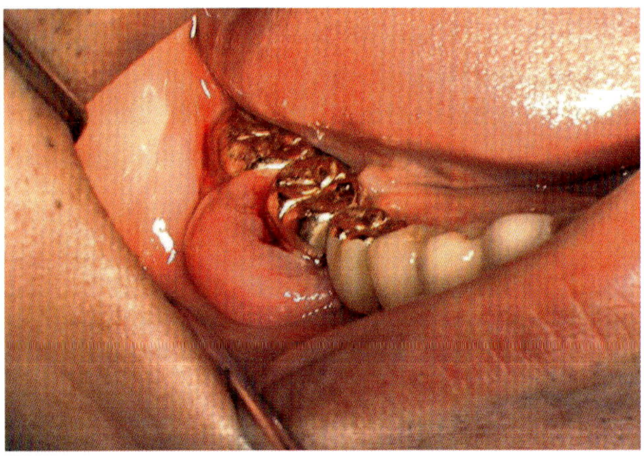

Fig. 6.14 A swollen mass caused by marginal periodontitis of the lower gingiva

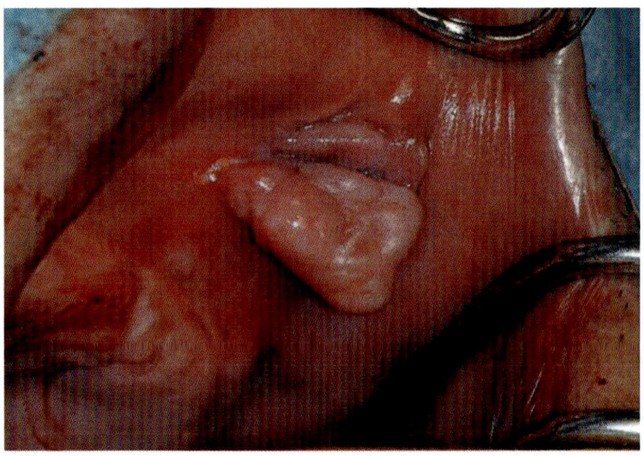

Fig. 6.17 A denture fibroma of the upper alveolus caused by the full denture

Ulcerative stomatitis, especially decubitus and tuberculous ulcers, may occasionally show ambiguous shape or induration (Figs. 6.18 and 6.19) and are thus indistinguishable from ulcerative types of oral cancers. If the potential source of the irritation is removed and topical steroid is then applied, the oral mucosa will revert to normal. However, the observational period should take place within a couple of weeks.

Leukoplakia, erythroplakia, oral lichen planus, and chronic hyperplastic candidiasis should be distinguished from the leukoplakic or ulcerative types of oral cancers, but considerable attention must be given to the premalignant potential of these lesions as is mentioned regarding precancerous lesions later in the chapter.

Benign tumors, such as papilloma, are generally sharply demarcated or pedunculated and without digital induration (Figs. 6.20 and 6.21) and, thus, should be clinically distinguishable from the papillary type of oral cancers. In addition, benign salivary gland tumors may develop in the oral cavity. The tumors are usually covered with normal oral mucosa and well demarcated. Ulceration of the covering oral mucosa is hardly seen, but can be exposed by mechanical irritation, for example, hard food or a broken denture (Fig. 6.22). Benign salivary gland tumors, as well as malignant salivary gland tumors, may thus present similar masses to those of the indurative type of oral cancers.

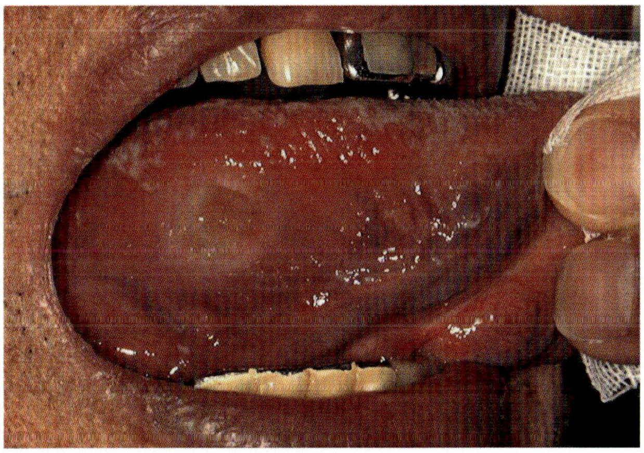

Fig. 6.18 A decubitus ulcer of the tongue

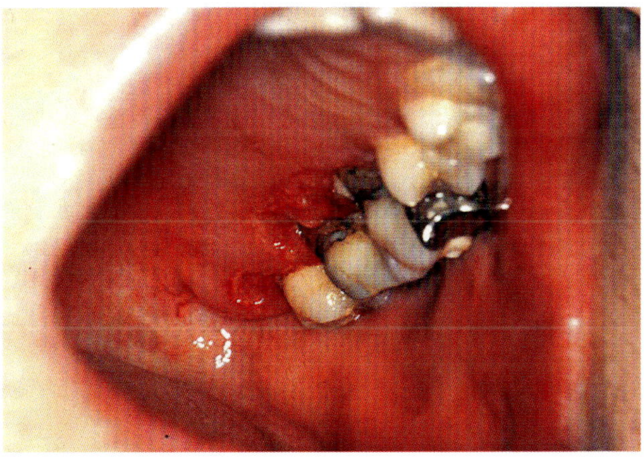

Fig. 6.19 A tuberculous ulcer of the upper gingiva

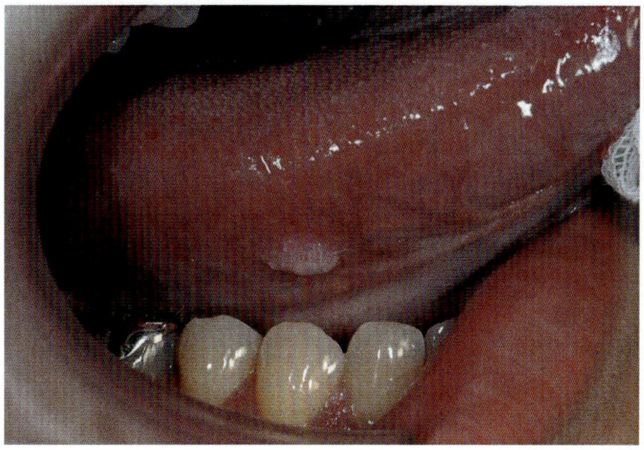

Fig. 6.20 A papilloma of the tongue

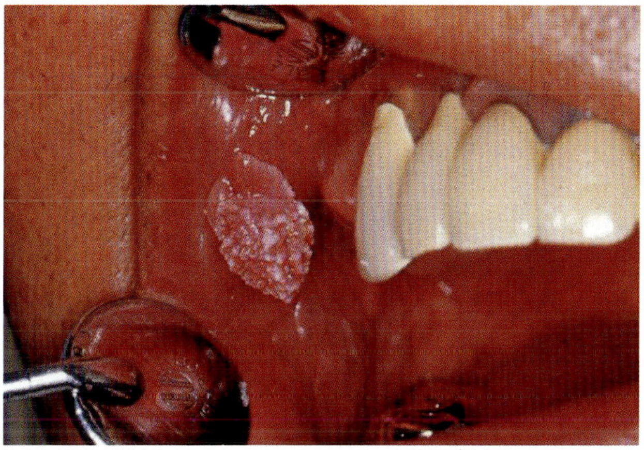

Fig. 6.21 A papilloma of the buccal mucosa

Finally, if malignancy is undeniable and definite and differential diagnosis is required in any suspicious lesions, it is extremely important that a biopsy be performed without hesitation.

6.1.2.2 Precancerous Lesions and Conditions

Leukoplakia and erythroplakia are generally considered precancerous lesions. Erythroplakia takes the form of a bright red and velvety patch and histologically has the appearance of epithelial atrophy with pronounced epithelial dysplasia or carcinoma in situ. As this lesion has the highest risk of cancerization among precancerous lesions, it is always recommended to excise them surgically. In contrast, leukoplakia takes various forms of white and keratotic patches. Most leukoplakias are flat and smooth-surfaced: a

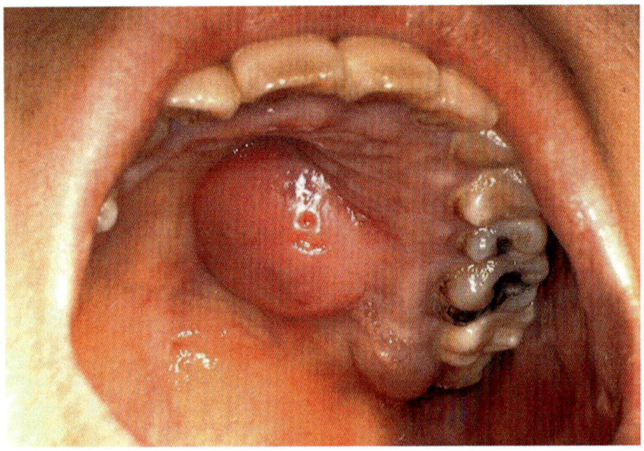

Fig. 6.22 A pleomorphic adenoma of the hard palate with small ulceration of the covering mucosa

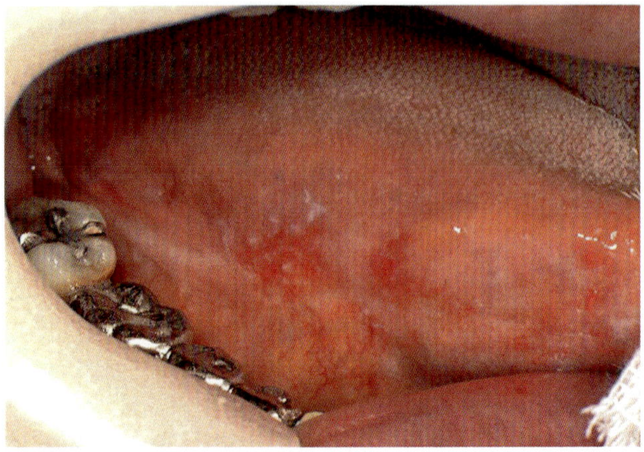

Fig. 6.23 A leukoplakia of the tongue with partial reddening

homogeneous leukoplakia. This type of leukoplakia histologically appears hyperkeratotic without epithelial dysplasia. A nonhomogeneous leukoplakia may be pronounced, nodular, or verrucous and have a low premalignant potential but higher than that of homogeneous leukoplakias. The surface may have a so-called "ebbing tide" appearance, and the lesion may be a mixture of white and red lesions: a speckled leukoplakia. Speckled leukoplakias have the highest premalignant potential of the leukoplakias. As leukoplakias have various premalignant potentials, surgical excision is usually recommended for some lesions with higher malignant potential. For other lesions with lower malignant potential or widespread lesions, regular and careful follow-up is alternatively recommended. In case of the latter lesions, it is extremely important not to overlook malignant changes such as reddening, ulceration, fissuring, nodularity, and digital induration at follow-up and then to biopsy any suspicious area in the leukoplakic patch immediately (Figs. 6.23 and 6.24).

In other precancerous lesions and conditions, including oral lichen planus, submucous fibrosis, chronic hyperplastic candidiasis, leukoedema, and white sponge nevus, rare but such possible malignant changes, like those in leukoplakias mentioned above, must be clinically examined with care and any suspicious area should be biopsied.

6.1.2.3 Other Malignancies in the Oral Cavity

Malignancies in the oral cavity account for 1–3 % of all malignancies in Western and most Asian countries including Japan, and more than 90 % of them are carcinomas. Most of the carcinomas are pathologically squamous cell carcinomas originating in the covering mucosa in the oral cavity, so-called oral cancer, while carcinomas may also arise from salivary glands and rarely within the bone of the mandible or maxilla. The remaining malignancies, other than the carcinomas, are malignant melanomas, hematological malignancies such as malignant lymphomas and leukemias, and various kinds of sarcomas. Here,

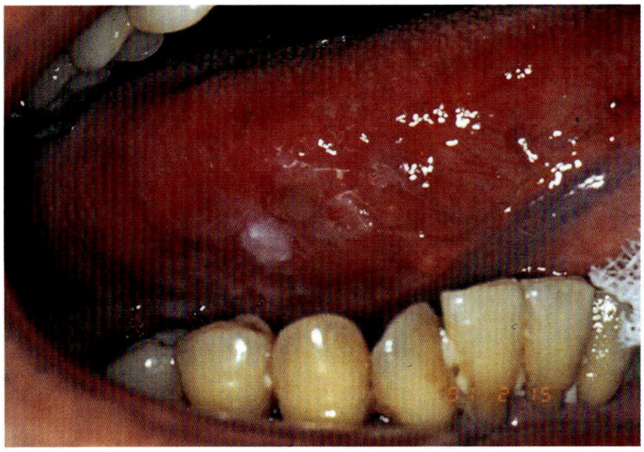

Fig. 6.24 A leukoplakia of the tongue with partial ulceration and whitish nodularity

only primary malignant melanoma in the oral cavity is described. In addition, malignancies of the lip and the maxillary sinus, which are adjacent to the oral cavity, are described, as they may frequently involve the oral cavity.

Malignancies of the Salivary Gland

Salivary gland tumors show a great variety of histological appearances and make up a complex group of neoplasms. The current WHO classification includes 23 different types and subtypes [12]. Almost any type of tumor may develop in intraoral glands but there is a considerably higher proportion of malignancies in these salivary glands. Intraoral salivary gland malignancies often originate in sublingual glands and minor salivary glands in the palate. Rare intraosseous salivary gland tumors may develop in the mandible. Most of the malignancies are carcinomas and are followed, in the order of incidence, by mucoepidermoid carcinomas, adenoid cystic carcinomas, carcinoma ex pleomorphic adenomas, and acinic cell carcinomas. The tumors are usually covered with normal oral mucosa and are well demarcated, but occasionally develop an ulcer of the covering oral mucosa and then present similar masses to those of the indurative type of oral cancers (Figs. 6.25, 6.26, 6.27, 6.28, and 6.29).

Malignancies Within the Bone

Malignant odontogenic tumors and malignancies originating in odontogenic epithelial cells, including the odontogenic cyst lining, may arise within the bone of the mandible or maxilla. As mentioned above, salivary gland malignancies may also develop intraosseously. The early symptom of a malignancy within the bone is a painless swelling that characteristically involves both the buccal and lingual or buccal and palate sulci. If teeth are present, they may become loose and painful. If the patient is edentulous, a previously satisfactory denture may no longer fit and may be displaced, or it may cut into soft tissues and then ulcerate or produce a localized denture fibroma or granuloma. Anesthesia of the upper or lower lip is quite common.

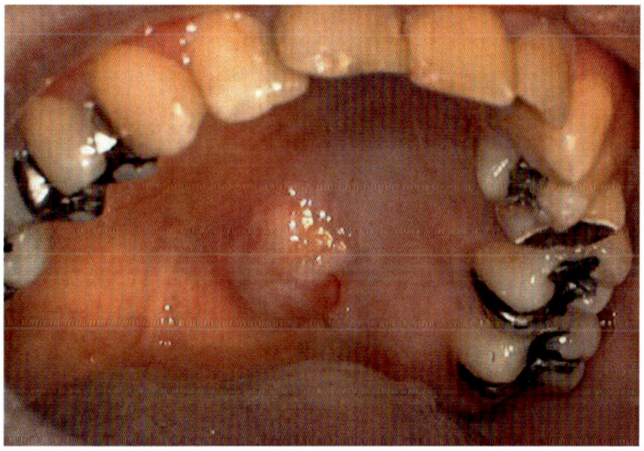

Fig. 6.25 A mucoepidermoid carcinoma (highly differentiated type with low grade malignancy) of the palatine gland

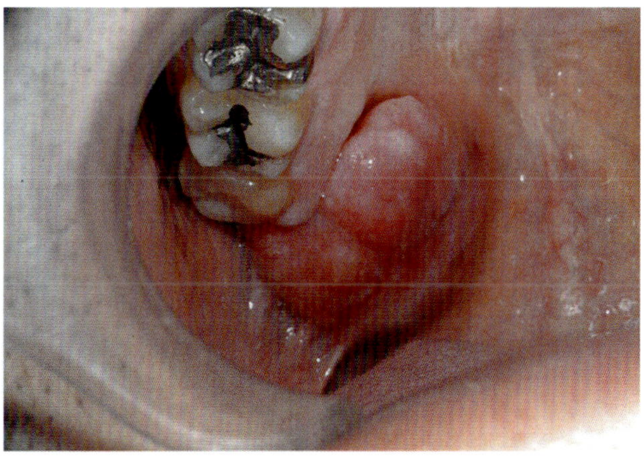

Fig. 6.26 A mucoepidermoid carcinoma (poorly differentiated type with high grade malignancy) of the palatine gland

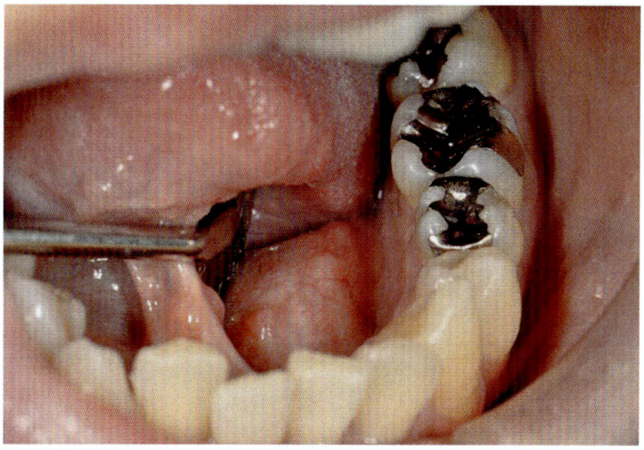

Fig. 6.27 An adenoid cystic carcinoma of the sublingual gland

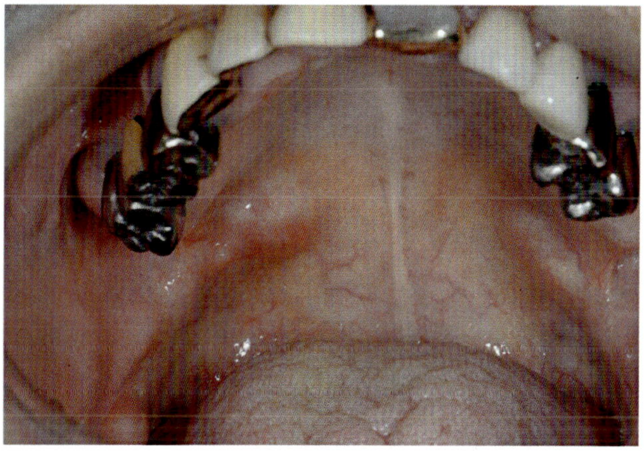

Fig. 6.28 A carcinoma ex pleomorphic adenoma of the palatine gland

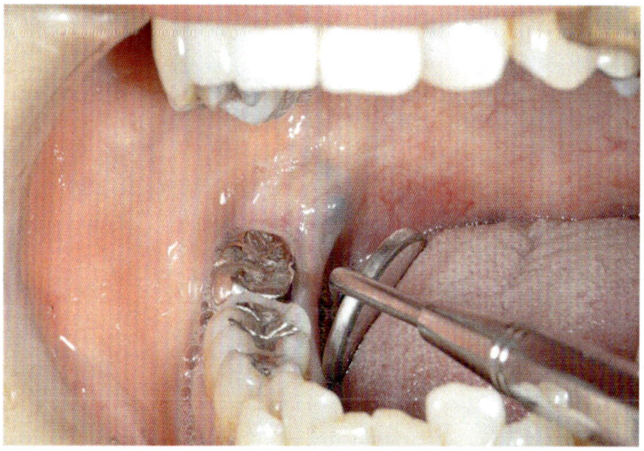

Fig. 6.29 An acinic cell carcinoma of the molar minor salivary gland

Malignant Melanoma

Malignant melanoma may first arise in the oral cavity and the prognosis is very poor. The tumor presents as a raised, soft, vascular, dark brown, or black mass and often destroys adjacent bone and loosens teeth in its vicinity (Fig. 6.30).

Bleeding and ulcerations from the tumor are relatively common. It has a strong tendency to invade blood vessels and lymph nodes, and thus nodal involvement and distant metastasis are frequently found. Although histological evidence is usually required, biopsy should not be performed without careful preparation to avoid its invasion. A frozen section for rapid diagnosis is strongly advocated to embark on treatment as soon as the diagnosis is confirmed.

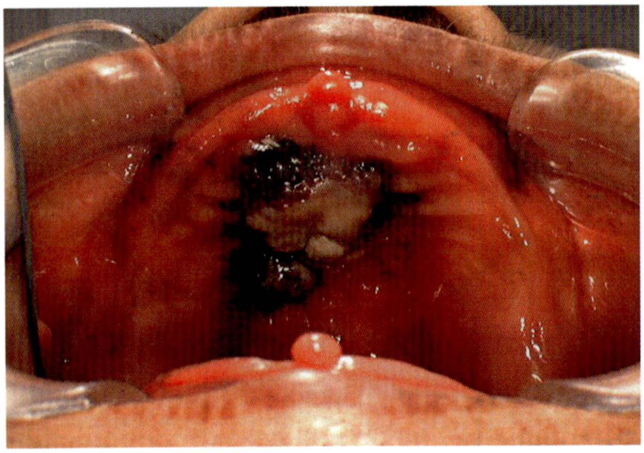

Fig. 6.30 A malignant melanoma of the hard palate

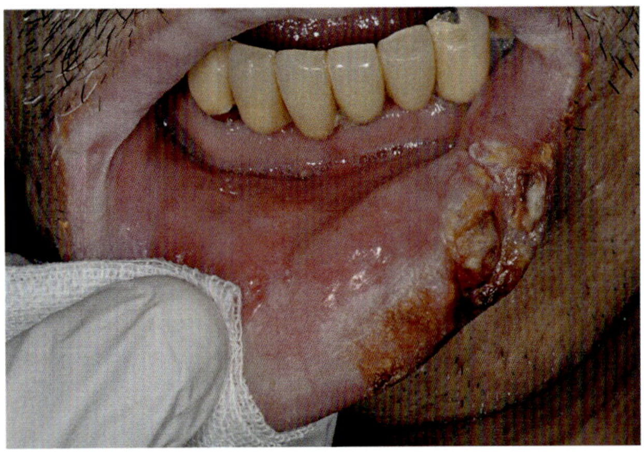

Fig. 6.31 A squamous cell carcinoma of the lip with scabbing ulcer

Malignancies of the Lip

The most common malignancy of the lip is carcinoma. Carcinomas of the lip often arise in the vermillion border of the lower lip and are pathologically highly differentiated squamous cell carcinomas in most cases. Carcinoma of the lip is common in occupations and countries where the patient is subjected to intense solar radiation, and many of the patients have a history of blistering cheilitis due to sunlight. Patients also tend to have dirty, jagged, or stained teeth, and sometimes the tumor arises at a site irritated by such a tooth. Common precipitating factors may be some form of irritation and leukoplakic change due to hot tobacco smoke. The tumor usually begins as a small, painless scabbing ulcer, which arises in the substance of the lip and, if not treated, spreads to the buccal mucosa and gingiva (Fig. 6.31).

Malignancies of the Maxillary Sinus

Malignancies of the maxillary sinus may destroy the bony walls of the antrum and then present as a swelling in the mouth. Squamous cell carcinoma accounts for more than 90 % of the malignancies. All degrees of differentiation are found, but many of them are anaplastic. Other malignancies such as adenocarcinoma, lymphoepithelioma, and sarcoma may arise in the maxillary sinus, but their incidence is obviously small. The earliest presenting symptom is often a unilateral serosanguineous discharge or frank epistaxis. The established tumor may produce unilateral swelling of the cheek, buccal sulcus, alveolus, or palate. Intraoral swelling may dislodge a denture that has fitted satisfactorily up until that time and present a denture fibroma or granuloma or ulcerate along with the edge of the denture (Fig. 6.32). If teeth are present in relation to the floor of the maxillary sinus, they may become loose, painful, and periostitic.

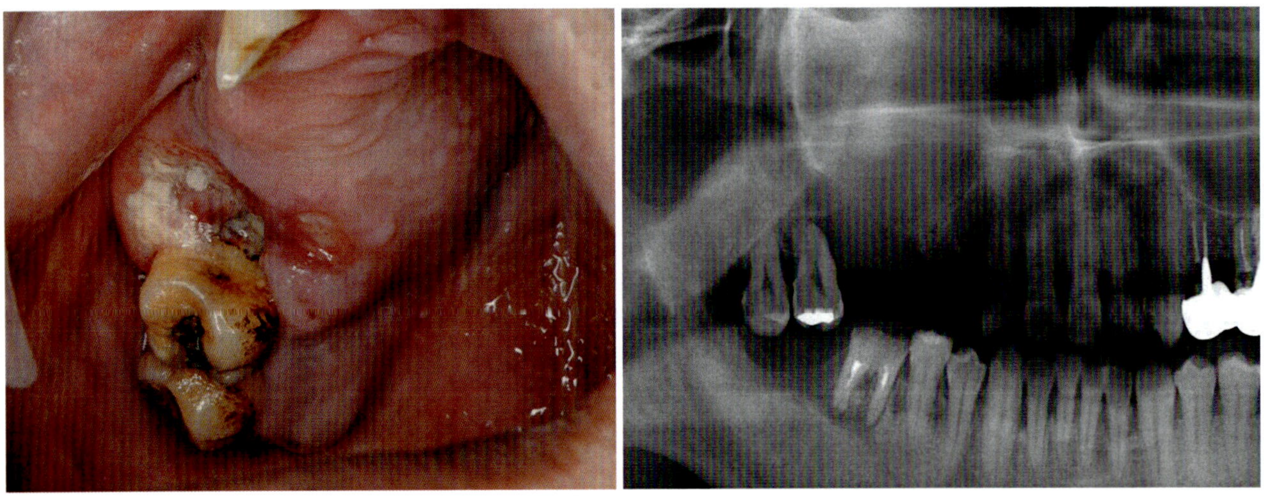

Fig. 6.32 A squamous cell carcinoma of the maxillary sinus producing swelling and ulceration of the alveolus

References

1. UICC (2009) TNM classification of malignant tumours, 7th edn. Wiley-Blackwell, London
2. Paymaster JC (1956) Cancer of the buccal mucosa: a clinical study of 650 cases in Indian patients. Cancer 9:431–435
3. Stones HH (1957) Oral and dental diseases. Livingstone, Edinburgh
4. Fletcher GH, MacComb WS (1962) Radiation therapy in the management of cancer of the oral cavity and oropharynx. Springfield, Chicago
5. Gardner AF, Hamburger S, Love S (1963) Oral carcinoma: analysis of one hundred and eighty-nine cases. J Am Dent Assoc 66:456–465
6. Paterson P (1963) The treatment of malignant disease by radiation. Edward Arnold, London
7. McCarthy PL, Shklar G (1964) Diseases of the oral mucosa. Mcgraw-Hill, New York
8. Spiessl B (1966) Plattenepithelkarzinom der Mund-höhle. Georg Thieme Verlag, Stuttgart
9. Sandler HC (1970) A retrospective study of a head and neck cancer control program. Cancer 25:1153–1161
10. Ueno T (1969) Studies on treatment and results of cancer of the buccal cavity. J Jpn Stomatol Soc 36:4–10
11. Izumo T, Kirita T, Ariji E, Ozeki S, Okada N, Okabe S et al (2012) General rules for clinical and pathological studies on oral cancer: a synopsis. Jpn J Clin Oncol 42:1099–1109. doi:10.1093/jjco/hys141
12. Barners L, Eveson JW, Reichart P, Sidransky D (2005) Pathology and genetics of the head and neck tumours. IARC, Lyon

Surgical Approaches to the Oral Cavity

7

Masanori Shinohara

Abstract

The surgical managements concerning oral cancer are described in this chapter. At first, the principles of surgical treatment of oral cancer are commented. Then, when performing surgical therapy, the standard of the safety margin of oral cancer is commented. Furthermore, vital staining with iodine solution for determining of the safety margin is described. The surgical method is commented every each part of the oral cavity, because the oral cavity is divided into six sites. At first, the anatomical features for surgical approaches are described. Then, the surgical method in each part (tongue, oral floor, buccal mucosa, upper and lower gingiva, and hard palate) is explained using the figure. About the indication of the operation method in each part, the selection criteria for the surgical method that followed TNM classification are commented. Finally, the points to note when performing surgical resection of tumor are described. In addition, the basic approaches for oral cancer are described about squamous cell carcinoma mainly.

Keywords

Glossectomy • Mandibulectomy • Maxillectomy • Safety margin • Surgical approach • Vital staining

7.1 Introduction

Oral cancer refers to a malignant tumor that arises in any of the following six sites: the tongue, the oral floor, the buccal mucosa, the upper gingiva and alveolus, the lower gingiva and alveolus, and the hard palate. Types of malignant tumors that arise in the oral cavity include squamous cell carcinomas, salivary gland carcinomas, and sarcomas among others, but squamous cell carcinomas account for the majority of cases. Surgical therapies concerning squamous cell carcinomas are described below, but the surgical basics for the other malignant tumors are almost the same.

M. Shinohara (✉)
Department of Oral and Maxillofacial Surgery, Kumamoto University School of Medicine,
1-1-1, Chuo-ku, Kumamoto 860-8556, Japan
e-mail: shinora@kumamoto-u.ac.jp

Oral cancers tend to occur on the tongue and gingiva, but can occur at any of the other sites as well. They also readily metastasize to cervical lymph nodes, and so cervical lymph node metastasis is an important prognostic factor for determining not only the treatment of the primary lesion but also for overall prognosis [1]. Therefore, at the time of therapy, it is important to treat metastatic lymph nodes of the cervical region at the same time as the primary lesion. Surgical resection is the general rule for radical therapy targeting the primary lesion; however, the operative procedures differ between cases where resection of bone is necessary, such as upper and lower gingival and hard palate carcinomas, and cases of soft tissue resection, such as tongue, floor of the mouth, and buccal mucosa carcinomas. In addition, surgical therapies bring about tissue damage and subsequent functional disturbances, and there are many factors to consider depending on the structure of the tissue adjacent to the oral carcinoma. The oral cavity is involved in many functions, and post-therapy functional disturbances severely reduce

T. Kirita and K. Omura (eds.), *Oral Cancer: Diagnosis and Therapy*,
DOI 10.1007/978-4-431-54938-3_7, © Springer Japan 2015

patients' post-therapy quality of life (QOL). For that reason, what is desirable at the time of surgical therapy is not only the complete resection of the tumor but also surgery that causes the least functional disturbance possible. Moreover, functional reconstruction aimed at restoring postoperative function is necessary. In addition, the first choice of treatment for lymph node metastasis is neck dissection.

Superficial type : Those primarily showing superficial growth
Exophytic type : Those primarily showing exophytic growth
Endophytic type: Those primarily showing endophytic growth

Fig. 7.1 Clinical growth pattern

When performing surgical therapy, it is first necessary to have a correct understanding of the extent of the tumor's progression and its metastatic condition, as well as its characteristics. Clinical, imaging, and histopathological diagnoses must be made correctly to achieve this goal. For clinical diagnosis, the clinical growth pattern (Fig. 7.1) is correlated with local recurrence, rate of cervical lymph node metastasis, rate of distance metastasis, and 5-year survival rate, making it useful as a predictor of pathological condition [2–9] (Figs. 7.2, 7.3, and 7.4). Through imaging diagnosis, the

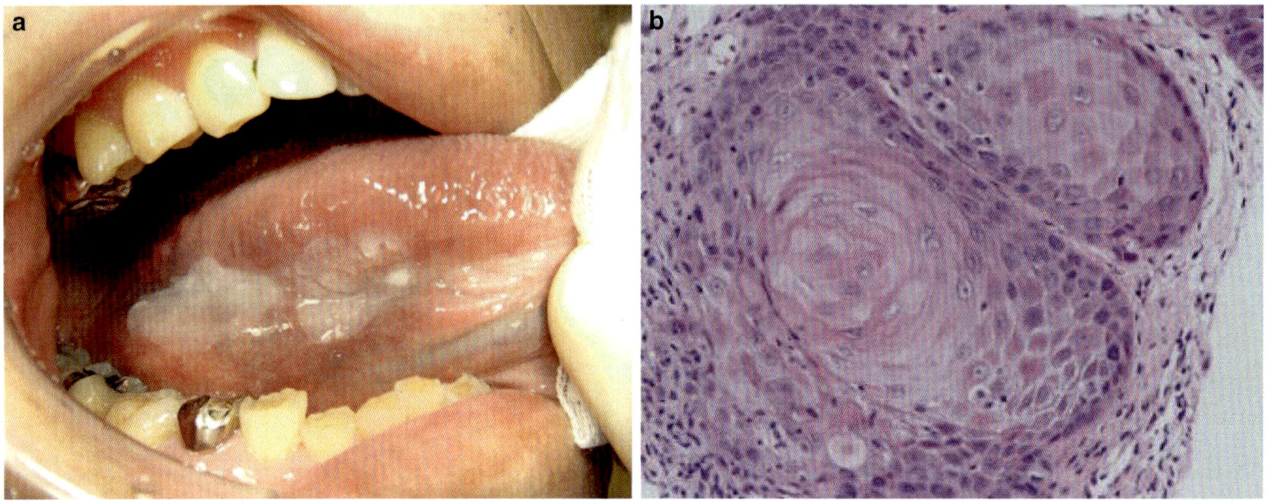

Fig. 7.2 Clinical growth pattern: superficial type of tongue, (**a**) clinical finding, (**b**) histological finding; squamous cell carcinoma. Tumor shows superficial growth

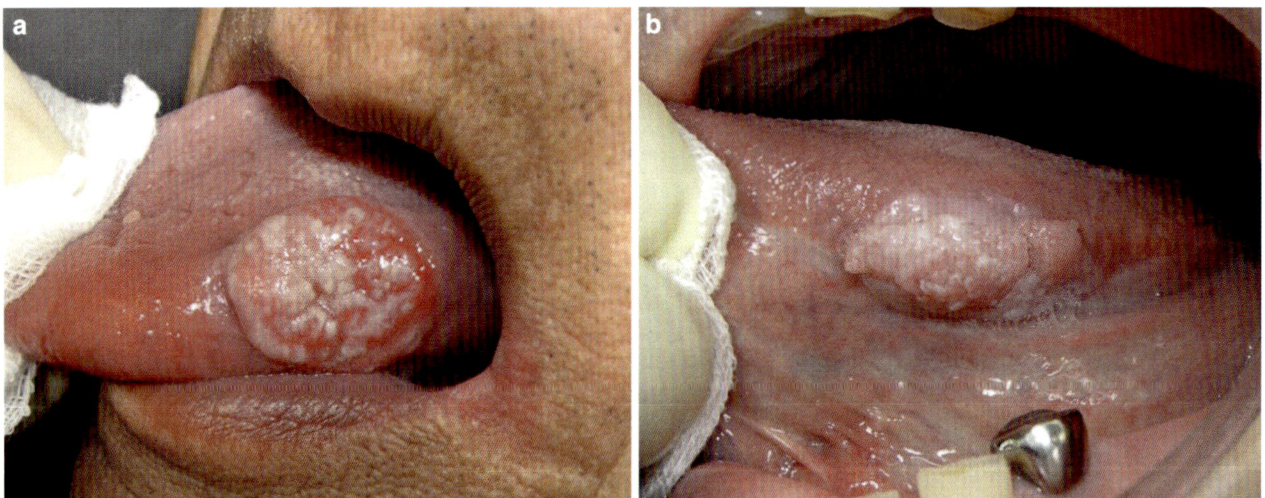

Fig. 7.3 Clinical growth pattern; exophytic type of tongue. Tumor shows exophytic growth

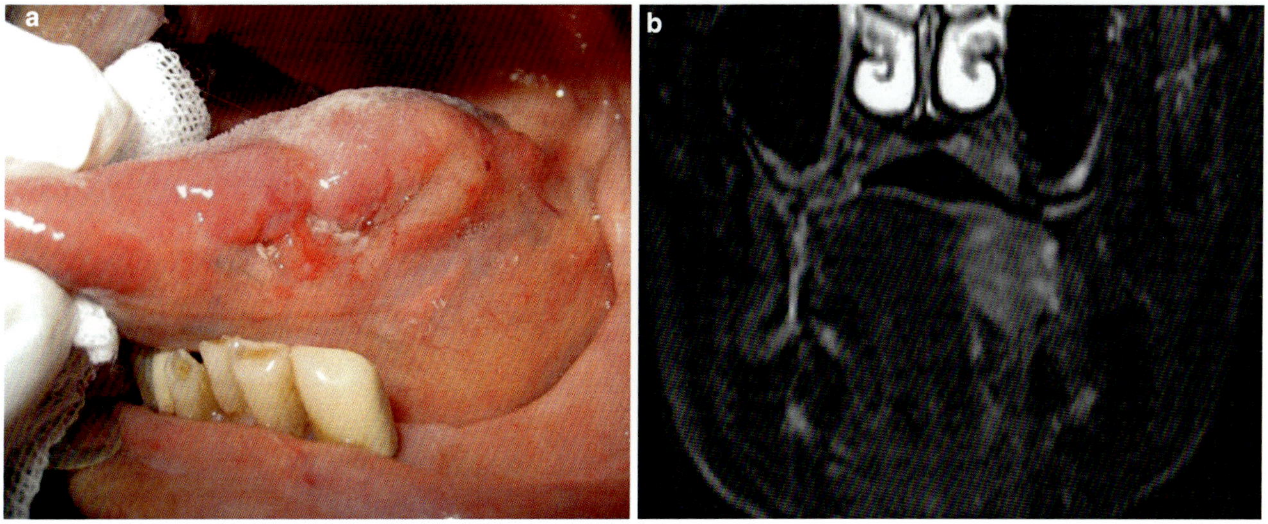

Fig. 7.4 Clinical growth pattern: endophytic type of tongue. (**a**) Clinical finding, (**b**) MRI finding. Tumor shows endophytic growth

YK-1: Well defined borderline
YK-2: Cords, less marked borderline
YK-3: Groups of cells, no distinct borderline
YK-4C: Diffuse invasion, cord-like type invasion
YK-4D: Diffuse invasion, diffuse type invasion

Fig. 7.5 Mode of tumor invasion

extent of tumor progression as well as cervical lymph node metastatic state can be clearly grasped. Practitioners should take advantage of the imaging exams of CT, MRI, and ultrasound, as well as the more recent technologies of FDG-PET and sentinel lymph node detection [10–13]. Additionally, indications of treatment selection and assessments of histological grade and type should be made according to histopathological diagnoses [14–16] (Fig. 7.5).

It is necessary to judge a tumor's progression state and characteristics accurately and to determine the surgical margin using the above-described kinds of information before performing surgical therapy. Practitioners must also predict the functional impairments resulting from resection and furthermore consider reconstruction methods to address them.

7.2 The Safety Margin During Tumor Resection

The oral cavity is located adjacent to vital organs, and hard and soft tissues are mixed in it to form a complex shape. Thus, determining the surgical margin of oral cancer is not simple. There are many reports concerning the establishment of the surgical margin [16–23]. With a safety margin of 5 mm or less from the tumor, the postoperative local recurrence rate is no different from cases with a positive margin [23]. However, the recurrence rate for a margin of 5 mm or less has been observed to be five times higher than a margin of over 5 mm (10 %) [20], and samples show that local tumor recurrence rate drops reliably when there is a distance of 5 mm or more from the tumor margin. From these reports, a safety margin of 10 mm or more at the time of resection can be considered reasonable [21, 24–26]. However, in the oral cavity, local recurrence occurs at a higher frequency for the endophytic and superficial types of clinical growth patterns compared with the exophytic type [1]. Additionally, since recurrence tendencies are high for cases where the histopathological mode of tumor invasion is bad, it is necessary to consider various factors when establishing the safety margin [14–16]. Furthermore, it is important to perform a suitable mandibulectomy in accordance with the invasion into the bone in cases where the oral cancer is adjacent to the mandible [17, 18].

7.3 Vital Staining with Iodine Solution

Vital staining with iodine solution has become an indispensable auxiliary diagnostic method for the detection of early-stage cancer and it is widely used in the upper gastrointestinal region. In the oral cavity, iodine staining allows visualization of epithelial dysplasia and can identify malignant and potentially malignant lesions [27–30] (Figs. 7.6 and 7.7). Further, the accuracy of iodine staining compared with visual examination in discriminating between normal and epithelial dysplastic oral mucosa has been demonstrated [28–31]

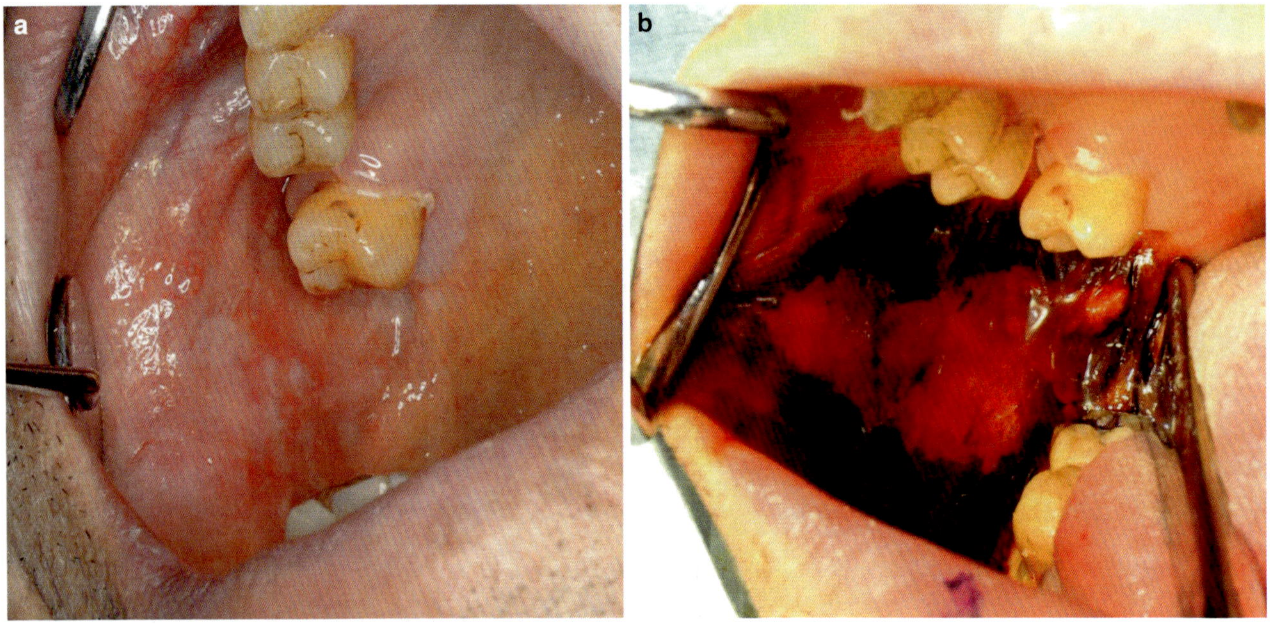

Fig. 7.6 Vital staining with iodine solution: (**a**) prestaining and (**b**) poststaining. Dysplastic lesion of buccal mucosa is unstained

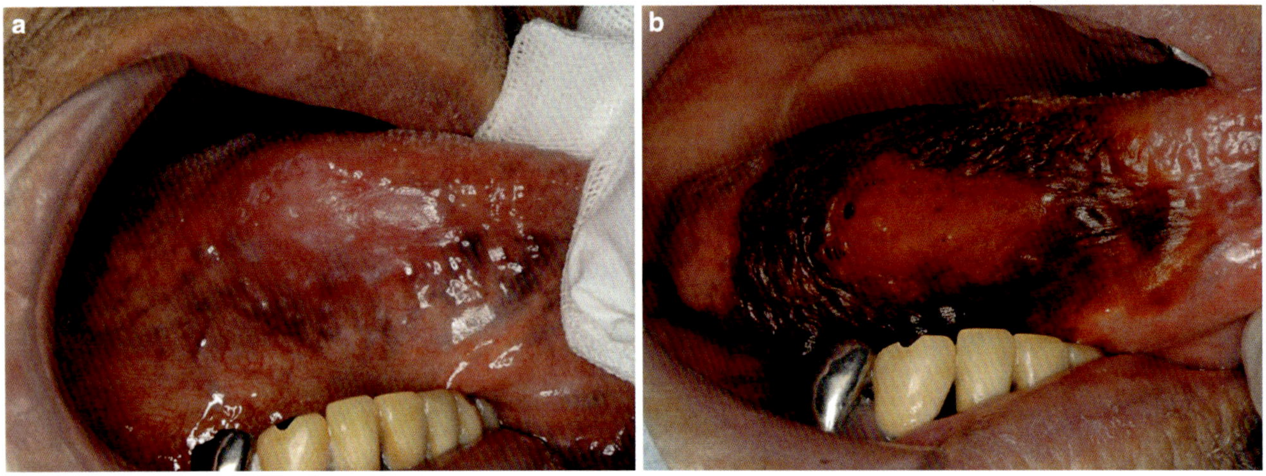

Fig. 7.7 Vital staining with iodine solution: (**a**) prestaining and (**b**) poststaining. Dysplastic lesion is unstained

(Fig. 7.8). In an examination of primary lesion recurrence rate in cases of partial resection that considered the presence or absence of iodine staining, the group that utilized iodine staining was shown to have a significantly lower primary lesion recurrence rate. Consistent with these results, it has also been reported that, for superficial T1 or early T2 lesions, medical cases for which the surgical margin was determined by performing vital staining with iodine solution had a clearly lower local recurrence rate compared with cases where it was not performed (Fig. 7.9). Hence, determining the surgical margin by performing vital staining with iodine solution is useful for superficial lesions. However, there are also cases where the unstained area covers a large range, and so judgments of where to resect to can be difficult for such cases [32, 33] (Figs. 7.10 and 7.11).

7.4 Tongue Carcinomas

Looking at the tongue anatomically, it is organized into the intrinsic and extrinsic muscles of the tongue. The intrinsic muscles are the superior longitudinal muscle, the inferior longitudinal muscle, the transverse muscle, and the vertical muscle; the extrinsic muscles are the genioglossus muscle, the hyoglossus muscle, and the styloglossus muscle. For surgery, the practitioner judges the invasion status of these

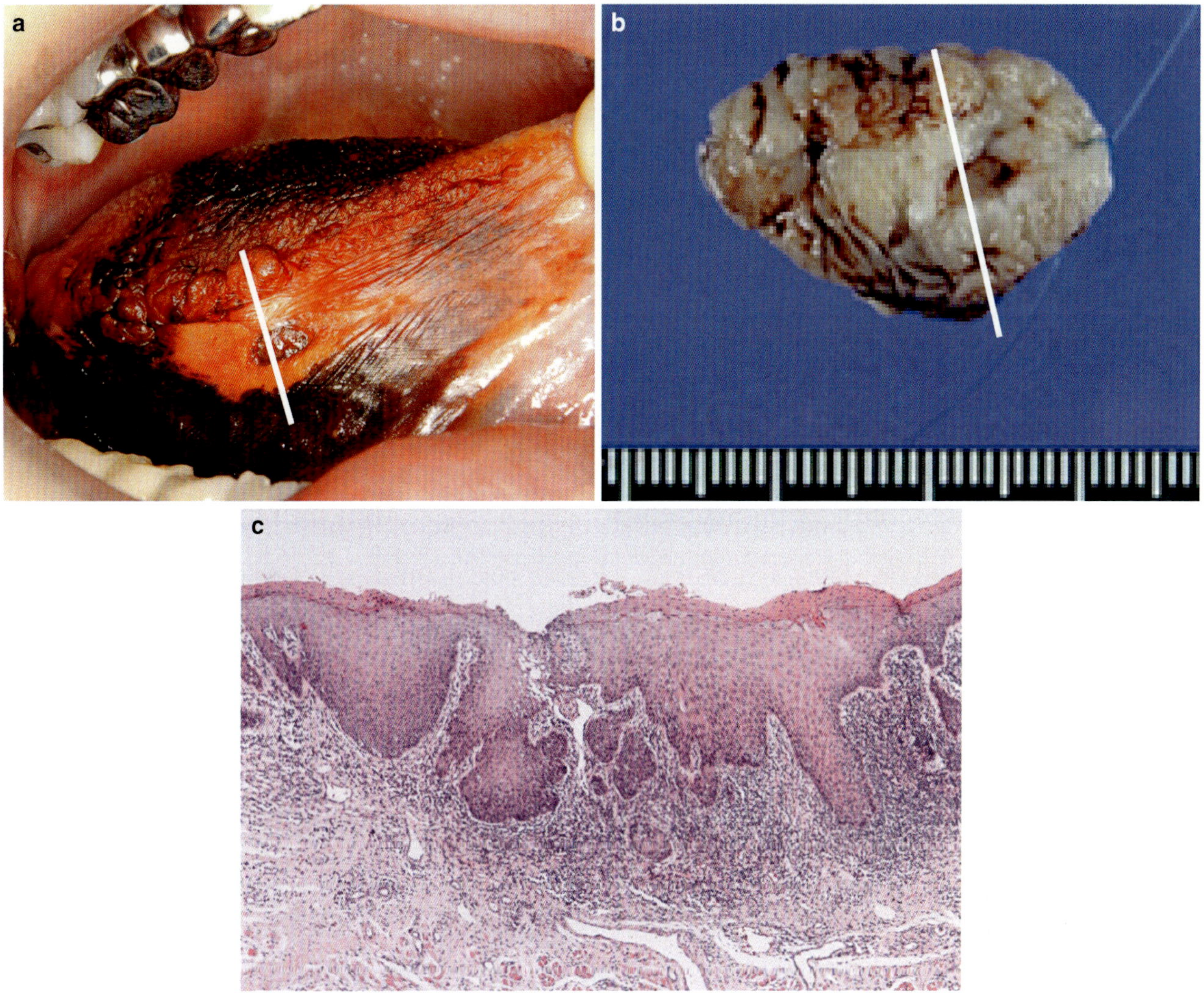

Fig. 7.8 Vital staining with iodine solution. (**a**) Precancerous lesion is unstained; (**b**) surgical material. (**c**) HE staining; early invasive carcinoma is found a part of the epithelial dysplasia

muscle groups and the tumor to determine the surgical margin. Also, resection at a shallow depth is not problematic for tumors with superficial or exophytic clinical growth patterns, but performing vital staining with iodine solution is useful to judge the extent of dysplastic epithelium in the tumor periphery. When resecting endophytic tumors, careful attention should be paid to the deep parts of the surgical margin [17]. It is commonly necessary to resect not only the intrinsic but also the extrinsic muscles of the tongue. Furthermore, the tongue is adjacent to the floor of the mouth, the lower gingiva and alveolus, and the buccal mucosa; because a tumor can easily invade these tissues, accurate diagnosis of the extent of tumor progression at the time of surgery is important [34–38]. The histopathological malignancy of such tumors must also be considered (Fig. 7.12). It is unnecessary to take a wide safety margin for tumors with low malignancy, but a safety margin of 1 cm or more must be taken for those with high malignancy or invasiveness. Therefore, the surgical margin for a tongue carcinoma will change depending on the primary lesion's size, the depth of invasion [17], and the invasive state and histopathological malignancy with regard to the floor of the mouth [34], the base of the tongue, and the mandible [35–38]. Furthermore, it may be necessary to perform neck dissection concurrently via a pull-through operation because tongue carcinomas result in a high frequency of cervical lymph node metastasis.

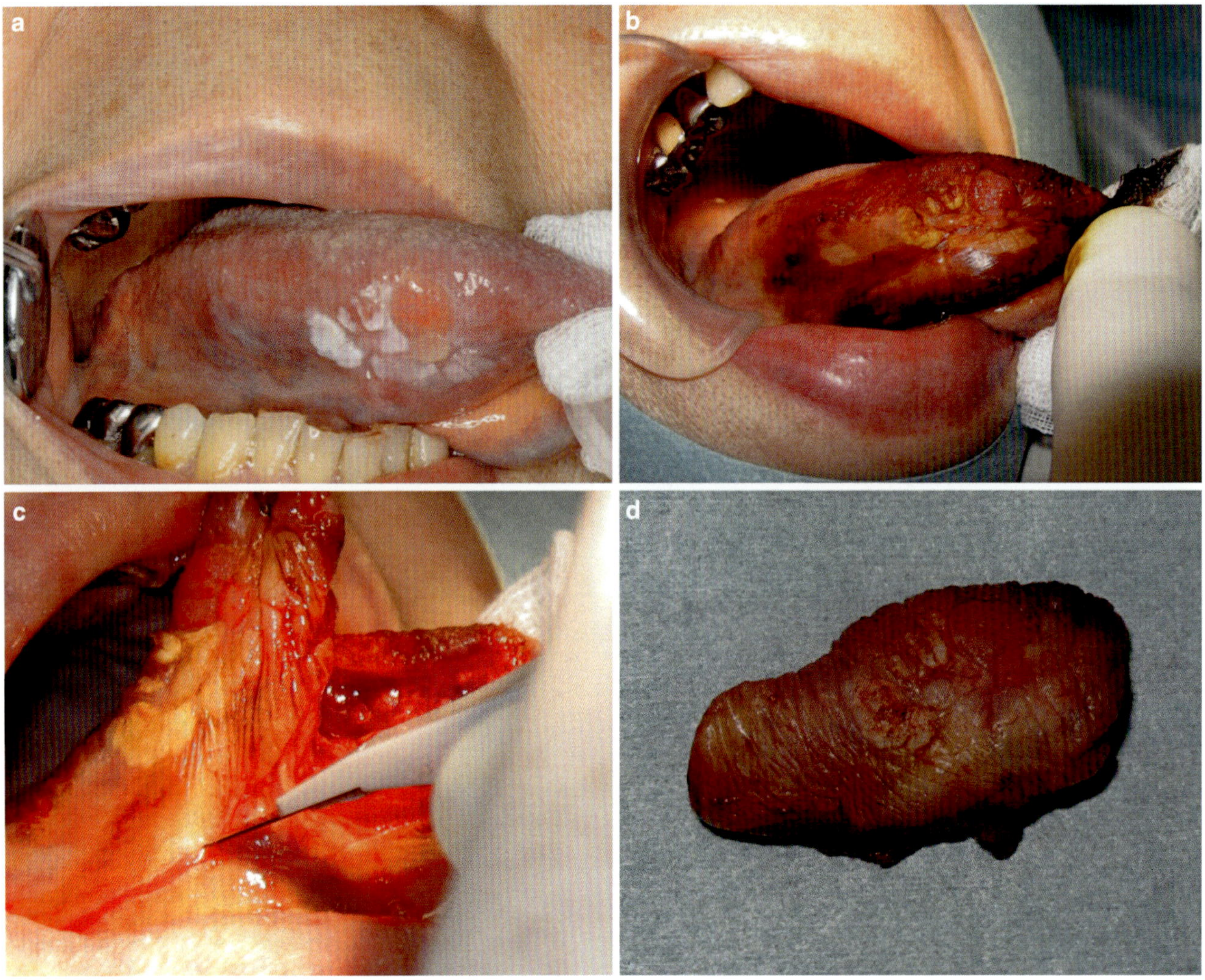

Fig. 7.9 Vital staining with iodine solution: (**a**) early carcinoma with precancerous lesion, (**b**) vital staining with iodine solution, (**c**) excision of lesion, and (**d**) removal tissue

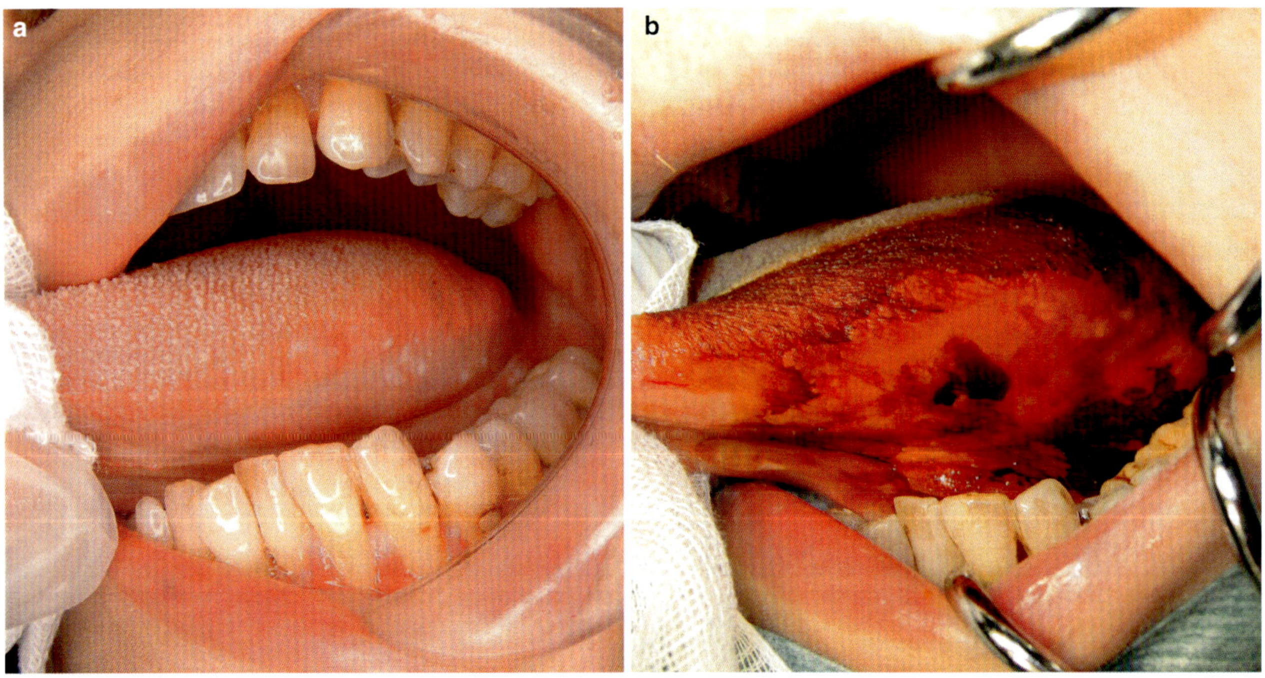

Fig. 7.10 Vital staining with iodine solution: (**a**) prestaining and (**b**) poststaining. The unstained area covers a large range

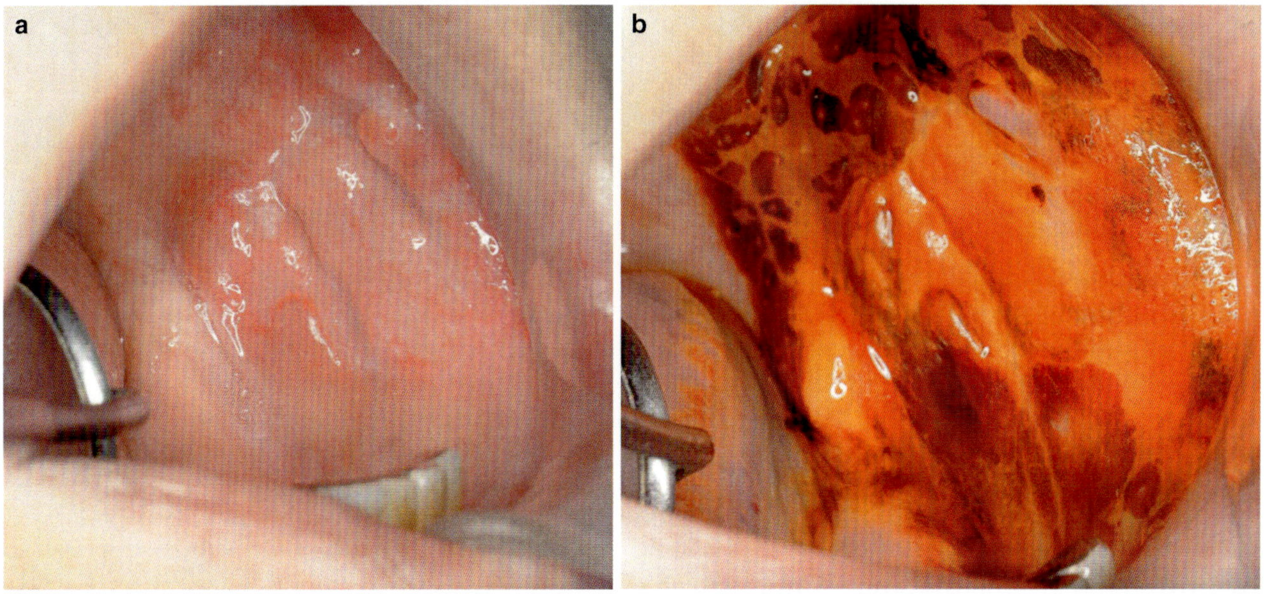

Fig. 7.11 Vital staining with iodine solution. (**a**) Prestaining and (**b**) poststaining. The unstained area of buccal mucosa covers a large and irregular range

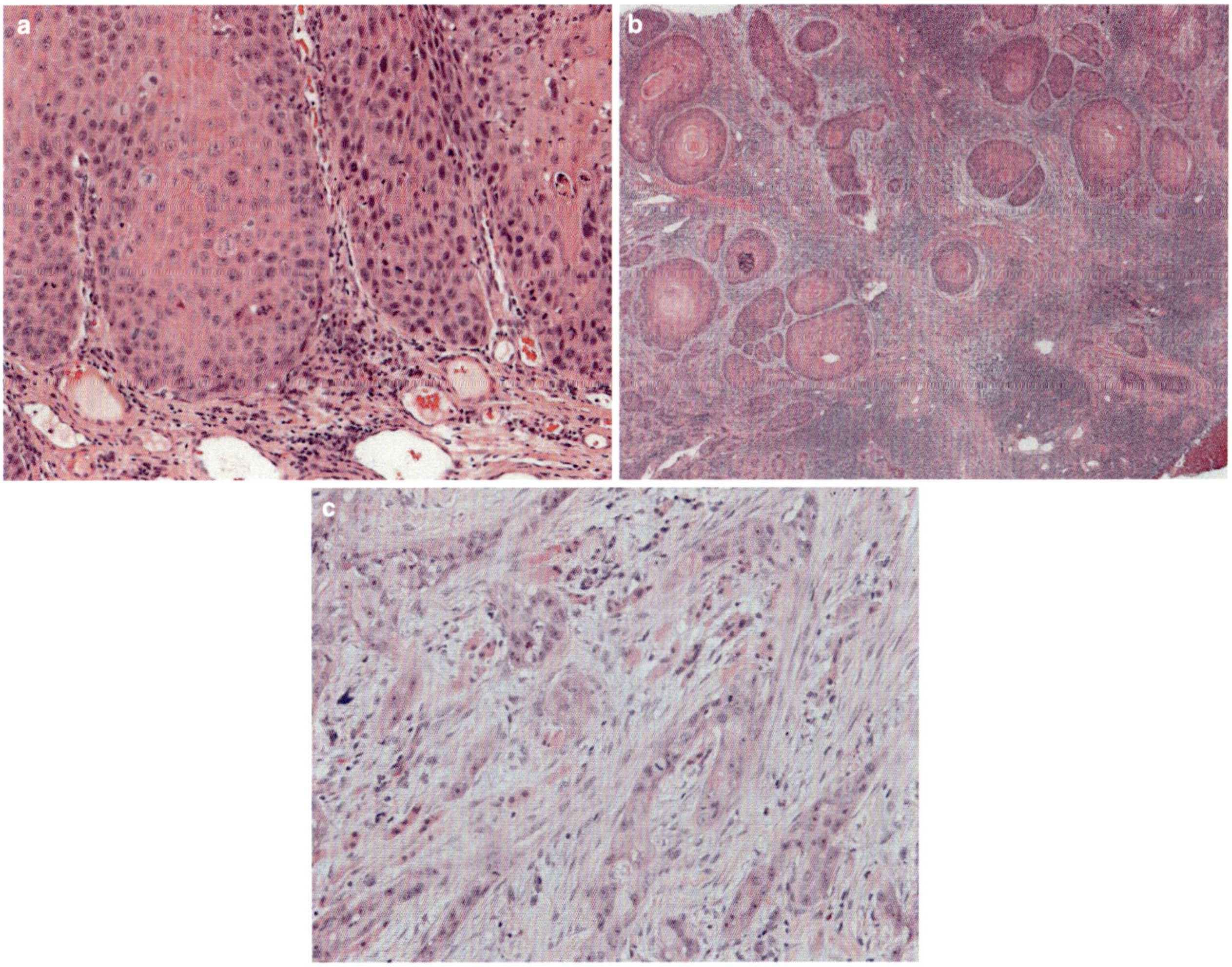

Fig. 7.12 Mode of tumor invasion: (**a**) YK-2, cords, less marked borderline; (**b**) YK-3, groups of cells, no distinct borderline; and (**c**) YK-4C, diffuse invasion, cord-like-type invasion

Footnote

A "pull-through operation" refers to the surgical technique in which—in consideration of the lymph vessels running from the primary lesion to the submandibular tissue or metastatic lymph nodes of the cervical region—the primary lesion is resected en bloc with dissected cervical tissue and pulled out from the submandibular region through the floor of the mouth [39–41] (Figs. 7.13 and 7.14). A pull-through operation is conducted in addition to resection of the primary lesion in cases of N1 and N2b carcinomas of the tongue or floor of the mouth, cases of cervical metastatic lymph node metastasis with multiple lesions, cases of distant metastasis, and N2a/N3 cases. On the other hand, if the primary lesion is late T2 (3–4 cm) or greater and resection through the intraoral approach is difficult, the pull-through operation can be conducted at the same time as neck dissection [42, 45]. For T1 or early T2 at N0, resection of the primary lesion through the intraoral approach will not be problematic for the most part. However, when neck dissection is conducted concurrently because cervical metastasis is suspected upon imaging, the appropriateness of the pull-through operation becomes an issue. The majority opinion mostly supports conducting the pull-through operation, but there are also those who deem it unnecessary.

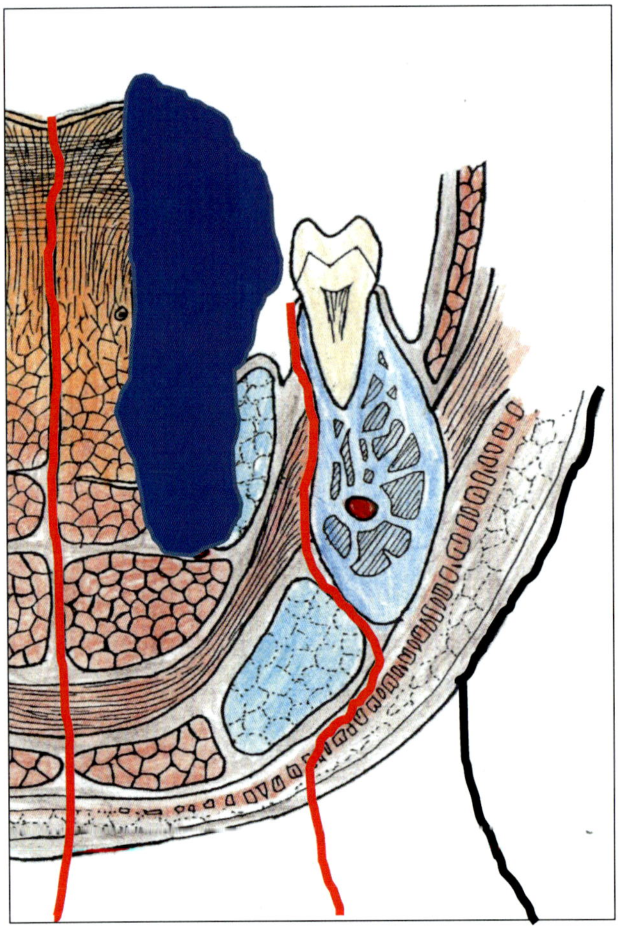

Fig. 7.13 Schema of pull-through operation; primary lesion is resected en bloc with dissected cervical tissue

7.4.1 Surgical Resection of Tongue Carcinomas (Figs. 7.15 and 7.16)

1. Partial Glossectomy Performed for T1/Early T2 N0
   Partial glossectomy refers to the resection of a part or less than half of the oral tongue (Fig. 7.17). The surgery is performed via the intraoral approach. It is important to bear in mind not only the horizontal safety margin but also the vertical safety margin at the time of resection. It is also necessary to perform resection taking into account the tumor's clinical growth pattern and histopathological malignancy. Resection of deep muscle tissue will be considerable for tumors that have deeply invaded the muscle layers. Hence, sufficient postoperative hemostasis on the wound and primary suturing are conducted (Fig. 7.18). A skin graft should be performed when there is a possibility that suturing will cause functional disturbance of the tongue. Impairment of oral function after partial glossectomy is mild.
   Note: Sometimes the term "early T2" is used for tongue carcinomas with a maximum diameter of between 2 and 3 cm, and the term "late T2" (or "advanced T2") for those with a maximum diameter of between 3 and 4 cm; for tongue carcinomas there are some who consider the classification significant.
2. Partial Glossectomy Performed for Late T2/T3 (Superficial Type)
   Because the surgical margin and resection depth become deep for these tumors, it is important that the safety margin be sufficiently verified. There are also cases where primary suturing cannot be performed, and a skin graft or, depending on the case, flap transplantation becomes necessary (Fig. 7.19). There are also cases where a safe resection cannot be made via the intraoral approach, and surgery must be performed via the extraoral approach.
3. Partial Glossectomy, Oral Tongue Hemiglossectomy, Oral Tongue Subtotal-Total Glossectomy, Hemiglossectomy, and Subtotal-Total Glossectomy Performed for Late T2/T3/T4 N0 Oral tongue hemiglossectomy refers to a resection to the lingual septum by a hemiglossectomy of only the oral tongue (Figs. 7.20 and 7.21). Oral tongue subtotal-total glossectomy refers to a resection of over half (subtotal) or all of the oral tongue (Fig. 7.22). Hemiglossectomy refers to a hemiglossectomy that includes the base of the tongue (Figs. 7.23 and 7.24). Subtotal-total glossectomy refers to a resection of over half (subtotal) or all of the tongue including the base of the tongue (Fig. 7.25).
   There are cases where performing these resections via the intraoral approach is possible, but performing them via

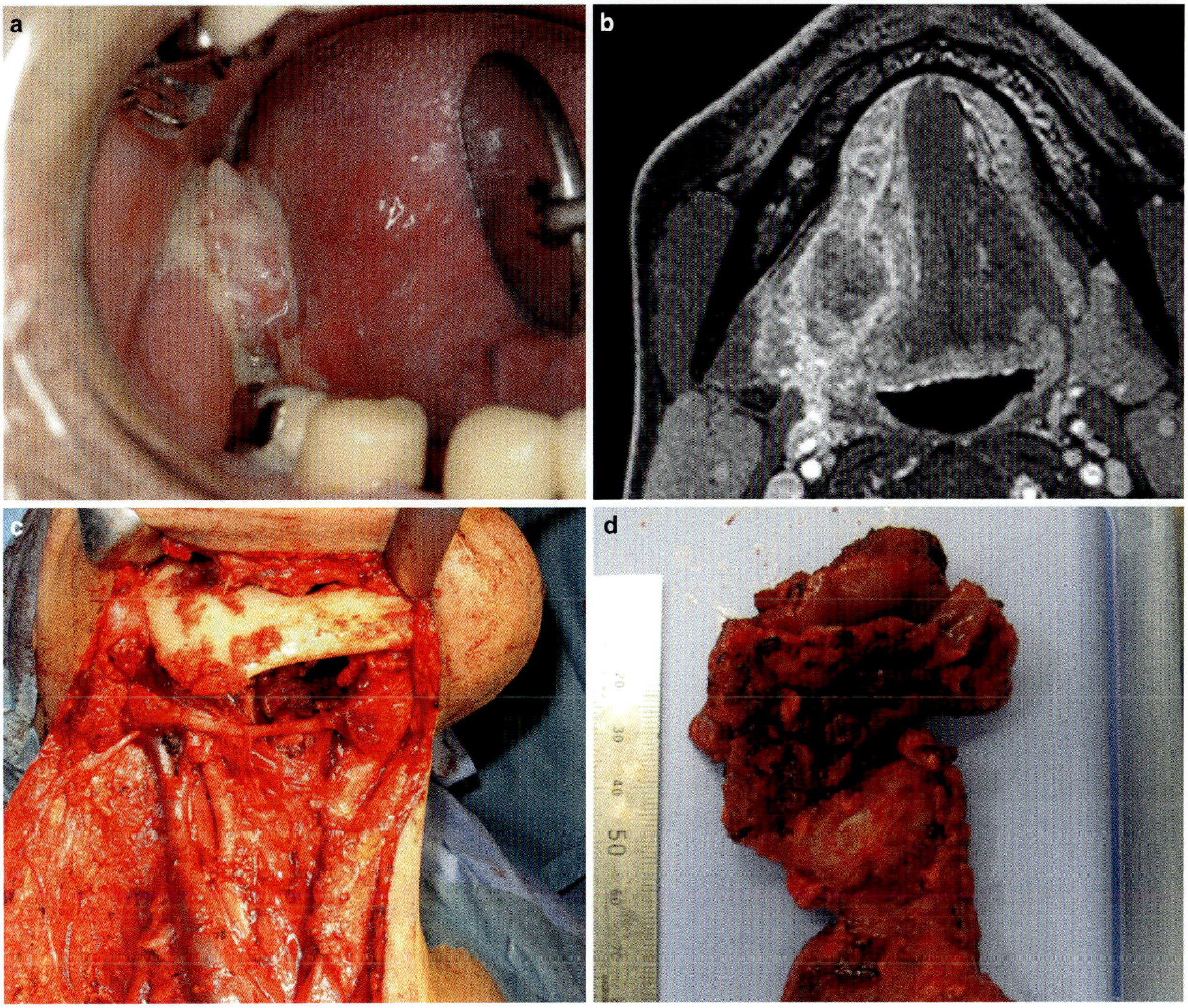

Fig. 7.14 Pull-through operation. (**a**) Tongue carcinoma (T2N1M0) and (**b**) MRI; tumor occupies the part of less than half of the oral tongue. (**c**) Hemiglossectomy with radical neck dissection. (**d**) Primary lesion is resected en bloc with dissected cervical tissue

Partial glossectomy:
Resection of a part or less than half of the oral tongue

Oral tongue hemiglossectomy:
Resection to the lingual septum by a hemiglossectomy of only the oral tongue

Oral tongue subtotal-total glossectomy:
Resection of over half (subtotal) or all of the oral tongue

Hemiglossectomy :
Resection to the lingual septum by a hemiglossectomy of the oral tongue and the base of the tongue

Subtotal-total glossectomy:
Resection of over half (subtotal) or all of the tongue including the base of the tongue

Fig. 7.15 Surgical resection of tongue carcinomas

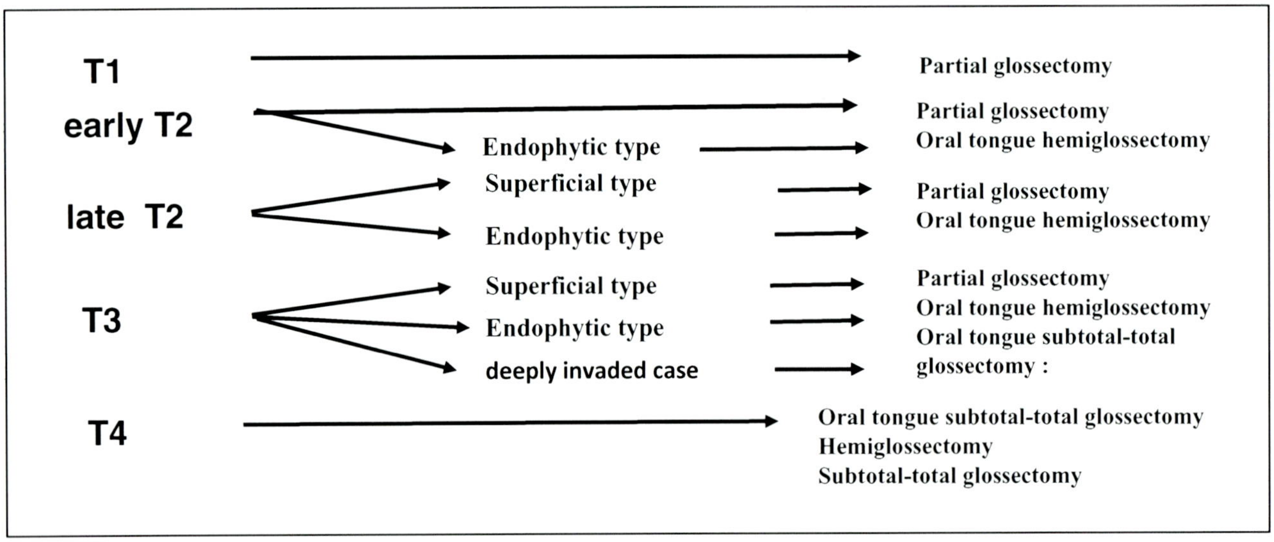

Fig. 7.16 Algorithm of the surgical treatment of tongue carcinoma

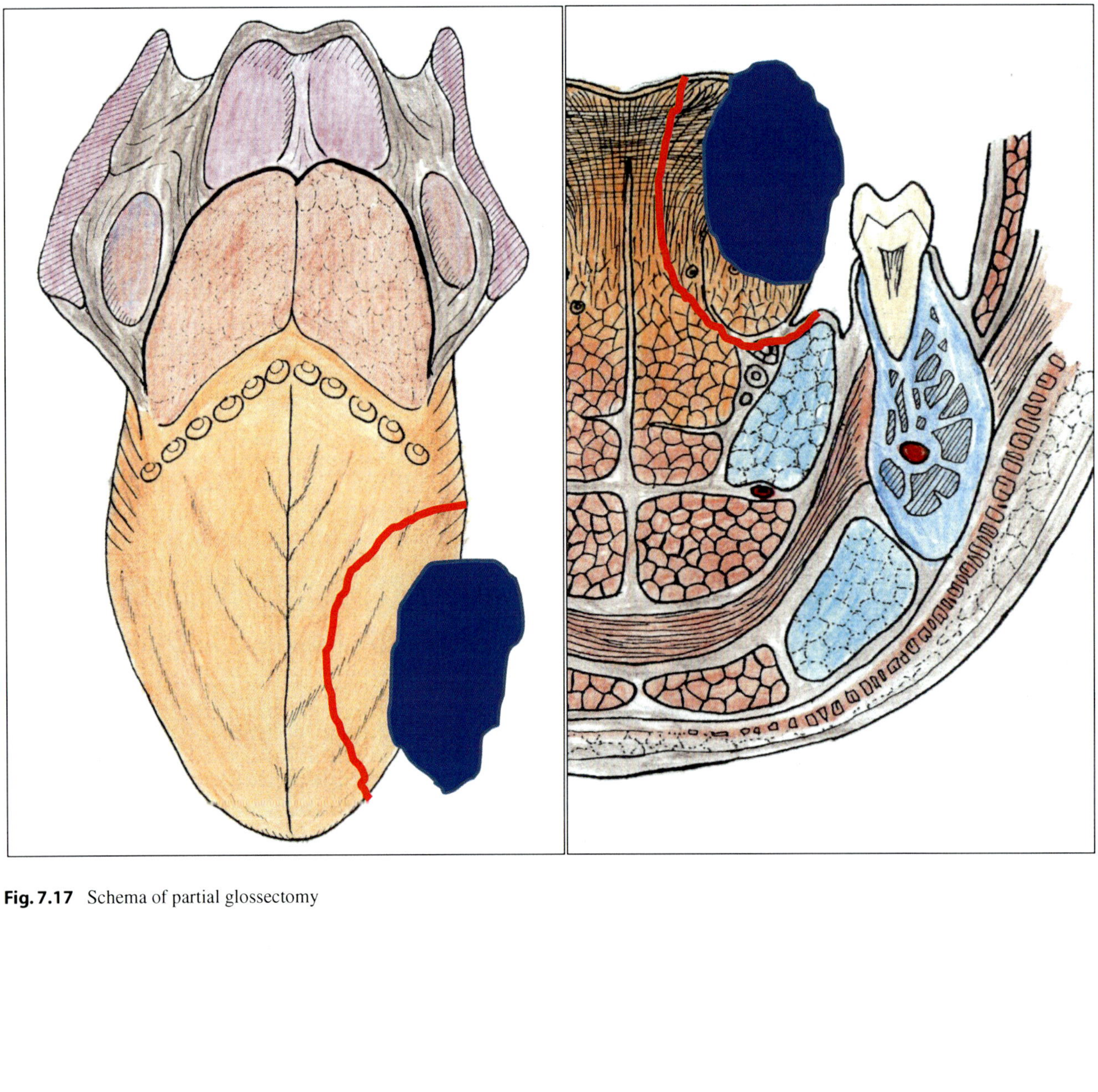

Fig. 7.17 Schema of partial glossectomy

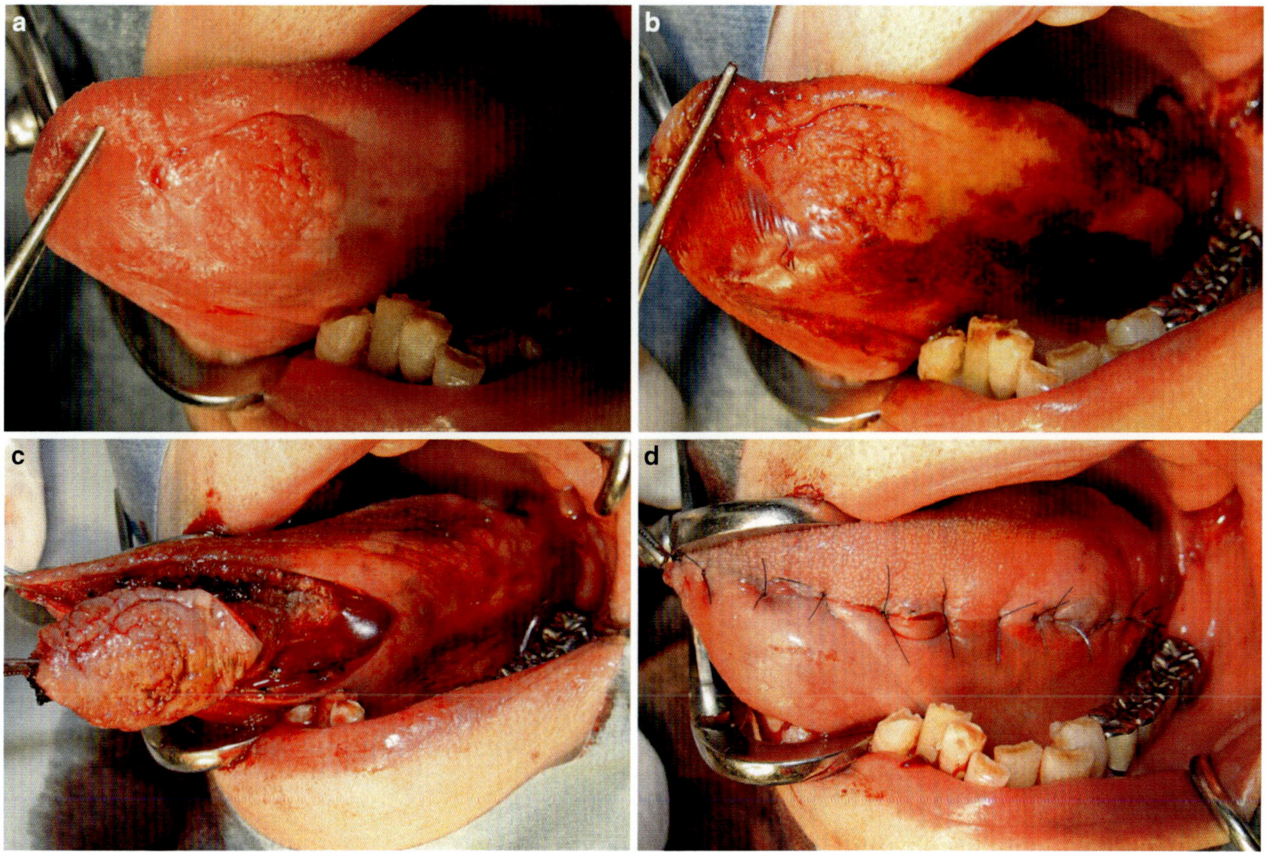

Fig. 7.18 Partial glossectomy. (**a**) Tongue carcinoma (T1), (**b**) vital staining with iodine solution, (**c**) partial glossectomy, and (**d**) primary suturing

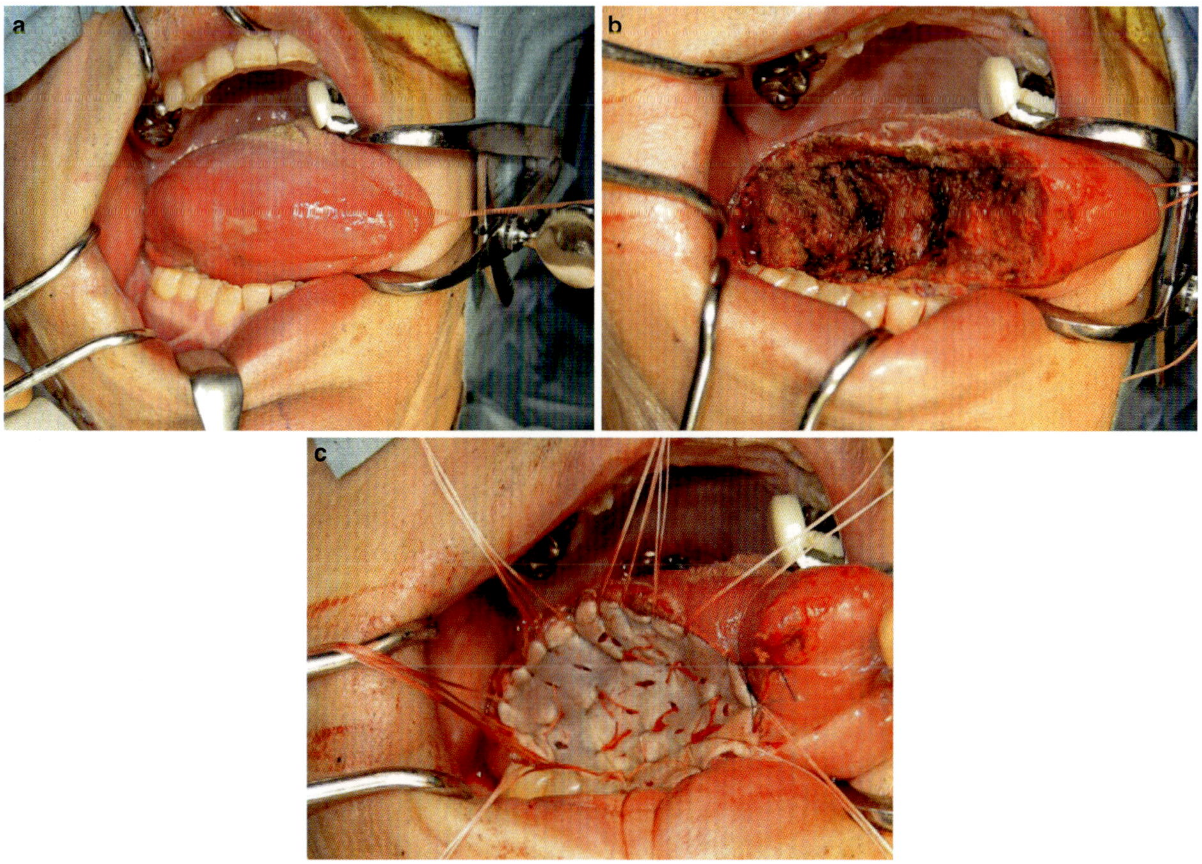

Fig. 7.19 Partial glossectomy. (**a**) Tongue carcinoma (T2), (**b**) partial glossectomy, and (**c**) surgical defect is covered with shin graft

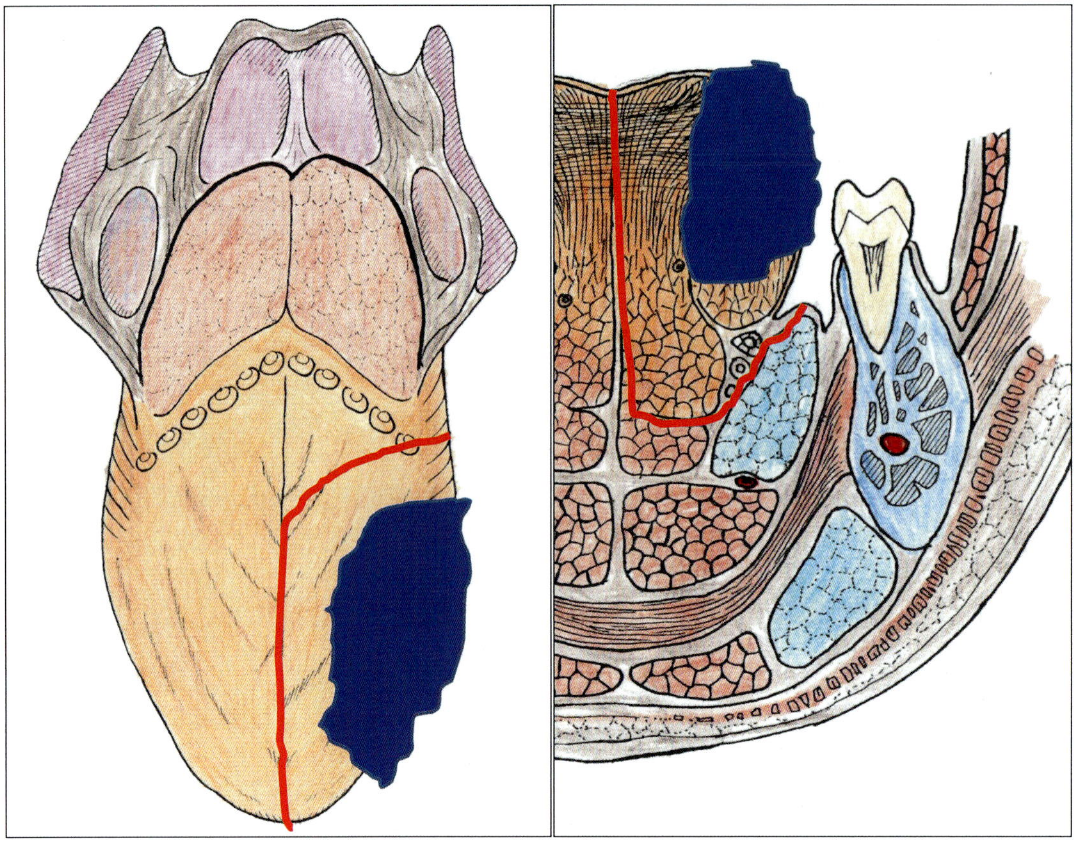

Fig. 7.20 Hemiglossectomy of the oral tongue

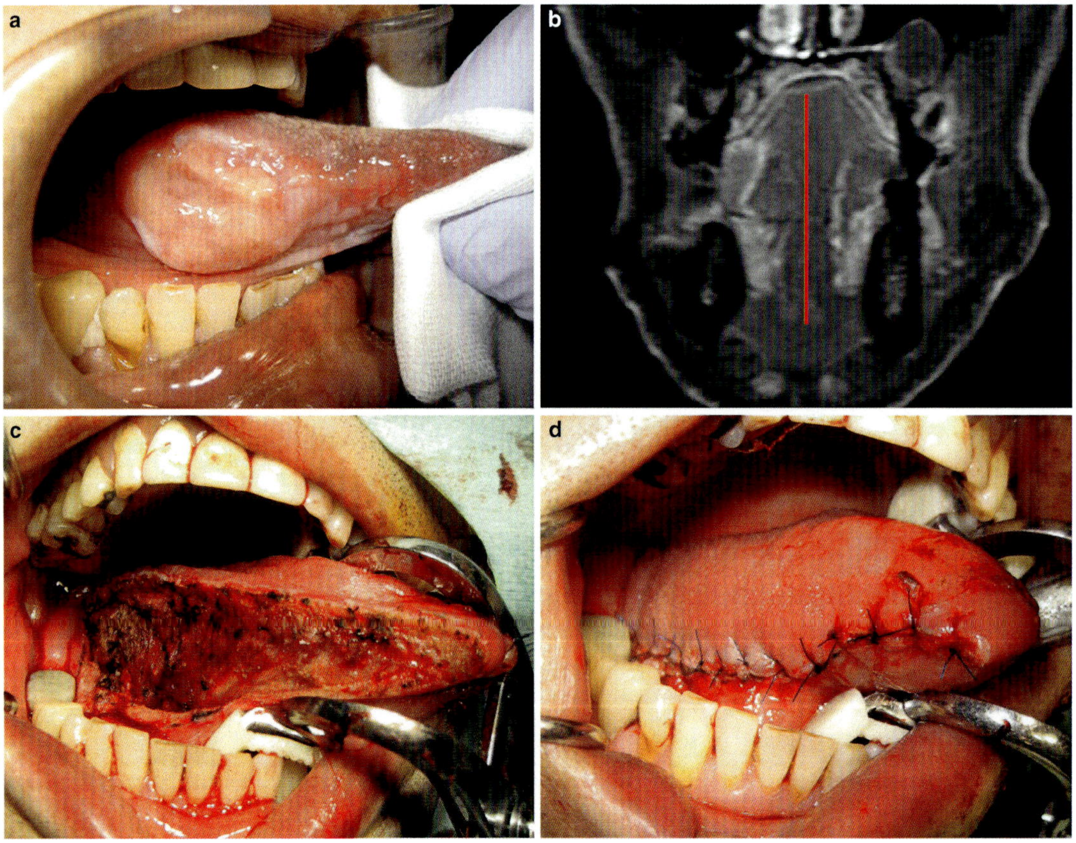

Fig. 7.21 Hemiglossectomy of the oral tongue. (**a**) Tongue carcinoma (T2) and (**b**) MRI; tumor occupies the part of less than half of the oral tongue. (**c**) Resection to the lingual septum of the oral tongue. (**d**) Primary suturing

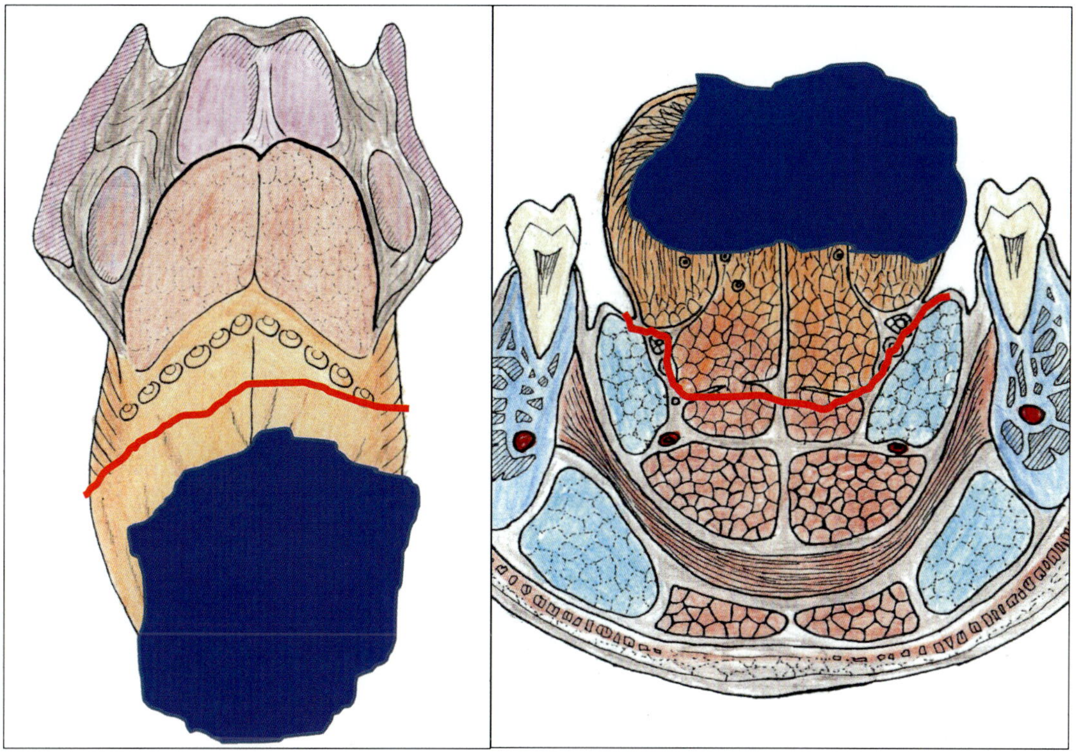

Fig. 7.22 Subtotal-total glossectomy of the oral tongue. Resection of over half (subtotal) or all of the oral tongue

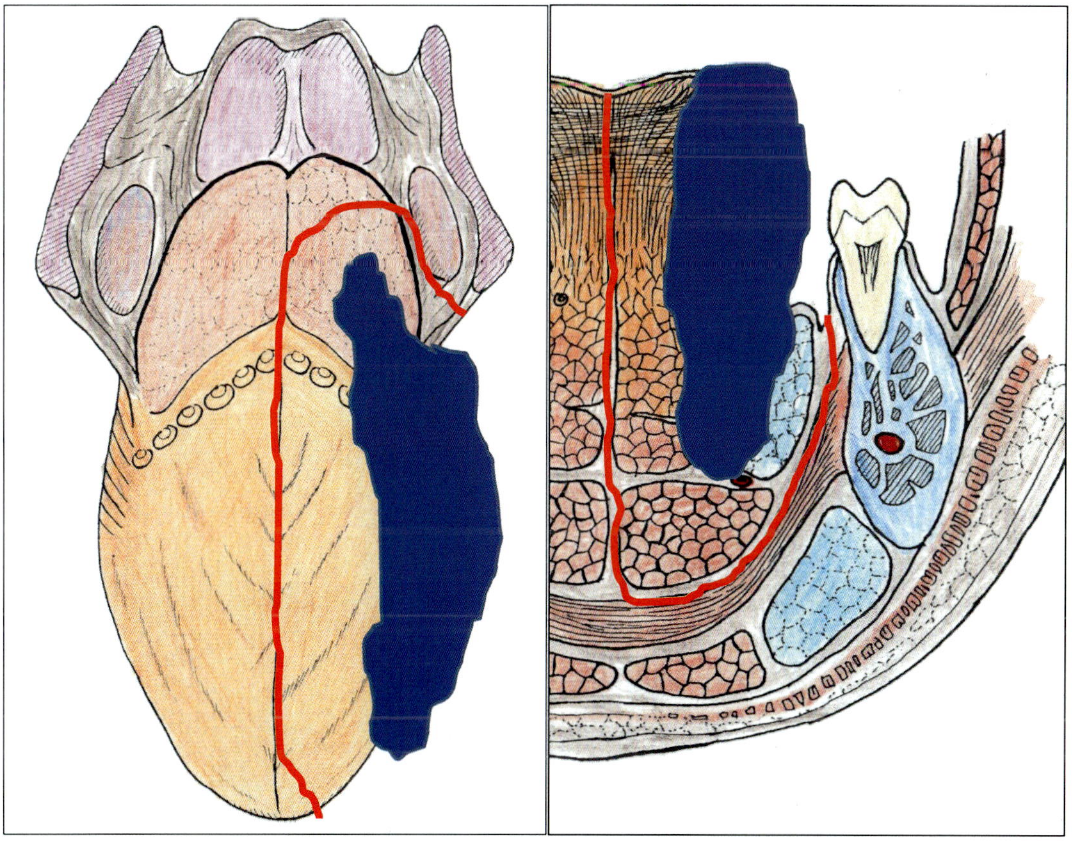

Fig. 7.23 Hemiglossectomy that includes the base of the tongue

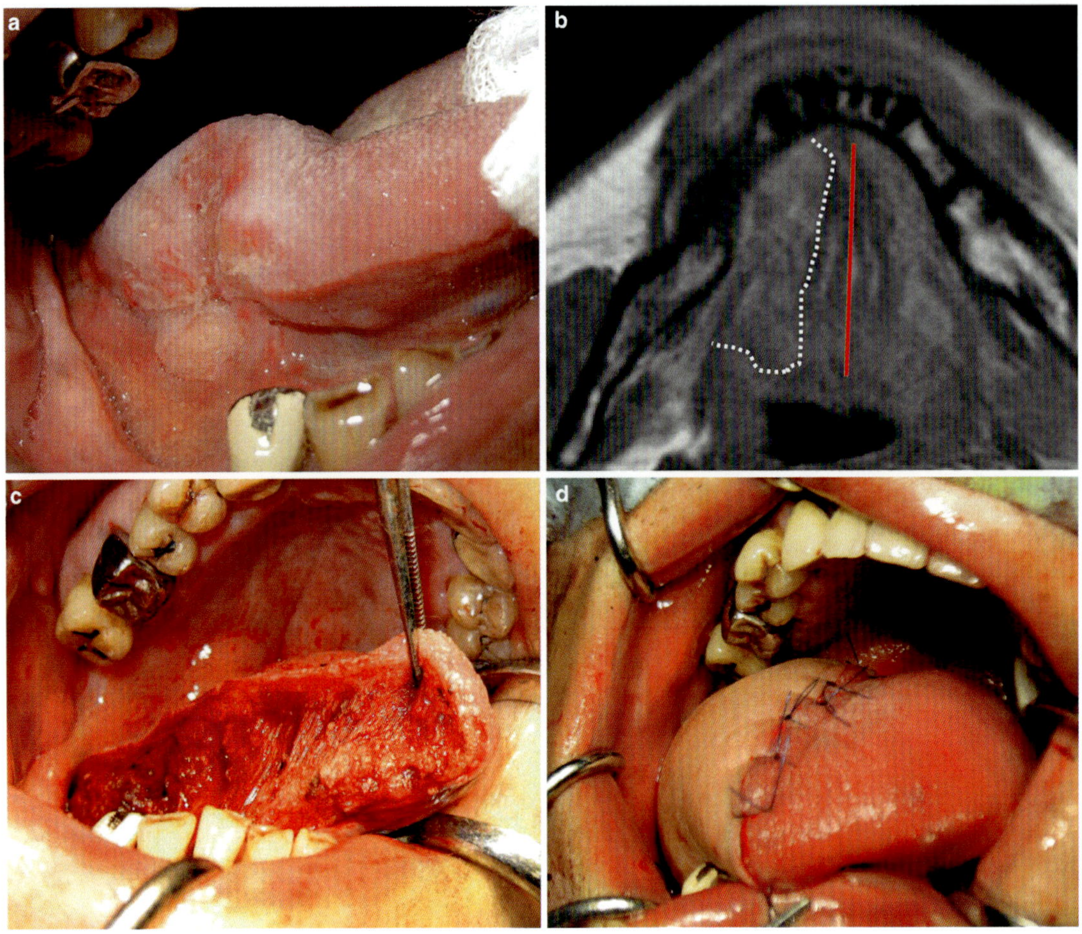

Fig. 7.24 Hemiglossectomy. (**a**) Tongue carcinoma (T3) and (**b**) MRI; tumor includes the base of the tongue. (**c**) Resection to the lingual septum by a hemiglossectomy with base of the tongue. (**d**) Reconstruction with forearm flap

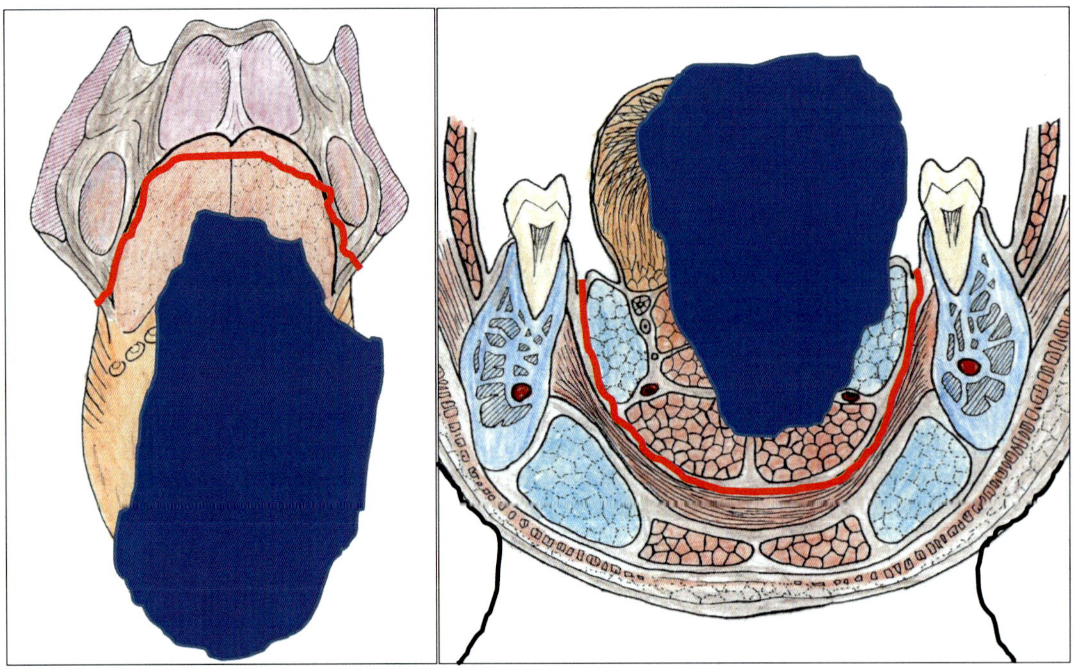

Fig. 7.25 Subtotal-total glossectomy: resection of over half (subtotal) or all of the tongue including the base of the tongue

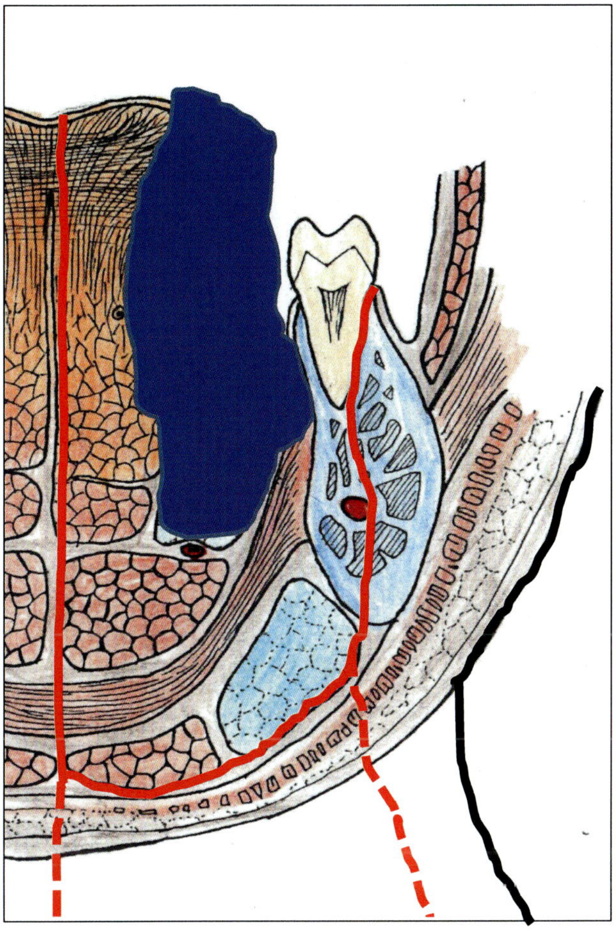

Fig. 7.26 Command operation. Hemiglossectomy with the cortical bone on the lingual side by sagittal splitting osteotomy and/or neck dissection

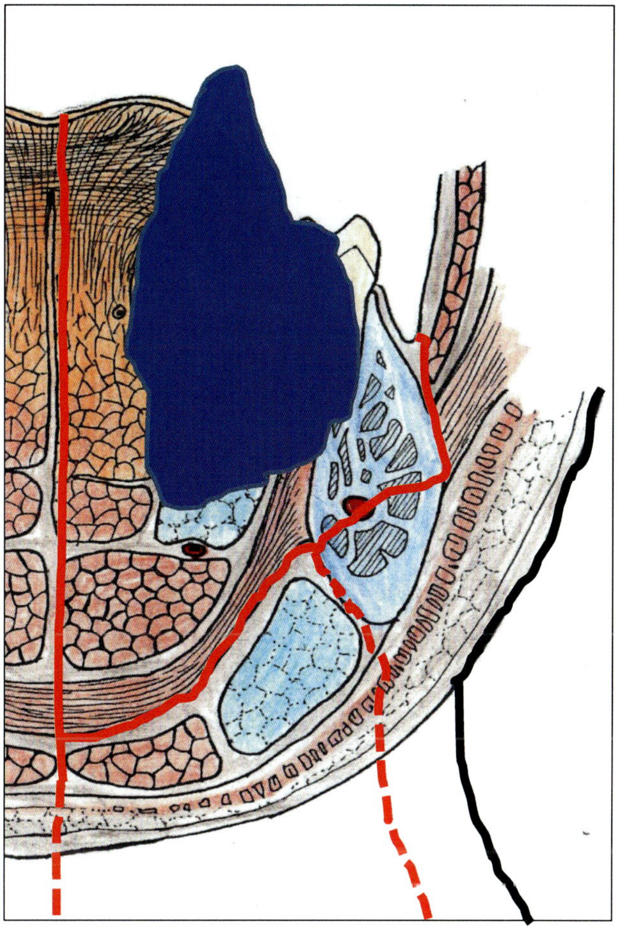

Fig. 7.27 Command operation. Hemiglossectomy with marginal mandibulectomy and/or neck dissection

the extraoral approach is preferable in order to reliably ensure the safety margin of the deep parts of the tumor.

For cases in which the extraoral approach is used, preventative neck dissection is sometimes performed concurrently (via the pull-through method) to sufficiently resect deep tissue or to accompany soft tissue reconstructive surgery [42–45].

Oral tongue hemiglossectomy method is as follows. (1) From the neck, use the fingers to separate the left and right geniohyoid muscles and genioglossus muscles and divide the lingual septum into left and right. (2) From inside the oral cavity, make an incision from the exact center of the floor of the mouth to the exact center of the tongue and detach the lingual septum. (3) From the neck, cut the geniohyoid and mylohyoid muscles on the affected side near the submental hyoid bone. (4) From inside the oral cavity, detaching parallel with the lingual septum in the center of the tongue dorsum, cut the intrinsic muscles of the tongue and the styloglossus muscle posteriorly, cut the genioglossus muscle anteriorly, and resect the floor of the mouth.

4. Partial Glossectomy Performed Concurrently with Neck Dissection for Cases of T1/Early T2 N1–3 (via the Pull-Through Method)

For late T2/T3/T4N1 3, neck dissection is performed concurrently with resection of the primary lesion. This involves a compound operation of partial glossectomy, hemiglossectomy, oral tongue subtotal-total glossectomy, etc., and the mandible and surrounding tissues, depending on the extent of tumor invasion. Concerning tumor progression towards the mandible, if the distance of the tumor from the mandible is 1 cm or more, then a mandibulectomy is not necessary[5].

5. Surgical Treatment of T4 Cases [46–48]
   (a) In cases of invasion into the floor of the mouth or into the mandibular bone marrow, the practitioner resects the mandible while concurrently ensuring the safety margin. One performs a marginal mandibulectomy if the tumor has yet to reach the mylohyoid muscle. In this situation, if the tumor is limited to the cortical bone on the lingual side of the mandible, one resects the cortical bone on the lingual side by sagittal splitting osteotomy (Fig. 7.26). One resects the upper portion of the bone if the tumor has only infiltrated the upper portion of the mandible (Fig. 7.27).

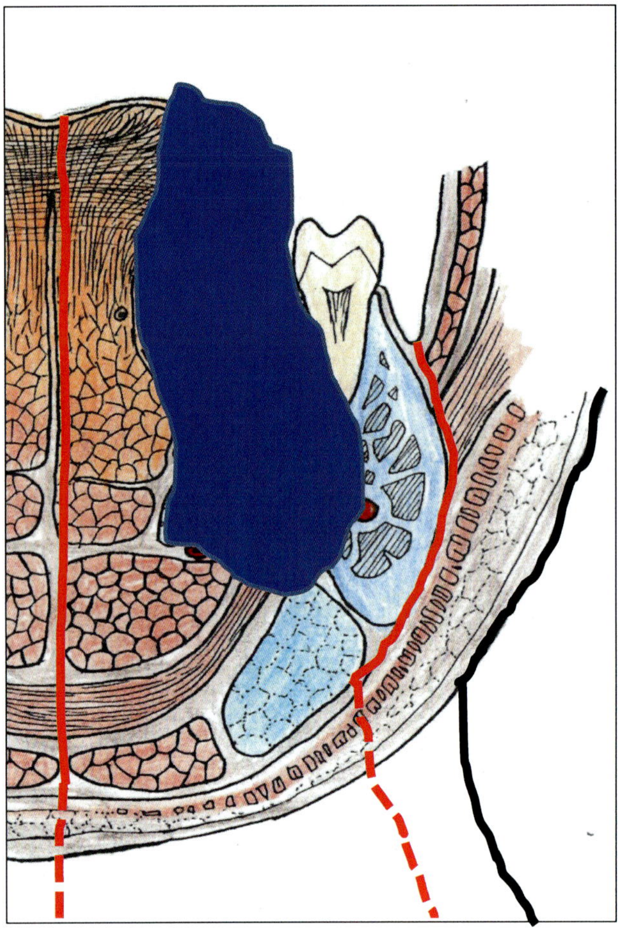

Fig. 7.28 Command operation. Hemiglossectomy with segmental mandibulectomy and/or neck dissection

A segmental mandibulectomy is performed in cases where the tumor exceeds the mylohyoid muscle or invades into the mandibular bone marrow, into the submandibular space, or into the extrinsic muscles of the tongue (Figs. 7.28, 7.29, and 7.30).

(b) In cases involving invasion posterior to the lingual margin to the base of the tongue, the base of the tongue, the palatoglossal arch, and the tonsillar fossa are resected in addition to a total glossectomy. Furthermore, if the tumor has invaded inferiorly, then a laryngectomy is also performed (Fig. 7.31). Determining the surgery indicated is difficult in cases where invasion is observed in the masticatory muscle space, the pterygoid process, the base of the skull, or the internal carotid artery and its surroundings.

7.5 Surgical Therapy for Lower Gingival Carcinomas

Lower gingival carcinomas invade the mandible relatively quickly in many cases, causing bone destruction. In the establishment of surgical margins, because the tumor progression into the bone cannot be directly probed physically, it is diagnosed via diagnostic imaging techniques such as dental X-ray, panoramic X-ray, CT, and MRI scans. It is important to have a complete picture of the depth and type of bone resorption and invasion to adjacent structures and to establish a treatment plan [49–51].

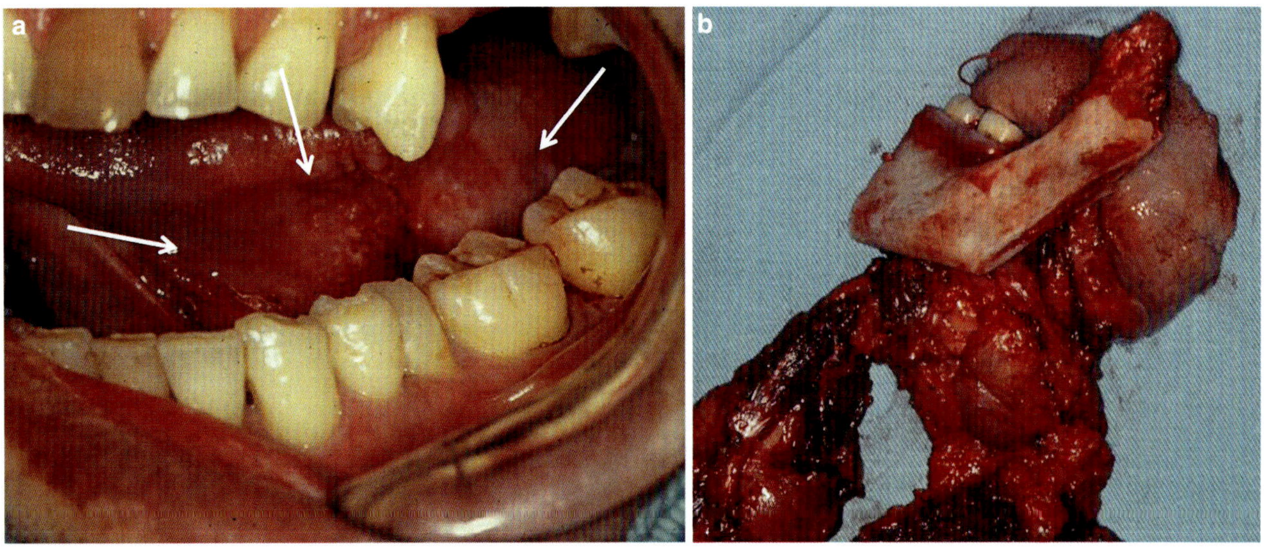

Fig. 7.29 Command operation of tongue carcinoma. (**a**) Tongue carcinoma invades the mandible (T4N2cM0). (**b**) Total glossectomy with segmental mandibulectomy and bilateral neck dissection

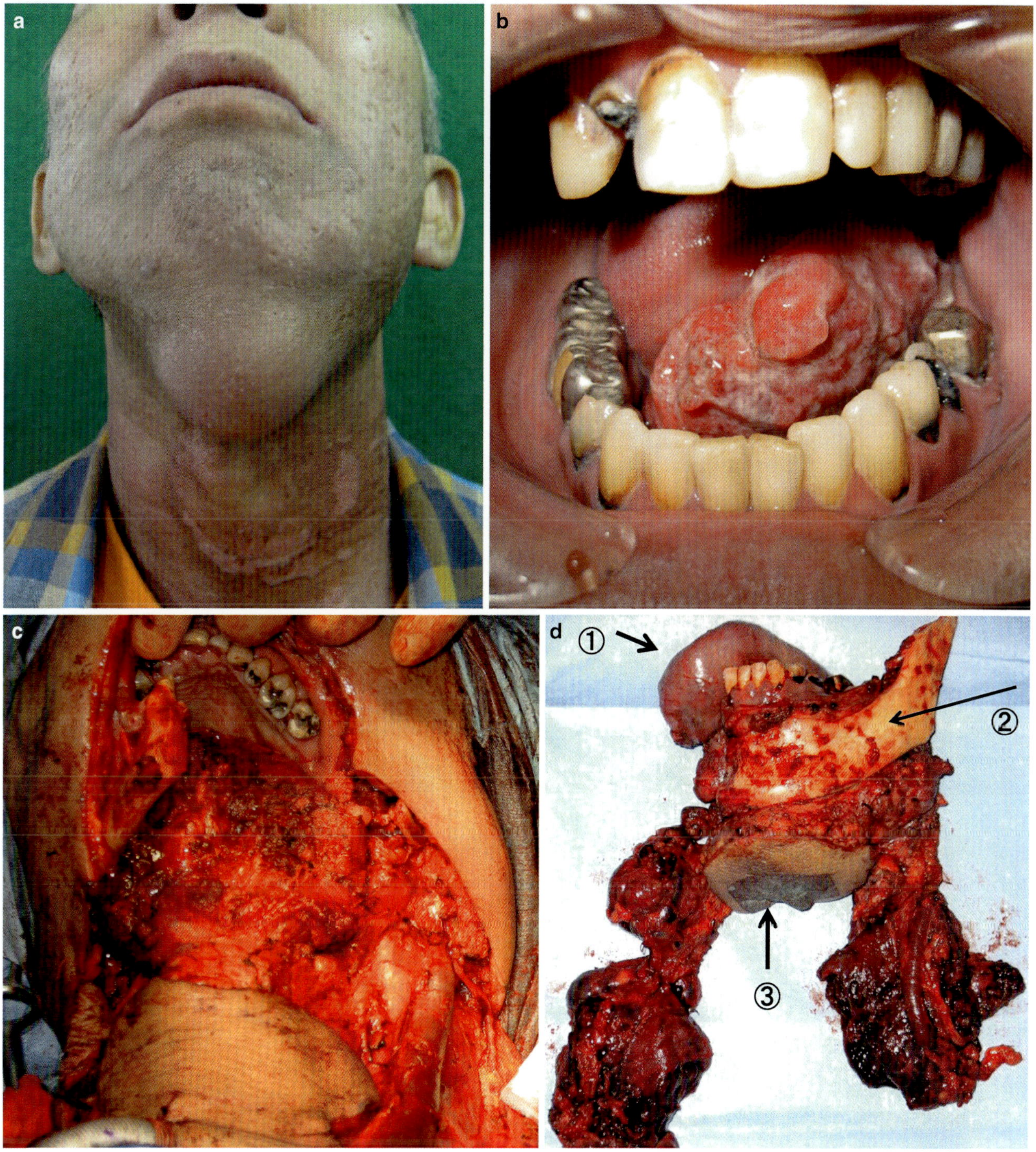

Fig. 7.30 Tongue carcinoma with mandibular invasion and cervical metastasis: (**a**) cervical metastasis and (**b**) tongue carcinoma invades into the mandible. (**c**) Hemiglossectomy, segmental mandibulectomy, bilateral neck dissection, and skin resection of submental region. (**d**) Surgical specimen: (1) tongue, (2) mandible, and (3) skin

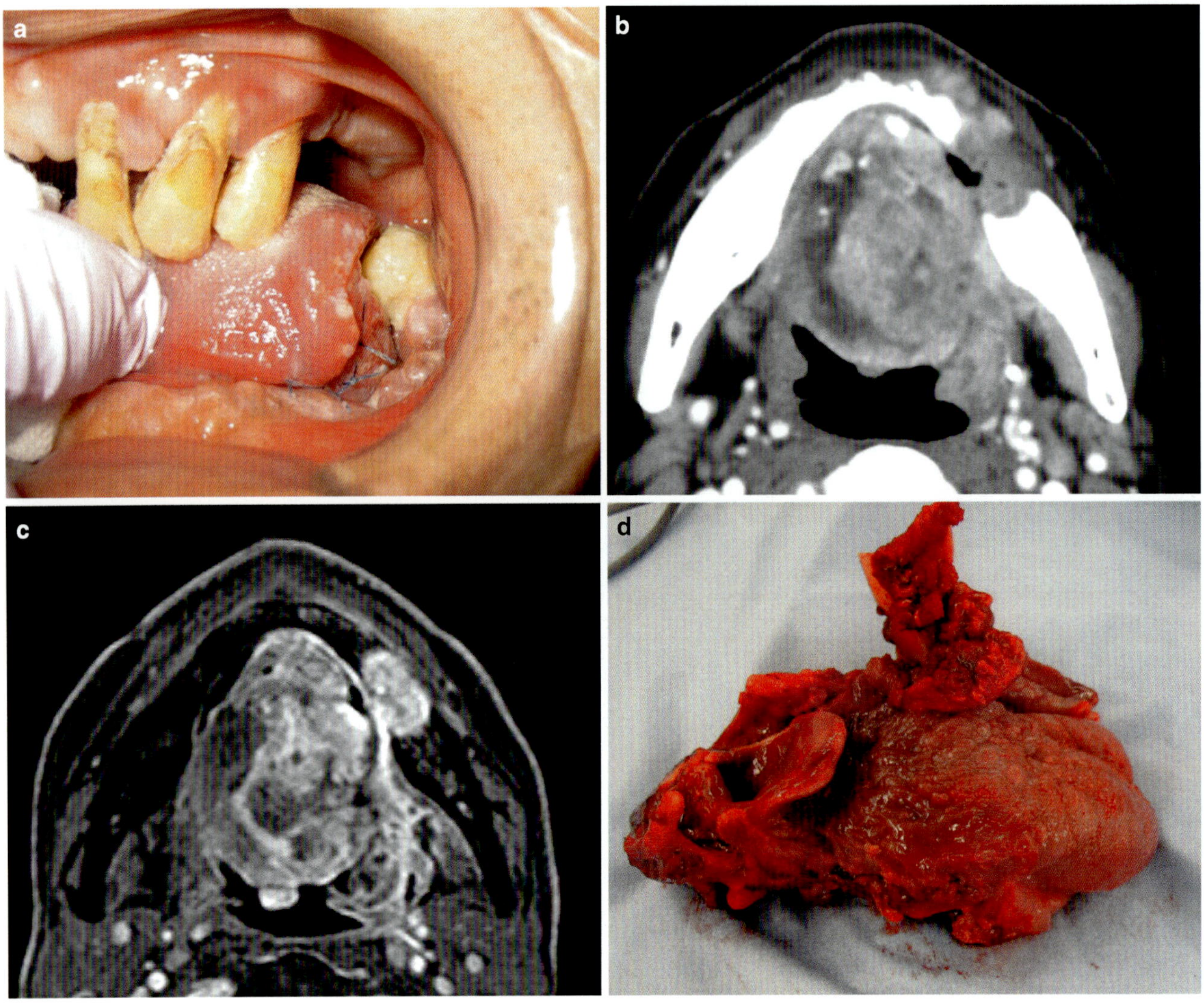

Fig. 7.31 Total glossectomy. (**a**) Tongue carcinoma (T4) and (**b**) CT; tumor invades the base of the tongue and mandible. (**c**) MRI; tumor invades the base of the tongue and mandible. (**d**) Total glossectomy with laryngectomy

7.5.1 Surgical Methods for Lower Gingival Carcinomas (Fig. 7.32)

Concerning the treatment standards for T4 in "General Rules for Clinical and Pathological Studies on Oral Cancer" the T classification is currently widely utilized as the diagnostic criteria of the mandibular canal in Japan [1]: i.e., an invasion reaching the mandibular canal is classified as T4. This differs from the UICC classification, whereby T4 refers to invasion beyond the alveolar bone. Surgical treatment of a lower gingival carcinoma in principle requires a mandibulectomy, and the basic operative procedure differs depending on the surgical margin.

A gingivectomy is a method during which only the gingival mucosa and periosteum are resected, and the alveolar bone is not. This method is indicated for precancerous lesions and in situ carcinoma of the gingiva.

Marginal mandibulectomy refers to a resection of the only lingual cortex and/or alveolar process (Figs. 7.33, 7.34, and 7.35). Segmental mandibulectomy refers to a resection of under half (subtotal) of the mandible without condyle (Figs. 7.36 and 7.37). Hemi-mandibulectomy refers to a resection of half of the mandible with one-side condyle (Fig. 7.38). Subtotal mandibulectomy(with/without condylectomy)refers to a resection of over half (subtotal) of the mandible with/without condyle (Fig. 7.39). Total mandibulectomy refers to a resection of all of the mandible including the both side condyle.

Marginal mandibulectomy is performed for cases of T1 where the invasion into the bone is light. For T2 and T3, the

Fig. 7.32 Surgical resection of lower gingival carcinoma

Gingivectomy :
Resection of only the gingival mucosa and periosteum, and the alveolar bone is not resected.

Marginal mandibulectomy:
Resection of the only lingual cortex and/or alveolar process

Segmental mandibulectomy
Resection of under half (subtotal) of the mandible without condyle

Hemi-mandibulectomy
Resection of half of the mandible with one side condyle

Subtotal mandibulectomy (with/without condylectomy)
Resection of over half (subtotal) of the mandible with/without condyle

Total mandibulectomy
Resection of all of the mandible including the both side condyle

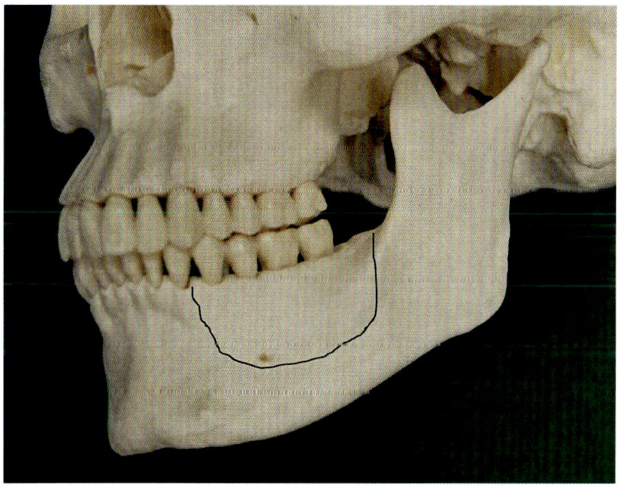

Fig. 7.33 Surgical resection of lower gingival carcinoma. Marginal mandibulectomy

relationship between mandibular resorption type (Fig. 7.40) and depth is especially important [52]. In these cases, marginal resection or segmental resection of the mandible can be chosen, but that judgment is determined by the extent of tumor progression [42–45, 49–52] (Figs. 7.41, 7.42, 7.43, and 7.44).

In cases of T4a, for invasions reaching the mandibular canal, into the buccal space or subcutaneous fat, into the submandibular space, and into the extrinsic muscles of the tongue, segmental resection (Fig. 7.45), hemi-mandibulectomy (Fig. 7.46), subtotal mandibulectomy, and total mandibulec-

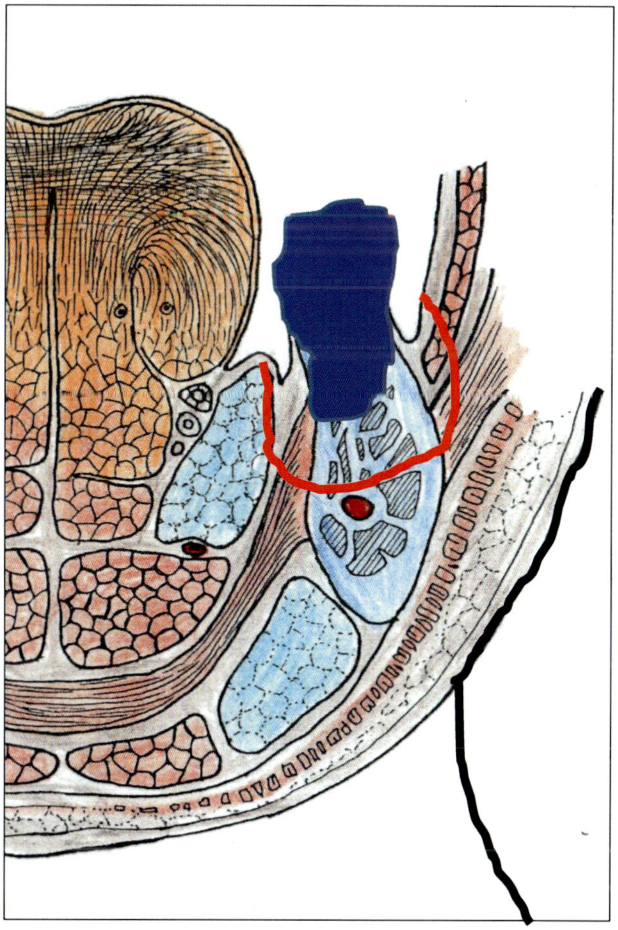

Fig. 7.34 Schema of marginal mandibulectomy

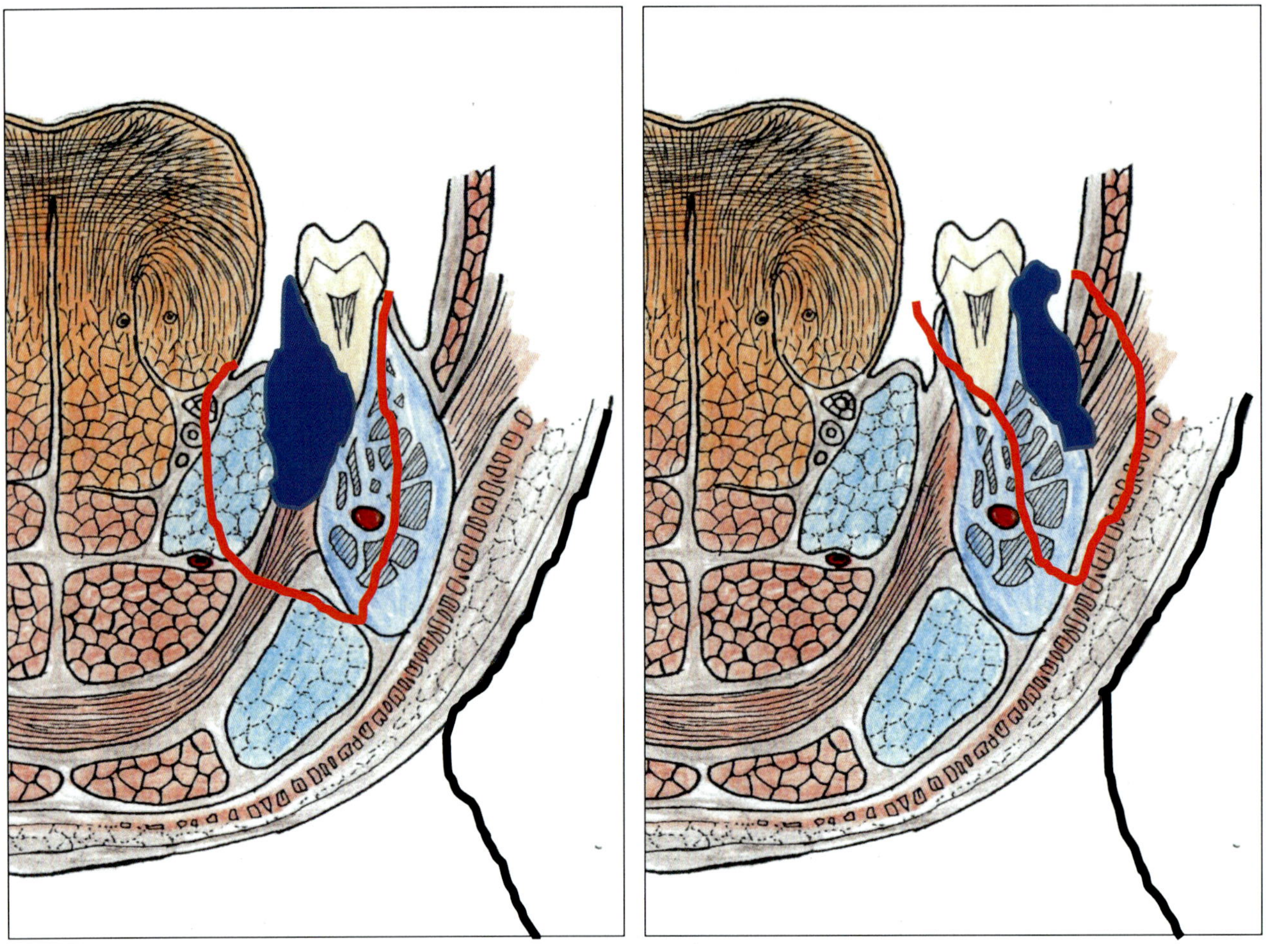

Fig. 7.35 Schema of marginal mandibulectomy (sagittal splitting)

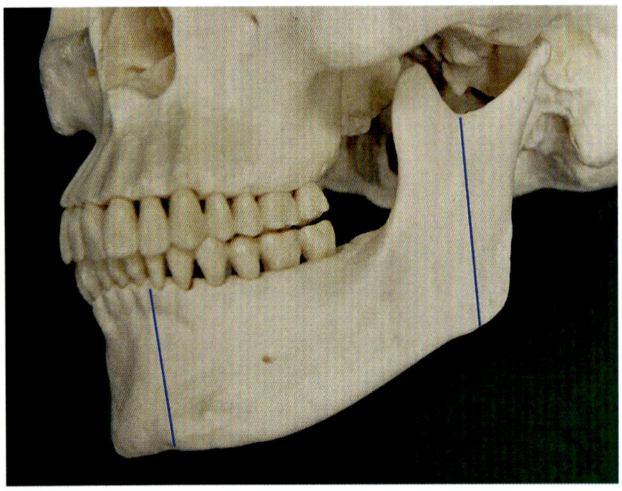

Fig. 7.36 Surgical resection of lower gingival carcinoma. Segmental mandibulectomy

tomy can be performed. For these cases, making an excision on the lower lips and expanding them increase the practitioner's field of vision and an accurate resection can be performed (Fig. 7.47). In cases of T4b, for invasions into the masticatory muscle space, into the pterygoid process, into the base of the skull, and into the periphery of the internal carotid artery, a hemi-mandibulectomy or subtotal mandibulectomy is necessary, but difficulties in resection may occur.

7.5.2 Selection Criteria of Marginal Mandibulectomy and Segmental Mandibulectomy (Fig. 7.48)

In terms of postoperative QOL, marginal mandibulectomy surpasses segmental mandibulectomy in both aesthetic and functional respects. On the other hand, segmental mandibu-

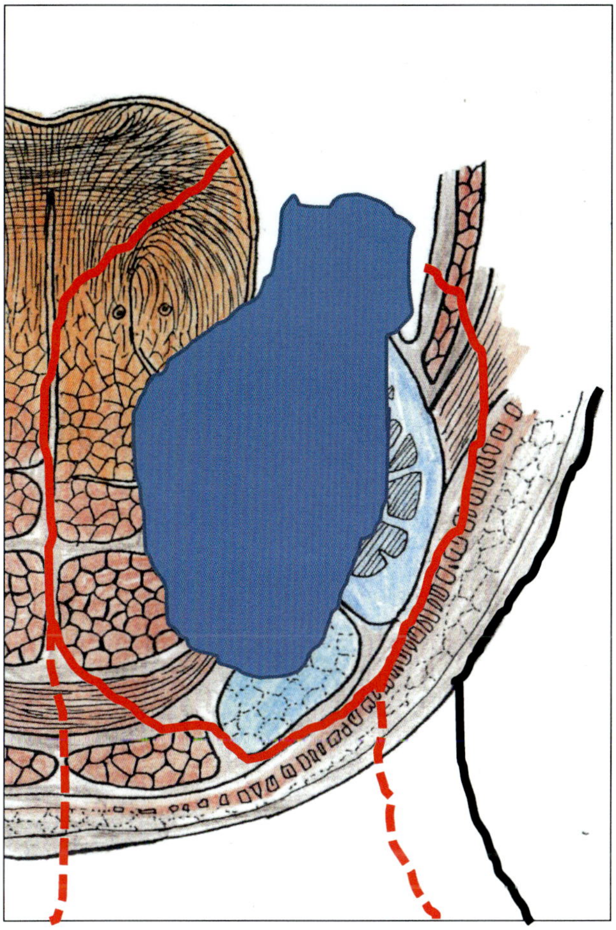

Fig. 7.37 Schema of segmental mandibulectomy

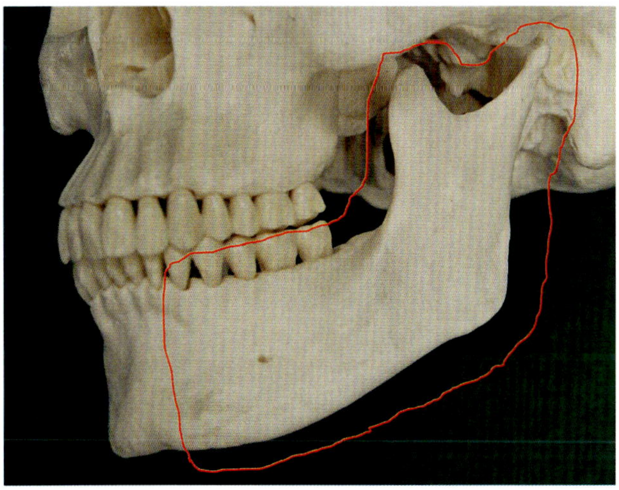

Fig. 7.38 Surgical resection of lower gingival carcinoma. Hemi-mandibulectomy

lectomy is preferable with regard to the certainty of tumor resection; practitioners often waver over selection between the two. Tentatively, as a general rule, practitioners should perform a marginal mandibulectomy or less for T1 and a segmental mandibulectomy or more for T4. For T2 and T3, for cases limited to the alveolus and not reaching the mandibular canal, if the bone resorption pattern is the expansive type, then marginal resection is recommended.

1. Invasion to Adjacent Soft Tissue and Surgical Methods
   There are many reports of local recurrence arising more often in the surrounding soft tissue than in the surgical margin of bone post-resection [50, 51, 53–56]. Segmental mandibulectomies that include soft tissue are considered appropriate for targeting cases of tumor progression into the soft tissue surrounding the mandible bone, especially progressing towards the mylohyoid muscle and pharynx (Figs. 7.49 and 7.50).
2. Bone Resorption Depth and Surgical Treatment
   Segmental mandibulectomy including the mandibular canal is necessary for tumor invasion clearly reaching the mandibular canal. In histological examinations of resected samples to the present [57], tumors were not observed in sites 1 cm removed from areas where bone resorption was radiographically observed. This fact means that taking a minimum safety margin of 1 cm from the radiographic bone resorption site is necessary and that segmental mandibulectomy is indicated for cases where the safety margin extends past the mandibular canal (Figs. 7.51 and 7.52).
3. Bone Absorption Type and Surgical Treatment
   The concordance rate of radiographic bone resorption and pathological bone invasion ranges are high in the expansive type and low in the invasive type [49, 58] (Figs. 7.53, 7.54, and 7.55). For the invasive type, predicting the tumor's bone invasion from X-ray images of bone resorption is difficult, and furthermore, it is necessary to establish a large surgical margin because of the high amount of residual tumor [59]. Marginal mandibulectomy ought to be limited to cases where bone invasion is slight and inside the alveolar bone. On the other hand, segmental mandibulectomy is more appropriate for cases that present with images of bone resorption of the invasive type or for cases that present with bone resorption adjacent or leading to the mandibular canal of the expansive type [49–51]. However, some opinions hold that even for cases that present as the invasive type on X-ray imaging, marginal mandibulectomy is possible if it is restricted to the alveolar part.

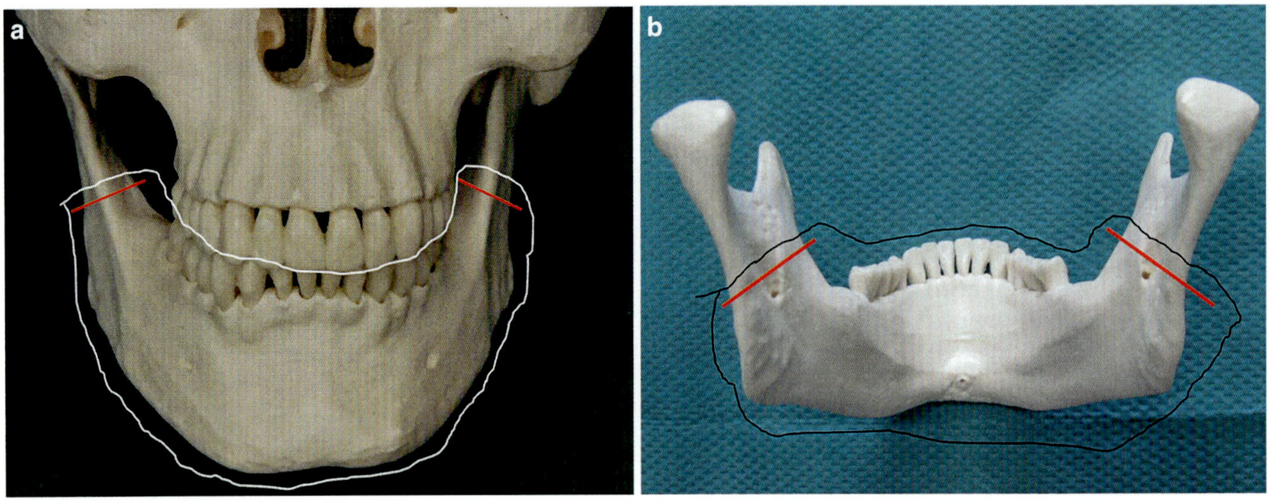

Fig. 7.39 Subtotal mandibulectomy

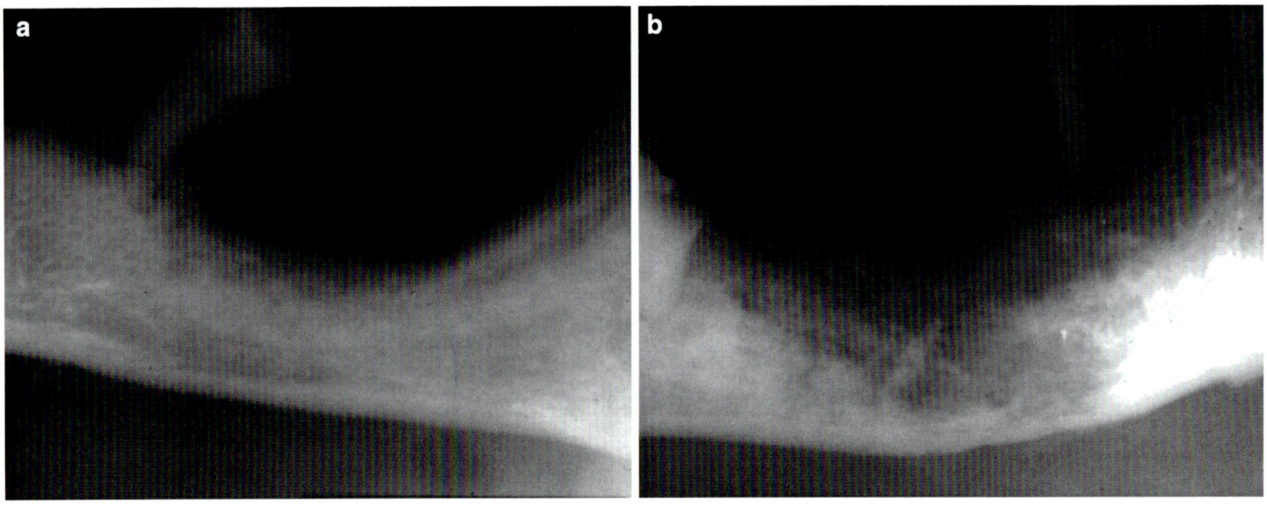

Fig. 7.40 Mandibular absorption type. (**a**) Expansive type and (**b**) invasive type

4. Vertical Height of the Mandible and Surgical Methods
   For a marginal mandibulectomy, the possibility of bone fracture has been noted when a minimum of 1 cm of bone is not left at the mandibular lower edge. Therefore, in edentulous case, segmental mandibulectomy is selected, because of not enough vertical height of mandible [56, 57] (Fig. 7.56).
5. Histopathological Malignancy and Surgical Methods
   Recurrence rates are high for histological high-grade malignancy cases, and poor prognoses are common. Additionally, there are reports showing a relationship between the histological mode of tumor invasion and the mode of mandibular invasion by X-ray imaging[25]. These issues must be considered when establishing treatment strategies (Fig. 7.57).

7.6 Upper Gingival Carcinomas and Hard Palate Carcinomas

Upper gingival carcinomas appear at a lower frequency compared with lower gingival carcinomas and hard palate carcinomas at a frequency that is lower still. Similar to lower

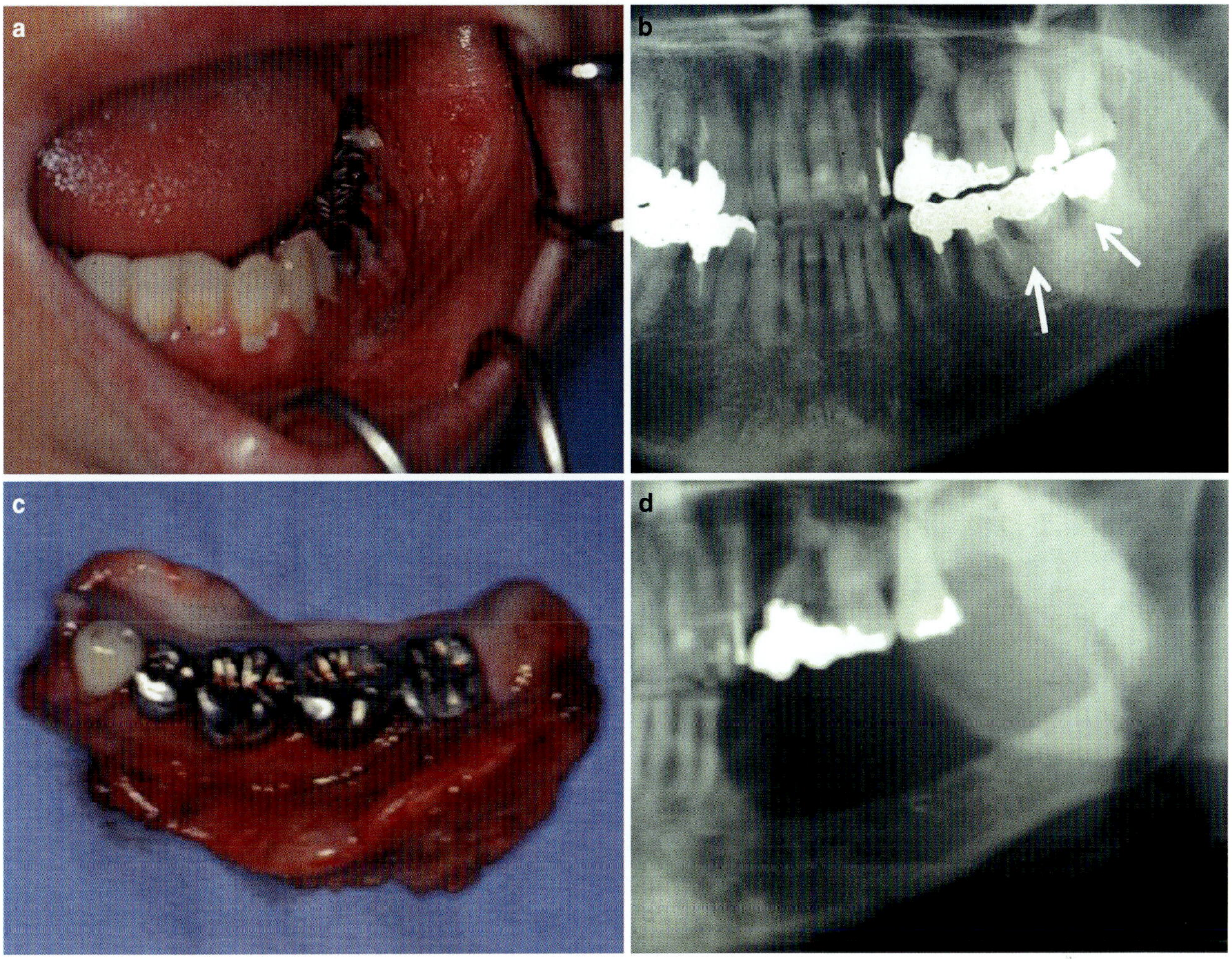

Fig. 7.41 Marginal mandibulectomy. (**a**) Clinical finding, gingival carcinoma (T2N0M0). (**b**) Tumor invades only the alveolar bone. (**c**) Surgical specimen. (**d**) X-ray finding

gingival carcinomas, upper gingival and hard palate carcinomas rapidly invade towards the bone from mucous membranes. As anatomical features for surgical therapies, there is superior progression to cavities such as the maxillary sinus and nasal cavity and inferior progression to the pterygopalatine fossa. Hard palate carcinomas progress to the soft palate and have a large effect on oral function. Moreover, unlike other types of oral cancer, they possess the anatomical feature of being unsuitable for an en bloc resection of the primary lesion and metastatic lymph nodes of the cervical region; however, their frequency of cervical lymph node metastasis is generally lower than for lower gingival carcinomas[1]. Since chemotherapy (e.g., selective intra-arterial chemotherapy from the superficial temporal artery) is easy to implement for upper gingival and hard palate carcinomas, and since radical resection of the maxillary bone causes aesthetic impairment, especially for advanced carcinomas, not just surgical therapy alone but multidisciplinary treatment

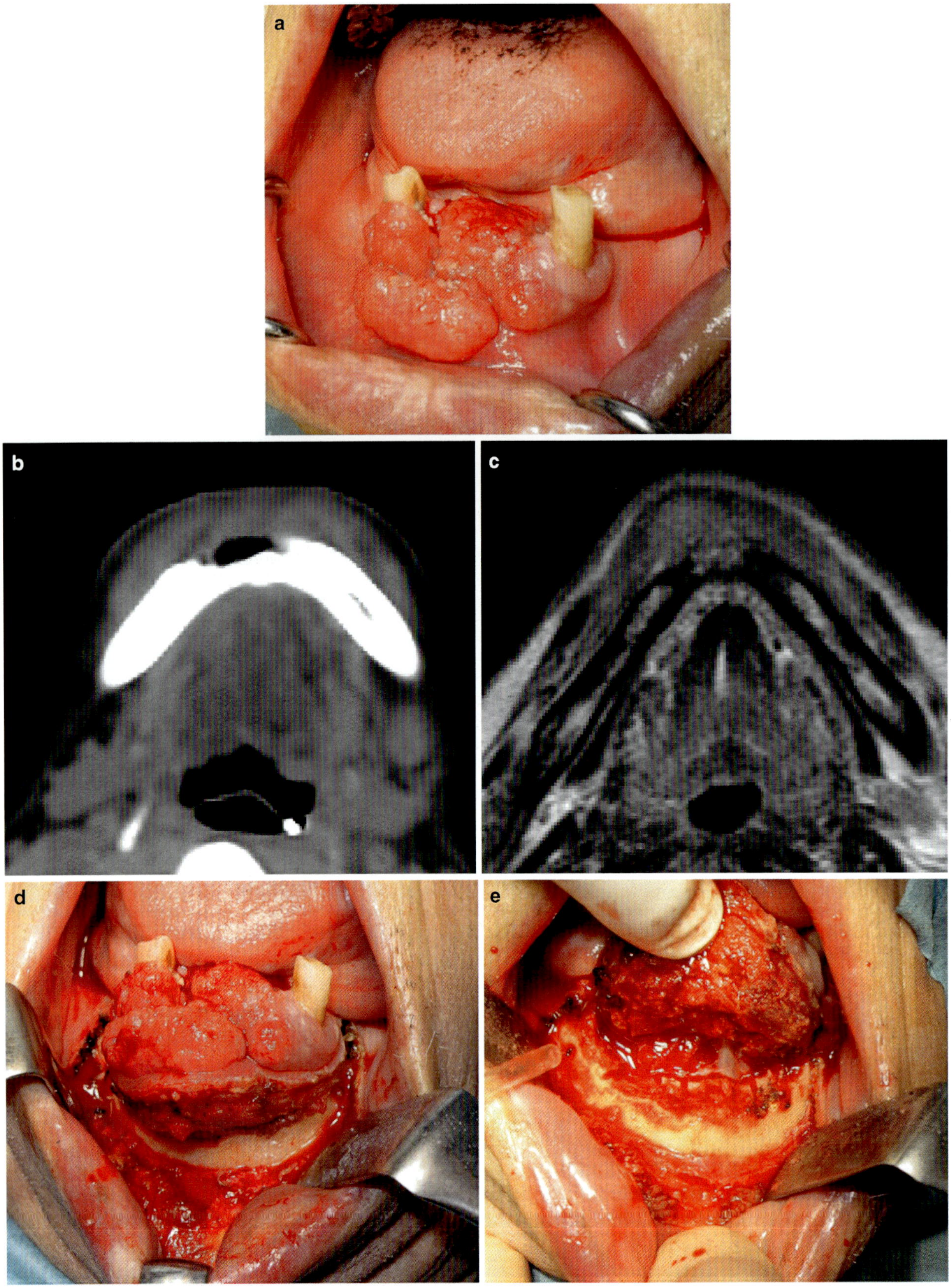

Fig. 7.42 Marginal mandibulectomy (intraoral approach). (**a**) Clinical finding; gingival carcinoma (T2N0M0). (**b**) CT finding; tumor invades just the alveolar bone. (**c**) MRI finding; tumor invasion remains in the alveolar bone. (**d**) Resection of soft tissue. (**e**) Removal of the tumor with alveolar bone

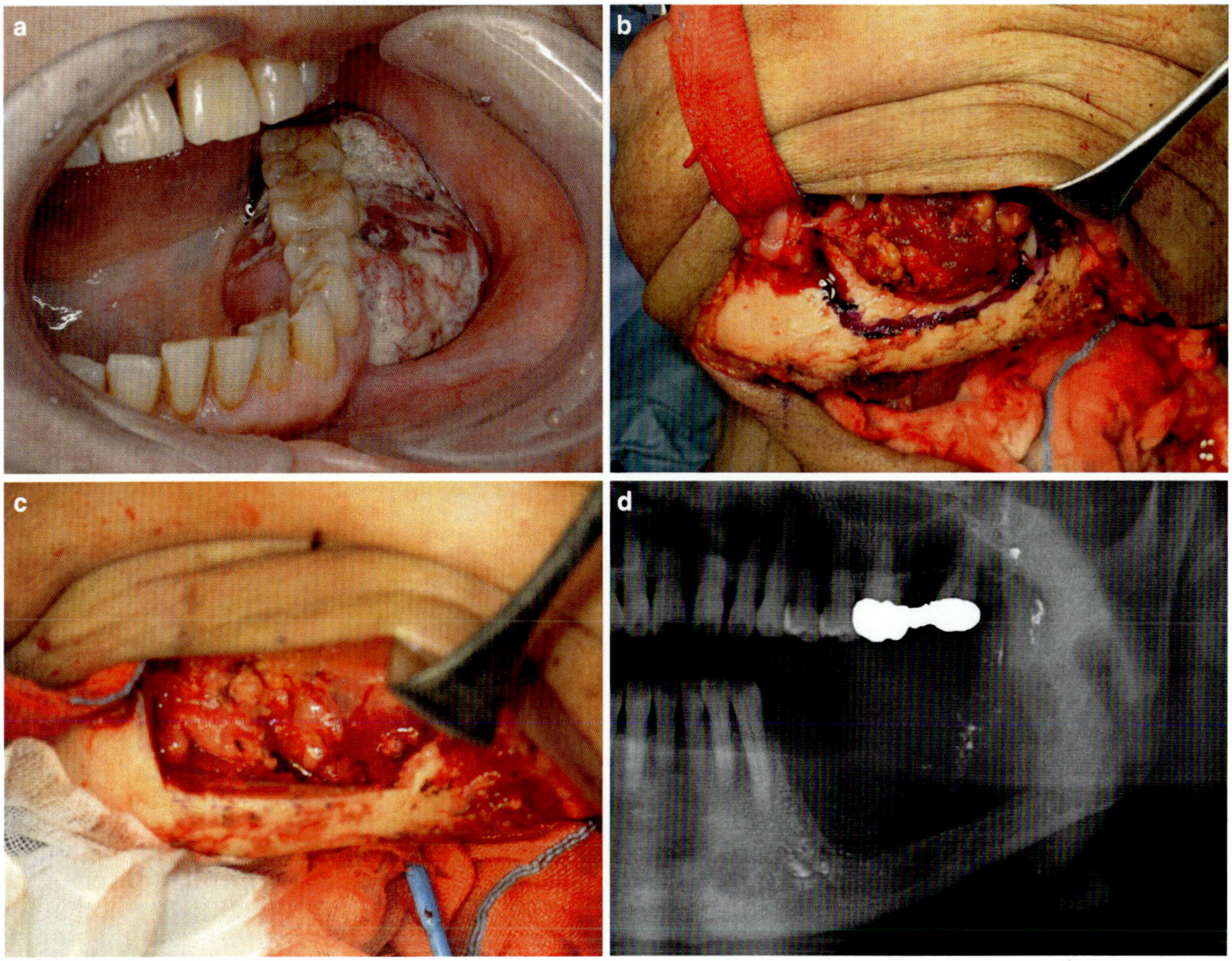

Fig. 7.43 Marginal mandibulectomy (extraoral approach). (**a**) Clinical finding; gingival carcinoma (T3N0M0). (**b**) Cut line for marginal mandibulectomy. (**c**) Removal of tumor (marginal mandibulectomy). (**d**) X-ray finding

that jointly uses irradiation therapy and chemotherapy is widely utilized. In surgical resection, because the anatomical structure of the region is complex, close examination of progression into the surrounding tissue of the mandible bone, nasal cavity, maxillary sinus, etc., by diagnostic imaging is important.

7.6.1 Surgical Resection of Upper Gingival Carcinomas and Hard Palate Carcinomas (Fig. 7.58)

1. Gingivectomy is indicated by precancerous lesions and carcinomas in situ.

   The bone is not resected; only the lesion and the surrounding gingiva and periosteum are resected.
2. Partial maxillectomy is indicated by early-stage exophytic-type carcinomas.

From inside the oral cavity, the procedure is intended to resect a part of the maxillary bone from the upper gingiva and alveolus, hard palate, or internal or external walls of the maxillary sinus (Figs. 7.59, 7.60, 7.61, 7.62, and 7.63).

Since the cavities of the nasal cavity as well as the maxillary sinus are superior to the carcinoma, functional impairments can be diminished if the nasal mucosa and sinus mucosa can be saved. However, cases of antrostomy of the maxillary sinus are typical. At these times, beyond the resection of the bone, it is essential to ensure a sufficient safety margin and to have a complete picture of the invasion state towards the buccal soft tissue.

Footnote: Basic Operative Procedure for Partial Maxillectomy (1) Skin incision: Ensure a wide surgical field (Fig. 7.64). (2) While being mindful of the safety margin, make an incision in the buccal mucosa above the gingiva, and cut away the soft tissue of the buccal site away from the maxillary bone. (3) Dissect the mucous

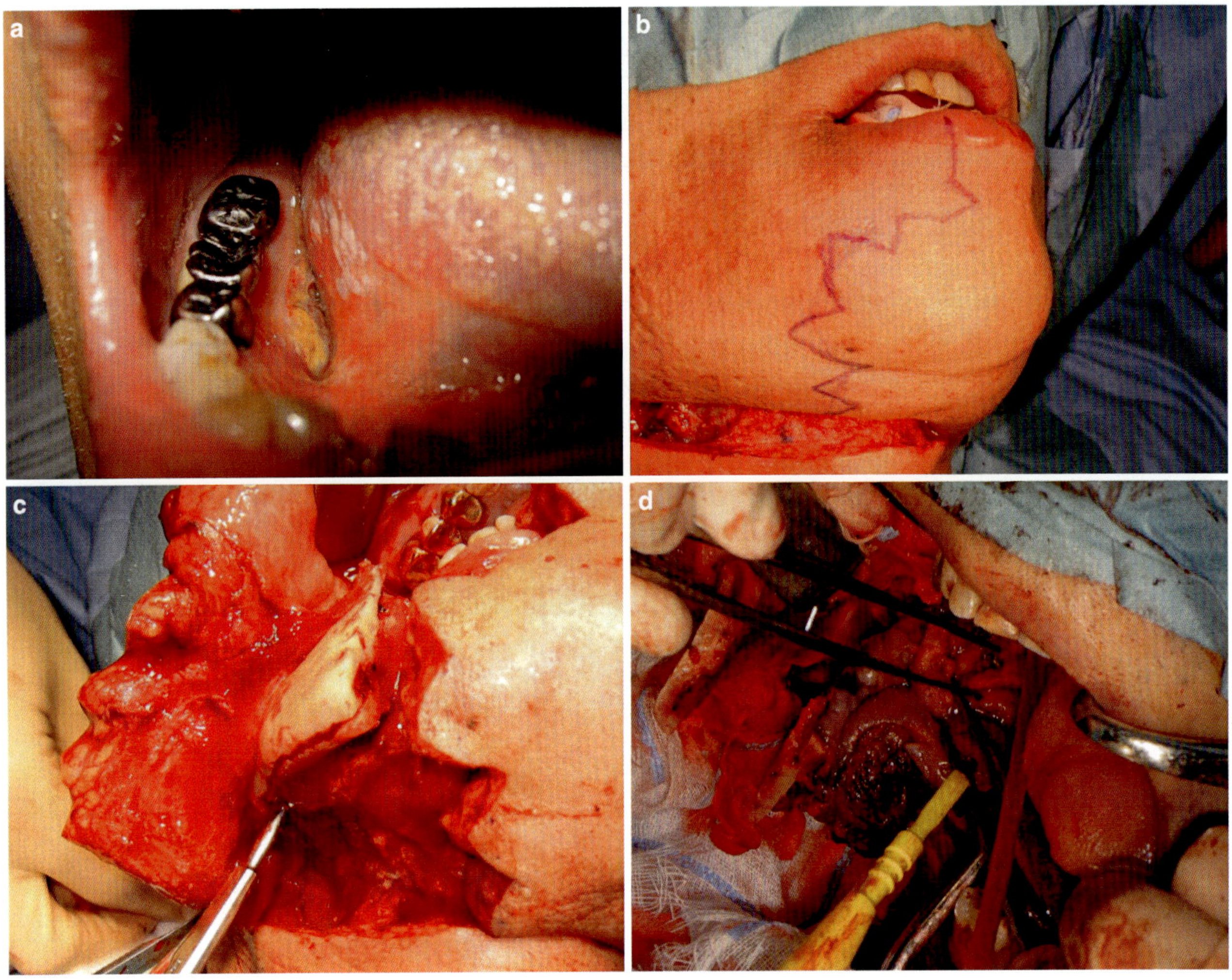

Fig. 7.44 Marginal mandibulectomy (sagittal splitting). (**a**) Clinical finding; lower gingival carcinoma. (**b**) Excision line on the lower lips. (**c**) Sagittal splitting of mandible. (**d**) Removal of tumor that invades into the tongue. (**e**) Tumor is removed. (**f**) Removal of tissue. (**g**) Bone fixation by miniplate. (**h**) Postoperative condition

membrane of the hard palate with an electric scalpel, exposing the palatine process. Cut with a saw. (4) In the event the carcinoma has advanced, resect to the palatal bone. It is necessary to deal with the great palatal artery and vein. (5) Cut off the anterior and posterior walls of the maxillary sinus. Cut off the lateral walls of the nasal cavity. At this time, check for progression in the superior direction from the buccal gingiva parallel with the periosteum or towards the buccal area or in the case of an anterior primary lesion, for progression towards the anterior wall of the maxillary sinus, the pterygopalatine fossa, as well as the medial pterygoid muscle.

3. Subtotal and total maxillectomies are indicated in cases of maxillary sinus carcinomas that have advanced greatly within the maxillary sinus [60].

A subtotal maxillectomy is intended to resect the maxillary bone while preserving only the orbital bone (Figs. 7.65, 7.66, and 7.67). A total maxillectomy is intended to remove the zygoma, frontal bone, palatal bone, and pterygoid process from the maxillary bone and constitutes a complete removal of the maxillary bone.

In these cases, it is necessary to expand the buccal area to ensure the operative field. Additionally, directions of tumor progression that should be noted as requiring caution regarding the surgical margin are (1) progressions in the superior direction or the buccal area from the buccal gingiva along the periosteum and (2) progressions towards the anterior wall of the maxillary sinus and the pterygopalatine fossa, as well as the medial pterygoid muscle.

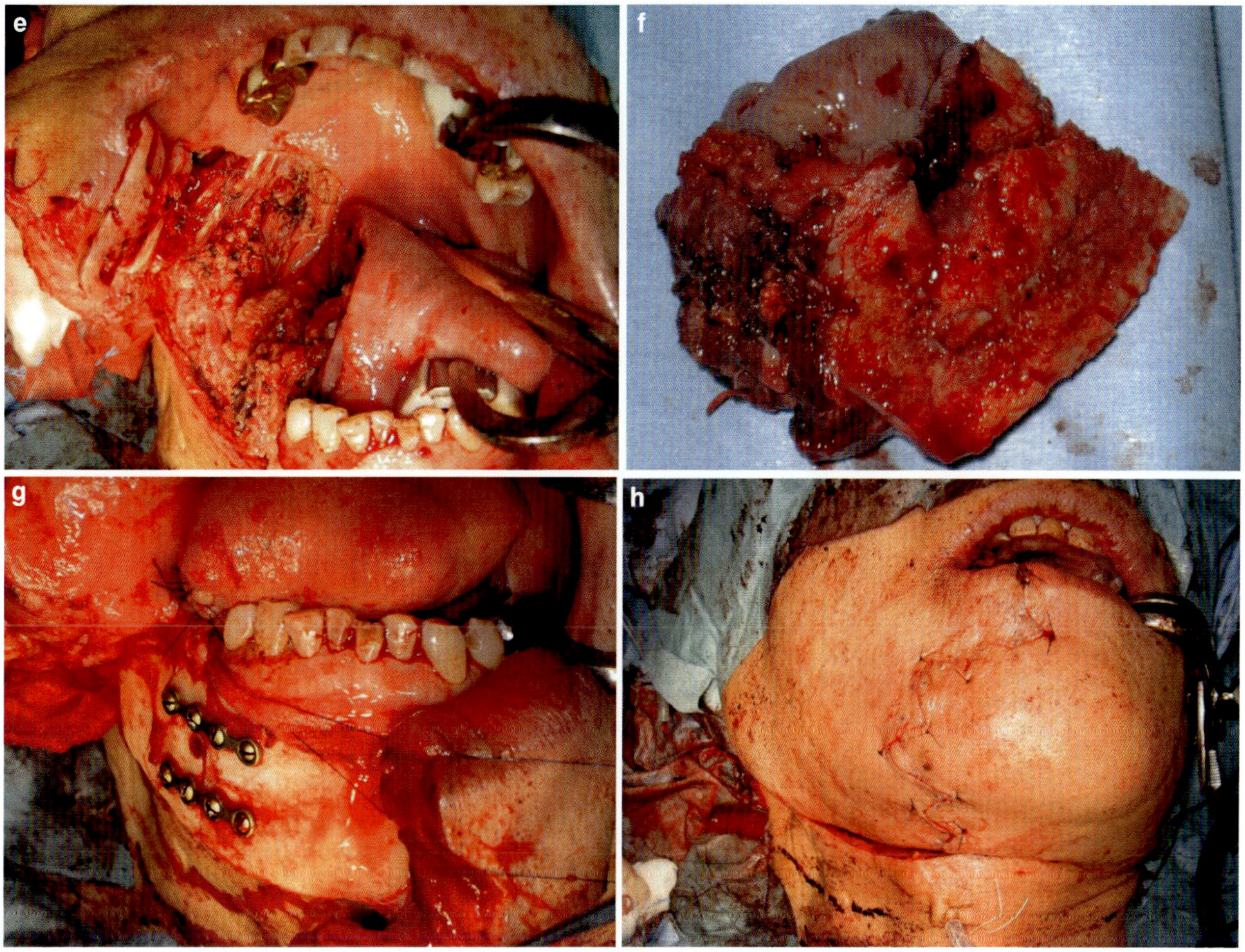

Fig. 7.44 (continued)

4. Extended maxillectomies are indicated for cases where the carcinoma has extensively destroyed the maxillary bone and invaded the surrounding tissue.
   In addition to all of the maxillary bone, the surgical margin is intended to remove the zygoma, the mastication muscle groups attached to the bone periphery, the nasal bone, characteristic nasal cavity contents, ethmoid cells, orbital contents, the skull base, etc. (Fig. 7.68).

7.7 Carcinoma of the Floor of the Mouth

Carcinomas of the floor of the mouth are characterized by horizontal progression of the carcinoma and its ease of invasion into the surrounding tissue and by its ease of invasion into the deep parts of loose connective tissue under the mucous membrane of the mouth floor. Many carcinomas appear 2 cm anterior to the center of the floor of the mouth. Primary lesion subsites are divided into the median type (corresponding to the anterior teeth) and lateral type (corresponding to the molar region) (Fig. 7.69). The median type is located in the anterior floor of the mouth, mesial to the corresponding area between the canine teeth and the mandibular first premolars. Tumors in this area often have spread to the contralateral mucous membrane of the mouth floor. The lateral type is located in the posterior floor of the mouth, distal to the corresponding area between the canine teeth and the mandibular first premolars. Tumors in this area often include the lingual margin and the base of the tongue. However, identification of the primary site is sometimes difficult in advanced cases.

When carcinomas of the floor of the mouth progress in the superior direction, they invade the inferior aspect of the tongue; when they do in the anterior or lateral direction, they invade the mandible. In the inferior direction, it causes invasion into the genioglossus muscle, the hyoglossus muscle, and the mylohyoid muscle. In the posterior direction, it

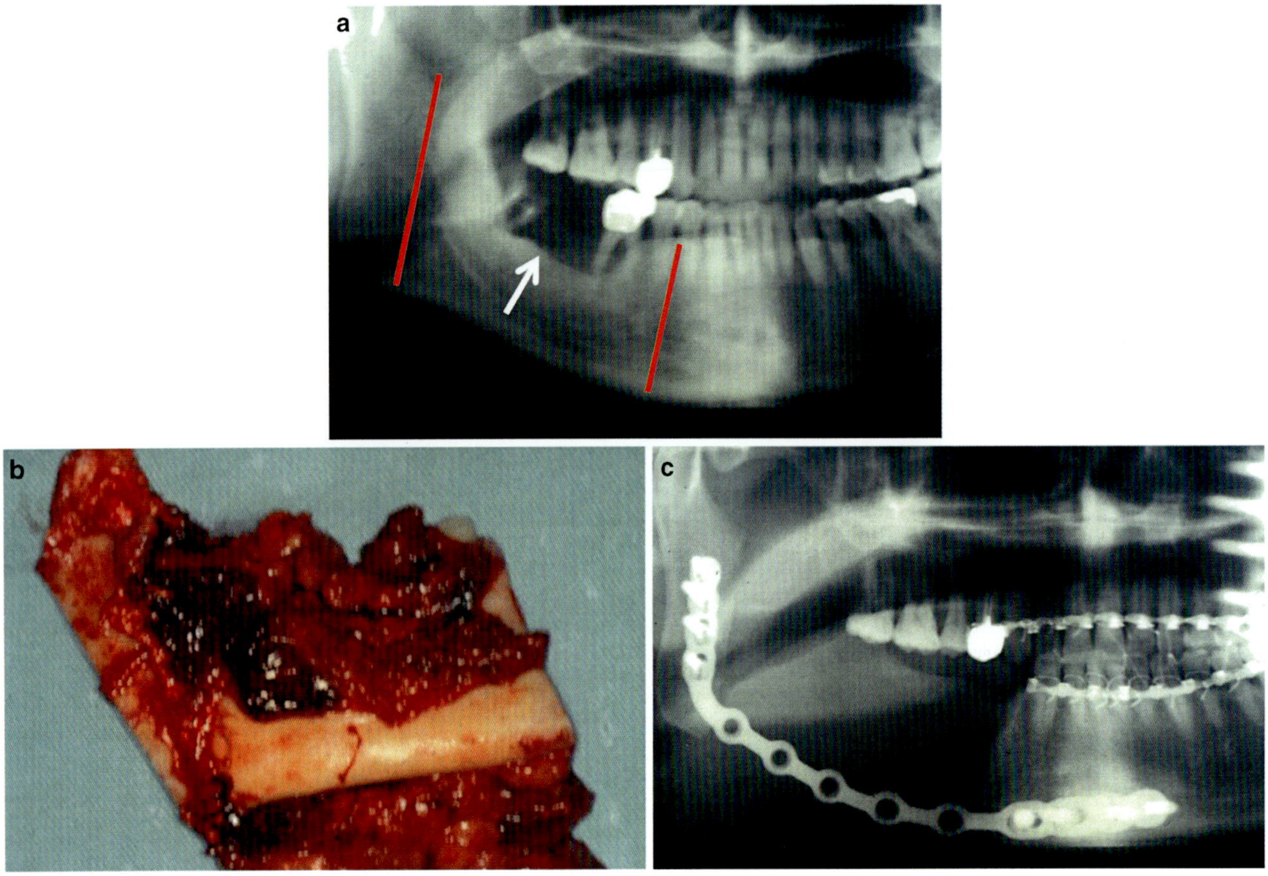

Fig. 7.45 Segmental mandibulectomy. (**a**) X-ray finding; tumor invades into the mandible (*up arrow*). (**b**) Removal of tissue. (**c**) Reconstruction by titanium plate

causes invasion into the intrinsic muscles of the tongue (i.e., the inferior longitudinal muscle, the transverse muscle, and the vertical muscle) and simultaneous invasion towards the base of the tongue (oropharynx). Infiltration to the deep lingual artery, sublingual artery, lingual nerve, and hypoglossal nerve and their periphery can occur. There is a possibility of gland carcinomas invading along the nerves, and further, bilateral cervical lymph node metastasis easily arises.

7.7.1 Surgical Resection of Carcinoma of the Floor of the Mouth [47, 48, 61–63]

1. In cases of T1/early T2 N0 carcinomas of the floor of the mouth, a partial resection of the floor of the mouth is performed (Fig. 7.70).
2. In cases of late T2/T2/T4 N0, a total resection of the floor of the mouth is performed concurrently with preventative neck dissection (via the pull-through method) (Fig. 7.71). For cases where the tumor is in contact with the lingual gingiva or the alveolar mucosa, but has not invaded into the mandible, resection of the tumor and alveolar part (marginal mandibulectomy) is performed (Fig. 7.72).
3. In cases of T4, combined resection is performed to resect the tumor. Here, tumor resection and segmental mandibulectomy are performed for cases where the tumor has advanced to the gingiva or buccal mucosa and invaded the mandible. For cases where the tongue has been invaded, partial glossectomy is performed on the invaded part (Fig. 7.73).
4. In cases of early T2 N1–N3, floor of the mouth resection and neck dissection are performed concurrently (via the pull-through method).
5. For late T2–T3/T4N1–3, resection of the primary lesion (a compound operation of the tissue surrounding the tongue and mandible as well as the total resection of the floor of the mouth) and neck dissection (via the pull-through method) are performed concurrently. Also, for function-sparing surgery, preoperative chemoradiotherapy is usually performed.

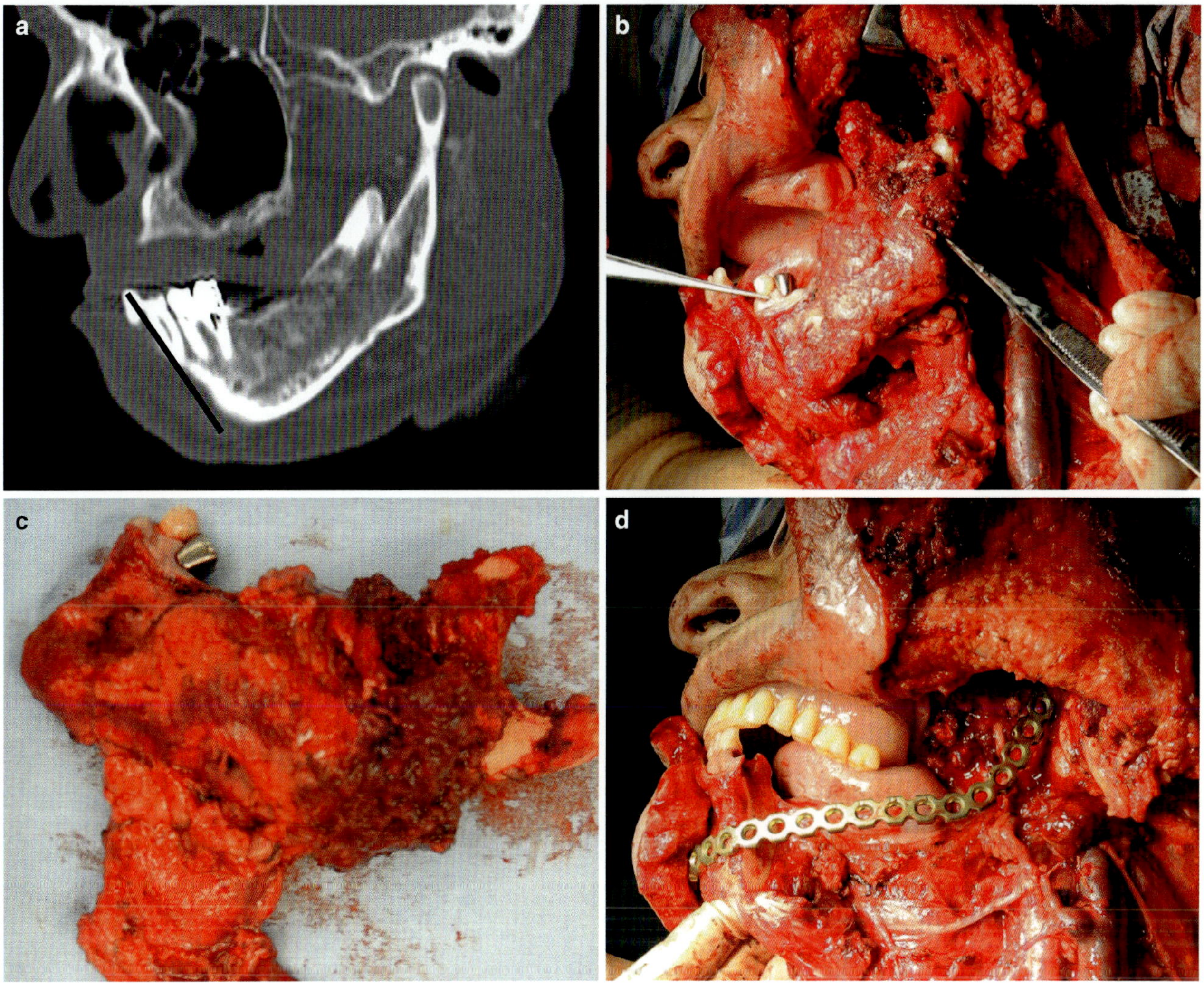

Fig. 7.46 Hemi-mandibulectomy. (**a**) CT finding; tumor invades into the mandible. Bone absorption is invasive type. (**b**) Hemi-mandibulectomy. (**c**) Hemi-mandibulectomy with neck dissection. (**d**) Reconstruction by titanium plate

7.7.2 Selection Criteria for Combined Mandibular Resection for Carcinomas of the Floor of the Mouth [64, 65]

1. Cases with a layer of normal tissue interposed between the tumor and the mandible: mandible resection can be avoided by attaching the lingual periosteum to the resection side [66] (Fig. 7.71).
2. Cases with tumor invasion limited to the periosteum or cortical bone: the continuity of the mandible is preserved by means of marginal mandibulectomy [45, 55, 67, 68]. For marginal resection, there are the methods of partial resection at the center of the so-called alveolar crest and sagittal splitting of the lingual cortex [68, 69] (Figs. 7.72, 7.73, and 7.74). If 1 cm or more remains at the lingual margin, resection of the alveolar crest part is strongly preferable to sagittal splitting [70].
3. Cases with observed bone invasion or destruction of the mandible: compound operation of the mandible is indicated, by the marginal resection or segmental resection methods [44, 66] (Fig. 7.73).
4. Cases with progression to the mandibular canal or invasion of the carcinoma into the bone marrow, cases with tumor invasion into the deep parts of the perimandibular space, and cases with marked alveolar ridge resorption in edentulous jaw even to the degree that bone invasion is suspected: segmental mandibulectomy is performed [56].

7.8 Buccal Mucosa Carcinomas [61–63]

The cheek is the outer wall of the oral cavity and is composed of the buccal muscles, subcutaneous adipose tissue, and skin. The buccal mucosa extends from the upper and

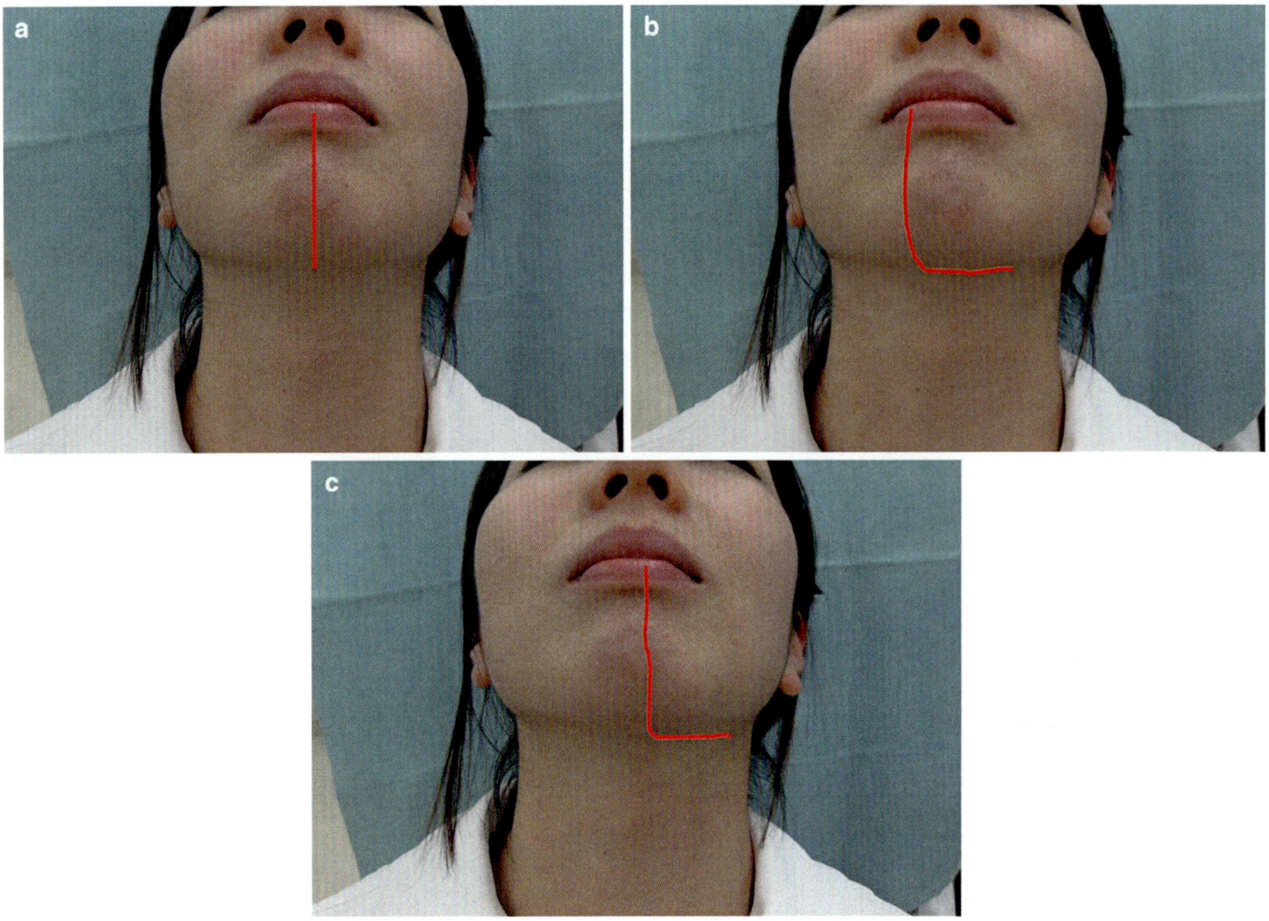

Fig. 7.47 (a) Sedillot-Kocher incision. (b) v. Langenbeck incision. (c) Fritz-König incision

lower gingiva to the commissure of the mouth and leads to the surface of the mandibular ramus.

Subsites of buccal mucosa carcinoma onset can be classified into (1) the upper and lower lip mucosa, (2) the buccal mucosa, (3) the posterior acetabulum, and (4) the upper and lower alveolar ridges. Lateral progression of buccal mucosa carcinomas involves invasion of the buccinator muscle, the subcutaneous area, and the skin. Medial progression involves invasion of the upper and lower gingiva and alveola, the maxillary bone, and the mandible. Anterior progression involves invasion of the commissure of the mouth, whereas posterior progression from the rear acetabulum causes invasion of the mandible and pterygomandibular space along the lower mucosa. Similarly, superior progression causes infiltration to the tuber maxillae and pterygopalatine fossa, whereas inferior progression causes infiltration of the soft palate and the base of the tongue.

1. Partial resection: Applies to cases with a light degree of invasion into the muscle layer for T1–T3 superficial tumors. Resection of the tumor including the surrounding healthy tissue is performed (Fig. 7.75).
2. Full-thickness buccal resection (through-and-through operation): Indicated for cases where T1–T4 tumor invasion is deep and has reached the subcutaneous tissue or the skin. Resection is performed to hollow out the area including the buccal mucosa and skin (Fig. 7.76).
3. Combined resection applies to cases where a T4 tumor has widely invaded the surrounding tissue. The buccal tumor is resected en bloc with the surrounding tissue (maxillary bone, mandible, tongue, floor of the mouth, etc.). For the surgical margin, resection of the buccal mucosa, mandible, maxillary bone, skin, or a resection enlarged in the superior or anterior directions from the retromolar triangle is performed (Fig. 7.77).

7.9 Points to Note When Performing Surgical Resection of Tumors

When surgery is indicated, practitioners should be able to completely image the intracranial resection area preoperatively. Further, they should prepare by intracranial simulations

Fig. 7.48 Selection criteria of marginal mandibulectomy and segmental mandibulectomy

Marginal mandibulectomy

Invasion to Adjacent Soft Tissue :
Tumor is limited to the alveolar tissue and not invaded the mylohyoid muscle

Bone Resorption Depth :
Tumor is limited to the alveolus and not reached the mandibular canal,

Bone Absorption Type : X-ray images of bone is expansive type,

Histopathological Malignancy : low-grade malignancy cases

Segmental mandibulectomy

Invasion to Adjacent Soft Tissue :
Tumor is invaed into the buccal space or subcutaneous fat, into the submandibular space, and into the extrinsic muscles of the tongue.

Bone Resorption Depth : Tumor invade into the mandibular canal

Bone Absorption Type : X-ray images of bone is the invasive type

Histopathological Malignancy : high-grade malignancy cases

Vertical Height of the Mandible : edentulous case,
not enough vertical height of mandible

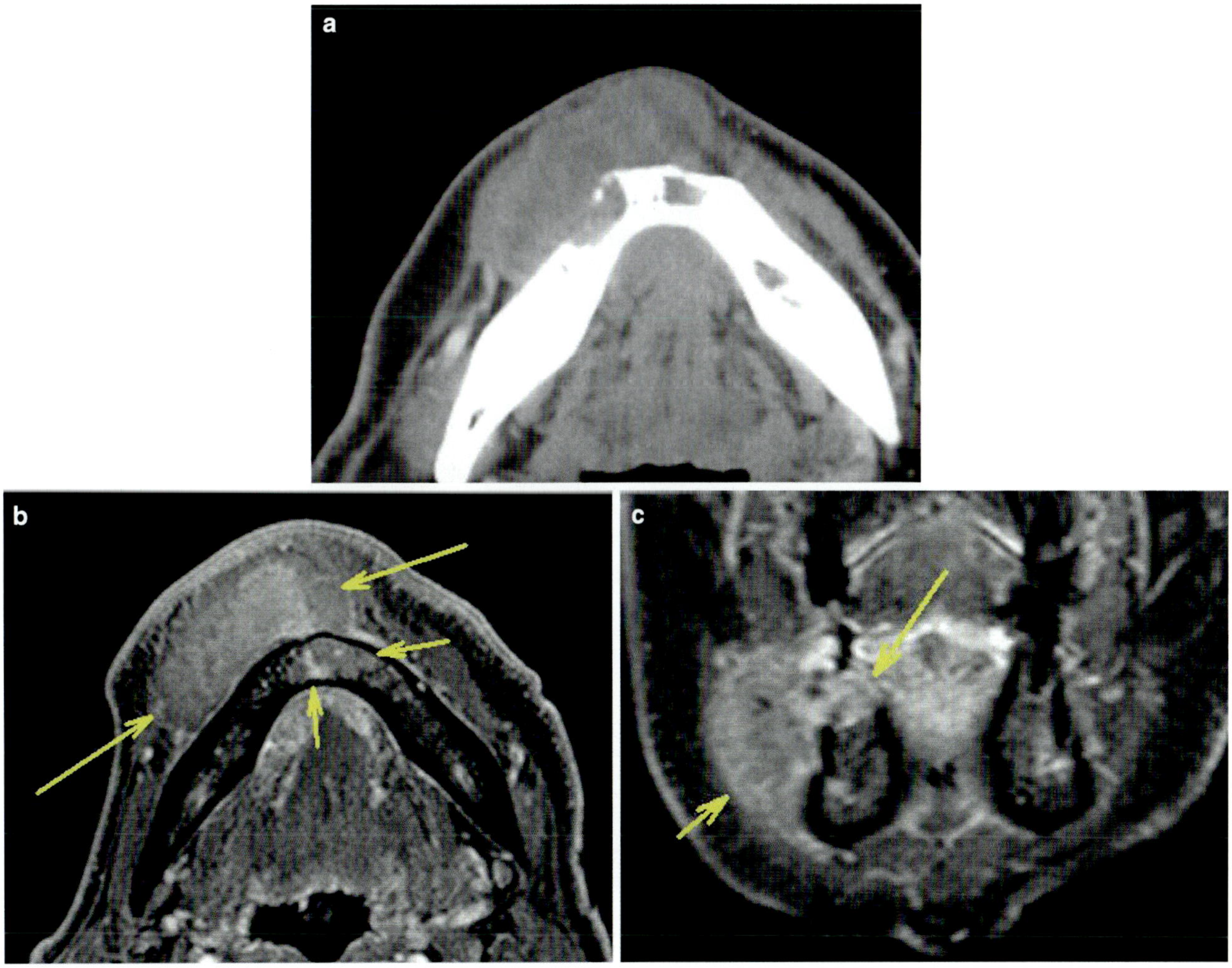

Fig. 7.49 Lower gingival carcinoma(T4N2M0). (**a**) CT imaging, tumor destructs the mandible and invades surrounding tissue until the skin. (**b, c**) MR imaging, tumor invades into the mandible and expounds surrounding tissue until the skin (*up arrow*). (**d**) Incision line of the skin (command operation). (**e**) Segmental mandibulectomy (*up arrow*). (**f**) Tumor with mandible (*up arrow*) and skin tissue is removed. (**g**) Removal of tissue (*up arrow*); skin

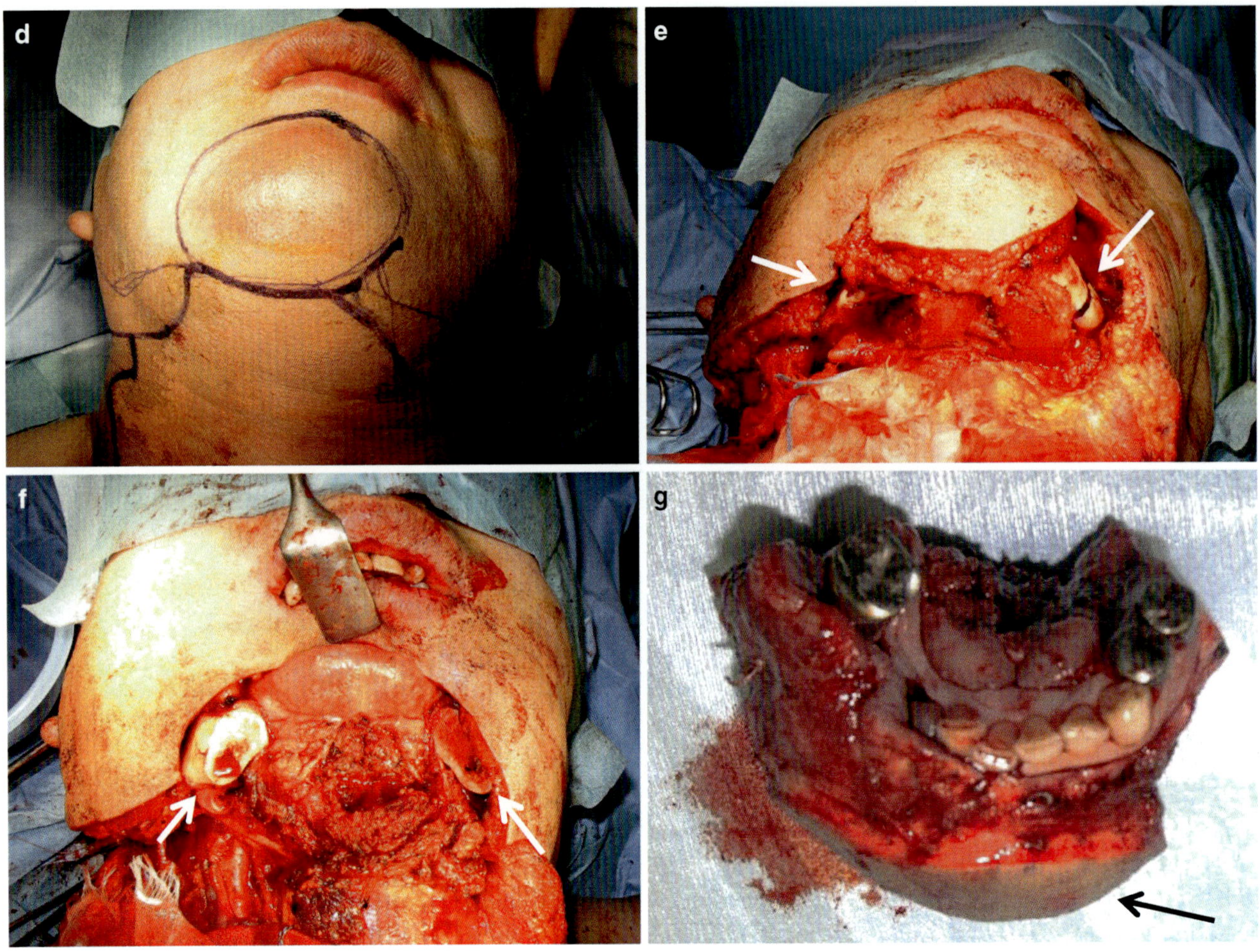

Fig. 7.49 (continued)

including any potential accidents that may happen during the length of the surgical procedure. Since pathology differs for each patient, the optimum treatment must be considered individually for all patients. For this reason, it is necessary to be thoroughly familiar with the anatomy of the head and neck, to comprehend the extent of tumor progression accurately by means of preoperative imaging diagnosis, and further to understand tumor characteristics through histopathological evidence.

Practitioners must make use of various operative procedures to perform the optimal treatment. Surgical principles are a combination of basic techniques. For this reason, it is essential to master these basic techniques precisely, to deepen one's knowledge to make flexible and practical use of them on a case-by-case basis, and to prepare by training in these surgical procedures.

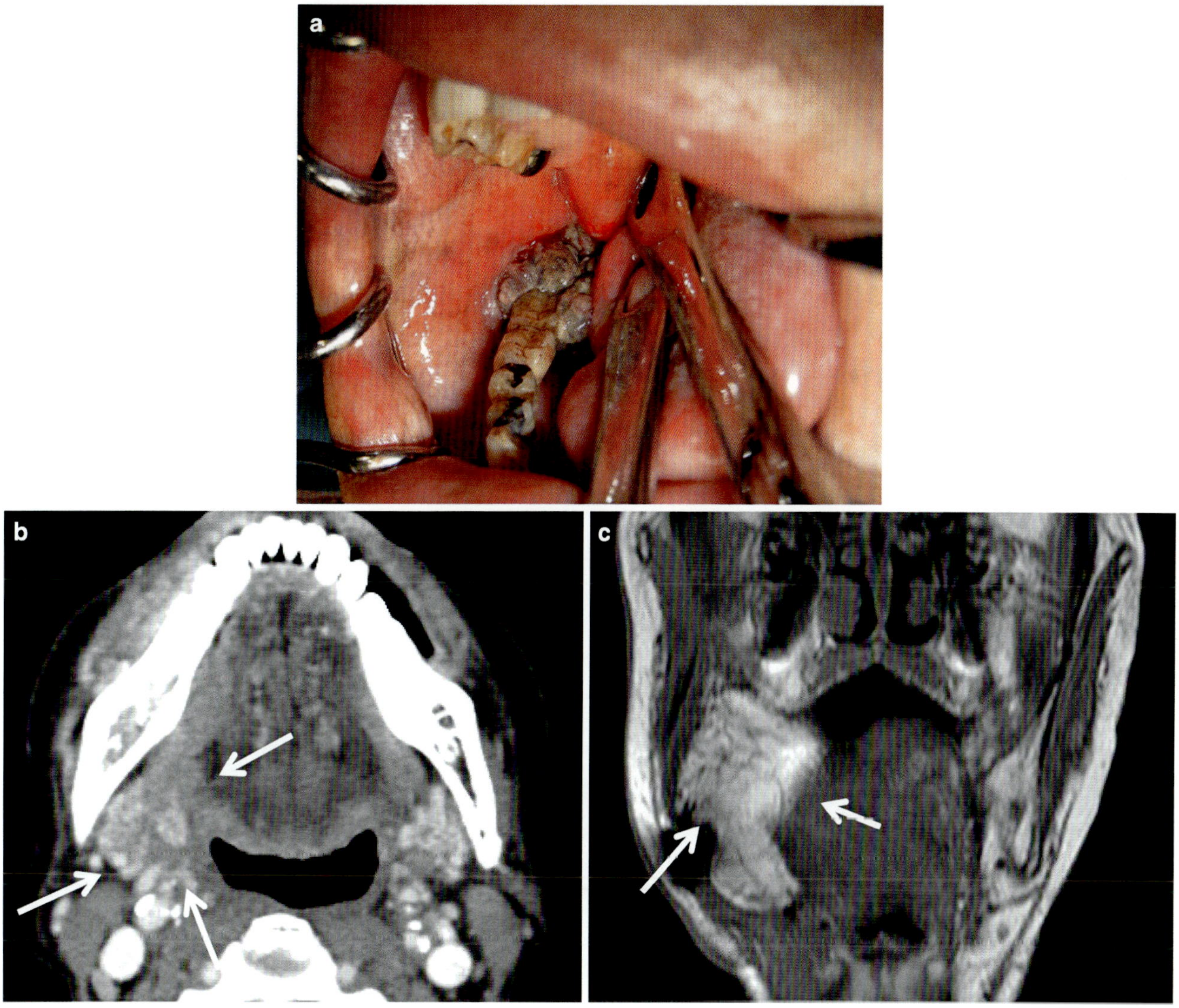

Fig. 7.50 Lower gingival carcinoma (T4N2bM0). (**a**) Clinical finding and (**b**) CT imaging; tumor invades into the pharyngeal space (*up arrow*). (**c**) MR imaging; tumor invades into the pharyngeal space (*up arrow*). (**d**) Incision line of skin (Fritz König Incision). (**e**) Segmental mandibulectomy (*up arrow*). (**f**) Tumor with mandible (*up arrow*), pharyngeal tissue and a part of tongue is removed. (**g**) Removal of tissue

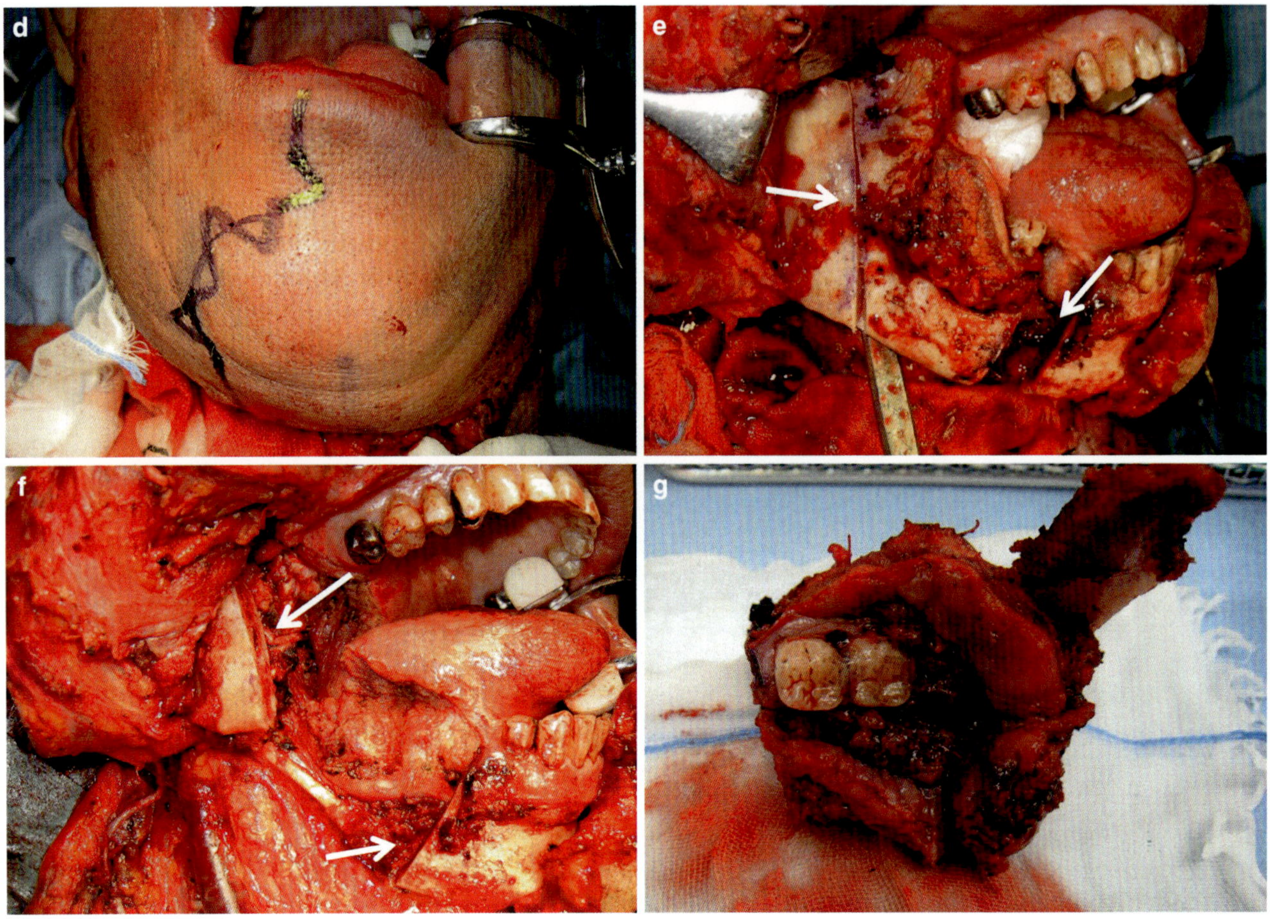

Fig. 7.50 (continued)

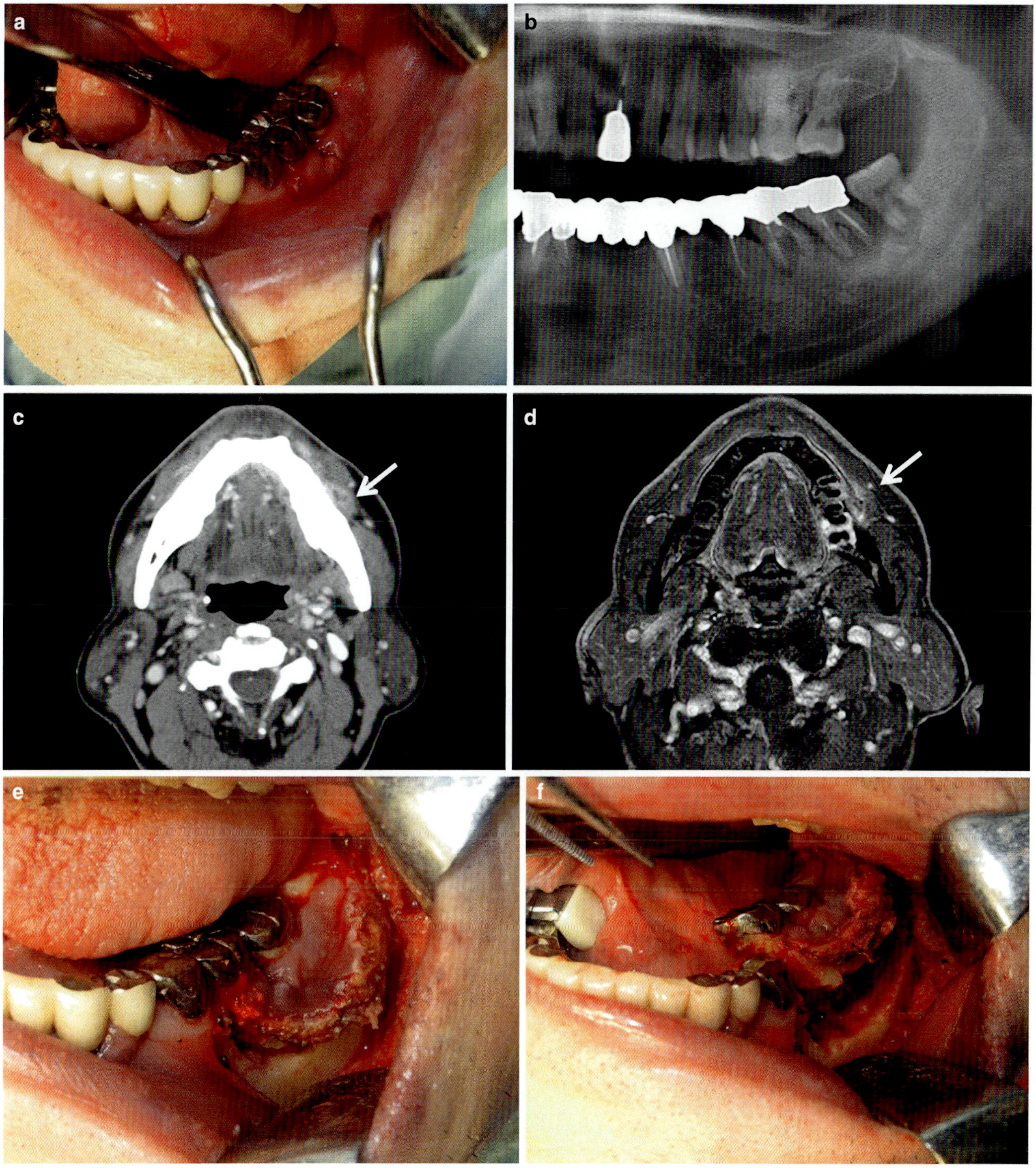

Fig. 7.51 Marginal mandibulectomy. (**a**) Lower gingival carcinoma (T2N0M0). (**b**) X-ray finding; tumor invasion is limited to the alveolar bone and does not invade until the mandibular canal (——). (**c**) CT imaging, tumor invades around the mandible (*up arrow*). (**d**) MR imaging, tumor invades around the mandible (*up arrow*). (**e**) Incision of oral mucosa. (**f**) Marginal mandibulectomy

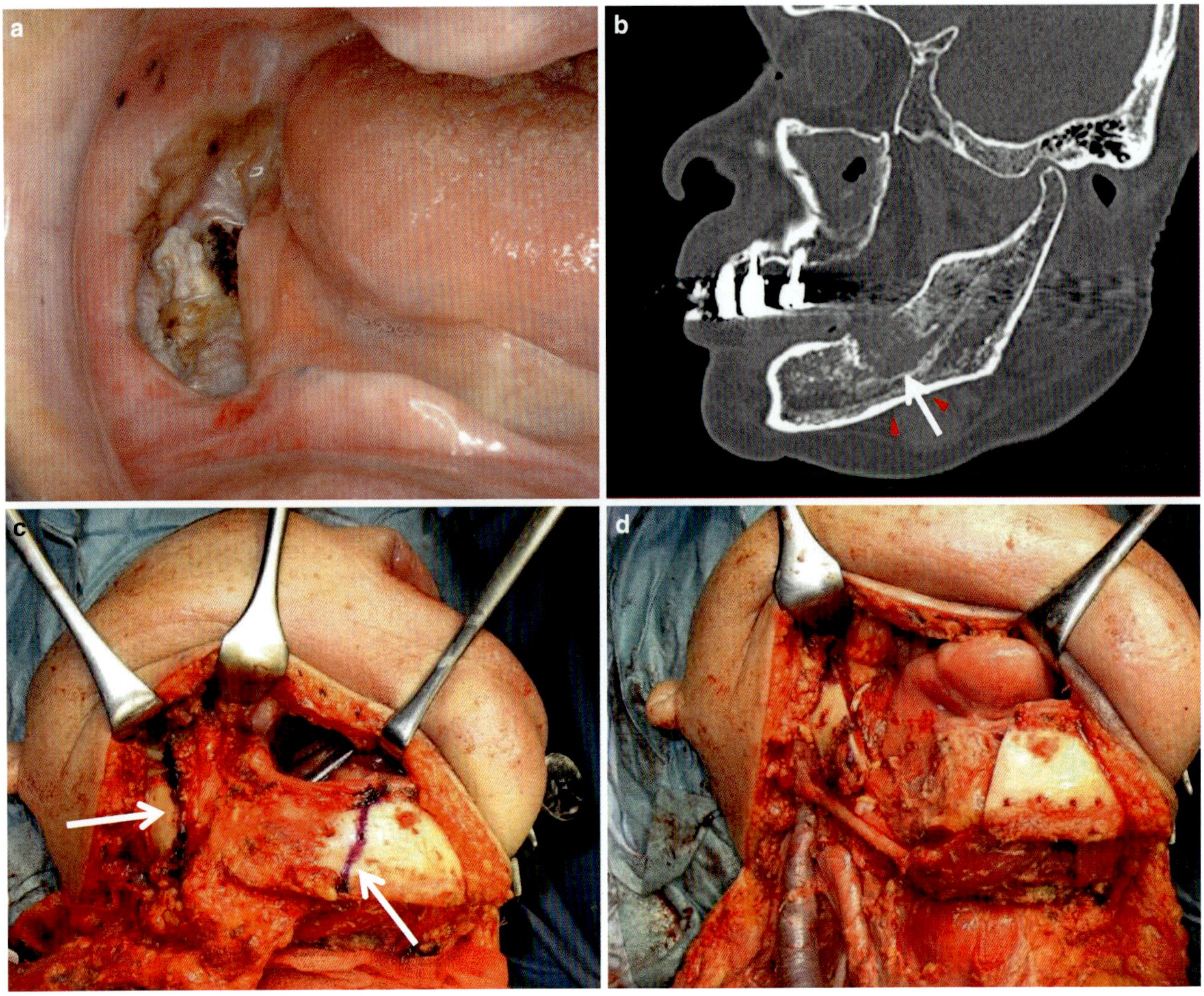

Fig. 7.52 Segmental mandibulectomy. (**a**) Lower gingival carcinoma (T4N1M0). (**b**) CT imaging, tumor invades into the mandibular canal (*up arrow*). (**c**) Segmental mandibulectomy (*up arrow*) with neck dissection. (**d**) Tumor is removed with the mandible

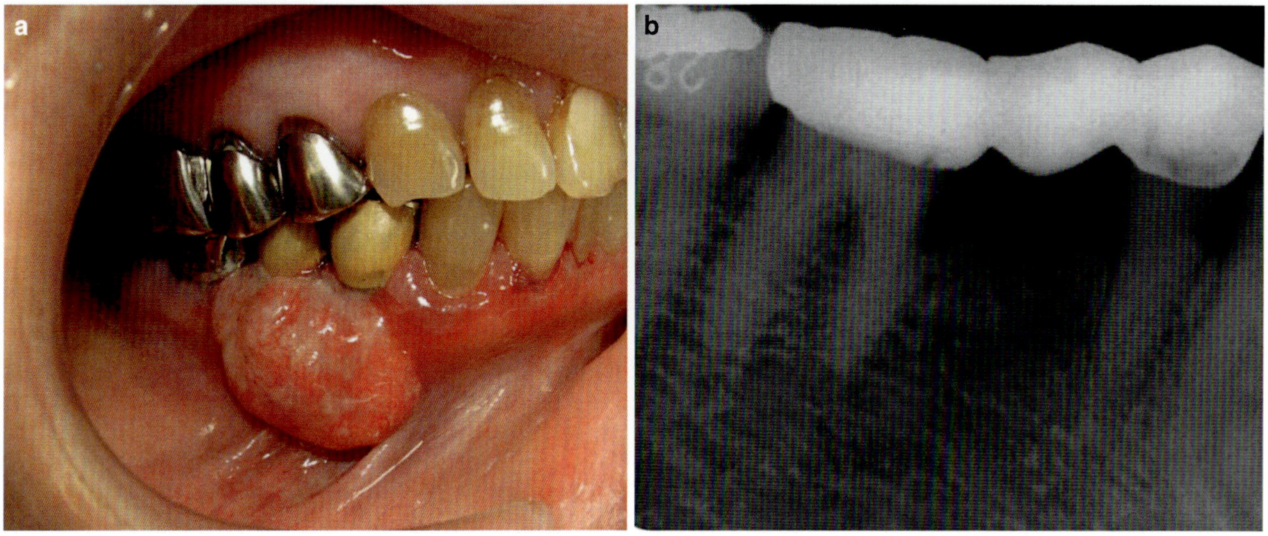

Fig. 7.53 (**a**) Tumors show exophytic growth. (**b**) X-ray imaging, no finding of bone destruction

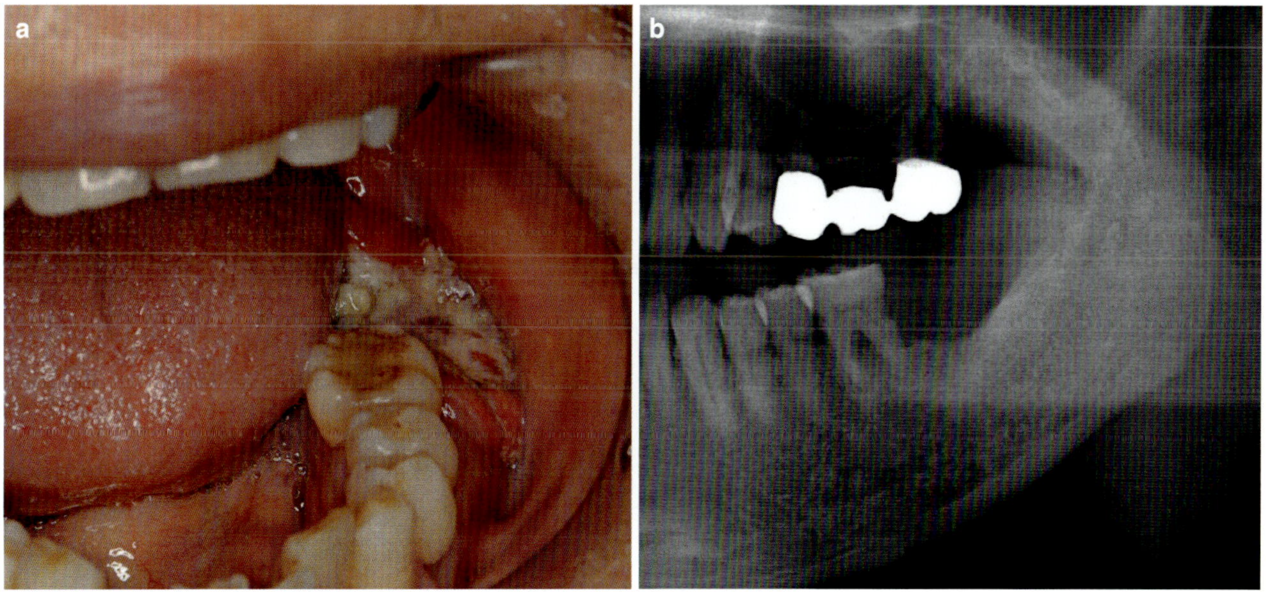

Fig. 7.54 Mandibular absorption type. (**a**) Lower gingival carcinoma (T2N0M0). (**b**) X-ray finding, expansive type

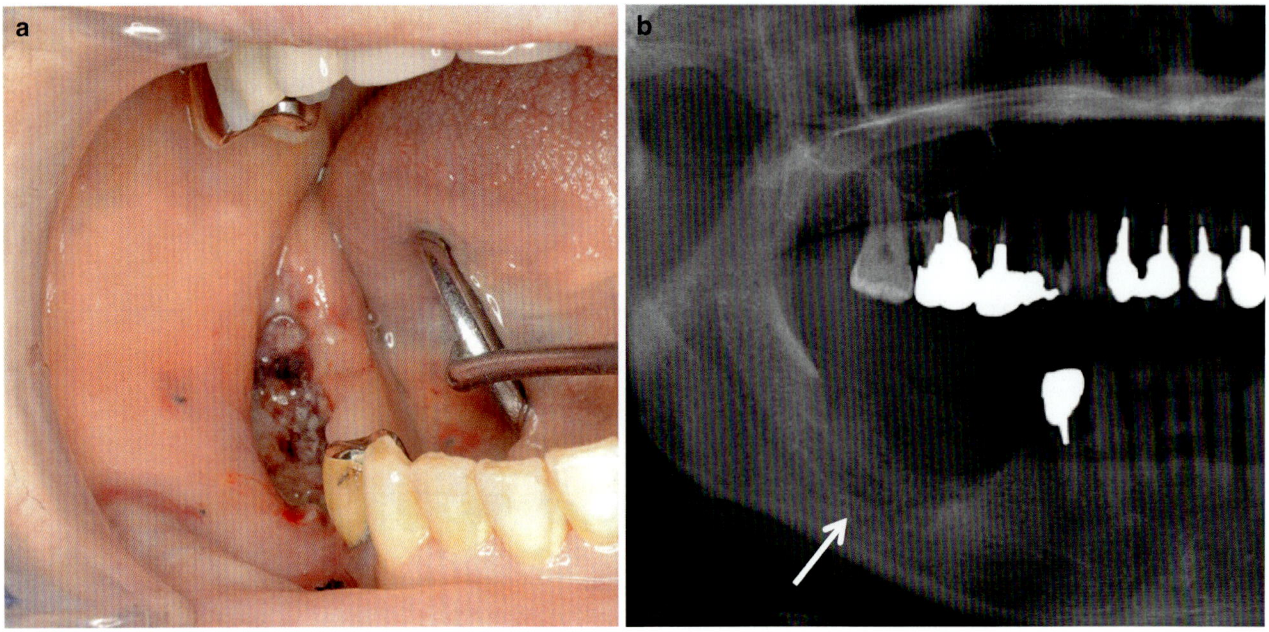

Fig. 7.55 Mandibular absorption type. (**a**) Lower gingival carcinoma (T4N1M0). (**b**) X-ray finding, invasive type (*up arrow*)

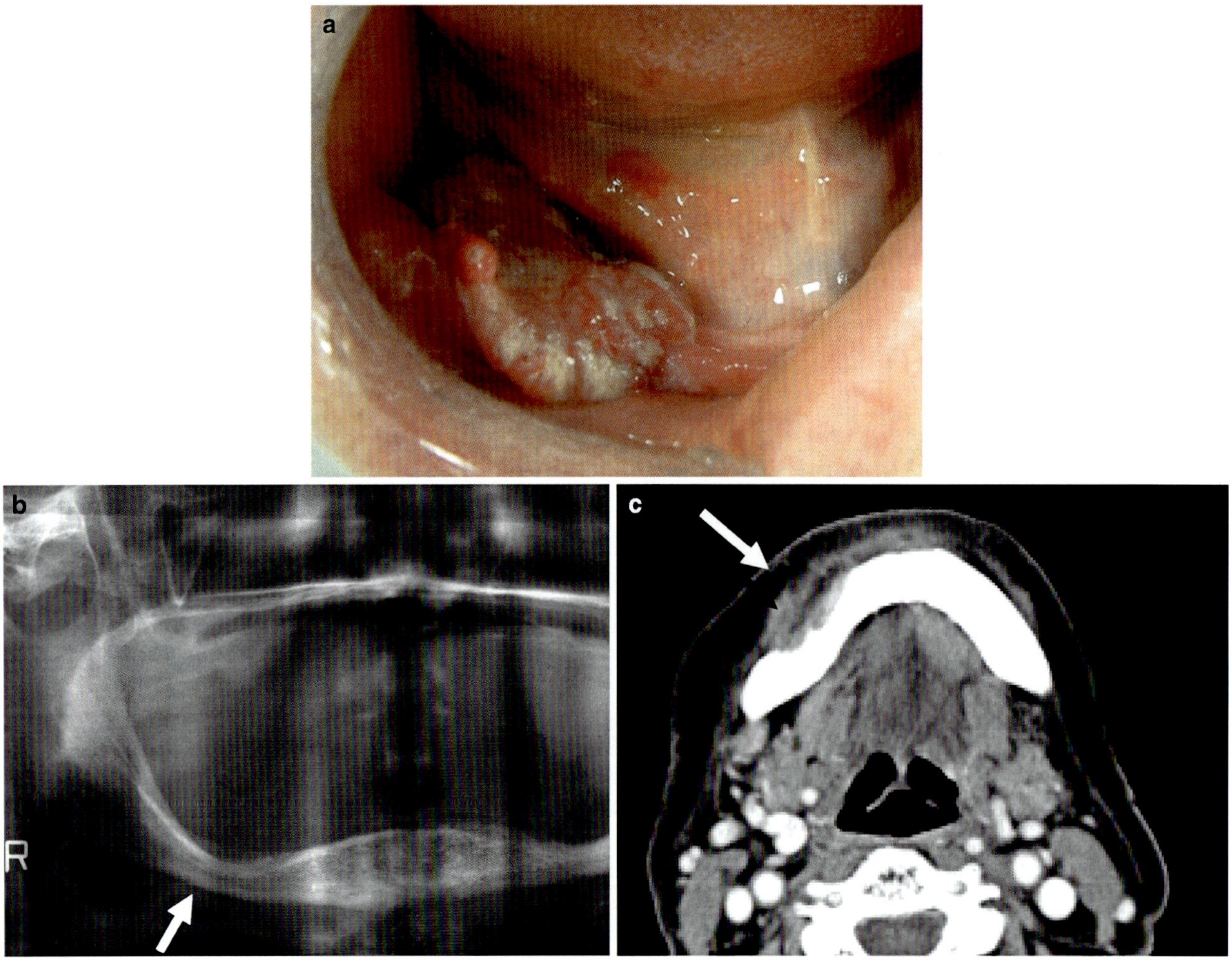

Fig. 7.56 Lower gingival carcinoma of the edentulous jaw. (**a**) Tumors show exophytic growth. (**b**) There are no enough vertical height of the mandible. (**c**) CT imaging, bone destruction is limited to the bone surface (*up arrow*)

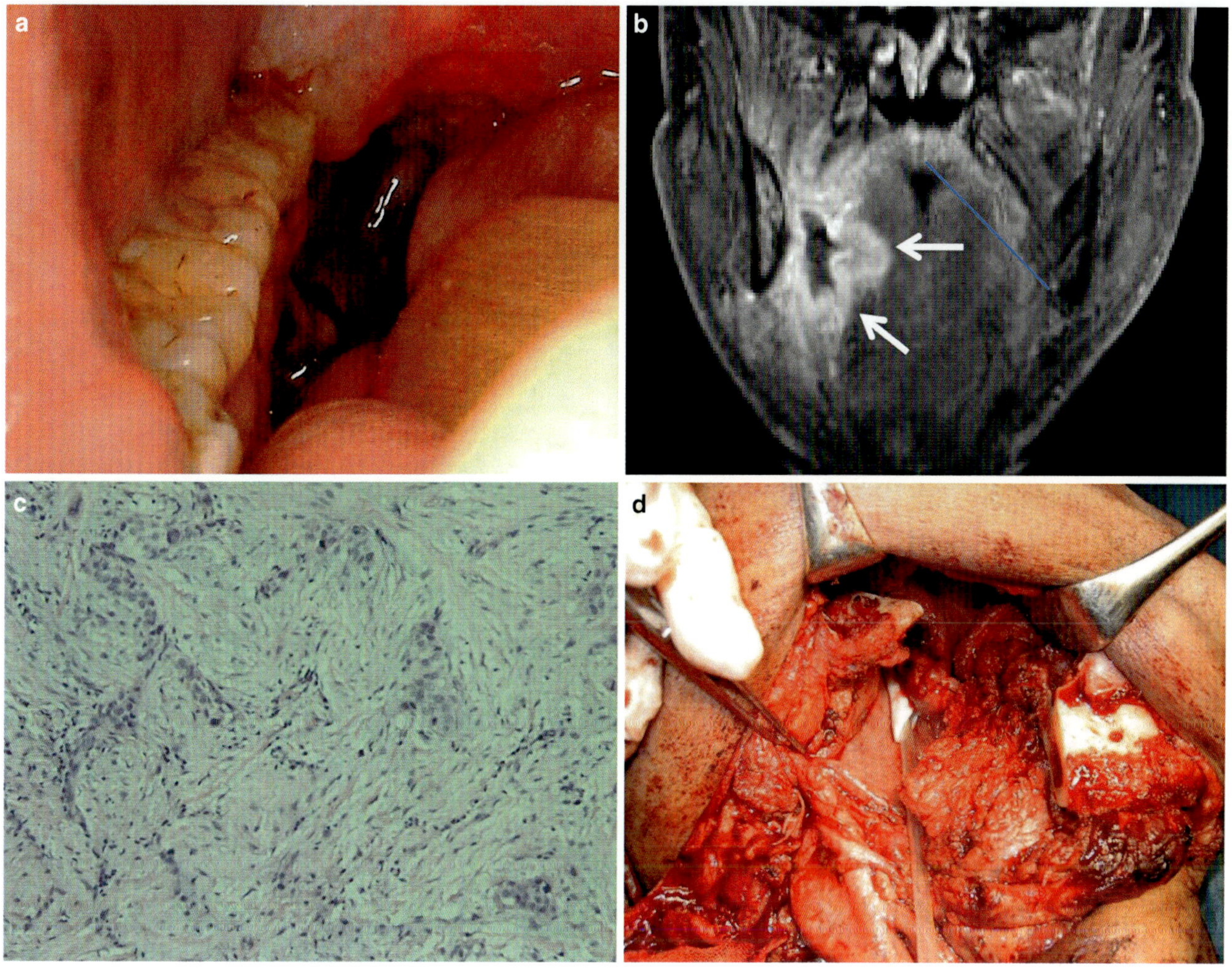

Fig. 7.57 Histological malignancy and surgical methods. (**a**) Lower gingival carcinoma (T4N1M0). (**b**) MR imaging, tumor invades into the mandible and surrounding tissue. (**c**) Histological finding, tumor cell shows cord-like-type invasion. (**d**) Segmental mandibulectomy with neck dissection

Fig. 7.58 Surgical resection of upper gingival carcinomas

Gingivectomy:
Resection of only the gingival mucosa and periosteum, and the alveolar bone is not resected.

Partial maxillectomy:
Resection of a part of the maxillary bone from the upper gingiva and alveolus, hard palate, or internal or external walls of the maxillary sinus

Subtotal maxillectomies:
Reseciont the maxillary bone without the orbital bone.

Total maxillectomies:
Resection of the zygoma, frontal bone, palatal bone, and pterygoid process from the maxillary bone, and constitutes a complete removal of the maxillary bone.

Extended maxillectomies:
In addition to all of the maxillary bone, remove of ethmoid cells, orbital contents, the skull base, etc.

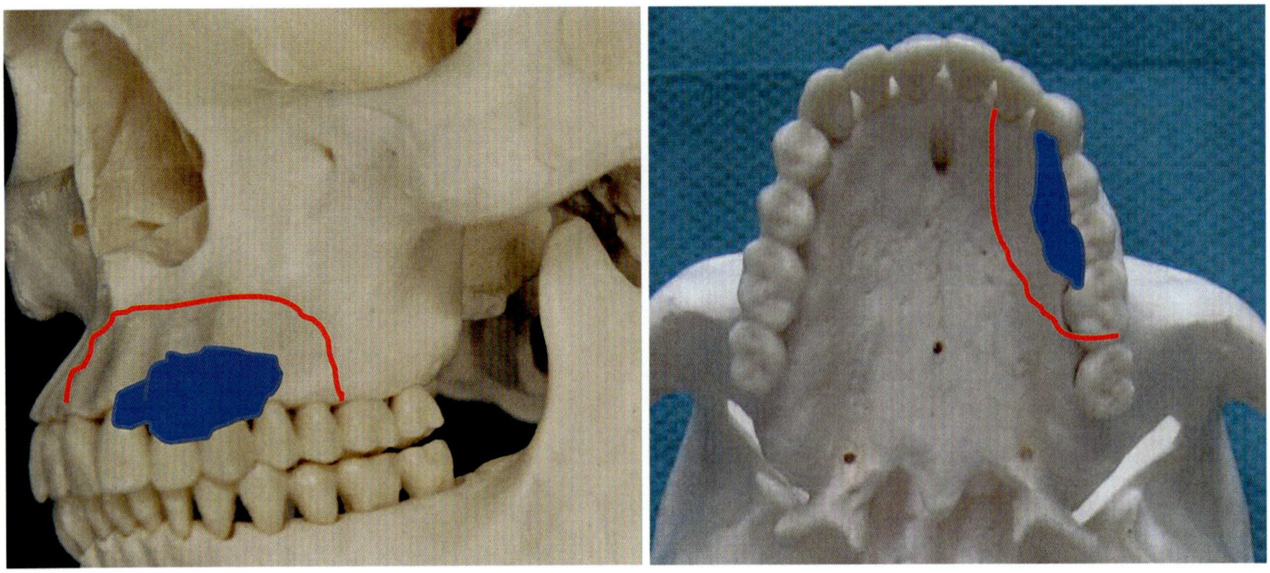

Fig. 7.59 Surgical resection of upper gingival carcinoma. Partial maxillectomy (only alveolectomy)

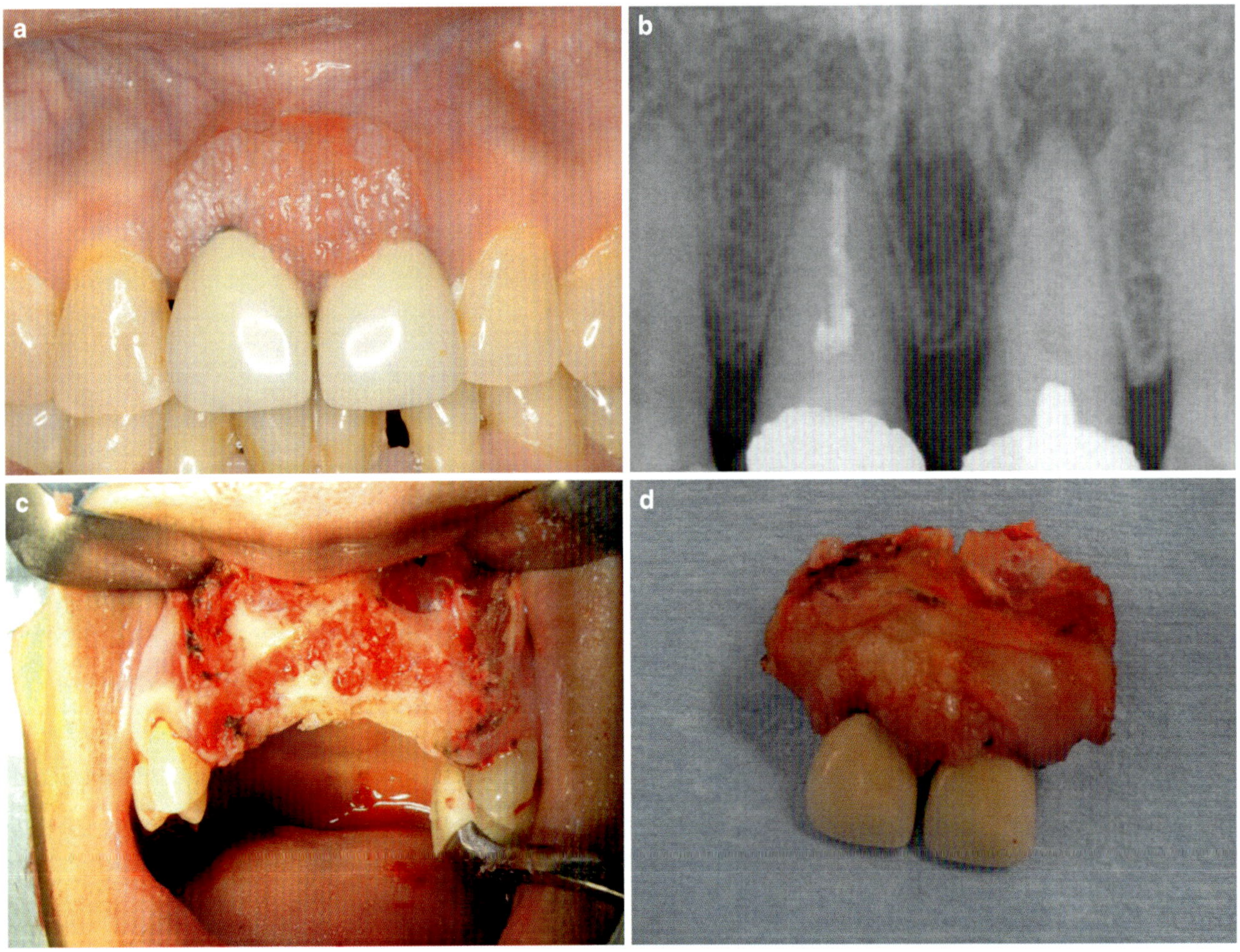

Fig. 7.60 Partial maxillectomy (only alveolectomy). (**a**) Clinical finding. (**b**) X-ray imaging, no finding of bone destruction. (**c**) Partial maxillectomy. (**d**) Removal of tissue

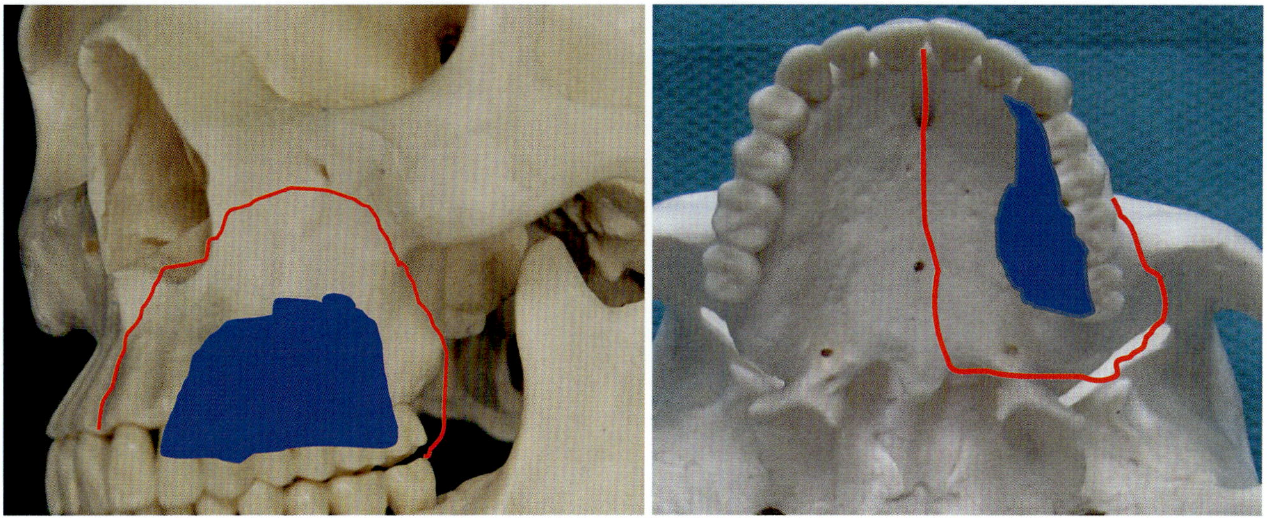

Fig. 7.61 Surgical resection of upper gingival carcinoma partial maxillectomy

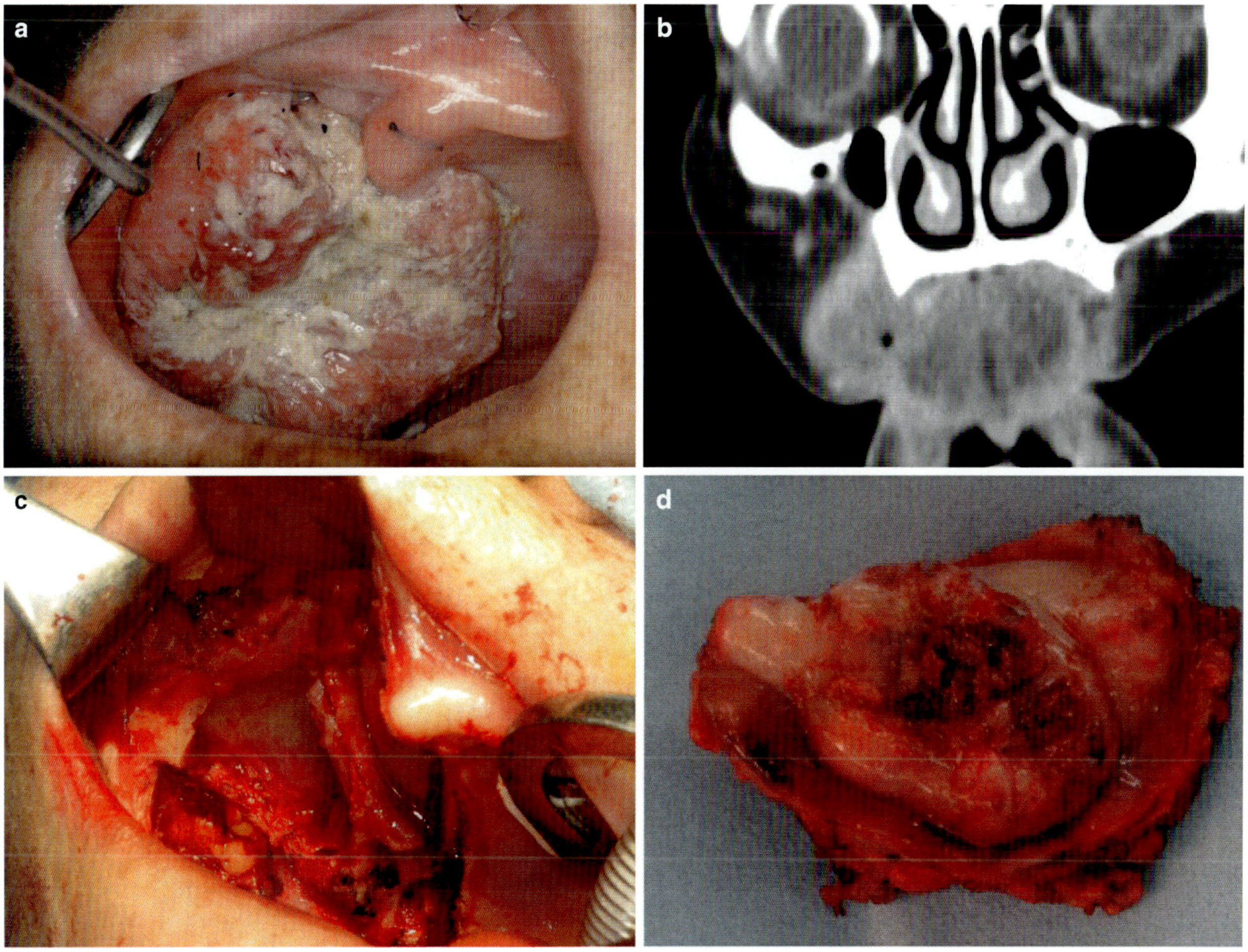

Fig. 7.62 Partial maxillectomy. (**a**) Clinical finding, upper gingival carcinoma (T3N0M0). (**b**) CT imaging, tumor does not invade into the maxillary sinus. (**c**) Partial maxillectomy. (**d**) Removal of tissue

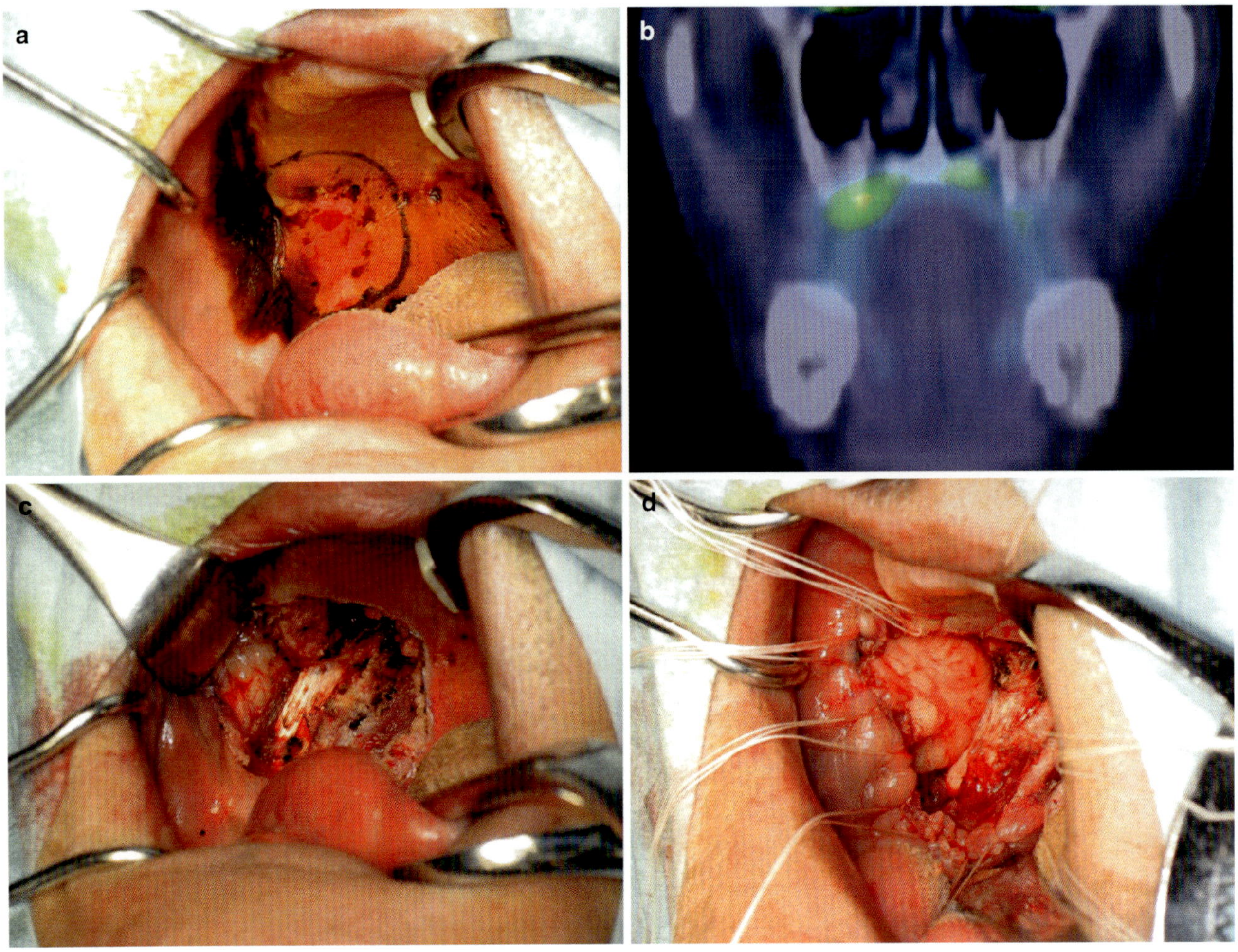

Fig. 7.63 Partial maxillectomy. (**a**) Clinical finding, upper gingival carcinoma (T2N0M0). (**b**) PET-CT imaging, tumor does not invade into maxillary sinus. (**c**) Partial maxillectomy. (**d**) Surgical defect is covered with buccal fat tissue

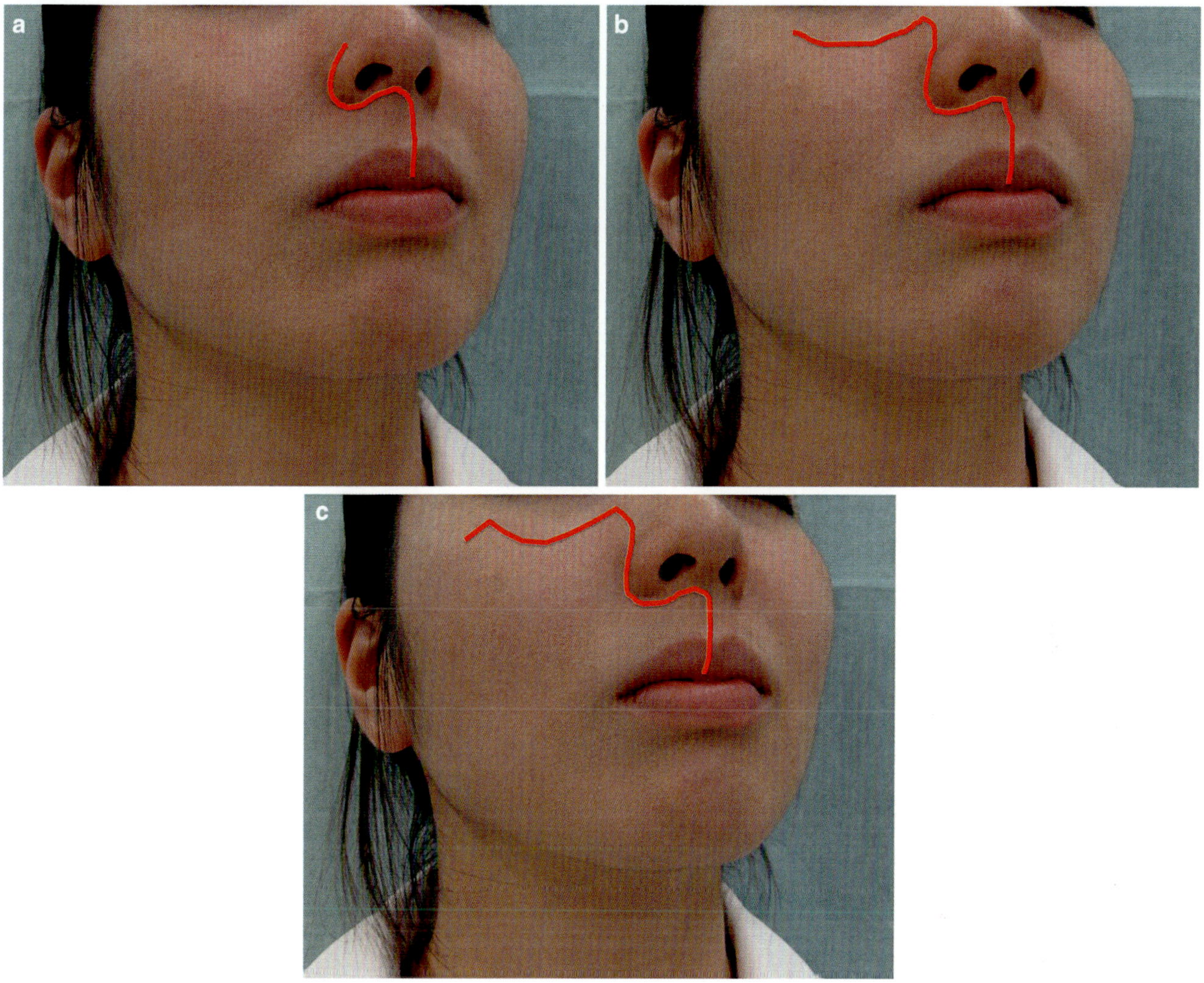

Fig. 7.64 (**a**) Matis incision. (**b**) Weber incision. (**c**) Weber-Kocher incision

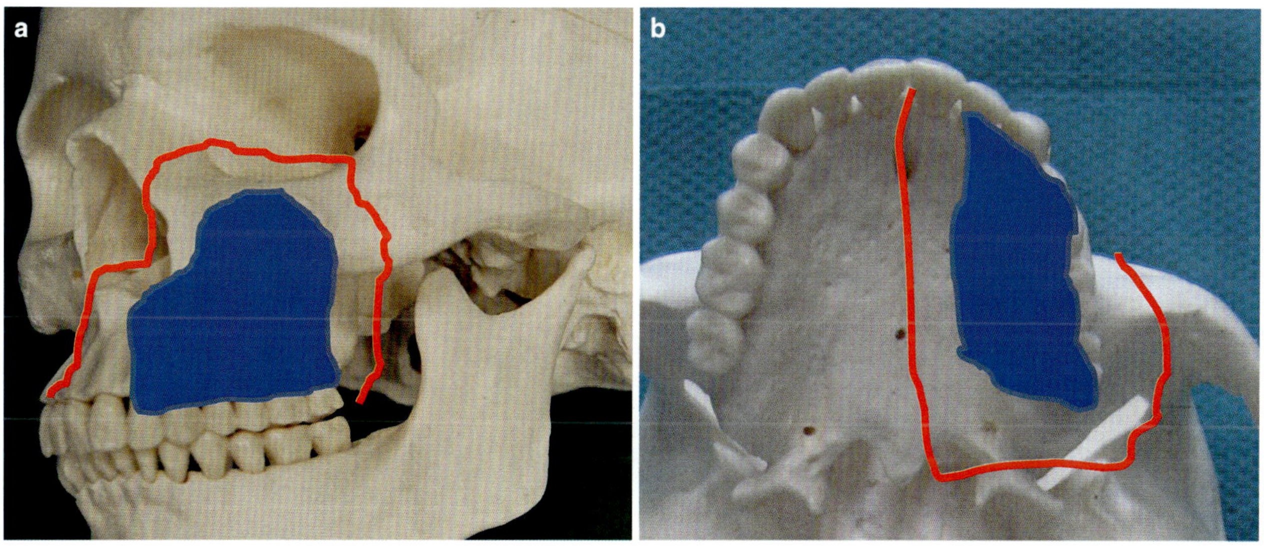

Fig. 7.65 Surgical resection of upper gingival carcinoma. Total maxillectomies

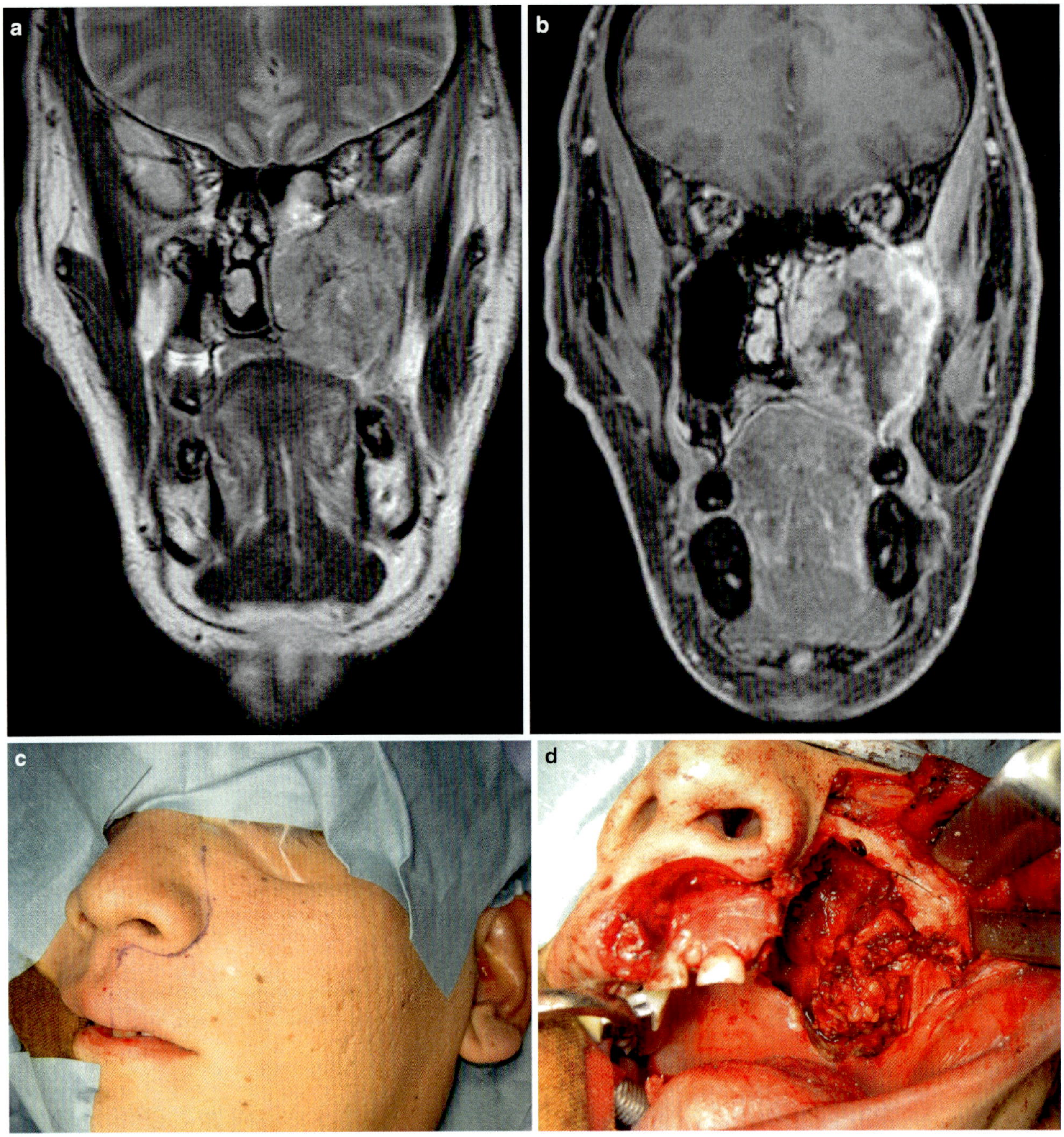

Fig. 7.66 Total maxillectomy. (**a**, **b**) MR imaging, tumor invades into the maxillary sinus. (**c**) Matis incision. (**d**) Total maxillectomy

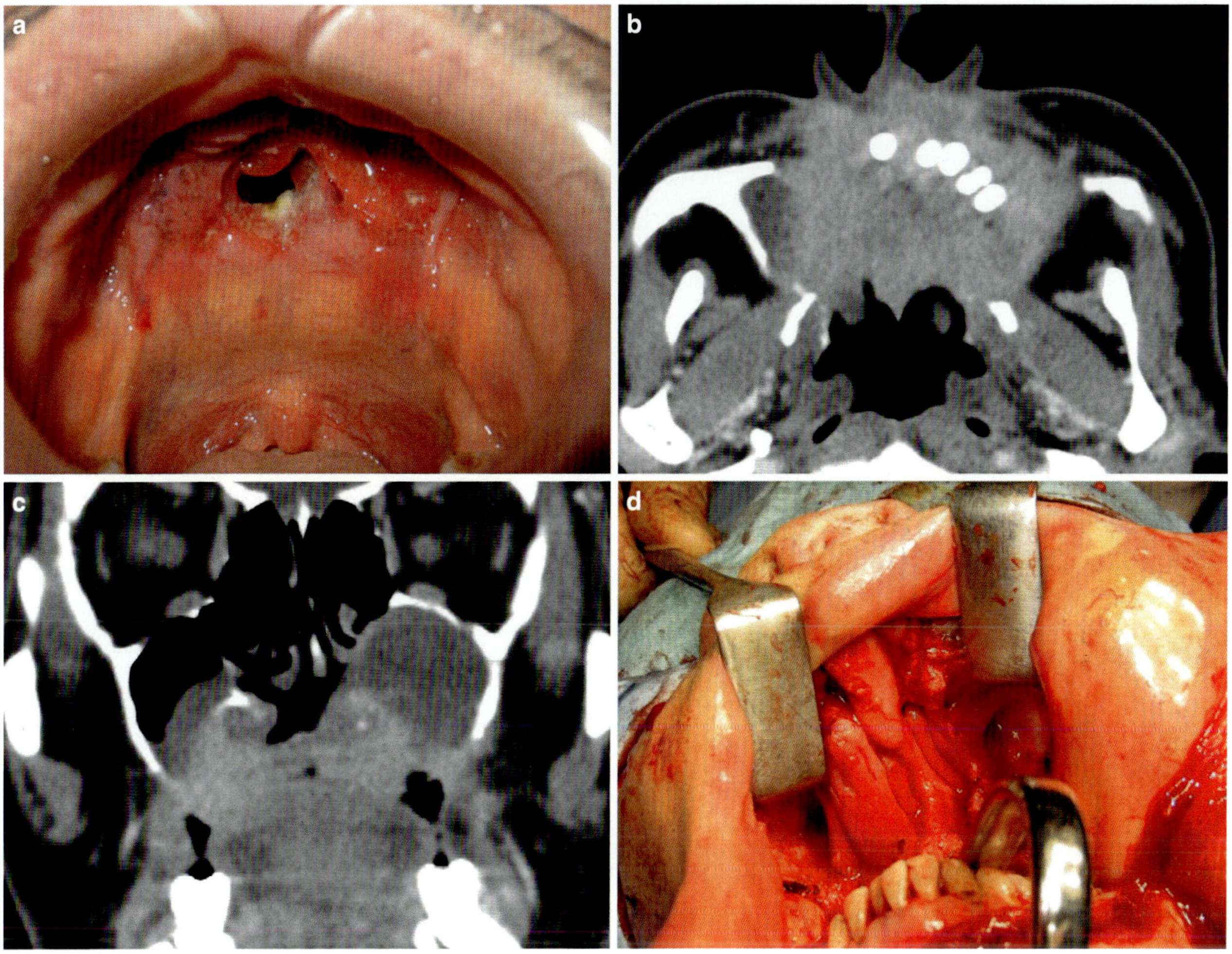

Fig. 7.67 Total maxillectomy. (**a**) Clinical finding, upper gingival carcinoma (T4N0M0). (**b**, **c**) CT finding, tumor invades into the maxillary bone and surrounding tissue. (**d**) total maxillectomy

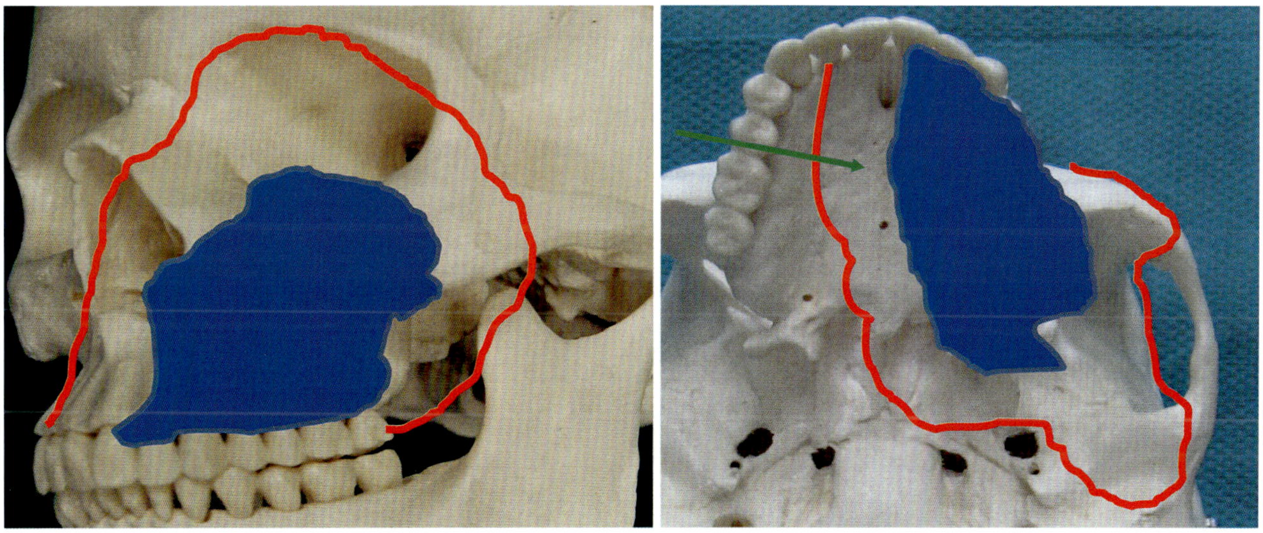

Fig. 7.68 Surgical resection of upper gingival carcinoma extended maxillectomy

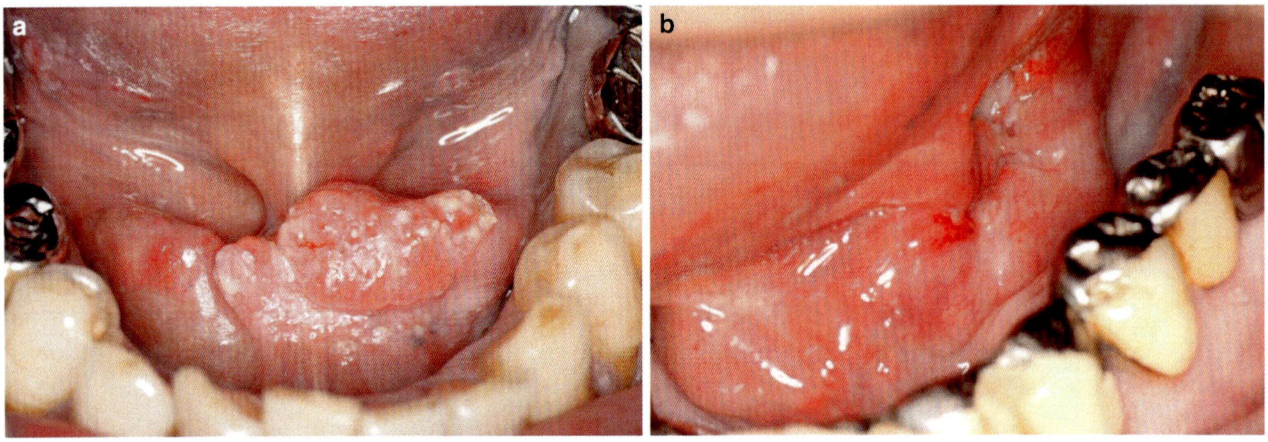

Fig. 7.69 Carcinoma of the floor of the mouth. (**a**) Median type. (**b**) Lateral type

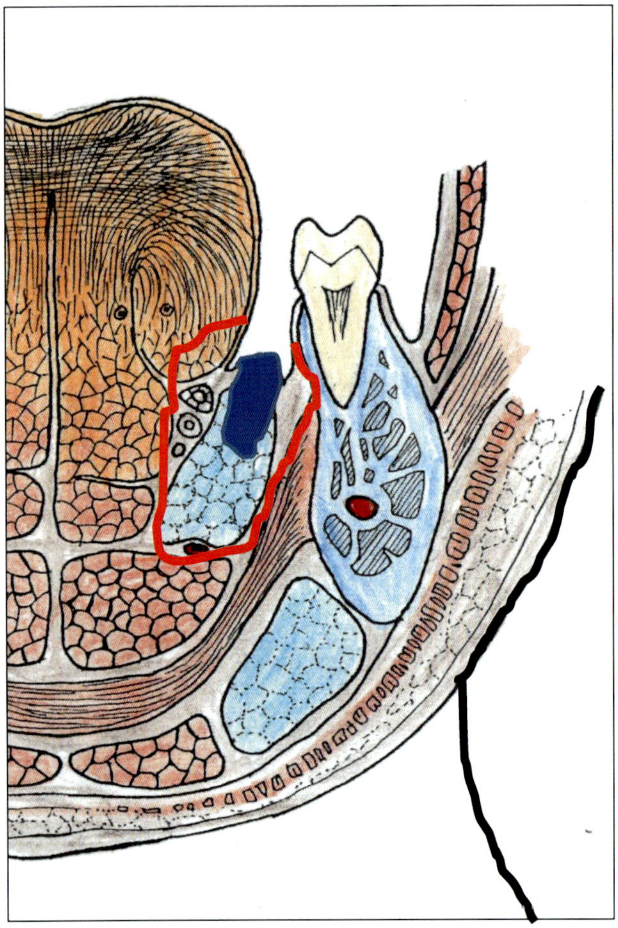

Fig. 7.70 Schema of a partial resection of the floor of the mouth

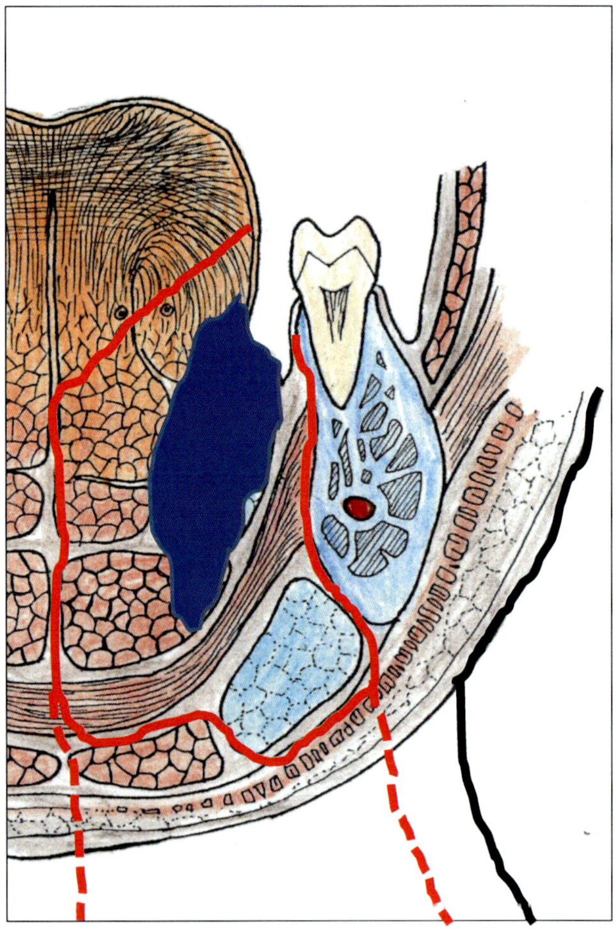

Fig. 7.71 Schema of a partial resection of the floor of the mouth and neck dissection by pull-through method

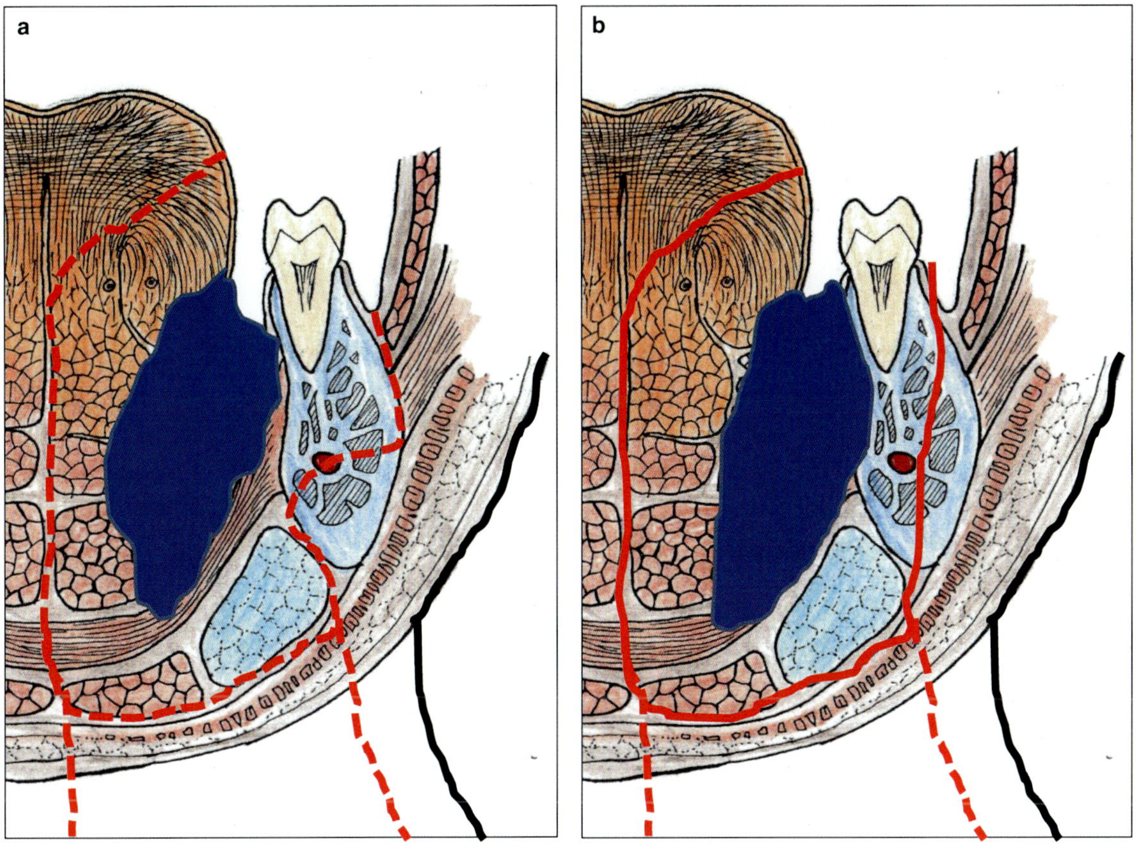

Fig. 7.72 Command operation. (**a**) Tumor resection with marginal mandibulectomy and/or neck dissection; (**b**) tumor resection with the cortical bone on the lingual side by sagittal splitting osteotomy and/or neck dissection

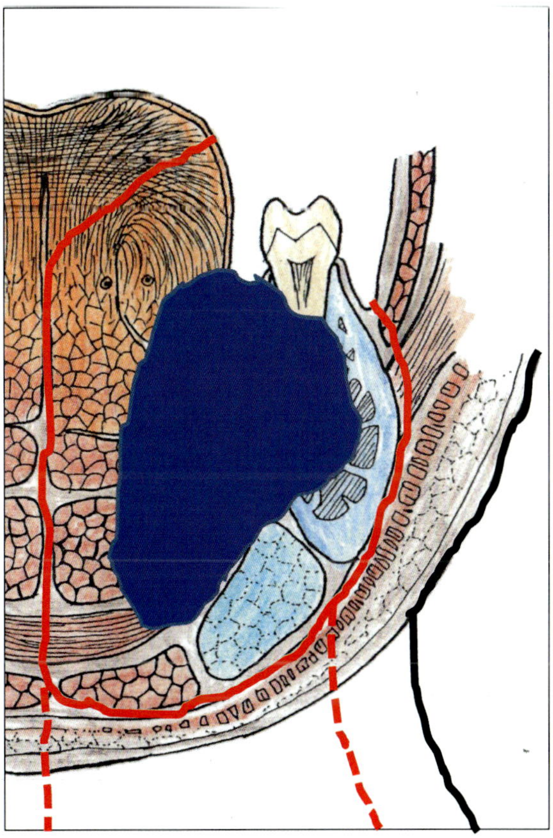

Fig. 7.73 Schema of a tumor resection of the floor of the mouth with segmental mandibulectomy and neck dissection by pull-through method

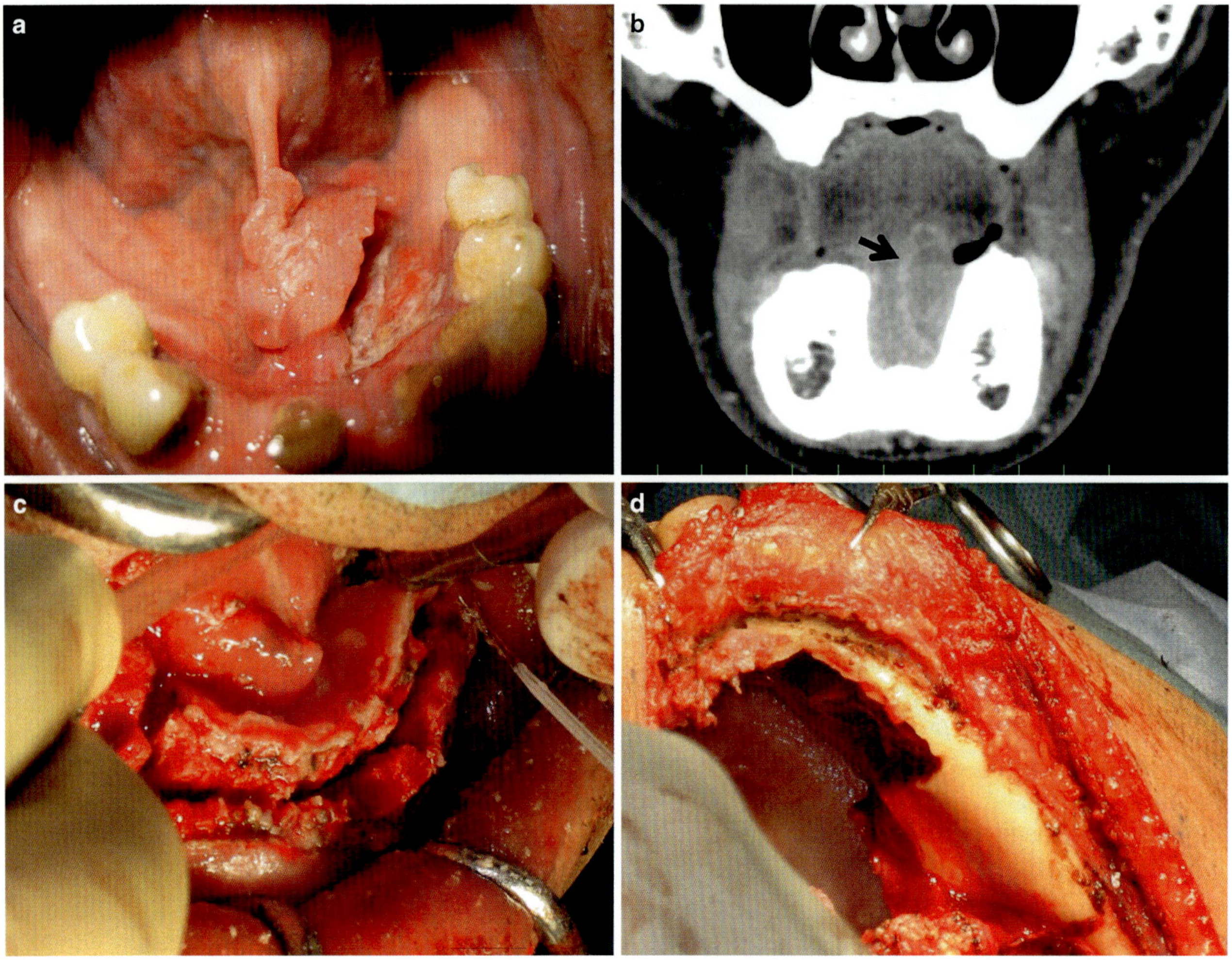

Fig. 7.74 Tumor resection with the cortical bone on the lingual side by sagittal splitting osteotomy. (**a**) Clinical finding, carcinoma of the floor of the mouth. (**b**) CT finding, tumor invades the cortical bone. (**c**) Segmental mandibulectomy. (**d**) Tumor is removed with the cortical bone

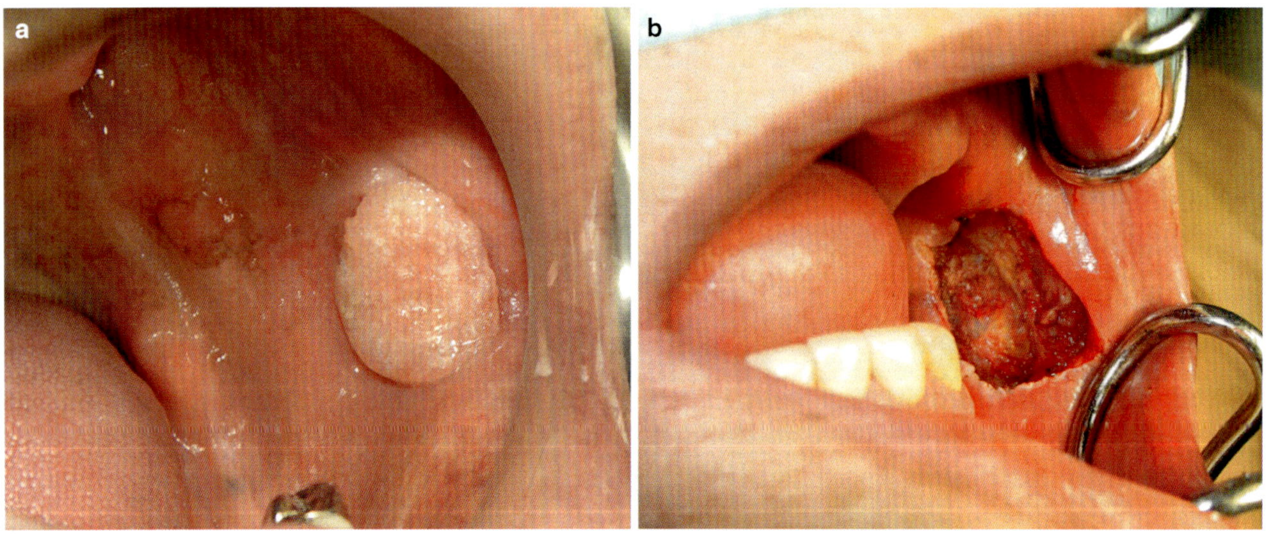

Fig. 7.75 Buccal mucosa carcinoma. (**a**) Clinical finding, buccal mucosa carcinoma (T2N0M0). (**b**) Tumor is removed from the buccal mucosa

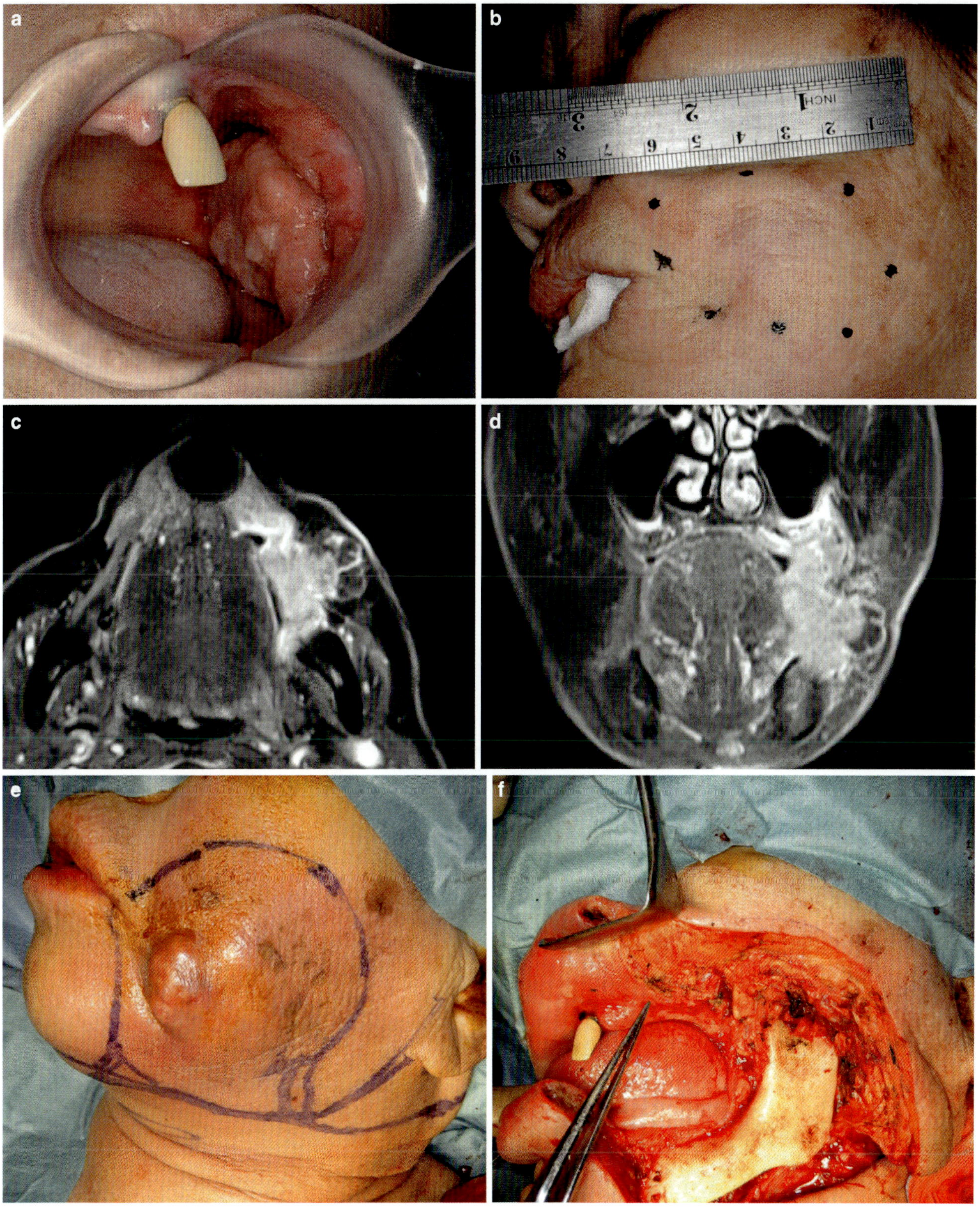

Fig. 7.76 Full-thickness buccal resection (through-and-through operation). (**a**) Clinical finding, buccal mucosa carcinoma (T4N1M0). (**b**) Clinical finding, tumor invades the buccal skin. (**c**, **d**) MR imaging, tumor invades into the skin tissue. (**e**) Excision line for through-and-through operation. (**f**) Full-thickness buccal resection

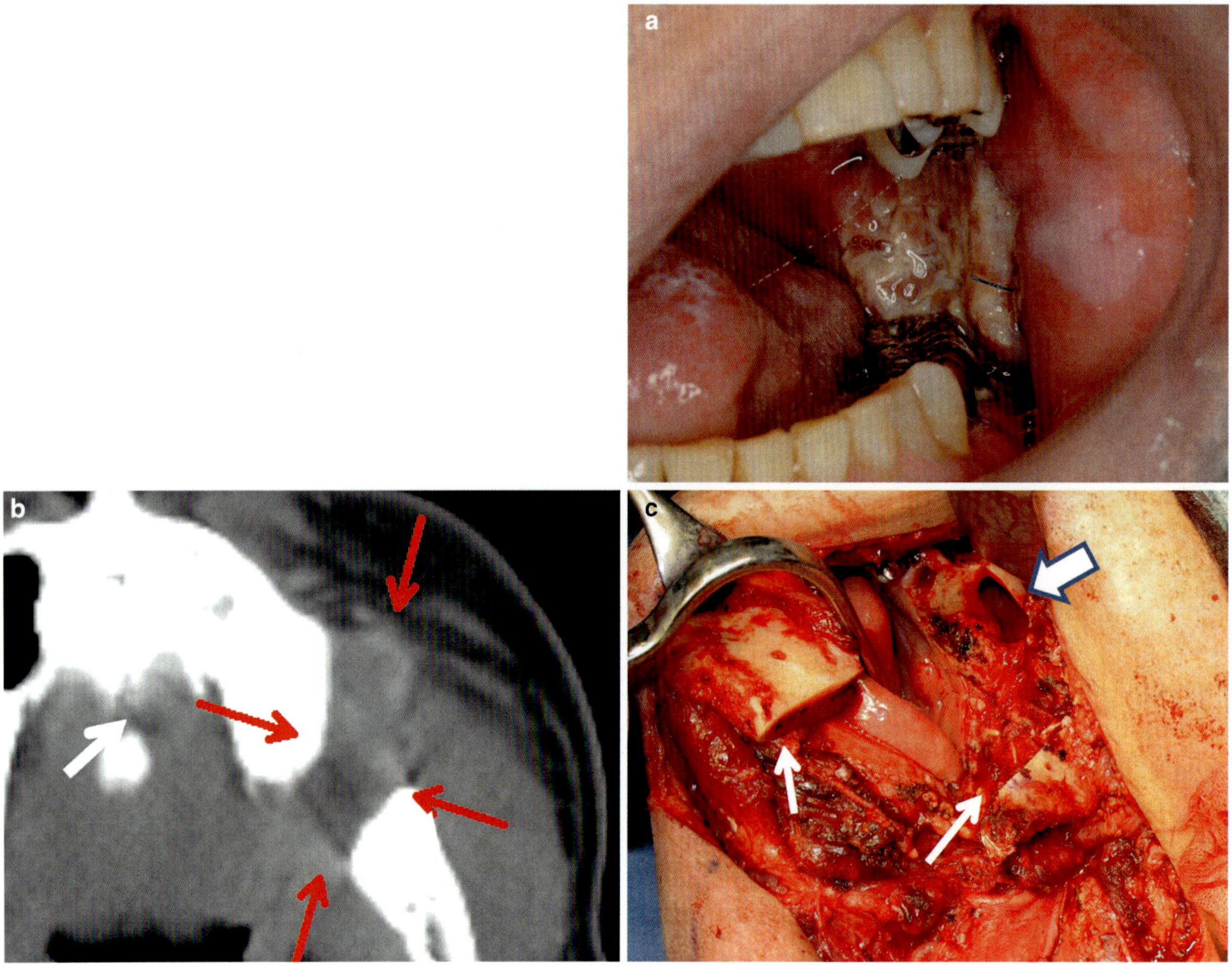

Fig. 7.77 Command operation. (**a**) Clinical finding, buccal mucosa carcinoma (T4N2M0). (**b**) CT imaging, tumor invades into the mandible and maxilla. (**c**) Tumor is removed with the mandible (*up arrow*) and maxilla (*open up arrow*)

References

1. Izumo T, Kirita T et al (2012) General rules for clinical and pathological studies on oral cancer: a synopsis. Jpn J Clin Oncol 42:1099–1109
2. Bell RB, Kademani D, Potter BE et al (2007) Is there a difference in survival compared with other subsites in the oral cavity? J Oral Maxillofac Surg 65:229–236
3. Garzino-Demo P, Dell'Acqua A et al (2006) Clinicopathological parameters and outcome of 245 patients operated for oral squamous cell carcinoma. J Craniomaxillofac Surg 34:344–350
4. Kademani D, Bell RB et al (2005) Prognostic factors in intraoral squamous cell carcinoma: the influence of histologic grade. J Oral Maxillofac Surg 63:1599–1605
5. Pericot J, Escriba JM et al (2000) Survival evaluation of treatment modality in squamous cell carcinoma of the oral cavity and oropharynx. J Craniomaxillofac Surg 28:49–55
6. Eckardt A, Barth EL et al (2004) Recurrent carcinoma of the head and neck: treatment strategies and survival analysis in a 20-year period. Oral Oncol 40:427–432
7. Po Wing Yuen A, Lam KY, Lam LK et al (2002) Prognostic factors of clinically stage I and II oral tongue carcinoma-a comparative study of stage, thickness, shape, growth pattern, invasive front malignancy grading, Martinez-Gimeno score, and pathologic features. Head Neck 24:513–520
8. Spiro RH, Guillamondegui O Jr et al (1999) Pattern of invasion and margin assessment in patients with oral tongue cancer. Head Neck 21:408–413
9. Kirita T, Okabe S et al (1994) Risk factors for the postoperative local recurrence of tongue carcinoma. J Oral Maxillofac Surg 52:149–154
10. Leslie A et al (1999) Staging of squamous cell carcinoma of the oral cavity and oropharynx: a comparison of MRI and CT In t- and N staging. J Comput Assist Tomogr 23:43–49
11. Lucchichenti G et al (2004) Computed tomography and magnetic resonance features of carcinoma of the tongue. Radiol Med 108:394–403
12. Sarvanan K, Bapuraj JR et al (2002) Computed tomography and ultrasonographic evaluation of metastatic cervical lymph nodes with surgicoclinicopathologic correlation. J Laryngol Otol 116:194–199
13. Shoaib T, Soutar DS et al (2001) The accuracy of head and neck carcinoma sentinel lymph node biopsy in the clinically N0 neck. Cancer 91:2077–2083
14. Jakobsson PA et al (1973) Histological classification and grading of malignancy in carcinoma of the larynx. Acta Radiol 12:1–8

15. Anneroth G et al (1987) Review of the literature and a recommended system of malignancy grading in oral squamous cell carcinoma. Scand J Dent Res 95:229–249
16. Yamamoto E, Kohama G (1983) Mode of Invasion. Bleomycin sensitivity and clinical course in squamous cell carcinoma of oral cavity. Cancer 15:2175–2180
17. Aksu G, Karadeniz A et al (2006) Treatment results and prognostic factors in oral tongue cancer: analysis of 80 patients. Int J Oral Maxillofac Surg 35:506–513
18. Guerra MFM, Gias LN et al (2003) Marginal and segmental mandibulectomy in patients with oral cancer: a statistical analysis of 106 cases. J Oral Maxillofac Surg 61:1289–1296
19. Lee JG (1974) Detection of residual carcinoma of the oral cavity oropharynx, hypopharynx, and larynx: a study of surgical margins. Trans Am Acad Opthalmol Otolaryngol 78:ORL49–ORL53
20. Vikram B, Strong EW et al (1984) Failure at the primary site following multimodality treatment in advanced head and neck cancer. Head Neck Surg 6:720–723
21. Mistry RC, Qureshi SS et al (2005) Post-resection mucosal margin shrinkage in oral cancer: quantification and significance. J Surg Oncol 91:131–133
22. Johnson RE, Sigman JD et al (1997) Quantification of surgical margin shrinkage in the oral cavity. Head Neck 19:281–286
23. Looser KG, Shah JP et al (1978) The significance of "positive" margins in surgically resected epidermoid carcinomas. Head Neck Surg 1:107–111
24. Nason RW, Binahmed A et al (2009) What is the adequate margin of surgical resection in oral cancer? Oral Surg Oral Med Oral Pathol Oral Radiol Endod 107:625–629
25. Kurita H, Nakanishi Y et al (2010) Impact of different surgical margin conditions on local recurrence of oral squamous cell carcinoma. Oral Oncol 46:814–817
26. Binahmed A, Nason RW et al (2007) The clinical significance of the positive surgical margin in oral cancer. Oral Oncol 43:780–784
27. Epstein JB, Scully C et al (1992) Toluidine blue and Lugol's iodine application in the assessment of oral malignant disease and lesions at risk of malignancy. J Oral Pathol Med 21:160–163
28. Umeda M, Shigeta T et al (2011) Clinical evaluation of Lugol's iodine staining in the treatment of stage I-II squamous cell carcinoma of the tongue. Int J Oral Maxillofac Surg 40:593–596
29. Izumo T (2011) Oral premalignant lesions: from the pathological viewpoint. Int J Clin Oncol 16:15–26
30. Petruzzi M, Lucchese A et al (2010) Use of Lugol's iodine in oral cancer diagnosis: an overview. Oral Oncol 46:811–813
31. Kurita H, Kurashina K et al (1996) Vital staining with iodine solution in delineating the border of oral dysplastic lesions. Oral Surg Oral Med Oral Pathol Oral Radiol Endod 81:275–280
32. Kerawala CJ, Beale V et al (2000) The role of vital tissue staining in the marginal control of oral squamous cell carcinoma. Int J Oral Maxillofac Surg 29:32–35
33. Martin IC, Kerawala CJ et al (1998) The application of toluidine blue as a diagnostic adjunct in the detection of epithelial dysplasia. Oral Surg Oral Med Oral Pathol Oral Radiol Endod 85:444–446
34. Asakage T, Yokose T et al (1997) Tumor thickness predicts cervical metastasis in patients with stage I/II carcinoma of the tongue. Cancer 82:1443–1448 [IV]
35. Bova R, Cheung I et al (2003) Total glossectomy: is it justified? ANZ J Surg 74:134–138
36. Yuen AP, Lam KY et al (2000) A comparison of the prognostic significance of tumor diameter, length, width, thickness, area, volume, and clinicopathological features of oral tongue carcinoma. Am J Surg 180:139–143
37. Karakida K, Ota Y et al (2002) Examination of factors predicting occult metastasis of the cervical lymph nodes in T1 and T2 tongue carcinoma. Tokai J Exp Clin Med 27:65–71
38. Al-Rajhi N, Khafaga Y et al (2000) Early stage carcinoma of oral tongue: prognostic factors for local control and survival. Oral Oncol 36:508–514
39. Lim YC, Choi EC (2007) Unilateral, clinically T2N0, squamous cell carcinoma of the tongue: surgical outcome analysis. Int J Oral Maxillofac Surg 36:610–614
40. Jahnke V (1985) Surgery for squamous cell carcinoma of the tongue and floor of the mouth. Auris Nasus Larynx 12(Suppl 2):S5–S9
41. Jahnke V (1975) Surgery of the tongue and floor of the mouth. Arch Otorhinolaryngol 210:275–291
42. Wax M, Bascom D et al (2002) Marginal mandibulectomy vs segmental mandibulectomy, indication and controversies. Arch Otolaryngol Head Neck Surg 128:600–603
43. Wong RJ, Keel SB et al (2000) Histological pattern of mandibular invasion by oral squamous cell carcinoma. Laryngoscope 110:65–72
44. Werning JW, Byers RM et al (2001) Preoperative assessment for and outcomes of mandibular conservative surgery. Head Neck 23:1024–1030
45. Genden EM, Rinaldo A et al (2005) Management of mandibular invasion: when is a marginal mandibulectomy appropriate? Oral Oncol 41:776–782
46. Guerra MFM, Gias LN et al (2003) Marginal and segmental mandibulectomy in patients with oral cancer: a statistical analysis of 106 cases. J Oral Maxillofac Surg 61:1289–1296
47. Ash CS, Nason RW et al (2000) Prognostic implications of mandibular invasion in oral cancer. Head Neck 22:794–798
48. Brown JS, Lowe D et al (2002) Patterns of invasion and routes of tumor entry into the mandible by oral squamous cell carcinoma. Head Neck 24:370–383
49. Politi M, Costa F et al (2000) Review of segmental and marginal resection of the mandible in patients with oral cancer. Acta Otolaryngol 120:569–579
50. Totsuka Y, Usui Y et al (1991) Results of surgical treatment for squamous carcinoma of the lower alveolus: segmental vs. marginal resection. Head Neck 13:114–120
51. Tei K, Totsuka Y et al (2004) Marginal resection for carcinoma of the mandibular alveolus and gingiva where radiologically detected bone defects do not extend beyond the mandibular canal. J Oral Maxillofac Surg 62:834–839
52. Swearingen AG, McGraw JP et al (1966) Roentgenographic pathologic correlation of carcinoma of the gingival involving the mandible. Am J Roentgenol Radium Ther Nucl Med 96:15–18
53. Notani K, Yamazaki Y et al (2003) Management of mandibular osteoradionecrosis corresponding to the severity of osteoradionecrosis and the method of radiotherapy. Head Neck 25:181–185
54. Nomura T, Shibahara T et al (2005) Patterns of mandibular invasion by gingival squamous cell carcinoma. J Oral Maxillofac Surg 63:1489–1493
55. Ord RA, Sarmadi M et al (1997) A comparison of segmental and marginal bony resection for oral squamous cell carcinoma involving the mandible. J Oral Maxillofac Surg 55:470–477
56. O'Brien CJ, Adams JR et al (2003) Influence of bone invasion and extent of mandibular resection on local control of cancers of the oral cavity and oropharynx. Int J Oral Maxillofac Surg 32:492–497
57. Lam KH, Lam LK et al (1999) Mandibular invasion in carcinoma of the lower alveolus. Am J Otolaryngol 20:267–273
58. Totsuka Y, Usui Y et al (1991) Mandibular involvement by squamous cell carcinoma of the lower alveolus. Analysis and comparative study of histologic and radiologic features. Head Neck 13:40–50
59. Hong SX, Cha IH et al (2001) Mandibular invasion of lower gingival carcinoma in the molar region: its clinical implications on the surgical management. Int J Oral Maxillofac Surg 30:130–138
60. Imai J, Uno T et al (1998) Squamous cell carcinoma of the maxillary sinus treated with radiation therapy and conservative surgery. Cancer 82:104–107

61. Chong V (2005) Oral cavity cancer. Cancer Imaging 5:S49–S52
62. Sieczka E, Datta R et al (2001) Cancer of the buccal mucosa are margins and T-stage accurate predictors of local control? Am J Otolaryngol 22:395–399
63. Inagi K, Takahashi H et al (2003) Treatment effects in patients with squamous cell carcinoma of the oral cavity. Acta Otolaryngol Suppl 547:25–29
64. Wolff D, Hassfeld S et al (2004) Influence of marginal and segmental mandibular resection on the survival rate in patients with squamous cell carcinoma of the inferior parts of the oral cavity. J Craniomaxillofac Surg 32:318–323
65. Shaha AR (1992) Marginal mandibulectomy for carcinoma of the floor of the mouth. J Surg Oncol 49:116–119
66. Machetta FC, Sako K et al (1971) The periosteum of the maxilla and intraoral carcinoma. Am J Surg 122:711–713
67. Dubner S, Heller KS (1993) Local control of squamous cell carcinoma following marginal and segmental mandibulectomy. Head Neck 15:29–32
68. Guerra MF, Campo FJ et al (2003) Rim versus sagittal mandibulectomy for the treatment of squamous cell carcinoma: two types of mandibular preservation. Head Neck 25:982–989
69. Barttelbort SW, Bahn SL et al (1987) Rim mandibulectomy for cancer of the oral cavity. Am J Surg 154:423–428
70. Barttelbort SW, Ariyan S et al (1993) Mandible preservation with oral cavity carcinoma. Rim mandibulectomy versus sagittal mandibulectomy. Am J Surg 166:411–415

Management of the Neck

8

Ken Omura

Abstract

Regional nodal status is one of the most significant prognostic factors in patients with oral squamous cell carcinoma; therefore, diagnosis and treatment of cervical nodal disease is one of the most highly debated topics among head and neck surgeons. Imaging modalities currently available in clinical practice include ultrasonography, computed tomography, magnetic resonance imaging, and positron emission tomography. However, none of these methods can independently confirm occult metastasis. A patient's risk of regional metastasis is determined through clinicopathological evaluation of the primary tumor. Elective management of the neck is warranted when the risk of occult metastasis is >20 %. In these situations, the modality of elective treatment is influenced by that selected to treat the primary tumor. When surgery is indicated, selective neck dissection (SND [I–III)] is generally required; however, SND (I–IV) is recommended for patients with tongue squamous cell carcinoma. Modified radical neck dissection is the gold standard for the N-positive neck; however, SND is applicable in selected patients. For patients with multiple node metastases or extracapsular spread, postoperative radiotherapy or chemoradiotherapy is recommended as soon as possible after surgery.

Keywords

Extracapsular spread of tumor • Level • Neck dissection • Occult node metastasis • Postoperative radiotherapy/chemoradiotherapy

8.1 Introduction

Oral squamous cell carcinomas (OSCCs) that are localized to the primary tumor site without regional metastatic disease have excellent cure rates with either surgery or radiation therapy. The presence of regional metastatic disease decreases the cure rate by approximately 50 % [1, 2]. The status of the cervical lymph nodes is one of the most significant prognostic factors for patients with OSCC; therefore, diagnosis and treatment of cervical nodal disease is one of the most highly debated topics among head and neck surgeons. This chapter examines various approaches used to evaluate and treat patients with regional nodal disease.

K. Omura, D.D.S., Ph.D. (✉)
Tokyo Medical and Dental University, Tokyo, Japan

Oral Cancer Center, Tokyo General Hospital, Tokyo, Japan
e-mail: omura.osur@tmd.ac.jp

8.2 Regional Lymph Nodes

The cervical lymphatic system is a rich network of lymphatic channels that drain into numerous lymph nodes scattered throughout the face and neck. There are approximately 300 lymph nodes in the face and neck region [3]. Cervical lymph nodes are categorized into six nodal groups or levels from I through VI; levels I, II, and V are further divided into sublevels A and B [4, 5] (Table 8.1). This classification does not

T. Kirita and K. Omura (eds.), *Oral Cancer: Diagnosis and Therapy*,
DOI 10.1007/978-4-431-54938-3_8, © Springer Japan 2015

Table 8.1 Cervical lymph node levels

Level	Lymph node group	Boundary			
		Superior	Inferior	Anterior (medial)	Posterior (lateral)
IA	Submental nodes	Symphysis of mandible	Body of hyoid bone	Anterior belly of the contralateral digastric muscle	Anterior belly of the ipsilateral digastric muscle
IB	Submandibular nodes	Body of mandible		Anterior belly of the digastric muscle	Stylohyoid muscle
IIA	Upper jugular nodes, anterior to XI nerve	Skull base	Horizontal plane defined by the inferior border of the hyoid bone	Stylohyoid muscle	Vertical plane defined by the spinal accessory nerve
IIB	Upper jugular nodes, posterior to XI nerve (submuscular recess)	Skull base	Horizontal plane defined by the inferior border of the hyoid bone	Vertical plane defined by the spinal accessory nerve	Lateral border of the sternocleidomastoid muscle
III	Middle jugular nodes	Horizontal plane defined by the inferior border of the hyoid bone	Horizontal plane defined by the inferior border of the cricoid cartilage	Lateral border of the sternohyoid muscle	Lateral border of the sternocleidomastoid muscle or sensory branches of the cervical plexus
IV	Lower jugular nodes	Horizontal plane defined by the inferior border of the cricoid cartilage	Clavicle	Lateral border of the sternohyoid muscle	Lateral border of the sternocleidomastoid muscle or sensory branches of the cervical plexus
VA	Posterior triangle nodes (spinal accessory group)	Apex of the convergence of the sternocleidomastoid and trapezius muscles	Horizontal plane defined by the inferior border of the cricoid cartilage	Lateral border of the sternocleidomastoid muscle or sensory branches of the cervical plexus	Anterior border of the trapezius muscle
VB	Posterior triangle nodes (transverse cervical artery group, supraclavicular group)	Horizontal plane defined by the inferior border of the cricoid cartilage	Clavicle	Lateral border of the sternocleidomastoid muscle or sensory branches of the cervical plexus	Anterior border of the trapezius muscle
VI	Central (anterior) compartment lymph nodes (paratracheal, perithyroidal, Delphian)	Hyoid bone	Superior edge of the manubrium sternum bone	Common carotid artery	Common carotid artery

include the facial and retropharyngeal nodes, which rarely harbor metastases from the oral cavity [6–8].

- Level I contains the submental (IA) and submandibular (IB) nodes; it is bounded by the body of the mandible superiorly, the anterior belly of the contralateral digastric muscle anteriorly, the hyoid bone inferiorly, and the stylohyoid muscle posteriorly.
- Level II contains the upper jugular lymph nodes; it extends from the skull base superiorly to the hyoid bone (clinical definition) or the carotid bifurcation (surgical definition) inferiorly; this group consists of the following two sublevels: nodes anterior to the spinal accessory nerve (IIA) and nodes posterior to the spinal accessory nerve (IIB).
- Level III contains the middle jugular lymph nodes; it extends from the hyoid bone (clinical definition) or the carotid bifurcation (surgical definition) superiorly to the cricoid cartilage (clinical definition) or the omohyoid muscle (surgical definition) inferiorly.
- Level IV contains the lower jugular lymph nodes; it extends from the cricoid cartilage (clinical definition) or the omohyoid muscle (surgical definition) superiorly to the clavicle inferiorly.
- Level V contains the lymph nodes in the posterior triangle; it is bounded by the anterior border of the trapezius muscle posteriorly, the posterior border of the sternocleidomastoid muscle anteriorly, and the clavicle inferiorly; this group consists of the following two sublevels: nodes superior to the level of the cricoid cartilage (VA, spinal accessory group) and nodes inferior to the level of the cricoid cartilage (VB, transverse cervical group).
- Level VI contains the anterior lymph nodes from the hyoid bone superiorly to the suprasternal notch inferiorly, and the lateral border is formed by the common carotid artery.

8.3 Patterns of Regional Node Metastases

OSCCs are likely to present with nodal metastases in levels I, II, and III. Initial involvement of level IV is quite uncommon; metastatic spread to level V nodes is even more infrequent [9]. However, "skip metastases" or metastases to the inferior cervical nodes in level III or IV without demonstrable involvement of levels I and II are currently of concern [10, 11].

8.4 Evaluation of Regional Nodal Status

All patients with OSCC require careful assessment of their cervical nodal status for optimal treatment planning and determination of their prognosis.

8.4.1 Physical Examination

Palpation remains the first step in evaluating the neck of patients with OSCC. However, the diagnostic accuracy of this method varies depending on the body habitus of the patient and experience of the examiner. Both the specificity and sensitivity of the palpation method for diagnosing nodal disease are reportedly 60–70 % [12, 13]. In addition, some nodal regions are inaccessible to palpation, such as the parapharyngeal and retropharyngeal areas.

8.4.2 Imaging Studies

Imaging modalities currently available in routine clinical practice include ultrasonography (US), computed tomography (CT), magnetic resonance imaging (MRI), and positron emission tomography (PET) with or without CT.

US is a useful diagnostic imaging modality, which has been reported to have high sensitivity but low specificity for evaluating nodal diseases [14, 15]. US is advantageous because of its relatively low cost, its ability to capture accurate measurements of nodal size, and its compatibility with guided fine-needle aspiration (FNA); however, its usefulness is dependent on the experience of the clinician.

Cross-sectional imaging studies play a large role in the evaluation of nodal status. Although both MRI and CT can provide valuable supplemental information, CT appears to be slightly superior when appropriate criteria are used [15–18]. Regardless of the type of imaging studies performed, clinicians use the following criteria that were developed as an aid to determine whether a node is metastatic: (1) a node >1.0 cm (or >1.5 cm in the jugulodigastric region, >0.8 cm in the retropharyngeal region), especially when round; (2) decreased central attenuation in the node; (3) a poorly defined mass in the lymph node-bearing region; and (4) the combination of ill-defined borders and structures. If any of these criteria are present, the node must be considered to harbor metastasis [19, 20].

PET differs from other imaging modalities in that it evaluates metabolic activity rather than anatomical structures. PET has a lower resolution compared with CT or MRI, but this has been overcome with the advent of fusion-imaging technology, which combines the physiological data observed on a PET scan with the anatomical detail observed on a CT scan (PET/CT) [21, 22].

Although recent advances in modern technology have led to the development of various diagnostic imaging modalities as discussed above, none of these modalities alone can confirm a cervical lymph node metastasis (Fig. 8.1, Table 8.2).

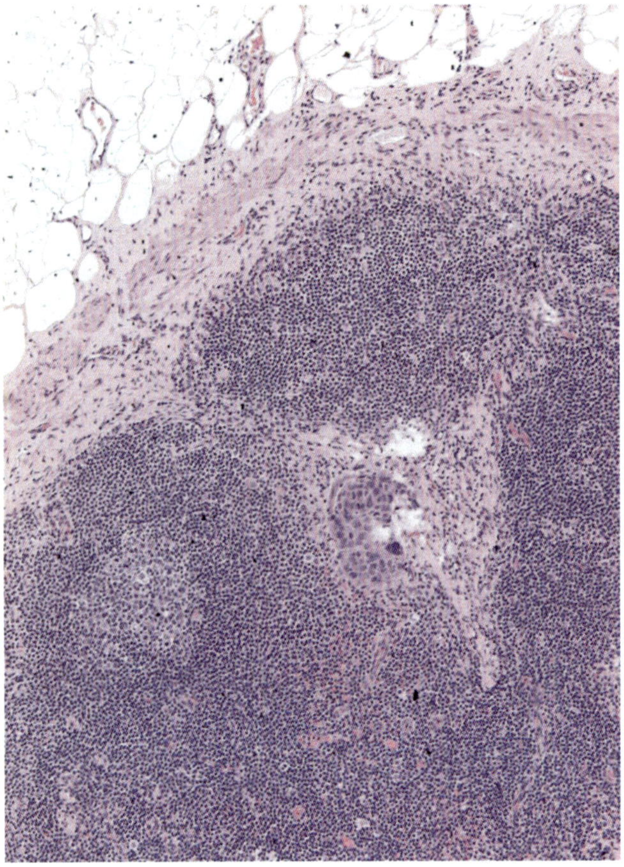

Fig. 8.1 Occult metastasis (micrometastasis)

Table 8.2 Sensitivity and specificity of imaging modalities used in evaluation of neck disease

Modality	Sensitivity (%)	Specificity (%)
US	50–58	75–82
CT	40–68	78–92
MRI	55–80	82–92
PET/CT	57–79	82–96

8.4.3 Pathological Examination

A patient's cervical node status can be pathologically evaluated; however, pathological confirmation should be obtained only for clinically and radiologically suspicious nodes.

8.4.3.1 FNA

FNA is an accurate and reliable procedure with minimal morbidity that allows for a quick cytological diagnosis of suspicious nodes. For nodes that are difficult to access, guidance with US or CT is helpful [15, 23]. Sensitivity and specificity of FNA for masses of the head and neck have been reported as 97 % and 96 %, respectively [24]. The accuracy of FNA is directly related to the diagnostic capability of the cytopathologist and the quality of the material obtained. If a definitive diagnosis cannot be determined after repeated FNAs, the patient may require an open biopsy procedure.

8.4.3.2 Open Biopsy

The prognostic impact of an open biopsy of a suspicious lymph node remains controversial. Some reports have stated that an open biopsy increases the rates of local complications, local recurrences, and distant metastasis [20]. However, other reports indicate that biopsy of the neck does not imply a poor prognosis as long as adequate treatment is subsequently administered [25–27]. Currently, from a practical standpoint, an open biopsy of a suspicious node is rarely recommended for patients with OSCC.

8.4.3.3 Sentinel Lymph Node Biopsy

Currently, sentinel lymph node biopsy receives considerable attention as a procedure for assessing the stage of regional disease. Although this technique is promising, it is under investigation [28–30].

8.5 Staging of Regional Node Metastasis

The staging system of regional lymph node metastases established by the UICC (outlined in Table 8.3) considers factors such as size, number, and laterality of the involved nodes.

8.6 Prognostic Implications of Regional Node Metastasis

The presence of clinically apparent, histologically confirmed lymph node metastasis is the single most significant prognostic factor in patients with OSCC. In general, it has been observed that patients with lymph node metastasis have a 50 % lower overall survival rate than patients with early-stage disease, owing to neck metastases [1, 2]. However, the unfavorable impact of metastasis on survival varies depending on several factors.

The presence of extracapsular spread (ECS) of tumor, which is usually considered one of the most important predictor of poor prognosis, is not included in N-staging system (Fig. 8.2). ECS has been associated with higher rates of regional nodal recurrence, as well as significantly lower survival rates [31, 32]. As expected, ECS correlates with the size of the metastatic node and is typically found in cases of nodal metastases >3 cm [33]. However, it must be kept in mind that approximately 20 % of all lymph node metastases with ECS are <1 cm in diameter [31, 33]. Although a correlation between the degree of ECS and prognosis has not yet been established, Cater et al. have reported that macroscopic ECS carries a poorer prognosis than that of microscopic ECS

Table 8.3 N-staging system for carcinoma of the oral cavity

Nx	Regional lymph nodes cannot be assessed
N0	No regional lymph node metastases
N1	Metastasis in a single ipsilateral lymph node, 3 cm or less in greatest dimension
N2	Metastasis in a single ipsilateral lymph node, more than 3 cm but not more than 6 cm in greatest dimension; or in multiple ipsilateral lymph nodes, none more than 6 cm in greatest dimension; or in bilateral or contralateral lymph nodes, none more than 6 cm in greatest dimension
N2a	Metastasis in a single ipsilateral lymph node more than 3 cm but not more than 6 cm in greatest dimension
N2b	Metastasis in multiple ipsilateral lymph nodes, none more than 6 cm in greatest dimension
N2c	Metastasis in bilateral or contralateral lymph nodes, none more than 6 cm in greatest dimension
N3	Metastasis in a lymph node more than 6 cm in greatest dimension

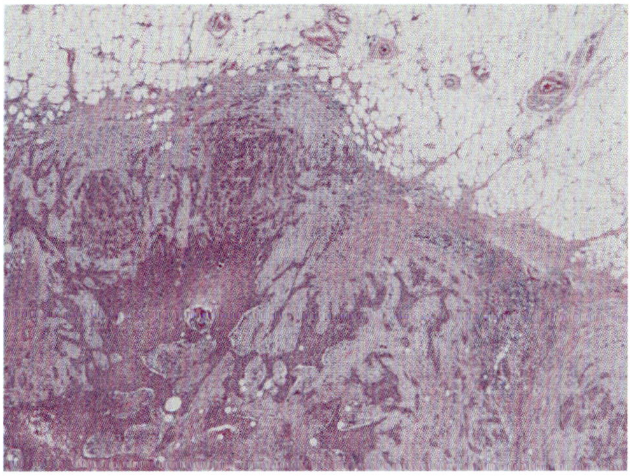

Fig. 8.2 Extracapsular spread of tumor

[34]. In addition, the number of involved nodes affects the patient's survival, i.e., survival rates are significantly lower when multiple nodes are involved [2]. The level in which the neck metastases occur, which is also not included in N-staging system, also is a significant factor in patient survival. Several studies have suggested that survival decreases as lymph nodes in lower levels of the neck become involved [35, 36].

8.7 Principles of Neck Treatment

Early-stage regional node metastasis (clinically N1) can be treated with equal success by using either surgery or radiation therapy. In general, the choice of treatment modality is dictated by the modality selected to treat the primary tumor. For advanced cervical metastases (clinically N2 or N3), a combined approach of surgery and postoperative radiation or chemoradiation therapy is usually indicated. Management of the clinically negative (N0) neck is a subject of controversy.

8.7.1 Classification of Neck Dissection

Since the original description of radical neck dissection (RND) given by Crile in 1906, neck dissection has been the accepted standard treatment for regional metastases [37]. RND was popularized by Martin et al. in the 1950s [38], and since that time, surgical treatment of regional node metastases has mainly been RND. However, during the past few decades, RND has been modified in various ways on the basis of our increased understanding of the pattern of lymph node metastasis and the need to decrease postoperative morbidity [39].

The most recent classification of neck dissection was published in 2002 as a consensus statement proposed by the American Head and Neck Society and the American Academy of Otolaryngology – Head and Neck Surgery and was primarily driven by the need to refine the selective neck dissection (SND) nomenclature [4] (Table 8.4).

- RND is the standard basic procedure for the dissection of cervical lymph node levels I–V with simultaneous resection of the sternocleidomastoid muscle, internal jugular vein, and accessory nerve.
- In modified radical neck dissection (MRND), levels I–V are also dissected, but with the preservation of one or more nonlymphatic structures (sternocleidomastoid muscle, spinal accessory nerve, and internal jugular vein) routinely removed in RND (Figs. 8.3 and 8.4).
- In SND, one or more lymph node groups/levels routinely removed in RND are preserved (Figs. 8.5 and 8.6).
- The operation is called extended neck dissection (END) when additional lymph node groups or nonlymphatic structures (muscles, blood vessels, and nerves) are dissected (Figs. 8.7 and 8.8).

In the current classification of neck dissection revised in 2002, surgery is no longer referred to as supraomohyoid neck dissection (SOHND), but rather as SND (I–III). The same applies for extended SOHND or anterolateral neck dissection—now referred to as SND (I–IV). This classification system is also intended to include notation that accounts for

Table 8.4 Classification of the neck dissection

Radical neck dissection (RND)
Modified radical neck dissection (MRND)
Selective neck dissection (SND)
SND (I–III)
SND (I–IV)
SND (II–IV)
Extended neck dissection (END)

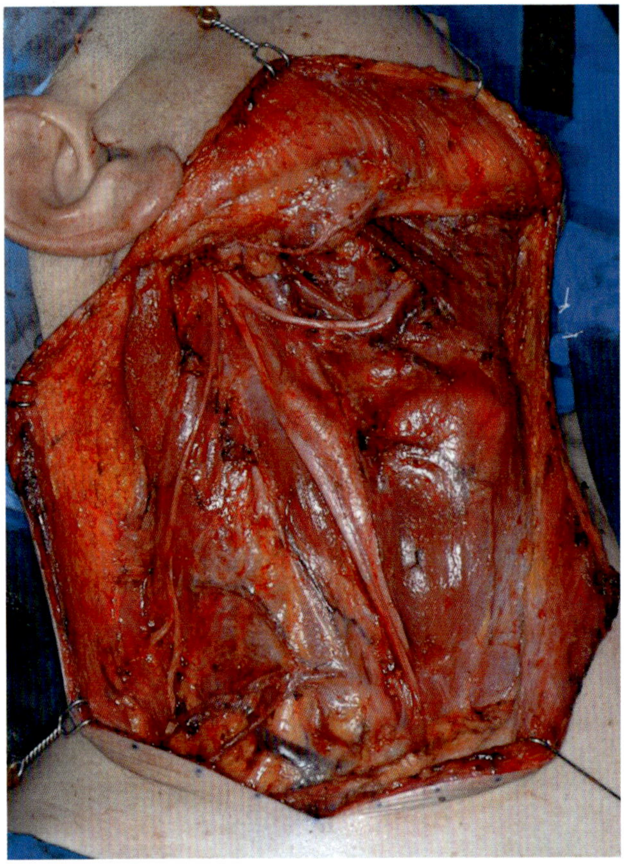

Fig. 8.3 Lateral view of the surgical field after MRND (spinal accessory nerve preserved: digastric and stylohyoid muscles included in the surgical specimen)

other regional nodal groups that are removed during neck dissection, such as the facial or retropharyngeal nodes, for example, which would be indicated by using SND (I–III facial nodes or I–III retropharyngeal nodes).

8.7.2 Neck Node Management

It is well known that cervical lymph node status is one of the most important prognostic factors in patients with OSCC.

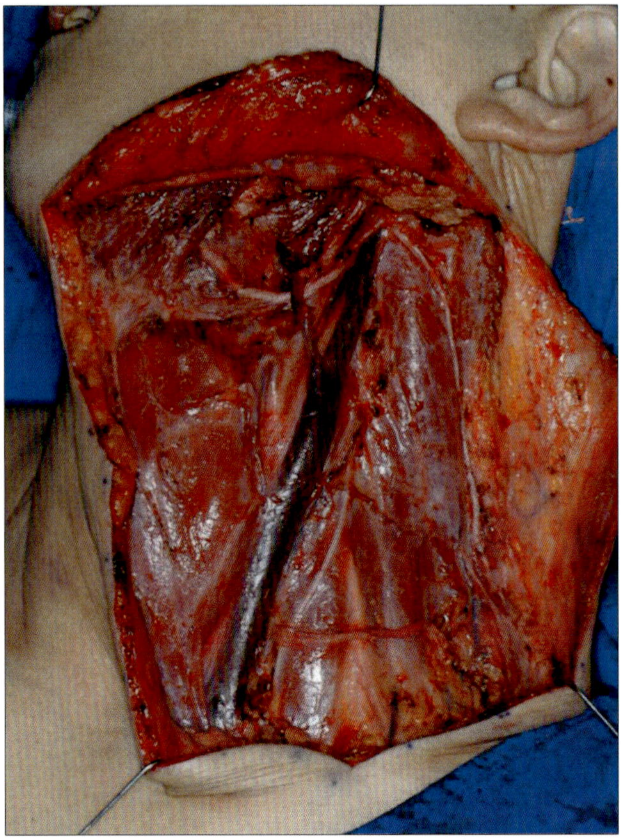

Fig. 8.4 Lateral view of the surgical field after MRND (spinal accessory nerve and internal jugular vein preserved: digastric and stylohyoid muscles included in the surgical specimen)

8.7.2.1 Characteristics of Primary Tumor Influencing Nodal Metastasis

Various characteristics of the primary tumor such as the location, size, T stage, and other clinicopathological features influence the risk of regional node metastasis. SCCs of the floor of the mouth and tongue are more likely to metastasize to cervical nodes than those of the hard palate. Larger tumor size or advanced T stage increases the risk for nodal metastasis [40]. Morphological characteristics of the primary tumor that increase the risk of nodal metastasis include an endophytic rather than exophytic pattern of growth and an increased depth of invasion [41]. Predisposing histological factors that indicate a higher risk of nodal metastasis include a poorer degree of differentiation, lymphovascular invasion by the tumor, and perineural infiltration, as well as a higher grade of malignancy or invasiveness of the tumor front [42–46].

8.7.2.2 Management of N0 Neck

Management of the clinically N0 neck in patients with OSCC is currently a controversial issue, specifically in terms of whether patients should undergo observation or elective treatment.

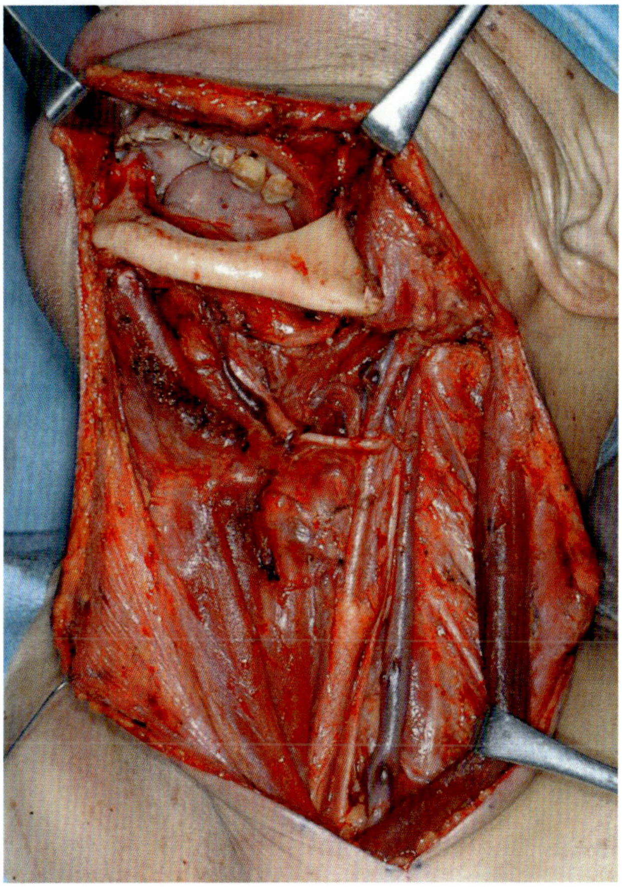

Fig. 8.5 Lateral view of the surgical field after marginal mandibulectomy and SND (I–IV) (digastric, stylohyoid and mylohyoid muscles included in the surgical specimen)

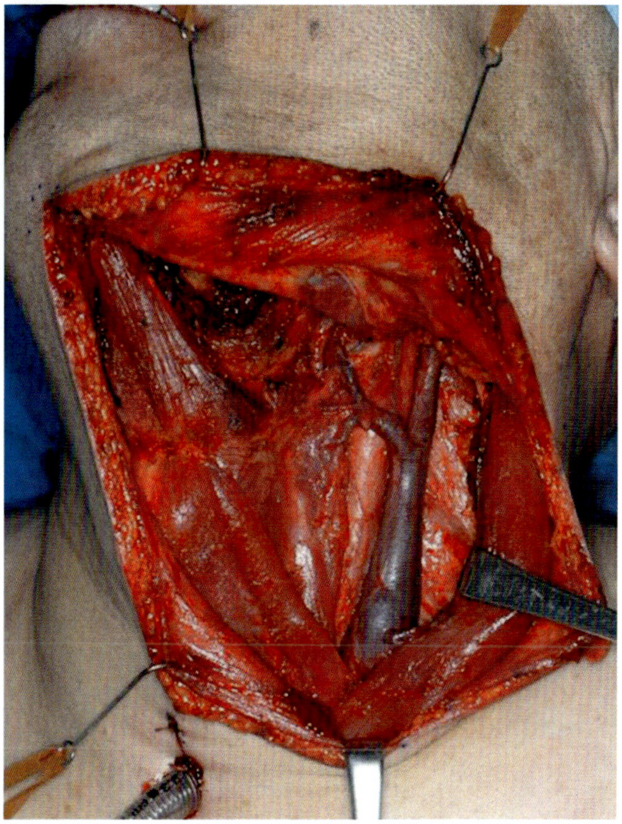

Fig. 8.6 Lateral view of the surgical field after partial glossectomy and SND (I–III) (digastric, stylohyoid, and mylohyoid muscles included in the surgical specimen)

Elective management of the neck is based on the following premises: (1) untreated occult metastasis invariably progresses to clinically evident metastasis; (2) occult metastasis increases the patient's risk of developing additional regional metastases and distant metastases; and (3) regional metastases may be unresectable when they are detected [47, 48]. For these reasons, elective treatment for the neck is often considered. However, there are no definite guidelines for the treatment of the clinically N0 neck. Therefore, in most institutions, elective management of the neck is warranted when the risk of occult metastasis is >20 % [49]. Treatment is also indicated when the patient is unlikely to return for close follow-up. Furthermore, elective neck dissection is indicated when the neck has need to be entered either for resection of the primary tumor (e.g., mandibulotomy) or reconstruction (e.g., free tissue transfer).

The modality of elective treatment is dictated by the modality selected to treat the primary tumor, which may include neck dissection or external beam irradiation. Elective neck dissection offers a distinct advantage over observation or elective neck irradiation, i.e., it provides important prognostic information that can be used for treatment planning, such as the need for adjuvant treatment [50]. When neck dissection is indicated, SND (I–III) is generally required. However, because "skip metastasis" to level IV nodes has been documented in up to 15 % of patients with tongue SCC, SND that addresses levels I–IV is advocated in such cases [10]. Recent prospective multi-institutional studies have demonstrated that sublevel IIB is rarely involved by isolated metastasis from OSCCs, except in some tongue SCC cases. Thus, it is justifiable to omit the dissection of sublevel IIB in the elective treatment of most OSCC cases [51].

Elective neck irradiation is generally performed when the primary tumor is treated by using radiotherapy. Radiation portals usually cover levels I to III as with neck dissection, with a minimum dose equivalent to 45–50 Gy over 4.5–5 weeks [52, 53].

8.7.2.3 Management of N1–3 Neck

The generally accepted approach to treating regional node metastasis is surgery, usually with postoperative radiotherapy. The type and extent of neck dissection performed is influenced by several factors, including the site of the primary tumor, treatment modality for the primary tumor, extent of nodal metastasis, and invasion of nonlymphatic structures.

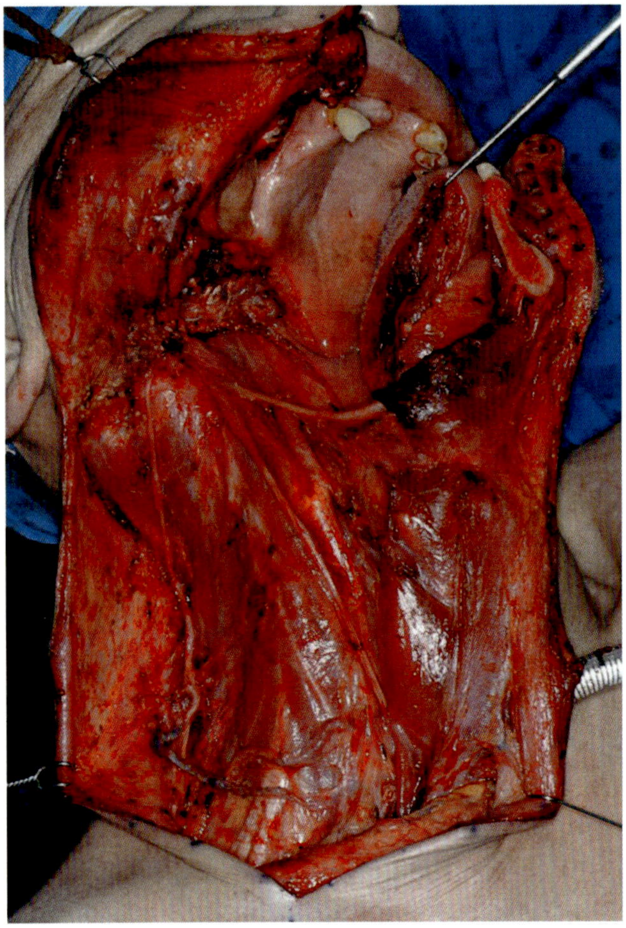

Fig. 8.7 Anterolateral view of the surgical field after partial glossectomy, lateral pharyngectomy, and END (retropharyngeal nodes dissected: digastric and stylohyoid muscles included in the surgical specimen)

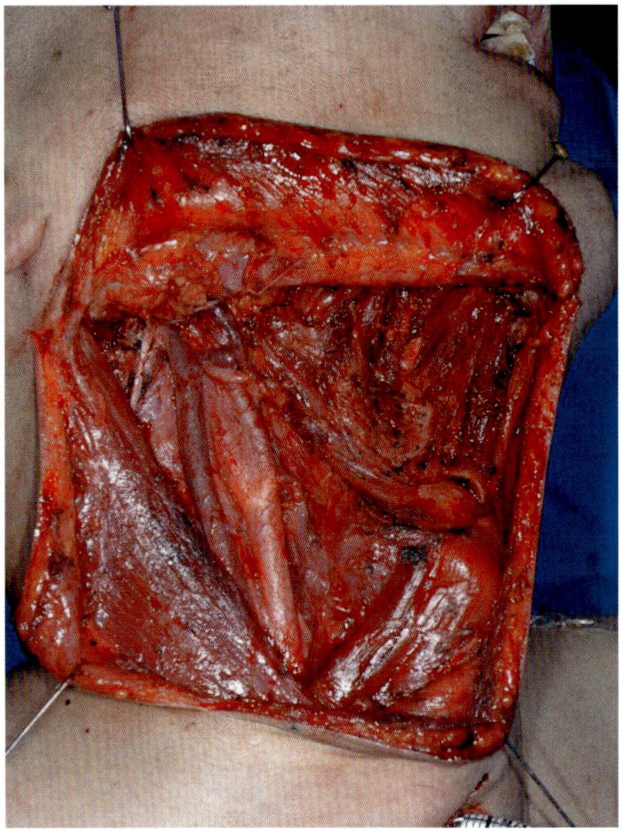

Fig. 8.8 Lateral view of the surgical field after partial glossectomy and END (right half of the hyoid bone removed: digastric, stylohyoid, and mylohyoid muscles included in the surgical specimen)

In general, for the clinically N1 neck, MRND is usually performed [54]. However, SND (I–III or I–IV) may be also indicated for patients with a single mobile node in level I or II [55, 56]. Usually, postoperative radiation therapy is recommended if multiple nodes are involved or ECS is present [57].

For patients with the clinically N2 neck, RND or MRND is recommended with postoperative radiotherapy or chemoradiotherapy. In some selected cases, SND (I–IV) is applicable. In N2c cases, MRND or SND (I–III or I–IV) should be considered for the less involved side of the neck.

In the treatment of the clinically N3 neck, MRND can be attempted, but usually RND is required in combination with adjuvant radiotherapy or chemoradiotherapy.

OSCCs can also metastasize to the nodes situated outside the region treated by using RND. These include the facial nodes and retropharyngeal nodes [6–8], and they are dissected in combination with some type of ND procedure (END).

Because patients with multiple node metastases or ECS often present with neck failure and/or distant metastasis after neck dissection, postoperative radiotherapy or concomitant chemoradiotherapy is recommended [58, 59]. In such cases, the dose of radiation therapy should be at least 60 Gy to the entire operative field, and 66 Gy to the site at increased risk for recurrence, such as the site wherein ECS was detected. Concomitant cisplatin (100 mg/m^2) is usually administered every 3 weeks. Moreover, radiation therapy should begin as soon as possible, no later than 6 weeks after surgery [60, 61].

8.7.2.4 Treatment Outcome

Regional recurrence rates in the pathologically N0 neck are consistently low, at 3–7 %, irrespective of the treatment modality. Recurrence rates following neck treatment vary depending on other factors, such as control of the primary tumor, ECS, and the pathological N stage. In cases where the primary tumor has been controlled, overall recurrence rates are approximately 10–15 % for N1 disease without ECS, 20–30 % for N2 disease, and as high as 70 % for N3 disease [62, 63]. Adjuvant radiotherapy decreases the regional recurrence rate by approximately half for all stages of the disease.

Conclusions

Management of regional disease in patients with OSCC remains one of the most challenging issues for head and neck surgeons. Appropriate management requires a full understanding of the incidence, patterns, evaluation methods, and prognostic implications of regional metastasis as well as the available treatment, consisting of surgery, radiotherapy, and/or chemotherapy.

References

1. Schuller DE, McGuirt WF, McCabe BF et al (1980) The prognostic significance of metastatic cervical lymph nodes. Laryngoscope 90: 557–570
2. O'Brien CJ, Smith JW, Soong SJ et al (1986) Neck dissection with and without radiotherapy: prognostic factors, patterns of recurrence and survival. Am J Surg 152:456–463
3. Ferito A, Robbins KT, Medina JE et al (2002) Is it time to eliminate confusion regarding cervical lymph node levels according to the scheme originated at the Memorial Sloan-Kettering Cancer Center? Acta Otolaryngol 122:805–807
4. Robbins KT, Clayman G, Levine PA et al (2002) Neck dissection classification update. Revisions proposed by the American Head and neck society and the American academy of otolaryngology-head and Neck surgery. Arch Otolaryngol Head Neck Surg 128: 751–758
5. Robbins KT, Shaha AR, Medina JE et al (2008) Consensus statement on the classification and terminology of neck dissection. Arch Otolaryngol Head Neck Surg 134:536–538
6. Sheahan P, Colreavy M, Toner M et al (2004) Facial node involvement in head and neck cancer. Head Neck 26:531–536
7. Harada H, Omura K (2009) Metastasis of oral cancer to the parotid node. Eur J Surg Oncol 35:890–894
8. Umeda M, Shigeta T, Takahashi H et al (2004) Metastasis to the lateral retropharyngeal lymph node from squamous cell carcinoma of the oral cavity: report of three cases. Int J Oral Maxillofac Surg 38:1004–1008
9. Shah JP (1990) Patterns of cervical lymph node metastasis from squamous cell carcinomas of the upper aerodigestive tract. Am J Surg 160:405–409
10. Byers RM, Weber RS, Andrews T et al (1997) Frequency and therapeutic implications of 'skip metastases' in the neck from squamous cell carcinoma of the oral tongue. Head Neck 19:14–19
11. Rapoport A, Ortellado DK, Dedivitis RA (2009) Rationale for selective neck dissection in N+oral cancer. Int Surg 94:339–343
12. Sako K, Pradier RN, Marchetta FC et al (1964) Fallibility of palpation in diagnosis of metastasis to cervical nodes. Surg Gynecol Obstet 118:989–990
13. Ali S, Tiwari RM, Snow GB (1985) False positive and false negative neck nodes. Head Neck 8:78–82
14. Baatenburg De Jong RJ, Rongen RJ, Lameris JS et al (1989) Metastatic neck disease. Palpation vs ultrasound examination. Arch Otalaryngol Head Neck Surg 115:689–690
15. van den Breckel MW, Castelijns JA, Stel HV et al (1993) Modern imaging techniques and ultrasound-guided aspiration cytology for assessment of neck node metastases: a prospective comparative study. Eur Arch Otorhinolaryngol 250:11–17
16. Stern WB, Silver CE, Zeifer BA et al (1990) Computed tomography of the clinically negative neck. Head Neck 12:109–113
17. Friedman M, Shelton VK, Mafee M et al (1984) Metastatic neck disease. Evaluation by computed tomography. Arch Otolaryngol 110:443–447
18. Yucel T, Saatci I, Sennaroglu L et al (1997) MR imaging in squamous cell carcinoma of the head and neck with no palpable lymph nodes. Acta Radiol 38:810–814
19. Curtin HD, Ishwaran H, Mancuso AA et al (1998) Comparison of CT and MR imaging in staging of neck metastases. Radiology 207:123–130
20. Curtin HD, Weissman JL (1996) Radiologic evaluation of head and neck cancer. In: Myers EN, Suen JY (eds) Cancer of the Head and Neck, 3rd edn. WB Saunders, Philadelphia
21. Ng SH, Yen TC, Chang JT et al (2006) Prospective study of [18 F] fluolodeoxyglucose positron emission tomography and computed tomography and magnetic resonance imaging in oral cavity squamous cell carcinoma with palpably negative neck. J Clin Oncol 24:4371–4376
22. Nahmias C, Carlson ER, Duncan LD et al (2007) Positron emission tomography/computerized tomography (PET/CT) scanning for preoperative staging of patients with oral/head and neck cancer. J Oral Maxillofac Surg 65:2524–2535
23. de Bondt RB, Nelemans PJ, Hofman PA et al (2007) Detection of lymph node metastases in head and neck cancer: a meta-analysis comparing US, USgFNAC, CT and MR imaging. Eur J Radiol 64:266–272
24. Peters BR, Schnadig VJ, Quinn FB Jr et al (1989) Intraobserver variability in the interpretation of fine-needle aspiration biopsy of head and neck masses. Arch Otolaryngol Head Neck Surg 115: 1438–1442
25. McGuirt WF, McCabe BF (1978) Significance of node biopsy before definitive treatment of cervical metastatic carcinoma. Laryngoscope 88:594–597
26. Robbins KT, Cole R, Marvel J et al (1991) The violated neck: cervical node biopsy prior to definitive treatment. Otolarygol Head Neck Surg 117:60–61
27. Ellis ER, Mendenhall WM, Rao PV et al (1991) Incisional or excisional neck-node biopsy before definitive radiotherapy, alone or followed by neck dissection. Head Neck 13:177–183
28. Terada A, Hasegawa Y, Yatabe Y et al (2011) Follow up after intra operative sentinel node biopsy of N0 neck oral cancer patients. Eur Arch Otorhinolaryngol 268:429–435
29. Melkane AE, Mamelle G, Wycisk G et al (2012) Sentinel node biopsy in early oral squamous cell carcinomas: a 10-year experience. Laryngoscope 122:1782–1788
30. Broglie MA, Haerle SK, Huber GF et al (2013) Occult metastases detected by sentinel node biopsy in patients with early oral and oropharyngeal squamous cell carcinomas: impact on survival. Head Neck 35:660–666
31. Snow GB, Annyas AA, van Slooten EA et al (1982) Prognostic factors of neck node metastasis. Clin Otolaryngol 7:185–192
32. Johnson JT, Barnes EL, Myeres EN et al (1981) The extracapusular spread of tumors in cervical node metastasis. Arch Otolaryngol 107:725–729
33. Carter RL (1993) The pathologist's appraisal of neck dissection. Eur Arch Otorhinolaryngol 250:429–431
34. Carter RL, Barr LC, O'Brien CJ (1985) Transcapsular spread of metastatic squamous cell carcinoma. Am J Surg 150:495–499
35. Spiro RH, Alfonso AE, Farr HW et al (1974) Cervical node metastasis from epidermoid carcinoma of the oral cavity and oropharynx. A critical assessment of current staging. Am J Surg 128:562–567
36. Mendelson BC, Woods JE, Beahrs OH (1976) Neck dissection in the treatment of carcinoma of the anterior two thirds of the tongue. Surg Gynecol Obstet 143:75–80
37. Crile G (1906) Excision of cancer of the head and neck. With special reference to the plan of dissection based on one hundred and thirty-two operation. JAMA 47:1780–1786

38. Martin H, Del Valle B, Ehrlich H et al (1951) Neck dissection. Cancer 4:441–449
39. Robbins KT, Medina JE, Wolfe GT et al (1991) Standardizing neck dissection terminology. Official report of the academy's committee for head and neck surgery and oncology. Arch Otolaryngol Head Neck Surg 117:601–605
40. Byers RM, El-Naggar AK, Lee YY et al (1998) Can we detect or predict the presence of occult nodal metastases in patients with squamous cell carcinoma of the tongue? Head Neck 20:138–144
41. Spiro RH, Huvos AG, Wong GY et al (1986) Predictive value of tumor thickness in squamous carcinoma confined to the tongue and floor of the mouth. Am J Surg 152:345–350
42. Rubio Bueno P, Naval Gias L, Garcia Delgado R et al (1998) Tumor DNA content as a prognostic indicator in squamous cell carcinoma of the oral cavity and tongue base. J Sci Spec Head Neck 20:232–239
43. Fagan JJ, Collins B, Barnes L et al (1998) Perineural invasion in squamous cell carcinoma of the head and neck. Arch Otolaryngol Head Neck Surg 124:637–640
44. Woolgar JA, Scott J (1995) Prediction of cervical lymph node metastasis in squamous cell carcinoma of the tongue/floor of mouth. J Sci Spec Head Neck 17:463–472
45. Yamamoto E, Miyakawa A, Kohama G (1984) Mode of invasion and lymph node metastasis in squamous cell carcinoma of the oral cavity. Head Neck 6:938–947
46. Bryne M, Koppang HS, Lilleng R et al (1992) Malignancy grading of deep invasive margins of oral squamous cell carcinomas has high prognostic value. J Pathol 166:375–381
47. Shasha D, Harisson LB (1998) Elective irradiation of the N0 neck in squamous cell carcinoma of the upper aerodigestive tract. Otolaryngol Clin North Am 31:803–813
48. Andersen PE, Cambronero E, Shaha AR et al (1996) The extent of neck disease after regional failure during observation of the N0 neck. Am J Surg 172:689–691
49. Weiss MH, Harrison LB, Isaacs RS (1994) Use of decision analysis in planning a management strategy for the stage N0 neck. Arch Otolaryngol Head Neck Surg 120:699–702
50. Greenberg JS, El Naggar AK, Mo V et al (2003) Disparity in pathologic and clinical lymph node staging in oral tongue carcinoma. Implication for therapeutic decision making. Cancer 98:508–515
51. Ferlito A, Silver CE, Rinaldo A (2009) Elective management of the neck in oral cavity squamous carcinoma: current concepts supported by prospective studies. Br J Oral Maxillofac Surg 47:5–9
52. Fletcher GH (1972) Elective irradiation of subclinical disease in cancers of the head and neck. Cancer 29:1450–1454
53. Mendenhall WM, Million RR, Cassisi NJ (1980) Elective neck irradiation in squamous-cell carcinoma of the head and neck. Head Neck 3:15–20
54. Byers RM, Wolf PF, Ballantyne AJ (1988) Rationale for elective modified neck dissection. Head Neck 10:160–167
55. Byers RM (1985) Modified neck dissection: a study of 967 cases from 1970 to 1980. Am J Surg 150:414–421
56. Traynor SJ, Cohen JI, Gray J et al (1996) Selective neck dissection and the management of the node-positive neck. Am J Surg 172: 654–657
57. Amdur RJ, Parson JT, Mendenhall WM et al (1989) Postoperative irradiation for squamous cell carcinoma of the head and neck: An analysis of treatment results and complications. Int J Radiat Oncol Biol Phys 16:25–36
58. Bernier J, Domenge C, Ozsahin M et al (2004) Postoperative irradiation with or without concomitant chemotherapy for locally advanced head and neck cancer. N Engl J Med 350:1945–1952
59. Cooper JS, Pajak TF, Forastiere AA et al (2004) Postoperative concurrent radiotherapy and chemotherapy for high-risk squamous-cell carcinoma of the head and neck. N Engl J Med 350:1937–1944
60. Peters LJ, Goepfert H, Ang KK et al (1993) Evaluation of the dose for postoperative radiation therapy of head and neck cancer: First report of a postoperative randomized trial. Int J Radiat Oncol Biol Phys 26:3–11
61. Huang J, Barbera L, Brouwers M et al (2003) Does delay in starting treatment affect the outcomes of radiotherapy? A systematic review. J Clin Oncol 21:555–563
62. Mastronikolis NS, Fitzgerald D, Owen C et al (2005) The management of squamous cell carcinoma of the neck. The Birmingham UK experience. Eur J Surg Oncol 31:461–466
63. Chan SW, Mukesh BN, Sizeland A et al (2003) Treatment outcome of N3 nodal head and neck squamous cell carcinoma. Otolaryngol Head Neck Surg 129:55–60

9 Oral and Maxillofacial Reconstruction

Satoshi Yokoo and Tadaaki Kirita

Abstract

The content of this chapter does not include general textbook or ordinary items understandable by everyone. No general flap elevation or reconstruction method is described. Described are practices of pre- and postoperative management of oral and maxillofacial reconstructive surgery and in the operation room. The sole objective of the practices is to clarify how to prepare reconstruction materials reliably, safely, and efficiently, to restore defecting oral and maxillofacial regions, and maintain the reconstructed condition. This chapter has been written for reconstructive surgeons already performing surgeries at the forefront of the field of oral and maxillofacial reconstructive surgery.

Keywords

Biological life and Social life • Step-Surgery Concept • Functional Unit Reconstruction • Stereolithographic mandibular model (SLMN)

9.1 General Principles

9.1.1 Disability/Rehabilitation Medicine and Maintenance of Social Life

Considering the importance of maintaining QOL in recent medical care and its social implications, resection of a lesion with the aim of only prolonging life has become a thing of the past, even in cancer therapy. The oral and maxillofacial system is important for not only the maintenance of life, such as food ingestion, mastication, and swallowing, but also communication through conversation and facial expression, i.e., social interaction. Although resection of oral cancer lesions prolongs and maintains the "biological life" of patients, impairment causes economic difficulty attributed to inability to work and social isolation. Oral and maxillofacial reconstruction and rehabilitation, i.e., resumption of "social life," has to be carried out with the aim of "disability medicine"-based "holistic rehabilitation (right to live a normal life)" [1, 2] (Fig. 9.1).

Impairment of function after extensive resection of oral cancer can be anticipated when "cancer" is diagnosed, surgery can be planned upon the occurrence of impairment [1, 2], and a rehabilitation plan can be designed before the impairment. These steps provide a clear advantage not available upon sudden onset of cerebrovascular disorders or accidents.

After surgical treatment of oral cancer, subsequent pre- and postoperative rehabilitation by specialists (otorhinolaryngology-head and neck surgeons, oral and maxillofacial surgeons, plastic and reconstructive surgeons, speech-language-hearing therapists, nurses, and clinical psychologists) is essential. It is therefore necessary for medical professionals to cooperate with one another for the benefit of the patients to whom they provide medical care and to facilitate their return to normal social life.

S. Yokoo, D.M.D., D.M.Sc
Department of Stomatology and Maxillofacial Surgery, Gunma University Graduate School of Medicine, 3-39-22 Showa-machi, Maebashi, Gunma 371-8511, Japan
e-mail: syokoo@gumma-u.ac.jp

T. Kirita, D.D.S., D.M.Sc. (✉)
Department of Oral and Maxillofacial Surgery, Nara Medical University, 840 Shijo-cho, Kashihara, Nara 634-8521, Japan
e-mail: tkirita@naramed-u.ac.jp

T. Kirita and K. Omura (eds.), *Oral Cancer: Diagnosis and Therapy*,
DOI 10.1007/978-4-431-54938-3_9, © Springer Japan 2015

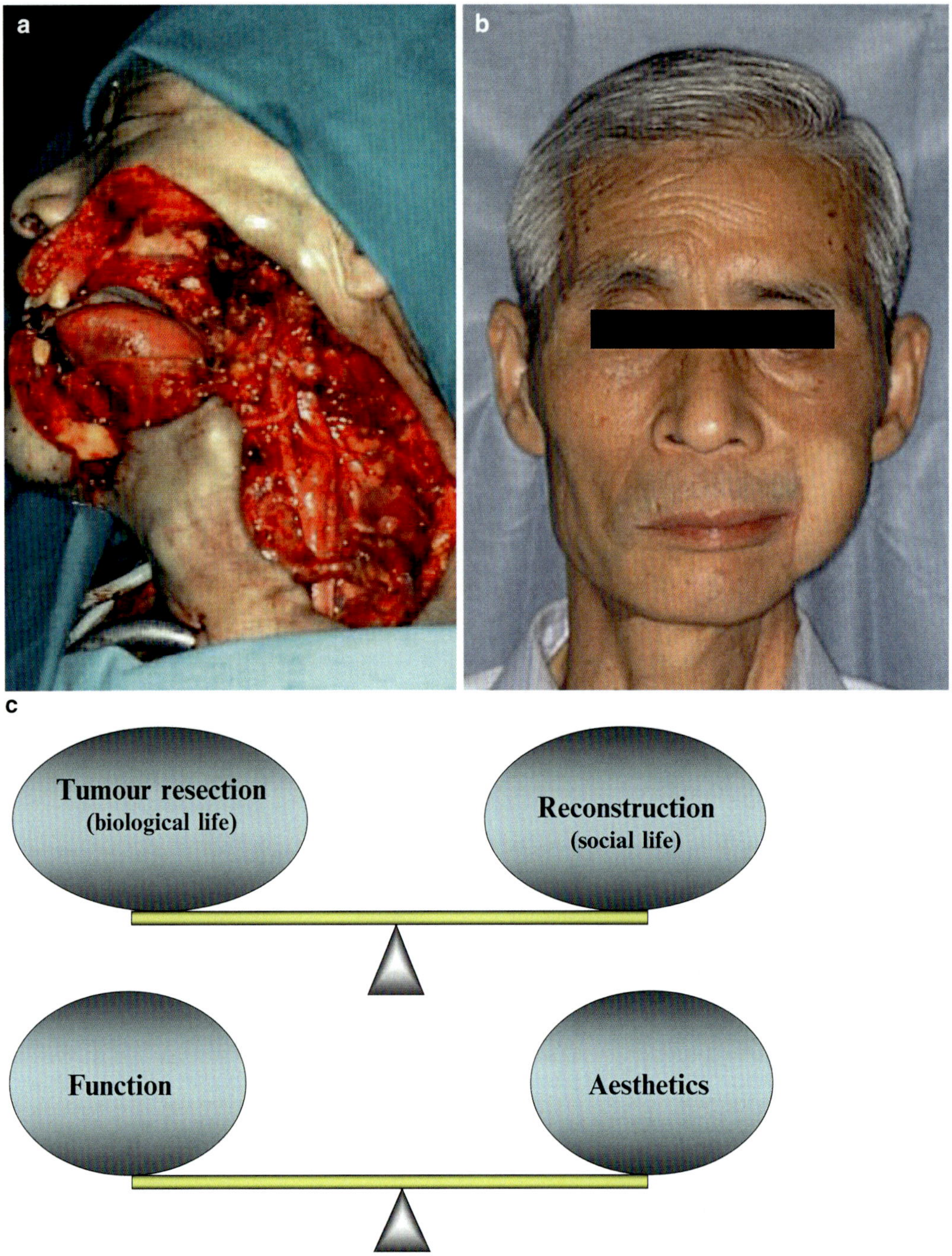

Fig. 9.1 Disability/rehabilitation medicine and maintenance of social life. (**a**) Tumor resection: maintenance of biological life. (**b**) Reconstruction and disability/rehabilitation medicine: maintenance of social life. (**c**) Oral cancer therapy today: treatment of the cancer itself and disability/rehabilitation medicine for any resulting impairment are essential, just like a set of wheels, and reconstructive surgery fills the role of an axle connecting these wheels

In cancer treatment, "treatment of the cancer itself" and "disability/rehabilitation medicine" for any resulting impairment are essential, just like a set of wheels, and reconstructive surgery fills the role of an axle connecting these wheels.

Reconstructive surgery is a science and an art. To achieve favorable outcomes, surgeons need to select transplantation procedures through which they can perform to their best and utilize their skills. Oral and maxillofacial reconstruction requires both functionality and aesthetics to which due consideration is requisite, despite the difficulties of the reconstruction.

9.1.2 Step-Surgery Concept

In oral and maxillofacial reconstructive surgery, there are two concepts regarding the principle of facial reconstruction methodology: (1) restoration of defects with facial and neck tissue, particularly with adjacent tissue if possible, and (2) unit principle, that is, reconstruction of each facial unit with color and texture. The former is feasible with regard to color and texture compatibility. The latter is subdivided from the aesthetic units [3] to sub- [4, 5] and mini-units [6]. Initial reconstruction with adjacent facial and neck tissue (applying the unit principle as needed) is conducive to acceptable outcomes for small facial defects. For moderate or more severe defects, however, the outcome of this initial reconstruction with adjacent tissue has often been unsatisfactory. Particularly, when the defect extends over 2 or more units or full thickness, reproducing the outline of each unit and its three-dimensional contour using the skin flap and graft is challenging because predicting and controlling three-dimensional changes induced by postoperative contracture and gravity is difficult. Moreover, when the optimum adjacent tissue for the reconstruction of the defect has already been used in the initial surgery, the most desirable outcome cannot, in many cases, be obtained by repeated revisions.

As a therapeutic policy for moderate or more severe full-thickness facial defects, we propose the step-surgery concept: (1) In *the initial step*, only filling and transplantation of minimum supporting tissue necessary for the restoration of function by free flap transplantation is carried out, and the surrounding tissue is conserved, (2) in *the touch-up step*, aesthetic surgery by transplantation of necessary supporting tissue is carried out with the use of a local facial/neck flap and skin graft, (3) as much cutaneous surface exposed on the face as possible is replaced with the facial/neck skin in *the touch-up step*, and (4) all the steps are planned as a series before surgery. Treatment based on this concept provides two advantages: (1) the free skin and musculocutaneous flaps transplanted in *the initial step* serve as a host side with abundant blood circulation, making secondary aesthetic surgery with a local skin flap easy, and (2) since the exposed cutaneous surface is resected after confirming time-course changes in the transplanted free flap, and since secondary surgery is carried out accordingly, the outline and contour are readily reproduced. When the cutaneous surface of the free flap is exposed on the face, differences of color match, texture, and thickness between the flap and the surrounding tissue present serious aesthetic problems; replacing the free flap with skin of the face/neck is desirable [7, 8]. When free flaps are used in reconstructive surgery, the importance of aesthetic outcomes should be taken into consideration.

The case presented here is of a 51-year-old man with recurrent squamous cell carcinoma of the left buccal mucosa after external irradiation (65 Gy). Resection of the full-thickness cheek, oral commissure, and vermilion was carried out. The number of defective units was 3, and there was no supporting tissue. The defects of full thickness of the cheek, upper lip, and oral commissure were reconstructed with free forearm and vermilion advancement flaps *in the initial step*, and aesthetic revision with a malar flap and a skin graft was carried out in the *touch-up step*. The outcome was acceptable. For patients who receive ≥50-Gy of irradiation, as in the present case, *the initial step* with the use of free skin or musculocutaneous flaps is very important (Fig. 9.2).

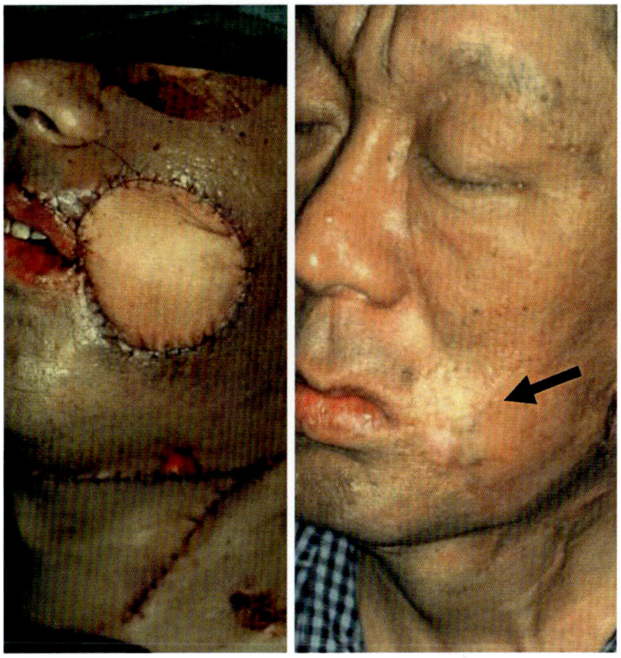

Fig. 9.2 Step-surgery concept. A 51-year-old man with recurrent squamous cell carcinoma of the left buccal mucosa after external irradiation (65 Gy). The defects of full thickness of the cheek, upper lip, and oral commissure (the number of defective units was 3, and there was no supporting tissue) were reconstructed with free forearm and vermilion advancement flaps in *the initial step*, and aesthetic revision with a malar flap and a skin graft was carried out in *the touch-up step*. For patients who receive ≥50 Gy of irradiation, as in the present case, *the initial step* with the use of free skin and musculocutaneous flaps is very important

9.2 Practice of and Strategy for Oral and Maxillofacial Reconstruction

9.2.1 Free Radial Forearm Flap

9.2.1.1 Role of Perforating Vein in Vascular Pedicle

The vascularized free forearm flap reported by Yang et al. [9] is now recognized as one of the most useful means for reconstructive surgery. Because of its long length, the large diameter of the blood vessel, and the flexibility of the cutaneous portion, it is widely used, particularly for head and neck, oral, and maxillofacial reconstruction [10–12]. The radial artery is generally used as the feeding artery. Two options for the drainage vein are the cephalic vein and radial comitant vein [9, 13]. The cephalic vein is generally selected because

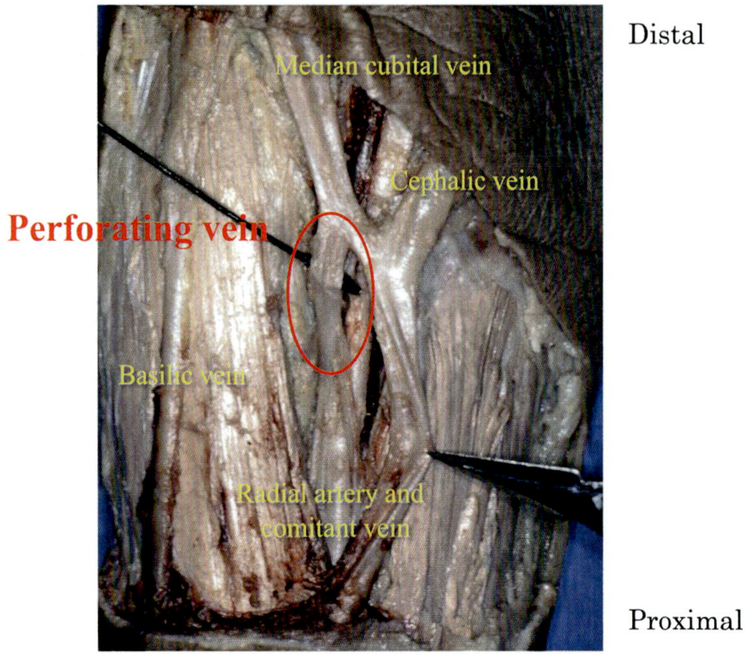

Fig. 9.3 Perforating vein. The perforating vein communicates between the radial comitant and cutaneous venous system

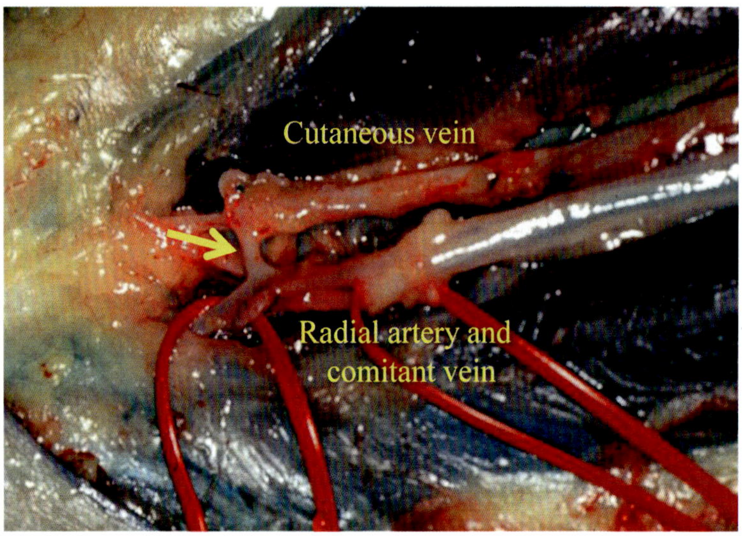

Fig. 9.4 Vascular pedicle of the forearm flap. The *arrow* indicates the perforating vein communicates between two venous systems

comitant veins in the forearm are very thin and not necessarily useful for vascular anastomosis. We have focused on the perforating vein connecting the deep venous and cutaneous venous systems since 1987 and have elevated it included in the vascular pedicle of forearm flaps. The perforating vein is situated anterior to the cubital fossa and is described in the first edition of Grant's Atlas of Anatomy (1943). It branches from the radial comitant vein at a site slightly distal to the bifurcation of the radial and ulnar arteries and joins the medial cubital or radial cephalic vein (Fig. 9.3). The deep venous system comprises the radial comitant vein and comitant vein of the proximal brachial artery. The cutaneous venous system comprises the cephalic, medial cubital, and basilic veins. Thus, the perforating vein connects the deep and cutaneous venous systems (Fig. 9.4).

In conventional elevation of the forearm flap, only one of the two drainage vein systems is used—the cutaneous or deep venous system. By including the perforating vein in the vascular pedicle, however, both systems can be used for drainage through single venous anastomosis. Soutar et al. [11] have pointed out that the two venous systems of the forearm are connected through a vein flowing into the medial cubital vein. In this context, Evans et al. [14] have also pointed out that when the vascular pedicle is dissected at a

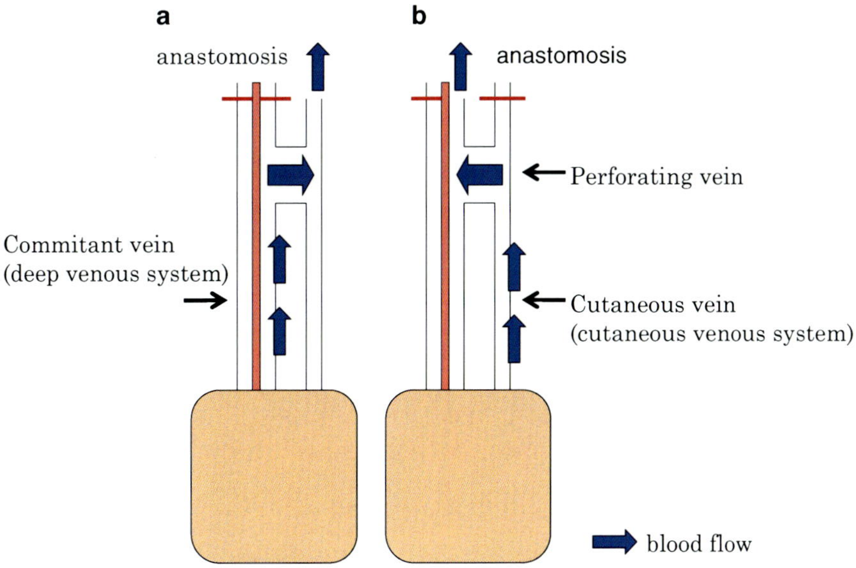

Fig. 9.5 Perforating vein as "oscillating vein." Venous drainage through the two systems is possible by anastomosis of either the cutaneous and deep vein. The absence of venous valve in the perforating vein and its surroundings has been confirmed. The blood flow of the perforating vein may differ between cutaneous and deep vein anastomosis. This corresponds to the "oscillating vein"

site more proximal than at the perforating vein, circulation of the two systems is achieved by a single venous anastomosis. Timmons et al. [15] also have described the anatomical presence of a vein with a large diameter connecting the two venous systems. Thoma et al. [16] have demonstrated that the vena comitans generally joins the cephalic vein through another vein with a large diameter at a site anterior to the cubital fossa: a venous drainage pattern connecting the two venous systems through this other vein has been shown in 65 % of head and neck reconstruction cases with forearm flaps. These anastomosed veins are identical to the perforating vein described by us.

The usefulness of the perforating vein is summarized below. Venous drainage through the two systems is possible by anastomosis of either the cutaneous or deep vein. We have confirmed the absence of a venous valve in the perforating vein and its surroundings. Therefore, blood flow in the perforating vein may differ between cutaneous and deep vein anastomosis (Fig. 9.5). This corresponds to the "oscillating vein" proposed by Taylar et al. [17]. Timmons et al. [15] have demonstrated anatomically that, generally, the direction of venous valves in the comitant vein is determined so as to maintain the direction of blood flow from the deep to the cutaneous venous system, suggesting that this is the standard direction. Accordingly, inclusion of the comitant vein in the drainage system may provide a more advantageous circulatory condition, particularly for initial drainage after reperfusion. We have demonstrated this experimentally [18, 19]. Even when only the cutaneous vein is anastomosed, the perforating vein is capable of maintaining drainage through the comitant vein and reducing congestion of the flap in the initial phase after reperfusion, compared with drainage through only the cutaneous vein. Even when a flap is elevated with the radial artery and vein, excluding the cutaneous vein in the distal forearm, the cutaneous vein with a large diameter in the cubital fossa can be used for vascular anastomosis due to the connection through the perforating vein (Fig. 9.6). For example, women with very thin cutaneous veins difficult to identify and patients with unusable forearm cutaneous veins because of chemotherapy are good candidates for this method.

The drawbacks of this method are: (1) vascular ligation up to the brachial artery and vein is complex, (2) ligation and division of a vein with a large diameter in the cubital fossa may cause edema [16], and (3) a slightly long scar is unavoidable because the skin incision is extended to the cubital fossa.

9.2.1.2 Simple Dressing Technique Using Polyurethane Foam for Fixture of Skin Grafts

Various methods of grafting skin, including tie-over dressing, are used depending on the location, area, and shape of the graft [20–23]. We use polyurethane foam (Allevyn Hydrocellular Dressing® (AHD®), Smith & Nephew, Largo, FL) and polyurethane film (Tegaderm®, 3M, St Paul, MN) to affix a skin graft to the flap-donor region of the forearm. The procedure

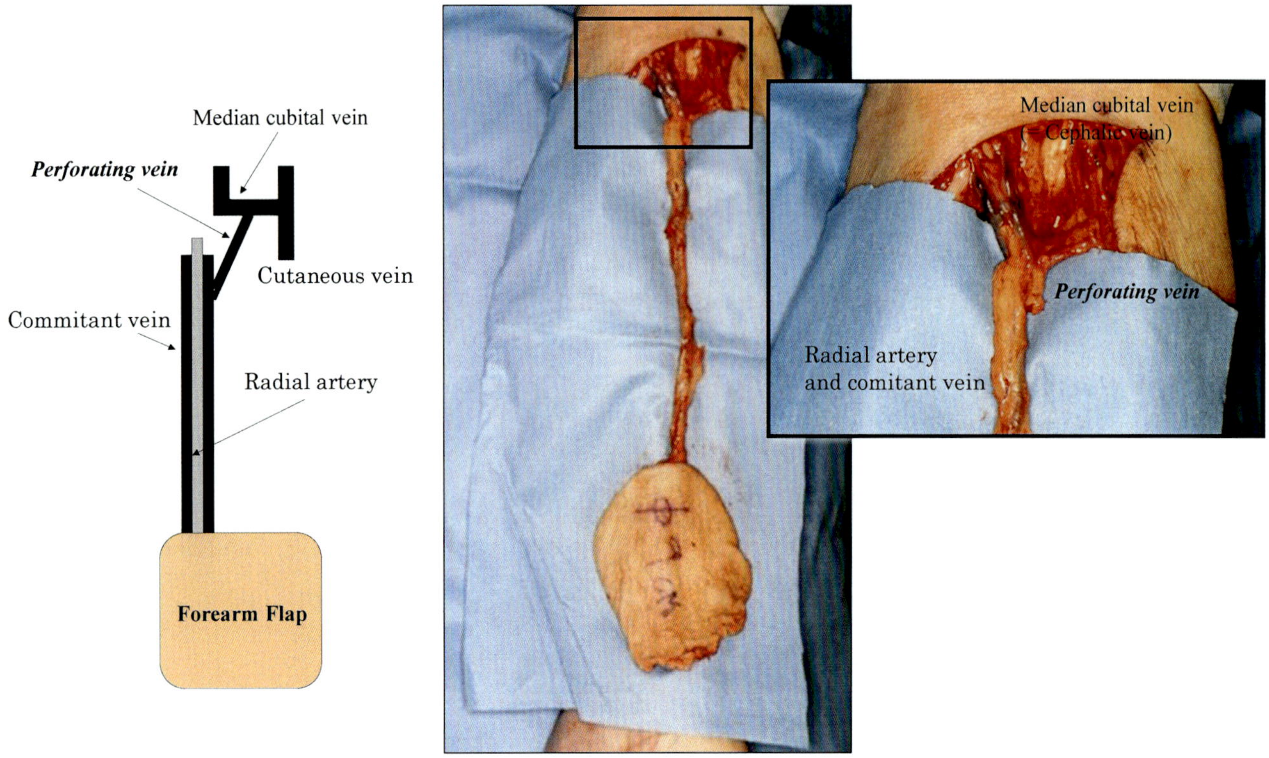

Fig. 9.6 Usefulness of the perforating vein. Even when only the cutaneous vein is anastomosed, the perforating vein is capable of maintaining drainage through the comitant vein (deep venous system). Even when a flap is elevated with the radial artery and vein, excluding the cutaneous vein in the distal forearm, the cutaneous vein with a large diameter in the cubital fossa can be used for vascular anastomosis due to the connection through the perforating vein

comprises four steps: (1), a skin graft is sutured to the wound remaining elevating a forearm flap, and the donor bed is washed well with physiological saline, and a small hole for drainage is made or a quilted suture is used, as needed (Fig. 9.7a), (2) a sheet of polyurethane foam (AHD)® of almost the same size as that of the skin graft is placed over the skin graft and covered with another sheet about 1–2 cm wider (Fig. 9.7b), (3) the two AHD® sheets are affixed with adhesive polyurethane film (Tegaderm®), and (4) the procedure is completed with bandage.

The duration of fixture is the same as that for tie-over dressing, but this is not strictly specified because the fixture can be readily repeated at bedside. When grafting skin to the forearm, heed should be paid to the formation of hematoma and to partial necrosis attributed to overpressure [24, 25]. Favorable grafts are obtained by fixtures at about 10 mmHg [26]. The surface of the wound on the forearm flap-donor region becomes uneven because of exposure of the tendon. Application of even pressure onto the wound surface is difficult, and the conventional method may exert overpressure on convex regions. In our method, elastic AHD exerts appropriate pressure on the graft. Also, since two AHD sheets are tiered, the lower sheet fits the morphology of the skin defect and rules out dead space; the slightly larger upper sheet prevents detachment of the skin graft, and the polyurethane film (Tegaderm®) fortifies the fixture. The region of the skin graft heals flawlessly under a moist healing condition, and the postoperative treatment period is short (Fig. 9.7c).

9.2.1.3 Reflex Sympathetic Dystrophy After Free Radial Forearm Flap Elevation

Reflex sympathetic dystrophy (RSD) is an intractable chronic pain syndrome whereby persistent pain, edema, and abnormal sweating develop after trauma and surgery, mainly in the injured region, and the tissue finally atrophies [27]. Clinical symptoms are observed over the entire upper limb of the forearm flap-donor region—a complication after elevating a forearm flap—to which due attention should be paid.

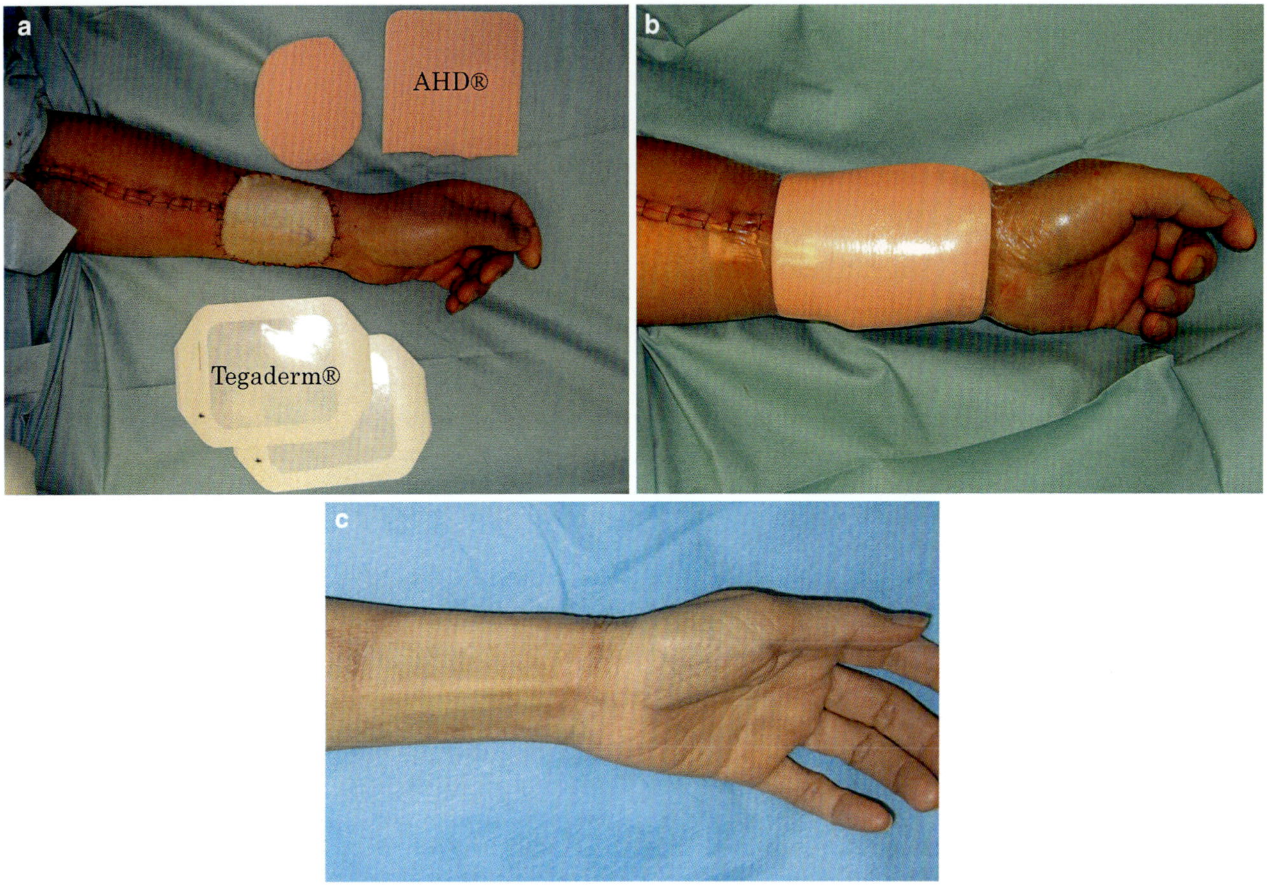

Fig. 9.7 Surgical procedure using polyurethane foam for fixture of skin graft. (**a**) The skin graft is fixed with 5-0 nylon suture and two sheets of polyurethane foam (AHD®) are placed on the skin graft: the first is one of the same size as the graft, and the second is one size larger to overlap by 1–2 cm the edges of the first sheet. (**b**) The ADHs are fixed with adhesive polyurethane film (Tegaderm®). Dressing is simple and easy without an assistant. The same procedure can be repeated at any time. (**c**) The region of the skin graft heals flawlessly, under a moist healing condition, and the postoperative treatment period is short

In the patient presented here, numbness and spontaneous pain developed mainly in the flap-donor region about 3 months after surgery (Fig. 9.8a, b). The range of symptoms gradually increased, and skin redness and edema appeared throughout the upper left limb about 6 months after surgery. One year after surgery, the patient developed a severe burning sensation throughout the limb induced by even a slight touch of clothing in the area, and then pain began to radiate to the left shoulder (Fig. 9.8c). Diagnosed with RSD at the Department of Anesthesia, the patient was treated with stellate ganglion block with 6 ml of 1 % lidocaine 3–4 times a month at a pain clinic. Skin redness and edema of the forearm remitted after 20 cycles of the treatment and were mostly resolved after 40 cycles (about 1 year)

In artificial synapse formation, a theory of the developmental mechanism of RSD, a synapse is artificially formed between nerve fibers in an injured peripheral nerve region, and sympathetic distal impulses are transmitted as pain to pain-transmitting fibers [28]. In this patient, an artificial synapse may have formed between the lateral antebrachial cutaneous nerve and the superficial branch of the radial nerve in the injured region of the forearm, inducing pain. Clinical diagnosis of RSD is based on a score established by Gibbons et al. [29] (Table 9.1). The patient's score was 5 based on the symptoms of pain hypersensitivity, burning sensation, skin color tone, and fluctuations in skin temperature, leading to our diagnosis of RSD. The principle of the management of RSD is early diagnosis and treatment, especially that progression to the chronic phase makes recovery difficult by any method of treatment. For RSD of the upper limbs, stellate ganglion block is the most effective. Edema and color change associated with the sympathetic nerve may be improved by

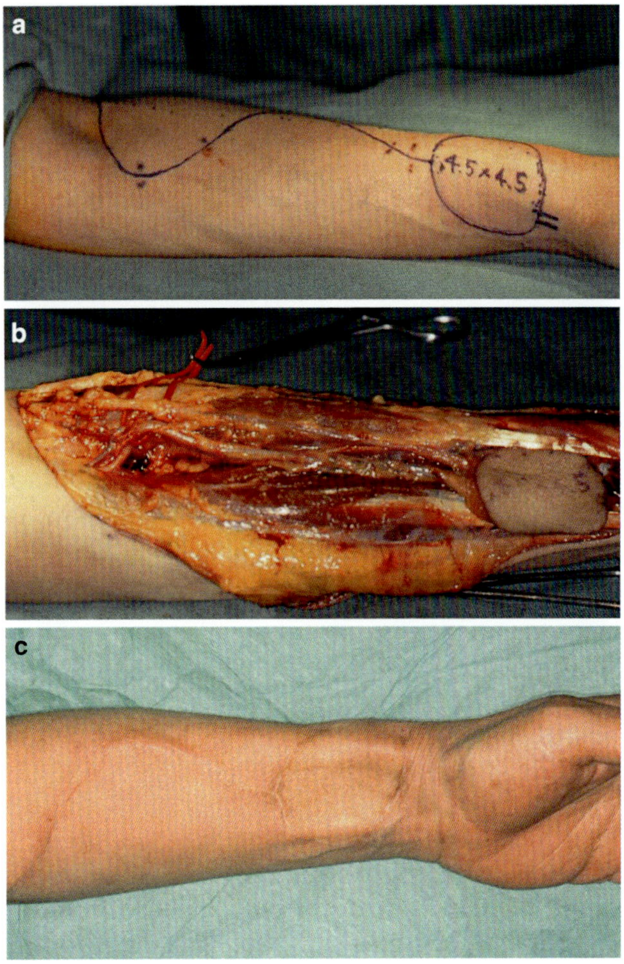

Fig. 9.8 A case of RSD after forearm flap elevation. (**a**) Design of forearm flap. (**b**) Elevation of forearm flap: lateral antebrachial cutaneous nerve and superficial branch of the radial nerve were resected in this case. (**c**) Severe burning sensation and tenderness were found at the left forearm, which rapidly spread to the upper limb after surgery

Table 9.1 RSD score

1. Allodynia or hyperpathia	1.0
2. Burning pain	1.0
3. Edema	0.5
4. Color or hair growth change	1.0
5. Sweating change	0.5
6. Temperature change	0.5
7. Radiographic change (demineralization)	0
8. Quantitative measurement of vasomotor/sudomotor disturbance	0
9. Bone scan consistent with RSD	0
10. Response to sympathetic block	0.5

For each criterion, the patient was assigned one point of positive, half-points for equivocal, and no points if the criterion was negative or not mentioned. Patients with a total RSD score of <3 were considered not to have RSD. Those with a score of 3–4.5 were considered possible RSD patients. Those with scores of ≥5 were considered probable RSD patients [21]

stellate ganglion block, but peripheral nerve block has in some studies been described as more effective.

9.2.2 Vascularized Free Rectus Abdominis Musculocutaneous Flap in the Oromandibular Region in Terms of Efficiency of the Anterior Rectus Sheath

The anterior rectus sheath is one of the firm lateral abdominal aponeuroses of the abdominal external oblique muscle. The efficiency of the sheath in reconstructive surgery has been demonstrated in the repair of full-thickness right ventricular defects after mediastinitis or sternal dehiscence [30], in the treatment of bronchopleural fistulas complicated by empyema [31], in pleural reconstruction of the chest wall [32], dural reconstruction [33], and breast reconstruction after subcutaneous mastectomy [34]. We have utilized this sheath in oromandibular reconstruction with the vascularized free rectus abdominis musculocutaneous flap (RAM). The RAM is effective in the maintenance of the formed bulge of the oral floor, prevention of the sinking of the reconstructed tongue, and prevention of the exposure of reconstruction plates after the resection of the mandibular continuity. Therefore, we consider that RAMs are absolutely indicated for these types of reconstruction (Table 9.2). As is important, the muscle attached to the rectus sheath is harvested with a 3- to 4-cm extension superiorly and inferiorly (Fig. 9.9). Extensive resection of the anterior rectus sheath caused no problems.

In the preparatory phase of swallowing, the tongue margin and the oral floor elevate, retaining the alimentary bolus in the oral cavity with glossopalatal closing function [35] (Fig. 9.10). In reconstructive flaps, however, this function is impaired: the bolus on the reconstructed oral floor cannot be moved to the dorsum of the tongue. When the oral floor is reconstructed with a thin flap, as with a forearm flap to reform it to the pre-resection state, a wide depression results, where saliva and food residues become awkwardly trapped. This makes smooth food transfer difficult, causing a time lag between glossopalatal closure and bolus transfer, as well as mistimed swallowing as a whole resulting in misswallowing [36]. For an efficient swallowing function, it is essential to raise the oral floor to a height similar to that of the tongue margin, thereby forming the preparatory phase of swallowing statically. In other words, the nonfunctioning oral floor should not be depressed. Even when the bulge of the floor is formed with thick and bulky reconstructive materials, like the musculocutaneous flap, the cutaneous and muscular portion, in time, generally sags because of gravity, resulting

Table 9.2 Purpose and devices of reconstruction with RAM

Resection procedure of primary tumor	Purpose of reconstruction	Device
Resection of the oral floor with hemiglossectomy	Preservation of swallowing	*Hammock technique*[a]
Total resection of the mobile tongue or more extensive resection	Preservation of swallowing and articulation	Money-pouch-like reconstruction[b] + *hammock technique* + cricopharyngeal myotomy + laryngeal suspension[c] + neuroanastomosis[d]
Resection of the mandibular continuity with oral defect	Prevention of reconstruction plate exposure	*Reinforcement of the muscular portion*

Italics: reconstruction on devices with anterior rectus sheath

[a]Mylohyoid muscle-like structure was reconstructed by attaching the anterior rectus sheath to the anterior and posterior mandible and hanging it in a hammock pattern

[b]Reconstructed tongue was rounded and markedly raised like a money pouch

[c]Fixation with mandible, hyoid bone, and thyroid cartilage

[d]Neuroanastomosis with the tenth intercostal and the hypoglossal nerves

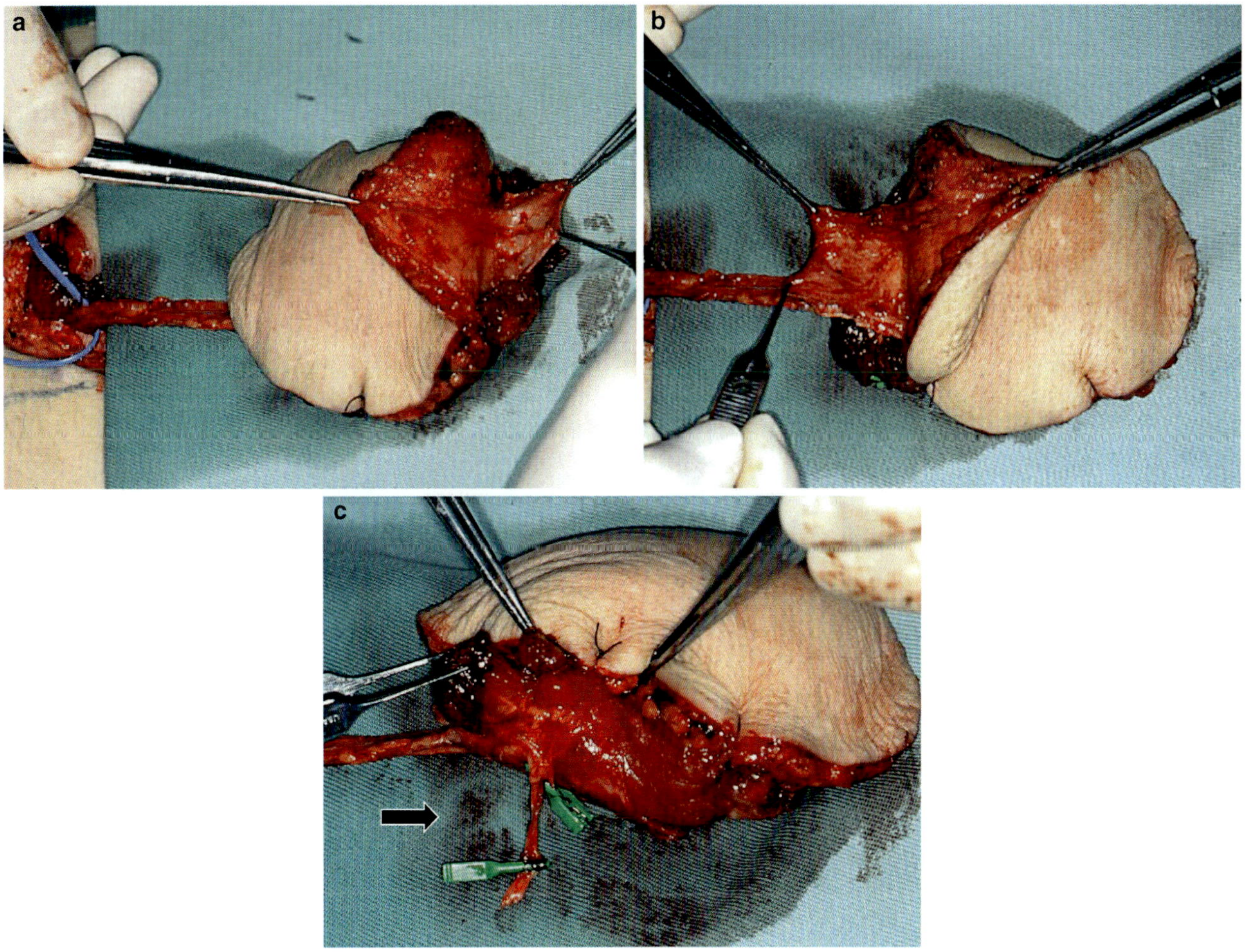

Fig. 9.9 Preparation of anterior rectus sheath and tenth intercostal nerve. Raising the RAM is designed so that the center of the flap is positioned at the paraumbilical region. The rectus sheath is obtained with proximal and distal extensions of about 3–4 cm each, which is particularly important to attain the final goal of reconstruction with the sheath (**a**, **b**). When the intercostal nerve is used in reconstruction, the tenth intercostal nerve as a motor nerve of the lower abdominal rectus abdominis muscle is carefully distinguished from the paraumbilical region (*arrow*: the tenth intercostal nerve) (**c**)

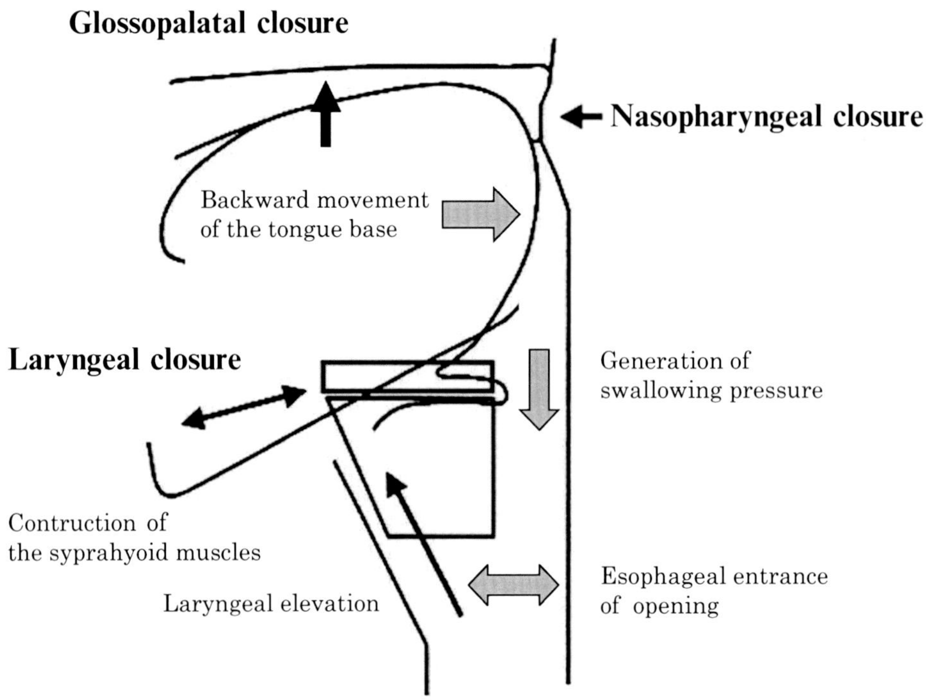

Fig. 9.10 Ideal static reconstruction of the oral and the pharyngeal phase of swallowing

in the depression of the oral floor. Therefore, we developed a method of forming the mylohyoid muscle-like tissue by fixing the anterior rectus sheath anteriorly and posteriorly to the mandibular areas in a hammock pattern. This protects the muscle from the influence of gravity, allowing the maintenance of the bulge and preventing the sinking of the reconstructed oral floor and tongue. We have termed this method *the hammock technique*, where a musculocutaneous flap with a firm anterior sheath is indispensable and where RAM is the optimal material. Although the mylohyoid muscle attaches to the hyoid bone, and elevates the oral floor and hyoid bone, in reconstructive surgery, the anterior sheath is not fixed at the hyoid bone because recovering the function by elevating the reconstructed oral floor is not possible even if such fixation is done. Conversely, fixation to the hyoid bone results in flap pulling and, consequently, in hindering the formation of the bulge of the reconstructed oral floor and the raising of the reconstructed tongue by the money-pouch-like reconstruction [37] (Figs. 9.11 and 9.12)

After total resection of the mobile tongue or more extensive resection, it is essential for the purpose of generating swallowing pressure to build the reconstructed tongue with height and roundness, to make the oropharyngeal space narrow, to provide the glossopalatal closing function, to maintain the mobility of the tongue base, and to avoid forming a gap to the posterior pharyngeal wall (Fig. 9.10). To achieve this outcome, the following techniques are essential: (1) *the hammock technique* (the bulge of the reconstructed oral floor is maintained, and the depression of the reconstructed tongue is prevented), (2) *the money-pouch-like reconstruction method* [37] (the tongue is reconstructed to give it height and roundness), (3) *neuroanastomosis* [35] [38] (the reinnervated muscle is used to maintain the bulk of the muscular portion of the RAM), (4) *cricopharyngeal myotomy*, and (5) *resection of the infrahyoid muscles* and *thyroid cartilage/hyoid bone/mandible fixation*. With these serial reconstruction procedures, the anatomical and functional structures of swallowing from the preparatory phase to the pharyngeal phase are statically reconstructed. Therefore, the residual tissues easily assist in the swallowing function.

In reconstruction after the resection of the mandibular continuity with oral defects, vascularized free osteocutaneous flaps are usually the first choice. When bone reconstruction is not possible because of insufficient conditions, however, mandibular continuity is restored with a reconstruction plate. The muscular portion and the anterior sheath are wrapped around the plate, whereby the anterior rectus sheath firmly reinforces the muscular portion. The flap margin is deepithelialized and submucosally inserted into the oral cavity; consequently the sheath on the muscular portion is further reinforced by the dermis. We term this method *the wrap-around technique* for mandibular reconstruction. To date, plate exposure has not been observed in any of the

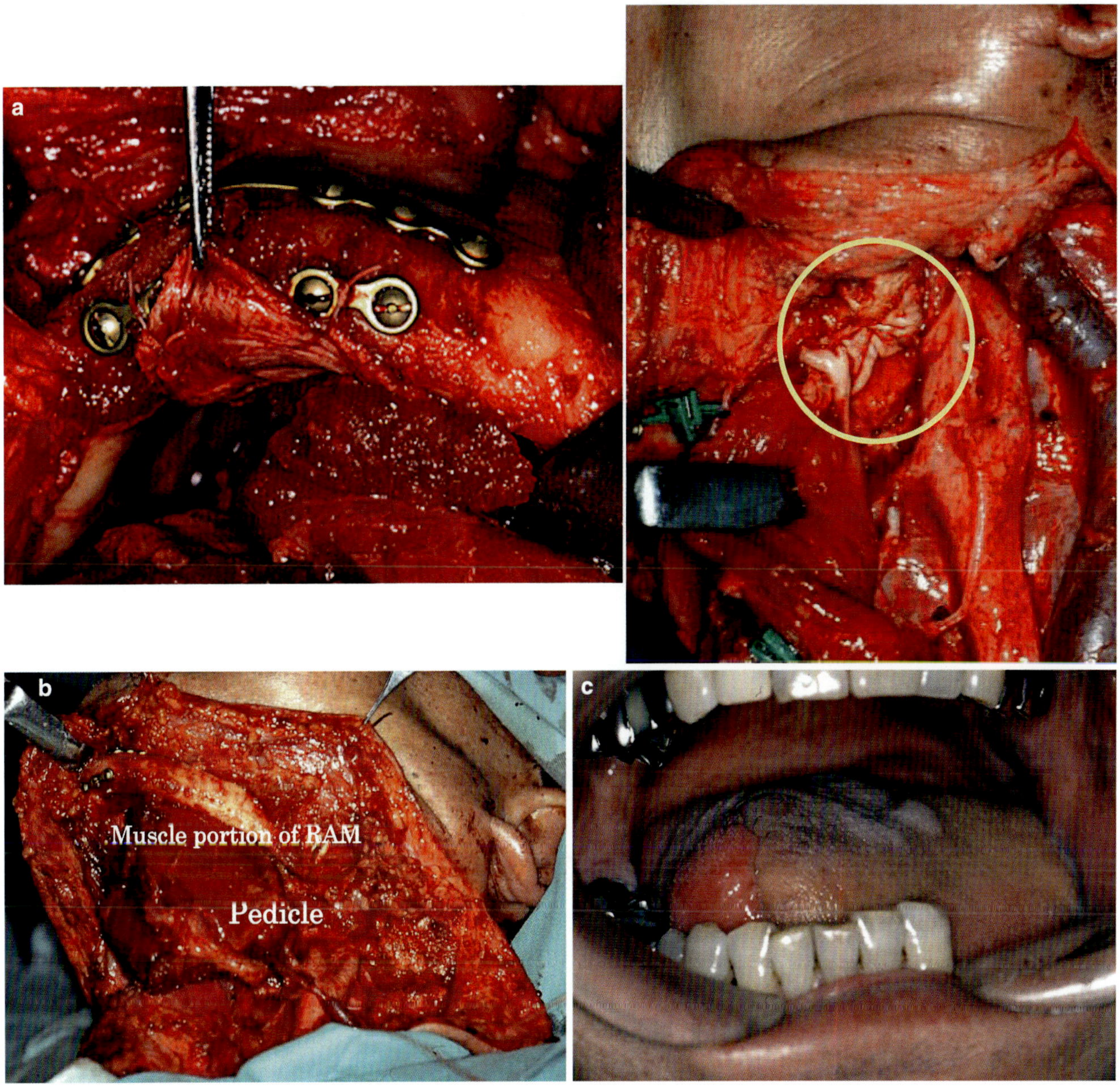

Fig. 9.11 Reconstruction after resection of oral floor with hemiglossectomy. A 67-year-old man with squamous cell carcinoma of the left oral floor (T3N1M0) underwent resection of the oral floor with hemiglossectomy and right radical neck dissection. *Hammock technique*: the anterior rectus sheath was fixed anteriorly and posteriorly to the mandible and hung in a hammock pattern (**a**, *round*: mandibular angle), forming a mylohyoid muscle-like structure (**b**). Simultaneously, the oral floor was reconstructed to form a bulge. Seven years after the operation, the bulge of the reconstructed oral floor was maintained without gravity-induced depression (**c**)

patients who underwent the procedures of this technique with the anterior rectus sheath (Fig. 9.13). After primary reconstructive surgery, usually 6 months thereafter, secondary generative mandibular reconstruction was carried out by implanting titanium mesh and particulate cancellous bone and marrow (PCBM) in the mandibular defect. A 3D model was prepared from CT images, and the mandibular morphology on the healthy side was reproduced in the defective side using the titanium mesh as a scaffold. PCBM collected from the posterior iliac crest was then buried in the rectus abdominis muscle. New bone formation was usually confirmed 3 months after the surgery, and regenerative mandibular reconstruction was completed in the next 6 months (Fig. 9.14).

Alternative to the muscle sheath alone, the tensor fascia lata flap may also serve as material for these reconstructions

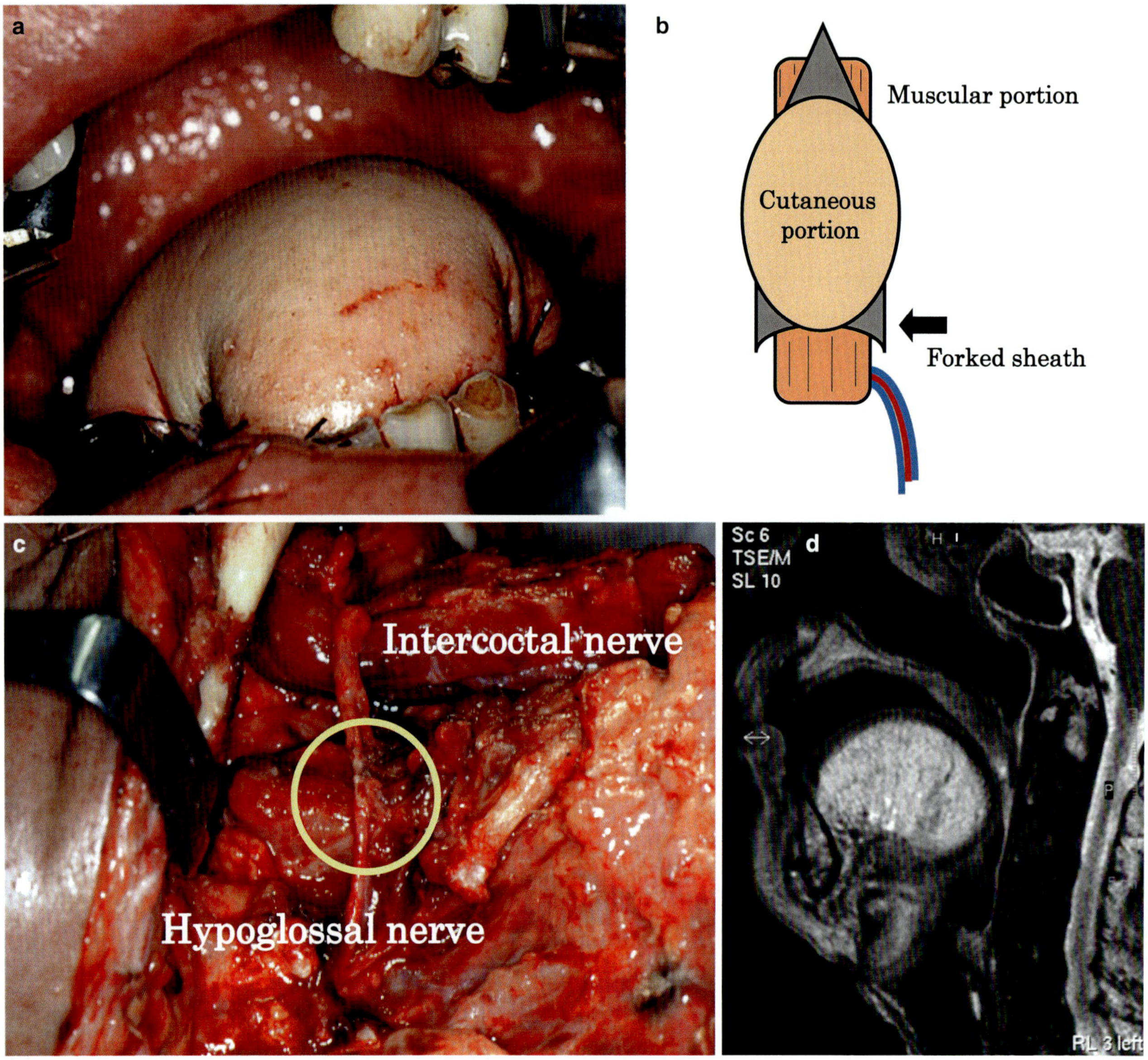

Fig. 9.12 Reconstruction after total glossectomy. A 51-year-old man with advanced squamous cell carcinoma of the right tongue (T3N2cM0) underwent total glossectomy and bilateral radical neck dissection. *Money-pouch-like reconstruction*: the reconstructed tongue was rounded and markedly raised by the money-pouch-like reconstruction method. This technique gave the reconstructed tongue glossopalatal closing, and the mobility of the tongue base was preserved (**a**). *Preparation of the proximal anterior rectus sheath*: the anterior rectus sheath was fixed anteriorly and posteriorly to the mandible, in a hammock pattern, to form a mylohyoid muscle-like structure and to prevent flap sinking. Since the posterior area is sutured to the bilateral sides of the molar areas, the sheath should be prepared in a *forked shape* (**b**). *Neuroanastomosis*: the intercostal nerve is anastomosed to the hypoglossal nerve to reinnervate the rectus abdominis muscle and to prevent fatty degeneration and atrophy (*round*: neuroanastomosis) (**c**). MRI after 6 months showing the absence of flap sinking of fatty degeneration and of atrophy of the rectus abdominis muscle (**d**)

[39]; however, RAM appears to be the most efficacious in terms of the facility of flap elevation, the wide caliber and long length of the pedicle, the flexibility of the cutaneous portion (especially, the application to three-dimensional reconstruction), and the maintenance of the bulk of the muscular portion by reinnervation.

9.2.3 Double Pedicled (DOP) and Supercharged (SUP) Pectoralis Major Musculocutaneous Flap

Although free tissue transfer is the preferred reconstruction option in most major oral and maxillofacial reconstructions, the pectoralis major musculocutaneous (PMMC) flap is

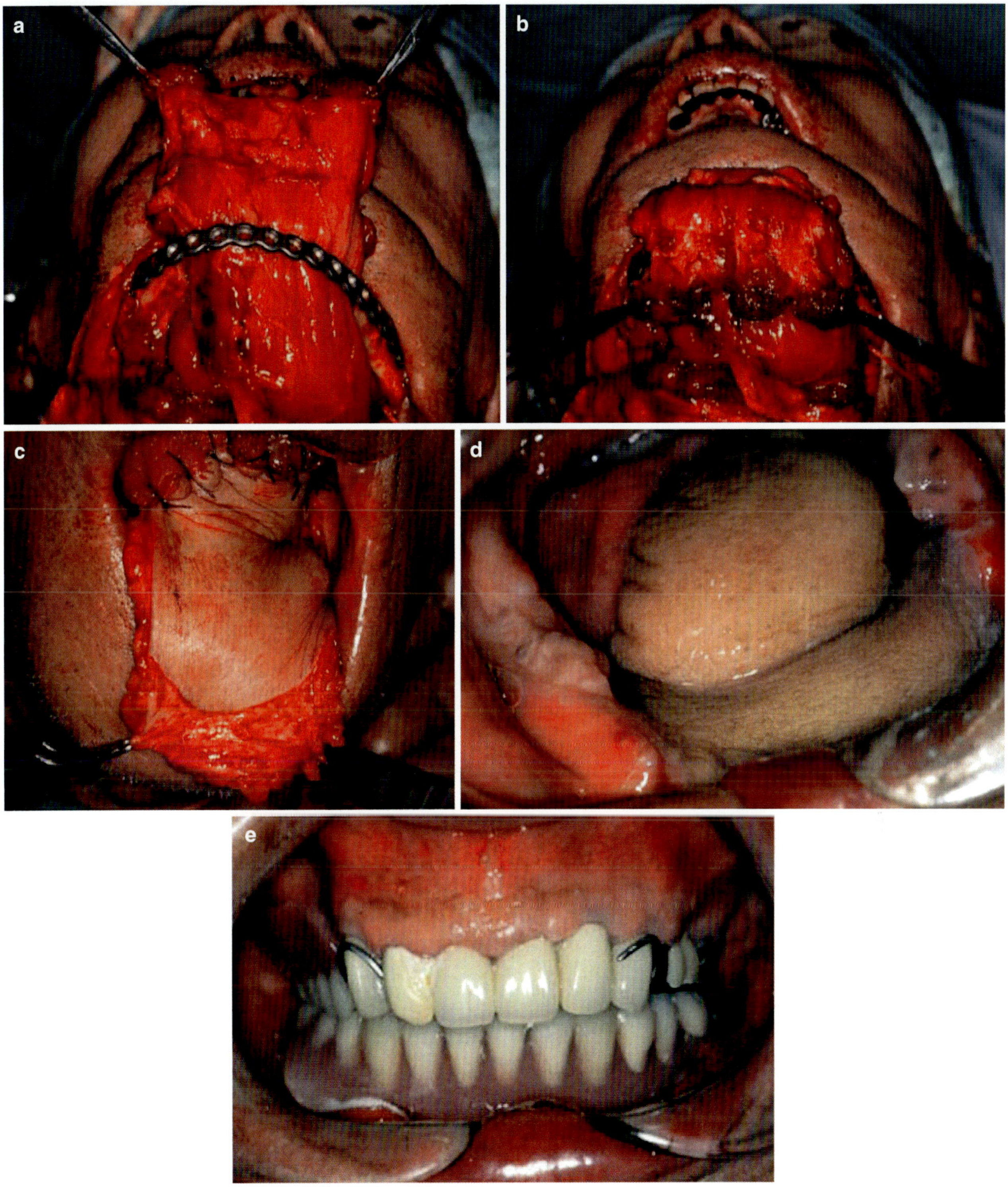

Fig. 9.13 The wrap-around technique for mandibular reconstruction. A 65-year-old man with squamous cell carcinoma of the left oral floor (T4N2bM0) underwent resection of the tumor, anterior hemoglossectomy, resection of the anterior mandibulectomy, and left radial and right supraomohyoid neck dissection. The muscular portion with the anterior rectus sheath was wrapped around the reconstruction plate. The anterior rectus sheath firmly reinforced the muscular portion (**a**, **b**). The flap margin was deepithelialized and submucosally inserted into the oral cavity, by which the sheath on the muscular portion was further reinforced by the dermis (**c**). No plate exposure was observed 4 years after operation (**d**). After mandibular denture application, masticatory function recovered (**e**)

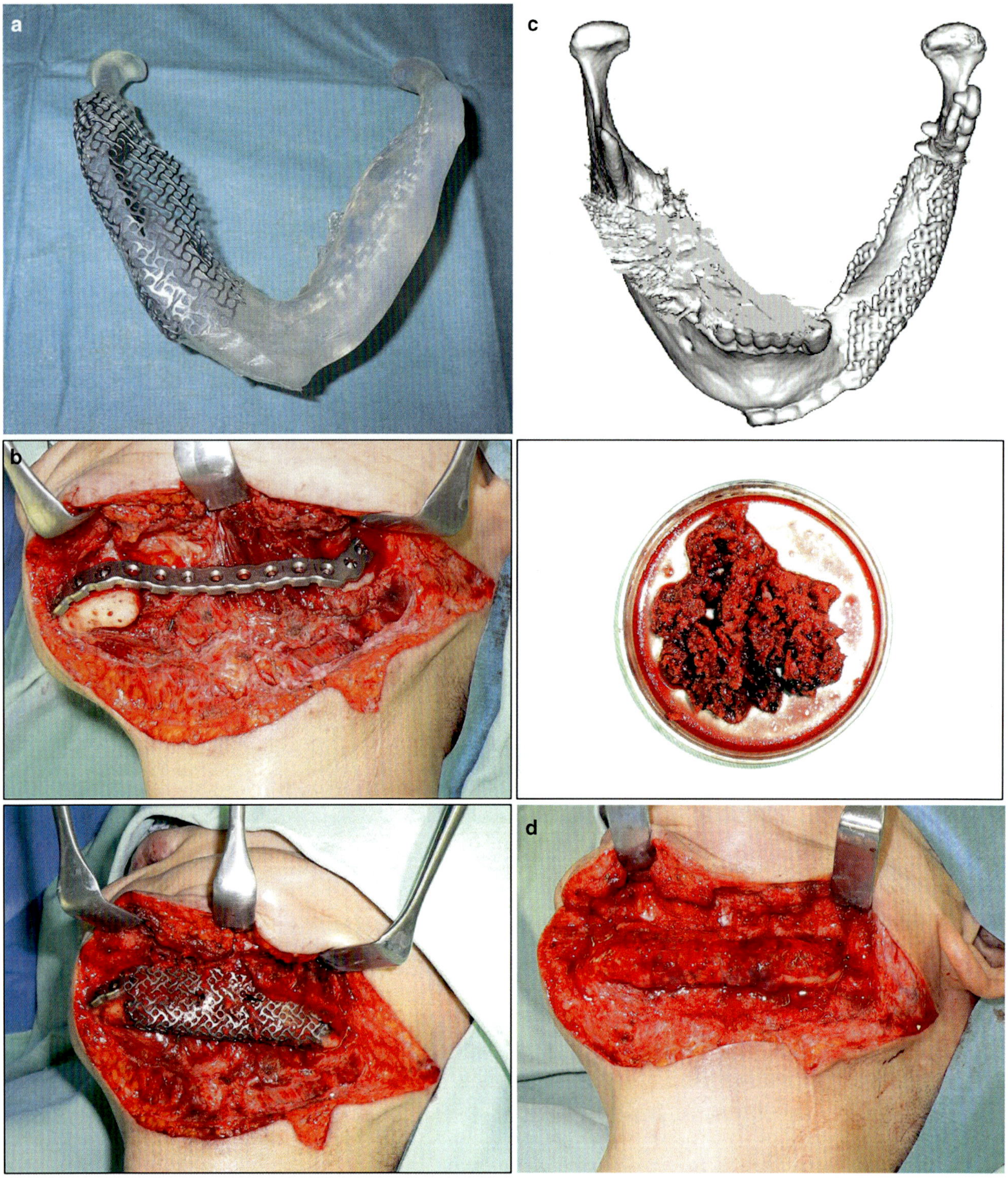

Fig. 9.14 Regenerative mandibular reconstruction. (**a**) A 3D model was prepared from CT images, and the mandibular morphology on the healthy side was reproduced in the defective side using the titanium mesh as a scaffold. (**b**) PCBM collected from the posterior iliac crest was buried in the rectus abdominis muscle. (**c**) New bone formation was confirmed 3 months after surgery. (**d**) Regenerative mandibular reconstruction was completed in the next 6 months

commonly used in the salvage of necrotic free flaps and is the first choice for patients who are not candidates for free flaps. The PMMC flap has a high incidence of distal skin necrosis, however, because of vascular insufficiency resulting in partial to total flap loss and fistula formation [40]. The pectoral branch of the thoracoacromial artery is the main blood supply to the skin island overlaying the upper part of the pectoralis major muscle. The lateral thoracic artery and the anterior

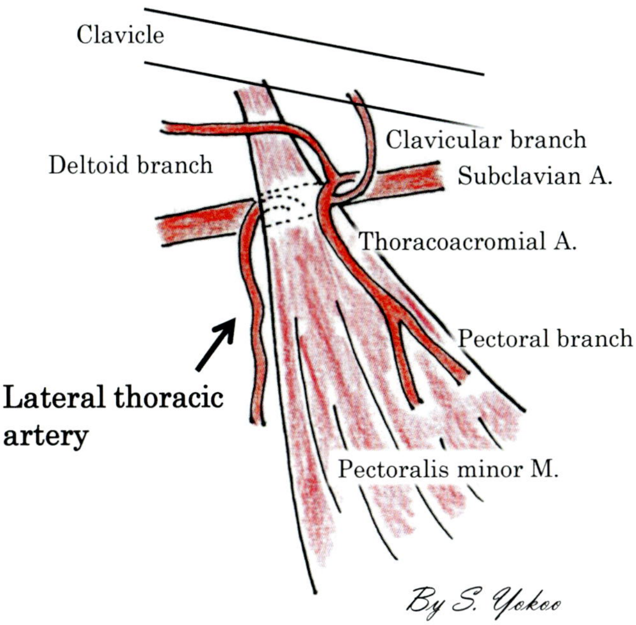

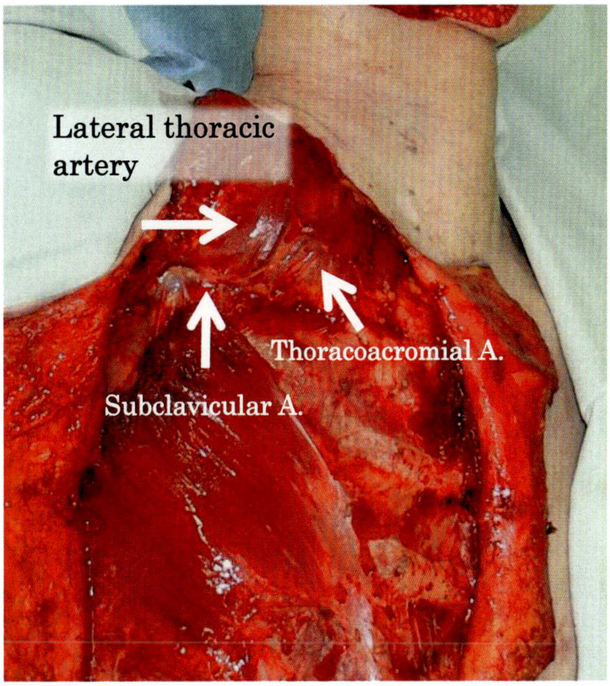

Fig. 9.15 Vascular anatomy of pectoralis major muscle. The thoracoacromial axis classically divides into four main branches: the clavicular, deltoid, pectoral, and acromial arteries. The lateral thoracic artery may also arise from this system, but, more commonly, branches out separately from the axillary artery. The thoracoacromial artery commonly divides into two major branches: the pectoral and deltoid. The acromial and clavicular arteries variably arise from either division. The deltoid arteries run in the deltopectoral groove with the cephalic vein, supplying both the pectoralis major and deltoid. It gives off a cutaneous perforator in the midpoint of the deltopectoral groove. The acromial branch contributes to a vascular plexus along with branches from the deltoid, suprascapular, and posterior humeral circumflex vessels. The clavicular branch runs a cephalad and medial course toward the sternoclavicular joint. The pectoral branch pieces the clavipectoral fascia and then runs a cephalocaudal course on the deep surface of the pectoralis major muscle, which it supplies

intercostals branches of the internal mammary artery supply the skin region overlaying the lower part of the pectoralis major muscle [41–43]. The skin island must be designed in the lower chest to attain a pedicle length sufficient for oral and maxillofacial reconstruction. In the conventional harvesting method for oral and maxillofacial reconstruction, the lateral thoracic artery and all intercostal branches from the internal mammary vessel are cut to avoid compromise of arc of rotation of the flap. The dissections of these two dominant sources of blood supply to the skin island overlaying the lower PMMC flap poses a high risk of distal flap necrosis. The PMMC flap preserves the lateral thoracic vessels in addition to the pectoral branches of the thoracoacromial artery and is, therefore, a very valid choice from the viewpoint of blood supply [41, 44] (Fig. 9.15). Cadaver dissection has also shown that the lateral thoracic artery is a more dominant pedicle of the PMMC flap than the pectoral branch of the thoracoacromial artery in approximately 6 % of all cases studied. This percentage was very close to the total rate of skin necrosis of PMMC flaps [45]. Dissecting the lateral thoracic artery as a routine harvesting technique in such cases could result in total loss of the pectoralis major skin flap.

A skin island designed in the lower chest to reach the oral and maxillofacial defect includes the fourth intercostal perforating branches [43]. The muscle is elevated from the chest wall inferiorly to superiorly. The pectoral branch of the thoracoacromial artery is included in the flap as in the conventional harvesting method of the PMMC flap. The lateral thoracic artery, identified underneath the lateral border of the pectoralis muscle in the region of the maxilla, comes out underneath the lateral border of the pectoralis minor muscle and enters the lateral part of the pectoralis major muscle [46]. The pectoralis minor muscle overlying the lateral thoracic artery is dissected completely to release the lateral thoracic artery up to the clavicle [42]. The lateral thoracic vessels are kept pedicled, not cut, if the length of the pedicle is not compromised. This is called "double pedicled pectoralis major musculocutaneous flap" or "DOP-PMMC flap." Lateral thoracic vessels should be preserved with the pedicle, not dissected, when the length of the pedicle is not compromised in oral and maxillofacial reconstruction; the flap could reach the oral cavity without limitation, when the pectoralis minor muscle is completely dissected. Compromise of pedicle length is often experienced, especially when wrapping the muscle of the PMMC flap around the titanium reconstruction plate used in segmental mandibulectomy (*wrap-around procedure*), even when the pectoralis minor muscle is completely dissected. The compromise may be due to the long distance between the thoracoacromial artery and the lateral thoracic at the bifurcation of the subclavian artery, to the short length of the lateral thoracic artery from the bifurcation of the subclavian artery to the point of entry into the pectoralis major muscle, or to the constitution of the patient—a long neck compared with the chest. In such cases, the lateral thoracic vessels are cut at the bifurcation of subclavian vessels, and then microvascular anastomosis is carried out between lateral thoracic vessels and the transverse cervical artery and external jugular vein. We named our new procedure "supercharged pectoralis major musculocutaneous flap (SUP-PMMC flap)." Thus, the lateral thoracic artery is preserved without any compromise of pedicle length, which takes into consideration the blood supply of the lower part of PMMC flaps. Lateral thoracic vessels are suitable for microvascular anastomosis as described for the free lateral thoracic flap and for the lateral thoracic perforator flap [47, 48]. It should be noted that a deficit of the lateral thoracic artery has been reported in approximately 15 % of cases [47, 49]. Although we have not been able to fully resolve the issue of compromised distal skin blood supply because of the necessity of dissecting the branches of the internal mammary artery, it is worthwhile to preserve the lateral thoracic vessel that is the major contribution to the lateral and distal PMMC flap (Fig. 9.16).

9.2.4 Platysma Flap and Cervical Island Flap

The application of a cervical skin flap to oral and cervical defects, subject of many reports, was initially described as "the apron flap" by Ward et al. in 1950 [50]. In 1969, Farr et al. [51] have described a similar flap as a cervical island skin flap. In both studies, blood circulation is described as

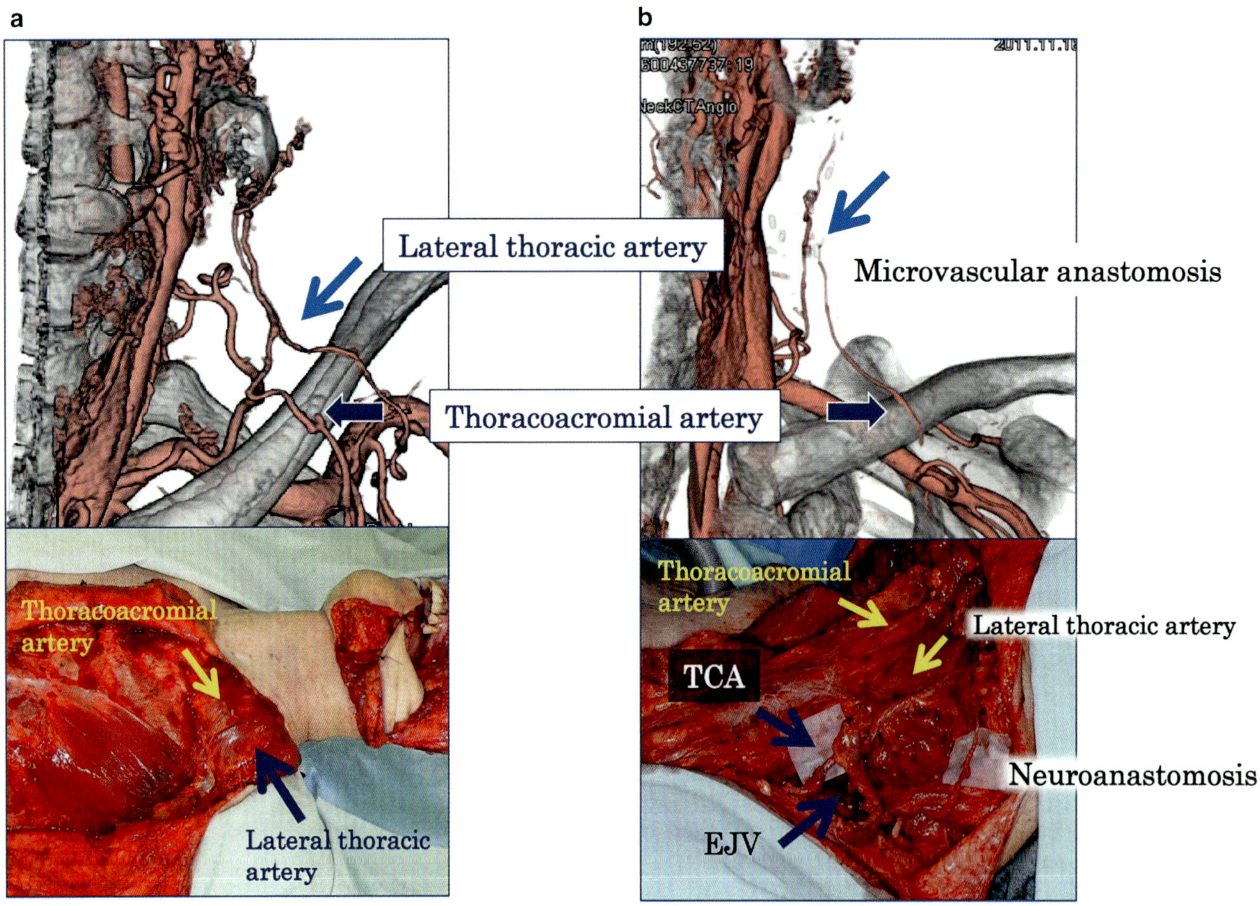

Fig. 9.16 Computer tomographic angiography of DOP- and SUP-PMMC flap. Computer tomographic angiography shows the lateral thoracic artery and pectoral branch of the thoracoacromial artery of DOP- (**a**) and SUP-PMMC flap (**b**) one year after surgery. The great auricular nerve is also anastomosed to the medial pectoral nerve to prevent muscle atrophy. *TCA* transverse cervical artery, *EJV* external jugular vein

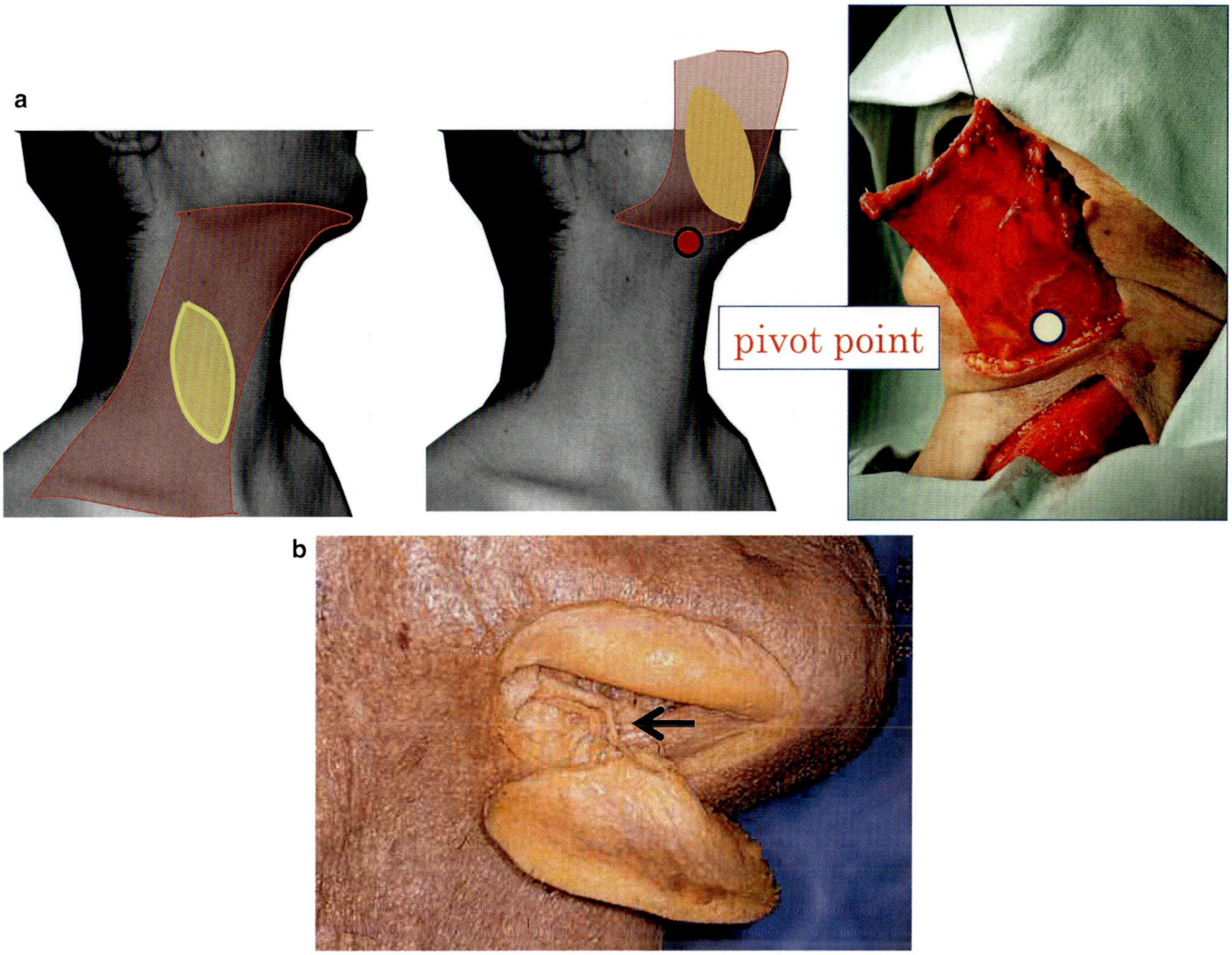

Fig. 9.17 Design of platysma flap and pivot point. Since the platysma flap is of an axial pattern that uses the submental branch of the facial artery, the arc of rotation and the pivot point is determined by this artery. (**a**) Design, arc of rotation, and pivot pointand (**b**) submental branch of the facial artery

being of a random pattern. In 1978, Futrell et al. [52] have described an axial-pattern flap by using the submental branch of the facial artery, the dominant pedicle of the platysma, for feeding the platysma musculocutaneous flap and have used it in oral reconstruction. Although the platysma flap and cervical island flaps are very similar, their circulation systems are totally different and should be clearly differentiated, yet they are still being confused in many studies [53]. By taking the circulation systems into consideration, a platysma flap can be elevated safely.

Since the platysma flap is of an axial pattern that uses the submental branch of the facial artery as the dominant pedicle, the skin flap is a complete island. The suprasternal branch of the suprascapular artery and the platysma branch of the suprathyroid artery are minor pedicles; therefore, their circulation system is Mathes's type II [54, 55]. When a skin flap is used for oral reconstruction, cutting the minor pedicle is requisite, and the skin flap is fed only by the dominant pedicle present in the upper region. Thus, the arc of rotation is determined by this artery (Fig. 9.17). The anterior region in neck skin receives blood supply from the submental branch of the facial artery, with the anterior margin of the sternocleidomastoid muscle regarded as the boundary [56]. Accordingly, a skin island of the platysma flap should be set in this region or in a region from where subcutaneous (dermal) blood flow is foreseen (Fig. 9.18). The submental branch of the facial artery and its arborization are distributed in the deep adipofascial layer and extend perforators to the platysma and skin. Thus, no axial-pattern circulation is obtainable unless this layer is conserved. Imanishi et al. [57] have shown that the dominant pedicle extends a long branch to the deep adipofascial layer and forms a vascular plexus, but it extends only a small vessel to the platysma, and no vascular plexus is formed between the platysma and skin. Thus, elevating a platysma flap as a musculocutaneous flap is risky; it should be elevated

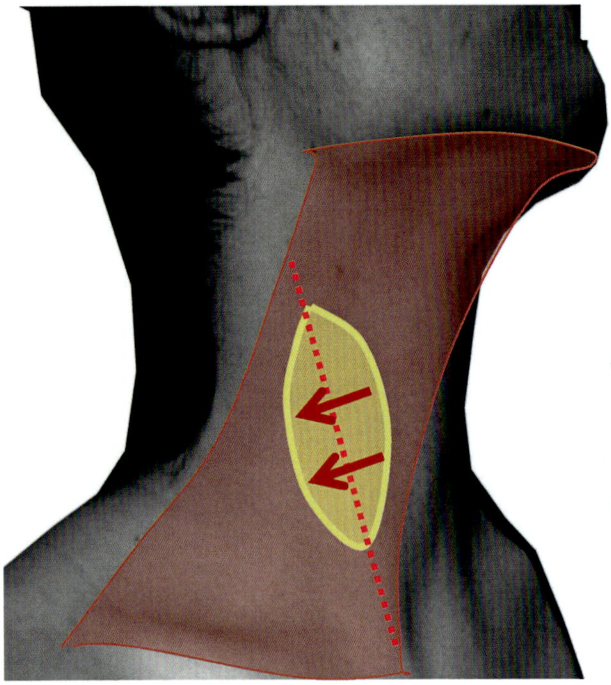

Fig. 9.18 Vascular territory of the submental branch of the facial artery and setting region of the platysma flap in the neck. The anterior region in neck skin receives blood supply from the submental branch of the facial artery, with the anterior margin of the sternocleidomastoid muscle regarded as the boundary. Accordingly, a skin island of the platysma flap should be set in this region or in a region from where subcutaneous (dermal) blood flow is foreseen

as an adipofasciomusculocutaneous flap. This anatomical fact is very important when elevating a platysma flap (Fig. 9.19). Venous circulation in the platysma flap is retrogradely drained by including the external jugular vein [56]. The deep adipofascial layer into which the jugular vein distributes is important for venous circulation. Skin loss has been reported in 20–70 % of platysma flaps [58], but has occurred in only 3 % with the use of our method of elevation. From the viewpoint of cervical lymph flow based on Harnsberger's fascia classification [59], a platysma flap destroys the structure of the cervical fascia. Moreover, since the deep adipofascial layer is present in the superficial space [59], the platysma flap includes the superficial cervical lymph node. Taken together, these conditions may induce a late neck lymph node metastasis-like abnormality. Nonetheless, we have not encountered any late metastatic case assumed to have induced an abnormality in cervical lymph flow (Fig. 9.20).

For a cervical island flap, a peninsula design is prepared in anticipation of a random pattern in the cervical region. The rule of cervical skin flap preparation (width/length = 1:2–3) is observed. The main platysma-feeding artery is the submental branch of the facial artery, and its branch is distributed in the deep adipofascial layer. Thus, no axial-pattern circulation of the platysma flap can be obtained unless this layer is conserved and unless there is a marked difference in the circulation system and flap stability from those of a cervical island flap dissected and elevated in this layer. Furthermore, since a cervical island flap is a random-pattern flap receiving blood supply from the skin pedicle, only the skin and superficial adipofascial layer, not including the platysma muscle, may be elevated. From the viewpoint of circulation, a cervical island flap can be concomitantly used with neck dissection. A cervical island flap, in combination with a sternocleidomastoid muscle flap by separate elevation, can also be used for reconstruction after subtotal glossectomy. By including the deep adipofascial layer and the submental branch of the facial artery in a cervical island flap, similar to those in a platysma flap, both axial and random circulatory patterns can be constructed, facilitating the preparation of a skin flap with more favorable circulation (Fig. 9.21).

With regard to the surgical procedure, a platysma flap may be more difficult to prepare because it requires conservation of the long branch in the deep adipofascial layer. Since the pivot point of a platysma flap is located around the center of the submandibular gland in which the submandibular branch bifurcates from the facial artery, the arc of rotation is limited. Therefore, to reconstruct the tongue is very challenging with the use of the lingual side of the mandible as the route for the flap to reach the target. In a systematic review of cases between 1982 and 2002 (Szudek et al. [53]), the platysma flap has been applied to the mobile tongue and the base of the tongue in 37 % of 190 cases, but these include cases treated with a cervical island flap that is actually a random-pattern skin flap just including the platysma and is termed a platysma myocutaneous flap.

An 80-year-old woman (Patient 1) underwent tumor resection of squamous cell carcinoma of the right buccal mucosa (T2N0M0, WHO grade I, INFa). The region down to the subcutaneous fat layer, including the buccinator muscle, was the vertical resection range. A 5×4 cm platysma flap was elevated. The buccinator muscle was reconstructed by filling the platysma muscle sheet. Reconstruction while maintaining flexibility was possible by applying the deep adipofascial layer to the fat layer and the skin flap region (skin and superficial adipofascial layer) to the buccal mucosal defect. Since the cervical branch of the facial artery was conserved due to its distribution in the deep adipofascial layer, the platysma muscle has been maintained without fatty change for 8 years after surgery. No disturbance of mouth opening attributed to scar contracture in the reconstructed region has been noted, and favorable functioning of the oral cavity prevails (Fig. 9.22).

A 68-year-old woman (Patient 2) underwent reconstruction with a PMMC flap after resection of squamous cell

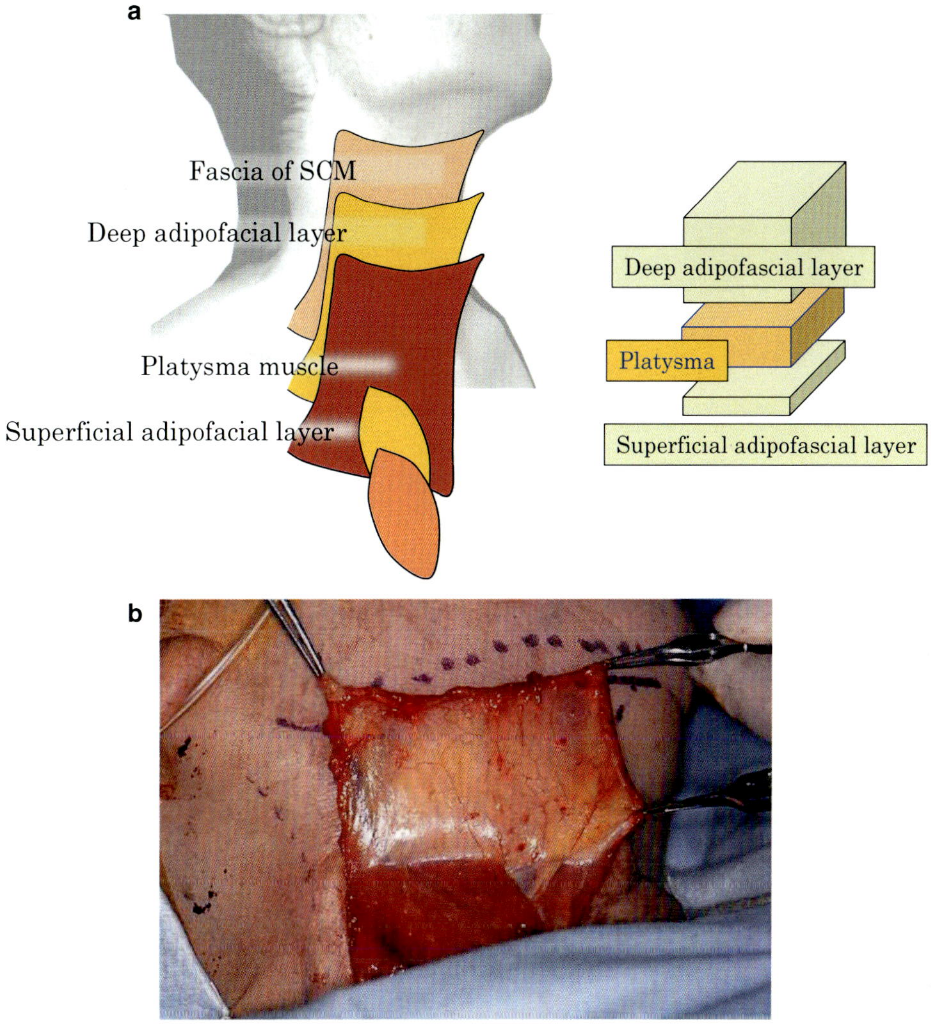

Fig. 9.19 The platysma adipofasciomusculocutaneous flap. The submental branch of the facial artery and its arborization are distributed in the deep adipofascial layer and extend perforators to the platysma and skin (**a**). Thus, no axial-pattern circulation is obtainable unless this layer is conserved. The dominant pedicle extends a long branch to the deep adipofascial layer and forms a vascular plexus, but extends only a small vessel to the platysma, and no vascular plexus is formed between the platysma and skin (**b**). Thus, elevating a platysma flap as a musculocutaneous flap is risky; it should be elevated as an adipofasciomusculocutaneous flap

carcinoma of the oral floor, but an orocervical fistula formed because of poor blood circulation. A moderate tissue defect after fistula resection was reconstructed with a platysma flap prepared from the collateral nonsurgical side. Having an appropriate volume, the platysma flap was very useful in closing the fistula (Fig. 9.23).

In a 60-year-old woman (Patient 3) with disturbed mouth opening (7 mm) resulting from scar contracture after resection of carcinoma of buccal mucosa, the contracture was eliminated by cicatrectomy wherewith mouth opening increased to about 30 mm. As in Patient 1, the buccinator muscle region was reconstructed with a platysma muscle sheet, the fat layer with the deep adipofascial layer, and the buccal mucosal defect with the skin flap region. Since the cervical branch of the facial artery was conserved, the platysma muscle has been maintained for 4 years after surgery, sustaining flexibility of the buccal mucosal region. Mouth opening has increased to 35 mm (Fig. 9.24).

An 80-year-old woman (Patient 4) underwent modified radical neck dissection and resection of squamous cell carcinoma of the left oral floor (T2N1M0, WHO grade I, INFb). The patient's condition was complicated by cardiovascular disease, necessitating cutting operating time short. Therefore, the floor of the mouth was reconstructed with a cervical island flap. Submandibular reconstruction

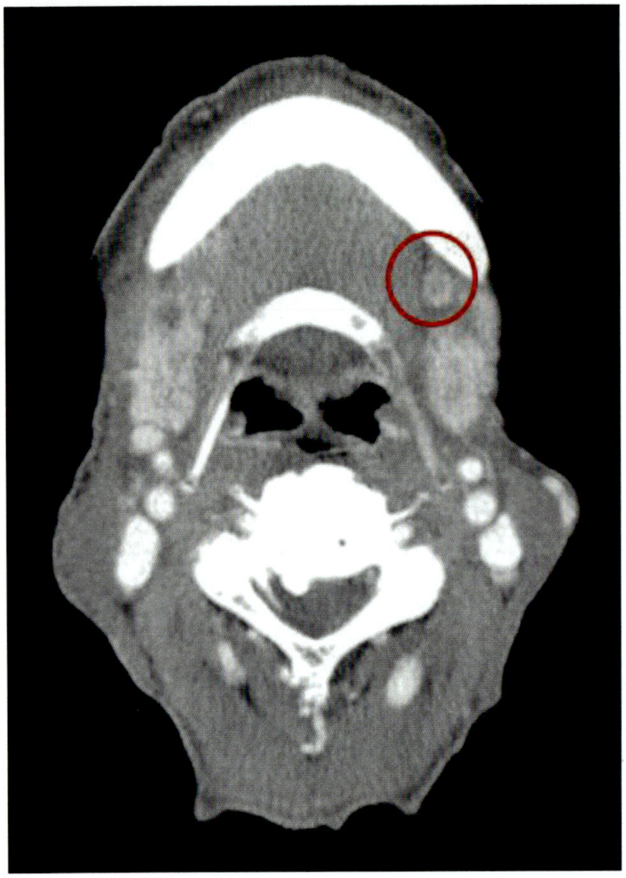

Fig. 9.20 Late cervical metastasis after reconstruction with platysma flap (squamous cell carcinoma of buccal mucosa). From the viewpoint of cervical lymph flow, a platysma flap destroys the structure of the cervical fascia. Moreover, since the deep adipofascial layer is present in the superficial space, the platysma flap includes the superficial cervical lymph node. Taken together, these conditions may induce a late neck lymph node metastasis-like abnormality. Nonetheless, we have not encountered any late metastatic case assumed to have induced an abnormality in cervical lymph flow

was carried out while preventing formation of dead space in this region by plication of the mylohyoid muscle and the digastric muscle and by inserting the cervical island flap through the submandibular region. The postoperative result was good (Fig. 9.25).

An 85-year-old woman (Patient 5) underwent elective supraomohyoid neck dissection and subtotal glossectomy for squamous cell carcinoma of the left tongue; the carcinoma was suspected of having infiltrated the mylohyoid muscle and was by histopathology diagnosed as infiltration factor (INF) type C (T4aN0M0, WHO grade II). Since the patient's age and cardiovascular disease necessitated cutting operating time short, the submandibular defect was reconstructed with a sternocleidomastoid muscle flap and the tongue with a cervical island flap. The postoperative result was good (Fig. 9.26).

9.2.5 Functional and Aesthetic Reconstruction of Full-Thickness Cheek, Oral Commissure, and Vermilion Defects

Full-thickness cheek defects arise as a result of resecting buccomucosal squamous cell carcinomas. In terms of direct tumor invasion or safety margins, even the vermilion including the oral commissure has to be resected in some cases where patients demonstrate massive defects involving the cheek, oral commissure, and vermilion. Various vascularized free flaps have previously been reported for reconstructing the cheek [60–67]. The vermilion was reconstructed by tissue-expanding vermilion musculocutaneous flaps (vermilion advancement flaps) as described by Goldstein [68]. Both functional and aesthetic problems can be resolved by using both procedures in combination.

A tumor resection team resected the cheek, oral commissure, and vermilion (Fig. 9.27a). Neck dissection was carried out according to the status of each case. A reconstruction team raised a flap (radial forearm flap or rectus abdominis musculocutaneous flap) commensurate with the size of the defect. Microvascular anastomoses were carried out with arterial branches from the external carotid system and venous branches from the external or internal jugular system. After vascular anastomosis, the flap was transplanted into the oral cavity (Fig. 9.27b), and the distal portion of the flap was sutured to the oral mucosa. When the suture advanced to the vicinity of the oral commissure, the flap was folded to the facial side. Subsequently, repair of the cheek-skin defect was carried out. Then a portion of the folded flap was deepithelialized, corresponding to the neovermilion (Fig. 9.27c). Rectus abdominis musculocutaneous flaps were used for larger defects than radial forearm flaps. When reconstruction was carried out with a rectus abdominis musculocutaneous flap, the contour of the cheek was reconstructed with the muscle portion and the oral cavity and the cheek skin were lined with the cutaneous portion. A cutaneous portion elevated was twice as large as the muscle portion, because the folding was done in the cutaneous portion alone (Fig. 9.27d). Mucosal lining of the vermilion and the oral commissure was carried out with vermilion advancement flaps raised by incising the residual vermilion along the white roll up to the contralateral oral commissure including the labial artery and orbicularis oris muscle (Fig. 9.27e). The upper and lower vermilion advancement flaps were advanced to the point of the putative new oral commissure. The flap ends were then sutured to the deepithelialized skin flap to form both the vermilion and the neocommissure (Fig. 9.27f).

Vermilion reconstruction is considered successful only when both sphincteric and sensory functions are reestablished. Full-thickness cheek defects have been repaired with various vascularized free flaps without eliminating postoperative

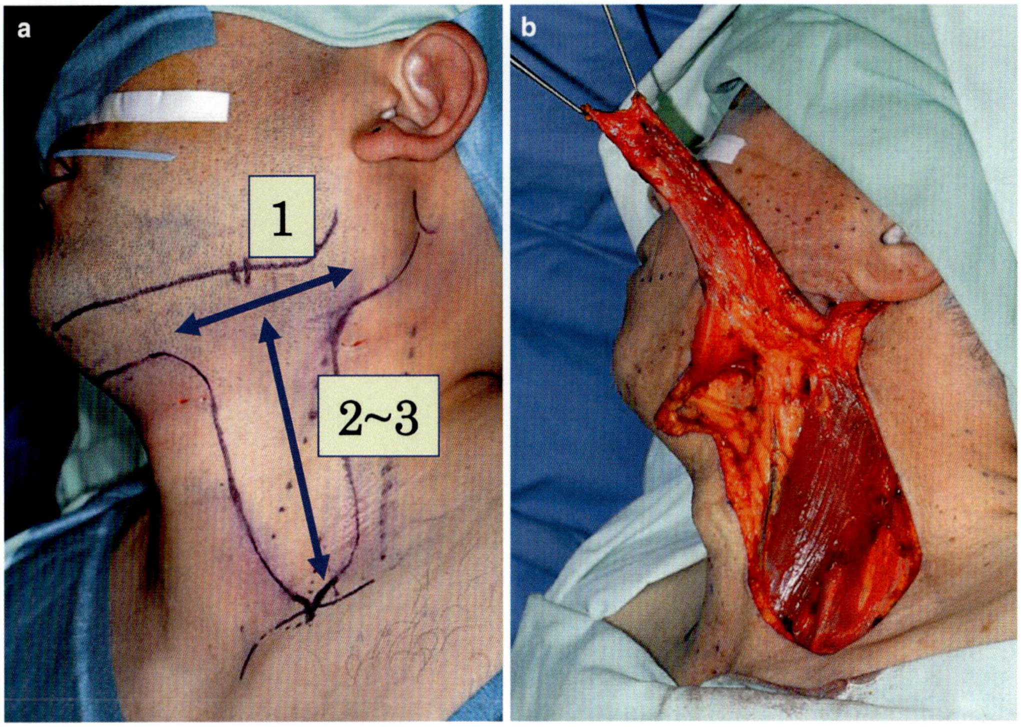

Fig. 9.21 Design and elevation of cervical island flap. A peninsula design is prepared in anticipation of a random pattern in the cervical region for the cervical island flap. The rule of cervical skin flap preparation (width/length = 1:2–3) is observed. The main platysma-feeding artery is the submental branch of the facial artery, and its branch is distributed in the deep adipofascial layer. Thus, no axial-pattern circulation of the platysma flap can be obtained unless this layer is conserved and unless there is a marked difference in the circulation system and flap stability from those of a cervical island flap dissected and elevated in this layer. Furthermore, since a cervical island flap is a random-pattern flap receiving blood supply from the skin pedicle, only the skin and superficial adipofascial layer, not including the platysma muscle, may be elevated. From the viewpoint of circulation, a cervical island flap can be concomitantly used with neck dissection

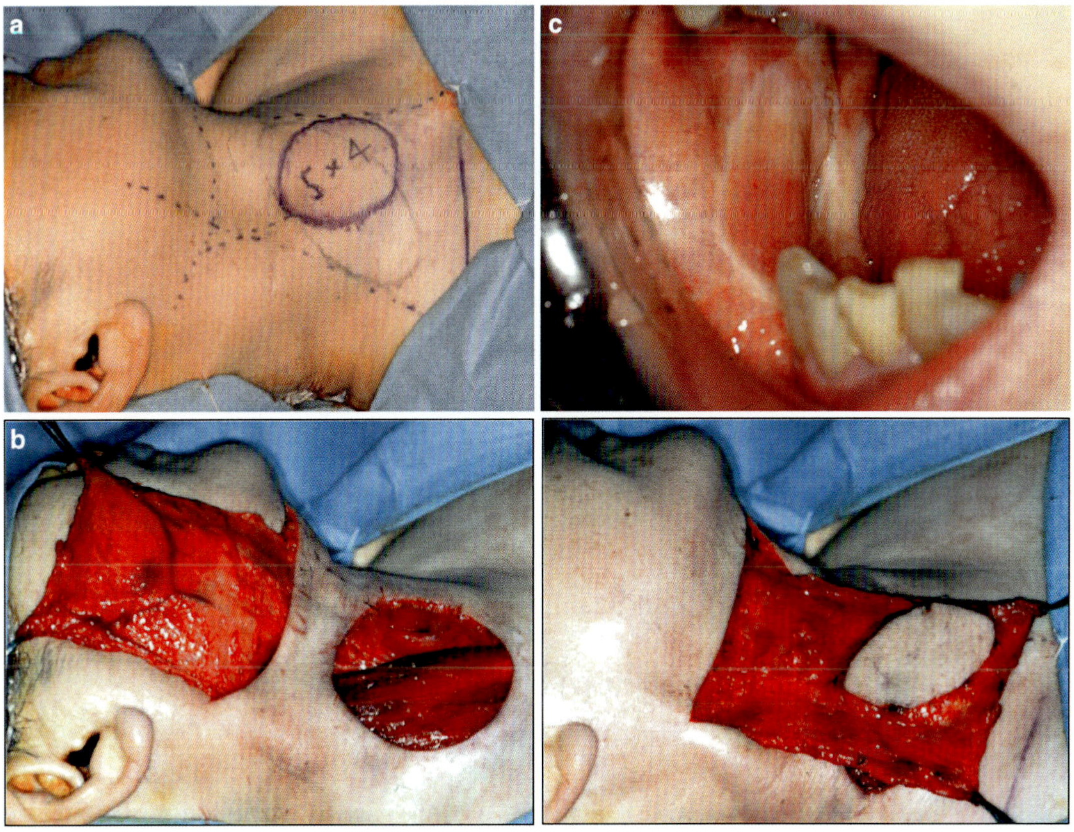

Fig. 9.22 Patient 1: platysma flap reconstruction after resection of squamous cell carcinoma of buccal mucosa. (**a**) Design of platysma flap, (**b**) elevation of flap, (**c**) 8 years after surgery

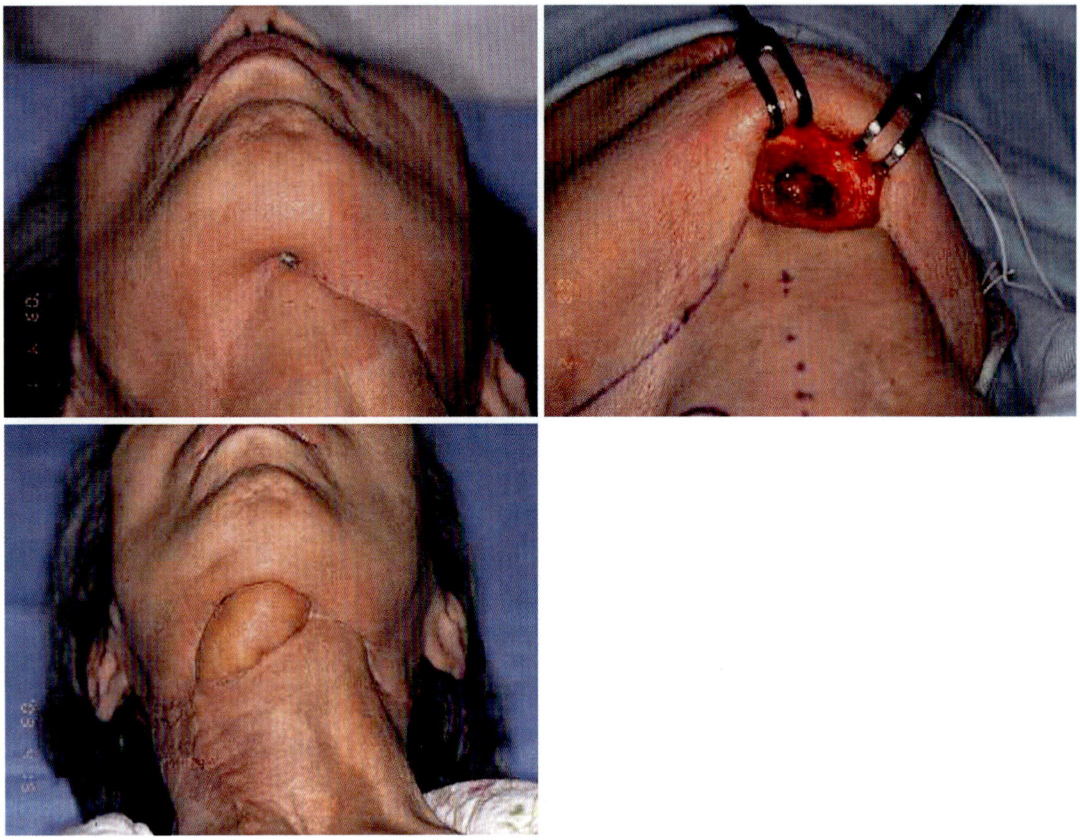

Fig. 9.23 Platysma flap reconstruction of cervical fistula. (**a**) Orocervical fistula after reconstruction with PMMC flap, (**b**) moderate defect after fistula resection, (**c**) closing the fistula

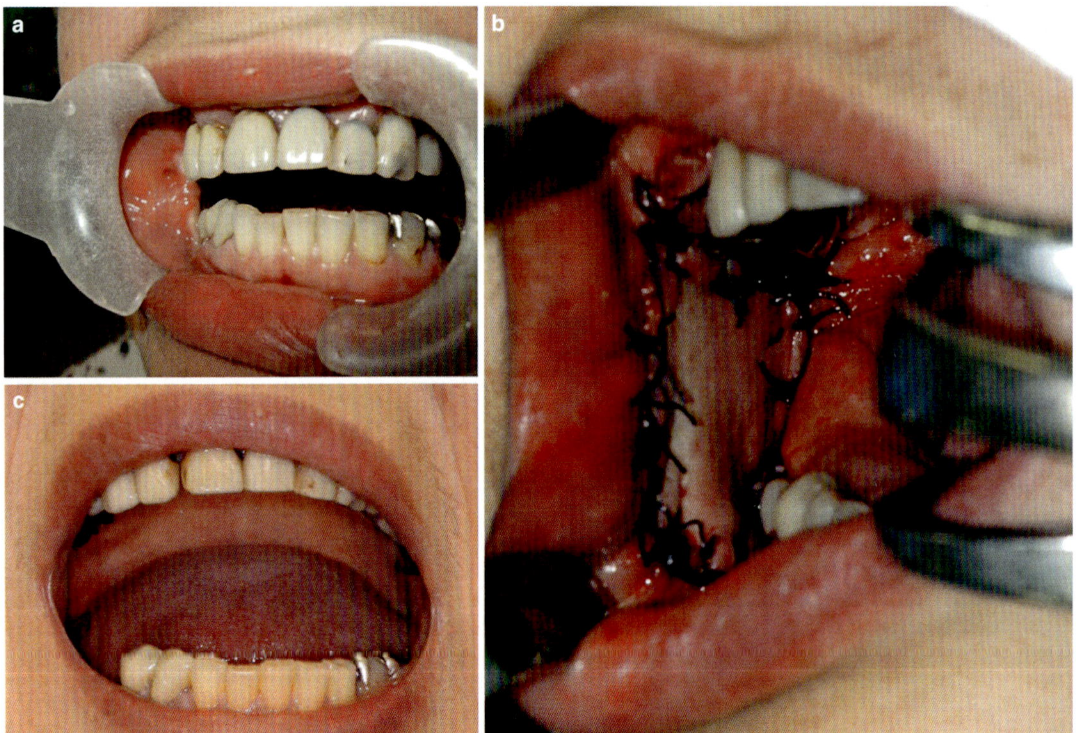

Fig. 9.24 Platysma flap reconstruction after cicatrectomy. (**a**) 7 mm mouth opening before surgery, (**b**) platysma flap reconstruction after cicatrectomy, (**c**) 35 mm mouth opening 1 year after surgery

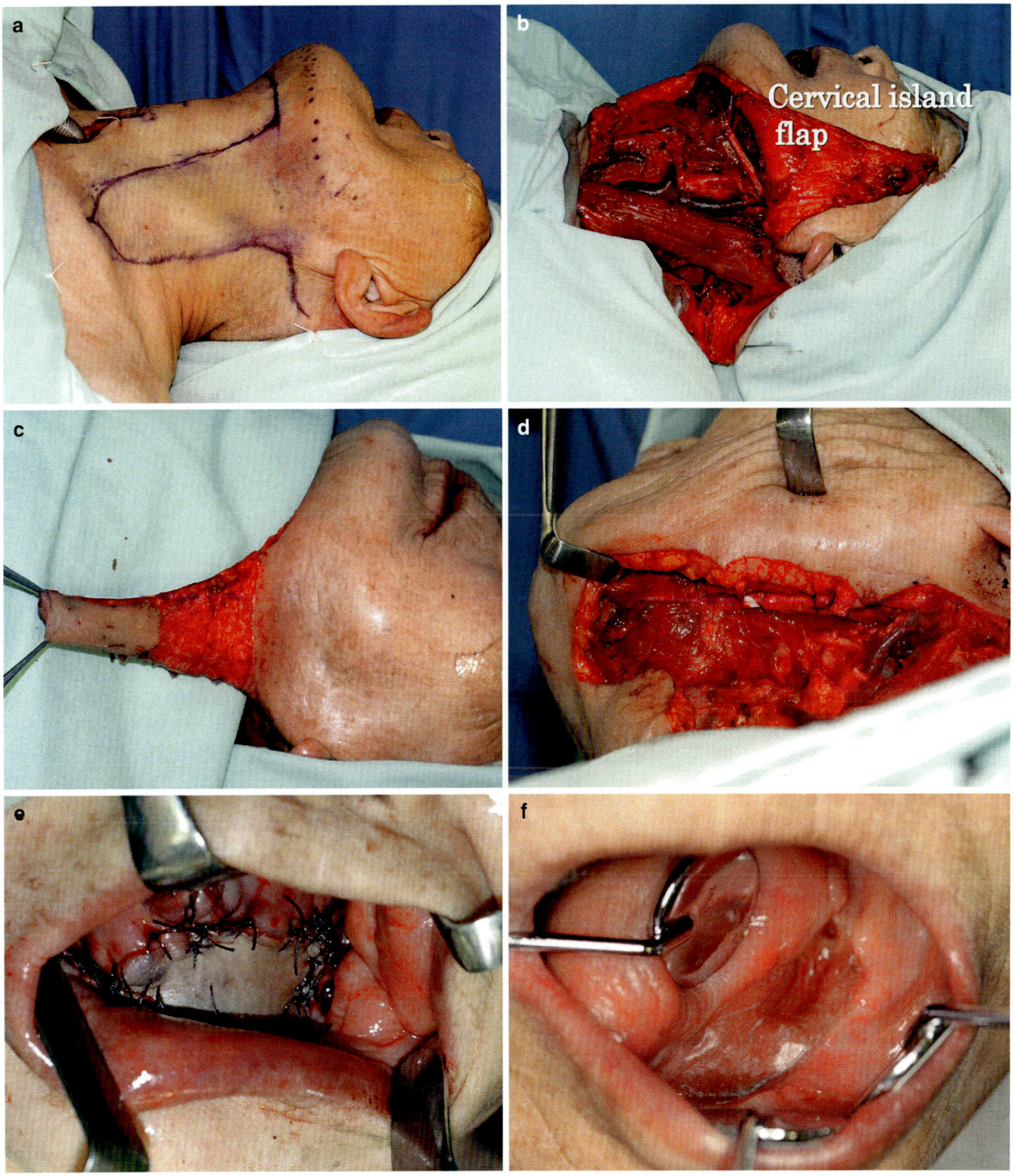

Fig. 9.25 Cervical island flap reconstruction after resection of squamous cell carcinoma of the floor of the mouth. (**a**) Design, (**b**) cervical island flap elevation and supraomohyoid neck dissection, (**c**) deepithelization of flap, (**d**) reconstruction of submandibular region (formation of mylohyoid structure), (**e**) reconstruction of the floor of the mouth, (**f**) 4 years after surgery

functional disorders such as trismus due to scar contracture [60–67].

In our procedure in this presentation, the reconstructed cheek was soft and supple, demonstrating no scar contracture, because a radial forearm flap or a rectus abdominis musculocutaneous flap of good blood supply was used. Since continuity of the orbicularis oris muscle ring and configuration of the vermilion were reconstructed using a combination of these soft and supple skin flaps and a vermilion advancement flap as described by Goldstein [68], sphincteric function was

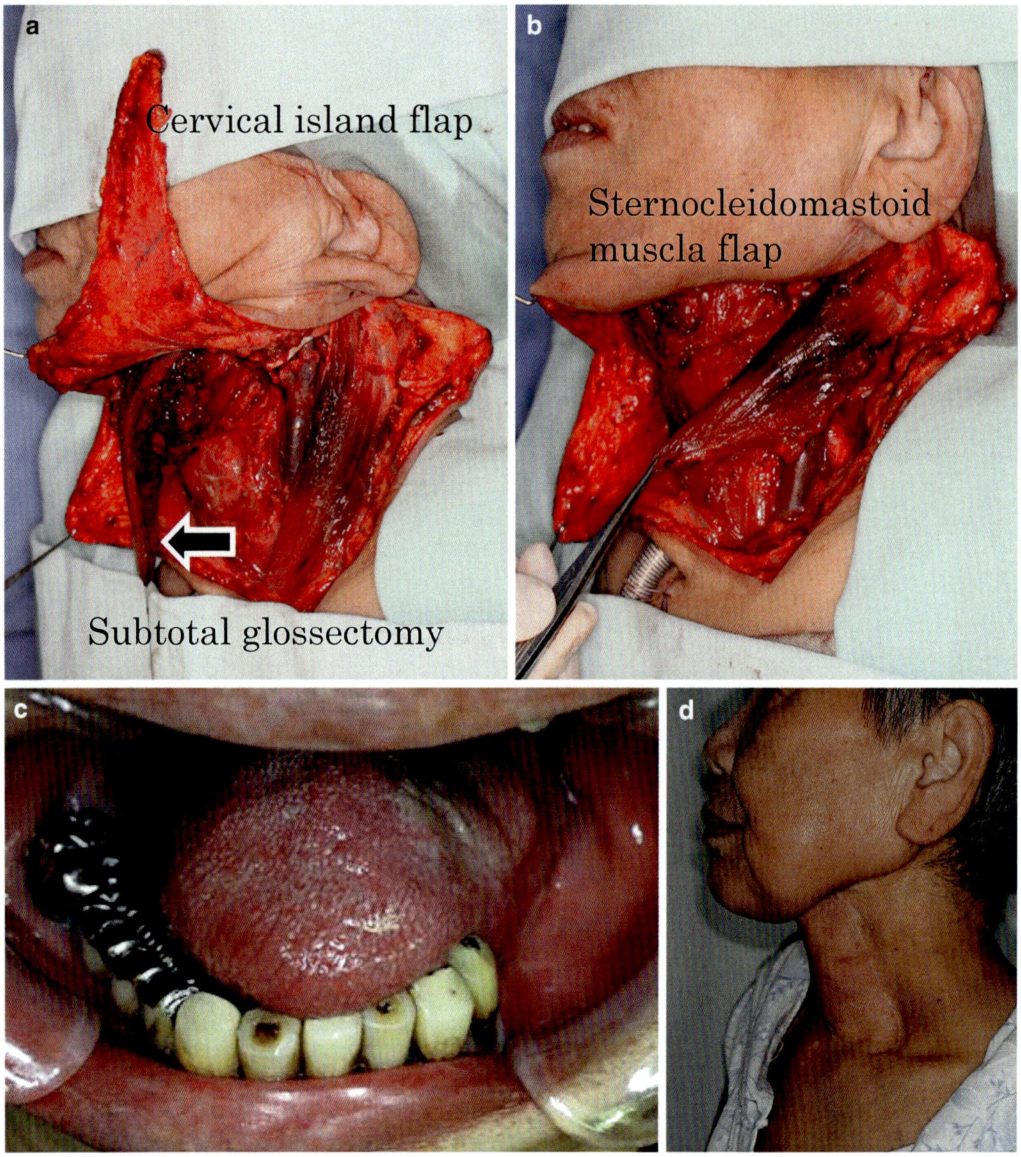

Fig. 9.26 Reconstruction after subtotal glossectomy with combination with cervical island flap and sternocleidomastoid muscle flap. (**a**) Cervical island flap elevation and modified radical neck dissection, (**b**) reconstruction of the floor of the mouth and submandibular dead space with sternocleidomastoid muscle flap, (**c**) reconstruction of the floor of the mouth, and (**d**) condition of submandibular and cervical region

restored. It is particularly essential to retain or restore sensory function in lip reconstruction in order to avoid insufficient lip closure and drooling. As suggested by Goldstein [68], the sensory function of the vermilion can be retained because the musculocutaneous flap (vermilion advancement flap) is innervated. Corderio and Santamaria [69] have reported that in large defects of the midface, orbit, and maxilla that include the upper lip and oral commissure, the midface is reconstructed and sphincteric function and sensory function of the lip and oral commissure are reestablished with a combination of a rectus abdominis musculocutaneous flap and a lip switch flap. The same concept was applied in our patients for the reconstruction of the oral commissure and lips (Fig. 9.28).

9.2.6 Maxillomandibular Reconstruction

9.2.6.1 Introduction

Among osseous reconstruction materials for mandibular and maxillary defects, vascularized free bone is highly resistant to infection because it is a living bone—an advantage when blood supply to the recipient site is poor due to radiotherapy and when the bone defect is large [70]. Fibular and scapular

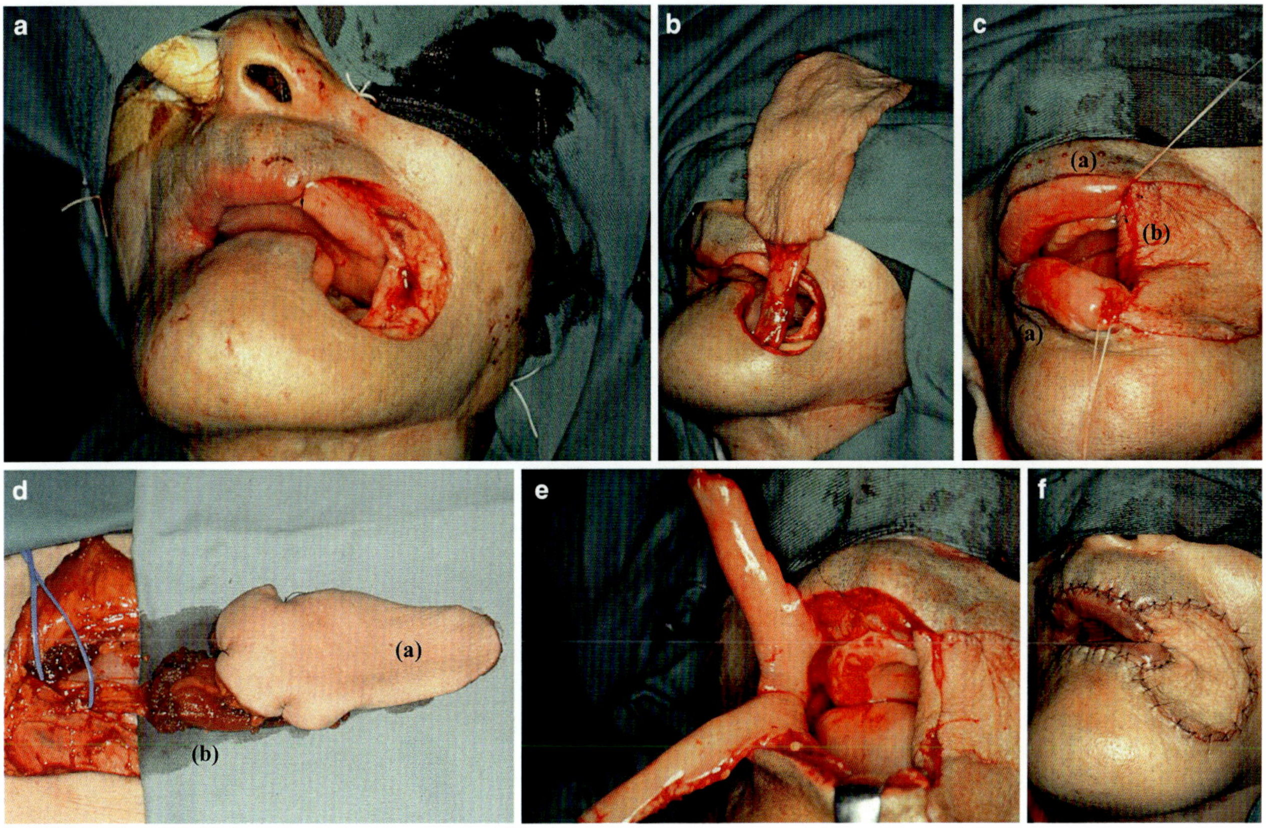

Fig. 9.27 Operative procedure. (**a**) The full-thickness cheek including the upper and lower lips and the oral commissure were resected. (**b**) A free radial forearm flap was grafted for repair of the cheek defect. (**c**) (*a*) Design of the vermilion advancement flap. (*b*) The free radial forearm flap deepithelialized at the folded portion and formation of the neovermilion and neocommissure. (**d**) Rectus abdominis musculocutaneous flaps were used for larger defects than radial forearm flaps. When reconstruction was carried out with a rectus abdominis musculocutaneous flap, the contour of the cheek was reconstructed with the muscle portion, and the oral cavity and the cheek skin were lined with the cutaneous portion. The elevated cutaneous portion was twice as large as the muscle portion because the folding was done in the cutaneous portion alone. (*a*) Cutaneous portion. (*b*) Muscular portion. (**e**) Raising the vermilion advancement flap. (**f**) Completed reconstruction

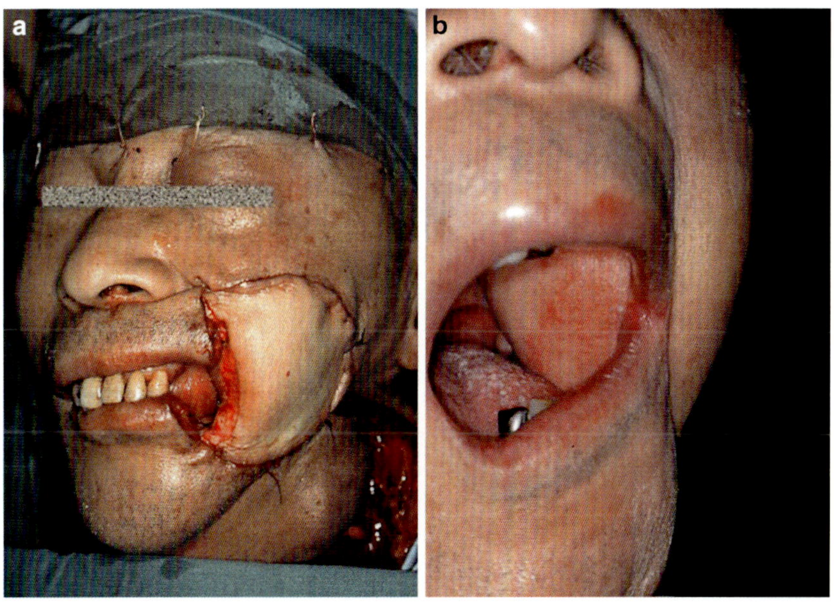

Fig. 9.28 Vermilion advancement flap and rectus abdominis musculocutaneous flap. (**a**) The full-thickness cheek including 10 % of the lower lip and the oral commissure were resected. The contour of the cheek was reconstructed with the muscle portion, and the oral cavity and the cheek skin were lined with the cutaneous portion of the rectus abdominis musculocutaneous flap. Vermilion advancement flap repaired for the lower lip alone. (**b**) One year postoperatively: good form of the oral commissure was reestablished

bones are frequently used for maxillomandibular reconstruction, and while there are no clear criteria for choosing grafts, it is essential that the selection be based on a full understanding of the characteristics of the kind of bone [71–73]. In surgery for oral cancer, soft tissue is often widely resected with the maxilla and the mandible, and bone is transplanted as a complex tissue graft, such as fibular and scapular flaps and vascularized LD musculocutaneous flaps with scapular bone (scapular tip flap) (Fig. 9.29).

Iliac bone bloc and PCBM are used for shaping autologous bone grafts that are collected from anterior and posterior iliac crests. A titanium mesh (metal) and poly-L-lactic acid (PLLA) mesh (artificial biomaterial) are used as scaffolding for PCBM. A titanium plate is used as temporary reconstruction material until bone grafting, but may sometimes be placed for a long time [74, 75].

For mandibular reconstruction, alveolar ridge plasty combined with secondary bone grafting and distraction osteogenesis may be applied at final occlusal reconstruction with dental implants and resection dentures after marginal mandibular resection [76]. Since the continuity of the mandible is lost after segmental mandibular resection, masticatory disturbance and facial deformity occur because of mandibular deviation. Currently, vascularized free bone flap grafts are widely used for primary reconstruction of the mandible; also used is the combined graft of a reconstruction plate and soft tissue (skin and musculocutaneous flaps) or one of soft tissue alone (skin or musculocutaneous flap) [1, 77–81]. Since reliable closure of the oral mucosal side is an essential prerequisite to a successful autologous bone graft, the risk of infection is high in immediate reconstruction. An autologous bone or a vascularized free bone graft is mainly used for secondary reconstruction. Although primary operative time can be shortened, multiple surgeries may be requisite, and positioning and morphological restoration of the mandible may become difficult due to scar contracture. Moreover, reconstruction with a vascularized free bone graft may not be possible when no blood vessel is available for anastomosis at the recipient site, a crucial issue to be investigated for secondary reconstruction. The level of functional recovery after

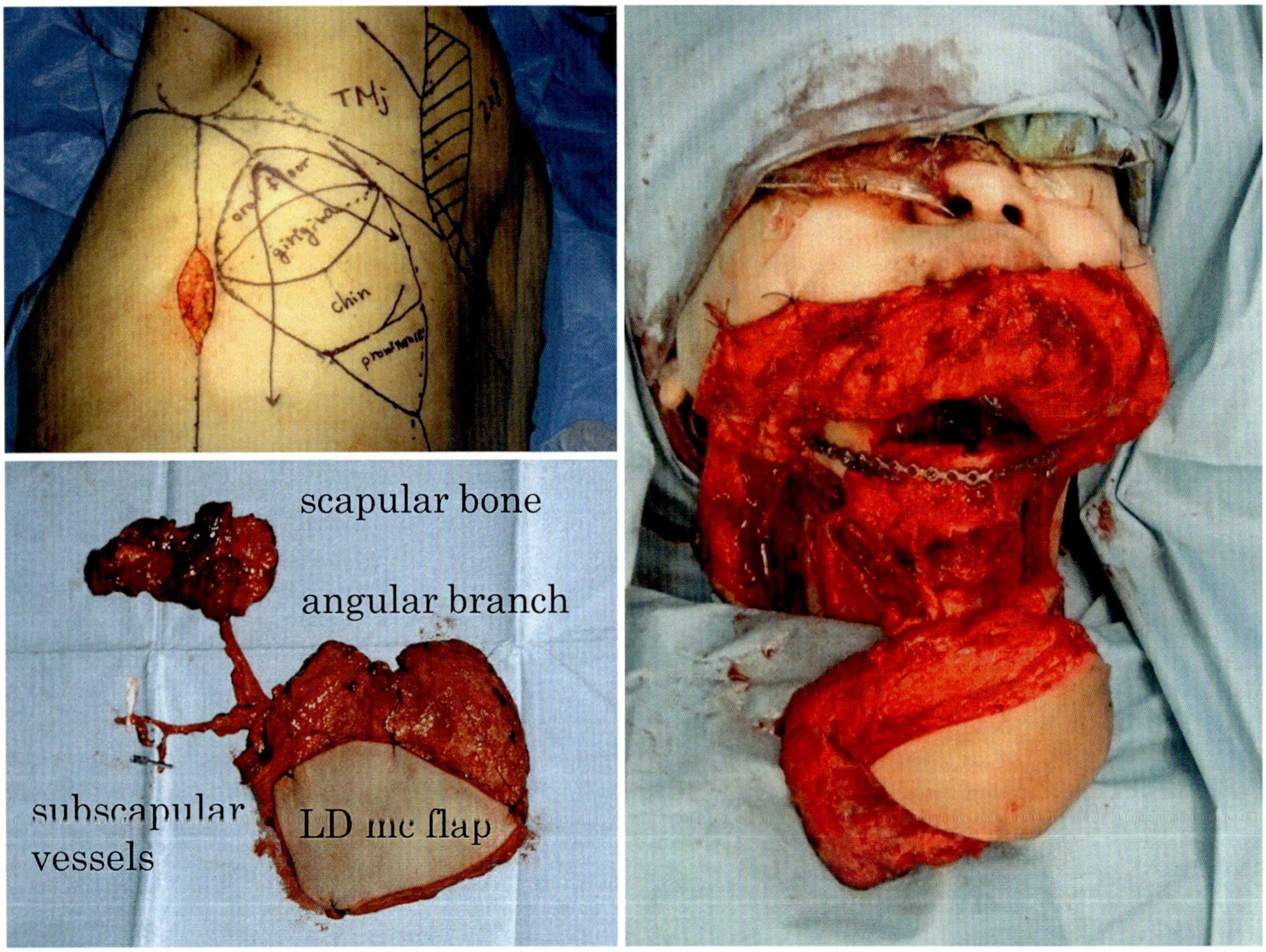

Fig. 9.29 Vascularized LD musculocutaneous flap with scapular bone (scapular tip flap)

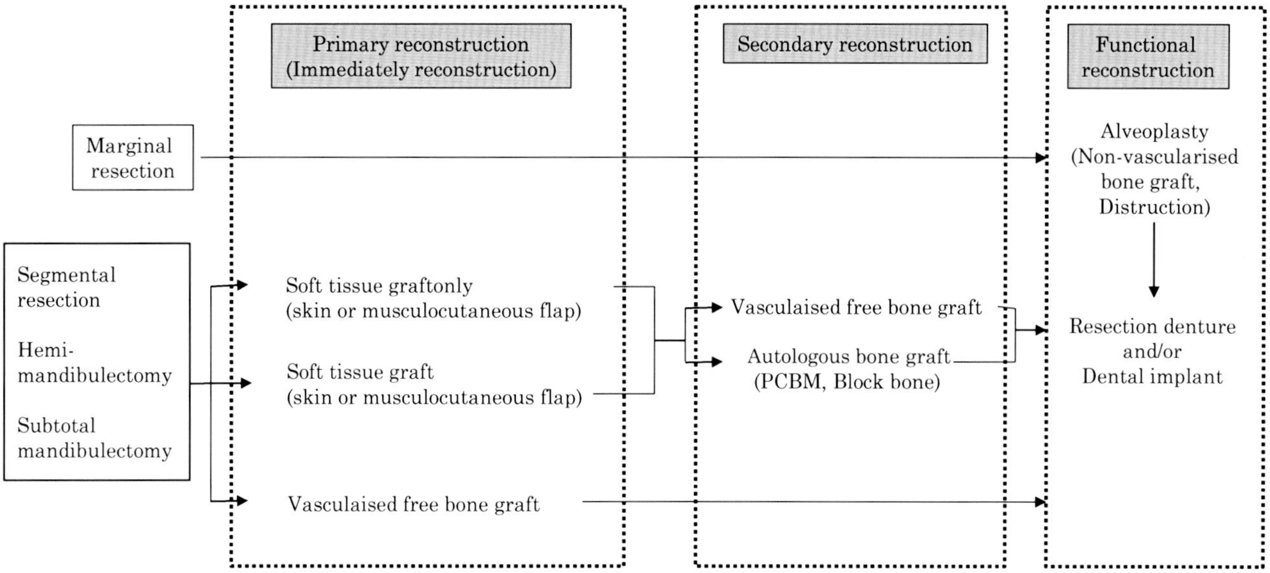

Fig. 9.30 Algorithm of mandibular reconstruction

mandibular reconstruction, and when mandibular continuity is restored, varies, because the occlusal relation among the upper and lower dentitions, the mobility of surrounding soft tissue, and the number of residual teeth are strongly reflected (Fig. 9.30).

For maxillary reconstruction, when the defect was large, instability of resection dentures due to sagging or an excessive volume of a musculocutaneous flap in cases with soft tissue reconstruction alone was an issue [82, 83]. Therefore, osseous reconstruction with a vascularized free bone flap has been introduced, which, with dental implants, markedly increases the stability of resection dentures. After subtotal or less extensive maxillectomy producing a hard palate/unilateral alveolar defect or a smaller defect with residual teeth, resection dentures may be more effective than closure with flaps (Figs. 9.31, 9.32, and 9.33) [82, 84–88].

9.2.6.2 Strategy of Mandibular Reconstruction

In our department, a 5 cm or smaller segmental defect is treated with a graft comprising a combination of a non-vascularized free iliac bone block and PCBM (Strategy 1) (Fig. 9.34). For segmental defects larger than 5 cm, a vascularized free bone graft (Strategy 2) with fibular or scapular bone (Figs. 9.29 and 9.35) is applied, or, more recently, regenerative mandibular reconstruction is carried out, in which a wrap-around procedure with a reconstruction plate and musculocutaneous flap is used before secondary reconstruction with a PCBM graft (Strategy 3). For hemi- and posterior mandibular defects, basically the methods of Kroll et al. [80] and Bulter et al. [89] are used. Instead of a free-end saddle reconstruction with a bone flap or a reconstruction plate, aesthetic contour reconstruction with a musculocutaneous flap alone is carried out (Strategy 4).

Strategy 2: Vascularized Osteocutaneous Flap (Scapular Osteocutaneous Flap)

A 47-year-old man with mandibular invasion of the right oral floor by squamous cell carcinoma (T4N1M0) underwent tumor excision involving left radical neck dissection, resection of the right oral floor tumor, subtotal glossectomy of the mobile tongue, and right segmental mandibular resection (from the right mandibular ramus to the right lower canine region), before oromandibular reconstruction with a free scapular osteocutaneous flap. For vascular anastomosis, the right subscapular and suprathyroid arteries were anastomosed end to end with the right subscapular and external jugular veins, respectively, and the scapular bone was fixed with mini plates. The oral floor and the tongue were reconstructed with a scapular flap (Fig. 9.35).

Strategy 3: Regenerative Mandibular Reconstruction

A 54-year-old woman with left squamous cell carcinoma of the lower gingiva (T2N2bM0) underwent primary tumor excision involving left modified radical neck dissection and segmental mandibular resection. In the primary reconstruction after resection, a titanium reconstruction plate was wrapped with a vascularized free rectus abdominis musculocutaneous flap to reproduce mandibular morphology. In the secondary reconstruction 6 months thereafter, regenerative mandibular reconstruction of the defective

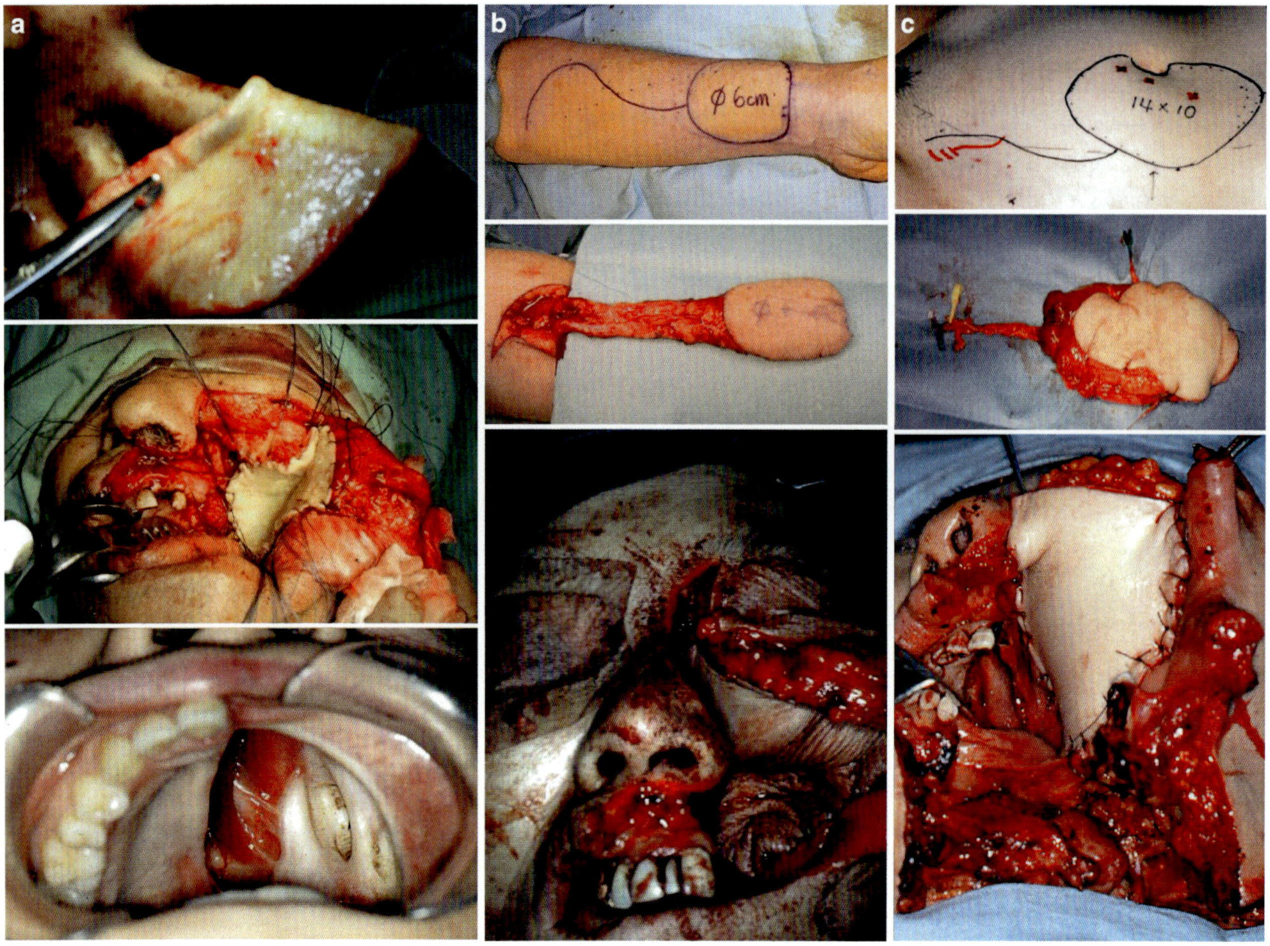

Fig. 9.31 Soft tissue reconstruction of maxilla. (**a**) Skin graft. (**b**) Vascularized free forearm flap. (**c**) Vascularized free rectus abdominis musculocutaneous flap

region was carried out with a titanium mesh and PCBM. A 3D model was constructed from CT images, and the mandibular morphology on the healthy side was reproduced with a titanium mesh on the defective side. With the titanium mesh as a scaffold, PCBM collected from the posterior iliac crest was buried in the muscular portion of abdominis musculocutaneous flap. New bone formation was confirmed after 3 months, and regenerative mandibular reconstruction was completed 6 months postoperatively. An aesthetically and functionally favorable outcome was attained (Fig. 9.36).

Strategy 4: Reconstruction After Hemimandibulectomy: A Strategy Not Necessarily Requiring Osseous or Plate Reconstruction

Viewpoints on osseous reconstruction or free-end saddle reconstruction with a plate after hemimandibulectomy vary markedly among institutions, and no conclusion has been reached: some institutions report no functional improvement after surgery, while others describe improvement of postoperative QOL and facial appearance [89–91]. Basically, we use the reconstruction method established by the MD Anderson Cancer Center for hemimandibular and posterior defects [80, 89]. Instead of free-end saddle reconstruction with a bone flap or reconstruction plate, the contour is reconstructed with a musculocutaneous flap alone (Fig. 9.37). The most important aspect of this procedure is maintenance of the facial contour, i.e., preventing reduction of the volume of the musculocutaneous flap and facial asymmetry over time. Rectus abdominis musculocutaneous flaps are advantageous in that (1) reduction of whole total tissue volume is small because atrophy of subcutaneous fat and muscle with fatty change is mild due to the good blood supply, (2) muscular atrophy is delayed by reformation of the intercostal nerve to nerve suturing, and (3) modification can be carried out with the use of an anterior sheath of the abdominis muscle to prevent gravity-induced sinking of the musculocutaneous flap. Thus, a vascularized free rectus abdominis musculocutaneous flap is the specified standard flap for this reconstruction

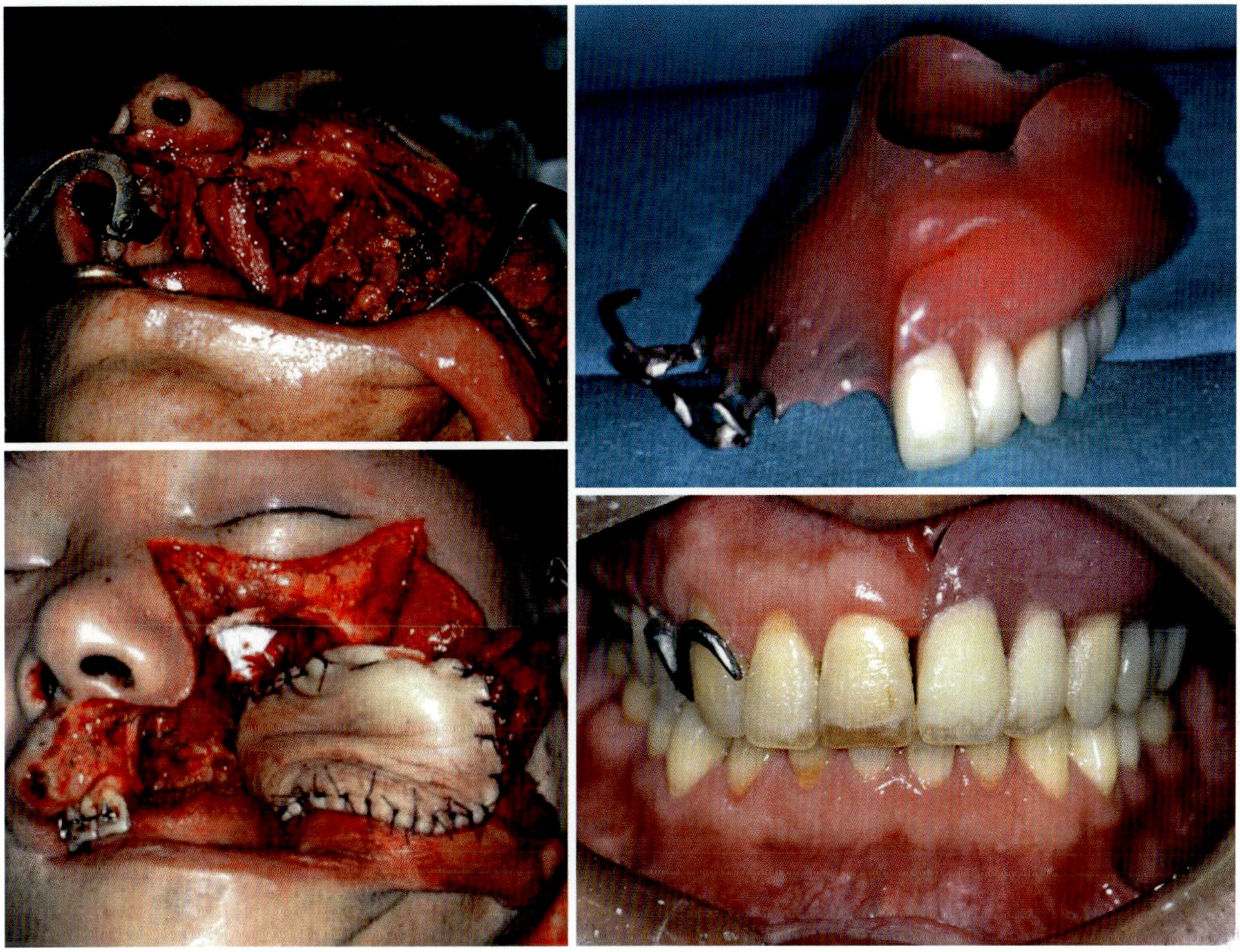

Fig. 9.32 Reconstruction with free forearm flap and resection denture after subtotal maxillectomy

(Figs. 9.37 and 9.38) [1]. When an abdominis musculocutaneous flap cannot be used, a pectoralis major musculocutaneous flap is selected (Figs. 9.39 and 9.40), for which conservation or reformation of a motor nerve, the medial pectoral nerve, is essential. This reconstruction also requires strict body weight management to maintain the overall volume of tissue (Figs. 9.38 and 9.40). MaCraw [92] reported that, when muscle is cut at its origin or end together with the dominant nerve, the muscle volume decreases to 50 % and fatty change occurs rapidly. Poor blood supply is also a major cause of fatty change in the muscle. Therefore, clinical and histopathological analyses are used in our institution to ascertain that early volume reduction of a musculocutaneous flap is prevented and a favorable facial contour is attained and maintained over a long period of time. A rectus abdominis musculocutaneous flap or a pectoralis major musculocutaneous flap incorporates an abundant blood supply; thus, subcutaneous fat does not markedly change over time, and the motor nerve can be reformed. Moreover, fixation of musculocutaneous flaps, particularly the muscle portion, is crucial for maintaining the motor function of the muscle and preventing its atrophy.

Trismus, which occurs in many cases of mandibular free-end saddle reconstruction when using a plate with an artificial condylar head, was not observed in cases treated with aesthetic contour reconstruction incorporating a musculocutaneous flap, and no major difference was noted in the eating function. Interestingly, some patients from whom a reconstruction plate with an artificial condylar head was removed on a patient's request, the patients' satisfactions with the function increased, indicating that the functions of the masticatory muscles, mandibular ligament, and temporomandibular joint structures, such as the articular disk and capsule, were not reconstructed after mandibular resection, and the simple insertion of a free bone flap and plate did not reconstruct functionally. Moreover, it is possible that trismus, which frequently develops in cases treated with free-end saddle reconstruction, is a functional disorder due to scar

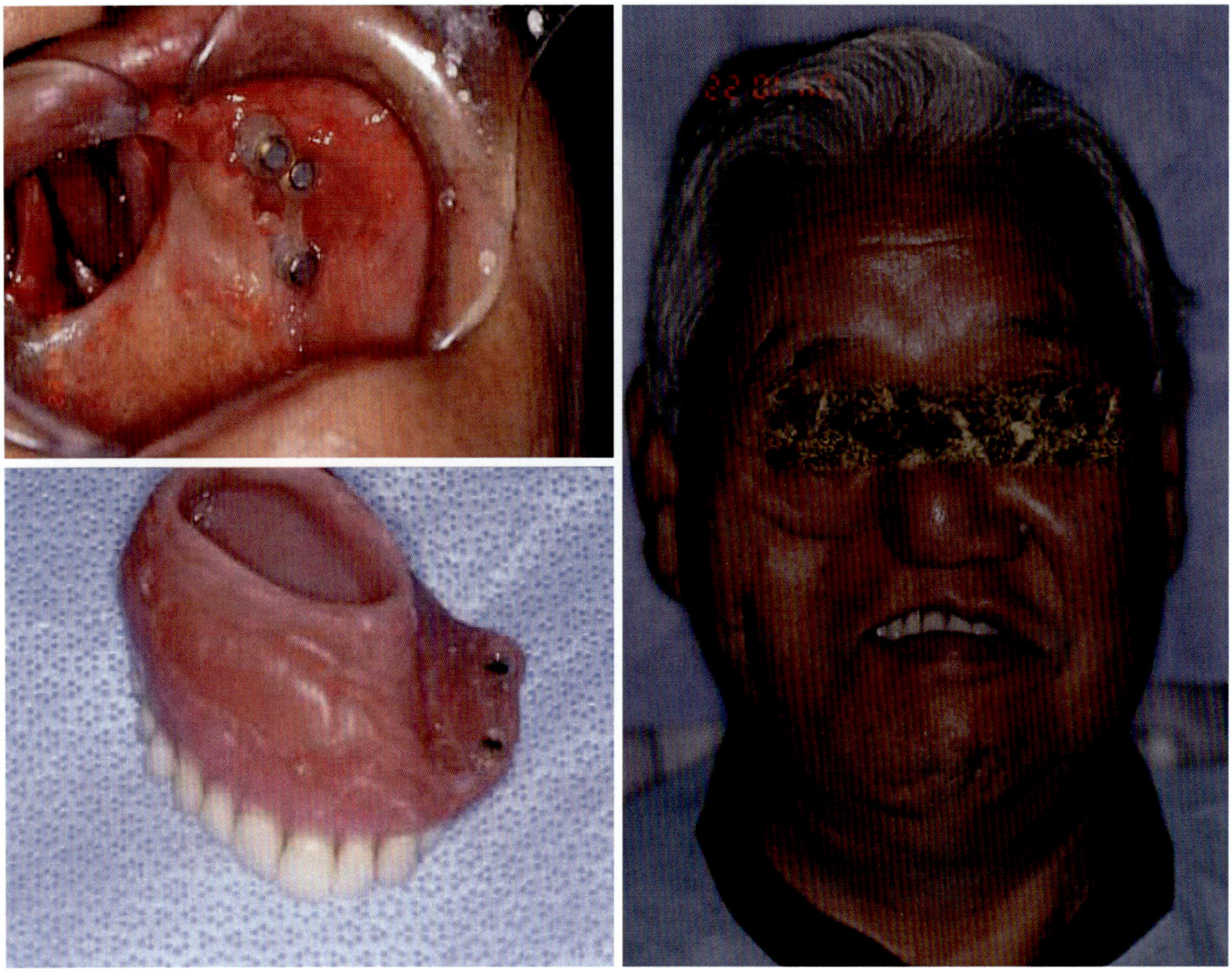

Fig. 9.33 Reconstruction with dental implants and resection denture after subtotal maxillectomy

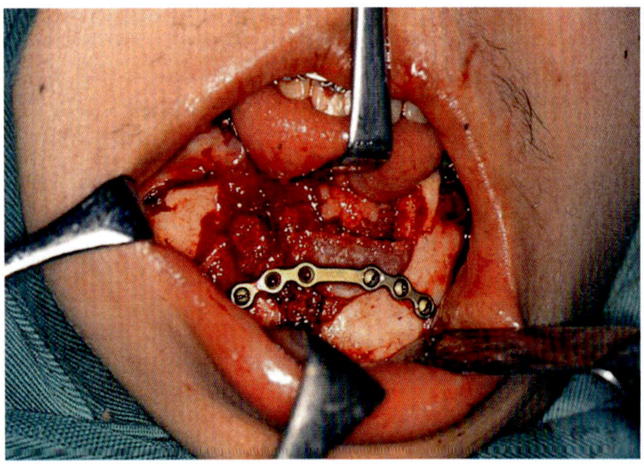

Fig. 9.34 Strategy 1 for mandibular reconstruction: reconstruction of 5 cm or smaller segmental mandibular defect with non-vascularized free iliac bone block and PCBM

contracture on the reconstructed side and fatigue caused by overstress of the temporomandibular joint on the non-reconstructed side.

In aesthetic contour reconstruction with a musculocutaneous flap, marked deviation of the residual mandible toward the resected side is problematic for occlusal reconstitution, and a jaw that is nearly or completely edentulous makes it more difficult. To overcome this, we regard postoperative modification of the prosthesis as essential and requisite for maintaining mandibular function with a musculocutaneous flap alone. Ten patients with osseous or plate reconstruction after hemimandibulectomy and eleven with only soft tissue reconstruction, evaluated with the use of the performance status scale (PSS), functional assessment of cancer treatment in general (FACT-G), and disease-specific questions, have demonstrated that osseous reconstruction or free-end saddle

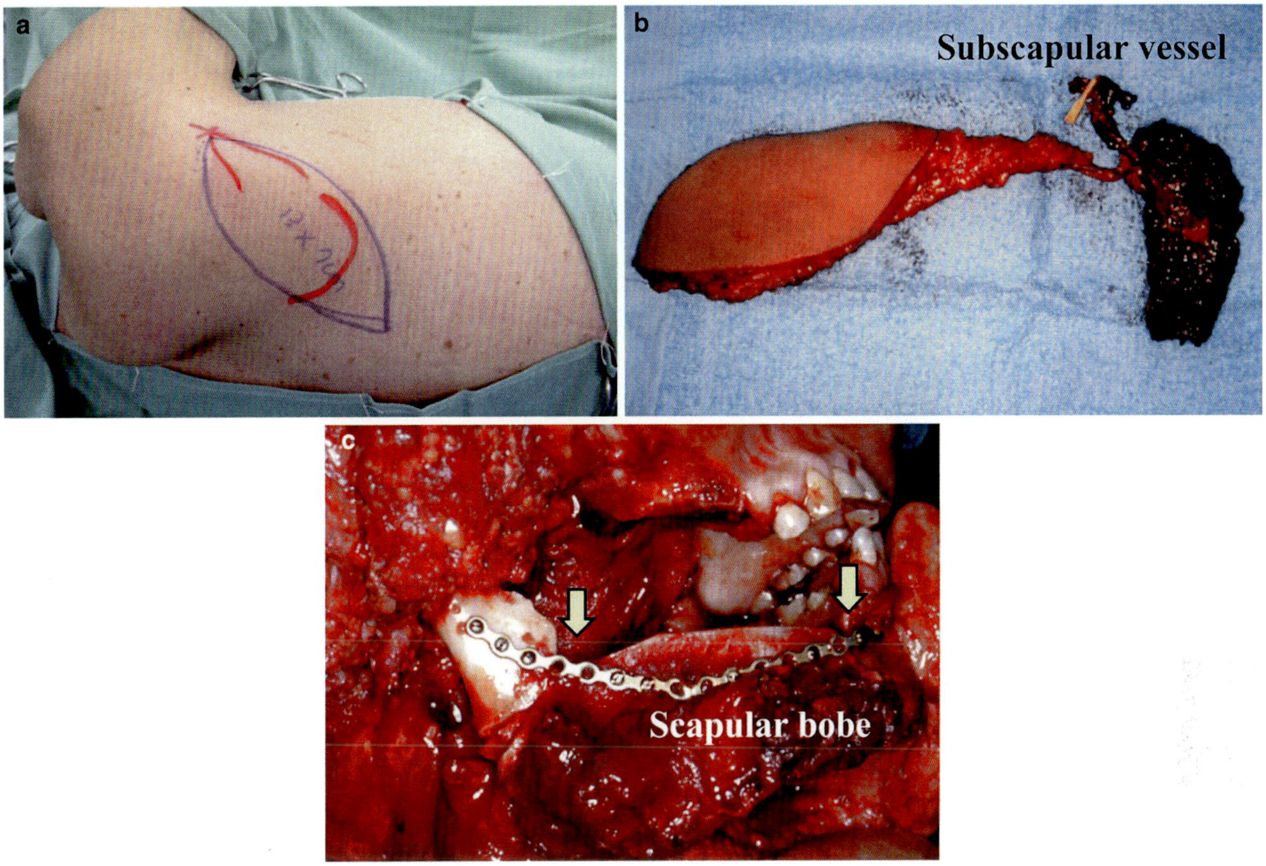

Fig. 9.35 Strategy 2 for mandibular reconstruction: vascularized osteocutaneous flap (scapular osteocutaneous flap)

reconstruction with a plate improves patient QOL [93]. No description of postoperative prosthetic treatment of the soft tissue reconstruction has been mentioned, however. We consider that aesthetic hemimandibular reconstruction with a musculocutaneous flap alone is effective only when modifications of the prosthesis, such as the application of dental implants to the residual bone and prosthetic appliances with palatal lump, and strict management of occlusion, are carried out (Fig. 9.41).

Dental implant placement in reconstructed bone improves the masticatory function, and some oral and maxillofacial surgeons consider that free-end saddle reconstruction of the mandible with a bone flap is a prerequisite to dental implant placement. On the other hand, the sensory perception of peri-implant soft tissue is crucial for dental implants to improve masticatory function [94]. In our experience, if the reconstructed region does not sense stimuli, dental implants, although placed into the grafted bone, do not improve masticatory function.

9.2.6.3 Maxillomandibular Reconstruction and Functional Unit Reconstruction

When maxillomandibular reconstruction, particularly reconstruction of the masticatory function, is considered, many oral and maxillofacial surgeons, plastic surgeons, and oral and maxillofacial prosthodontists carry it out with the percept that occlusion = mastication. Mastication is a collective term comprising three functions: manipulation, trituration, and consolidation. The role of occlusion is only trituration; the others are effected by tongue movement. Occlusion is just one of the functional units of the masticatory system, along with the tongue, mouth floor, and buccal mucosal movements; that is why the reconstruction of occlusion alone does not restore the masticatory function. Occlusal reconstruction causes swallowing disorders, and the resection of the tongue alone sometimes leads to the inability of chewing. Based on the principle of functional unit reconstruction, it is not possible to effectively reconstruct the oral function by reconstructing individual units,

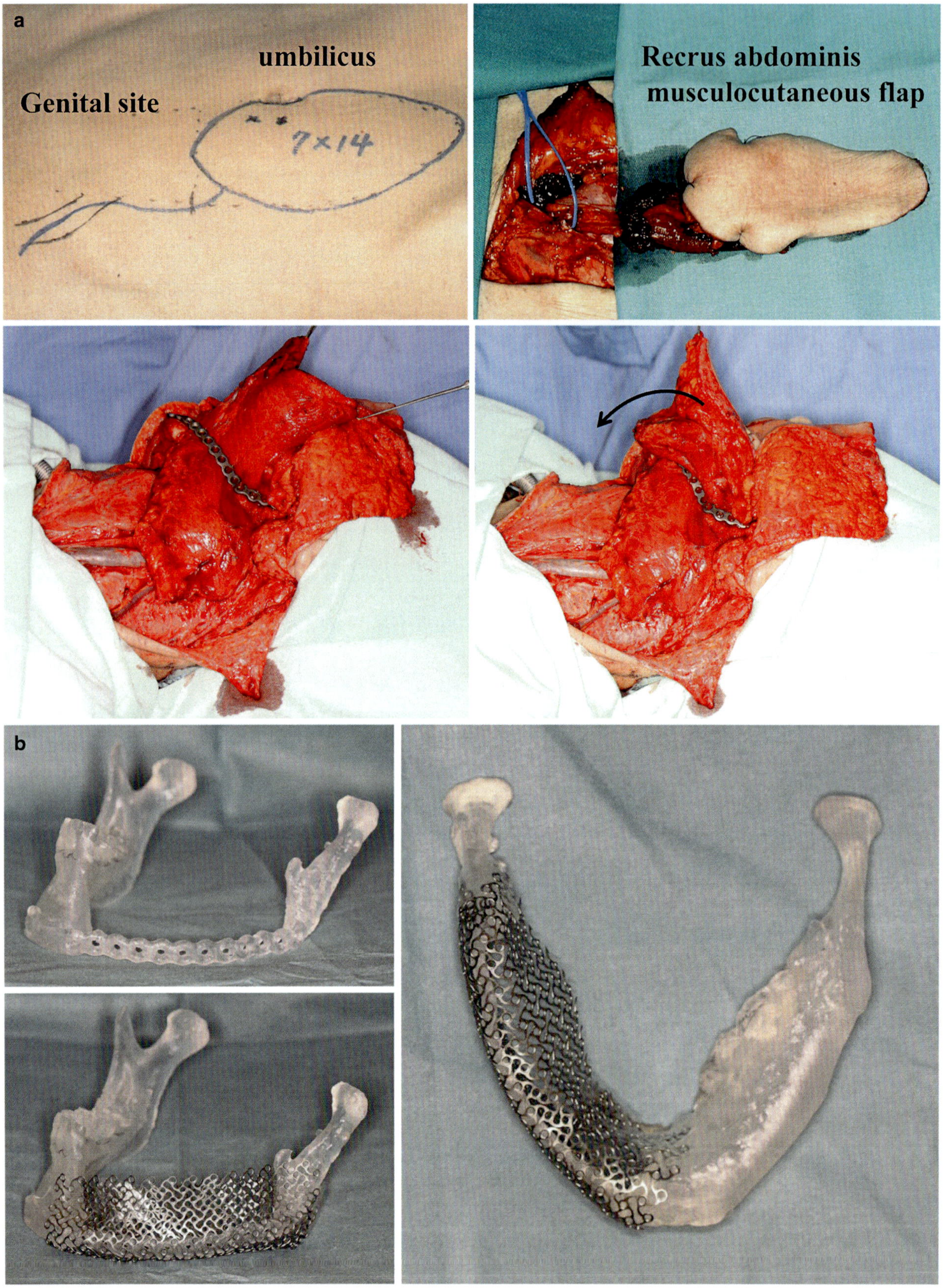

Fig. 9.36 Strategy 3 for mandibular reconstruction: regenerative mandibular reconstruction. (**a**) The primary reconstruction, so-called wrap-around procedure, in which a titanium reconstruction plate was wrapped with a muscular portion of the vascularized free rectus abdominis musculocutaneous flap, was carried out to restore the contour of the lower face. (**b**) A 3D model was constructed from CT images, and the mandibular morphology on the healthy side was reproduced with a titanium mesh on the defective side. (**c**) Six months thereafter, secondary regenerative mandibular reconstruction was carried out with PCBM and titanium mesh as a scaffold. PCMB collected from the posterior iliac crest was then buried in the rectus abdominis muscle of the flap. (**d**) Regenerative mandibular reconstruction was completed in the next 6 months

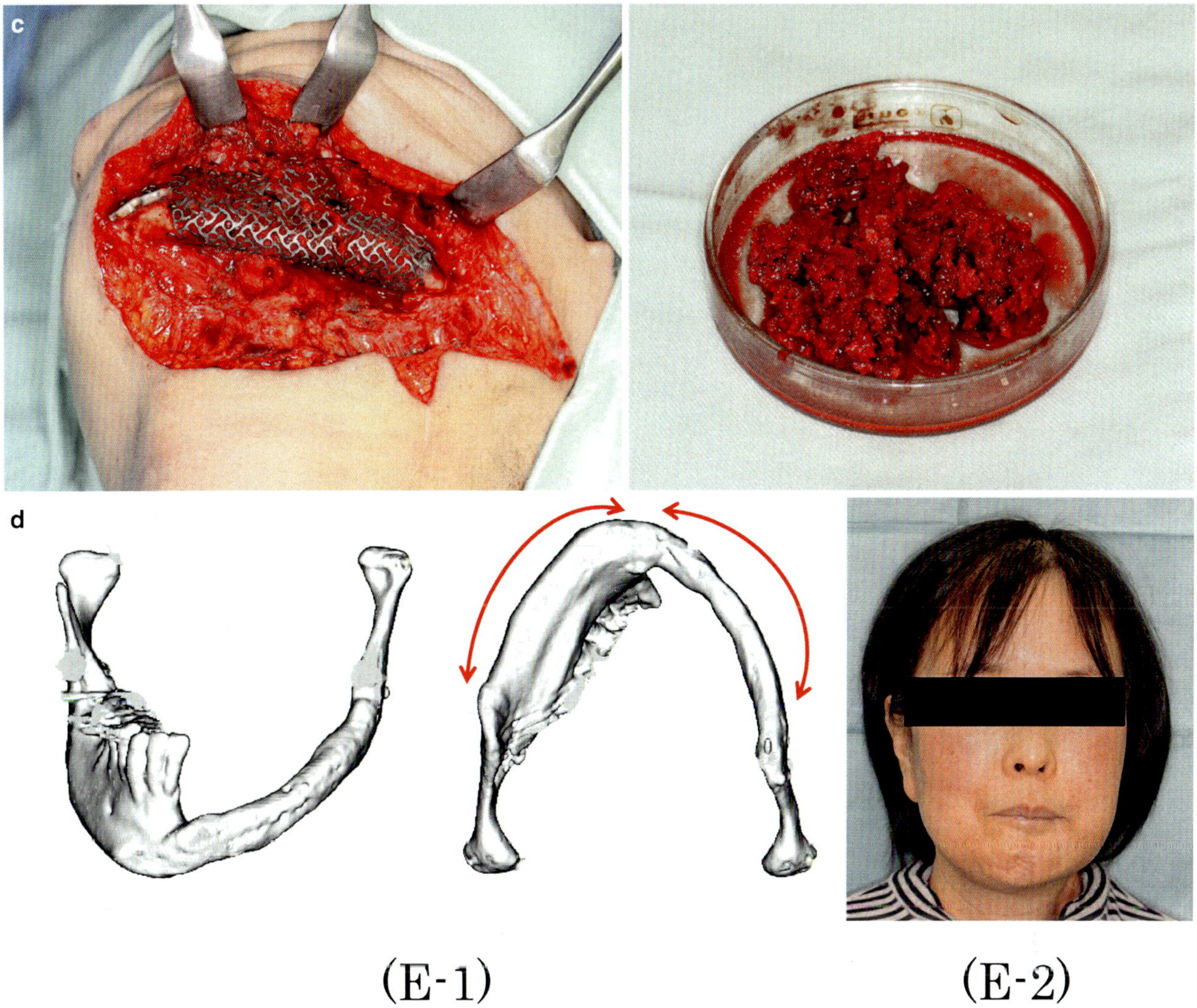

Fig. 9.36 (continued)

such as the tongue, oral floor, buccal mucosa, and mandible. The goal of functional reconstruction comprises diverse elements: not only the extent of resection (residual function) and the reconstruction method, but also the patient's potential (laryngeal function and residual teeth) and motivation (positive attitude toward rehabilitation). The consistency of postoperative meals desired by patients also varies. Since easily ingestible therapeutic diets are better than normal diets that sometimes cause distress, it is important to set an optimal method and goal based on each patient's potential and residual function. Moreover, it is difficult to evaluate functions after reconstruction. Evaluation of the movement of individual units, such as the tongue and mandible, is often not reflected in postoperative meal consistency, which is not directly linked to the degree of satisfaction. To make eating an enjoyable activity, not just to maintain life, it is necessary to evaluate the ease of eating and the savoring of food. Functional oral and oropharyngeal reconstruction including maxillomandibular reconstruction is a challenge toward answering the crucial question: What is eating?

9.2.6.4 Mandibular Reconstruction with a Prefabricated Osseous Free Flap Using a Three-Dimensional Digital Model

For successful mandibular reconstruction, it is important that the continuity lost in the mandibular bone due to mandibulectomy be restored precisely and for donor bone shaping to complement the mandibular defect. The vascularized fibula first reported by Hidalgo [95] has been a preferred donor site because of its length and versatility, and many hospitals and medical centers mainly use vascularized fibular osteocutaneous flaps for mandibular reconstruction.

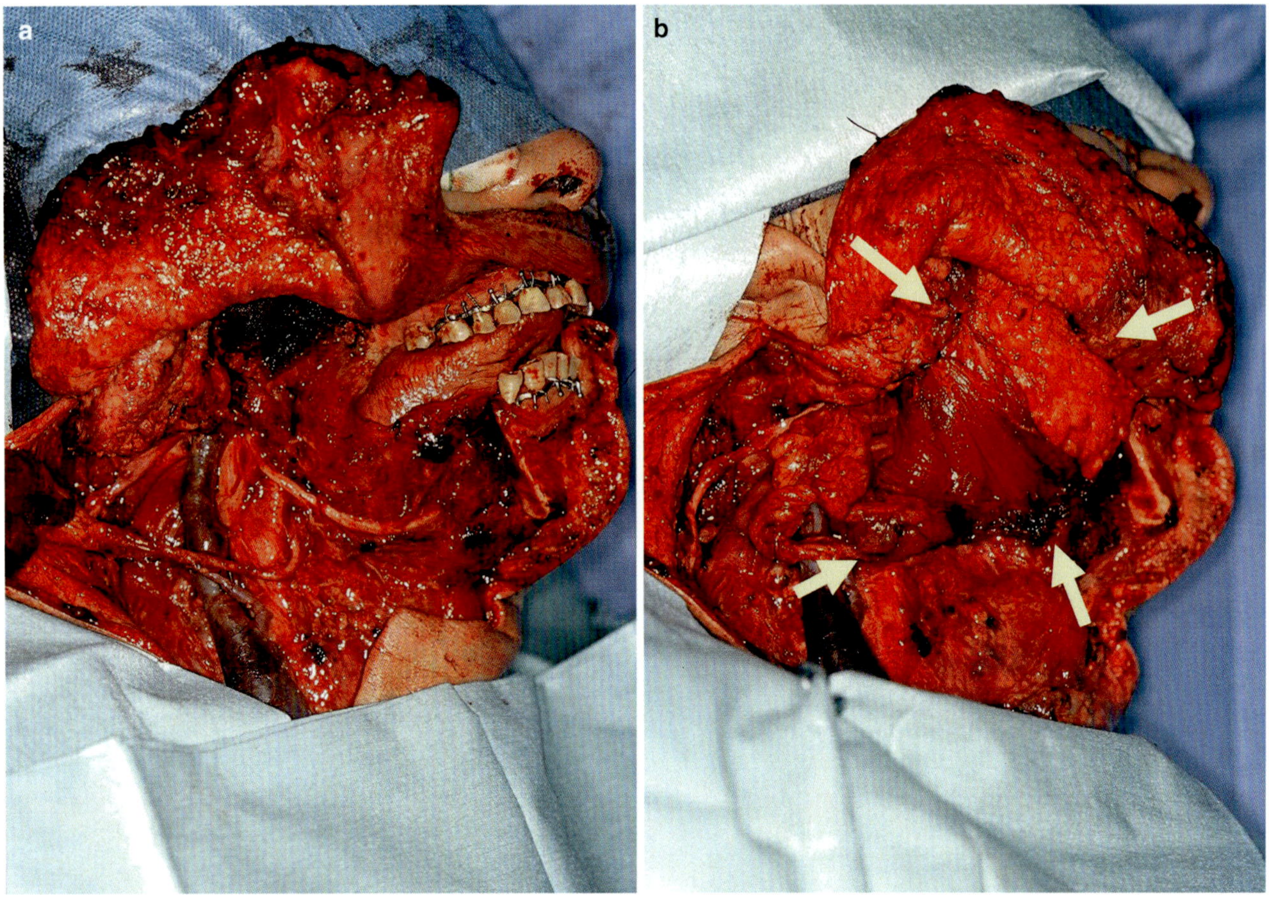

Fig. 9.37 Strategy 4 for mandibular reconstruction: reconstruction after hemimandibulectomy. (**a**) Hemimandibulectomy. (**b**) Aesthetic facial contour reconstruction with a rectus abdominis musculocutaneous flap alone

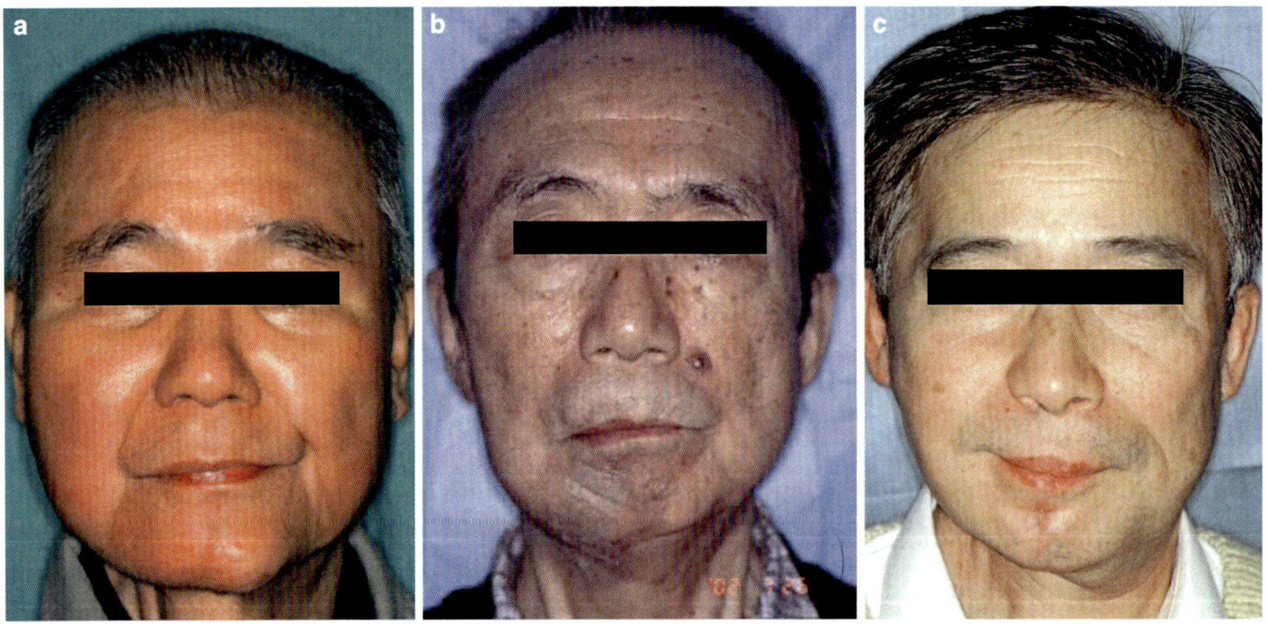

Fig. 9.38 Results of aesthetic facial contour reconstruction after hemimandibulectomy with a rectus abdominis musculocutaneous flap. (**a**) Seven years postoperative. (**b**) One year postoperative. (**c**) One year postoperative

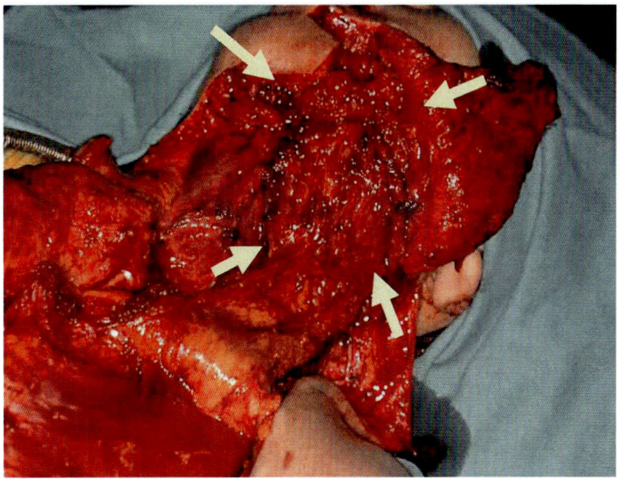

Fig. 9.39 Aesthetic facial contour reconstruction with a pectoralis major musculocutaneous flap alone

Unlike reconstruction of some other defects, mandibular reconstruction demands a high degree of precision because of the spatial and functional constraints of the mandible. When fibular osteotomies are required for a mandibular defect, mandibular reproduction at the time of reconstruction is difficult, the operation time is long, and the manipulation requires high-level proficiency. In an attempt to overcome these problems, preoperative surgical planning (model-based surgery) using a prefabricated stereolithographic mandibular model (SLMM) is a useful technique. Furthermore, computer-aided design software can be used to not only maximize the precision of bony osteotomies, which helps to recreate the shape of the mandibular arch, but also improve the overall efficiency of the reconstructive process (Fig. 9.42a, b). The prefabricated model clarifies the form and state of the diseases, shortens the operation time, and reduces operative blood loss [96–99].

In the preoperative state, a prefabricated SLMM constructed preoperatively by three-dimensional (3D)-CT and computer-aided virtual preplanning is used to accurately and promptly perform mandibulectomy and fibular osteotomies. Replicas of the mandible and fibula (acrylic plastic or plaster of Paris) are also made preoperatively using a 3D printer for model-based surgery (Fig. 9.43). Surgical guides are also prefabricated to decide on the line of mandibular resection (Fig. 9.44). A precisely simulated, postreconstructive mandibular model with fibular replacement is also made using model-based surgery (Fig. 9.45), and the number and lengths of harvested fibula can be planned.

During the operation, in order to avoid malocclusion and displacement of the condylar head after mandibulectomy, a 3D adjustable fixation device is applied to fix the parts of the mandible to be preserved, and, then, the surgical guide is matched to the mandibular bone by setting it preoperatively (Fig. 9.44). Segmental mandibulectomy is performed according to the planned line of resection with the surgical guide. Segmental mandibulectomy and fibular harvesting are performed simultaneously by maxillofacial and orthopedic or plastic microsurgical teams. After mandibulectomy, the harvested fibula is shaped with several osteotomies to fit the mandibular defect using a prefabricated reconstruction model

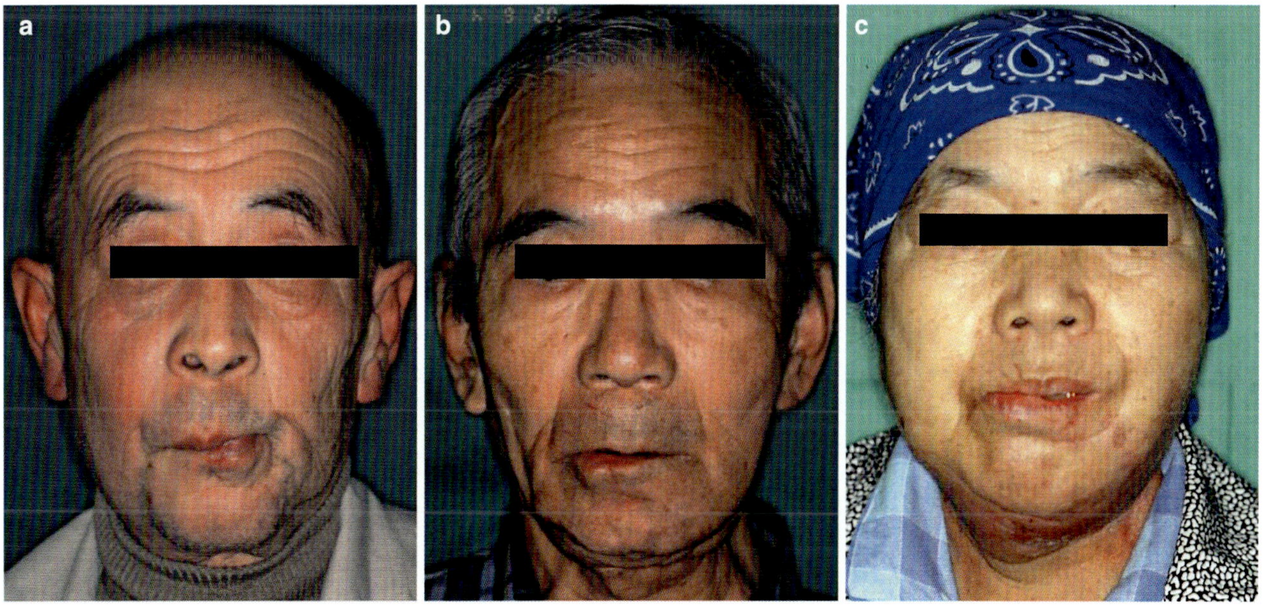

Fig. 9.40 Results of aesthetic facial contour reconstruction after hemimandibulectomy with a pectoralis major musculocutaneous flap. (**a**) Six years postoperative. (**b**) Five years postoperative. (**c**) One year postoperative

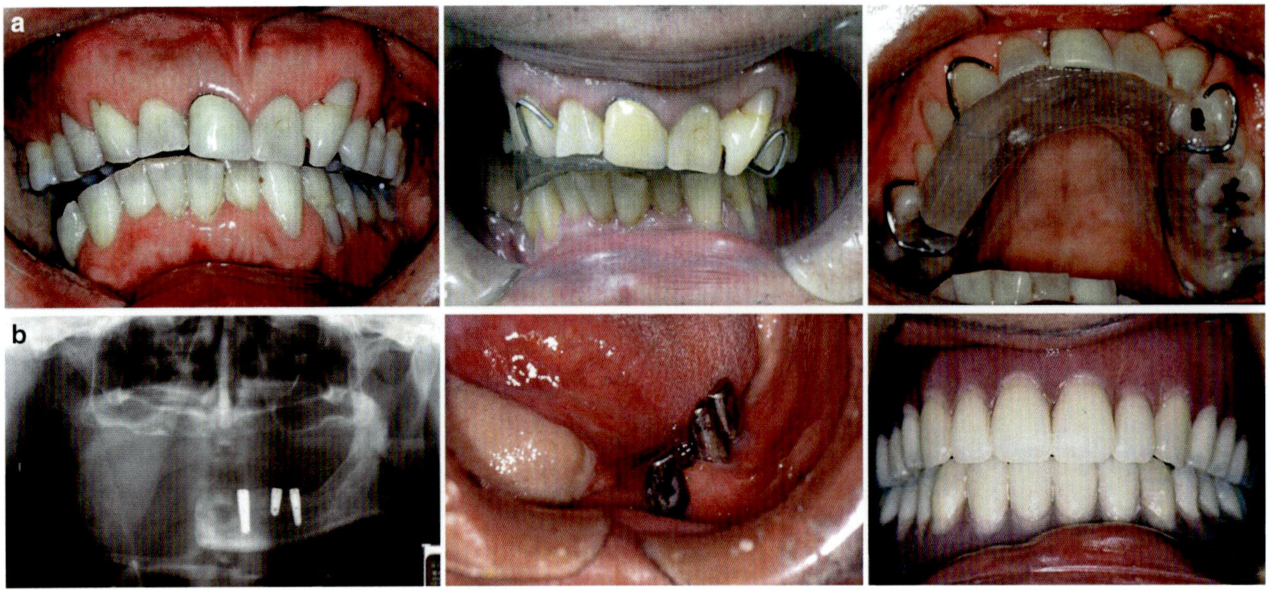

Fig. 9.41 Application of dental implants or palatal lump. (**a**) Palatal lump. (b) Dental implants

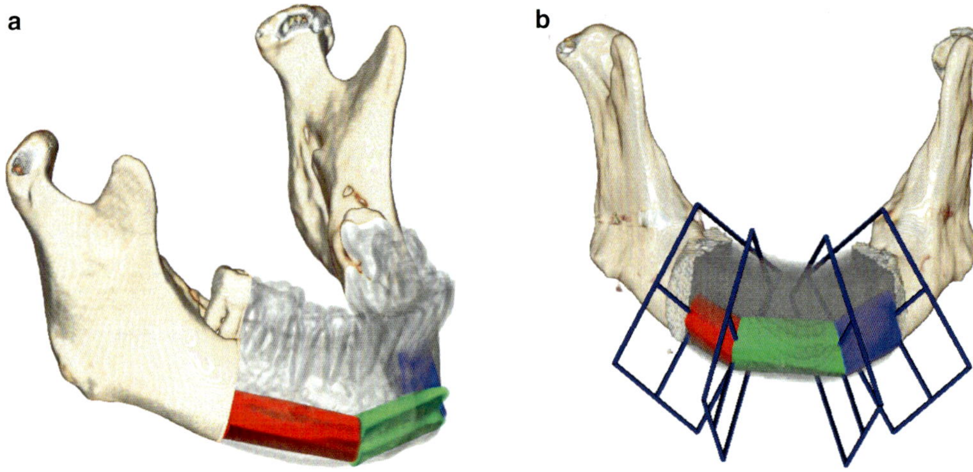

Fig. 9.42 (**a**) Computer-aided virtual surgical planning. (**b**) Planned resection margin with surgical guides

and fibular osteotomy guide template (Fig. 9.46a, b), and it is fixed to the remaining mandibular bone with a titanium mini plate (Fig. 9.47). Next, the graft is anastomosed to the recipient site vessels after fixing the grafted bone (Fig. 9.48).

The SLMM technique has been reported to be useful [97–99]. Using it, we can perform model-based surgery to simulate the resection range and fibular osteotomies and facilitate accurate and prompt mandibulectomy and fibular osteotomy during the operation. In addition, the prefabricated reconstructed model is helpful for recreating the symmetry of the mandible postoperatively.

The mandibulectomy is performed according to the planned line of resection with a surgical guide, and the mandible is reconstructed with more accurate shaping of the harvested fibula, in accordance with the configuration of the virtual graft in the prefabricated SLMM.

This procedure using a SLMM can effectively facilitate mandibular reconstruction surgery, and it is useful to increase the accuracy and shorten the operation time, achieving satisfactory aesthetic results. This technique is simple, effective, and helpful for surgeons performing not only mandibular but also maxillofacial reconstructions [100].

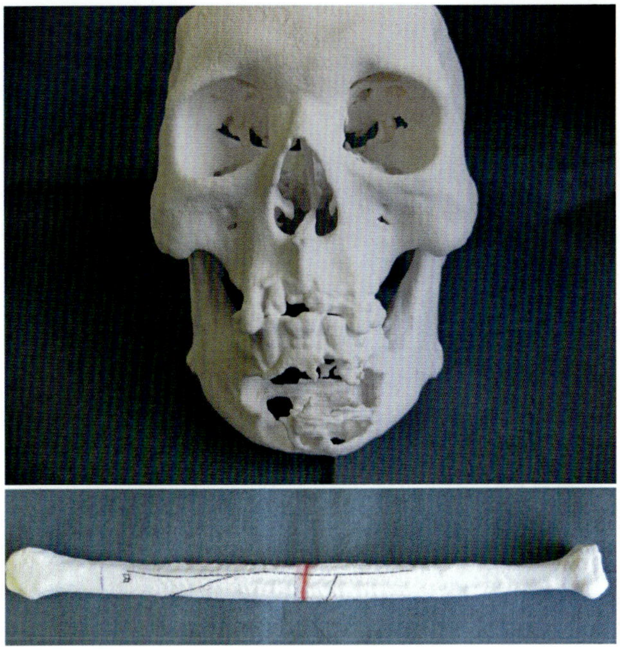

Fig. 9.43 Craniofacial skeleton and fibula models (acrylic plastic or plaster of Paris) were made preoperatively based on 3D-CT

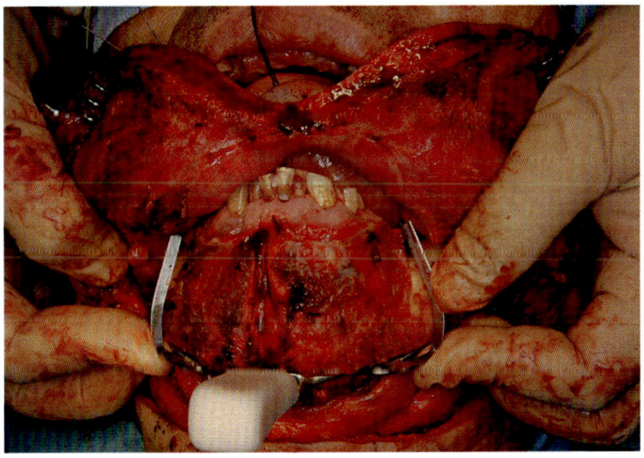

Fig. 9.44 A surgical guide was also prefabricated to decide on the line of mandibular resection

9.2.6.5 Double-Barreled Vascularized Fibula Graft for Mandibular Reconstruction

The vascularized fibula flap is ideal for mandibular reconstruction and has become the most popular reconstruction method after mandibular resection, because it generally provides adequate bone graft length and can be easily contoured by multiple osteotomies to recreate the proper mandibular curvature and osseointegrated implant insertion is easy.

However, the main disadvantage of the fibula is its limited width, which is not suitable for patients with a large difference in height between the neomandible and the dentulous or nonatrophic mandible [101, 102]. Using the single

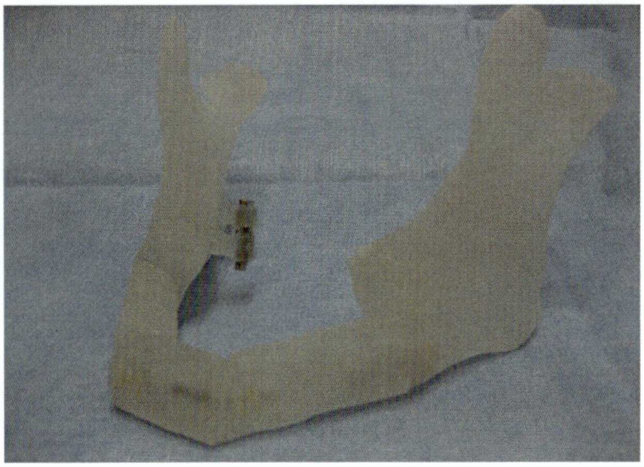

Fig. 9.45 A precisely simulated postreconstructive mandibular model with fibular replacement was also made employing model-based surgery

fibula bone may produce a height discrepancy between the native mandible and the grafted fibula that results in subsequent difficulty in wearing conventional dentures or osseointegrated implants [103]. Because the low height of the reconstructed segment creates a large distance to the occlusal plane and a large vertical dimension for the prosthetic device, this evokes high leverage forces, which can be detrimental to the implants in cases of solely implant-borne superstructures, as well as to supporting teeth in free-end hybrid situations, especially if the crown/fixture ratio is greater than 1:1 [104]. Moreover, patients are not satisfied with the postoperative facial appearance after reconstruction of the symphysis because of the collapse of the cheilion and lower lip [105].

Then, to avoid a large vertical dimension of the prosthetic superstructure, it is good to use a long fibula graft that is halved and folded onto itself to increase the height of the neomandible [106]. The basis for the use of the double-barreled graft is that the height of the mandible is at least twice the diameter of the fibula; otherwise, the reconstructed segment would be too high. If the mandible is within twice the diameter of the fibula, the fibula will be segmented and used as a one-and-a-half fibula. The average thickness of the fibular diaphysis is about 10 mm, and the height of the segment is established from the panoramic radiograph and 3D-CT scans of the head and neck.

Surgical Planning

Preoperatively, a prefabricated stereolithographic or plaster of Paris mandibular model (replica) of the mirror images of the contralateral unaffected mandible is prepared using CT data and computer-aided design/computer-aided manufacturing technology. The extent of the mandibulectomy, the length of fibula required, the osteotomy sites of the fibula,

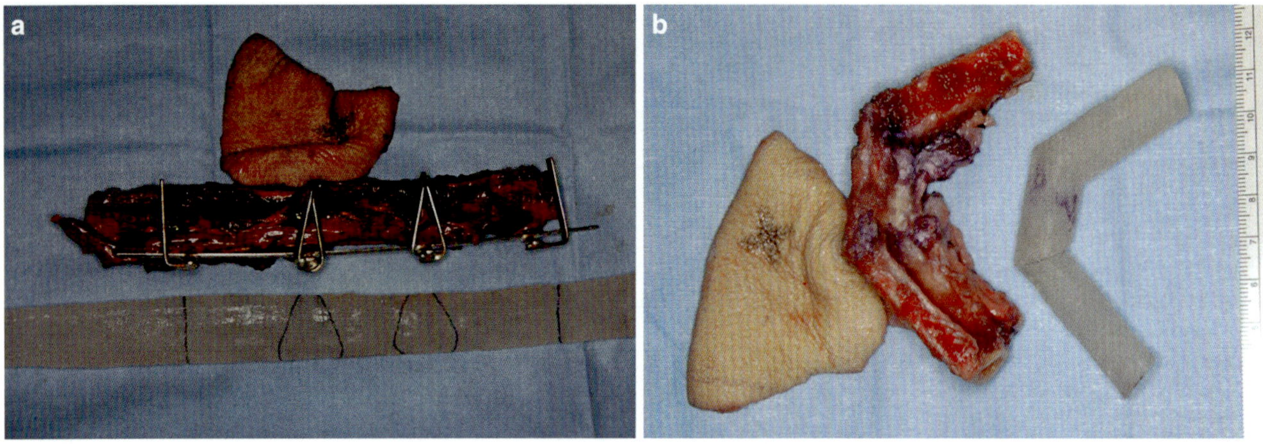

Fig. 9.46 After mandibulectomy, the harvested fibula was shaped with several osteotomies to fit the mandibular defect using a prefabricated reconstruction model and fibular osteotomy guide template (**a**, **b**)

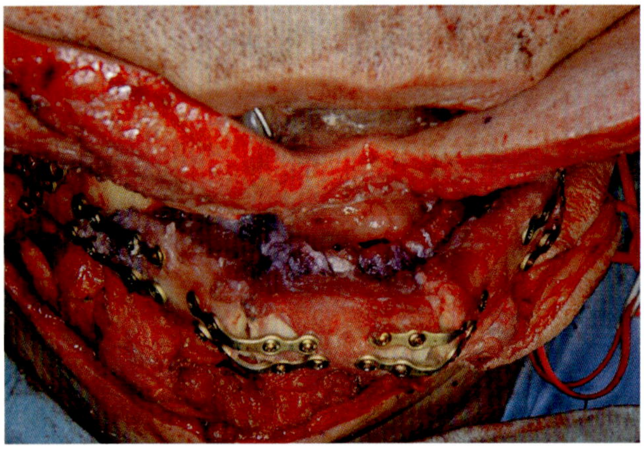

Fig. 9.47 Shaped harvested fibula was fixed to the remaining mandibular bone with a titanium mini plate

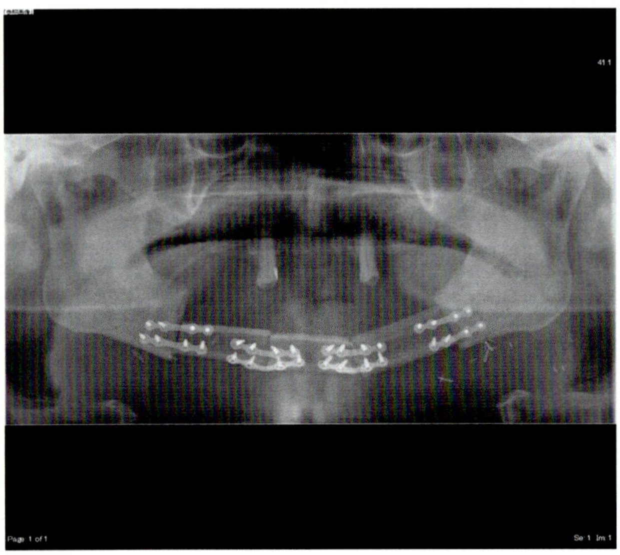

Fig. 9.48 Panoramic radiograph of the reconstructed mandible at 12 months postoperatively

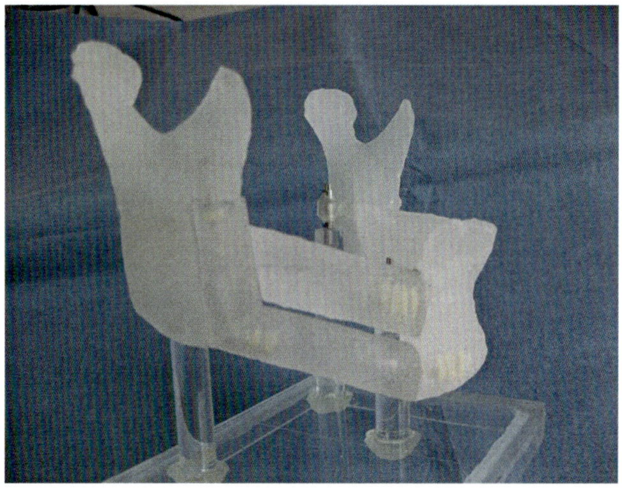

Fig. 9.49 A prefabricated stereolithographic or plaster of Paris mandibular model (replicas) is prepared preoperatively by use of the CT data and computer-aided design/computer-aided manufacturing technology. Postreconstructive mandibular model with fibular replacement was also made

and the site of double barreling are determined with these replicas (Fig. 9.49).

Operative Procedure

Segmental mandibulectomy, harvesting of the fibula osteocutaneous flap, and mandibular reconstruction are performed according to the presurgical planning. In cases in which the soft tissue defect is in the intra- or extraoral region and requires reconstruction at the same time, a fibula flap is harvested including the skin paddle in the distal third of the lower limb with careful protection of the perforators. The harvested fibula is formed with some osteotomies to fit the mandibular defect without damaging the vascular bundle, using the prefabricated reconstruction model. The anterolateral

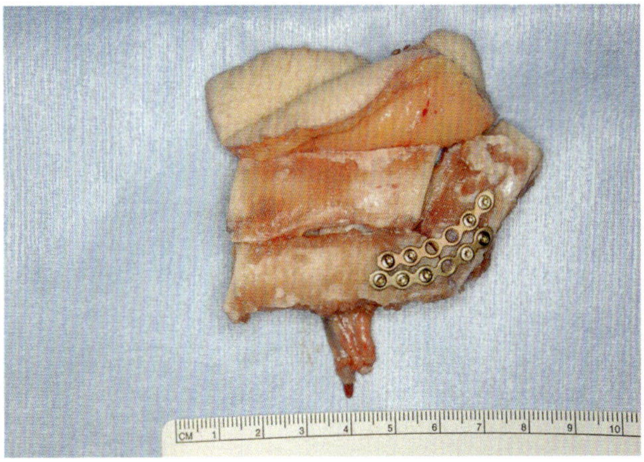

Fig. 9.50 The double-barrel fibula graft was shaped with several osteotomies to fit the mandibular defect using a prefabricated reconstruction model and fibular osteotomy guide template

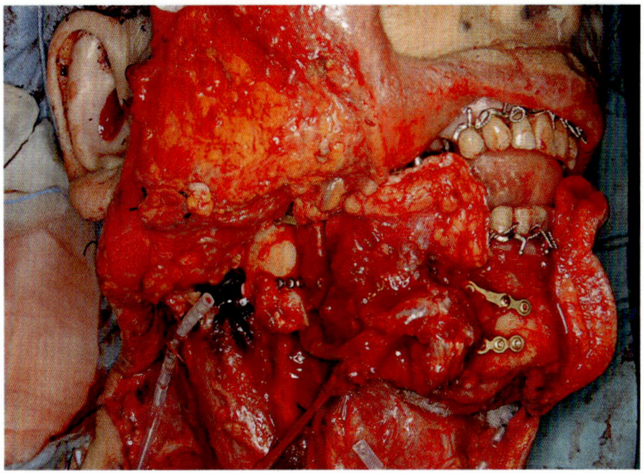

Fig. 9.51 The lower barrel of the osteotomized fibula is partially fixed into the defect with mini plates so that the locations of osseointegrated dental implants can be planned on the upper barrel

surfaces of two osteotomized bones are folded into contact to form the double barrel. At the folding point, an approximately 1 cm portion of the fibula is discarded, and periosteal continuity is maintained to prevent stretching, compressing, kinking, or twisting of the vascular bundle (Fig. 9.50). It is also possible that the segmentalization of the fibula at the folding point by using a single vertical osteotomy and reflection of about 2 cm of periosteum at this point without the removal of any bony segment will reduce the operative time and the risk of injury to the vascular pedicle with no loss of bone stock. At the curving point, the fibula is contoured by wedge osteotomies and fit to the mandibular defect using a prefabricated reconstruction model. The lower barrel of the osteotomized fibula is then partially fixed into the defect with mini plates so that the locations of osseointegrated dental implants can be planned on the upper barrel [102, 105]. At that time, the upper barrel is located slightly more lingually than the lower barrel to avoid a crossbite. After the neomandible is created, anastomoses are performed between recipient and peroneal vessels (Figs. 9.51 and 9.52).

Microsurgically anastomosed bone grafts can develop a solid union by 4 weeks after transfer so that functional loading of implants is possible 4–6 weeks postoperatively [107]. The fibula is a long bone, with a thick cortex. It has a denser structure than the scapula, radius, or iliac bone, and it is therefore more suitable for supporting dental implants [108]. The implant-bearing bone of the double-barreled graft is a more suitable distance to the occlusal plane of the adjacent dentate mandible than the bone of the conventional single fibula graft (Fig. 9.53). This reduces the height of the prosthetic superstructure and diminishes unfavorable lever arm forces on the implants in cases of solely implant-borne superstructures, as well as to the supporting teeth in free-end hybrid situations [106].

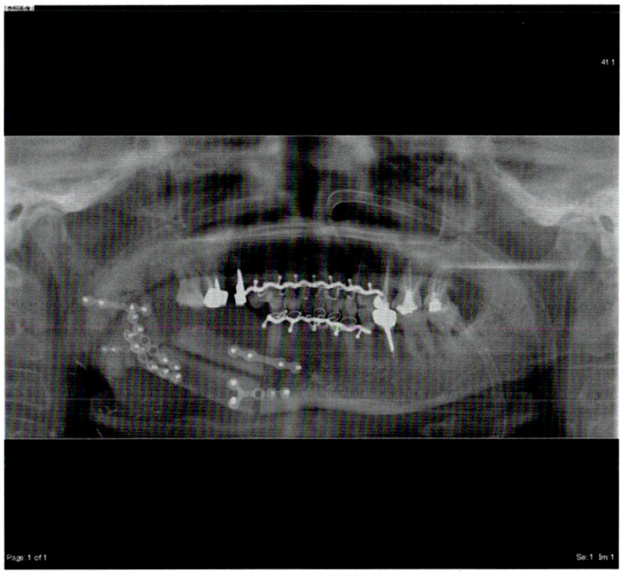

Fig. 9.52 Panoramic radiograph of the reconstructed mandible with double-barrel fibula graft at 6 months postoperatively

In the case of a mandibular defect larger than 10 cm, the double-barreled technique is not suitable, because the fibula length usually required during bone harvest is 24 cm, which would result in higher risk of donor site morbidity. In the case of a larger defect, as for reconstruction of the mandibular body and ramus, the partial double-barreled fibula graft can be applied. The mandibular body and ramus are reconstructed with a medial fibular fragment, and the remaining fibula is halved and folded into part of the medial fibula to increase the vertical height [109]. In the symphysis, the partial double-barreled fibula graft is performed to support the lower lip and cheilion (Fig. 9.54). For patients with

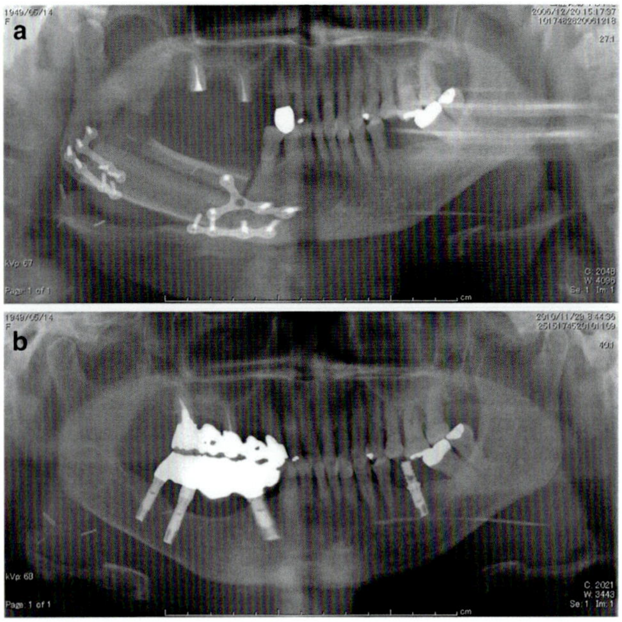

Fig. 9.53 Panoramic radiograph reveals the bone union of the native mandible and the double-barrel fibula graft 6 months after surgery (**a**) and positive osseointegration between the dental implants and fibula 12 months after initial surgery (**b**)

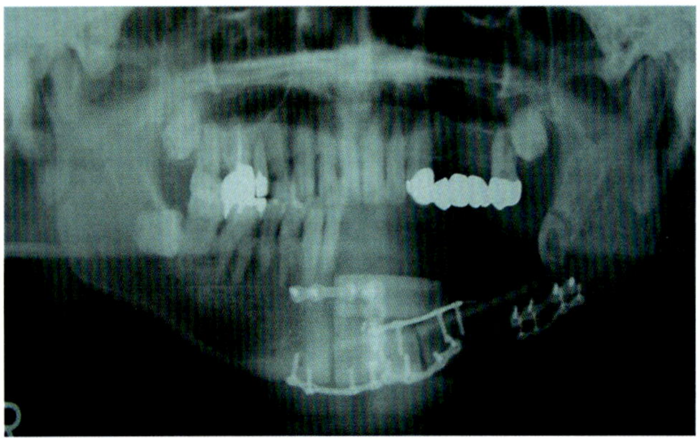

Fig. 9.54 In the symphysis, the partial double-barrel fibula graft is performed to support the lower lip and cheilion

preservation of the mandibular lower border, a double-barreled fibula graft is used as an onlay graft instead, with enough vertical allowance for dental rehabilitation.

The advantages of using the double-barreled fibula graft in mandibular reconstruction can be summarized as follows: (1) the greatest bone length to fold in the double barrel; (2) no delayed operation compared with the onlay bone graft and distraction of the fibula for achieving the height of the native mandible; (3) greater suitability for osseointegrated implantation than the iliac bone graft; (4) a unique blood supply that allows folding of bone struts and does not affect blood flow through the supplying vessels and the medullary cavity; and (5) low donor site morbidity and the possibility of using a skin paddle in the reconstruction of a composite defect [103, 110].

References

1. Yoloo S, Komori T, Furudoi S, Shibuya Y, Umeda M, Ichinose A, Nomura T, Terashi H, Tahara S, Nibu K (2003) Indications for vascularised free rectus abdominis musculocutaneous flap in oromandibular region in terms of efficiency of anterior rectus sheath. Microsurgery 23:96–102
2. Yokoo S, Minamikawa T, Furudoi S, Shibuya Y, Umeda M, Komori T (2008) Reconstruction using rectus abdominis musculocutaneous flap for maintenance of eating and swallowing function after advanced oral oncologic surgery. J Jpn Stomatol Sci 57:1–18
3. Gonzalez-Ulloa M (1956) Restoration of the face covering by means of selected skin in regional aesthetic units. Br J Plast Surg 9:212–221
4. Burget GC, Menick FJ (1985) The submit principle in nasal reconstruction. Plast Reconstr Surg 76:239–247
5. Menick FJ (1987) Aristry in aesthetic surgery. Aesthetic perception and the subunit principle. Clin Plast Surg 14:723–735
6. Iwahira Y, Maruyama A, Yoshitake M (1994) A miniunit approach to lip reconstruction. Plast Reconstr Surg 93:1282–1285
7. Mureau MA, Posch NA, Meeuwis CA et al (2005) Anterolateral thigh flap reconstruction of large external facial skin defects: a follow-up study on functional and aesthetic recipient- and donor-site outcome. Plast Reconstr Surg 115:1077–1086
8. Silfen R, Ritz M, Morgan D et al (2005) Can aesthetic facial reconstruction be judged in black and white? Aesthetic Plast Surg 29:6–9
9. Song R, Gao Y, Sing Y (1982) The forearm flap. Plast Reconstr Surg 9:21–26
10. Harii K, Ebihara S, Ono I et al (1985) Pharyngoesophargeal reconstruction using a fabricated forearm flap. Plast Reconstr Surg 75:463–474
11. Souter DS, MaGregor IA (1986) The radial forearm flap in intraoral reconstruction: the experience of 60 consecutive cases. Plast Reconstr Surg 78:1–8
12. Tahara S, Suzuki T, Sagara S (1989) Eye socket reconstruction with free radial forearm flap. Ann Plast Surg 21:112–116
13. Mühlbauer W, Herndl E, Stock W (1985) The forarm flap. Plast Reconstr Surg 70:336–342
14. Evans HB (1991) The radial forearm flap, microsurgery. In: Bunke HJ (ed) Transplantation-replantation. Lea & Febiger, Philadelphia/London
15. Timmons MJ (1986) The vascular basis of the radial forearm flap. Plast Reconstr Surg 77:80–92
16. Thoma A, Archiald S, Jackson S et al (1994) Surgical patterns of venous drainage of the free forearm flap in head and neck reconstruction. Plast Reconstr Surg 93:54–59
17. Taylor GI, Caddy CM, Watterson PA et al (1990) The venous territories (venosome) of human body: experimental study and clinical implication. Plast Reconstr Surg 86:185–188
18. Yokoo S, Tahara S, Hashikawa K, Ichinose A (2000) Reliability of the deep system in venous drainage of the free radial forearm flap. J Jpn PRS 20:597–602
19. Ichinose A, Tahara S, Yokoo S et al (2002) Importance of the deep vein in the drainage of radial forearm flap. A haemodynamic study. Scand J Plast Reconstr Surg Hand Surg 37:145–149
20. Fleurg AL, Ress TD (1956) The use of foam rubber in pressure dressings. Plast Reconstr Surg 18:309–311

21. Burd DA (1984) The pressure button: a refinement of the traditional "tie-over" dressing. Br J Plast Surg 37:127–129
22. Niranjan NS (1985) A modified tie-over dressing for skin grafts. Br J Plast Surg 38:415–418
23. Lapid O, Thomson HC (2005) The speed tie-over dressing. Ann Plast Surg 54:215–217
24. Flowers RS (1970) Unexpected postoperative problems in skin grafting. Surg Clin North Am 50:439
25. Converse MJ (1977) Transplantation of skin: grafts and flaps. In: Reconstructive plastic surgery, vol 1, 2nd edn. Sanders, Philadelphia
26. Ganong WF (1973) Review of medical physiology, 6th edn. Maruzen Co Ltd, Tokyo
27. Bonica JJ (1990) Causalgia and other sympathetic dystrophies. In: The management of pain, 2nd edn. Lea and Febiger, Philadelphia
28. Seltzer Z, Devor M (1978) Ephaptic transmission in chronically damaged peripheral nerves. Neurology 29:1061–1064
29. Gibbons JJ, Wilson PR (1992) RSD score; criteria for the diagnosis of reflex sympathetic dystrophy and causalgia. Clin J Pain 8:260–263
30. Landin DA, Smith DP, Izenberg PH, Deschner P (1992) Acute repair of a full-thickness right ventricular defect with a composite myofascial pedicle flap. Plast Reconstr Surg 90:310–313
31. Aoki T, Watanabe T, Tsuchida M, Yamato Y, Hayashi J, Souma T (1999) Successful treatment of bronchopleural fistula complicated by empyema with reconstruction using isolated rectus sheath and omentopexy. Jpn J Chest Surg 13:152–155
32. Ueda K, Inoue T, Tanaka I (1991) Chest wall reconstruction by a rectus abdominis myocutaneous composite flap attached with the external oblique fascia. Br J Plast Surg 44:538–540
33. Ueda K, Inoue T, Harada T (1992) Dura and cranial base reconstruction using the external oblique fascia and rectus abdominis muscle flap. J Reconstr Microsurg 8:427–432
34. Sakai S, Suzuki I, Izawa H (1992) Adipofascial (anterior rectus sheath) flaps for breast reconstruction. Ann Plast Surg 29:173–177
35. Zhang F, Lineaweaver WC, Ustuner T (1997) Comparison of muscle mass preservation in denervated muscle and transplanted muscle flap after motor and sensory reinnervation and neurotization. Plast Reconstr Surg 99:803–808
36. Lund WS (1987) Deglutition. In: Wright D (ed) Scott-Brown's otolaryngology, Basic science. Butterworth, London
37. Kiyokawa K, Tai Y, Inoue Y, Yanaga H, Mori K, Nakashima T (1999) Functional reconstruction of swallowing and articulation after total glossectomy without laryngectomy: money pouch-like reconstruction method using rectus abdominis myocutaneous flap. Plast Reconstr Surg 104:2015–2020
38. Yokoo S, Komori T, Umeda M, Takenono I, Hashikawa K, Hanagaki H, Tahara S (2001) Functional reconstruction of mobile tongue and suprahyoid muscles after resection of cancer of the tongue. Br J Oral Maxillofac Surg 39:252–255
39. Mattes SJ, Nahai F (1997) Reconstructive surgery. In: Principles, anatomy & technique. Churchill Livingstone, New York
40. Lui R, Gullane P, Brown D et al (2001) Pectoralis major myocutaneous flap in head and neck reconstruction: retrospective review of indications and results in 244 consecutive cases at Toronto General Hospital. J Otolaryngol 30:e34–e40
41. Yang D, Marshall G, Morris SF (2003) Variability in the vascularity of the pectoralis major muscle. J Otolaryngol 32:e12–e15
42. Po-Wing Yuen A (2006) Preservation of lateral thoracic artery to improve vascular supply of distal skin without compromising pedicle length in harvesting pectoralis major myocutaneous flap. J Plast Reconstr Aesthet Surg 59:1433–1435
43. Rikimaru H, Kiyokawa K, Inoue Y et al (2005) Three-dimensional anatomical vascular distribution in the pectoralis major myocutaneous flap. Plast Reconstr Surg 115:1342–1352
44. Ishikawa Y (1990) Study on the vascular pattern of the pectoralis major musculocutaneous flap. Jpn J Oral Maxillofac Surg 36:1037–1055
45. Ord RA (1996) The pectoralis major myocutaneous flap in oral and maxillofacial reconstruction: a retrospective analysis of 50 cases. J Oral Maxillofac Surg 54:1292–1295
46. Urken ML, Biller HF (1995) Pectoralis muscle. In: Urken ML, Cheney ML et al (eds) Atlas of regional and free flaps for head and neck reconstruction. Ranem Oress, New York
47. Harii K, Torii S, Sekiguchi J (1978) The free lateral thoracic flap. Plast Reconstr Surg 62:212–222
48. Kim JT, Ng SW, Naidu S et al (2011) Lateral thoracic perforator flap: additional perforator flap option from the lateral thoracic region. Plast Reconstr Aesthet Surg 64:1596–1602
49. Taylor GI, Daniel RK (1975) The anatomy of several free flap site. Plast Reconstr Surg 56:243–253
50. Ward GE, Hendrick JW (1950) Malignant epithelial tumors of the skin of head and neck. Am J Surg 79:771–786
51. Farr HW (1969) Cervical island flap repair of oral and pharyngeal defects in the composite operation for cancer. Am J Surg 72:759–763
52. Futrell JW, Johns ME (1978) Platysma myocutaneous flap for intraoral reconstruction. Am J Surg 136:504–507
53. Szudek J, Taylor M et al (2007) Systemic review of the platysma myocutaneous flap for head and neck reconstruction. Arch Otolaryngol Head Neck Surg 133:655–661
54. Mathes SJ (1981) Classification of the vascular anatomy of muscles: experimental and clinical correlation. Plast Reconstr Surg 67:177–187
55. Mathes SJ, Nahai F (1997) Platysma flap. In: Mathes SJ (ed) Reconstructive surgery, principles, anatomy, & technique. Churchill Livingstone and Quality medical publishing Inc, New York
56. Hurwitz DJ, Rabson JA et al (1983) The anatomic basis for the platysma skin flap. Plast Reconstr Surg 72:302–313
57. Imanishi N, Nakajima H, Kishi K, Chang H, Aiso S (2005) Is the platysma flap musculocutaneous? Angiographic study of the platysma. Plast Reconstr Surg 115:1018–1024
58. Coleman JJ III, Jurkiewicz MJ et al (1983) The platysma musculocutaneous flap. Plast Reconstr Surg 72:315–321
59. Harnsberger HR (2011) Surahyoid and infrahyoid neck overview. In: Harnsberger HR (ed) Diagnostic imaging head and neck. Amirsys, Atlanta
60. Baser B, Pradhan KA (1988) Bipedal myocutaneous flap for one-stage reconstruction of the cheek after cancer surgery. J Laryngol Otol 102:601–602
61. Bhathena HM, Kavarana NM (1988) Bipaddled, retrograde radial extended forearm flap with microarterial anastomosis for reconstruction in oral cancer. Br J Plast Surg 41:354–357
62. Sakai S, Endo T (1989) A compound radial artery forearm flap for the reconstruction of lip and chin defects. Br J Plast Surg 42:337–338
63. Naasan A, Quaba AA (1990) Reconstruction of the oral commissure by vascularised toe web transfer. Br J Plast Surg 43:376–378
64. Freedman AM, Hidalgo DA (1990) Full-thickness cheek and lip reconstruction with the radial forearm free flap. Ann Plast Surg 25:287–294
65. Zide BM (1990) Deformities of the lips and cheeks. In: McCarthy JG (ed) Plastic surgery, vol 3. Saunders, Philadelphia
66. Sadove RC, Luce EA, McGrath PC (1991) Reconstruction of lower lip and chin with the composite radial forearm-palmaris longus free flap. Plast Reconstr Surg 88:209–214
67. Cabrera RC, Zide BM (1997) Cheek reconstruction. In: Aston SJ, Beasley RW, Thorne CHM (eds) Grabb and Smith's plastic surgery, 5th edn. Lippincott-Raven, Philadelphia
68. Goldstein MH (1984) A tissue-expanding vermilion myocutaneous flap for lip repair. Plast Reconstr Surg 73:768–770
69. Cordeiro PG, Santamaria E (1999) Primary reconstruction of complex midfacial defects with combined lip-switch procedure and free flaps. Plast Reconstr Surg 103:1850–1856

70. Pogrel MA, Podlesh S et al (1997) A comparison of vascularised and nonvascularised bone graft for reconstruction of mandibular continuity defects. J Oral Maxillofac Surg 55:1200–1206
71. Takushima A, Harii K et al (2001) Mandibular reconstruction using microvascular free flaps: a statistical analysis of 178 cases. Plast Reconstr Surg 108:1555–1563
72. Cordeiro PG, Disa JJ et al (1999) Reconstruction of the mandible with osseous free flaps: a 10-year experience with 150 consecutive patients. Plast Reconstr Surg 104:1314–1320
73. Disa JJ, Cordeiro PG (2000) Mandible reconstruction with microvascular surgery. Semin Surg Oncol 19:226–234
74. Schöning H, Emshoff R (1998) Primary temporary AO plate reconstruction of the mandible. Oral Surg Oral Med Oral Pathol Oral Radiol Endod 86:667–672
75. Wei FC, Celik N (2002) Complications after reconstruction by plate and soft-tissue free flap in composite mandibular defects and secondary salvage reconstruction with osteocutaneous flap. Plast Reconstr Surg 112:37–42
76. Hirota M, Mizuki N et al (2008) Vertical distraction of a free vascularized scapular flap in the reconstructed mandible for implant therapy. Int J Oral Maxillofac Surg 37:481–483
77. Boyd JB, Mulholland RS et al (1995) The free flap and plate in oromandibular reconstruction: long-term review and indications. Plast Reconstr Surg 112:1018–1028
78. Chepeha DB, Teknos TN (2008) Lateral oromandibular defect: when is it appropriate to use a bridging reconstruction plate combined with soft tissue. Head Neck 30:709–717
79. Disa JJ, Pusic AL (2001) Simplifying microvascular head and neck reconstruction: a rational approach to donor site selection. Ann Plast Surg 47:385–389
80. Kroll SS, Rabb GL et al (1998) Reconstruction of posterior mandibular defects with soft tissue using the rectus abdominis free flap. Br J Plast Surg 51:503–507
81. Bianchi B, Ferri A et al (2010) Reconstruction of anterior through and through oromandibular defects following oncological resection. Microsurgery 30:97–104
82. Brown JS, Jones DC et al (2002) Vascularized iliac crest with internal oblique muscle for immediate reconstruction after maxillectomy. Br J Oral Maxillofac Surg 40:183–190
83. Hu YJ, Hardianto A et al (2007) Reconstruction of a palatomaxillary defect with vascularized iliac bone combined with a superficial inferior epigastric artery flap and zygomatic implants as anchorage. Int J Oral Maxillofac Surg 36:854–857
84. Okay DJ, Genden E et al (2001) Prosthodontic guidelines for surgical reconstruction of the maxilla: a classification system of defects. J Prothet Dent 86:352–363
85. Cordeiro PG, Santamaria E (2000) A classification system and algorithm for reconstruction of maxillectomy and midfacial defects. Plast Reconstr Surg 105:2331–2346
86. Mukohyama H, Haraguchi M et al (2005) Rehabilitation of a bilateral maxillectomy patient with a free fibula osteocutaneous flap. J Oral Rehabil 32:541–544
87. Shestac KC, Schusterman MA et al (1988) Immediate microvascular reconstruction of combined palatal and midfacial defects. Am J Surg 156:252–255
88. Davison SP, Sherris DA et al (1998) An algorithm for maxillectomy defect reconstruction. Laryngoscope 108:215–219
89. Bulter CE, Lewin JS (2003) Reconstruction of large composite oromandibulomaxillary defects with free vertical rectus abdominis myocutaneous flaps. Plast Reconstr Surg 223:499–507
90. Schimmele SR (2001) Delayed reconstruction of continuity defects of mandible after tumor surgery. J Oral Maxillofac Surg 59:1340–1344
91. Komisar A (1990) The functional result of mandibular reconstruction. Laryngoscope 100:364–374
92. MaCraw JB, Dibbell DG, Carraway JH (1977) Clinical dentition of independent myocutaneous vascular territories. Plast Reconstr Surg 60:341–352
93. Keith MW, Nabil MR, Shanna LRNA et al (1998) Effects of hemimandibulectomy on quality of life. Laryngoscope 108:1574–1577
94. Schmelzeisen R, Neukan FW, Shirota T et al (1996) Postoperative function after implant insertion in vascularized bone grafts in maxilla and mandible. Plast Reconstr Surg 97:719–725
95. Hidalgo DA (1989) Fibula free flap: a new method of mandible reconstruction. Plast Reconstr Surg 84:71–79
96. Brown GA, Milner B, Firoozbakhsh K (2002) Application of computer-generated stereolithography and interpositioning template in acetabular fractures: a report of eight cases. J Orthop Trauma 16(5):347–352
97. Cunningham LL Jr, Madsen MJ, Peterson G (2005) Stereolithographic modeling technology applied to tumor resection. J Oral Maxillofac Surg 63(6):873–878
98. Yeung RW, Samman N, Cheung LK, Zhang C, Chow RL (2007) Stereomodel-assisted fibula flap harvest and mandibular reconstruction. J Oral Maxillofac Surg 65:1128–1134
99. Yamanaka Y, Yajima H, Kirita T, Shimomura H, Aoki K, Yamakawa N, Imai Y (2010) Mandibular reconstruction with vascularized fibular osteocutaneous flaps using prefabricated stereolithographic mandibular model. J Plast Reconstr Aesthet Surg 63:1751–1753
100. Rohner D, Bucher P, Hammer B (2013) Prefabricated fibular flaps for reconstruction of defects of the maxillofacial skeleton: planning, technique, and long-term experience. Int J Oral Maxillofac Implants 28:e219–e221. doi:10.11607/jomi.te01
101. Klesper B, Wahn J, Koebke J (2000) Comparisons of bone volumes and densities relating to osseointegrated implants in microvascularly reconstructed mandibles: a study of cadaveric radius and fibula bones. J Craniomaxillofac Surg 28:105–110
102. Chang YM, Tsai CY, Wei FC (2008) One-stage, double-barrel fibula osteoseptocutaneous flap and immediate dental implants for functional and aesthetic reconstruction of segmental mandibular defects. Plast Reconstr Surg 122:143–145. doi:10.1097/PRS.0b013e3181774135
103. He Y, Zhang ZY, Zhu HG, Wu YQ, Fu HH (2011) Double-barrel fibula vascularized free flap with dental rehabilitation for mandibular reconstruction. J Oral Maxillofac Surg 69:2663–2669. doi:10.1016/j.joms.2011.02.051, Erratum in: J Oral Maxillofac Surg 70(1):251 (2012)
104. Saadoun AP, LeGall M (1992) Implant positioning for periodontal, functional, and aesthetic results. Pract Periodontics Aesthet Dent 4:43–54
105. Shen Y, Sun J, Li J, Shi J, Ow A (2012) Long-term results of partial double-barrel vascularized fibula graft in symphysis for extensive mandibular reconstruction. J Oral Maxillofac Surg 70:983–991. doi:10.1016/j.joms.2011.02.125
106. Bähr W, Stoll P, Wächter R (1998) Use of the "double barrel" free vascularized fibula in mandibular reconstruction. J Oral Maxillofac Surg 56:38–44
107. Bitter K, Schlesinger S, Westerman U (1983) The iliac bone or osteocutaneous transplant pedicled to the deep circumflex iliac artery. II. Clinical application. J Maxillofac Surg 11:241–247
108. Serra JM, Paloma V, Mesa F, Ballesteros A (1991) The vascularized fibula graft in mandibular reconstruction. J Oral Maxillofac Surg 49:244–250
109. Guerra MF, Gías LN, Campo FJ, Pérez JS, de Artiñano FO, González FJ (2000) The partial double-barrel free vascularized fibular graft: a solution for long mandibular defects. Plast Reconstr Surg 105:1902–1903
110. Kirita T (2005) Recent advancement of therapy and research in oral cancer. In: Kuriyama S, Yoshiji H (eds) New perspectives in cancer research and therapy, 1st edn. Research Signpost, Kerala

Prosthetic Reconstruction for Oral Cancer Patients Using Dental Implants

10

Tetsu Takahashi, Yoshihiro Yamashita, Ikuya Miyamoto, Kensuke Yamauchi, So Yokota, Shinnosuke Nogami, and Kenko Tanaka

Abstract

Prosthetic reconstruction for patients who had ablative head and neck tumor surgery is still challenging because both soft and hard tissues are required. Use of dental implants in oral cancer reconstruction has become an important aspect of the reconstructive plan for these patients. For the mandibular defects, first, the continuity of the mandible should be restored according to tissue condition. In severe cases, free flap transfer should be performed. Relatively short segments or benign tumors with sufficient vascularity could possibly be treated with the bone-grafting procedure with particulate cancellous bone marrow (PCBM) combined with titanium mesh (PCBM-MESH). Second, facial contours and the final dental occlusion are simulated to determine the optimal base of the dental implant or conventional dentures. The final prosthetic treatment requires an intra-oral environment for the prosthesis, particularly enough alveolar ridge with good and healthy soft tissue around the prosthesis. For this purpose, PCBM-MESH is a useful technique to link between optimum facial contour and alveolar reconstruction. Local tissue management including thinning of the skin paddle and/or vestibuloplasty is often required. The choice of prosthesis depends on the condition of the reconstruction, the remaining dentition, the maxilla–mandibular relationship, and other factors.

Keywords

Dental implant • Free vascularized bone graft • PCBM • Reconstruction • Titanium mesh

10.1 Introduction

Oral cancer patients who undergo surgical treatment experience consequent severe functional impairment, including speech, swallowing, chewing, and esthetics. Prosthetic reconstruction for the patients who had ablative head and neck tumor surgery is challenging because both soft and hard tissues are required. Surgical treatment is often combined with radiotherapy, which further worsens oral functioning. The prosthetic rehabilitation of those patients may be difficult or sometimes may even be impossible because of the lack of stability when conventional complete or partial dentures are used. The use of dental implants can enhance the quality of life (QOL) of those patients by enabling use of an implant-supported/retained prosthesis. A proper choice of reconstruction techniques in

T. Takahashi (✉) • K. Yamauchi
S. Yokota • S. Nogami • K. Tanaka
Division of Oral and Maxillofacial Surgery,
Department of Oral Medicine and Surgery,
Tohoku University Graduate School of Dentistry,
4-1, Seiryo-machi, Aoba-ku, Sendai, Miyagi 980-8587, Japan
e-mail: tetsu@dent.tohoku.ac.jp

Y. Yamashita
Department of Oral and Maxillofacial Surgery,
Miyazaki University School of Medicine, Miyazyaki, Japan

I. Miyamoto
Department of Oral and Maxillofacial Surgery,
Kyushu Dental University, Kitakyushu, Japan

T. Kirita and K. Omura (eds.), *Oral Cancer: Diagnosis and Therapy*,
DOI 10.1007/978-4-431-54938-3_10, © Springer Japan 2015

combination with implant-supported/retained prosthetics can give better functional results in the oral rehabilitation of these patients [1]. There are numerous treatment modalities for mandibular defects after tumor surgery [2–4]. In this chapter, a strategy for mandibular reconstruction combined with dental implants for patients with oral cancer is discussed.

10.2 Necessity of Mandibular Reconstruction

Large segmental resection of both maxilla and mandible after ablative tumor surgery results in severe functional impairment and diminishes the QOL of the patients. The goals of mandibular reconstruction are to reestablish the form of the lower third of the face and to restore the patient's ability to eat in public, be intelligible to both trained and untrained listeners, and to maintain an unencumbered airway that allows the freedom to perform all activities [5]. Amputation of the mandible leads to lateral deviation of the chin and difficulties in performing prosthetic rehabilitation. Use of a reconstruction plate without any bony reconstruction may also result in difficulties in performing prosthetic rehabilitation and in plate fracture because of metal fatigue. Therefore, when the physical status of the patients is allowed, mandibular basal bone should be reconstructed; this will also facilitate the prosthetic restoration. The quality of prosthetic rehabilitation has long been pointed out as a very important factor for patient satisfaction [6]. Immediate reconstruction should be considered when head and neck ablative surgery is scheduled. Secondary reconstruction may also be proposed to the patient to enhance both functional and aesthetic outcomes and to avoid pathological fracture of the remaining mandible after amputation at initial ablative cancer surgery.

10.3 Strategy for Jaw Reconstruction Followed by Prosthetic Rehabilitation

Once jaw amputation is scheduled, the patient must be informed of the reconstruction possibilities associated with dental/occlusal reconstruction. The patient must be informed of the consequences of not undergoing basal bone reconstruction but must also understand that the full process of jaw reconstruction and prosthetic rehabilitation will be lengthy, necessitating several surgical procedures. After the amputation of the maxilla, use of obturators is still considered to be the gold standard in maxillary reconstruction [7]. Depending on the nature of the defect (size, vertical extent of maxillary resection, degree of soft tissue loss, involvement of soft palate) and the status of the patient's dentition, the conventional obturator can function quite well as a means of restoring the dentition and separating the oral and nasal cavities. Sometimes, however, the obturator is not favorable to function as a removable partial denture without optimal support provided by the remaining palatal bone, the obturated cavity, and remaining dentition (Fig. 10.1). On such occasions, endosseous and zygomatic implants can improve a patient's ability to wear these obturators by improving prosthetic stability and retention (Fig. 10.2) [7–9]. For the mandible, basal bone reconstruction is essential. Strategy for jaw reconstruction should be primarily considered for the mandible.

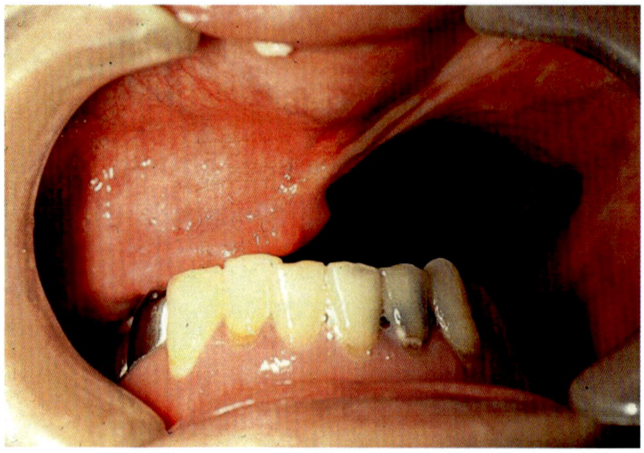

Fig. 10.1 Maxillary defect after amputation in an edentulous patient. In this situation, an obturator is not favorable to function as a removable partial denture without optimal support

First Step: Basal Bone Reconstruction Basal bone reconstruction should be considered either at the same time of mandibular amputation or after ablative surgery as a secondary reconstructive surgery. Depending on the reconstruction choice or prosthetic choice, alveolar bone reconstruction should be also considered.

Second Step: Evaluation of Oral Functions and Preparation for Prosthetic Rehabilitation In evaluation of oral functions such as swallowing ability, tongue movement, and mouth opening, mouth opening is a most important factor to fabricate the prosthesis. Dental and oral hygiene are also important factors.

Third Step: Prosthetic Rehabilitation After basal bone reconstruction, prosthetic rehabilitation is considered, that is, whether to use dental implants. If necessary, local soft tissue management should be performed before or after implant placement. Alveolar bone reconstruction is frequently necessary for prosthetic rehabilitation before implant placement.

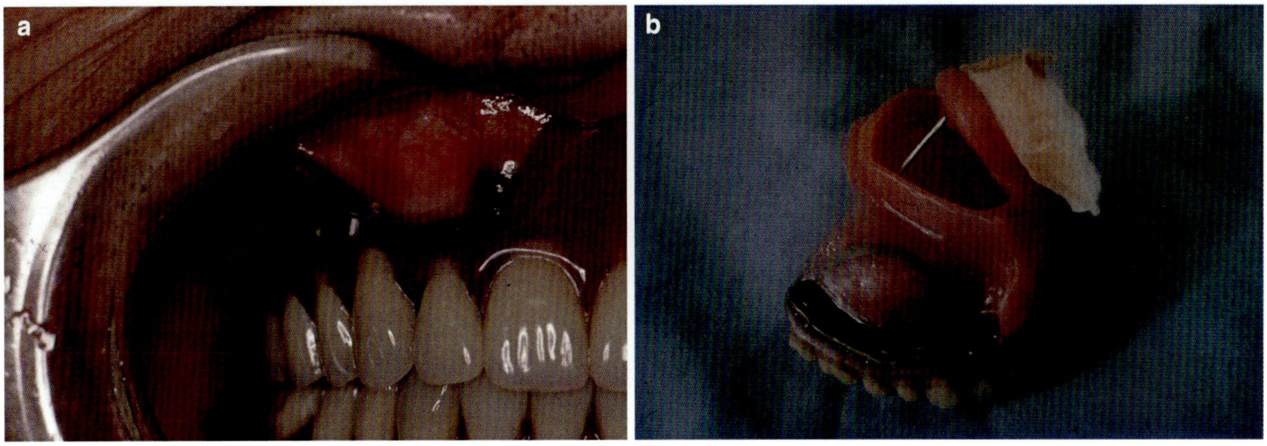

Fig. 10.2 **a** A maxillary implant-borne obturator supported by a milled bar attachment. **b** The facial prosthesis was retained by a magnetic attachment to the maxillary obturator prosthesis [9]

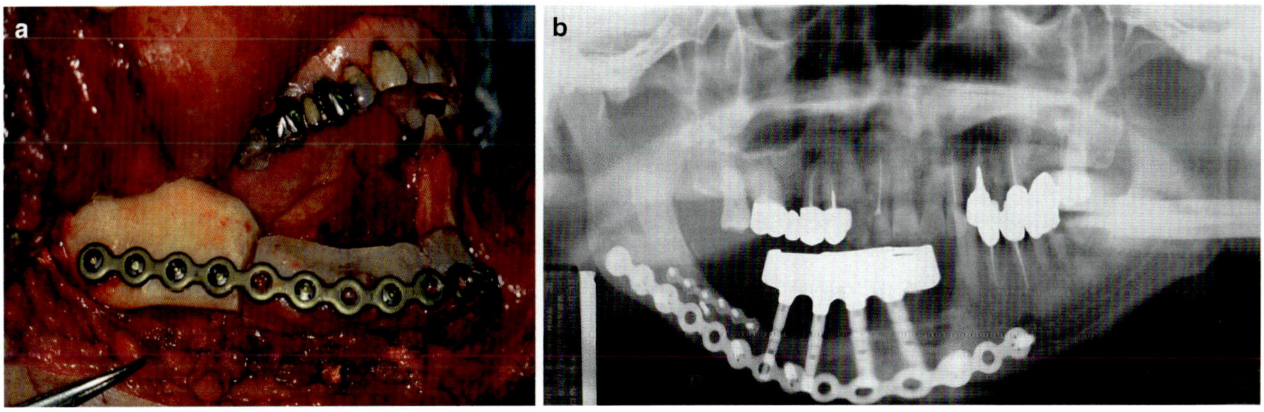

Fig. 10.3 **a** Use of nonvascularized free bone graft from the iliac crest for mandibular reconstruction following an ameloblastoma. **b** An implant-supported bridge was fabricated (at 5-year-follow-up)

10.4 Mandibular Reconstruction for Implant Placement

10.4.1 Nonvascularized Bone Graft

Harvest of free nonvascularized bone graft from the iliac crest is a well-established procedure for reconstruction of the mandible [7]. A block bone or cortico-cancellous bone harvested from the anterior or posterior iliac crest is used. Because of the nonvascular nature of these grafts, this procedure is generally performed as a secondary operation at least a year after the initial cancer ablation to avoid the high incidence of graft loss and infection when performed primarily. Indication of the nonvascularized bone graft is for the relatively short defects of the lateral mandible that do not cross the midline. This technique is especially effective following benign tumors such as ameloblastoma [7] (Fig. 10.3).

10.4.2 PCBM-MESH

Another procedure similar to free bone grafting is particulate cancellous bone marrow (PCBM) combined with titanium mesh (PCBM-MESH), which was first described by Boyne [10]. Several studies report successful results with this procedure [11–13]. PCBM was taken from the anterior and posterior iliac crest, respectively, as described by the authors in a previous publication [14]. With delayed reconstruction, the remaining mandible was exposed using an extra-oral approach to avoid entering the oral cavity. Dumbach and dynamic mesh plates [Dumbach Titanium Mesh-System, Titanium Dynamic Mesh, Micro-Titanium Augmentation Mesh (M-TAM); Stryker-Leibinger, Freiburg, Germany] were then adapted to the remaining bone by cutting and bending them into the desired shape. The mesh was fixated to each side of the host bone using titanium screws.

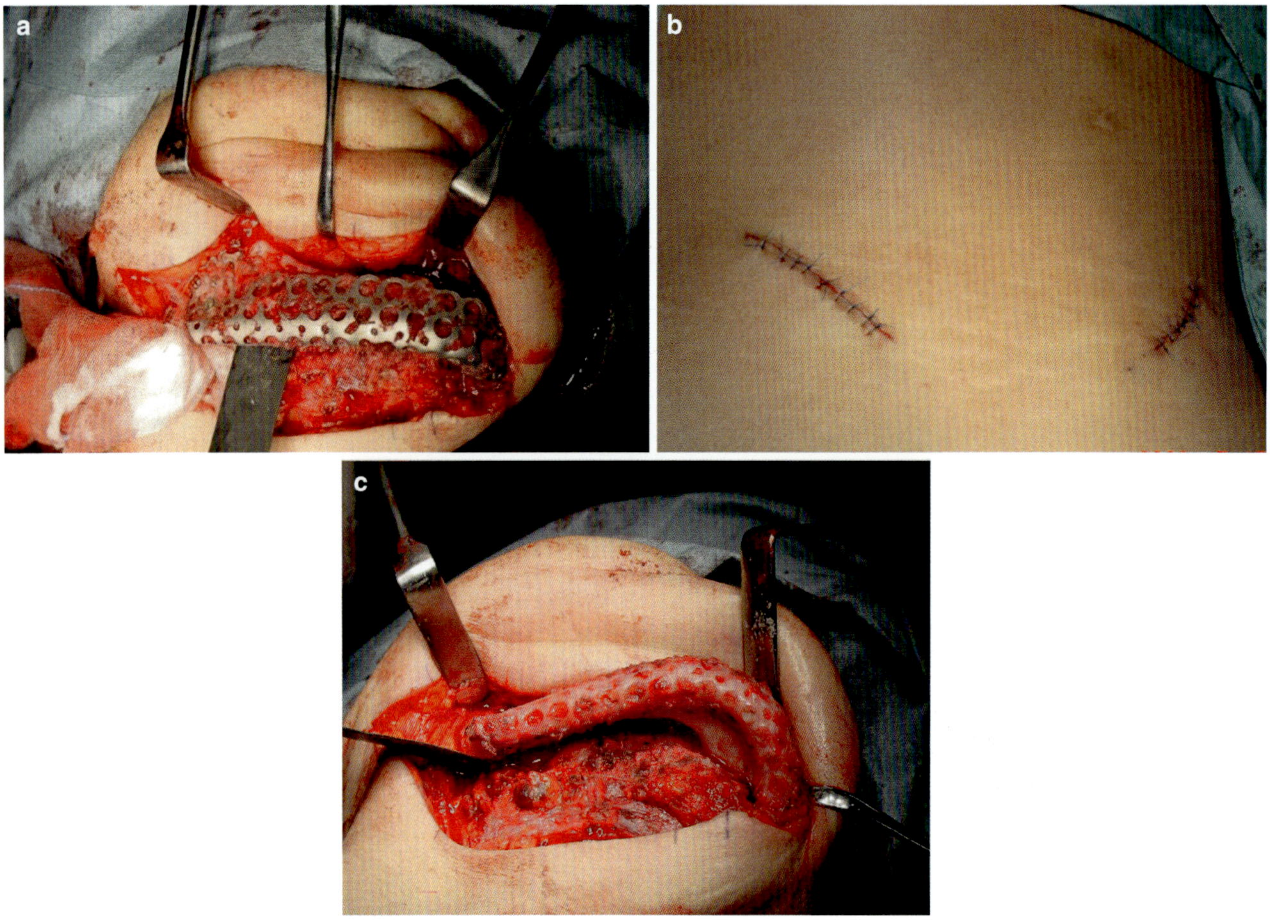

Fig. 10.4 **a** PCBM-MESH procedure. A Dumbach titanium mesh tray was adapted to the remaining bone. Then, particulate cancellous bone marrow (PCBM) was packed into the mesh tray. **b** PCBM was harvested from the bilateral posterior ilia. **c** Six months after bone graft. A very satisfactory amount of bone has formed in an ideal curve of the anatomical mandibular arch

The surrounding soft tissues including muscle, fatty, and fibrous tissue was then tightly sutured to the lateral, medial, and inferior surfaces of the tray to eliminate any dead space. The PCBM was loaded into the mesh and condensed to increase graft density. After adequate subcutaneous relaxation incisions were made, the overlying skin was sutured with minimal tension. The selection of the titanium mesh depends on the length and shape of the defect. Relatively large segmental defects need Dumbach; dynamic mesh was used for small defects and large alveolar defects; and titanium micromesh was applied to alveolar defects. Prosthetic rehabilitation started 6 months after implant insertion. PCBM-MESH has advantages for the reconstruction of facial contours in relatively difficult areas (e.g., the anterior part of the mandible) and the preparation of the bony bed for the application of dental implants (Figs. 10.4, 10.5). The risk factors for infection are reconstruction length, radiation therapy, and the existence of vascularity in the peripheral soft tissue [15].

10.4.3 Distraction Osteogenesis

Distraction osteogenesis (DO) is a unique technique that has been applied to the maxillofacial region. The main advantages of DO include circumventing donor site intervention for bone grafts, reducing morbidity, and elongating the soft tissues [16]. However, there are some disadvantages. First, DO is a very time-consuming technique and is burdensome for the patient to activate daily or twice daily by hand. Second, because the mandible is a three-dimensional curved structure, a curved DO is necessary [17], which is almost

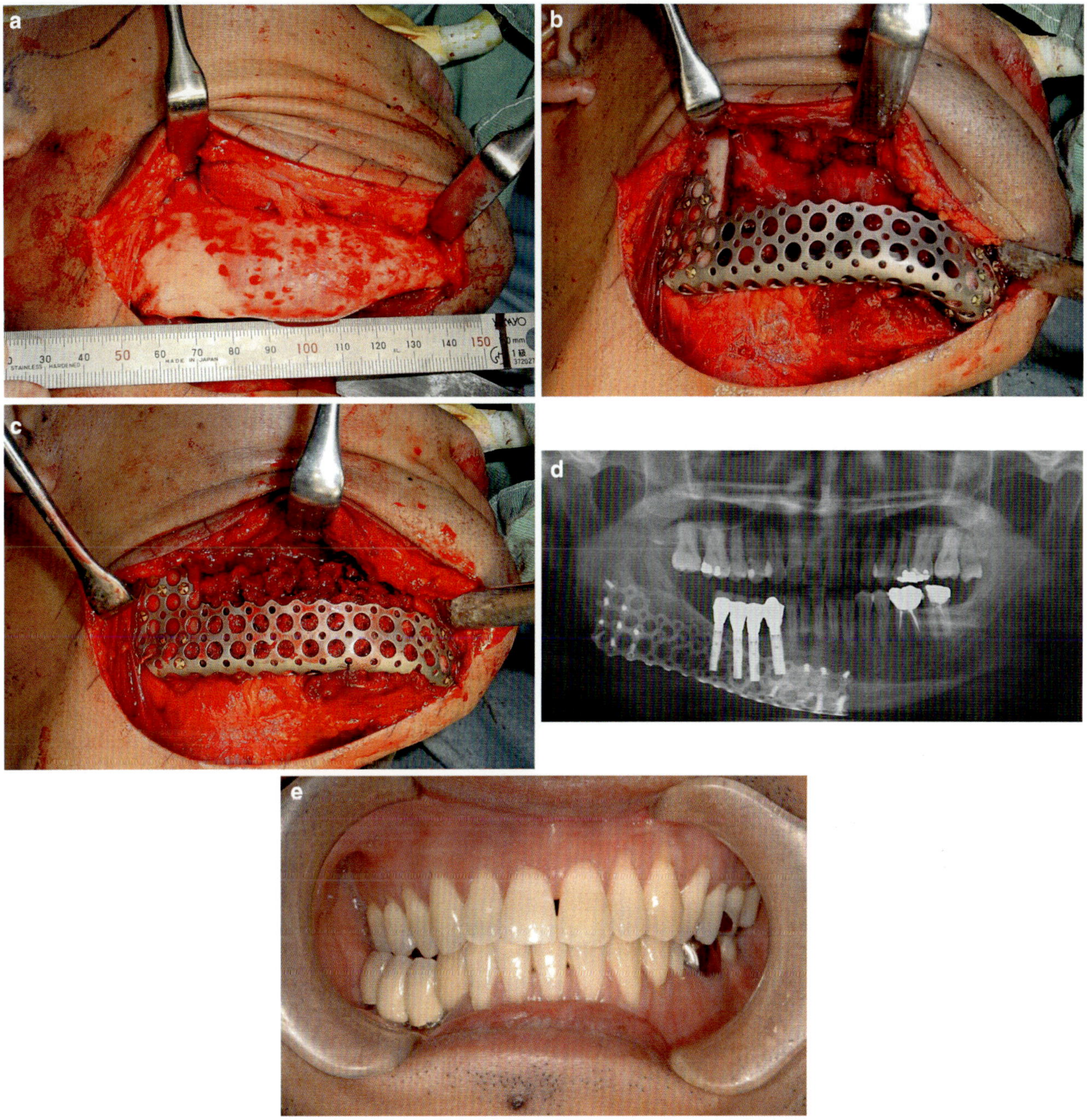

Fig. 10.5 **a** A case of mandibular reconstruction followed by the implant placement using PCBM-MESH method. A patient with a benign tumor (ossifying fibroma) underwent segmental resection. **b** A Dumbach titanium mesh tray was adapted to the remaining bone. **c** PCBM was packed into the mesh tray. **d** Implants were placed 6 months after PCBM grafting without removal of the mesh tray. **e** An implant-supported bridge was fabricated

impossible to apply in the anterior region. Therefore, DO could only be used in the posterior mandible. Third, when the bone transport technique is applied, a bone graft may be required to obtain continuity of the mandible at the end stage of the distraction [18] (Fig. 10.6).

10.4.4 Free Vascularized Bone Graft

Microvascular tissue transfer has revolutionized cancer reconstruction [19–22]. One of the advantages of this technique is that soft tissue can be transferred from a distant site

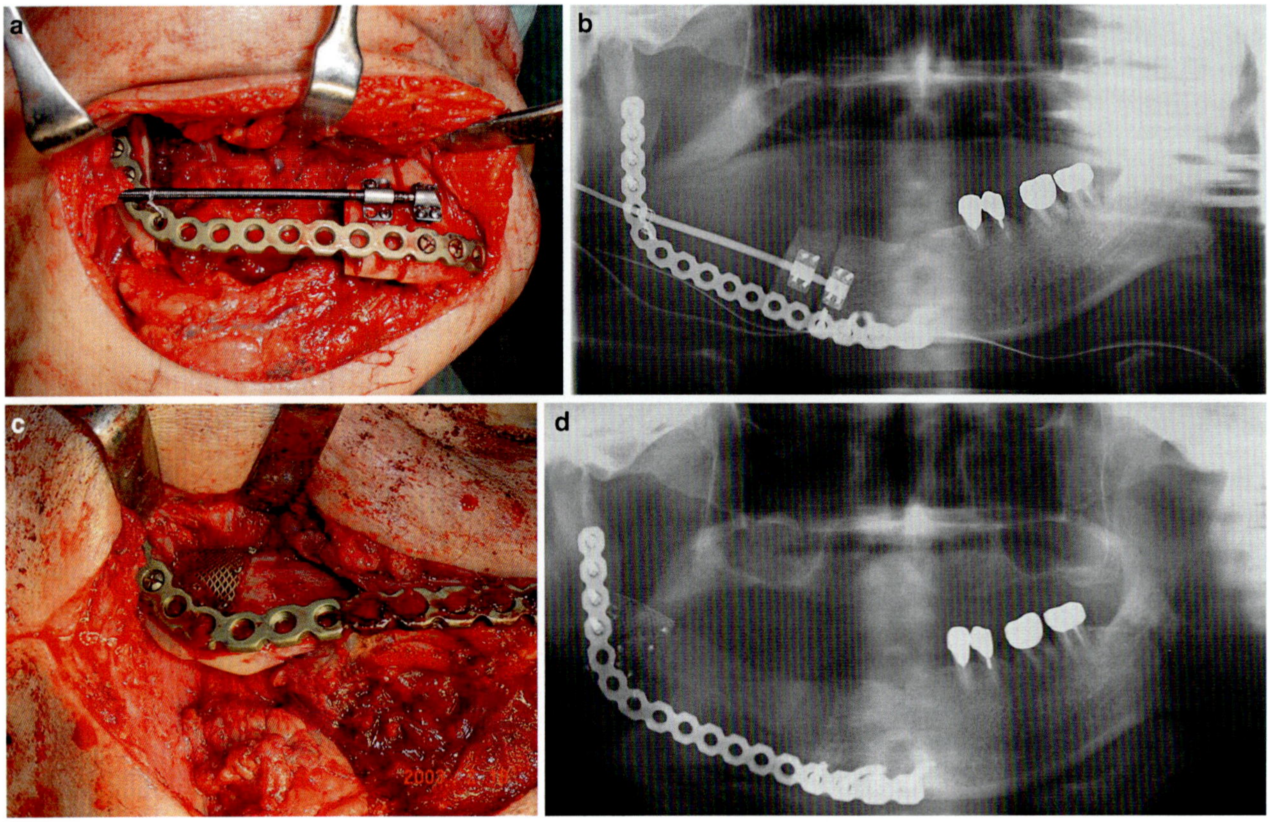

Fig. 10.6 **a** A case of mandibular reconstruction using distraction osteogenesis (DO). After amputation of the mandible, a reconstruction plate was placed. Simultaneously, a bone transport segment was fabricated and a distraction device was installed. **b** Panoramic X-ray after installation of the distraction device. **c** After the DO procedure, a small bone graft using a titanium mesh and autogenous cancellous bone was performed at the docking site of the transport segment and the remaining mandibular ramus. **d** A panoramic X-ray approximately 1 year after DO showed very good bone formation at the distracted area

in the same operative encounter as the ablative surgery and, in most instances, from a single donor site. There are three main donor sites for vascularized bone used in mandibular reconstruction: fibula, iliac, and scapula. Each donor site has its own advantages and disadvantages, and an ideal replacement for maxillary or mandibular bone and intraoral soft tissue does not yet exist [23] . The fibula can also be harvested as a bone-only, an osteoseptocutaneous, or a myo-osteocutaneous flap (soleus or flexor hallucis longus). The fibula flap is popular and has been the first choice for jaw reconstruction for many reconstructive surgeons because of the ease of the harvest, ability to work in two teams, availability of a long bone segment, and good pedicle length. One of the disadvantages is insufficient vertical height of the fibula. On average, the fibula's height is between 13 and 15 mm, which is similar to that of the edentulous mandible and is insufficient for that of the dentate mandible [7]; this accounts for the unfavorable implant axis and the space between the connection of the prosthesis and abutments. Various techniques to increase the height of the fibula have been proposed, including "double-barrelling"[24] and vertical distraction osteogenesis [25]. A relatively simple technique is to simply adapt the fibula to abut the native mandible in a slightly more superior position than the inferior border. The iliac crest is the only bone that provided sufficient bone volume [7]. This volume is crucial to both implant placement and stability of the tissue-borne prosthesis. The iliac crest offered advantages in height, width, and overall strength when harvested together with the internal oblique muscle and the cutaneous paddle, based on the deep circumflex iliac artery (DCIA) and the accompanying deep circumflex iliac vein (DCIV). Although the volume of the bone is good, the length of the available bone is somewhat limited, and the volume of soft tissue that must be included with this flap can be bulky [7]. The free scapula flap can provide a large amount of soft tissue connected with the bone. However, as was the case with fibula, the bone available is not the best choice for implant length. The available bone length is a maximum of 12 cm, but may be enhanced by harvesting the whole scapular tip and using it transversally for anterior reconstruction [26]. The scapula is also available for maxillary reconstruction. For implant placement, another augmentation procedure is necessary (Fig. 10.7).

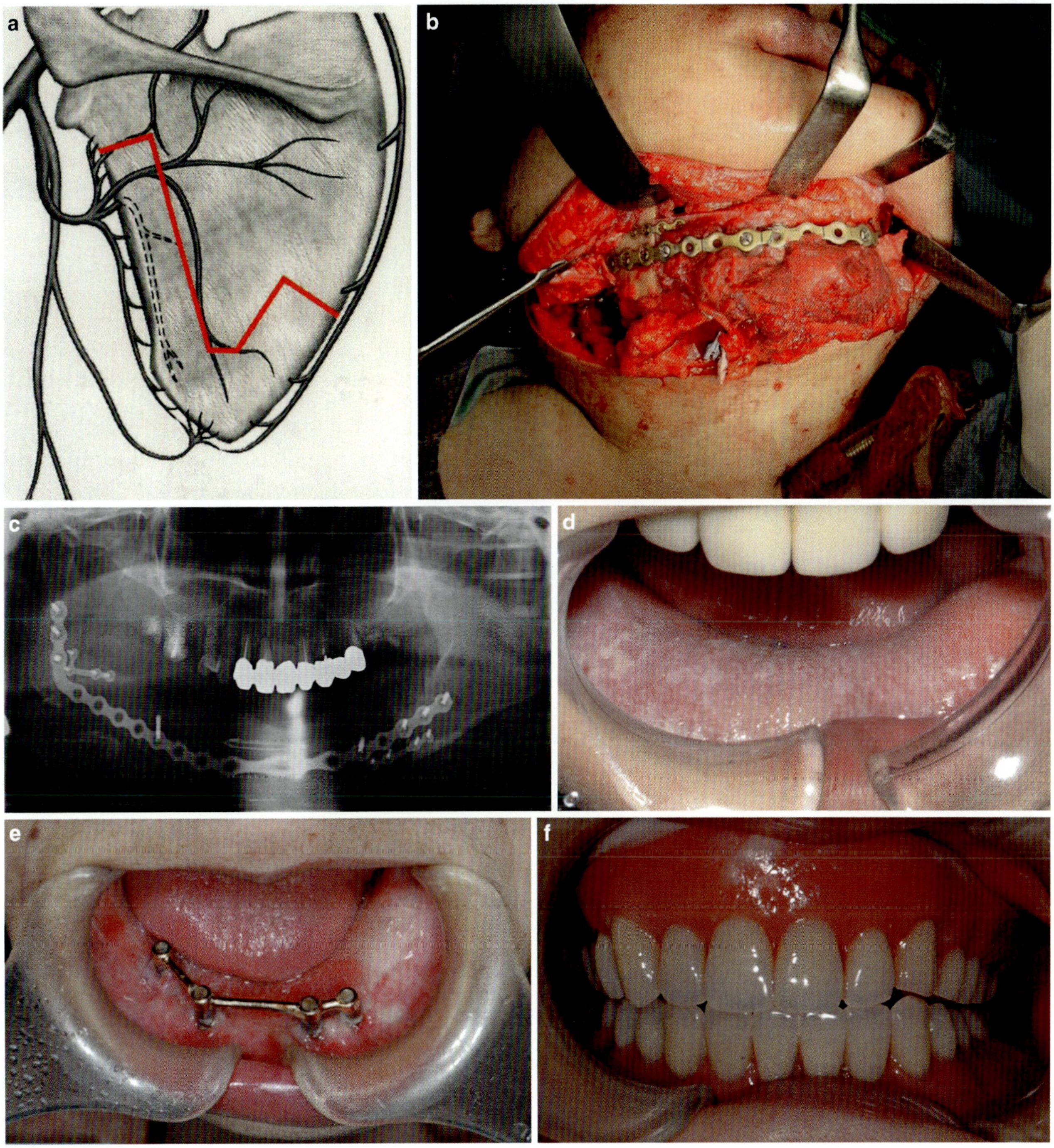

Fig. 10.7 **a** A vascularized scapula flap. When the bone flap is prepared as bipedicled, the bone may be cut into two or three pieces and fixed at the desired angle to simulate the contour of the mandible. **b** Use of a bipedicled scapula flap for the mandibular reconstruction. **c** Approximately two thirds of the mandible was reconstructed using a bipedicled scapula flap. **d** A subcutaneous flap is seen in the oral cavity. **e** Before the fabrication of a final prosthesis after implant placement, thinning of the skin paddle ("defatting") was performed, and a bar attachment was fabricated. **f** An implant-stabilized denture was fabricated

10.4.5 Choice for Bony Reconstruction of the Mandible

The anatomical reconstruction of the mandible is very difficult. Nonvascularized bone graft from the ilium is very simple with less donor site morbidity. However, it is only used for benign tumors because of the need for soft tissue coverage. PCBM-MESH is also primarily used for benign tumors. PCBM-MESH is excellent in forming the anatomical curved structure of the mandible, and is also available for defects of the mandible. DO is a unique technique that elongates both bone and soft tissues. However, it is very time consuming, and bone formation is sometimes compromised. Therefore, indication of DO for mandibular reconstruction is very limited. The free vascularized bone graft provides an adequate amount of both soft and hard tissues for restoration in various degrees of the mandible and is primarily used for malignant tumors. The fibula osteocutaneous flap is most versatile, because of its length, and is easy to adapt to the mandibular form using one or several osteotomies, bipartite or double-barreled gun fibula. However, other donor sites for vascularized bone reconstruction including the scapula and iliac crest are also feasible. The choice of bone reconstruction will be determined by donor site morbidity, the volume of transferred bone, and the length of the pedicle.

10.5 Preparation for Implant Placement After Reconstruction

10.5.1 Local Soft Tissue Management

After basal bone reconstruction, because of the inadequate volume and/or inadequate position of the flaps including the skin paddle, prosthetic rehabilitation is compromised, or is impossible. Therefore, local tissue management is always considered before implant placement followed by prosthetic rehabilitation [27]. Evaluation of the tongue mobility and sensitivity is an important factor for rehabilitation. Therefore, if tongue mobility is limited, tongue-associated tissue management should be performed to ensure tongue mobility. Lip competence is another important factor. Without lip coverage, saliva and leakage of food will hamper patient satisfaction. Therefore, surgical management to ensure lip competence is required to avoid this situation. Presence of skin paddles is often encountered after free flap reconstructions. "Defatting" or refinements and thinning of the skin paddle are always necessary before the implant-supported prosthesis is fabricated. The skin paddle would lead to peri-implant infection because of its thickness and lack of attached tissue. Ideally, performance of epithelialized palatal graft is considered or at least the implant/abutment area penetrating into the oral cavity. Vestibular groove management (vestibuloplasty) should also be considered. It is important to restore the vestibular groove, particularly if the floor of the mouth has been removed. If the vestibular groove is not deep enough, the prosthesis may cause pain in the surrounding tissue during chewing. Vestibuloplasty can also be performed with second-stage surgery or as a separate procedure (Fig. 10.8). A custom-fabricated splint should be used for several weeks to allow firm adaptation to the reconstructed jaw. This procedure can also address the common lack of vestibule depth that occurs after many reconstructions.

10.5.2 Alveolar Bone Reconstruction

Conventionally, an implant has been placed wherever sufficient bone is present without sufficient prosthodontic consideration. The "top-down theory" (restoration-driven implant placement) is to select the type and location of the prosthesis before placing the implant. Then, location of the implant is decided even if bone grafting is required to provide the patient with a prosthesis with superior functions, aesthetics, and long-term success. Therefore, to ensure perfect implant placement for a better prosthesis, an alveolar augmentation procedure may be required after base bone reconstruction. Alternatively, depending on the choice of prosthetic rehabilitation, that is, retained implant over dentures for an edentulous mandible, no alveolar bone augmentation is necessary. Nowadays, many alveolar ridge augmentation procedures are advocated for restoration-driven implant placement. An augmentation procedure depends on the type and the volume of the alveolar deficiency. Autogenous bone graft, PCBM-MESH, and DO are clinically used for this purpose. Although each procedure has advantages and disadvantages, in the clinical setting, PCBM-MESH has many advantages especially in large alveolar defects. PCBM-MESH is a useful technique to reconstruct large defects of the alveolar ridge for the optimal treatment in these morphologically unbalanced conditions (Fig. 10.9).

10.6 Implant Placement Followed by Prosthetic Rehabilitation

10.6.1 Timing for Implant Insertion

Although several groups have advocated simultaneous implant placement during reconstruction surgery, there is a general consensus that implant placement should be performed secondarily after reconstruction surgery to achieve better prosthetic rehabilitation. In secondary implant placement, no consensus exists for how long an interval is ideal between the primary reconstructive surgery and implant placement. However, some studies recommend a period of 1 year after cancer surgery to allow for complete bone healing, improved nutritional status, and monitoring of disease recurrence. In benign disease, implant reconstruction can proceed once it is determined that bone healing has been achieved (usually between 4 and 6 months) [7]. With regard to the irradiated bony flap, we must consider the radiation dose. Although there is no real consensus on that level of irradiation, when radiation therapy exceeds 55 Gy, it should be considered that the risk of osteoradionecrosis is too high, and implant insertion is not recommended [27].

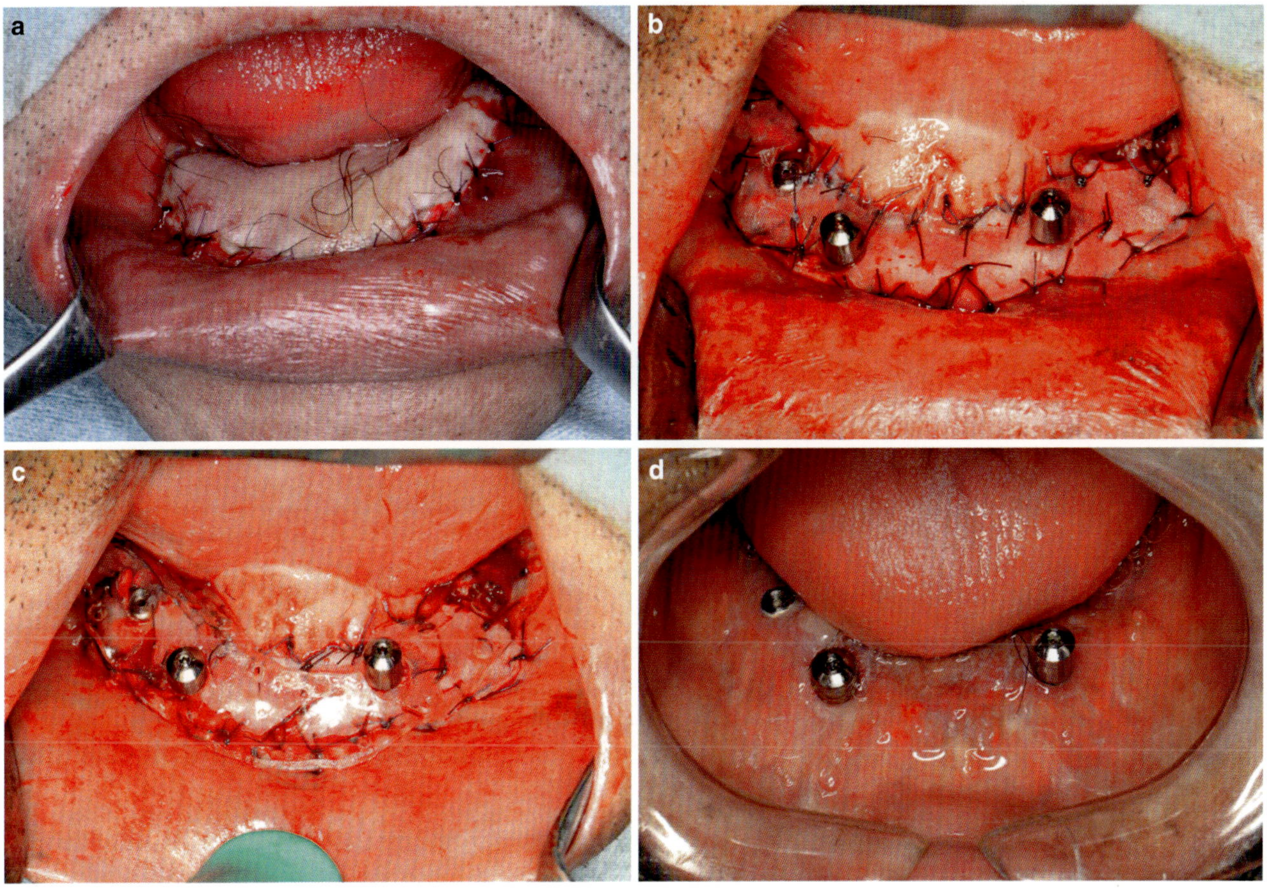

Fig. 10.8 **a** A case of vestibuloplasty for an implant-supported prosthesis. A bulky skin paddle was seen in the anterior mandible. Implants were placed and the flap was closed in the first implant operation. **b** At the secondary implant operation, vestibuloplasty was performed. After thinning of the skin paddle and removal of the excess tissue, the terdermis (Olympas Terumo Biomaterials) was sutured with surrounding mucosa and the remaining flap. **c** A splint was used to cover the terdermis around the implants and was fixed to the mandible by circumferential suture. **d** One month after vestibuloplasty

Some studies have suggested the use of therapy to improve the success of osseointegration in these patients [28]. However, there have been several reports denying the efficacy of HBO treatment [29, 30].

10.6.2 Implant Placement Procedure

The position, depth, and direction of implant placement are often planned based on the evaluation of radiographs and study casts. Insertion planned in such a manner may not be adequate for precise and safe surgery in some cases because of inadequate working clearance in the oral cavity. To obtain high initial stability and ensure osseointegration at the implant–bone interface, careful and precise drilling must be performed at the implant placement site. The SimPlant software program (Materialise) allows implants to be planned in two and three dimensions using data received from a computerized tomographic scan. The resulting implant plan can be transferred to the mouth and implemented by means of a stereolithographic surgical guide (SurgiGuide, Materialise) (Fig. 10.10).

10.6.3 Type of Prosthesis and Its Indications

There are several options of prosthesis including the implant-supported bridge, resin-bonded bridge, implant-borne denture, and implant-stabilized denture. Although a fixed denture is the best option, this may not be available because of the condition of the reconstructed dental arch. The bridge is the old standard, but it requires perfect alignment and a favorable crown-to-implant ratio. A resin-bonded bridge or a Maryland bridge is a bridge in which plastic teeth and gingiva are bonded to the metal framework. This type of prosthesis is used primarily when there is an unfavorable crown-to-implant ratio and a shifted implant axis when compared with the ideal prosthesis situation. An implant-borne denture uses a milled bar supporting a removable overdenture. The overdenture conceals and protects the bar, which is usually screwed in and permits perfect occlusion. Implant-borne dentures are useful for correcting poor implant alignment because the framework links all the implants and permits the distribution of biomechanical forces. Implant-stabilized dentures can be stabilized with as few as two implants. A bar-splinted or free-standing

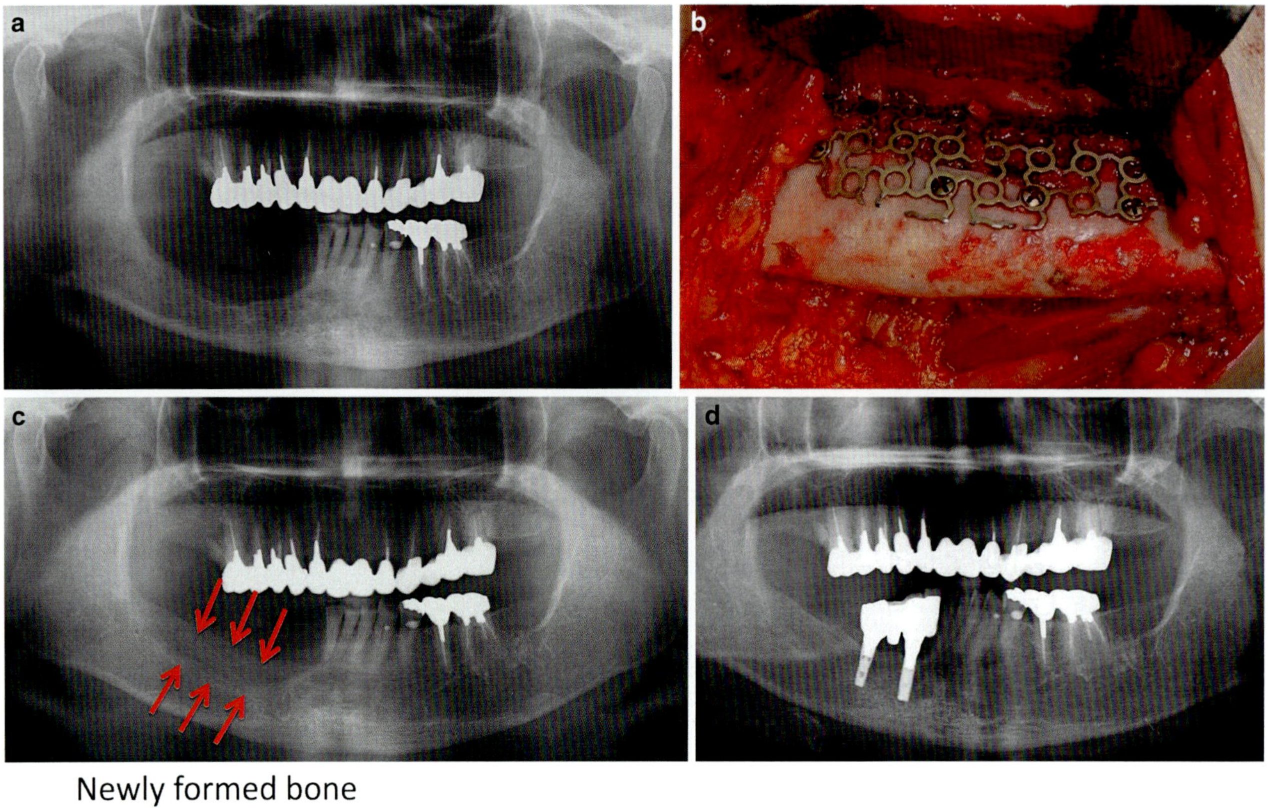

Fig. 10.9 **a** A case of alveolar bone reconstruction for prosthetic rehabilitation. Marginal bone resection was performed in a patient with mandibular gingival squamous cell carcinoma (SCC). Vertical height was insufficient for the final prosthesis. **b** PCBM-MESH method was used to reconstruct the alveolar bone. Titanium Dynamic Mesh was used, and PCBM was packed into the mesh tray. **c** A panoramic X-ray 6 months after the bone graft and removal of the mesh. Newly formed bone is shown as *arrows*. **d** An implant-supported bridge was fabricated

attachment may also be used. The advantages include the low forces transmitted to the implants, the small number of implants needed to stabilize the whole denture, and the ease of cleaning of components. However, the disadvantages include the removable denture and the mucosal support. The choice of prosthesis depends on the condition of the reconstruction, the remaining dentition, and the maxilla–mandibular relationship, among other factors.

10.7 Conclusions

Prosthetic reconstruction for patients who have had ablative head and neck tumor surgery is challenging because both soft and hard tissues are required. Use of dental implants in oral cancer reconstruction has become an important aspect of the reconstructive plan for these patients. For mandibular defects, first, the continuity of the mandible should be restored according to tissue condition. In severe cases, free flap transfer should be performed. Relatively short segments or benign tumors with sufficient vascularity could possibly be treated with PCBM-MESH. Second, facial contours and the final dental occlusion are simulated to determine the optimum base of the dental implant or conventional dentures. The final prosthetic treatment requires an intra-oral environment for the prosthesis, particularly sufficient alveolar ridge with good and healthy soft tissue around the prosthesis. For this purpose, PCBM-MESH is a useful technique to link between optimum facial contour and alveolar reconstruction. Local tissue management including thinning of the skin paddle or vestibuloplasty is often required. The choice of prosthesis depends on the condition of the reconstruction, the remaining dentition, the maxilla–mandibular relationship, and other factors.

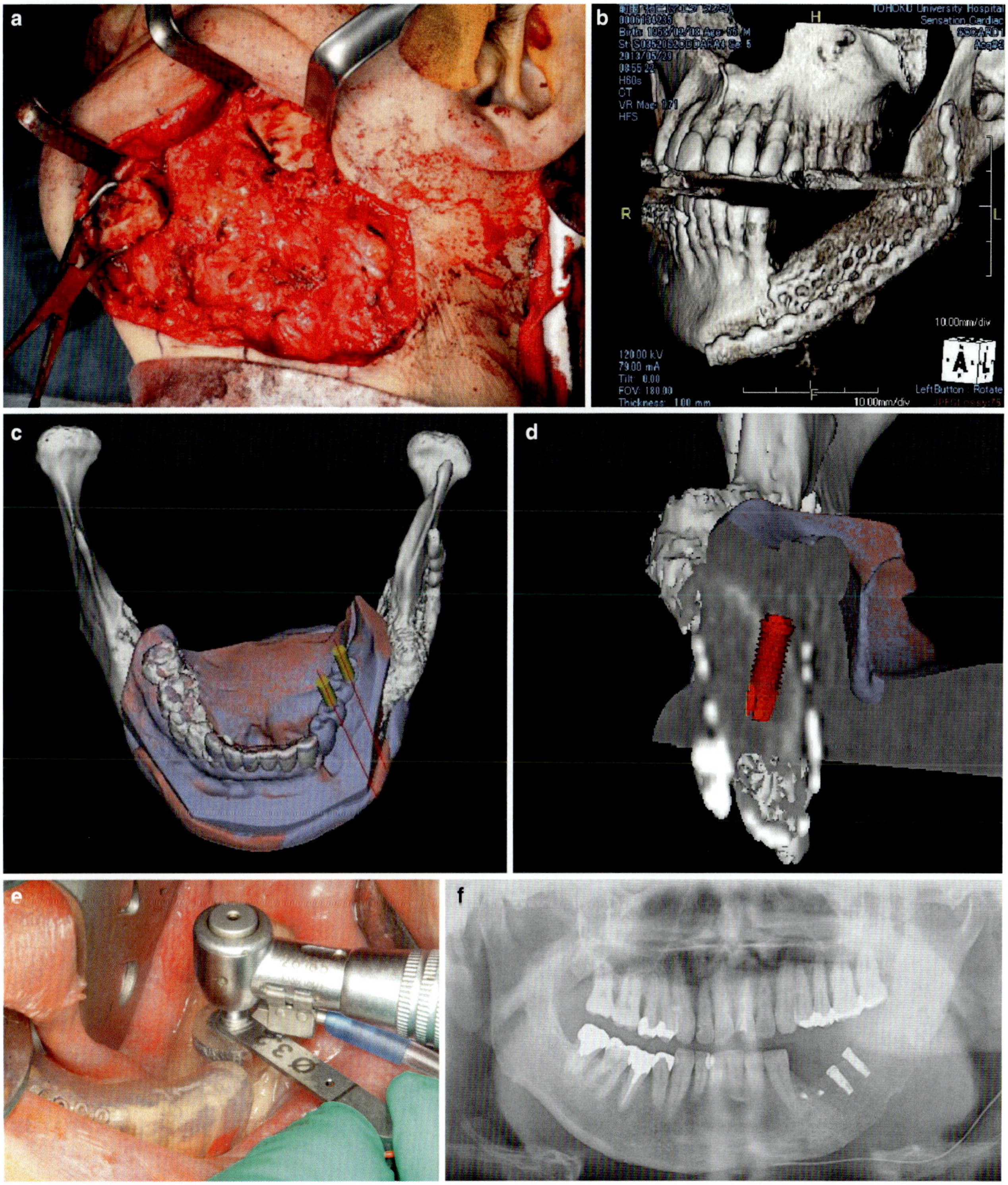

Fig. 10.10 **a** A case of implant placement using a stereolithographic surgical guide. Mandibular amputation was performed. **b** Mandibular reconstruction was performed using the PCBM-MESH procedure. At this time, a reconstruction plate combined with titanium mesh to reinforce the mesh tray. PCBM was paced into the mesh tray. A three-dimensional computed tomography (3D-CT) scan showed very good bone formation of the reconstructed area. **c** SimPlant software (Materialise) was used for the simulation of the implant placement. **d** Sagittal image of the reconstructed area. A virtual implant was used for simulation of implant placement. **e** Surge Guide was set on the remaining teeth, and a drill hole was making using for the precise and secure drilling. A "Longstop drill" was using with a certain stopper. **f** A panoramic X ray after implant placement

References

1. Shah JP, Gil Z (2009) Current concepts in management of oral cancer surgery. Oral Oncol 45:394–401
2. Goh BT, Lee S, Tideman H et al (2008) Mandibular reconstruction in adults: a review. Int J Oral Maxillofac Surg 37:597–605
3. Javed F, Al-Hezaimi K, Al-Rasheed A et al (2010) Implant survival rate after oral cancer therapy: a review. Oral Oncol 46:854–859
4. Mehta RP, Deschler DG (2004) Mandibular reconstruction in 2004: an analysis of different techniques. Curr Opin Otolaryngol Head Neck Surg 12:288–293
5. Bak M, Jacobson AS, Buckbinder D, Urken ML (2010) Contemporary reconstruction of the mandible. Oral Oncol 46: 71–76
6. Hakestam U, Karlsson T, Soderfeldt B et al (1997) Does the quality of advanced prosthetic dentistry determine patient satisfaction? Acta Odontol Scand 55:365–371
7. Kim DD, Gahli GE (2011) Dental implants in oral cancer reconstruction. Oral Maxillofac Surg Clin N Am 23:337–345
8. Fukuda M, Takahashi T, Nagai H, Iino M (2004) Implant-supported edentulous maxillary obturators with milled bar attachments after maxillectomy. J Oral Maxillofac Surg 62:799–805
9. Takahashi T, Fukuda M, Funaki K, Tanaka K (2006) Magnet-retained facial prosthesis combined with an implant supported edentulous maxillary obturator. A case report. Int J Oral Maxillofac Implants 21:805–807
10. Boyne PJ (1969) Restoration of osseous defects in maxillofacial casualties. J Am Dent Assoc 78:767–776
11. Carlson ER, Marx RE (1996) Mandibular reconstruction using cancellous cellular bone grafts. J Oral Maxillofac Surg 54: 889–897
12. Dumbach J, Rodemer H, Spitzer WJ et al (1994) Mandibular reconstruction with cancellous bone, hydroxylapatite and titanium mesh. J Craniomaxillofac Surg 22:151–155
13. Iino M, Fukuda M, Nagai H et al (2009) Evaluation of 15 mandibular reconstructions with Dumbach Titan mesh system and particulate cancellous bone and marrow harvested from bilateral posterior ilia. Oral Surg Oral Med Oral Pathol Oral Radiol Endod 107:e1–e8
14. Miyamoto I, Yamashita Y et al (2014) Evaluation of mandibular reconstruction with particulate cancellous bone and marrow and titanium mesh after mandibular reconstruction due to tumor surgery. Impl Dent 23:108–115.
15. Chiapasco M, Colletti G, Romeo E et al (2008) Long-term results of mandibular reconstruction with autogenous bone grafts and oral implants after tumor resection. Clin Oral Implants Res 19: 1074–1080
16. Samchukov ML, Cope JB, Cherkashin AM (2001) Craniofacial distraction osteogenesis. Mosby, St. Louis
17. Takahashi T, Fukuda M et al (2002) Distraction osteogenesis for reconstruction after mandibular segmental resection. Oral Surg Oral Med Oral Pathol Oral Radiol Endod 93:21–26
18. Sawaki Y, Hagino H et al (1997) Trifocal distraction osteogenesis for segmental mandibular defect: a technical innovation. J Craniomaxillofac Surg 25:310–315
19. Taylor GI, Townsend P, Corlett R (1979) Superiority of the deep circumflex iliac vessels as the supply for free groin flaps. Plast Reconstr Surg 64:595–604
20. Sanders R, Mayou BJ (1979) A new vascularized bone graft transferred by microvascular anastomosis as a free flap. Br J Surg 66: 787–788
21. Swartz WM, Banis JC et al (1986) The osteocutaneous scapular flap for mandibular and maxillary reconstruction. Plast Reconstr Surg 77:530–545
22. Hidalgo DA (1989) Fibula free flap: a new method of mandible reconstruction. Plast Reconstr Surg 84:71–79
23. Buckbinder D, Urken ML, Vickery C et al (1989) Functional mandibular reconstruction of patients with oral cancer. Oral Surg Oral Med Oral Pathol 68:499–504
24. Ruhin B, Menard P et al (2006) Double-barrel fibular free flap for mandibular reconstruction: beneficial alternative for dental implantation (5 cases). Rev Stomatol Chir Maxillofac 107:338–344
25. Chiapasco M, Brusati R, Galioto S (2000) Distraction osteogenesis of a fibular revascularized flap for improvement of oral implant positioning in a tumor patient: a case report. J Oral Maxillofac Surg 58:1434–1440
26. Hanasono NM, Skoracki RJ (2010) The scapular tip osseous free flap as an alternative for anterior mandibular reconstruction. Plast Reconstr Surg 125:164e–166e
27. Ferri J, Raoul G, Lauwers L (2011) Maxillo-mandibular amputations and implant rehabilitation. In: Ferri J, Hunziker EB (eds) Preprosthetic and maxillary surgery. Woodhead, Oxford
28. Barber HD, Seckinger RJ, Hayden RE et al (1995) Evaluation of osseointegration of endosseous implants in radiated, vascularized fibula flaps to the mandible: a pilot study. J Oral Maxillofac Surg 53:640–644
29. Eckert SE, Desjardins RP, Keller EE et al (1996) Endosseous implants in an irradiated tissue bed. J Prosthet Dent 76:45–49
30. Schoen PJ, Raghoebar GM, Bouma J et al (2007) Rehabilitation of oral function in head and neck cancer patients after radiotherapy with implant retained dentures: effects of hyperbaric oxygen therapy. Oral Oncol 43:379–388

Radiotherapy

11

Kanako Takayama, Yusuke Demizu, and Nobukazu Fuwa

Abstract

Radiotherapy has been used as a curative treatment for early-stage oral cavity cancer. Brachytherapy is performed by an experienced team, either alone or as a supplement to external beam radiation in selected small or superficial lesions. For more advanced lesions, a combined modality approach involving surgery followed by adjuvant radiation or chemoradiation has been performed. With the development of chemoradiotherapy in recent years, radiotherapy has been increasingly used as a radical treatment. However, the occurrence of adverse effects such as multiple caries and osteoradionecrosis after treatment is unavoidable. Intensity-modulated radiotherapy and particle beam radiation therapy have also been introduced for the treatment of oral cavity cancers. The accurate administration of doses to the tumor has become possible. Both can reduce normal tissue toxicities and can deliver high-dose radiation to the tumor. Therefore, better treatment results and reductions in late adverse events are expected. The role of chemoradiotherapy as a radical treatment is expected to progress along with chemotherapy. Intra-arterial chemoradiotherapy will be a particularly important modality for locally advanced oral cavity cancers.

Keywords

Brachytherapy • Chemoradiotherapy • Intensity-modulated radiation therapy • Particle therapy • Radiotherapy

11.1 Introduction

Oral cavity cancer is the most frequent head and neck cancer. The function of this region is extremely important, both functionally and aesthetically. Although the role of radiotherapy has been important, the radiosensitivity of oral cavity cancer is lower than that of other head and neck cancers. Therefore, the role of radiotherapy has been limited in cases of early-stage cancers. However, the role of radiotherapy has recently expanded along with the development of chemotherapy and new radiotherapy technologies.

11.2 General Treatment Strategies

11.2.1 Tongue Cancer

The optimal treatment for squamous cell carcinoma (SCC) of the oral tongue is dependent on the tumor size, location, and extension, as well as the cervical lymph node status. Surgical resection is generally performed in medically operable patients. Early-stage carcinoma can be treated with both radiotherapy and surgery, and both yield equally good results. Superficial T1-T2N0 lesions can be treated with

K. Takayama (✉)
Department of Radiation Oncology, Southern Tohoku Proton Therapy Center, Koriyama, Japan
e-mail: kanakotkym@gmail.com

Y. Demizu • N. Fuwa
Department of Radiology, Hyogo Ion Beam Medical Center, Tatsuno, Japan
e-mail: y_demizu@nifty.com

T. Kirita and K. Omura (eds.), *Oral Cancer: Diagnosis and Therapy*,
DOI 10.1007/978-4-431-54938-3_11, © Springer Japan 2015

brachytherapy or intraoral cone therapy. These methods yield good local control (LC) rates and fewer adverse effects. The 5-year LC rates were reported to range from 79 % to 93 % for T1 lesions and from 70 % to 83 % for T2 lesions treated with brachytherapy [1–3]. For brachytherapy with external radiation as a treatment for stage III–IV tongue cancers, the reported 5-year LC rates were 67 % and 35 % for T3N0 and T3N1 disease, respectively [4].

The outcomes for locally advanced lesions (T3, T4) were not satisfactory. The optimal treatment for patients with stage III–IV tongue cancer is surgical resection combined with radiotherapy. The incidence rates of occult nodal metastases of tongue cancer were reported to be 18 %, 39 %, and 46 % for T1N0, T2N0, and T3N0 clinically staged patients, respectively [5]. Occult nodal metastases have therefore been poor prognostic factors [6]. Postoperative radiotherapy is recommended for patients in the following situations: advanced lesions (large primary tumors, bone involvement, extensive perineural, or vascular invasion), positive or close surgical margins, the presence of multiple positive lymph nodes, or extracapsular extension (ECE) [7].

Radiotherapy for large primary lesions is generally performed for patients who refuse or are unable to undergo surgery. For inoperable advanced cancers, concurrent chemoradiotherapy has been recommended. Recently, good results have been reported for combined chemoradiotherapy by intra-arterial infusion; this method improved the LC rate and allowed patients to achieve a good quality of life without surgery [8]. This therapy will therefore play an important role in locally advanced tongue cancers.

11.2.2 Other Oral Cavity Cancers

Although early-stage cancers can be treated effectively with radiotherapy or surgery, surgery has remained the standard treatment. As the radiation tolerance of this region is lower than that of the tongue, it is difficult to administer efficient doses to this region.

Lesions with infiltration and deep ulceration are not good indications for radiation therapy because of the poor treatment effects and delayed healing. Brachytherapy is recommended for superficial tumors. Early-stage floor of the mouth, buccal mucosal, and retromolar trigone lesions can be treated effectively with radiotherapy that incorporates Au-198 (^{198}Au) seed implantation. Implanted cesium-137 (^{137}Cs) needles or iridium-192 (^{192}Ir) wires are used for tumors of the floor of the mouth. Carcinomas of the buccal mucosa and retromolar trigone are accessible to implantation techniques. However, it is difficult to insert sources or tubes into these areas, and therefore most patients undergo resection and postoperative radiation for these cancers. Because it is difficult to place the needles to treat tumors of the hard palate and upper alveolar ridge, lesions without bone invasion can also be treated with prostheses [9]. For lesions near the mandible, bone invasion requires special attention, and brachytherapy is contradicted because of the risk of osteoradionecrosis (ORN) and ulceration.

The 5-year LC rates have been reported as 90 % for T1 and 70–80 % for T2 lesions of the mouth floor and buccal mucosa after brachytherapy [10, 11]. The reported 5-year overall survival rate of early-stage tumor in the upper gingiva and palate is 80 % [9]. Regardless of the tumor stage, tumor thickness and depth of invasion should be included in estimating prognosis, planning therapy, and comparing results [12]. External radiotherapy is not used as the sole treatment modality for advanced oral cavity cancers. More advanced lesions or infiltrative invasion to the maxilla and mandibular bone should be treated with an approach that combines surgery and radiation or chemoradiation therapy. Intra-arterial chemoradiotherapy is also effective for some advanced cancers [13].

11.2.3 Management of Neck Lymph Node Metastases

For the treatment of cervical lymph node metastasis, the treatment results of external irradiation were not better than that of neck dissection. The standard treatment has been radical neck dissection. The most important prognostic factor of stage I–II oral cancer is occult cervical lymph node metastasis [14]. An additional 30–35 % of patients with carcinoma of the tongue, mouth floor, and buccal mucosa, clinically staged N0 disease at diagnosis, subsequently develop metastatic cervical adenopathy when only the primary site is treated [15].

Reportedly, elective neck irradiation can reduce the incidence of subsequent nodal metastases in the treated neck [16]. However, there is no clear evidence that elective neck dissection or elective neck irradiation improves survival. As the primary lesion size increases, the incidence of subsequent nodal metastases also increases. Patients with superficial lesions (<2 mm thick) and a negative neck can be placed under observation after primary therapy. Other N0 patients require close follow-up or may undergo a planned selective neck dissection or prophylactic radiotherapy. In lesions of the hard palate and upper gingiva, which have a low risk of occult lymph node involvement, elective treatment of the clinically negative neck should be considered only for high-grade tumors or advanced T-stage lesions.

The presence of multiple positive lymph nodes and ECE are poor prognostic factors. Postoperative neck irradiation is indicated in patients with lymph node metastases [17].

11.3 Radiation Techniques

11.3.1 External Radiotherapy

The radiosensitivity of oral cavity cancers is lower than that of other head and neck cancers. Therefore, external radiotherapy has been used as a palliative treatment for large tumors and for postoperative radiotherapy. Currently, the role of external radiotherapy is considered important with regard to the new technologies of intensity-modulated radiation therapy (IMRT) and particle therapy and the development of chemoradiotherapy.

11.3.1.1 Setting and Fixation

During simulation and treatment, the patient is commonly immobilized in a supine position with a thermoplastic mask (Fig. 11.1). Custom masking can facilitate optimal positioning in order to spare geographic misses from body motion. A spacer (bite block, intraoral stent) is used to open the mouth, depress the tongue away from the hard palate, and protrude the lower lip.

11.3.1.2 Target Volume

The gross tumor volume (GTV) encompasses the primary tumor and lymphadenopathy. The GTV is determined clinically by computed tomography (CT), magnetic resonance imaging (MRI), or positron emission tomography (PET). Basically, the clinical target volume (CTV) encompasses the GTV along with a 5–10-mm margin. The prophylactic irradiation range of oral cancer (CTV prophylactic) includes the regional lymph nodes (levels I–III). In cases with cervical lymph node metastasis above stage N2b, levels I–IV nodes are also included in the CTV prophylactic.

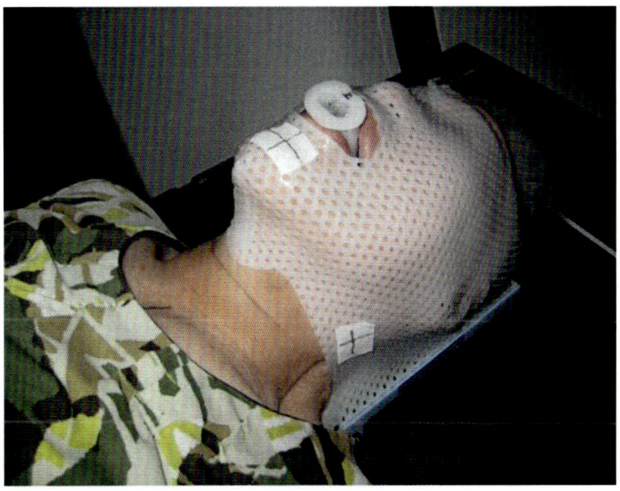

Fig. 11.1 Patient positioning and immobilization. External radiation treatment is generally performed with the patient in a supine position and wearing a custom-made thermoplastic mask

Regarding carcinoma of the tongue, the floor of mouth, and other advanced lesions (beyond the midline) or cases with cervical lymph node metastasis, prophylactic irradiation of both sides is required. In well-lateralized buccal mucosal lesions, the upper alveolar ridge and mandibular gingiva are treated by ipsilateral neck irradiation [18]. Well-lateralized tumors of the hard palate without lymph node metastases and bone invasion are low risk, and therefore only the primary tumor should be treated.

The planning target volume (PTV) includes a 5–10-mm margin around CTV. The organs at risk (OAR) include the spinal cord, mandible, and parotid glands.

11.3.1.3 Irradiation Method

Carcinoma of the oral cavity has traditionally been treated with opposed lateral fields, using CT-based two- or three-dimensional techniques. Beams of 4–6 MV are most suitable for the treatment of oral cavity cancers. For patients with N0-stage neck involvement and well-lateralized primary lesions, 40–50 Gy to the ipsilateral neck should be considered as elective nodal irradiation (Figs. 11.2 and 11.3). Mixed-beam or angled-wedge techniques are used depending on the tumor location. In cases with patients with N+neck staging, the dose to the involved lymph nodes should range from 66 Gy to 70 Gy over 6–7 weeks. Patients with advanced lesions and high-risk disease (multiple positive nodes) should receive external beam radiotherapy to the bilateral neck (Fig. 11.4). An additional boost that encompasses the tumor and palpable nodes with appropriate margins should be delivered to avoid a high dose to the spinal cord. For radical radiotherapy, the total dose should be 60–70 Gy over 6–7 weeks.

When external beam radiotherapy is used as the sole treatment modality, even small lesions require 66 Gy given in 33 fractions for reliable control. For large tumors, more than 70 Gy is required to achieve a good result, but there are increasingly significant consequences regarding normal tissue toxicity with doses in this range.

11.3.1.4 Postoperative Radiotherapy

There is no evidence of clinical significance regarding preoperative irradiation when used in conjunction with surgery; however, postoperative irradiation is common. Postoperative radiotherapy is required for advanced lesions (large primary tumors, bone involvement, extensive perineural, or vascular invasion), positive or close surgical margins, and the presence of multiple positive lymph nodes or ECE [7, 17]. In postoperative cases, the range of irradiation is determined by the pathological results of surgery.

In general, the radiation setup is the same as that for primary radiotherapy, but should be tailored individually depending on the location of the primary lesion. The radiation field should encompass the entire surgical bed and upper

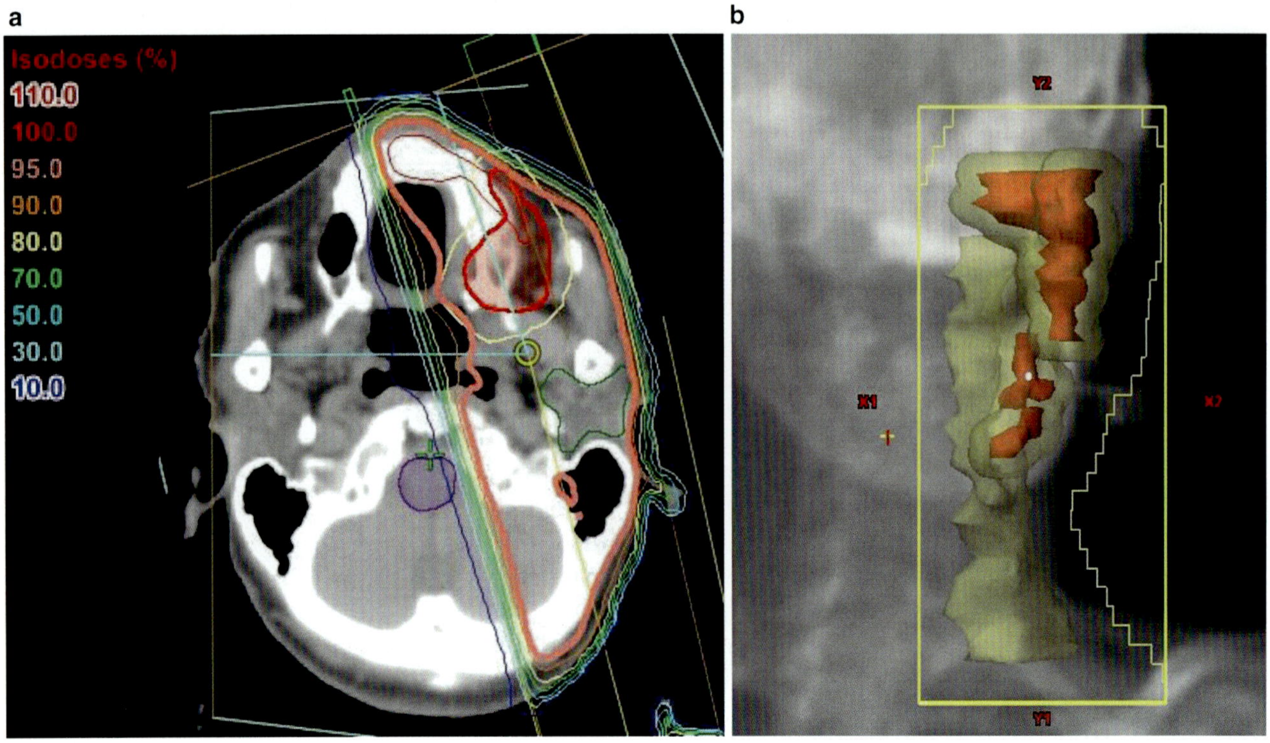

Fig. 11.2 Treatment plan for hemi-neck irradiation. Typical example of the irradiation fields for a carcinoma of the left upper gingiva and buccal mucosa (cT4aN1M0, SCC). The patient was treated ipsilaterally with parallel opposed oblique fields to avoid the spinal cord using CT-based three-dimensional techniques. With a spacer, the tongue could be excluded from the radiation field. (**a**) CT (*axial view*); showing the isodose lines, the *thick line* indicates the 95 % prescribed dose. (**b**) Beam's eye view, 340°. *Red*, tumor [gross tumor volume (GTV)]; *yellow*, clinical target volume (CTV) plus lymph node region; *purple*, brain stem

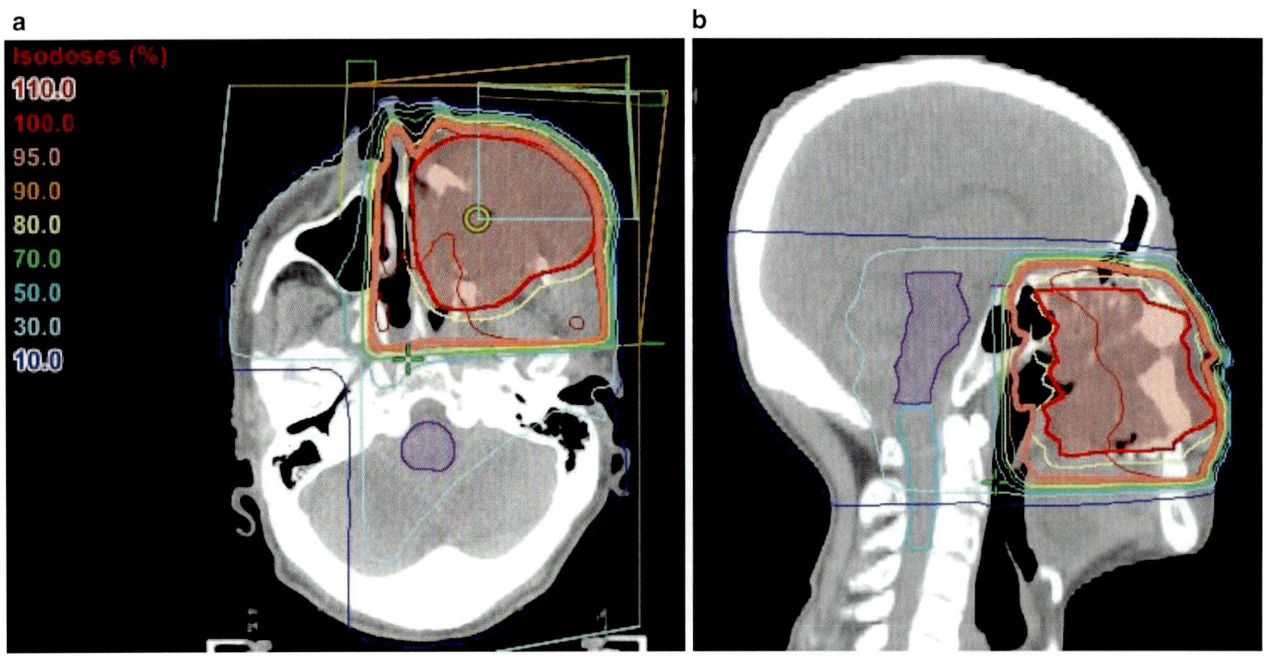

Fig. 11.3 Treatment plan incorporating the wedged-pair technique for anterior lesions of the maxillary gingiva. An example of the irradiation fields for a locally advanced carcinoma of the left upper gingiva (cT4aN0M0, SCC). The patient was vertically irradiated with two portals using angle wedges. Showing the isodose lines, the thick lines indicate the 95 % prescribed dose. (**a**) CT (*axial view*). (**b**) CT (*sagittal view*)

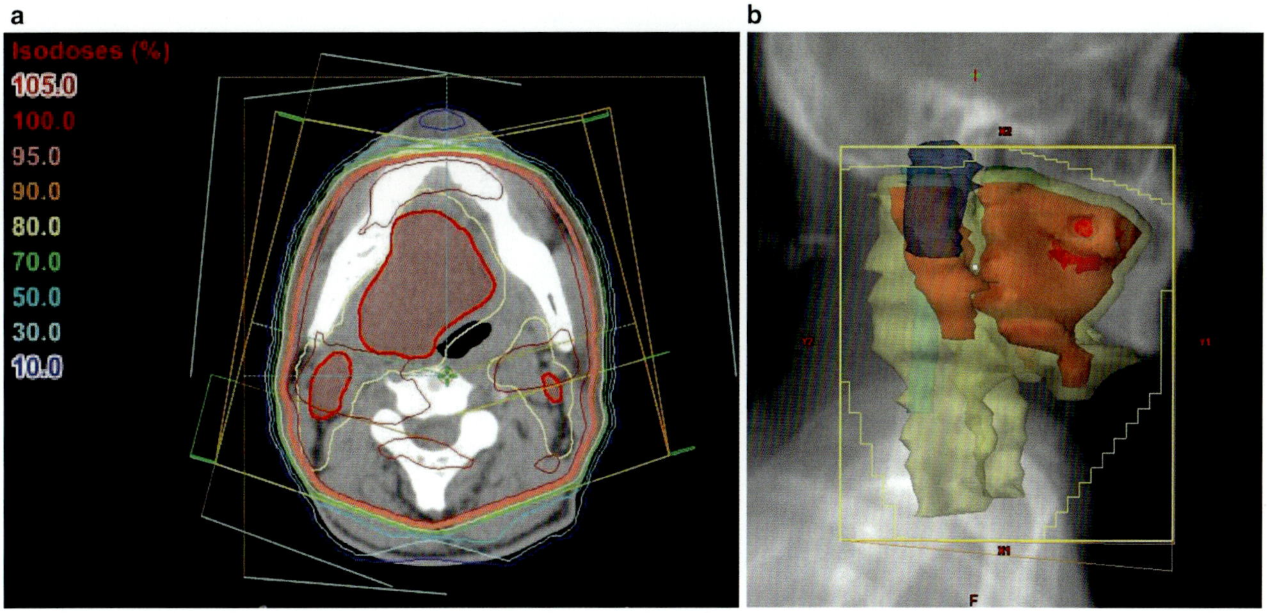

Fig. 11.4 Treatment plan for whole neck irradiation. An example of the irradiation fields for a carcinoma of the right tongue (cT4bN2cM0, SCC). The patient was treated with lateral opposed photon fields using a wedged-pair technique and "field-in-field" compensation. Two wedged beams at 150° were irradiated from the anterior oblique to avoid the shoulder. The primary site and neck levels I–IV were encompassed by the radiation field. (**a**) CT (*axial view*); showing the isodose lines, the *thick line* indicates the 95 % prescribed dose. (**b**) Beam's eye view, 285°. *Red*, GTV; *yellow*, CTV; *light blue*, spinal cord; *blue*, right parotid gland

neck nodes. In most cases, it is necessary to treat the patient with opposed lateral fields to cover the tumor bed and remaining tumors with appropriate surrounding margins (Fig. 11.5).

In cases with N0 neck staging, the regional lymph node (levels I–III) is irradiated. In the presence of multiple positive lymph nodes (more than 3) or ECE, the range from levels I to IV should be irradiated. If possible, to improve the quality of life of patients after treatment, dose reductions to the salivary glands and lower jaw are desirable.

If there is no gross residual tumor, the recommended dose is 40–50 Gy over 4–5 weeks. High-risk areas (positive primary surgical bed, close margins, ECE, perineural invasion) should receive an additional boost of up to 60–66 Gy over 6–6.5 weeks. In other immediate-risk areas, 56–60 Gy over 5.5–6 weeks should be administered.

It is ideal to start postoperative radiotherapy as soon as possible after surgical wound healing (usually 1 month after surgery) to reduce the potential risk of prolonged cumulative treatment time.

11.3.1.5 Intensity Modulated Radiation Therapy

IMRT is an advanced three-dimensional conformal treatment that uses a nonuniform beam intensity pattern with computer-aided optimization to achieve a superior dose distribution. The biggest advantage of IMRT is the ability to produce much higher dose distribution conformities than those achievable with conventional 3D conformal radiation therapy using uniform beam intensities. In particular, IMRT can produce concave-shaped isodose distributions that can more closely follow the shape or boundaries of the target and critical structures in three dimensions. The target volumes to receive various dosage levels are delineated, and the dosimetric plans are generated by inverse planning.

Figure 11.6 shows an example of treatment plan using IMRT for the oral cavity cancer. IMRT can reduce normal tissue toxicities including damage to the spinal cord, major salivary glands, and the mandible [19]. In the treatment of oral cavity cancer, salivary gland disorder becomes a problem. Figure 11.7 shows the difference in dose distribution between conventional radiotherapy and IMRT. In patients with bilateral neck disease, it may be difficult to effectively spare the parotid glands through conventional radiation therapy, particularly when the superior level II cervical lymph nodes are involved. Limiting the mean parotid dose to <25–30 Gy is associated with improved post-radiation salivary function [20]. IMRT is the preferred bilateral neck therapy for oral cancer for minimizing xerostomia. In addition, in oral cavity cancer, treatment with IMRT has contributed to improved survival rates of oral cavity cancer [21]; it is expected to be an excellent therapy.

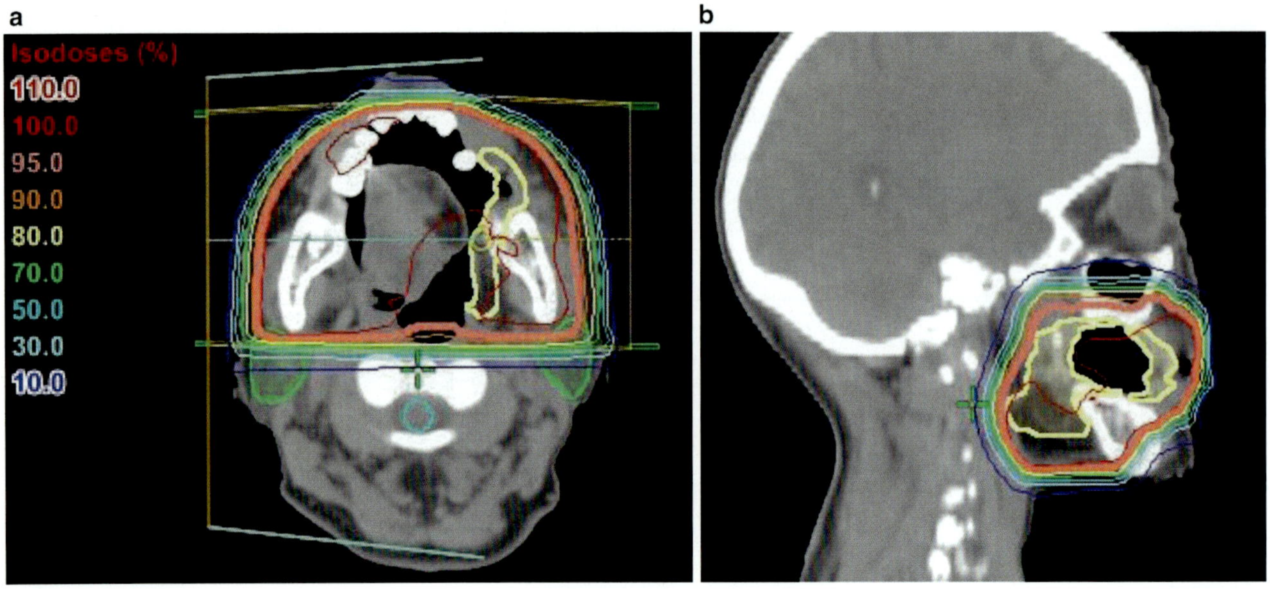

Fig. 11.5 Treatment plan for opposed lateral fields. An example of postoperative irradiation for a carcinoma of the buccal mucosa (cT2N0M0, SCC). The patient underwent partial resection and was treated with postoperative radiotherapy. The margin was free of tumor, and only the primary tumor was irradiated using parallel opposed lateral photon fields to avoid the spinal cord and parotid gland. A total dose of 50 Gy was delivered in 25 fractions. Showing the isodose lines, the *thick line* indicates the 95 % prescribed dose. (**a**) CT (*axial view*). (**b**) CT (*sagittal view*). *Yellow*, CTV; *light blue*, spinal cord; *green*, parotid glands

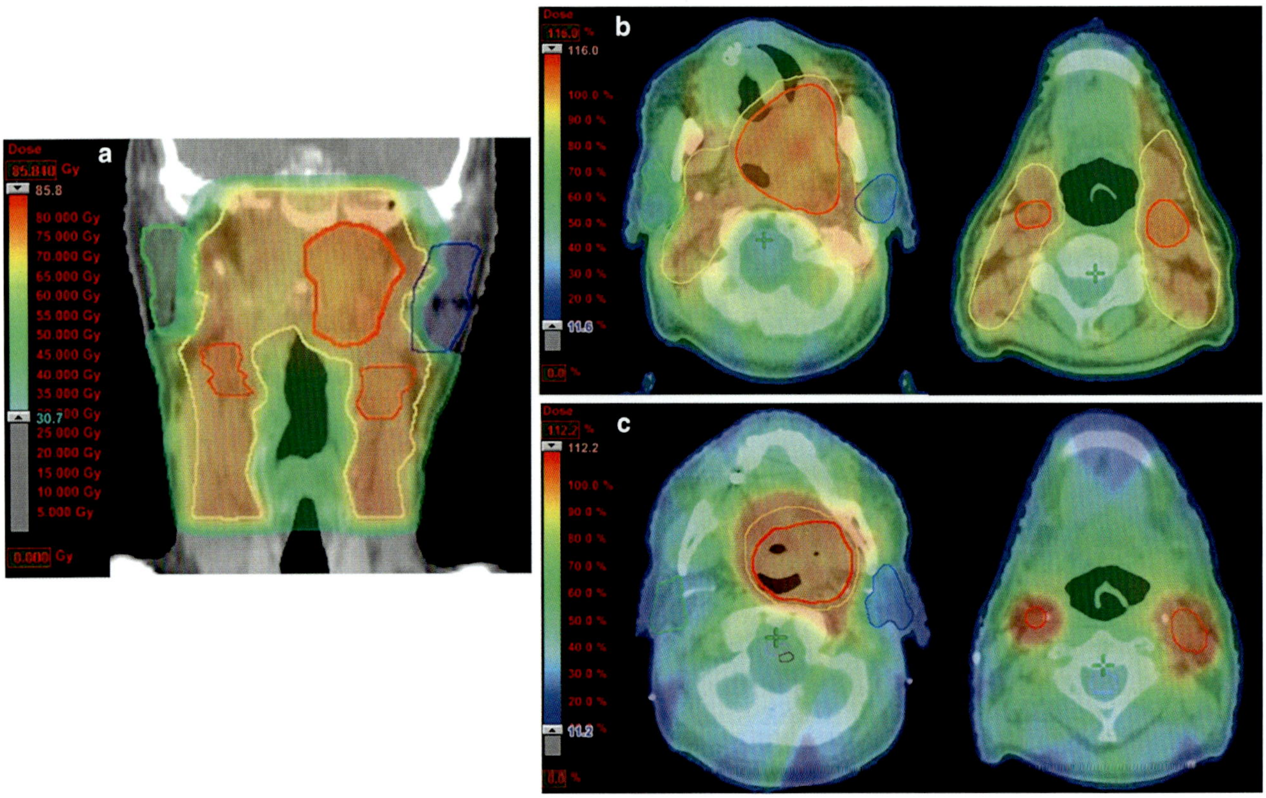

Fig. 11.6 Treatment plan for intensity-modulated radiation therapy (IMRT). An example of the irradiation fields for a carcinoma of the soft palate (cT4aN2cM0, SCC) that was treated with IMRT at a dose of 70 Gy in 35 fractions. (**a**) Total IMRT dose distribution using a 6-MV photon beam (*coronal view*). The patient was treated with nine portals to spare the spinal cord and parotid glands. (**b**) Dose distribution of the first plan using a dose color wash (*axial view*). The primary tumor and regional lymph node (levels I–III) with margin received 46 Gy in 23 fractions. (**c**) Dose distribution of the shrinking plan (*axial view*). The primary tumor and bilateral lymph nodes with 0.5–1-cm margins received a concomitant boost of 24 Gy in 12 fractions for a cumulative prescribed dose of 70 Gy. *Red*, GTV; *yellow*, CTV; *green*, right parotid gland; *blue*, left parotid gland

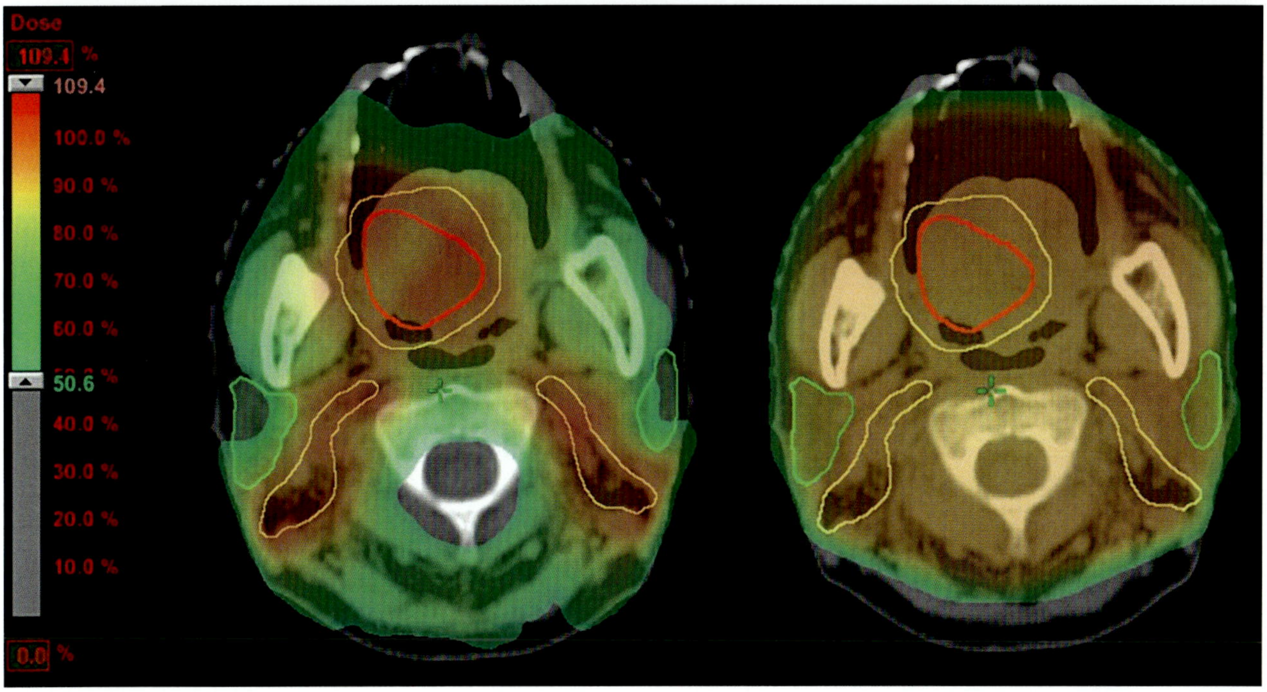

Fig. 11.7 Comparison of the dose distributions between IMRT and conventional radiotherapy. An example of the irradiation fields for a carcinoma of the right tongue (cT4aN2bM0, SCC). An image of the photon beam IMRT treatment plan is on the left, and the conventional radiation treatment plan is on the right. IMRT was successfully used to deliver the dose to the CTV and spare the organs at risk. *Red*, GTV; *yellow*, CTV; *green*, parotid glands

11.3.1.6 Electron Beam Therapy (Intraoral Cone Therapy)

Intraoral cone therapy is another option to enable radiation boosting and can be used in place of interstitial radioisotope implants or external radiation therapy for oral cancer.

The tumor must be located in a site accessible to cone placement. The tumor size should not exceed 3 cm at the greatest dimension. No deep invasion of the underlying tissues and no regional or distant metastasis should be present. This technique is suited for anterior oral cavity lesions in edentulous patients and well-differentiated, superficial lesions of the tongue, buccal mucosa, and oral lips. An example of intraoral cone therapy for a carcinoma of the tongue is shown in Fig. 11.8. Electron beam therapy is also effective for cervical lymph node metastases (Fig. 11.9).

The tumor should be tattooed before treatment. The target volume is the primary tumor with a 15–20-mm margin. The intraoral cone remains in constant contact with the oral mucosa during the treatment. Intraoral cone treatment involves electron beams in the 6–12-MeV range. The total dose is 60–70 Gy in 30–35 fractions when intraoral cone therapy is used alone. The boost doses vary between 20 and 30 Gy after a 40–50 Gy external beam radiotherapy course to the primary site and lymph node [22, 23].

Adverse events such as tongue ulcers have been reported with small-fractionated irradiation. However, it is possible to reduce side effects by inserting a lead plate between the tumor and the oral mucosa (such as the buccal mucosa, lips, gums, and tongue) during treatment. The 5-year LC rates and overall survival rates for all patients (T1-T3N0) were reported to be 52 % and 69 %, respectively [24].

11.3.2 Brachytherapy

Brachytherapy represents an effective treatment option and has played an important role in the treatment of oral cavity cancers. This irradiation only affects very localized areas around the radiation sources. Normal tissue exposure to radiation decreases with increasing distance away from the radiation source.

Brachytherapy has been used as a sole treatment modality for superficial early-stage tumors of the oral cavity, with good results. It has also been used to boost primary lesions treated with external beam radiation and can be used in combination with surgery or chemotherapy [25].

Regarding interstitial brachytherapy, the radioactive sources are placed directly in the target tissue. There are two main types of treatment, according to the level or intensity.

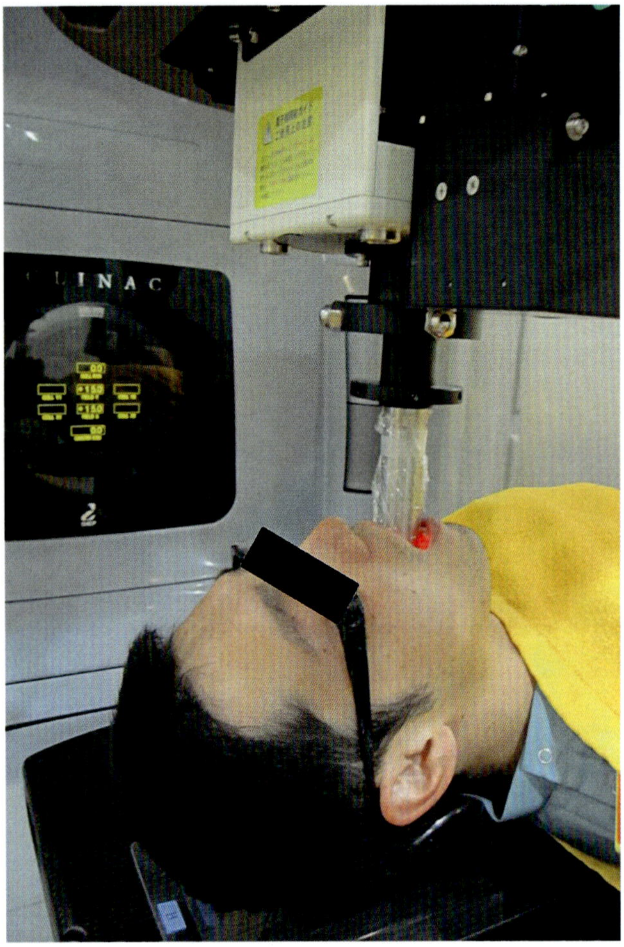

Fig. 11.8 Intraoral cone therapy for a carcinoma of the tongue

Low-dose-rate (LDR) brachytherapy involves implanting radiation sources that emit radiation at a rate of up to 2 Gy/h. High-dose rate (HDR) brachytherapy is used when the dose delivery rate exceeds 12 Gy/h.

The placement of radiation sources in the target area can be temporary or permanent. Temporary brachytherapy involves the placement of radiation sources for a set duration before withdrawal. Permanent brachytherapy, also known as seed implantation, involves the placement of small LDR radioactive sources in the tumor or treatment site, which are left permanently to gradually decay.

11.3.2.1 LDR Treatment Method

^{192}Ir wires or single pins, ^{137}Cs needles, and ^{198}Au seeds have been used as radiation sources (Fig. 11.10). The target volume should encompass the tumor with a margin of at least 5 mm. Radiation sources are arranged to cover the PTV, and dose calculations are performed with a dedicated treatment planning system [26]. Particularly for temporary implants, the treatment duration and removal date and time are determined by these calculations.

Radiation sources are usually implanted under local anesthesia. Depending on the lesion size, a single plane, double plane, or volume implant may be selected to cover the tumor with a 5-mm margin. Brachytherapy is usually performed for lesions less than 1 cm thick. For tumors of <1 cm thick, single-plane implants are adequate (Fig. 11.11). However, for tumors of <2 cm thick, double-plane implants are performed (Fig. 11.12). Further, for tumors of <2.5 cm thick, three-dimensional implantation may be possible (Fig. 11.13) [27].

Though the tongue mobility is limited by the rigidity of the cesium needles, ^{198}Au seeds are so small (2.5 × 0.8 mm) that patients can eat and speak during treatment. Figure 11.14 shows ^{198}Au seed implantation for tumor of the floor of the mouth. ^{198}Au seeds can be used for older patients with complications, but variations in dose distributions are likely to occur relative to the other two radiation sources. Therefore, it is used for superficial small lesions for the uniformity of the dose distribution [25, 28].

As a sole treatment modality, ^{192}Ir or ^{137}Cs temporary implants and ^{198}Au seeds permanent implants can be used to deliver 65–70 Gy in 5–7 days. In combination with 30 Gy of external beam therapy, doses of 50–70 Gy are often prescribed.

To reduce the risk of ORN, a custom-made plastic device is placed between the tongue and gum, which increase the distance between the radioactive sources and alveolar structures and decrease the radiation exposure to the normal tissues [25]. The risk of adverse effects is increased when combined with external beam radiation. Because LDR irradiation has a lower oxygen enhancement ratio (OER) and reoxygenation of the tumor cell occurs during treatment, the therapeutic ratio is high, and it has desirable properties. However, problems associated with LDR include isolation in the treatment room within a radiation-controlled area and exposure of the medical staff.

11.3.2.2 HDR Treatment Method

HDR brachytherapy is performed through a remote afterloading system (RALS) using an ^{192}Ir or cobalt ($_{60}$Co) microradiation source. First, guide needles are inserted from the submandibular region either freehand or with the aid of a custom template to facilitate optimal spacing. Applicators are then positioned in their places. Subsequently, the guide needles are removed and buttons were fastened on the skin side. Dose calculations are performed with a dedicated treatment planning system. The dose evaluation is defined as a plane 5 mm from the central applicator. Radiation sources are afterloaded using the tubes. Figure 11.15 shows an example of HDR interstitial brachytherapy using ^{192}Ir.

There is no need for an isolated treatment room and no risk of medical staff exposure, and it is easy to adjust the prescribed dose. However, the risk of ORN is reportedly higher with HDR than with LDR [29]. Fractionated irradiation

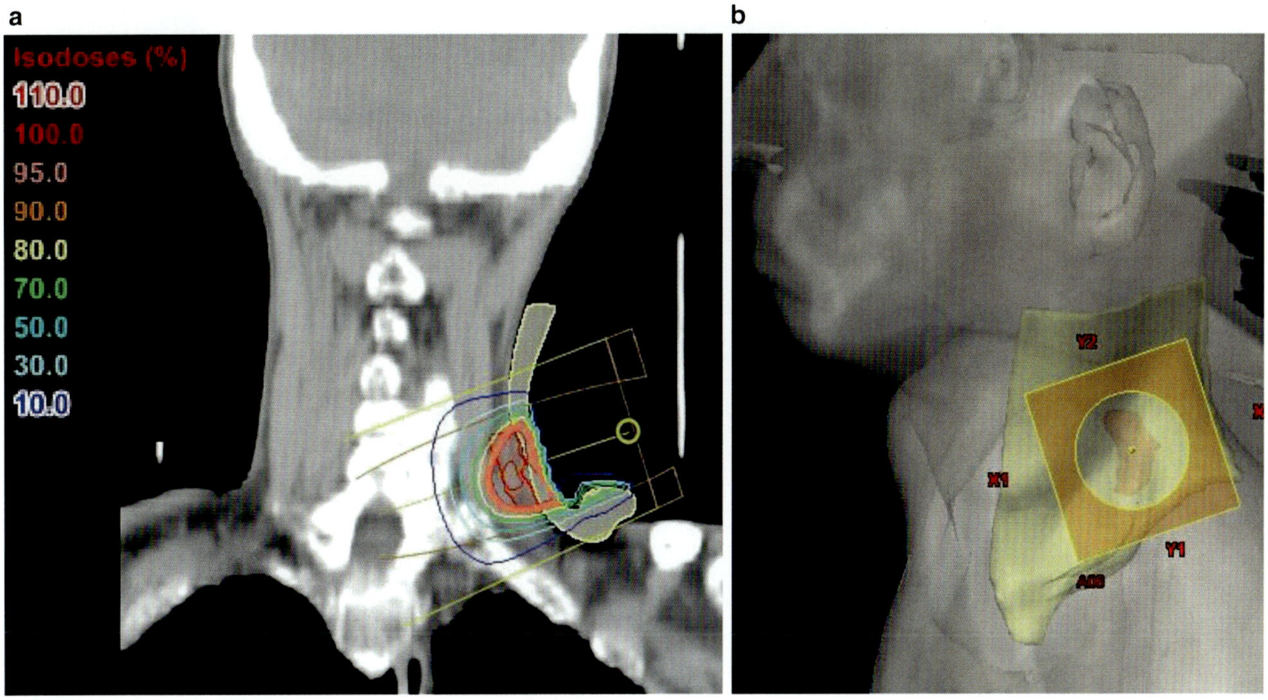

Fig. 11.9 A case of electron beam therapy for neck lymph node metastasis. During electron beam therapy, the use of an adequate bolus can increase the surface dose and attenuate the beam to protect underlying tissues. A 6- or 9-MeV electrons are often used. (**a**) CT (*coronal view*); showing the isodose lines, the *thick line* indicates the 95 % prescribed dose. (**b**) Digital reconstructed radiograph (*lateral*). *Red*, tumor (GTV); *yellow*, bolus; *orange*, lead plate

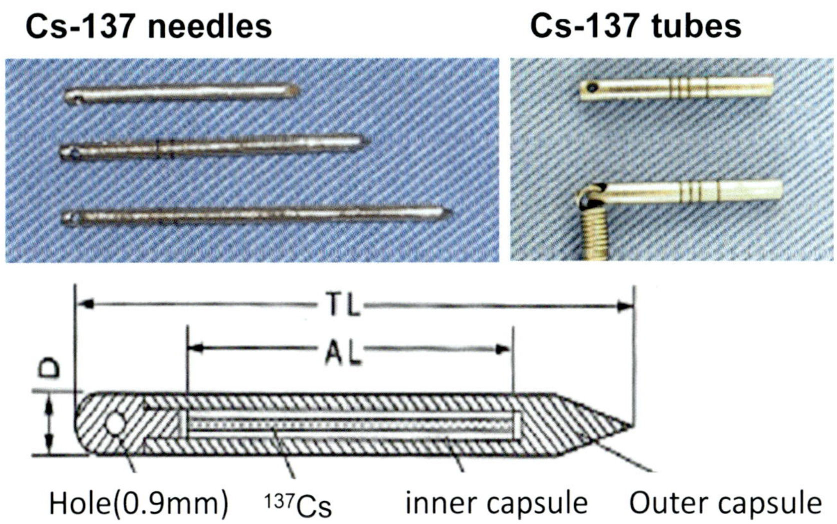

Fig. 11.10 ^{137}Cs radiation sources. ^{137}Cs seeds range from 1.5 to 4.5 cm in length. The γ-ray energy is 0.662 MeV, and the half-life is approximately 30.17 years (With permission from Okimoto T and Nishio M, Department of Radiology, Hokkaido Cancer Center)

is performed at doses of 10–12 Gy, given in 2 fractions per day, for a total dose of 55–60 Gy (9–10 fractions) in 5–7 days. The reported 5-year LC rates were 92.9 %, 81.9 %, and 71.8 % for T1, T2a, and T2b disease [2]. Other good therapeutic results with HDR have also been reported [30].

11.3.2.3 Mold Therapy

Although an interstitial implantation is difficult for lesions of the hard palate and alveolar ridge, surface mold radiation can also be considered for small superficial tumors of the lip, hard palate, lower gingiva, and floor of the mouth.

Brachytherapy with a customized intraoral mold is also effective for superficial oral cavity cancers. In order to reduce the doses to the normal tissues, a spacer with lead plates is effective. For radioactive sources, ^{192}Ir is used for HDR and ^{198}Au is usually used for LDR. Figure 11.16 shows an example of HDR blachytherapy with mold therapy using ^{198}Au, and an example of mold device is shown in Fig. 11.17.

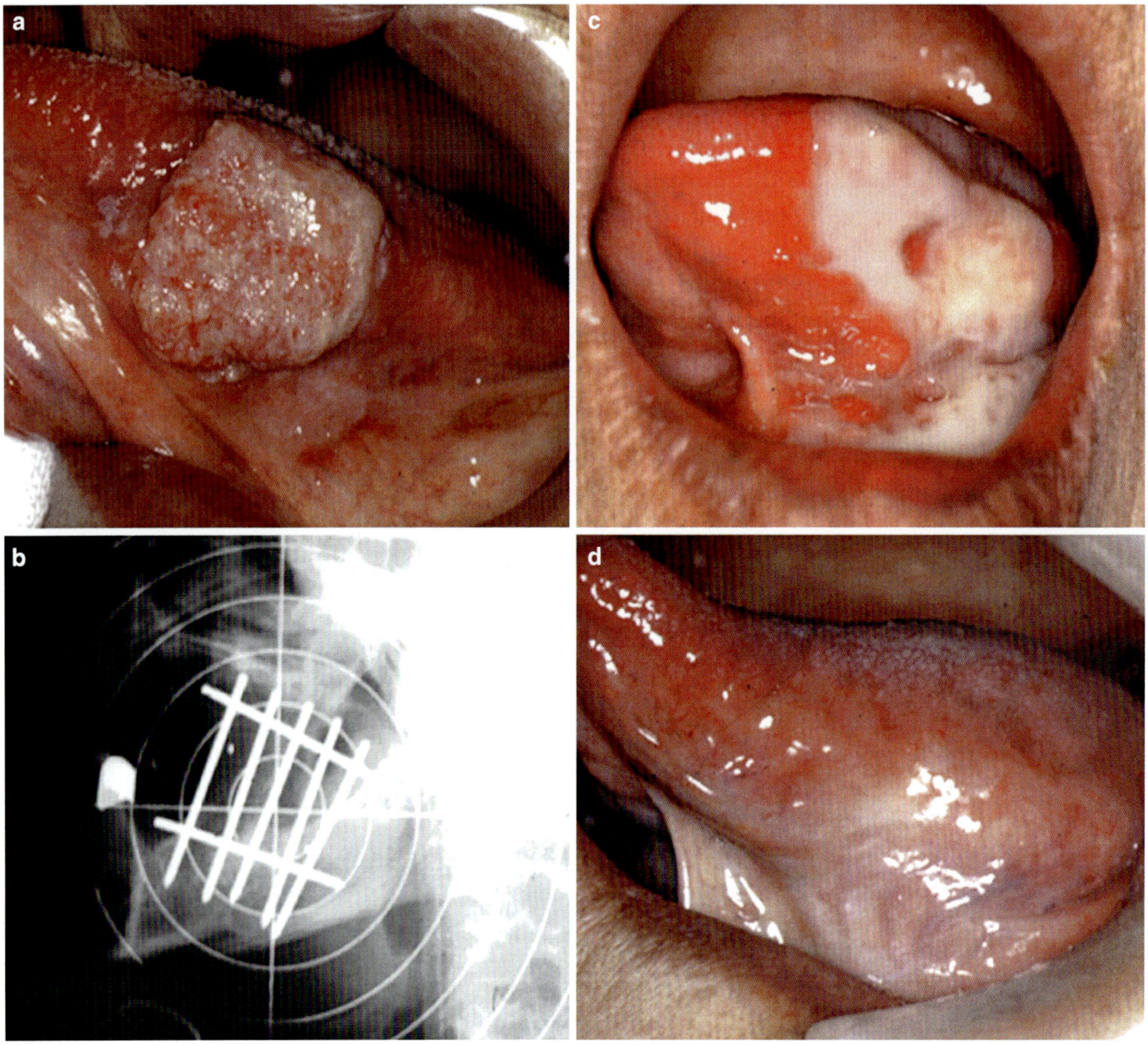

Fig. 11.11 Single-plane implant using ^{137}Cs needles. An example of low-dose-rate (LDR) brachytherapy with a ^{137}Cs source for a carcinoma of the left tongue (cT2N0M0, SCC). (**a**) Before treatment. (**b**) Single-plane implant (lateral X-ray). (**c**) Mucositis after treatment; the range of mucositis is limited to this area. (**d**) 5 years after treatment (With permission from Okimoto T and Nishio M, Department of Radiology, Hokkaido Cancer Center)

The intraoral mold technique is noninvasive and can minimize the risk of bone exposure. The treatment results are not inferior to those of other treatments, but it is used only for superficial tumors. For thicker tumors, external beam radiation is added before mold therapy [9].

11.4 Combination Therapy

11.4.1 Chemoradiotherapy

Cooper et al. reported the results of a randomized study that compared radiation alone to chemoradiation (radiation dose, 60–66 Gy; chemotherapy, three cycles of cisplatin at 100 mg/m^2) in patients with high-risk head and neck cancers after gross total resection [17]. The risk factors of concurrent chemoradiation are two or more involved lymph nodes, ECE of nodal disease, and microscopically involved resection margins. This study demonstrated benefits for loco-regional control and disease-free survival in the chemoradiation arm.

Bernier et al. also demonstrated the superiority of LC, progression-free survival, and overall survival in the chemoradiation arm [31]. These studies suggest that the addition of chemoradiation after surgery may be beneficial in selected patients with high-risk head and neck cancers, although this therapy features increased toxicity. Currently, concurrent chemoradiotherapy is the standard method for locally advanced cancers.

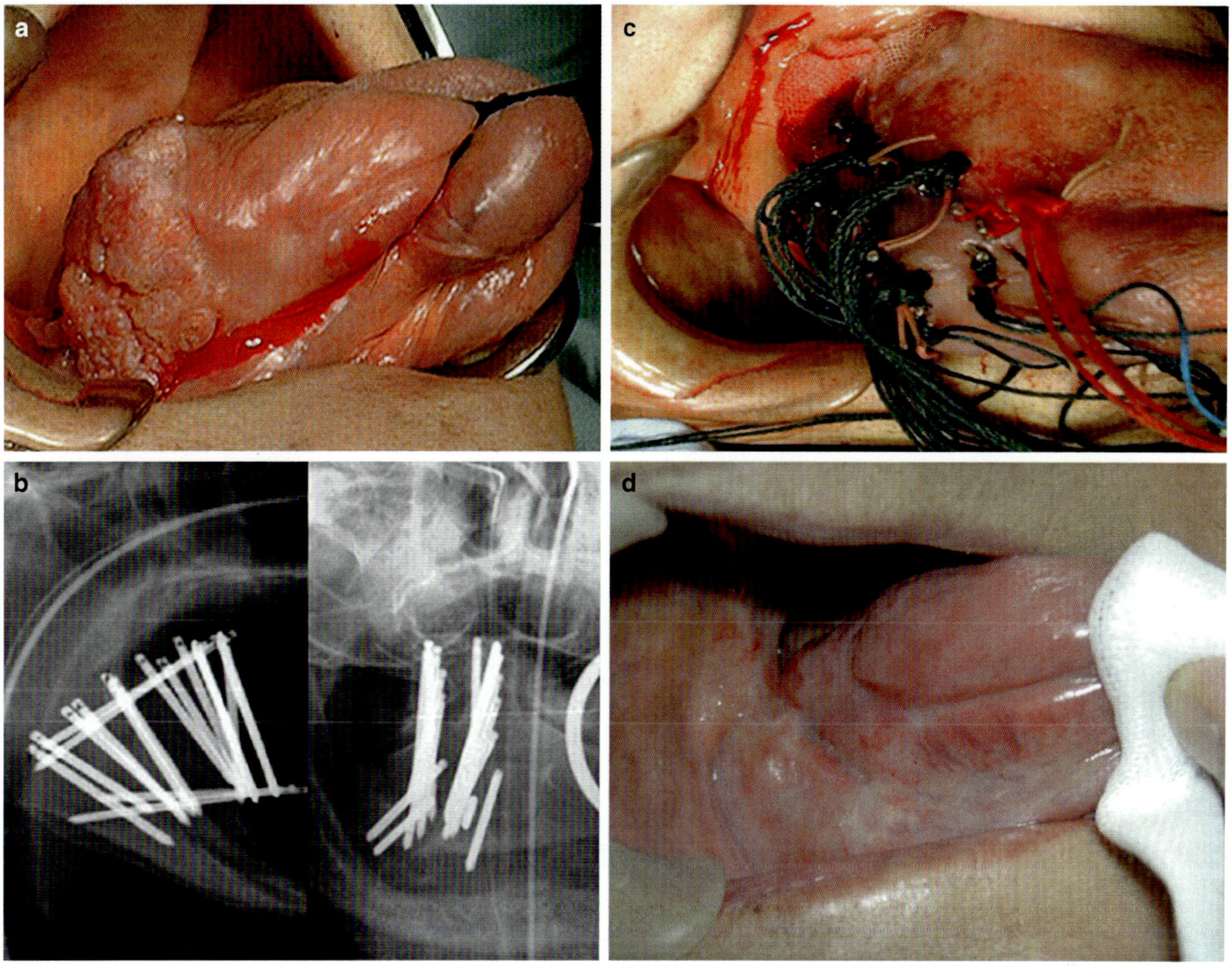

Fig. 11.12 Double-plane implant using ^{137}Cs needles and tumor-volume reduction brachytherapy. An example of LDR brachytherapy with a ^{137}Cs source for carcinoma of the right tongue (cT3N0M0). Before needle insertion, the tumor is trimmed with a laser to reduce the volume. This treatment aims to reduce the incidence of adverse events and improve the dose distribution. (**a**) Before treatment. (**b**) Double-plane implant. (**c**) Radiographs of ^{137}Cs implant. (**d**) 5 years after treatment (With permission from Okimoto T and Nishio M, Department of Radiology, Hokkaido Cancer Center)

11.4.2 Neoadjuvant Chemotherapy

Previously, neoadjuvant chemotherapy (NAC) was used widely to treat oral cavity cancers. Many randomized controlled studies of NAC and radiotherapy alone have shown no significant differences in the treatment results. Although the latest study, which included taxanes, yielded excellent treatment results [32], NAC is considered to be in the experimental stage.

11.5 Treatment of Recurrences

The management of recurrent oral cancer depends on the extent of disease, the history of therapy, and the occurrence of local, regional, or distant recurrences. Re-treatment, which usually involves additional surgery if possible, systemic therapy, re-irradiation, and palliative care are selected individually for each patient.

The risks and benefits of each therapy should be discussed with the individual patient. Palliative radiation treatments can also effectively reduce the pain associated with the tumor itself or with bone metastases and can prevent airway compression from neck metastases.

11.6 Prevention of Adverse Events

Various adverse events may occur during radiation therapy. Dermatitis, oral mucositis, salivary gland damage, and dysgeusia can arise during the acute phase. During the chronic phase, mucosal ulceration, neck edema, osteomyelitis, ORN, xerostomia, hardening of soft tissues, and trismus can occur in some cases (Fig. 11.18).

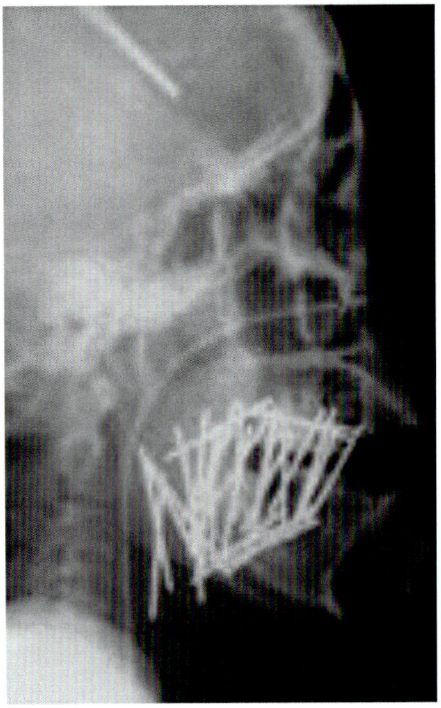

Fig. 11.13 Lateral X-ray of a volume implant using ^{137}Cs needles. An example of three-dimensional implantation of a ^{137}Cs source for a thick lesion

It is reported that the backscatter dose from dental filling materials caused upstream dose and may cause hot-spot mucositis. By removing metals or using intraoral spacer which absorb electron backscatter, a reduction in mucositis is expected [33]. Though acute adverse events often improve, late adverse events often become a sequela. In particular, in the radiotherapy for oral cancer, ORN becomes a severe problem.

To prevent ORN, the use of intraoral stents and spacers can help to increase the distance between the at-risk organ and the tumor. A distance of approximately 10 mm between the tumor and at-risk organ, using a removable spacer, is desired (Fig. 11.19). The occurrence of ORN has been reported to be reduced dramatically with the use of adequate spacers [34]. Acute reactions of the oral mucosa in response to radiation therapy usually begin within approximately 2 weeks and heal within 2–8 weeks.

Before radiotherapy for oral cancer, a careful oral and dental evaluation is required to reduce the subsequent risk of severe multiple caries and ORN. Dentition within the high-dose radiation volume, which introduces the possibility of significant periodontal disease, advanced caries, or abscess formation, or that in a state of disrepair should be extracted. In addition, impacted teeth, unopposed teeth, and opposed teeth with damaged oral mucosa should be considered for extraction.

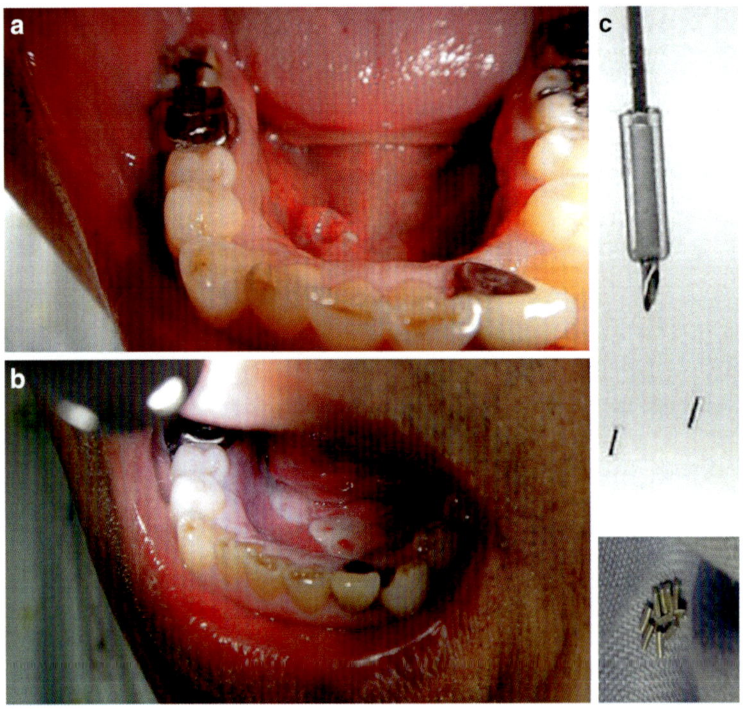

Fig. 11.14 Permanent implant using ^{198}Au seeds. An example of LDR brachytherapy with ^{198}Au seeds for a carcinoma of the floor of the mouth (cT2N0M0, 74 Gy/150 MBq, 15 seeds). ^{198}Au seeds are 2.5 × 0.8 mm in size. The γ-ray energy is 0.41 MeV, and the half-life is 2.7 days. (**a**) Before treatment. (**b**) 2 weeks after treatment; mucositis is locally observed. (**c**) ^{198}Au seeds and inserter (holder) (With permission from Okimoto T and Nishio M, Department of Radiology, Hokkaido Cancer Center)

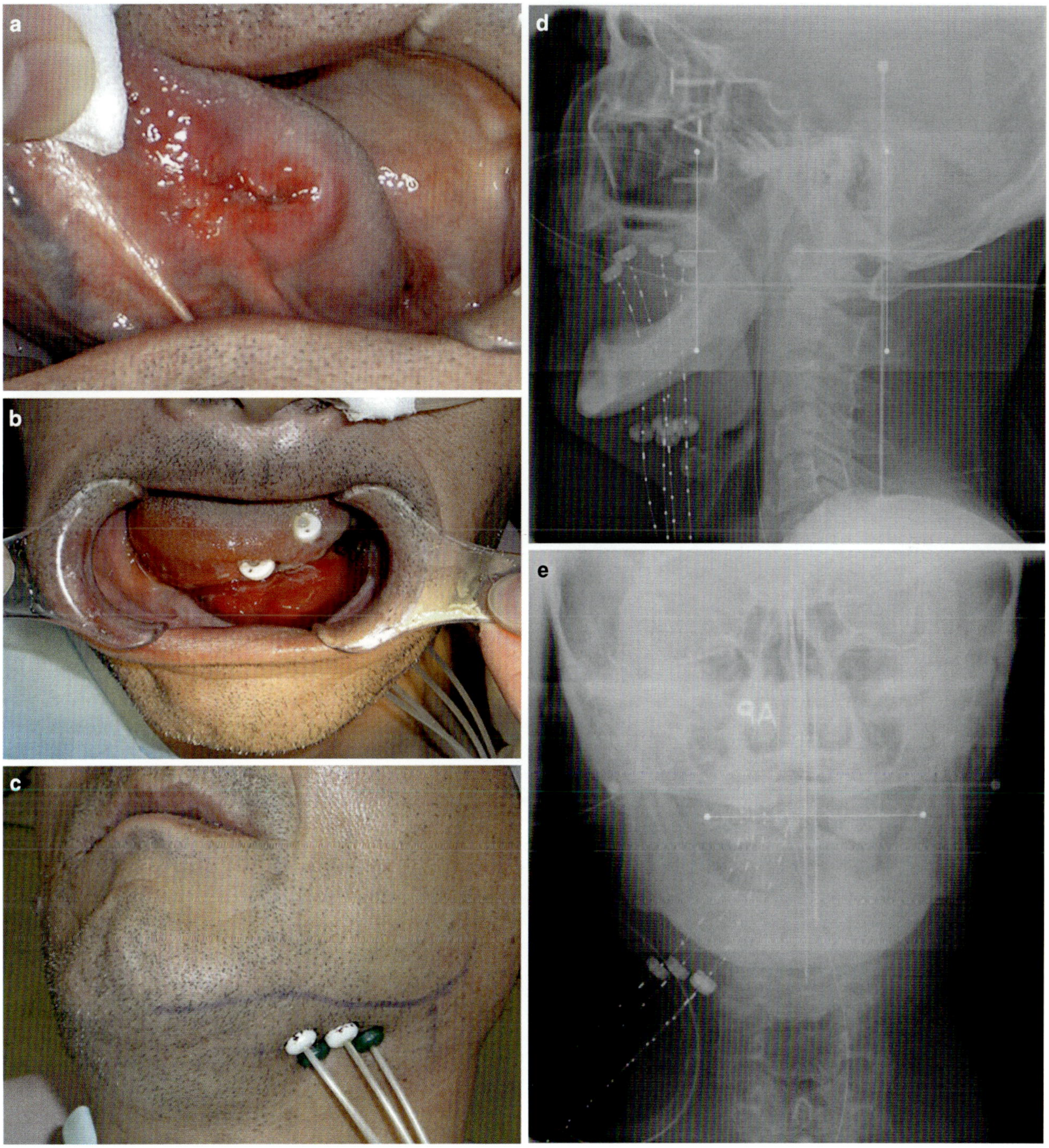

Fig. 11.15 High-dose-rate (HDR) brachytherapy through a remote afterloading system (RALS). An example of HDR interstitial brachytherapy with an ^{192}Ir source for a carcinoma of the left tongue (cT2N0M0). (**a**) Before treatment. (**b**, **c**) Using a submental approach, guide needles were inserted into the anterior floor of the mouth and oral tongue, and hollow tubes (applicators with buttons) were then positioned in their places. Subsequently, the guide needles were removed and buttons were fastened on the skin side. The ^{192}Ir radiation sources were afterloaded using the tubes. (**d**) Radiograph (lateral port). (**e**) Radiograph (anterior-posterior port)

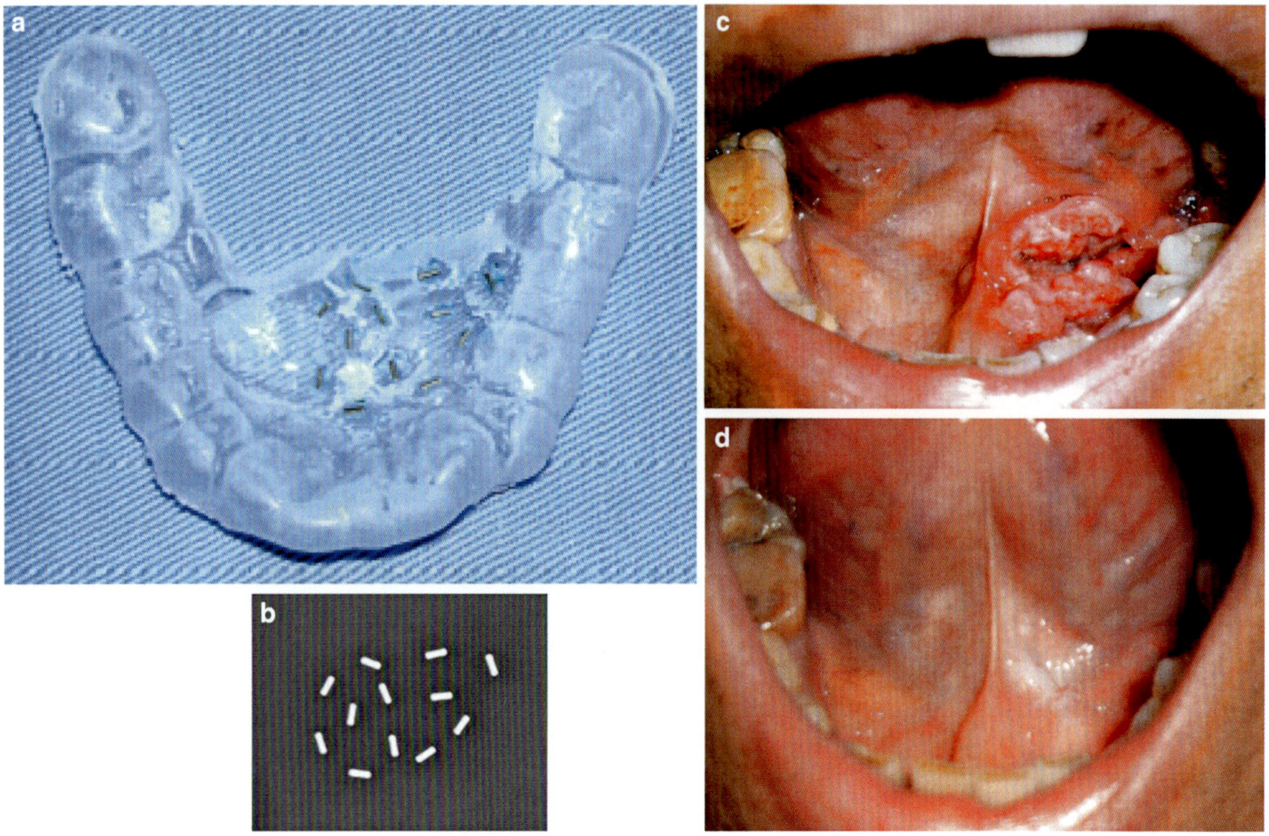

Fig. 11.16 Mold therapy with ^{198}Au seeds. An example of mold therapy with ^{198}Au seeds for a carcinoma of the floor of the mouth (cT2N0M0, 54 Gy/∞, 12 seeds). After external radiotherapy (33 Gy in 15 fractions), the mold apparatus was placed in the patient's oral cavity for 5 days. Dietary intake was possible during treatment. (A,B) Mold apparatus with embedded radioactive ^{198}Au seeds. (C) Before treatment. (D) 3 years after treatment (With permission from Okimoto T and Nishio M, Department of Radiology, Hokkaido Cancer Center)

The routine pre-irradiation extraction of all teeth is no longer recommended. However, the extraction of teeth expected to experience poor effects should be recommended to maintain adequate oral hygiene. All non-restorable teeth should be removed within 10–14 days before the radiation treatment to minimize the subsequent risk of ORN. Dental extractions in irradiated patients should be avoided if possible but, if required, should be accompanied by careful mucosal coverage of the gingiva.

Radiation impairs the capacities of bone healing and recovery after trauma. Therefore, surgical procedures after irradiation must be carefully considered. Radiation to the salivary glands decreases the nature of salivary secretions. Xerostomia increases the accumulation of plaque.

Continuous oral and dental care is very important for all patients receiving radiotherapy for oral cancer. After therapy, a lack of attention to dental hygiene can lead to advanced dental caries.

When ORN occurs after radiotherapy, it must be addressed conservatively. A small subset of ORN after brachytherapy may gradually be cured. However, extensive ORN after high-dose external beam radiation, severe necrosis, and osteomyelitis can spread widely.

In addition, when bilateral neck radiation is performed, permanently impaired salivary gland secretion is inevitable. If possible, the dose to at least one side of the parotid glands should be reduced by less than 40 Gy.

In rare cases, the occurrences of radiation-induced cancers and pseudotumors/pseudosarcomas have been reported as other late complications of radiation therapy [35].

11.7 Particle Therapy

11.7.1 Introduction

Particle therapy (also called particle beam radiation therapy) is a type of radiotherapy. While X-rays are used for conventional radiotherapy, beams with completely different characteristics such as protons and carbon ions are employed for particle therapy. Particle therapies that use protons and carbon ions are generally described as proton beam therapy (PBT) and carbon ion radiotherapy (CIRT), respectively. In current clinical practice, heavy ion radiotherapy is a synonym for CIRT.

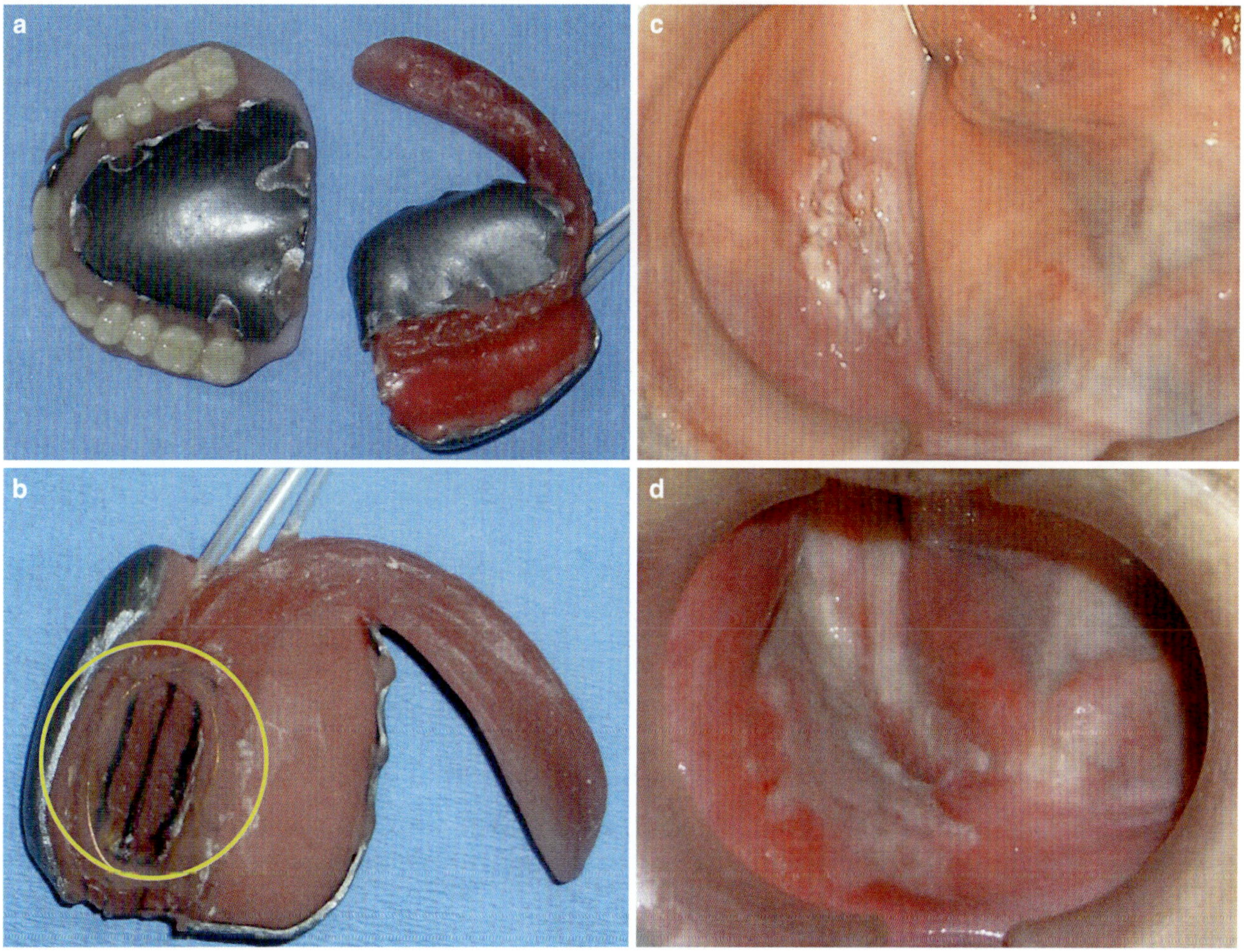

Fig. 11.17 HDR brachytherapy using a mold. An example of HDR mold therapy with a radioactive ^{192}Ir source for a carcinoma of the mandibular gingiva (cT2N0M0, SCC). Upon embedding the tubes in the dentures or molds, the ^{192}Ir radiation sources were afterloaded by RALS. A lead plate was used to protect the hard palate, right buccal mucosa, and tongue. (**a**, **b**) Mold apparatus. (**c**) Before treatment. (**d**) 1 month after treatment; regional mucositis is observed. *Yellow*, the site adjacent to the tumor

X-rays are waves of light or photons that do not possess electrical charges or masses, whereas charged particles such as protons and carbon ions possess both electric charges and masses (Fig. 11.20). Photons exert maximum energy near the body surface; this energy gradually decreases and passes through the entire thicknesses of the body structures. In contrast, charged particles show relatively low energy doses near the body surface and deposit maximum energy immediately before halting deep within the body (called the Bragg peak). By modifying this peak according to the tumor position and size (spread-out Bragg peak (SOBP)), charged particles can be used to deliver high-dose radiation to the tumor while minimizing the doses delivered to the organs at risk (Fig. 11.21).

Carbon ions, which are classified as high linear energy transfer (LET) radiation and demonstrate high ionization density and high rate of DNA damage induced by direct radiation activities, are likely to induce DNA double-strand breaks that are difficult to be repaired and can lead to cell death. Therefore, carbon ions possess the following biological characteristics and are expected to be effective even for X-ray-resistant tumors: a high relative biological effectiveness (RBE), with biological effects (depending on the position of SOBP) 1.2–3.5-fold greater than those obtained with equal physical X-ray doses; a low OER, which will be effective against X-ray-resistant hypoxic cells; and a low dependency on the cell cycle, which will be effective against X-ray-resistant late-S-phase cells. Meanwhile, the biological effects of protons are considered to be nearly identical to those of X-rays (RBE = 1.1).

Approximately 40 particle therapy centers are currently available worldwide. Only eight of these centers include carbon ion facilities (four in Japan, two in Germany, one in China, and one in Italy); the remaining centers include proton facilities. This is probably due because of smaller sizes and lower installation costs of proton facilities (70 million

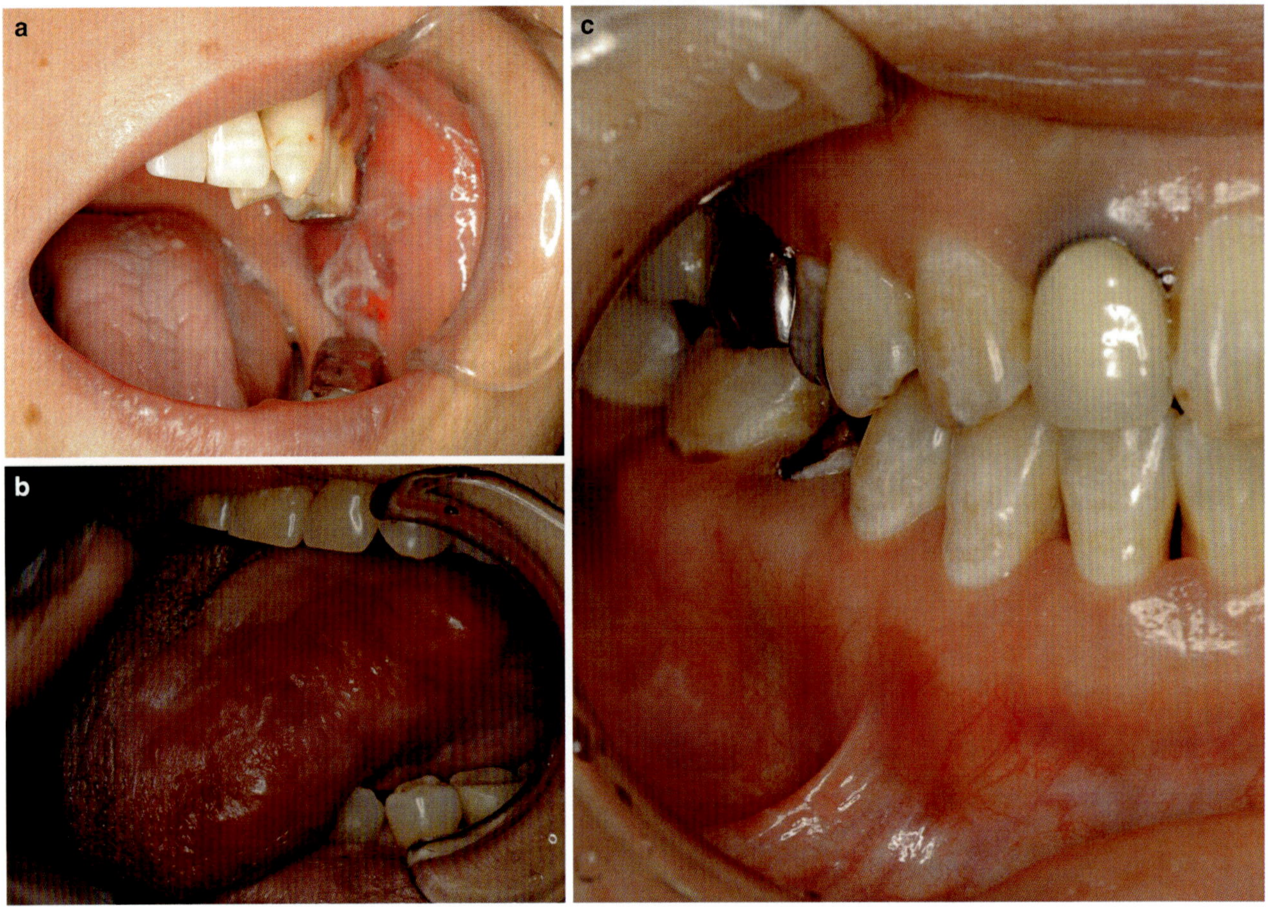

Fig. 11.18 Examples of late adverse effects of radiation therapy. (**a**) Mucositis from electron backscattering of a metal crown early in a course of external radiation therapy. (**b**) Xerostomia (6 months after treatment). (**c**) Tooth decalcification (6 months after treatment)

US dollars for a proton facility vs. 140 million US dollars for a carbon ion facility). In addition, the operation of rotating gantries, which feature 360° rotation and allow tumor irradiation from arbitrary angles, is only available at proton facilities.

11.7.2 Particle Therapy for Head and Neck Malignancies

11.7.2.1 SCC vs. Other Histological Types

With regard to head and neck malignancies, the efficacy of particle therapy has been primarily demonstrated for X-ray and chemoresistant tumors such as mucosal melanomas (MMs) [36, 37], adenoid cystic carcinomas (ACCs) [38–40], olfactory neuroblastomas [41], and sarcomas [42, 43], rather than for SCCs, which are both X-ray sensitive and chemosensitive. Figure 11.22 lists the histological types of 791 patients with head and neck malignancies who were treated at the Hyogo Ion Beam Medical Center (HIBMC) in Japan between 2001 and 2012. Although more than 90 % head and neck malignancies are epidemiologically diagnosed as SCCs, only 22 % tumors at the HIBMC were SCCs; the remaining 78 % were of other histological types.

Mizoe et al. [44], who reported the treatment outcomes of CIRT for head and neck malignancies according to histological types at the National Institute for Radiological Sciences in Japan, stated that SCCs had a significantly worse local control rate (61 % at 5 years) compared with those of MMs (75 %) and ACCs (73 %) and a significantly worse overall survival rate (17 % at 5 years) compared with that of ACCs (68 %). Although this difference was not significant,

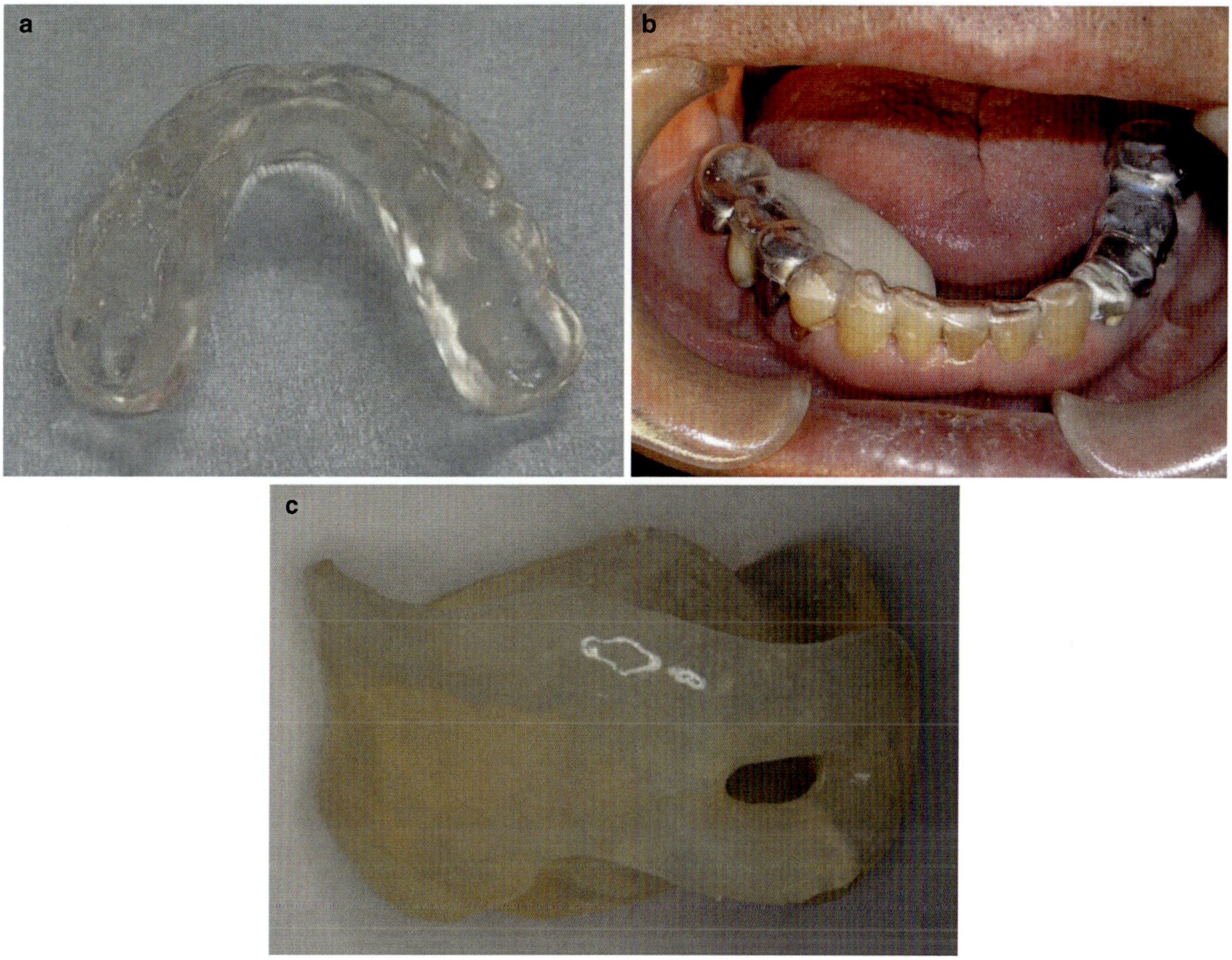

Fig. 11.19 Examples of custom-made intraoral spacers. Custom-made spacers help to protect the organs at risk from excess radiation exposure and avoid backscatter doses from dental materials. (**a**) Rigid acrylic resin spacers at sites adjacent to the tumor that require volume. (**b**) Mounting resin is used to add thickness between the tumor and organs at risk. (**c**) Soft silicon spacers induce little damage to the oral mucosa. An open breathing hole is located in the front. In addition to increasing the vertical and horizontal distances from the organs at risk, the spacer can fix the tongue and stabilize occlusion

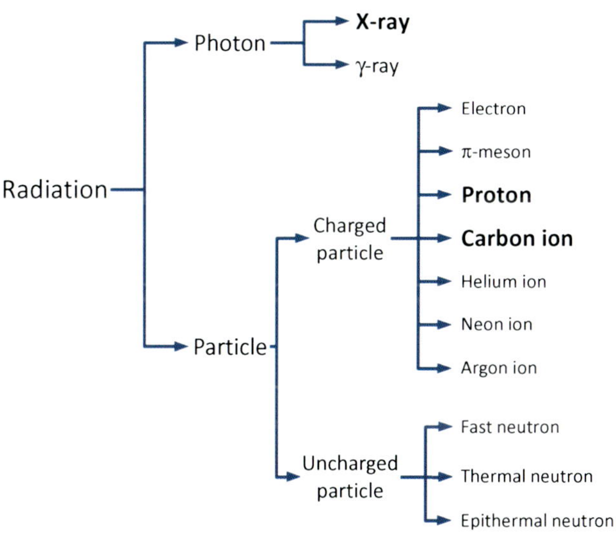

Fig. 11.20 Types of radiation

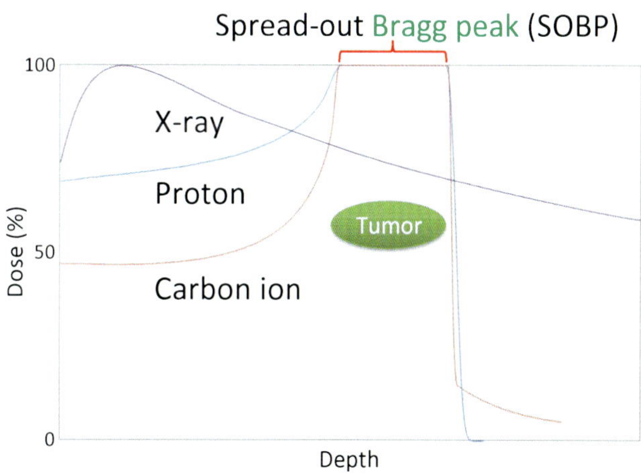

Fig. 11.21 Dose distributions of X-rays, protons, and carbon ions

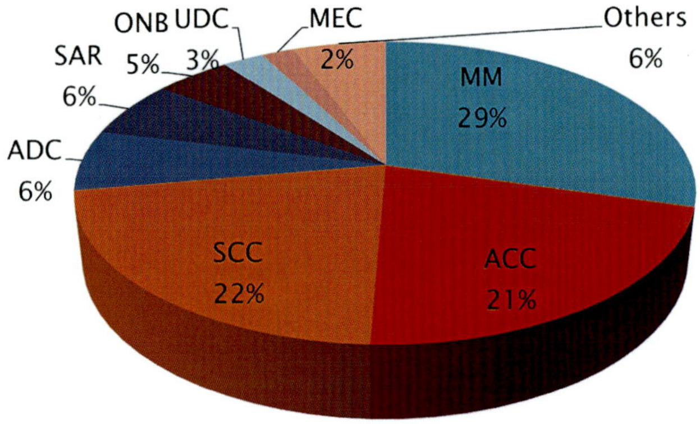

Fig. 11.22 Histological tumor types in 791 patients with head and neck malignancies who were treated during the period 2001–2012 at the Hyogo Ion Beam Medical Center, Japan. *MM* mucosal melanoma, *ACC* adenoid cystic carcinoma, *SCC* squamous cell carcinoma, *ADC* adenocarcinoma, *SAR* sarcoma, *ONB* olfactory neuroblastoma, *UDC* undifferentiated carcinoma, *MEC* mucoepidermoid carcinoma

commonly comprise hypofractionations (16–26 fractions) with large fraction size (2.5–4 GyE[1] per fraction), may be inadequate for rapidly growing SCCs. Second, the absence of concurrent chemotherapy (radiation alone is the mainstay of particle therapy) may be insufficient for chemosensitive SCCs.

11.7.2.2 PBT vs. CIRT

Although both PBT and CIRT are charged particle therapies, there are slight differences in their physical characteristics. With regard to the monoenergetic beam, carbon ions have the following features: a superior penumbra compared with that of protons and low-dose leakage (<10 %) on the distal side of the Bragg peak, which is not observed with protons (nuclear spallation reaction; Fig. 11.23). However, the latter issue does not practically matter because two or more portals are generally used in clinical settings. The largest difference in the mechanical aspects is in the availability of the rotating

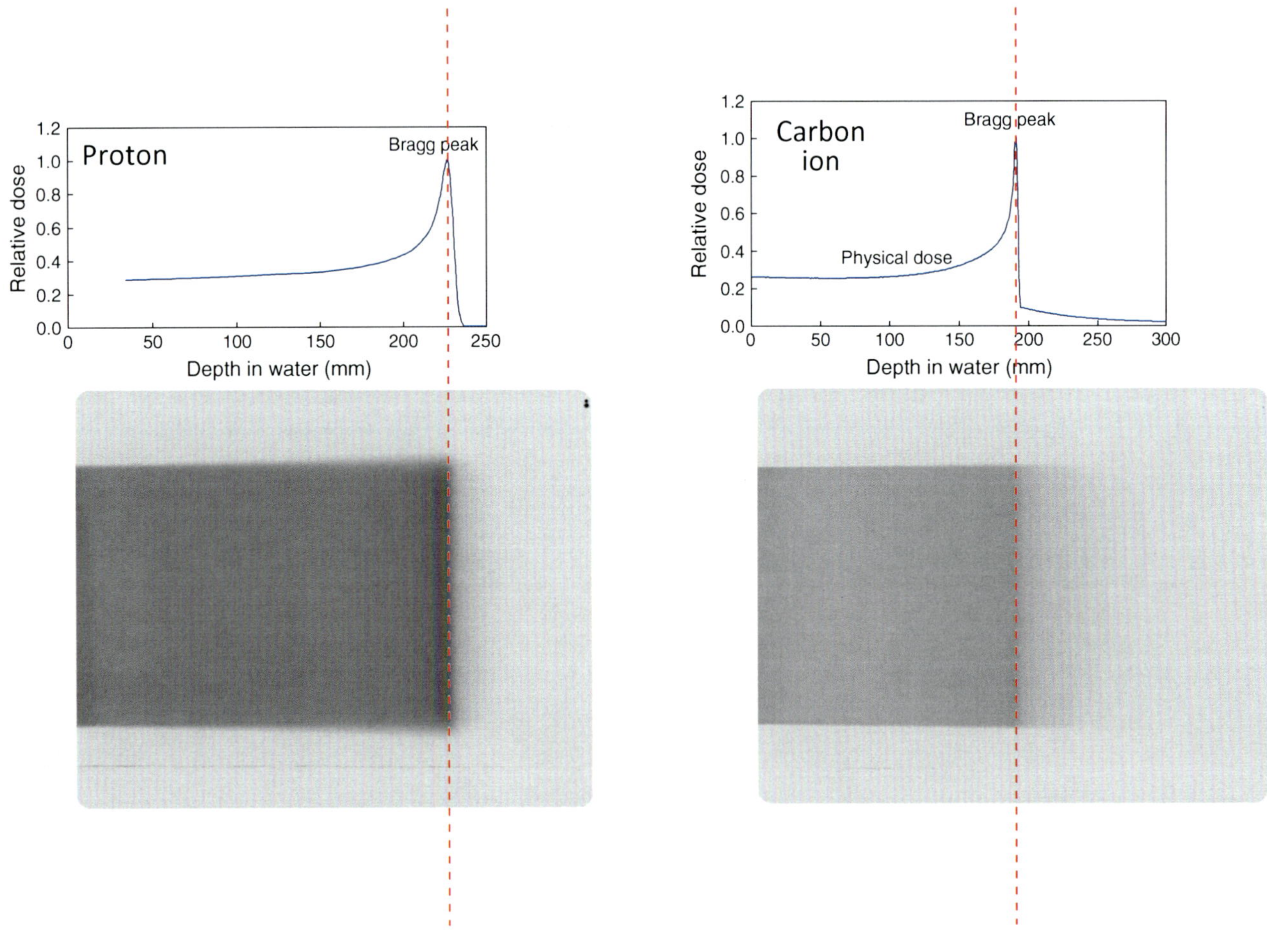

Fig. 11.23 Differences in dose distributions between proton (*left*) and carbon ion (*right*) monoenergetic beams (*upper*, calculated and measured depth-dose curves; *lower*, film densitometry)

the above overall survival rate for SCCs was even worse than that for MMs (35 %). Similar results have been obtained at the HIBMC (data not published).

The reasons behind the unfavorable outcomes of SCCs remain unknown. The authors speculate the following possibilities: first, particle therapy dose fractionations, which

[1]The particle beam doses are reported in gray equivalents (GyE), which are defined as the physical doses multiplied by the RBE of the protons or carbon ions. At HIBMC, the biological effects of both PBT and CIRT were evaluated in vitro and in vivo, and the RBE values for proton and carbon ion irradiation were determined to be 2–3.7 (depending on the SOBP depth) and 1.1, respectively [45].

Table 11.1 Comparison of protons and carbon ions

	Protons	Carbon ions
Rotating gantry	Available	Not available (fixed portals only)
Penumbra	Inferior	Superior
Range	Longer	Shorter

gantry. Table 11.1 shows a comparison between protons and carbon ions.

HIBMC was established in 2001 as the first institution worldwide to use both protons and carbon ions, and more than 5,900 patients have been treated by the end of September 2013. Our retrospective analyses have demonstrated no significant differences between PBT and CIRT in either efficacy or toxicity, despite the physical and biological differences mentioned above. As an example, the treatment outcomes of MMs are shown in Fig. 11.24.

11.7.3 Potential of Particle Therapy for Oral Malignancies

Thus far, the clinical outcomes of particle therapy for oral malignancies alone have not been published. However, particle therapy has great potential as a treatment for oral malignancies. Figure 11.25 shows a case of sublingual gland ACC (cT4aN0M0, cStage IVA) adjacent to the mandible that was treated with CIRT at a dose of 70.4 GyE using two portals. It is impossible for conventional photon therapy to sufficiently spare the mandible to avoid bone necrosis; however, CIRT could restrict the dose to most of the mandible to 60 GyE or less, thereby yielding a low possibility of bone necrosis [46]. A case of MM that was primarily situated on the left side of the soft palate with a solitary neck metastasis (cT3N1bM0, cStage IVA) is shown in Fig. 11.26. Both the primary lesion and neck metastasis were treated with PBT. PBT demonstrated great effects with acceptable toxicities.

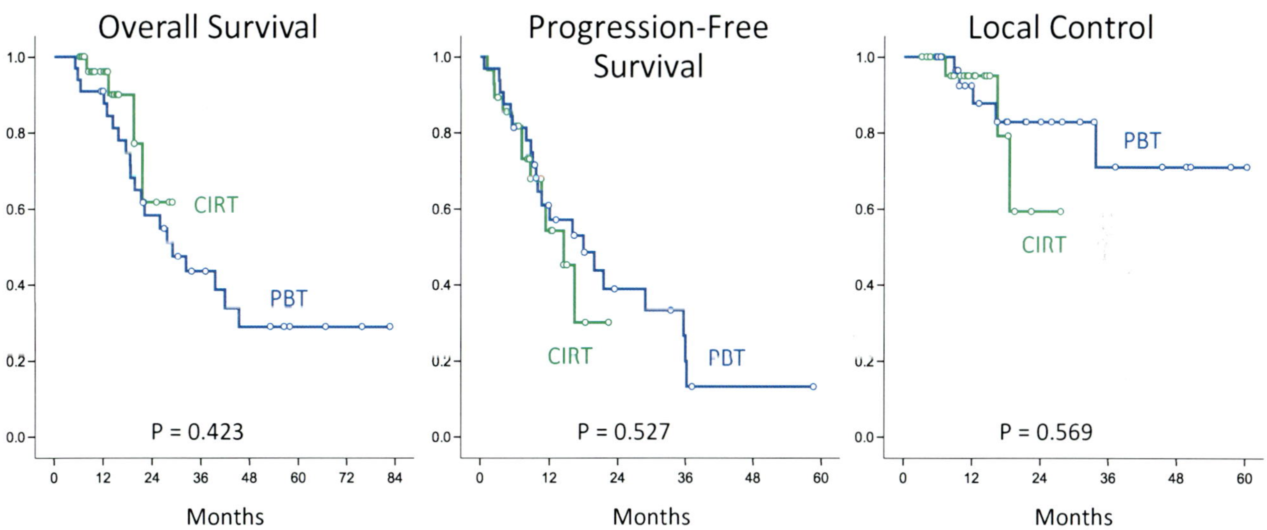

Fig. 11.24 Comparison of treatment outcomes between proton beam therapy (PBT) and carbon ion radiotherapy (CIRT) for mucosal melanoma of the head and neck at the Hyogo Ion Beam Medical Center

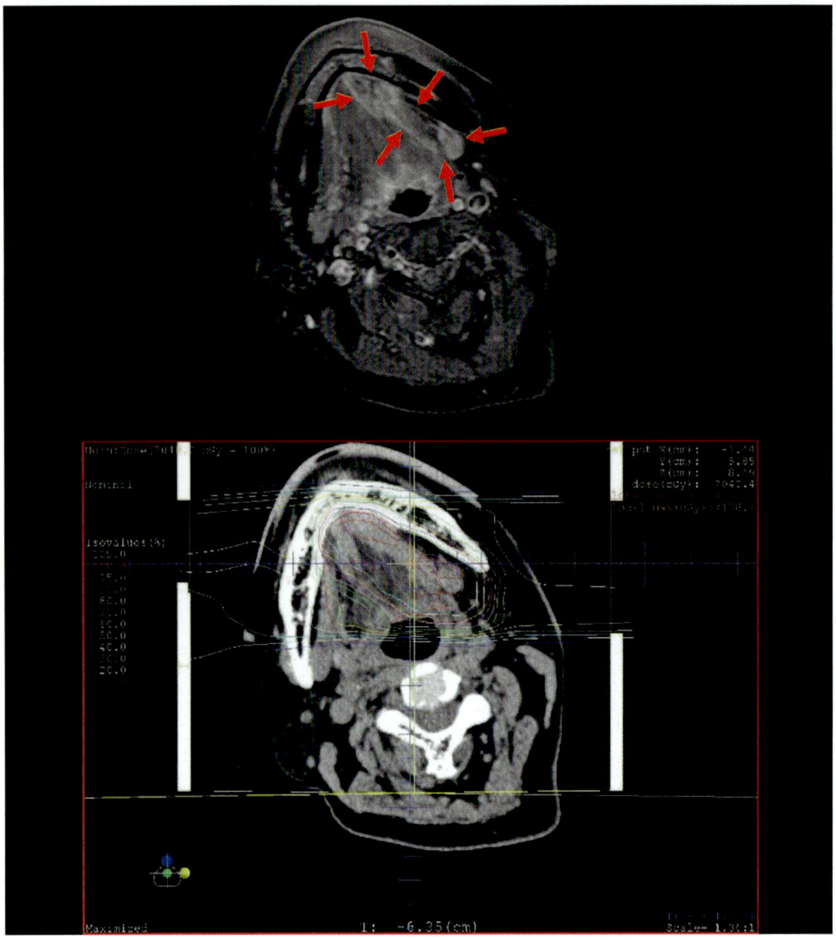

Fig. 11.25 A case of a 73-year-old female with an adenoid cystic carcinoma of the left sublingual gland (cT4aN0M0, cStage IVA). She was treated with carbon ion radiotherapy (CIRT) at a dose of 70.4 GyE in 32 fractions with two portals. *Upper*, magnetic resonance imaging (*arrows* indicate the tumor); *lower*, CIRT treatment planning

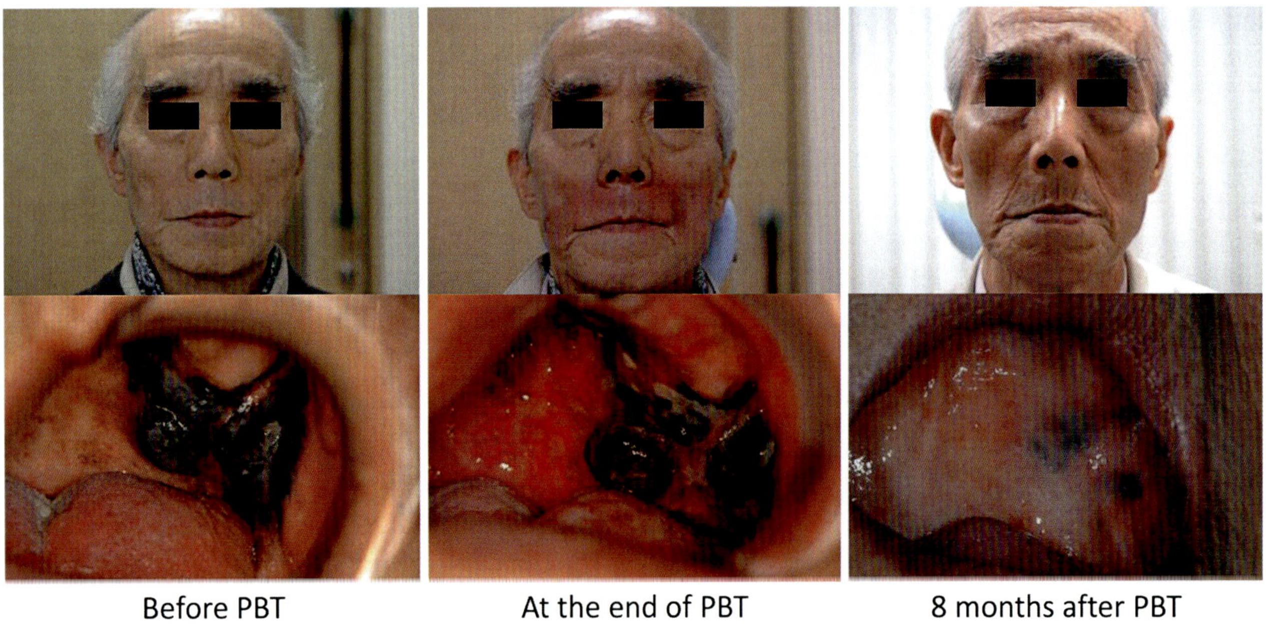

Fig. 11.26 A case of a 74-year-old male with a mucosal melanoma primarily situated in the *left side* of the soft palate with a solitary neck metastasis (cT3N1bM0, cStage IVA). Proton beam therapy (PBT) was performed for both the primary lesion (65 GyE in 26 fractions) and neck metastasis (56 GyE in 8 fractions). At the end of PBT, grade 3 oral mucositis and grade 1 dermatitis were observed, and the melanoma had already slightly diminished. Eight months after PBT, remarkable tumor regression was confirmed, and the patient recovered from his acute oral mucosal and skin reactions. The neck metastasis was also controlled

The usefulness of particle therapy for oral malignancies has not yet been sufficiently elucidated. However, the theoretical advantages of particle therapies are obvious, and the authors believe that particle therapy will certainly play an important role in the treatment of oral malignancies in the future.

References

1. Shibuya H, Hoshina M, Takeda M, Matsumoto S, Suzuki S, Okada N (1993) Brachytherapy for stage I and II oral tongue cancer: an analysis of past cases focusing on control and complications. Int J Radiat Oncol Biol Phys 26(1):51–58
2. Fujita M, Hirokawa Y, Kashiwado K, Akagi Y, Kashimoto K, Kiriu H, Matsuura K, Ito K (1999) Interstitial brachytherapy for stage I and II squamous cell carcinoma of the oral tongue: factors influencing local control and soft tissue complications. Int J Radiat Oncol Biol Phys 44(4):767–775
3. Inoue T, Inoue T, Teshima T, Murayama S, Shimizutani K, Fuchihata H, Furukawa S (1996) Phase III trial of high and low dose rate interstitial radiotherapy for early oral tongue cancer. Int J Radiat Oncol Biol Phys 36(5):1201–1204
4. Ihara N, Shibuya H, Yoshimura R, Oota S, Miura M, Watanabe H (2005) Interstitial brachytherapy and neck dissection for Stage III squamous cell carcinoma of the mobile tongue. Acta Oncol 44(7):709–716. doi:10.1080/02841860500267881
5. Decroix Y, Ghossein NA (1981) Experience of the Curie institute in treatment of cancer of the mobile tongue: II. Management of the neck nodes. Cancer 47(3):503–508
6. Nakagawa T, Shibuya H, Yoshimura R, Miura M, Okada N, Kishimoto S, Amagasa M, Omura K (2003) Neck node metastasis after successful brachytherapy for early stage tongue carcinoma. Radiother Oncol 68(2):129–135
7. Fletcher GH, Evers W (1970) Radiotherapeutic management of surgical recurrences and postoperative residuals in tumors of the head and neck. Radiology 95:185–188
8. Fuwa N, Kodaira T, Furutani K, Tachibana H, Nakamura T, Nakahara R, Tomoda T, Inokuti H, Daimon T (2008) Arterial chemoradiotherapy for locally advanced tongue cancer: analysis of retrospective study of therapeutic results in 88 patients. Int J Radiat Oncol Biol Phys 72(4):1090–1100. doi:10.1016/j.ijrobp.2008.02.021
9. Takeda M, Shibuya H, Inoue T (1996) The efficacy of gold-198 grain mold therapy for mucosal carcinomas of the oral cavity. Acta Oncol 35(4):463–467
10. Marcus RB Jr, Million RR, Mitchell TP (1980) A preloaded, custom-designed implantation device for stage T1-T2 carcinoma of the floor of mouth. Int J Radiat Oncol Biol Phys 6(1): 111–113
11. Chu A, Fletcher GH (1973) Incidence and causes of failures to control by irradiation the primary lesions in squamous cell carcinomas of the anterior two-thirds of the tongue and floor of mouth. Am J Roentgenol Radium Ther Nucl Med 117(3):502–508
12. Urist MM, O'Brien CJ, Soong SJ, Visscher DW, Maddox WA (1987) Squamous cell carcinoma of the buccal mucosa: analysis of prognostic factors. Am J Surg 154(4):411–414
13. Mitsudo K, Shigetomi T, Fujimoto Y, Nishiguchi H, Yamamoto N, Furue H, Ueda M, Itoh Y, Fuwa N, Tohnai I (2011) Organ preservation with daily concurrent chemoradiotherapy using superselective intra-arterial infusion via a superficial temporal artery for T3 and T4 head and neck cancer. Int J Radiat Oncol Biol Phys 79(5):1428–1435. doi:10.1016/j.ijrobp.2010.01.011
14. Hsu MY, Wang CC (2010) Elective radiotherapy or neck dissection for CT-staged T1-2N0 oral tongue cancer. Head Neck 32(10):1428–1430. doi:10.1002/hed.21525, author reply 1430
15. Teichgraeber JF, Clairmont AA (1984) The incidence of occult metastases for cancer of the oral tongue and floor of the mouth: treatment rationale. Head Neck Surg 7:15–21
16. Rabuzzi DD, Chung CT, Sagerman RH (1980) Prophylactic neck irradiation. Arch Otolaryngol 106(8):454–455
17. Cooper JS, Pajak TF, Forastiere AA, Jacobs J, Campbell BH, Saxman SB, Kish JA, Kim HE, Cmelak AJ, Rotman M, Machtay M, Ensley JF, Chao KS, Schultz CJ, Lee N, Fu KK, Radiation Therapy Oncology Group 9501/Intergroup (2004) Postoperative concurrent radiotherapy and chemotherapy for high-risk squamous-cell carcinoma of the head and neck. N Engl J Med 350(19): 1937–1944
18. Lin CY, Lee LY, Huang SF, Kang CJ, Fan KH, Wang HM, Chen EY, Chen IH, Liao CT, Cheng AJ, Chang JT (2008) Treatment outcome of combined modalities for buccal cancers: unilateral or bilateral neck radiation? Int J Radiat Oncol Biol Phys 70(5):1373–1381. doi:10.1016/j.ijrobp.2007.08.022
19. Nutting CM, Morden JP, Harrington KJ, Urbano TG, Bhide SA, Clark C, Miles EA, Miah AB, Newbold K, Tanay M, Adab F, Jefferies SJ, Scrase C, Yap BK, A'Hern RP, Sydenham MA, Emson M, Hall E; PARSPORT trial management group (2011) Parotid-sparing intensity modulated versus conventional radiotherapy in head and neck cancer (PARSPORT): a phase 3 multicentre randomised controlled trial. Lancet Oncol 12(2):127–136. doi:10.1016/S1470-2045(10)70290-4
20. Little M, Schipper M, Feng FY, Vineberg K, Cornwall C, Murdoch-Kinch CA, Eisbruch A (2012) Reducing xerostomia after chemo-IMRT for head-and-neck cancer: beyond sparing the parotid glands. Int J Radiat Oncol Biol Phys 83(3):1007–1014. doi:10.1016/j.ijrobp.2011.09.004
21. Chen PY, Chen HH, Hsiao JR, Yang MW, Hsueh WT, Tasi ST, Lin FC, Wu YH (2012) Intensity-modulated radiotherapy improves outcomes in postoperative patients with squamous cell carcinoma of the oral cavity. Oral Oncol 48(8):747–752. doi:10.1016/j.oraloncology.2012.02.010
22. Wang CC, Doppke KP, Biggs PJ (1983) Intra-oral cone radiation therapy for selected carcinomas of the oral cavity. Int J Radiat Oncol Biol Phys 9(8):1185–1189
23. Wang CC (1989) Radiotherapeutic management and results of T1N0, T2N0 carcinoma of the oral tongue: evaluation of boost techniques. Int J Radiat Oncol Biol Phys 17(2):287–291
24. Kakimoto N, Murakami S, Nakatani A, Yoshioka Y, Shimizutani K, Furukawa S (2012) Electron beam radiotherapy for tongue cancer using an intra-oral cone. Oral Oncol 48(5):463–468. doi:10.1016/j.oraloncology.2011.12.008
25. Kimura Y, Fuwa N, Kamata M, Matsumoto A, Nakamura PK, Nakamura T, Ariji E (2003) Stage I and II mobile tongue carcinomas treated by external radiation and gold seed implantation. Acta Oncol 42(7):763–770
26. Paterson R, Parker HM (1967) Interstitial treatment. In: Meredith WJ (ed) Radium dosage: the manchester system, 2nd edn. E. & S. Livingstone LTD, Edinbergh/London, pp 31–41
27. Nishio M (2005) General remarks on brachytherapy. Nihon Igaku Hoshasen Gakkai Zasshi 65(3):207–215
28. Matsumoto S, Takeda M, Shibuya H, Suzuki S (1996) T1 and T2 squamous cell carcinomas of the floor of the mouth: results of brachytherapy mainly using 198Au grains. Int J Radiat Oncol Biol Phys 34(4):833–841
29. Lau HY, Hay JH, Flores AD, Threlfall WJ (1996) Seven fractions of twice daily high dose-rate brachytherapy for node-negative carcinoma of the mobile tongue results in loss of therapeutic ratio. Radiother Oncol 39(1):15–18

30. Inoue T, Inoue T, Yoshida K, Yoshioka Y, Shimamoto S, Tanaka E, Yamazaki H, Shimizutani K, Teshima T, Furukawa S (2001) Phase III trial of high- vs. low-dose-rate interstitial radiotherapy for early mobile tongue cancer. Int J Radiat Oncol Biol Phys 51(1):171–175
31. Bernier J, Domenge C, Ozsahin M, Matuszewska K, Lefèbvre JL, Greiner RH, Giralt J, Maingon P, Rolland F, Bolla M, Cognetti F, Bourhis J, Kirkpatrick A, van Glabbeke M, European Organization for Research and Treatment of Cancer Trial 22931 (2004) Postoperative irradiation with or without concomitant chemotherapy for locally advanced head and neck cancer. N Engl J Med 350(19):1945–1952
32. Blanchard P, Bourhis J, Lacas B, Posner MR, Vermorken JB, Hernandez JJ, Bourredjem A, Calais G, Paccagnella A, Hitt R, Pignon JP; Meta-Analysis of Chemotherapy in Head and Neck Cancer, Induction Project, Collaborative Group (2013) Taxane-cisplatin-fluorouracil as induction chemotherapy in locally advanced head and neck cancers: an individual patient data meta-analysis of the meta-analysis of chemotherapy in head and neck cancer group. J Clin Oncol 31(23):2854–2860. doi:10.1200/JCO.2012.47.7802
33. Mail N, Albarakati Y, Ahmad Khan M, Saeedi F, Safadi N, Al-Ghamdi S, Saoudi A (2013) The impacts of dental filling materials on RapidArc treatment planning and dose delivery: challenges and solution. Med Phys 40(8):081714. doi:10.1118/1.4816307
34. Miura M, Takeda M, Sasaki T, Inoue T, Nakayama T, Fukuda H, Hoshi A, Hoshina M, Shibuya H (1998) Factors affecting mandibular complications in low dose rate brachytherapy for oral tongue carcinoma with special reference to spacer. Int J Radiat Oncol Biol Phys 41(4):763–770
35. Oota S, Shibuya H, Hamagaki M, Yoshimura R, Iwaki H, Kojima M, Takagi M (2003) Oral pseudotumor: benign polypoid masses following radiation therapy. Cancer 97(5):1353–1357
36. Yanagi T, Mizoe JE, Hasegawa A, Takagi R, Bessho H, Onda T, Kamada T, Okamoto Y, Tsujii H (2009) Mucosal malignant melanoma of the head and neck treated by carbon ion radiotherapy. Int J Radiat Oncol Biol Phys 74(1):15–20. doi:10.1016/j.ijrobp.2008.07.056
37. Zenda S, Kawashima M, Nishio T, Kohno R, Nihei K, Onozawa M, Arahira S, Ogino T (2011) Proton beam therapy as a nonsurgical approach to mucosal melanoma of the head and neck: a pilot study. Int J Radiat Oncol Biol Phys 81(1):135–139. doi:10.1016/j.ijrobp.2010.04.071
38. Pommier P, Liebsch NJ, Deschler DG, Lin DT, McIntyre JF, Barker FG 2nd, Adams JA, Lopes VV, Varvares M, Loeffler JS, Chan AW (2006) Proton beam radiation therapy for skull base adenoid cystic carcinoma. Arch Otolaryngol Head Neck Surg 132(11):1242–1249. doi:10.1001/archotol.132.11.1242
39. Schulz-Ertner D, Didinger B, Nikoghosyan A, Jakel O, Zuna I, Wannenmacher M, Debus J (2003) Optimization of radiation therapy for locally advanced adenoid cystic carcinomas with infiltration of the skull base using photon intensity-modulated radiation therapy (IMRT) and a carbon ion boost. Strahlenther Onkol 179(5):345–351. doi:10.1007/s00066-003-1071-7
40. Schulz-Ertner D, Nikoghosyan A, Jakel O, Haberer T, Kraft G, Scholz M, Wannenmacher M, Debus J (2003) Feasibility and toxicity of combined photon and carbon ion radiotherapy for locally advanced adenoid cystic carcinomas. Int J Radiat Oncol Biol Phys 56(2):391–398
41. Nishimura H, Ogino T, Kawashima M, Nihei K, Arahira S, Onozawa M, Katsuta S, Nishio T (2007) Proton-beam therapy for olfactory neuroblastoma. Int J Radiat Oncol Biol Phys 68(3):758–762. doi:10.1016/j.ijrobp.2006.12.071
42. Jingu K, Tsujii H, Mizoe JE, Hasegawa A, Bessho H, Takagi R, Morikawa T, Tonogi M, Tsuji H, Kamada T, Yamada S (2012) Carbon ion radiation therapy improves the prognosis of unresectable adult bone and soft-tissue sarcoma of the head and neck. Int J Radiat Oncol Biol Phys 82(5):2125–2131. doi:10.1016/j.ijrobp.2010.08.043
43. Yamaoka M, Akiyama M, Yokokawa Y, Terao Y, Yokoi K, Kato T, Fukushima T, Sakurai H, Ida H (2013) Multidisciplinary therapy including proton beam radiotherapy for an Ewing's sarcoma family tumor of maxillary sinus in a 4-year-old girl. Head Neck 35(12):E386–E390. doi:10.1002/hed.23352
44. Mizoe JE, Hasegawa A, Jingu K, Takagi R, Bessyo H, Morikawa T, Tonoki M, Tsuji H, Kamada T, Tsujii H, Okamoto Y (2012) Results of carbon ion radiotherapy for head and neck cancer. Radiother Oncol 103(1):32–37. doi:10.1016/j.radonc.2011.12.013
45. Kagawa K, Murakami M, Hishikawa Y, Abe M, Akagi T, Yanou T, Kagiya G, Furusawa Y, Ando K, Nojima K, Aoki M, Kanai T (2002) Preclinical biological assessment of proton and carbon ion beams at hyogo ion beam medical center. Int J Radiat Oncol Biol Phys 54(3):928–938
46. Emami B, Lyman J, Brown A, Coia L, Goitein M, Munzenrider JE, Shank B, Solin LJ, Wesson M (1991) Tolerance of normal tissue to therapeutic irradiation. Int J Radiat Oncol Biol Phys 21(1):109–122

Systemic Chemotherapy

12

Makoto Tahara and Tadaaki Kirita

Abstract

Systemic chemotherapy for oral squamous cell carcinoma is generally employed in the following situations: (a) postoperative adjuvant concurrent chemoradiotherapy for patients with high-risk features, (b) postoperative adjuvant chemotherapy, (c) preoperative concurrent chemoradiotherapy followed by surgery for advanced resectable patients, (d) concurrent chemoradiotherapy as primary treatment for cases unable to tolerate or unsuited for surgery or as salvage treatment in the persistent or recurrent disease setting, (e) neoadjuvant chemotherapy, and (f) palliative chemotherapy. The recent addition of cetuximab to radiotherapy or platinum-based chemotherapy has produced a significant improvement in overall survival for head and neck cancer. Further, numerous novel molecular targeting drugs are now under investigation for head and neck cancer.

Keywords

Chemoradiotherapy • Chemotherapy • Molecular targeting drug

12.1 Introduction

The mainstay of treatment for oral squamous cell carcinoma (OSCC) is surgery [1]. Primary radiotherapy with or without chemotherapy is not used routinely. Systemic chemotherapy is generally employed in the following situations: (a) postoperative adjuvant concurrent chemoradiotherapy (CRT) for patients with high-risk features, (b) postoperative adjuvant chemotherapy, (c) preoperative concurrent CRT followed by surgery for advanced resectable patients, (d) CRT as primary treatment for patients who are unable to tolerate or unsuited for surgery or as salvage treatment in the persistent or recurrent disease setting, (e) neoadjuvant chemotherapy, and (f) palliative chemotherapy.

12.2 Postoperative Adjuvant Concurrent Chemoradiotherapy

Stage III/IV resectable local advanced squamous cell carcinoma of the head and neck (SCCHN) has a poor prognosis. Known risk factors for recurrence are microscopic resection margin positive, extracapsular nodal extension positive, multiple cervical lymph node metastasis (≥2), lymph node metastasis with a diameter of 3 cm or more, perineural infiltration, level 4 (inferior internal jugular lymph node) or level 5 (accessory nerve lymph node) lymph node metastasis in oropharyngeal cancer/oral cavity cancer, and signs of vascular embolism.

In 1996, Bachaud et al. [2] reported the results of a randomized comparative study in 83 patients with postoperative high-risk relapse factors (extracapsular nodal extension positive) for cancers of the oral cavity, oropharynx, hypopharynx,

M. Tahara, M.D., Ph.D.
Division of Head and Neck Medical Oncology, National Cancer Center Hospital East, 6-5-1 Kashiwanoha, Kashiwa, Chiba 277-8577, Japan
e-mail: matahara@east.ncc.go.jp

T. Kirita, D.D.S., D.MSc. (✉)
Department of Oral and Maxillofacial Surgery, Nara Medical University, 840 Shijo-cho, Kashihara, Nara 634-8521, Japan
e-mail: tkirita@naramed-u.ac.jp

T. Kirita and K. Omura (eds.), *Oral Cancer: Diagnosis and Therapy*, DOI 10.1007/978-4-431-54938-3_12, © Springer Japan 2015

and larynx. The radiation monotherapy group had a 5-year overall survival (OS) rate of 13 % versus 36 % in the CRT (cisplatin 50 mg/body every week) group ($P<0.01$), showing the statistically significant superiority of CRT.

Smid et al. [3] compared radiation monotherapy with CRT using mitomycin and bleomycin in 114 patients with postoperative risk factors for recurrence (microscopic resection margin positivity, extracapsular nodal extension positivity, perineural infiltration, or signs of vascular infiltration) who had primary lesions in the oral cavity, oropharynx, hypopharynx, or larynx. Although this was a small randomized study, 2-year OS rate was 64 % in the radiation monotherapy group versus 74 % in the CRT group, showing that the latter was significantly superior ($P=0.036$).

The RTOG88-24 study (phase II), published in 1997, reported excellent results for postoperative adjuvant CRT (3-weekly cisplatin + RT) using cisplatin (100 mg/m^2, every 3 weeks), with a 3-year progression-free survival (PFS) rate of 39 % and 3-year OS rate of 47 % [4]. Based on these results, the EORTC and RTOG conducted the EORTC22931 study [5] and RTOG95-01 study [6], respectively, as phase III studies to compare 3-weekly cisplatin + RT with radiation monotherapy in patients with primary lesions in the oral cavity, oropharynx, hypopharynx, or larynx and postoperative risk factors for recurrence. The results of these studies were published in 2004.

The EORTC22931 study registered 334 patients with one or more risk factors for recurrence, namely microscopic resection margin positivity, extracapsular nodal extension positivity, stage III/IV disease, perineural infiltration, level 4 or level 5 lymph node metastasis (oropharyngeal and oral cavity cancer only), and signs of vascular embolism. Five-year PFS rate was 36 % in the radiation monotherapy group versus 47 % ($P=0.04$) in the CRT group and 5-year OS rate was 40 % versus 53 % ($P=0.02$), respectively, showing the superiority of CRT [5].

The RTOG95-01 study registered 416 patients with one or more postoperative risk factors for recurrence (microscopic resection margin positivity, extracapsular nodal extension positivity, or multiple cervical lymph node metastasis [≥2]). The 2-year local control rate (event: local relapse, cervical lymph node metastasis), the primary end point, was 72 % in the radiation monotherapy group versus 82 % ($P=0.003$) (Gray's test) in the CRT group, showing the superiority of CRT [6]. In addition, the 3-year disease-free survival (DFS) rate was 36 % versus 47 % ($P=0.04$), again showing the superiority of CRT. In contrast, the 3-year OS rate was 47 % versus 56 %, showing the superiority of radiation monotherapy, albeit without statistical significance ($P=0.19$). The results of the combined analysis were published in 2005 [7] and concluded that CRT with cisplatin (100 mg/m^2, every 3 weeks) greatly contributed to survival rate in radiation monotherapy, particularly in patients with the common high-risk relapse factors, namely microscopic resection margin positivity or extracapsular nodal extension positivity (HR = 0.702; see Fig. 12.1), whereas patients who only had the other risk factors for recurrence did not benefit from postoperative CRT (Table 12.1).

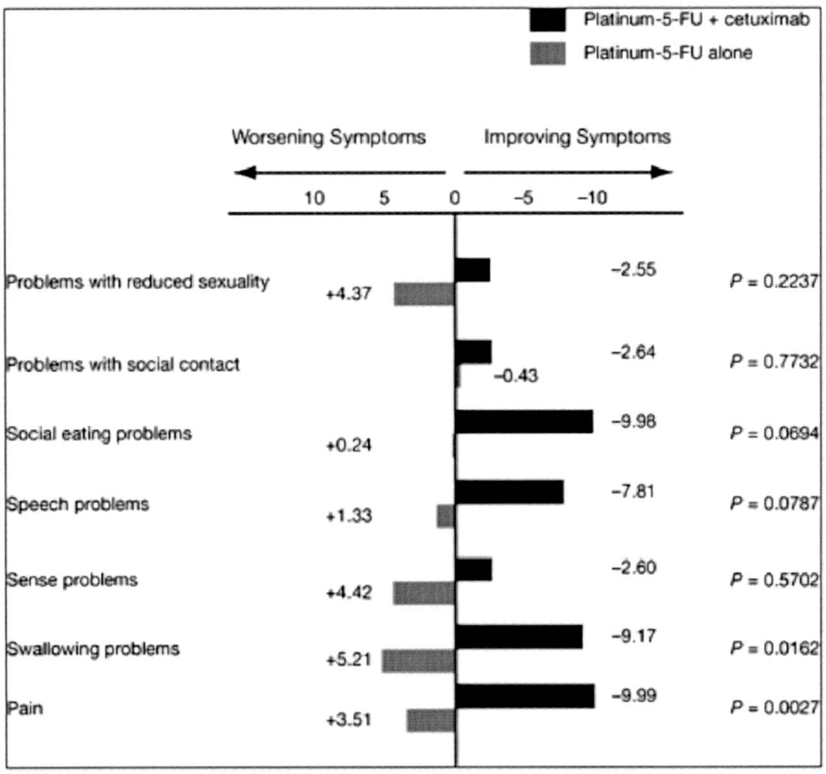

Fig. 12.1 EORTC QLQ-H&N 35 multi-item symptom scale score: mean change from baseline to worst post-baseline score [69]

Table 12.1 Percentage of risk reduction on overall survival for chemoradiotherapy compared with radiotherapy. (**a**) All patients in EORTC and RTOG trials; (**b**) subset analyses in patients eligible for both trials or one trial only

	Number	Risk reduction for CRT (%)	Probability
EORTC	334	30	0.04
ROG	416	16	0.19
Combined	750	28	<0.05
	Number	Risk reduction for CRT (%)	Probability
(Eligible for both studies)			
EORTC	233	33	Not described
RTOG	246	30	Not described
Combined	479	26	Not described
(Eligible for only one study)			
EORTC	101	25	0.06
RTOG	170	6	0.73

At the American Society of Clinical Oncology (ASCO) meeting of 2006, Fietkau et al. presented the results of the phase III part (ARO 96–3), which compared two postoperative adjuvant treatments, radiation monotherapy and 5-FU plus cisplatin CRT [8]. This study targeted 440 patients with postoperative risk factors for recurrence for head and neck squamous cell carcinoma (microscopic resection margin positivity, extracapsular nodal extension positivity, or multiple cervical lymph node metastasis [≥3]). Five-year DFS rate in the radiation monotherapy and CRT groups was 50 % versus 62 %, respectively ($P=0.023$), showing the statistically significant superiority of CRT, whereas 5-year OS rate was 49 % versus 58 %, respectively, showing no significant difference. These results failed to demonstrate the usefulness of postoperative 5-FU plus cisplatin CRT.

In 2008, Argiris et al. [9] reported the results of a phase III study of postoperative adjuvant treatment which compared radiation monotherapy and CRT using carboplatin in 72 patients with postoperative risk factors for recurrence (microscopic resection margin positivity, extracapsular nodal extension positivity, perineural infiltration, or signs of vascular infiltration) for SCCHN. In this study, the CRT group showed no superiority to the radiation monotherapy group in either 5-year DFS rate or 5-year OS rate, and thus the usefulness of postoperative CRT with carboplatin was not demonstrated.

Although no major meta-analysis of postoperative CRT has appeared, a meta-analysis of the above four phase III studies by Bachaud, Smid, Bernier, and Cooper and their colleagues demonstrated that CRT significantly contributes to survival compared with radiation monotherapy (relative risk, 0.80; 95 %CI, 0.71–0.90; $P=0.0002$) [10].

Based on the above results, CRT has been the standard postoperative adjuvant treatment for patients with postoperative high-risk relapse factors (microscopic resection margin positivity or extracapsular nodal extension positivity) for locally advanced SCCHN in Europe and the USA. Cisplatin 100 mg/m^2 every 3 weeks, as used in the EORTC22931 and RTOG95-01 studies, is believed to be the most commonly used standard regimen for concurrent monotherapy [5, 7, 10, 6].

12.3 Postoperative Adjuvant Chemotherapy

Although the role of postoperative adjuvant chemotherapy remains unclear, it is widely used in Japan. UFT was investigated in a randomized trial as adjuvant therapy after radical treatment of SCCHN in Japan [11]. Patients were randomly assigned to a UFT group or non-treatment group. The following three categories were included: (1) stages II–IV, receiving radical surgery ($n=424$); (2) stage II, receiving radical radiotherapy ($n=111$); and (3) nasopharyngeal cancer ($n=25$). In patients undergoing radical surgery, no significant difference was observed in 3-year overall survival (77.9 % for the UFT group vs. 72.9 % for the non-treatment group) or 3-year relapse-free survival (73.4 % vs. 66.2 %) between the two groups. In the patients receiving radical radiotherapy, furthermore, no significant difference was observed in either 3-year OS rate or 3-year relapse-free rate.

Recently, the results of a randomized phase III trial comparing S-1 with UFT as adjuvant chemotherapy after completion of definitive therapy for stages III–IVB SCCHN (ACTS-HC) were reported at the annual ASCO meeting of 2013 [12]. A total of 526 patients were enrolled and randomly assigned to UFT ($n=262$) or S-1 ($n=264$). Definitive therapy included surgery with or without adjuvant therapy, including radiotherapy or concurrent CRT ($n=149$ in the UFT group, $n=151$ in the S-1 group) and definitive radiotherapy or CRT with or without salvage surgery ($n=105$ in the UFT group, $n=100$ in the S-1 group). No significant difference was seen in DFS, the primary end point (3-year DFS: 60 % in the UFT group vs. 64.1 % in the S-1 group, HR 0.87; 95 % CI 0.66–1.16; $p=0.34$), whereas a significant difference was seen in OS (3-year OS: 75.8 % in the UFT group vs. 82.9 % in the S-1 group, HR 0.87; 95 %CI 0.44–0.94; $p=0.022$). Grade 3 or 4 toxicities were significantly more frequent in the S-1 group, including mucositis or stomatitis (2.4 % vs. 0 %), hyperpigmentation (3.6 % vs. 0 %), leukopenia (5.2 % vs. 0.8 %), neutropenia (3.6 % vs. 0 %), and thrombocytopenia (2.0 % vs. 0 %). Although S-1 was superior to UFT in terms of 3-year OS, this trial could not establish a role for adjuvant chemotherapy for a number of reasons: first, the choice of UFT as control arm was criticized because UFT did not demonstrate survival benefits compared with placebo in a previous study; second, the absence of a difference in DFS made it difficult to explain the improvement in OS; and third, subjects were not limited to patients with high-risk SCCHN, resulting in markedly prognoses in both groups than in previous trials of adjuvant therapy. In other words, there is concern that this study included patients who do not require adjuvant therapy.

12.4 Preoperative Concurrent Chemoradiotherapy

Combinations of surgery and radiotherapy with or without chemotherapy are used pre- or postoperatively [13], but there is no consensus regarding the sequence of surgery, radiotherapy, and/or chemotherapy for resectable advanced OSCC. The controversy about pre- or postoperative chemoradiotherapy continues for adjuvant therapy. However, in general, it is clear that radiotherapy and chemotherapy are more effective in unaffected and well-oxygenated tissue where the regional vasculature is intact, less hypoxic regions exist, and the drug delivery to the tumor may be better.

Preoperative concurrent chemoradiotherapy has been recently reported to be effective in advanced cases although the cases of postoperative radiotherapy or chemoradiotherapy outnumber those of preoperative concepts. These reports demonstrate that this approach is feasible with tolerable adverse events and that a high rate of completion of treatment regimen results in promising overall and disease-free survival rates [14–18]. Klug et al. [17] reviewed the survival data of 1,927 patients from 32 publications in the literature using a meta-analysis of preoperative CRT and radical surgery for advanced OSCC and SCC of the head and neck. They reanalyzed some reports and demonstrated that the mean 5-year survival rate was 62.6 % (58.4–66.8 %). This appears to be remarkably good when compared with the prospective randomized RTOG [6] and EORTC [5] studies with postoperative CRT (50 % and 53 %, respectively). Kirita et al. [19] also reported that the preoperative CRT followed by surgery for resectable advanced OSCC produced high clinical and histopathologic complete response and survival rates. In their study, the 5-year overall and progression-free survival rates were 87.1 % and 90.3 % for stage III patients and 70.0 % and 71.6 % for stage IV patients in all 154 patients. They also showed that the pathological CR in the primary tumors was seen in 89.1 % in the patients with CR (complete response) and in 73.1 % in the patients with good PR (partial response) and that 90.2 % of CR and 73.1 % of good PR patients have no residual tumor cells or viable tumor cells remained only within the central submucosa or shallow in the muscularis propria (central superficial portion). In the CR patients in the neck, pN+rate was 10.3 %, which was very low, and pathologically positive lymph nodes were only seen in levels IB (7.7 %) and IIA (7.7 %). In the PR and SD patients in the neck, pN+rate was 44.6 %, which was higher than that of the CR patients; pathologically positive lymph nodes were seen widely in several levels, especially in levels IB, IIA, and IIB.

Therefore, it is considered that even in advanced oral cancers, it could be possible to avoid extended resection and perform minimally invasive surgery in which the extent of resection on primary tumor and neck is reduced to preserve morphology and function in patients who achieve good response (CR and good PR in the primary tumor, CR in the neck) following preoperative CRT [19].

It is thought that the advantages of preoperative CRT followed by surgery for advanced but resectable OSCC patients are as follows. This treatment approach will produce better locoregional control rate and survival than postoperative CRT [20] and contribute to organ-function preservation with minimally invasive surgery, that is, less invasive surgery in the primary tumor and selective neck dissection for residual neck disease. Other advantages of this approach with a lower radiation dose would give better quality of life and reduce the critical complication of osteoradionecrosis. There is no evidence of a significantly higher rate of postoperative morbidity and more frequent occurrence of local complications such as wound infection, free flap failure, and prolonged duration of hospitalization from this treatment approach [15]. In case dental implants are used in OSCC patients for functional reconstruction, a lower radiation dose (<50 Gy) is reported to be significantly associated with improved implant survival compared with higher doses (>50 Gy), and no failures were observed with radiation doses <45 Gy [21].

12.5 Concurrent Chemoradiotherapy as Primary Treatment or Salvage Treatment

CRT for OSCC has been conducted either as primary treatment for patients who are unable to tolerate or who are unsuited for surgery or as salvage treatment in the persistent or recurrent disease setting.

A retrospective review of patients from four multi-institutional phase II studies with T4 OSCC aimed at evaluating long-term toxicity, locoregional control (LC), PFS, and OS of primary CRT [22] and identified 39 subjects, 16 (42 %) of whom had bony involvement. All regimens utilized concomitant 5-fluorouracil, hydroxyurea, and radiotherapy (FHX)-based regimens and added a third agent (cisplatin, paclitaxel continuous infusion, or paclitaxel 1-h infusion). Median radiotherapy dose delivered to the primary tumor was 74 Gy. Five-year OS, PFS, and LC rates were 56 %, 51 %, and 75 %, respectively. Sixty-nine percent of subjects with bony involvement never relapsed. Seven subjects developed osteoradionecrosis. Bone involvement with the primary tumor did not appear to be associated with an increased risk of death, relapse, or long-term complications. These data suggest that primary CRT is an effective treatment approach in patients with T4 OC tumors, including those with bone involvement. However, this study had several limitations, including its retrospective design and no control group for comparison; limited power of analysis due to a relatively small population; and specific subjects who were on a protocol with specific eligibility requirements. The results could not therefore be generalized into clinical practice, and further investigation is warranted.

In a meta-analysis of individual patient data from clinical trials comparing radiotherapy versus CRT (MACH-NC) in locally advanced head and neck cancers, OSCC accounted for 21 % of cases [23]. Result showed that CRT provided better survival than radiotherapy alone in OSCC (HR = 0.8). The results of his meta-analysis appear to suggest that concurrent chemotherapy may be a treatment option in patients unable to receive primary surgery.

Recently, numerous molecular targeted drugs have been investigated for cancer treatment, including head and neck cancer. Epidermal growth factor receptor (EGFR) has emerged as a promising target for cancer therapy. EGFR is a tyrosine kinase receptor of the ErbB family that is highly expressed and/or abnormally activated in many epithelial tumors, including SCCHN, colorectal cancer, and non-small-cell lung cancer [24–26]. EGFR ligand binding stimulates multiple cellular functions essential to tumor growth, including invasiveness, cell damage repair, and angiogenesis. EGFR expression in tumors is usually associated with more aggressive disease, increased resistance to chemotherapy and radiotherapy, increased metastasis, poor prognosis, and decreased survival [27, 28]. EGFR overexpression has been reported in more than 80 % of cases of SCCHN, and multivariate analyses have shown EGFR levels to be an independent predictor of a poor outcome in SCCHN [29].

Cetuximab, a chimeric monoclonal antibody that binds to the extracellular domain of EGFR [30], has shown both in vitro [31] and in vivo activity against SCCHN-derived cells and tumors [32]. Importantly, cetuximab has been shown to enhance the antitumor activity of radiotherapy [32, 33].

Bonner et al. conducted a multinational, randomized study to compare radiotherapy alone with radiotherapy plus cetuximab for locally advanced SCCHN, including in the larynx, hypopharynx, and oropharynx [34]. A total of 424 patients were randomly assigned to treatment with radiotherapy alone (213 patients) or radiotherapy plus weekly cetuximab (211 patients) at an initial dose of 400 mg/m^2, followed by 250 mg/m^2 weekly for the duration of radiotherapy. The addition of cetuximab to radiotherapy demonstrated a significant improvement in locoregional control (24.4 months in the cetuximab group vs. 14.9 months in the radiotherapy alone group, HR for locoregional progression or death, 0.68; $P = 0.005$), progression-free survival (17.1 months vs. 12.4 months, HR for disease progression or death, 0.70; $P = 0.006$), and overall survival (49.0 months vs. 29.3 months, HR for death, 0.74; $P = 0.03$). Based on this result, cetuximab plus radiotherapy is superior to radiotherapy alone in increasing both the duration of locoregional disease control and survival in locoregionally advanced SCCHN. None of the subjects in this trial had OSCC, and the role of cetuximab in combination with radiotherapy for OSCC therefore remains unclear.

12.6 Neoadjuvant Chemotherapy

The role of neoadjuvant chemotherapy prior to surgery remains controversial. In a randomized study of neoadjuvant chemotherapy with cisplatin and fluorouracil (PF) followed by surgery compared with surgery in OSCC [35], 195 patients with resectable, stage T2–T4 (>3 cm), N0–N2, M0 untreated, squamous cell carcinoma of the oral cavity were randomly assigned to three cycles of PF followed by surgery (chemotherapy arm) or surgery alone (control arm). In both arms, postoperative radiotherapy was reserved for high-risk patients. Postoperative radiotherapy was administered to 33 % of patients in the chemotherapy arm versus 46 % in the control arm. Mandible resection was performed in 52 % of patients in the control arm versus 31 % in the chemotherapy arm. In the chemotherapy arm, three toxic deaths were recorded. Five-year OS was 55 % for both arms, indicating that the addition of neoadjuvant chemotherapy with PF to standard surgery was unable to improve survival.

However, primary chemotherapy appeared to play a role in reducing the number of patients in this study who required mandibulectomy, radiation therapy, or both. Variations in the criteria used to select patients for these treatment options may hamper generalization of these results, but there appears to be room to use preoperative chemotherapy to spare destructive surgery or radiation therapy in patients with advanced, resectable oral cavity cancer.

Novel induction chemotherapy regimens which add docetaxel to PF (TPF) have shown promising results in two recent phase III trials (TAX323 and TAX324) in the setting of nonsurgical treatment of locally advanced SCCHN [26, 37, 38]. In both studies, patients were randomly assigned to receive PF versus TPF before radiotherapy (TAX323) or CRT (TAX324). Results showed a statistically significant improvement in OS in patients randomly assigned to the TPF arm, and TPF is accordingly suggested as the preferred combination chemotherapy regimen when induction treatment is used for nonsurgical management of patients with SCCHN. However, the potential benefits of TPF induction have recently been questioned: the DeCIDE and PARADIGM trials compared up-front chemoradiotherapy with TPF induction followed by CRT and failed to demonstrate a significant improvement in OS or disease-free survival (DFS) with TPF [39, 40]

Further, a recent randomized trial of neoadjuvant chemotherapy with TPF versus up-front surgery in patients with OSCC also failed to demonstrate a significant improvement in OS or DFS with TPF [41]. In this study, 256 patients with stage III or IVA locally advanced resectable OSCC were randomly assigned to two cycles of TPF followed by surgery and postoperative RT (54–66 Gy) or up-front surgery and postoperative RT. TPF consisted of two cycles of docetaxel 75 mg/m^2 on day 1, cisplatin 75 mg/m^2 on day 1, and 5-FU 750 mg/m^2 on days 1–5, repeated every 3 weeks. The clinical response rate to TPF was 80.6 %. TPF did not increase perioperative morbidity. After a median follow-up of 30 months, however, no significant difference was seen in either OS (HR 0.977; 95 % CI, 0.634–1.507; $p=0.918$) or DFS (HR 0.974; 95 % CI, 0.654–1.45; $p=0.897$).

Together, these findings suggest that neoadjuvant chemotherapy should not be recommended for clinical use in locally advanced OSCC.

12.7 Palliative Chemotherapy for Recurrent and/or Metastatic Setting

Despite aggressive surgery with or without adjuvant therapy, or multidisciplinary approaches, approximately 50 % of patients will develop incurable locoregional or distant recurrence. In this setting, chemotherapy is one treatment option. Because the prognosis of patients with recurrent and/or metastatic head and neck cancer is generally poor, the therapeutic goal is to extend survival without worsening quality of life.

The most common chemotherapy drugs used for advanced SCCHN include taxanes (paclitaxel and docetaxel), anthracyclines (adriamycin, epirubicin, and pirarubicin), platinums (cisplatin and carboplatin), and antimetabolites (e.g., methotrexate and 5-fluorouracil). However, no prospective clinical trial of chemotherapy drugs for recurrent or metastatic OSCC patients only has been conducted. Approximately 20–30 % of patients with recurrent or metastatic SCCHN who have enrolled in clinical trials to date had OSCC.

Cisplatin remains one of the most widely used standard agents in the recurrent and/or metastatic setting, with an average single-agent response rate of 28 %. Most single-agent studies have employed doses of 80–120 mg/m^2 administered as an intravenous bolus every 3–4 weeks. A small randomized trial compared cisplatin given as a single bolus of 120 mg/m^2 with 20 mg/m^2/day for 5 days, repeated every 3 weeks. In this study, antitumor activity was comparable between the two arms. Veronesi et al. [42] conducted a small randomized trial comparing 120 mg/m^2 versus 60 mg/m^2 of cisplatin administered as a bolus. Of 62 eligible patients, 59 were evaluable, with response rates in patients receiving high- and low-dose cisplatin of 16.1 % and 17.8 %, respectively. Median OS was 34 weeks, and survival in the two treatment arms was superimposable. These studies provided no evidence of dose dependency of cisplatin activity in advanced SCCHN.

Morton et al. [43] conducted a small randomized trial of cisplatin and bleomycin using a 2×2 factorial design for patients with recurrent or metastatic SCCHN. Of 116 enrolled patients, 30 % proved to be unfit for chemotherapy. Cisplatin significantly prolonged median survival by 10 weeks. This trial led to the widespread use of cisplatin alone.

Carboplatin is a second-generation platinum analog with a similar spectrum of activity against a number of solid tumors as cisplatin. Phase II studies of single-agent carboplatin have demonstrated a response rate of 20–26 % [44–47]. Although carboplatin is often considered to be less effective than cisplatin in SCCHN, little direct comparison has been done. In a Southwest Oncology Group (SWOG) study, 277 patients were randomly assigned to receive either cisplatin plus 5-FU, carboplatin plus 5-FU, or single-agent methotrexate [48]. Although no formal statistical comparison of cisplatin and carboplatin was performed, response rate was higher in the cisplatin arm than the carboplatin arm (32 % vs. 21 %), while median survival in these two arms was similar. Carboplatin may be preferred in some patients since it is associated with less neurotoxicity, nephrotoxicity, and nausea and vomiting than cisplatin, although it does cause more myelosuppression.

Docetaxel is a semisynthetic taxane analog that also possesses significant activity in SCCHN. Several single-agent phase II studies in chemotherapy-naïve patients with recurrent or metastatic SCCHN yielded response rate of 21–42 % [49–52]. Guardiola et al. [53] reported the results of a randomized phase II study which compared docetaxel with methotrexate in patients with recurrent SCCHN. Response rate was significantly higher in the docetaxel arm, with an objective response rate of 27 % vs. 15 % in the methotrexate arm. In contrast, no significant differences were seen between the arms in either OS or time to progression. Inuyama at al. employed a lower dose of docetaxel (60 mg/m^2, every 3–4 weeks). Response rate was 22 % in 59 evaluable patients and 17.4 % in 46 patients who received prior chemotherapy.

Paclitaxel is a diterpene plant-derived product that exerts cytotoxic effects by promoting microtubule assembly, ultimately leading to the disruption of mitosis and cell death. Single-agent activity for recurrent or metastatic SCCHN in phase II trials demonstrated an encouraging response rate range of 20–40 %. Previous studies of high-dose tri-weekly paclitaxel (200–250 mg/m^2) in patients with advanced or recurrent/metastatic SCCHN demonstrated an overall response of 35–40 %, which was associated with severe neuropathy and myelosuppression [54, 55]. A prospective phase II study of weekly paclitaxel for recurrent or metastatic head and neck cancer that paclitaxel showed acceptable toxicity but a poor response rate of 9.3 % (4/43) [56]. Japanese phase II trials, including an early and late phase II trial of weekly paclitaxel in patients with recurrent or metastatic head and neck cancer [57], enrolled a total of 74 patients. Overall

Table 12.2 Randomized trials of chemotherapy for recurrence or metastatic SCCHN

Author	Treatment	Number of patients	Response rate (%)	MST (months)
Morton et al. [43]	CDDP + bleomycin	116	13	4
	Bleomycin		14	2.8
	CDDP		24	4.2[a]
	No therapy		0	2.1
Forastiere et al. [48]	CDDP + 5-FU	87	32	6.6
	CBDCA + 5-FU	86	21	5.0
	MTX	88	10	5.6
Jacobs et al. [58]	CDDP + 5-FU	79	32[a]	5.5
	CDDP	83	17	5.0
	5-FU	83	13	6.1
Gibson et al. [84]	CDDP + 5-FU	104	41.4	8.7
	CDDP + paclitaxel	100	32.4	8.1

[a]Statistically significant difference

response rate was 29.0 % according to RECIST. The median duration of response, median time to progression, and median survival time were 7.4 months, 3.4 months, and 14.3 months, respectively. Together, these findings suggested that weekly paclitaxel has promising activity with acceptable toxicity in recurrent or metastatic head and neck cancer.

Numerous trials have compared various combinations of cytotoxic agents in patients with recurrent or metastatic SCCHN. One of the most widely used regimens is the combination of cisplatin plus 5-FU, with a response rate of approximately 30 % in this setting. Several phase III trials demonstrated a higher response rate but no significant prolongation of survival compared with single agents, including cisplatin and methotrexate [48, 58] (Table 12.2). The combination of cisplatin plus 5-FU has higher toxicity than the single agents alone, particularly in patients with a poor performance status or serious comorbidity, and any use of combination chemotherapy requires careful selection of both agents and patients.

Over the past decade, the combination of platinum plus a taxane analog, including paclitaxel and docetaxel, has demonstrated significant activity in recurrent or metastatic SCCHN. Several phase II trials of cisplatin plus paclitaxel yielded a response rate of 32–48 %. A randomized phase III trial of cisplatin plus 5-FU versus cisplatin plus paclitaxel, conducted as an intergroup trial of the ECOG and SWOG, reported no significant difference in response rate, survival, or quality of life measures (Table 12.2). Nevertheless, there is concern that the addition of paclitaxel to cisplatin increases the incidence and severity of neuropathy and combination treatment with carboplatin plus paclitaxel is now widely used.

Combination treatment with docetaxel plus cisplatin has also been investigated. Phase II studies in recurrent or metastatic SCCHN yielded response rates of 33–50 % with acceptable toxicity. These finding support the use of platinum plus taxane as a reasonable treatment option.

Molecular targeted drugs have been also investigated for recurrent or metastatic SCCHN. Cetuximab has been shown to enhance the antitumor activity of cisplatin [59] without any effect on its pharmacokinetic profile [60]. One of the most interesting aspects of cetuximab is that it appears to reverse tumor resistance to chemotherapy, such that the tumor again responds to therapy under which it previously progressed. This effect was initially noted in nonclinical studies with cetuximab plus irinotecan in irinotecan-refractory colorectal xenografts [61] and was subsequently confirmed in the clinical setting [62], leading many countries to approve the use of cetuximab in combination with irinotecan in patients with EGFR-expressing metastatic colorectal cancer that progressed on irinotecan-containing therapy

A phase IB study in patients with SCCHN demonstrated that the combination of cetuximab and cisplatin was active, even in a subset of patients who had been previously treated with cisplatin and had documented cisplatin resistance [63]. In patients with platinum-refractory recurrent and metastatic SCCHN, a combination of cetuximab plus cisplatin or carboplatin demonstrated response rates of 6–20 % in two phase II studies [64, 65], whereas single-agent cetuximab produced a major objective response rate of 13 % in a phase II study [66] (Table 12.3). These findings indicate that there is no clear evidence that cetuximab reverses platinum resistance in SCCHN.

The Eastern Cooperative Oncology Group completed a randomized placebo-controlled trial using cisplatin with or without cetuximab in recurrent or metastatic SCCHN as first-line therapy [67]. The addition of cetuximab to cisplatin resulted in significantly higher response rates in the cisplatin/cetuximab arm (26 %) than in the cisplatin-alone arm (10 %) ($P = 0.029$). Nevertheless, the two cohorts did not differ with respect to the primary end point of progression-free survival (4.1 vs. 3.4 months, $P = 0.27$) or secondary end point of overall survival (9.2 vs. 8 months, $P = 0.18$) (Table 12.3).

Table 12.3 Clinical trials of cetuximab for recurrent or metastatic SCCHN

Author	Phase	Subject	Therapy	*N*	RR	Median PFS (months)	Median OS (months)
Baselga et al. [64]	II	Platinum refractory	CDDP or CBDCA + CEX	98	10 %	[TTP 85 days]	183 days
Herbst et al. [65]	II	Platinum refractory	CDDP + CEX	25(PD/1)	20 %	3.0	6.1
				54(PD/2)	6 %	2.0	4.3
				51(SD)	18 %	4.9	11.7
Burtness et al. [67]	III	First line	CDDP + CEX	58	26 %	4.2	9.1
			CDDP + placebo	58	10 %	3.1	8.0
					$p=0.03$	$p=0.09$	$p=0.21$
Vermorken et al. [71]	III	First line	FP + CEX	222	35.6 %		10.1
			FP	220	19.5 %		7.4
					$p=0.0001$		$P=0.0362$

RR response rate = complete response + partial response, *PXL* paclitaxel, *CBDCA* carboplatin, *CEX* cetuximab, *PD/1* patients with documented progressive disease after chemotherapy administered according to the protocol (FP or PXL + CDDP), *PD/2* patients with documented disease recurrence and tumor progression within 3 months of platinum-based therapy, *SD* patients with stable disease after chemotherapy administered according to the protocol (FP or PXL + CDDP)

The EXTREME trial was a randomized phase III trial of platinum-based chemotherapy with or without cetuximab as first-line therapy for recurrent or metastatic SCCHN [68]. Four hundred and forty-two eligible patients were randomly assigned at a 1:1 ratio to receive cisplatin (100 mg/m^2 on day 1) or carboplatin (AUC 5 [check] on day 1) plus fluorouracil (1000 mg/m^2/day for 4 days) every 3 weeks for a maximum of six cycles, either alone (chemotherapy-alone group) or in combination with cetuximab (400 mg/m^2 initially, then 250 mg/m^2 per week) for a maximum of six cycles. Patients with stable disease who received chemotherapy plus cetuximab continued to receive cetuximab until disease progression or unacceptable toxic effects, whichever occurred first. The addition of cetuximab to platinum-based chemotherapy significantly prolonged median overall survival, from 7.4 months to 10.1 months (HR for death, 0.80; 95 % confidence interval, 0.64–0.99; $P=0.04$), and also prolonged median PFS from 3.3 months to 5.6 months (HR for progression, 0.54; $P<0.001$) and increased the response rate from 20 % to 36 % ($P<0.001$). The most common grade 3 or 4 adverse events in the chemotherapy-alone and cetuximab groups were anemia (19 % and 13 %, respectively), neutropenia (23 % and 22 %), and thrombocytopenia (11 % in both groups). For the most part, there was no significant difference in the overall incidence of grade 3 or 4 adverse events between the groups. Furthermore, QoL Questionnaire-Core 30 (QLQ-C30) demonstrated a significant improvement in global health status/QoL score in the cetuximab arm ($P=0.0415$) but no treatment differences in the social functioning scale [69]. For QLQ-Head and Neck 35 (QLQ-H&N35), the mean score in the cetuximab arm was not significantly worse than that in the chemotherapy arm for all symptom scales at all post-baseline visits. At cycle 3, some symptom scores significantly favored the cetuximab arm (pain, swallowing, speech problems, and social eating) (Fig 12.1). In other words, the addition of cetuximab to platinum–fluorouracil does not adversely affect the QoL of patients with recurrent or metastatic SCCHN, and platinum-based chemotherapy plus cetuximab is now considered to be a standard of care as first-line therapy for patients with recurrent or metastatic SCCHN.

Panitumumab is a fully human anti-EGFR monoclonal antibody that is used both as a single agent and in combination with chemotherapy for the treatment of metastatic colorectal cancer [70]. The SPECTRUM trial was a global phase 3 trial conducted at 126 sites in 26 countries to compare panitumumab plus cisplatin and 5-FU with chemotherapy alone as first-line treatment for recurrent or metastatic SCCHN [71]. Six hundred and fifty-seven patients were randomly assigned in a 1:1 ratio to chemotherapy plus panitumumab or chemotherapy alone. The addition of panitumumab to chemotherapy demonstrated a significant improvement in PFS (5.8 vs. 4.6 months; HR 0.780, 95 % CI 0.659–0.922; $p=0.0036$) but no statistically significant improvement in OS (11.1 vs. 9.0 months; HR 0.873; $p=0.1403$).

Zalutumumab is another monoclonal antibody targeting the EGFR. In a randomized phase III trial, 286 patients who had progressed on platinum-based chemotherapy were randomly assigned in a 2:1 ratio to zalutumumab or best supportive care [72]. PFS was longer in the zalutumumab group than in the control group (HR for progression or death, stratified by WHO performance status, was 0.63, 95 % CI 0.47–0.84; $p=0.0012$), while there was no statistically significant improvement in OS, the primary end point (6.7 vs. 5.2 months, hazard ratio 0.77, 95 % CI 0.57–1.05).

Several small molecule tyrosine kinase inhibitors targeting EGFR have been investigated, including gefitinib, erlotinib, lapatinib, and afatinib, but only afatinib has demonstrated clinically significant activity [73–76].

Afatinib is an oral ErbB family blocker that completely and irreversibly blocks signaling by all relevant ErbB family members, including EGFR, human epidermal growth factor receptor-2 (ErbB2), and ErbB4 and also blocks transphosphorylation of ErbB3 [77, 78]. The LUX-Lung 3 study, a prospective randomized trial in EGFR mutation-positive NSCLC patients, met its primary end point of PFS, with a median PFS of 11.1 months in afatinib-treated patients versus 6.9 months in chemotherapy-treated patients [79].

In SCCHN, afatinib has demonstrated preclinical activity in both in vitro and in vivo models [80, 81]. A randomized phase II study comparing afatinib with cetuximab in recurrent or metastatic SCCHN patients following failure of platinum-based chemotherapy showed that afatinib had clinical activity (response in stage I: 16.1 % in the afatinib arm and 6.5 % in cetuximab arm by investigator review, 8.1 % and 9.7 % by independent central review). Furthermore, in stage 2 of the study [82], after crossover to the opposite treatment arm, afatinib demonstrated a better disease control rate (33 % in patients who received cetuximab in stage I vs. 19 % in cetuximab-treated patients after crossover from afatinib) and median PFS (9.3 vs. 5.7 weeks), suggesting sequential therapy with afatinib may be beneficial in patients pretreated with an EGFR-targeted therapy. Afatinib is currently being evaluated in both a phase 3 trial comparing methotrexate in patients with recurrent or metastatic SCCHN who were pretreated with platinum-based chemotherapy and a phase 3 trial comparing placebo as adjuvant therapy after completion of definitive chemoradiotherapy in patients with locally advanced SCCHN.

Many novel molecular targets have been explored for head and neck cancer, including the phosphatidylinositol 3 kinase (PI3K), NOTCH, ALK1, and Hedgehog pathways [83]. Developing strategies to determine the optimal way to combine these novel agents with EGFR inhibitors or traditional cytotoxic drugs is an important new challenge for clinical and translational researchers.

References

1. Bessell A, Glenny AM, Furness S, Clarkson JE, Oliver R, Conway DI, Macluskey M, Pavitt S, Sloan P, Worthington HV (2011) Interventions for the treatment of oral and oropharyngeal cancers: surgical treatment. Cochrane Database Syst Rev (9):CD006205. 10.1002/14651858.CD006205.pub3
2. Bachaud JM, Cohen-Jonathan E, Alzieu C, David JM, Serrano E, Daly-Schveitzer N (1996) Combined postoperative radiotherapy and weekly cisplatin infusion for locally advanced head and neck carcinoma: final report of a randomized trial. Int J Radiat Oncol Biol Phys 36(5):999–1004
3. Smid L, Budihna M, Zakotonik B (2003) Postoperative concomitant irradiation and chemotherapy with mitomycin and bleomycin for advanced head and neck carcinoma. Int J Radiat Oncol Biol Phys 56:1055–1062
4. Al-Sarraf M, Thomas F, Roger W (1997) Postoperative radiotherapy with concurrent cisplatin appears to improve locoregional control of advanced respectable head and neck cancers: RTOG 88–24. Int J Radiat Oncol Biol Phys 37:777–782
5. Bernier J, Domenge C, Ozsahin M, Matuszewska K, Lefebvre JL, Greiner RH, Giralt J, Maingon P, Rolland F, Bolla M, Cognetti F, Bourhis J, Kirkpatrick A, van Glabbeke M (2004) Postoperative irradiation with or without concomitant chemotherapy for locally advanced head and neck cancer. N Engl J Med 350(19):1945–1952. doi:10.1056/NEJMoa032641
6. Cooper JS, Pajak TF, Forastiere AA, Jacobs J, Campbell BH, Saxman SB, Kish JA, Kim HE, Cmelak AJ, Rotman M, Machtay M, Ensley JF, Chao KS, Schultz CJ, Lee N, Fu KK (2004) Postoperative concurrent radiotherapy and chemotherapy for high-risk squamous-cell carcinoma of the head and neck. N Engl J Med 350(19):1937–1944. doi:10.1056/NEJMoa032646
7. Bernier J, Cooper JS, Pajak TF, van Glabbeke M, Bourhis J, Forastiere A, Ozsahin EM, Jacobs JR, Jassem J, Ang KK, Lefebvre JL (2005) Defining risk levels in locally advanced head and neck cancers: a comparative analysis of concurrent postoperative radiation plus chemotherapy trials of the EORTC (#22931) and RTOG (# 9501). Head Neck 27(10):843–850. doi:10.1002/hed.20279
8. Fietkau R, Lautenschlager C, Sauer R, Dunst J, Becker A, Baumann M (2006) Postoperative concurrent radiochemotherapy versus radiotherapy in high-risk SCCA of the head and neck: result of the German phase III trial ARO 96–3. Proc Am Soc Clin Oncol 24:5507 (abstr 5507)
9. Argiris A, Karamouzis MV, Johnson JT, Heron DE, Myers E, Eibling D, Cano E, Urba S, Gluckman J, Grandis JR, Wang Y, Agarwala SS (2008) Long-term results of a phase III randomized trial of postoperative radiotherapy with or without carboplatin in patients with high-risk head and neck cancer. Laryngoscope 118: 444–449
10. Winquist E, Oliver T, Gilbert R (2007) Postoperative chemoradiotherapy for advanced squamous cell carcinoma of the head and neck: a systematic review with meta-analysis. Head Neck 29(1):38–46. doi:10.1002/hed.20465
11. Tsukuda M, Ogasawara H, Kaneko S, Komiyama S, Horiuchi M, Inuyama Y (1994) A prospective randomized trial of adjuvant chemotherapy with UFT for head and neck carcinoma. Head and neck UFT study group. Gan To Kagaku Ryoho (Cancer Chemother) 21(8):1169–1177
12. Taguchi T, Kubota A, Yoshino K, Tomita K, Kohno N, Kawabata K, Fukushima M, Tsukahara K, Takemura H, Hasegawa Y, Terada T, Nagahara K, Nakatani H, Higaki Y, Iwae S, Beppu T, Hanamure Y, Teramukai S, Fujii M (2013) Adjuvant chemotherapy with S-1 after curative treatment in patients with head and neck cancer (ACTS-HNC). J Clin Oncol 31:suppl(abstr 6004)
13. Lung T, Tăşcău OC, Almăşan HA, Mureşan O (2007) Head and neck cancer, treatment, evolution and post therapeutic survival part 2: a decade's results 1993–2002. J Craniomaxillofac Surg 35: 126–131
14. Freier K, Engel M, Lindel K, Flechtenmacher C, Mühling J, Hassfeld S, Hofele C (2008) Neoadjuvant concurrent radiochemotherapy followed by surgery in advanced oral squamous cell carcinoma (OSCC): a retrospective analysis of 207 patients. Oral Oncol 44:116–123
15. Kirita T, Ohgi K, Shimooka H, Yamanaka Y, Tatebayashi S, Yamamoto K, Mishima K, Sugimura M (1999) Preoperative concurrent chemoradiotherapy plus radical surgery for advanced squamous cell carcinoma of the oral cavity: an analysis of long-term results. Oral Oncol 35:597–606
16. Kirita T, Shimooka H, Yamanaka Y, Tatebayashi S, Yamamoto K, Nishimine M, Sugimura M (2001) Prognostic value of response to preoperative chemoradiotherapy and residual tumor grades in

tongue carcinoma. Oral Surg Oral Med Oral Pathol Oral Radiol Endod 91:293–300

17. Klug C, Berzaczy D, Voracek M, Millesi W (2008) Preoperative chemoradiotherapy in the management of oral cancer: a review. J Craniomaxillofac Surg 36:75–88. doi:10.1016/j.jcms.2007.06.007
18. Mohr C, Bohndorf W, Carstens J, Härle F, Hausamen JE, Hirche H, Kimmig H, Kutzner J, Mühling J, Reuther J et al (1994) Preoperative radiochemotherapy and radical surgery in comparison with radical surgery alone. A prospective, multicentric, randomized DOSAK study of advanced squamous cell carcinoma of the oral cavity and the oropharynx (a 3-year follow-up). Int J Oral Maxillofac Surg 23:140–148
19. Kirita T, Yamanaka Y, Imai Y, Yamakawa N, Aoki K, Nakagawa Y, Yagyuu T, Hasegawa M (2012) Preoperative concurrent chemoradiotherapy for stages II-IV oral squamous cell carcinoma: a retrospective analysis and the future possibility of this treatment strategy. Int J Oral Maxillofac Surg 41:421–428. doi:10.1016/j.ijom.2011.12.003
20. Kessler P, Grabenbauer G, Leher A, Schultze-Mosgau S, Rupprecht S, Neukam FW (2004) Patients with oral squamous cell carcinoma. Long-term survival and evaluation of quality of life-initial results obtained with two treatment protocols in a prospective study. Mund Kiefer Gesichtschir 8:302–310
21. Colella G, Cannavale R, Pentenero M, Gandolfo S (2007) Oral implants in radiated patients: a systematic review. Int J Oral Maxillofac Implants 22:616–622
22. Cohen EE, Baru J, Huo D, Haraf DJ, Crowley M, Witt ME, Blair EA, Weichselbaum RR, Rosen F, Vokes EE, Stenson K (2009) Efficacy and safety of treating T4 oral cavity tumors with primary chemoradiotherapy. Head Neck 31(8):1013–1021. doi:10.1002/hed.21062
23. Pignon JP, le Maitre A, Maillard E, Bourhis J (2009) Meta-analysis of chemotherapy in head and neck cancer (MACH-NC): an update on 93 randomised trials and 17,346 patients. Radiother Oncol 92(1):4–14. doi:10.1016/j.radonc.2009.04.014
24. Mendelsohn J, Baselga J (2003) Status of epidermal growth factor receptor antagonists in the biology and treatment of cancer. J Clin Oncol 21(14):2787–2799. doi:10.1200/JCO.2003.01.504
25. Salomon DS, Brandt R, Ciardiello F, Normanno N (1995) Epidermal growth factor-related peptides and their receptors in human malignancies. Crit Rev Oncol Hematol 19(3):183–232
26. Rubin Grandis J, Melhem MF, Barnes EL, Tweardy DJ (1996) Quantitative immunohistochemical analysis of transforming growth factor-alpha and epidermal growth factor receptor in patients with squamous cell carcinoma of the head and neck. Cancer 78(6):1284–1292. doi:10.1002/(SICI)1097-0142(19960915)78:6<1284::AID-CNCR17>3.0.CO;2-X
27. Ang KK, Berkey BA, Tu X, Zhang HZ, Katz R, Hammond EH, Fu KK, Milas L (2002) Impact of epidermal growth factor receptor expression on survival and pattern of relapse in patients with advanced head and neck carcinoma. Cancer Res 62(24):7350–7356
28. Nicholson RI, Gee JM, Harper ME (2001) EGFR and cancer prognosis. Eur J Cancer 37(Suppl 4):S9–S15
29. Rubin Grandis J, Melhem MF, Gooding WE, Day R, Holst VA, Wagener MM, Drenning SD, Tweardy DJ (1998) Levels of TGF-alpha and EGFR protein in head and neck squamous cell carcinoma and patient survival. J Natl Cancer Inst 90(11):824–832
30. Goldstein NI, Prewett M, Zuklys K, Rockwell P, Mendelsohn J (1995) Biological efficacy of a chimeric antibody to the epidermal growth factor receptor in a human tumor xenograft model. Clin Cancer Res 1(11):1311–1318
31. Huang SM, Bock JM, Harari PM (1999) Epidermal growth factor receptor blockade with C225 modulates proliferation, apoptosis, and radiosensitivity in squamous cell carcinomas of the head and neck. Cancer Res 59(8):1935–1940
32. Harari PM, Huang SM (2001) Head and neck cancer as a clinical model for molecular targeting of therapy: combining EGFR blockade with radiation. Int J Radiat Oncol Biol Phys 49(2):427–433
33. Milas L, Mason K, Hunter N, Petersen S, Yamakawa M, Ang K, Mendelsohn J, Fan Z (2000) In vivo enhancement of tumor radioresponse by C225 antiepidermal growth factor receptor antibody. Clin Cancer Res 6(2):701–708
34. Bonner JA, Harari PM, Giralt J, Azarnia N, Shin DM, Cohen RB, Jones CU, Sur R, Raben D, Jassem J, Ove R, Kies MS, Baselga J, Youssoufian H, Amellal N, Rowinsky EK, Ang KK (2006) Radiotherapy plus cetuximab for squamous-cell carcinoma of the head and neck. N Engl J Med 354(6):567–578, 354/6/567 [pii] 10.1056/NEJMoa053422
35. Licitra L, Grandi C, Guzzo M, Mariani L, Lo Vullo S, Valvo F, Quattrone P, Valagussa P, Bonadonna G, Molinari R, Cantu G (2003) Primary chemotherapy in resectable oral cavity squamous cell cancer: a randomized controlled trial. J Clin Oncol 21(2):327–333
36. Vermorken JB, Remenar E, van Herpen C, Gorlia T, Mesia R, Degardin M, Stewart JS, Jelic S, Betka J, Preiss JH, van den Weyngaert D, Awada A, Cupissol D, Kienzer HR, Rey A, Desaunois I, Bernier J, Lefebvre JL (2007) Cisplatin, fluorouracil, and docetaxel in unresectable head and neck cancer. N Engl J Med 357(17):1695–1704
37. Posner MR, Hershock DM, Blajman CR, Mickiewicz E, Winquist E, Gorbounova V, Tjulandin S, Shin DM, Cullen K, Ervin TJ, Murphy BA, Raez LE, Cohen RB, Spaulding M, Tishler RB, Roth B, Viroglio Rdel C, Venkatesan V, Romanov I, Agarwala S, Harter KW, Dugan M, Cmelak A, Markoe AM, Read PW, Steinbrenner L, Colevas AD, Norris CM Jr, Haddad RI (2007) Cisplatin and fluorouracil alone or with docetaxel in head and neck cancer. N Engl J Med 357(17):1705–1715
38. Lorch JH, Goloubeva O, Haddad RI, Cullen K, Sarlis N, Tishler R, Tan M, Fasciano J, Sammartino DE, Posner MR (2011) Induction chemotherapy with cisplatin and fluorouracil alone or in combination with docetaxel in locally advanced squamous-cell cancer of the head and neck: long-term results of the TAX 324 randomised phase 3 trial. Lancet Oncol 12(2):153–159. doi:10.1016/S1470-2045(10)70279-5
39. Cohen E, Karrison T, Kocherginsky M (2012) DeCIDE: a phase III randomized trial of docetaxel (D), cisplatin (P), 5-fluorouracil (F) (TPF) induction chemotherapy (IC) in patients with N2/N3 locally advanced squamous cell carcinoma of the head and neck (SCCHN). J Clin Oncol 30(Suppl 15):356s (abstr 5500)
40. Haddad R, O'Neill A, Rabinowits G, Tishler R, Khuri F, Adkins D, Clark J, Sarlis N, Lorch J, Beitler JJ, Limaye S, Riley S, Posner M (2013) Induction chemotherapy followed by concurrent chemoradiotherapy (sequential chemoradiotherapy) versus concurrent chemoradiotherapy alone in locally advanced head and neck cancer (PARADIGM): a randomised phase 3 trial. Lancet Oncol 14(3):257–264. doi:10.1016/S1470-2045(13)70011-1
41. Zhong LP, Zhang CP, Ren GX, Guo W, William WN Jr, Sun J, Zhu HG, Tu WY, Li J, Cai YL, Wang LZ, Fan XD, Wang ZH, Hu YJ, Ji T, Yang WJ, Ye WM, Li J, He Y, Wang YA, Xu LQ, Wang BS, Kies MS, Lee JJ, Myers JN, Zhang ZY (2013) Randomized phase III trial of induction chemotherapy with docetaxel, cisplatin, and fluorouracil followed by surgery versus up-front surgery in locally advanced resectable oral squamous cell carcinoma. J Clin Oncol 31(6):744–751. doi:10.1200/JCO.2012.43.8820
42. Veronesi A, Zagonel V, Tirelli U, Galligioni E, Tumolo S, Barzan L, Lorenzini M, Comoretto R, Grigoletto E (1985) High-dose versus low-dose cisplatin in advanced head and neck squamous carcinoma: a randomized study. J Clin Oncol 3(8):1105–1108
43. Morton RP, Rugman F, Dorman EB, Stoney PJ, Wilson JA, McCormick M, Veevers A, Stell PM (1985) Cisplatinum and bleomycin for advanced or recurrent squamous cell carcinoma of the

head and neck: a randomised factorial phase III controlled trial. Cancer Chemother Pharmacol 15(3):283–289
44. Eisenberger M, Hornedo J, Silva H, Donehower R, Spaulding M, Van Echo D (1986) Carboplatin (NSC-241-240): an active platinum analog for the treatment of squamous-cell carcinoma of the head and neck. J Clin Oncol 4(10):1506–1509
45. de Andres BL, Lopez Pousa A, Alba E, Sampedro F (1986) Carboplatin, an active drug in advanced head and neck cancer. Cancer Treat Rep 70(10):1173–1176
46. Al-Sarraf M, Metch B, Kish J, Ensley J, Rinehart JJ, Schuller DE, Coltman CA Jr (1987) Platinum analogs in recurrent and advanced head and neck cancer: a Southwest oncology group and Wayne state university study. Cancer Treat Rep 71(7–8):723–726
47. Inuyama Y, Togawa K, Morita M, Takeoda S, Kaneko T, Takemiya S, Ono I, Nomura Y, Okuda M, Kikuchi K et al (1988) Phase II study of carboplatin in head and neck cancer. Gan To Kagaku Ryoho (Cancer Chemother) 15(7):2131–2138
48. Forastiere AA, Metch B, Schuller DE, Ensley JF, Hutchins LF, Triozzi P, Kish JA, McClure S, VonFeldt E, Williamson SK et al (1992) Randomized comparison of cisplatin plus fluorouracil and carboplatin plus fluorouracil versus methotrexate in advanced squamous-cell carcinoma of the head and neck: a Southwest oncology group study. J Clin Oncol 10(8):1245–1251
49. Catimel G, Verweij J, Mattijssen V, Hanauske A, Piccart M, Wanders J, Franklin H, Le Bail N, Clavel M, Kaye SB (1994) Docetaxel (Taxotere): an active drug for the treatment of patients with advanced squamous cell carcinoma of the head and neck. EORTC early clinical trials group. Ann Oncol 5(6):533–537
50. Dreyfuss AI, Clark JR, Norris CM, Rossi RM, Lucarini JW, Busse PM, Poulin MD, Thornhill L, Costello R, Posner MR (1996) Docetaxel: an active drug for squamous cell carcinoma of the head and neck. J Clin Oncol 14(5):1672–1678
51. Couteau C, Chouaki N, Leyvraz S, Oulid-Aissa D, Lebecq A, Domenge C, Groult V, Bordessoule S, Janot F, De Forni M, Armand JP (1999) A phase II study of docetaxel in patients with metastatic squamous cell carcinoma of the head and neck. Br J Cancer 81(3):457–462. doi:10.1038/sj.bjc.6690715
52. Inuyama Y, Kataura A, Togawa K, Saijo S, Satake B, Takeoda S, Konno A, Ebihara S, Sasaki Y, Kida A, Kanzaki J, Ichikawa G, Kono N, Moriyama H, Kamata S, Miyake H, Sakai M, Horiuchi M, Kubota A, Tsukuda M, Matsuura H, Baba S, Saito H, Matsunaga T, Taguchi T et al (1999) Late phase II clinical study of RP56976 (docetaxel) in patients with advanced/recurrent head and neck cancer. Gan To Kagaku Ryoho (Cancer Chemother) 26(1):107–116
53. Guardiola E, Peyrade F, Chaigneau L, Cupissol D, Tchiknavorian X, Bompas E, Madroszyk A, Ronchin P, Schneider M, Bleuze JP, Blay JY, Pivot X (2004) Results of a randomised phase II study comparing docetaxel with methotrexate in patients with recurrent head and neck cancer. Eur J Cancer 40(14):2071–2076. doi:10.1016/j.ejca.2004.05.019
54. Smith RE, Thornton DE, Allen J (1995) A phase II trial of paclitaxel in squamous cell carcinoma of the head and neck with correlative laboratory studies. Semin Oncol 22(3 Suppl 6):41–46
55. Forastiere AA, Shank D, Neuberg D, Taylor SG, DeConti RC, Adams G (1998) Final report of a phase II evaluation of paclitaxel in patients with advanced squamous cell carcinoma of the head and neck: an Eastern cooperative oncology group trial (PA390). Cancer82(11):2270–2274,10.1002/(SICI)1097-0142(19980601)82:11<2270::AID-CNCR24>3.0.CO;2-Q [pii]
56. Brotherton T Multicenter phase II trial of paclitaxel (taxol) (T): Weekly one-hour infusion in previously treated advanced head/neck cancer (AHNC). In: ASCO 2001, 2001. p abstract 921
57. Tahara M, Minami H, Hasegawa Y, Tomita K, Watanabe A, Nibu K, Fujii M, Onozawa Y, Kurono Y, Sagae D, Seriu T, Tsukuda M (2011) Weekly paclitaxel in patients with recurrent or metastatic head and neck cancer. Cancer Chemother Pharmacol 68(3):769–776. doi:10.1007/s00280-010-1550-3
58. Jacobs C, Lyman G, Velez-Garcia E, Sridhar KS, Knight W, Hochster H, Goodnough LT, Mortimer JE, Einhorn LH, Schacter L et al (1992) A phase III randomized study comparing cisplatin and fluorouracil as single agents and in combination for advanced squamous cell carcinoma of the head and neck. J Clin Oncol 10(2):257–263
59. Fan Z, Baselga J, Masui H, Mendelsohn J (1993) Antitumor effect of anti-epidermal growth factor receptor monoclonal antibodies plus cis-diamminedichloroplatinum on well established A431 cell xenografts. Cancer Res 53(19):4637–4642
60. Baselga J, Pfister D, Cooper MR, Cohen R, Burtness B, Bos M, D'Andrea G, Seidman A, Norton L, Gunnett K, Falcey J, Anderson V, Waksal H, Mendelsohn J (2000) Phase I studies of anti-epidermal growth factor receptor chimeric antibody C225 alone and in combination with cisplatin. J Clin Oncol 18(4):904–914
61. Prewett MC, Hooper AT, Bassi R, Ellis LM, Waksal HW, Hicklin DJ (2002) Enhanced antitumor activity of anti-epidermal growth factor receptor monoclonal antibody IMC-C225 in combination with irinotecan (CPT-11) against human colorectal tumor xenografts. Clin Cancer Res 8(5):994–1003
62. Cunningham D, Humblet Y, Siena S, Khayat D, Bleiberg H, Santoro A, Bets D, Mueser M, Harstrick A, Verslype C, Chau I, Van Cutsem E (2004) Cetuximab monotherapy and cetuximab plus irinotecan in irinotecan-refractory metastatic colorectal cancer. N Engl J Med 351(4):337–345. doi:10.1056/NEJMoa033025
63. Shin DM, Donato NJ, Perez-Soler R, Shin HJ, Wu JY, Zhang P, Lawhorn K, Khuri FR, Glisson BS, Myers J, Clayman G, Pfister D, Falcey J, Waksal H, Mendelsohn J, Hong WK (2001) Epidermal growth factor receptor-targeted therapy with C225 and cisplatin in patients with head and neck cancer. Clin Cancer Res 7(5):1204–1213
64. Baselga J, Trigo JM, Bourhis J, Tortochaux J, Cortes-Funes H, Hitt R, Gascon P, Amellal N, Harstrick A, Eckardt A (2005) Phase II multicenter study of the antiepidermal growth factor receptor monoclonal antibody cetuximab in combination with platinum-based chemotherapy in patients with platinum-refractory metastatic and/or recurrent squamous cell carcinoma of the head and neck. J Clin Oncol 23(24):5568–5577. doi:10.1200/JCO.2005.07.119
65. Herbst RS, Arquette M, Shin DM, Dicke K, Vokes EE, Azarnia N, Hong WK, Kies MS (2005) Phase II multicenter study of the epidermal growth factor receptor antibody cetuximab and cisplatin for recurrent and refractory squamous cell carcinoma of the head and neck. J Clin Oncol 23(24):5578–5587. doi:10.1200/JCO.2005.07.120
66. Vermorken JB, Trigo J, Hitt R, Koralewski P, Diaz-Rubio E, Rolland F, Knecht R, Amellal N, Schueler A, Baselga J (2007) Open-label, uncontrolled, multicenter phase II study to evaluate the efficacy and toxicity of cetuximab as a single agent in patients with recurrent and/or metastatic squamous cell carcinoma of the head and neck who failed to respond to platinum-based therapy. J Clin Oncol 25(16):2171–2177. doi:10.1200/JCO.2006.06.7447
67. Burtness B, Goldwasser MA, Flood W, Mattar B, Forastiere AA (2005) Phase III randomized trial of cisplatin plus placebo compared with cisplatin plus cetuximab in metastatic/recurrent head and neck cancer: an Eastern cooperative oncology group study. J Clin Oncol 23(34):8646–8654. doi:10.1200/JCO.2005.02.4646
68. Vermorken JB, Mesia R, Rivera F, Remenar E, Kawecki A, Rottey S, Erfan J, Zabolotnyy D, Kienzer HR, Cupissol D, Peyrade F, Benasso M, Vynnychenko I, De Raucourt D, Bokemeyer C, Schueler A, Amellal N, Hitt R (2008) Platinum-based chemotherapy plus cetuximab in head and neck cancer. N Engl J Med 359(11):1116–1127. doi:10.1056/NEJMoa0802656
69. Mesia R, Rivera F, Kawecki A, Rottey S, Hitt R, Kienzer H, Cupissol D, De Raucourt D, Benasso M, Koralewski P, Delord JP, Bokemeyer C, Curran D, Gross A, Vermorken JB (2010) Quality of life of patients receiving platinum-based chemotherapy plus cetuximab first line for recurrent and/or metastatic squamous cell carcinoma of

the head and neck. Ann Oncol 21(10):1967–1973. doi:10.1093/annonc/mdq077

70. Peeters M, Cohn A, Kohne CH, Douillard JY (2012) Panitumumab in combination with cytotoxic chemotherapy for the treatment of metastatic colorectal carcinoma. Clin Colorectal Cancer 11(1):14–23. doi:10.1016/j.clcc.2011.06.010
71. Vermorken JB, Stohlmacher-Williams J, Davidenko I, Licitra L, Winquist E, Villanueva C, Foa P, Rottey S, Skladowski K, Tahara M, Pai VR, Faivre S, Blajman CR, Forastiere AA, Stein BN, Oliner KS, Pan Z, Bach BA (2013) Cisplatin and fluorouracil with or without panitumumab in patients with recurrent or metastatic squamous-cell carcinoma of the head and neck (SPECTRUM): an open-label phase 3 randomised trial. Lancet Oncol 14(8):697–710. doi:10.1016/S1470-2045(13)70181-5
72. Machiels JP, Subramanian S, Ruzsa A, Repassy G, Lifirenko I, Flygare A, Sorensen P, Nielsen T, Lisby S, Clement PM (2011) Zalutumumab plus best supportive care versus best supportive care alone in patients with recurrent or metastatic squamous-cell carcinoma of the head and neck after failure of platinum-based chemotherapy: an open-label, randomised phase 3 trial. Lancet Oncol 12(4):333–343. doi:10.1016/S1470-2045(11)70034-1
73. Stewart JS, Cohen EE, Licitra L, Van Herpen CM, Khorprasert C, Soulieres D, Vodvarka P, Rischin D, Garin AM, Hirsch FR, Varella-Garcia M, Ghiorghiu S, Hargreaves L, Armour A, Speake G, Swaisland A, Vokes EE (2009) Phase III study of gefitinib compared with intravenous methotrexate for recurrent squamous cell carcinoma of the head and neck. J Clin Oncol 27(11):1864–1871. doi:10.1200/JCO.2008.17.0530
74. Soulieres D, Senzer NN, Vokes EE, Hidalgo M, Agarwala SS, Siu LL (2004) Multicenter phase II study of erlotinib, an oral epidermal growth factor receptor tyrosine kinase inhibitor, in patients with recurrent or metastatic squamous cell cancer of the head and neck. J Clin Oncol 22(1):77–85. doi:10.1200/JCO.2004.06.075
75. Argiris A, Ghebremichael M, Gilbert J, Lee JW, Sachidanandam K, Kolesar JM, Burtness B, Forastiere AA (2013) Phase III randomized, placebo-controlled trial of docetaxel with or without gefitinib in recurrent or metastatic head and neck cancer: an eastern cooperative oncology group trial. J Clin Oncol 31(11):1405–1414. doi:10.1200/JCO.2012.45.4272
76. de Souza JA, Davis DW, Zhang Y, Khattri A, Seiwert TY, Aktolga S, Wong SJ, Kozloff MF, Nattam S, Lingen MW, Kunnavakkam R, Stenson KM, Blair EA, Bozeman J, Dancey JE, Vokes EE, Cohen EE (2012) A phase II study of lapatinib in recurrent/metastatic squamous cell carcinoma of the head and neck. Clin Cancer Res 18(8):2336–2343. doi:10.1158/1078-0432.CCR-11-2825
77. Solca F, Dahl G, Zoephel A, Bader G, Sanderson M, Klein C, Kraemer O, Himmelsbach F, Haaksma E, Adolf GR (2012) Target binding properties and cellular activity of afatinib (BIBW 2992), an irreversible ErbB family blocker. J Pharmacol Exp Ther 343(2):342–350. doi:10.1124/jpet.112.197756
78. Li D, Ambrogio L, Shimamura T, Kubo S, Takahashi M, Chirieac LR, Padera RF, Shapiro GI, Baum A, Himmelsbach F, Rettig WJ, Meyerson M, Solca F, Greulich H, Wong KK (2008) BIBW2992, an irreversible EGFR/HER2 inhibitor highly effective in preclinical lung cancer models. Oncogene 27(34):4702–4711. doi:10.1038/onc.2008.109
79. Sequist L, Yang J-H, Yamamoto N, O'Byrne K, Hirsh V, Mok T, Geater S, Orlov S, Tsai C-M, Boyer M, Su W-C, Bennouna J, Kato T, Gorbunova V, Lee K, Shah R, Massey D, Zazulina V, Shahidi M, Schuler M (2013) Afatinib or cisplatin/pemetrexed in pulmonary adenocarcinoma patients with epidermal growth factor receptor mutations. J Clin Oncol 20;31(27):3327–3334
80. Schutze C, Dorfler A, Eicheler W, Zips D, Hering S, Solca F, Baumann M, Krause M (2007) Combination of EGFR/HER2 tyrosine kinase inhibition by BIBW 2992 and BIBW 2669 with irradiation in FaDu human squamous cell carcinoma. Strahlenther Onkol 183(5):256–264. doi:10.1007/s00066-007-1696-z
81. Solca F, Baum A, Krause M, Baumann M, Wong K, Greulich H, Guenther A (2007) Efficacy of BIBW 2992, a potent irreversible inhibitor of EGFR and HER2, in models of head and neck cancer. Eur J Cancer Suppl 5(4):326–327
82. Cupissol D, Seiwert T, Fayette J, Ehrnrooth E, Blackman A, Cong X, Cohen E (2013) A randomized, open-label, phase II study of afatinib versus cetuximab in patients (pts) with recurrent or metastatic (R/M) head and neck squamous cell carcinoma (HNSCC): analysis of stage 2 (S2) following crossover. J Clin Oncol 31(Suppl 15):363s (abstr 6001)
83. Psyrri A, Seiwert TY, Jimeno A (2013) Molecular pathways in head and neck cancer: EGFR, PI3K, and more. Am Soc Clin Oncol Educ Book 33:246–255. doi:10.1200/EdBook_AM.2013.33.246
84. Gibson MK, Li Y, Murphy B, Hussain MH, DeConti RC, Ensley J, Forastiere AA (2005) Randomized phase III evaluation of cisplatin plus fluorouracil versus cisplatin plus paclitaxel in advanced head and neck cancer (E1395): an intergroup trial of the Eastern cooperative oncology group. J Clin Oncol 23(15):3562–3567. doi:10.1200/JCO.2005.01.057

Chemotherapy

13

Iwai Tohnai and Kenji Mitsudo

Abstract

For patients with locally advanced head and neck cancer, including in the oral cavity, surgery with or without radiotherapy is widely accepted as the standard treatment and is thought to be the most effective curative therapy. However, extended surgery causes loss of oral function, including swallowing and speech, and reduces patient's quality of life. To preserve function while maintaining or improving locoregional control and survival rates, concurrent chemoradiotherapy represents one of the standard treatment modalities for definitive treatment of locoregionally advanced squamous cell carcinoma of the oral cavity, particularly in resectable advanced cases. Retrograde superselective intra-arterial chemotherapy and daily concurrent radiotherapy have the advantage of delivering a high concentration of the chemotherapeutic agents to the tumor bed, and they can be used to provide daily concurrent chemoradiotherapy to patients with advanced oral cancer. The treatment results of retrograde superselective intra-arterial chemoradiotherapy for locally advanced oral cancer have been reported to be similar to those of surgery, suggesting the usefulness of this treatment modality.

Oral cancer patients with advanced cervical lymph node metastases have a poor prognosis. Hyperthermia has generally been confined to treatment of cervical lymph node metastases accessible with a radiofrequency system using external application and in combination with synergistic chemoradiotherapy. Thermochemoradiotherapy using retrograde superselective intra-arterial infusion is used in patients with advanced cervical lymph node metastases, and not only the primary lesion but also cervical lymph node metastases are controlled.

In this chapter, the therapeutic results in patients with advanced oral cancer treated with retrograde superselective intra-arterial chemoradiotherapy and the effectiveness of thermochemoradiotherapy for patients with advanced cervical lymph node metastases are described.

Keywords

Chemoradiotherapy • Hyperthermia • Oral cancer • Organ preservation • Retrograde superselective intra-arterial infusion

13.1 Introduction

Radical surgery for patients with locally advanced oral cancer causes various dysfunctions such as dysmasesis, speech disorders, and dysphagia. Furthermore, the cosmetic result after surgery is of greater concern than with other cancers, such as gastric cancer and lung cancer. Therefore, organ preservation without surgery is desired for patients with

I. Tohnai (✉) • K. Mitsudo
Department of Oral and Maxillofacial Surgery, Yokohama City University Graduate School of Medicine, 3-9 Fukuura, Kanazawa-ku, Yokohama, Kanagawa 236-0004, Japan
e-mail: tohnai@yokohama-cu.ac.jp; mitsudo@yokohama-cu.ac.jp

T. Kirita and K. Omura (eds.), *Oral Cancer: Diagnosis and Therapy*,
DOI 10.1007/978-4-431-54938-3_13, © Springer Japan 2015

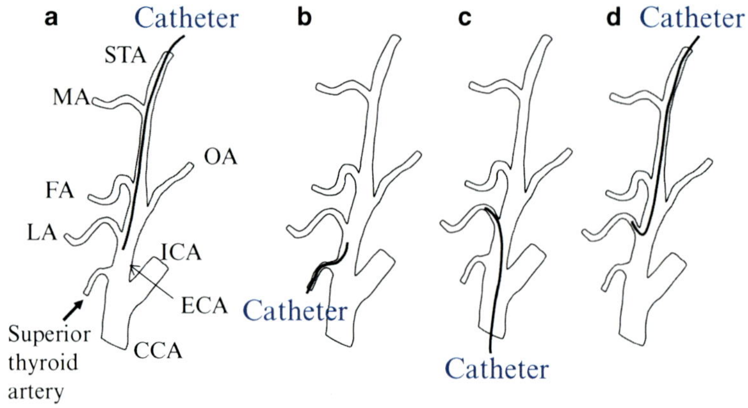

Fig. 13.1 The catheterization method for intra-arterial infusion. (**a**, **b**) Catheterization into ECA near a tumor-feeding artery via STA (**a**) or a superior thyroid artery (**b**) with a straight catheter. (**c**) Catheterization into the tumor-feeding artery via a femoral artery using the Seldinger method. (**d**) Catheterization into the tumor-feeding artery via STA with a hook-shaped catheter. *CCA* common carotid artery, *ICA* internal carotid artery, *ECA* external carotid artery, *LA* lingual artery, *FA* facial artery, *OA* occipital artery, *MA* maxillary artery, *STA* superficial temporal artery

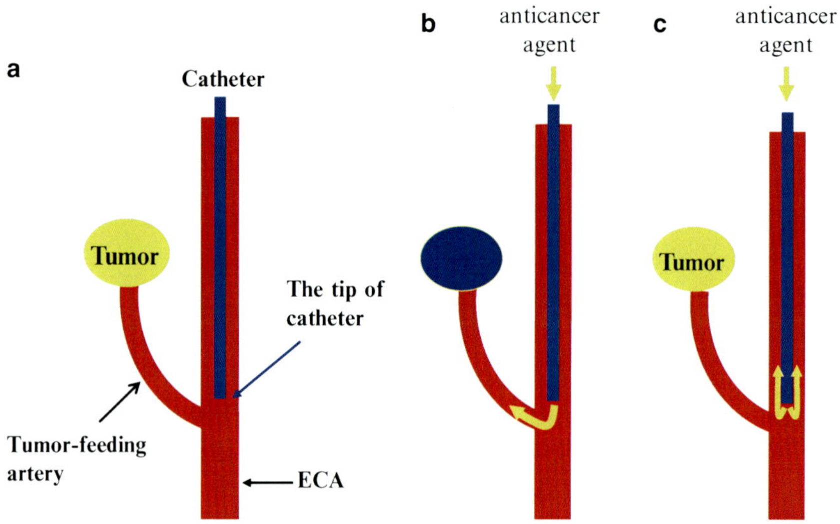

Fig. 13.2 (**a**) The tip of a straight catheter is located slightly peripheral to tumor-feeding artery. (**b**) The anticancer agents can be administered to the tumor with a manual one-shot injection of high pressure. (**c**) Anticancer agents cannot be administered to the tumor when a syringe pump is used because of low pressure

advanced oral cancer. One of the strategies of organ preservation therapy for advanced oral cancer patients is intra-arterial chemotherapy combined with radiotherapy.

Intra-arterial chemoradiotherapy (CRT) for head and neck cancer is historically classified into the following three groups. The oldest method is catheterization into the external carotid artery (ECA) near a target tumor-feeding artery via a superficial temporal artery (STA) or a superior thyroid artery using a straight catheter (Fig. 13.1a, b). The next method is catheterization into the tumor-feeding artery via a femoral artery using the Seldinger method (Fig. 13.1c). Superselective intra-arterial CRT using this method was found to be a beneficial treatment for advanced head and neck cancer. The third method is catheterization into the tumor-feeding artery via STA using a hook-shaped catheter (Fig. 13.1d). Superselective intra-arterial infusion using this method can be used to provide daily concurrent radiotherapy and chemotherapy for patients with advanced head and neck cancer, and it can be given safely without major complications, such as cerebral infarction. Intra-arterial chemotherapy for oral cancer using the three catheterization approaches is described below.

13.2 Conventional Intra-arterial Infusion via STA or a Superior Thyroid Artery (Catheterization into ECA)

Intra-arterial chemotherapy for head and neck cancer was first reported by Klopp et al. [1] and Sullivan et al. [2] in the 1950s. They reported insertion of a straight catheter into ECA via STA or a superior thyroid artery (Fig. 13.1a, b). The efficacy of treatment with intra-arterial chemotherapy has been reported [3–6].

Flow of the anticancer agents to the tumor bed is unstable with this method, because the tip of the catheter may be easily displaced near the tumor-feeding artery in ECA by neck extension. The tip of a straight catheter is located slightly peripheral to the tumor-feeding artery in ECA (Fig. 13.2a), and the anticancer agents can be administered to the tumor with a manual one-shot injection of high pressure (Fig. 13.2b). On the other hand, anticancer agents cannot be administered to the tumor when a syringe pump is used because of low pressure (Fig. 13.2c).

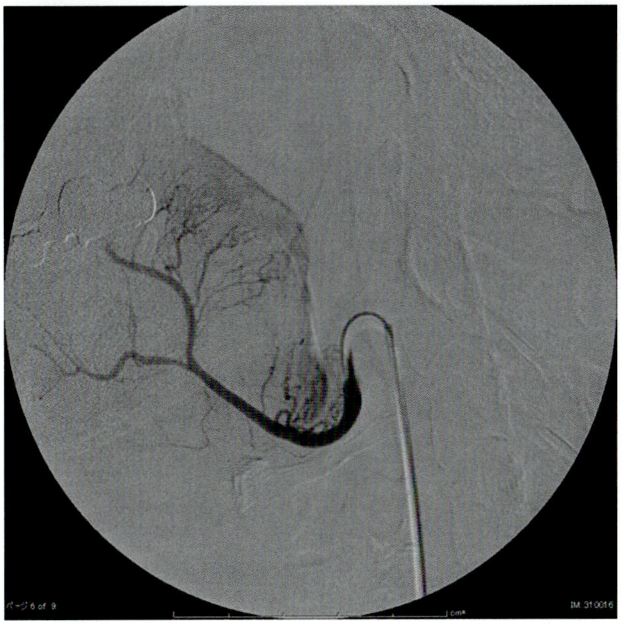

Fig. 13.3 Superselective intra-arterial infusion via a femoral artery by the Seldinger method. Tumor staining of the tongue from LA can be seen with use of contrast medium on digital subtraction angiography (DSA) (this figure was sponsored by Dr. Takamatsu S. at Fukui Prefectural Hospital)

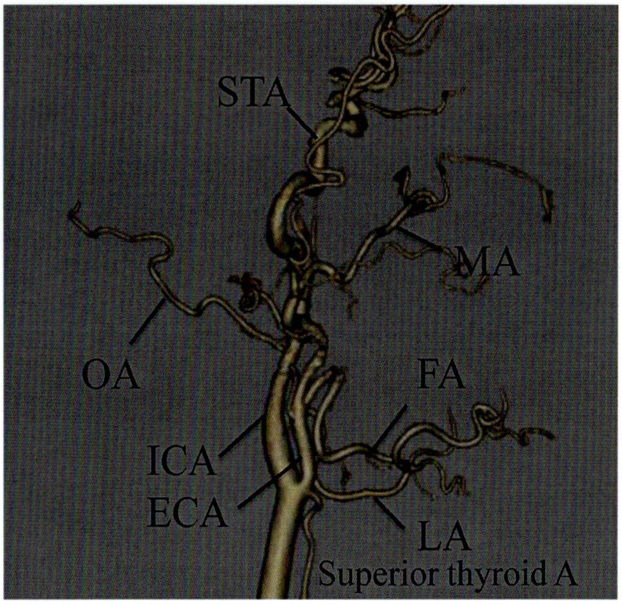

Fig. 13.4 Three-dimensional computed tomography angiography (3D-CTA) of the carotid artery

13.3 Superselective Intra-arterial Infusion via a Femoral Artery by the Seldinger Method

Lee et al. [7, 8] first reported superselective intra-arterial chemotherapy via a femoral artery using the Seldinger method (Fig. 13.3), and Robbins et al. [9–11] have developed a cisplatin (CDDP) delivery system in which extremely large amounts of anticancer agent with radiotherapy can be administered to patients with advanced head and neck cancer. Given the acronym "RADPLAT," this consists of rapid superselective intra-arterial infusions combined with intravenous sodium thiosulfate for systemic CDDP neutralization. They conducted a phase I study designed to determine the maximum-tolerated dose of CDDP that could be administered in intra-arterial chemotherapy. The maximum-tolerated dose was 150 mg/m^2/week for 4 weeks. In addition, this method has been found highly useful in the treatment of cervical lymph node metastasis [12, 13]. There have been many reports of RADPLAT for head and neck cancer [14–20], and RADPLAT has been widely accepted worldwide. However, Rasch et al. [21] reported that the local control rate and the survival rate of RADPLAT were no different from those of intravenous CRT in the Netherlands. Robbins questioned whether the result of this randomized trial was related to the technique used to deliver the intra-arterial infusions [22].

Catheterization via a femoral artery using the Seldinger method sometimes causes serious problems, such as cerebral infarction and sudden death [7, 8]. There is an interesting report that institutions inexperienced in the use of RADPLAT had a higher rate of grades 4 and 5 toxicities related to cerebral infarction than experienced institutions did [17].

13.4 Superselective Intra-arterial Infusion via STA and an Occipital Artery (OA)

This method was developed to overcome the disadvantages associated with the techniques mentioned above. A hook-shaped catheter is inserted from STA in retrograde fashion into a tumor-feeding artery; the usefulness of this method in combination with radiotherapy has been reported [23–27].

Before treatment, 3-dimensional computed tomography angiography (3D-CTA) of the carotid artery is necessary to identify the main tumor-feeding arteries and determine the morphology of the tumor-feeding artery originating from ECA (Fig. 13.4). Patients with severe calcification of the carotid artery or stenosis of the internal/external carotid artery are ineligible (Fig. 13.5a, b).

Catheterization from STA is performed according to the method of Hattori, Fuwa and Tohnai [23–25] (HFT method) [28] (Figs. 13.6, 13.7, and 13.8). STA is exposed by a 30-mm skin incision in the preauricular region of the affected side (Fig. 13.7a, b). Indwelling needle is inserted into STA (Fig. 13.7c), and an inner needle is removed from an outer needle A 0.016-inch guidewire (GT wire, Terumo Corp., Tokyo,

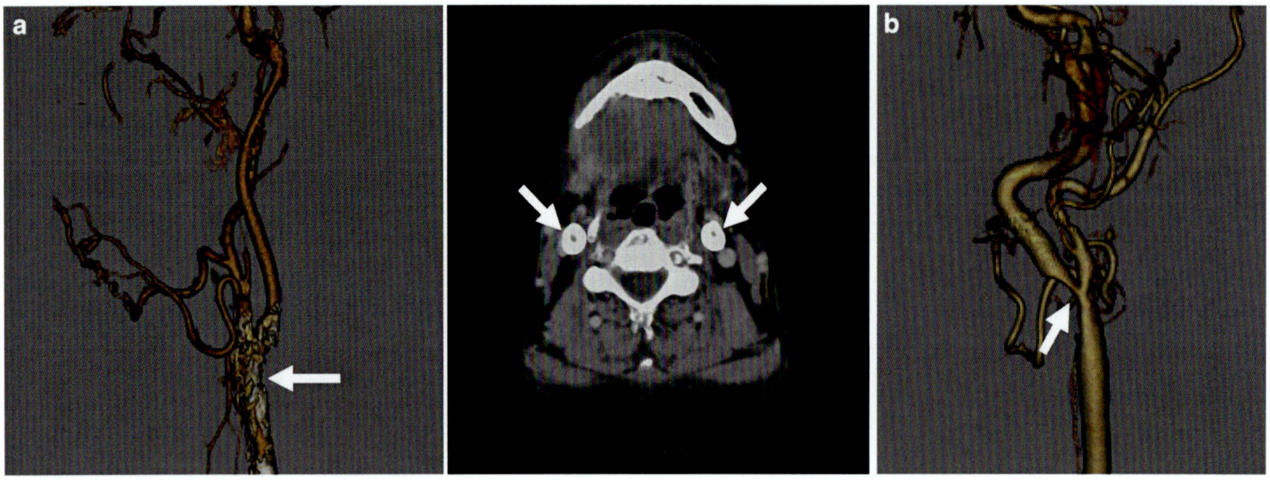

Fig. 13.5 Calcification of the external carotid artery (**a**: *arrowhead*) and stenosis of the internal carotid artery (**b**: *arrowhead*). Catheter insertion is contraindicated in these cases

Japan) (Fig. 13.6a) is inserted into the common carotid artery through an outer needle (Fig. 13.7d). A vinyl hook-shaped catheter (NECK, 4 Fr in outer diameter, Medikit Corp., Tokyo, Japan) (Fig. 13.6b) is inserted into STA along the guidewire (Fig. 13.7e) and placed below the bifurcation of the target artery (Fig. 13.7f). The tip of the catheter is then superselectively inserted into the target artery by drawing it back under fluoroscopic guidance (Fig. 13.7g, h), and the position of the catheter is checked by injection of contrast medium and blue dye (Fig. 13.7i, j). When catheterization using a hook-shaped catheter is not stable, the guidewire exchange method is used to replace it with a polyurethane straight catheter (Fig. 13.6c) [29].

When the tumor has two or more feeding arteries, catheters are inserted into the two arteries via STA and OA or bilaterally. Catheterization from OA is performed according to the method of Iwai et al. [30] (Fig. 13.8). OA is identified posterior of the mastoid process by an ultrasonic blood flow detector (Doppler ultrasound) (13.7d, and Fig. 13.8a). A 35-mm skin incision is made, and the sternocleidomastoid muscle and splenius capitis muscle are safely transected using the ultrasonic scalpel without OA injury (Fig. 13.7e, and 13.8b–e). Then, the catheter is superselectively inserted into the target artery under fluoroscopic guidance. The transected muscles, subcutaneous tissues, and skin are sutured, and the catheter is fixed to the skin around the mastoid process.

After catheterization, flow-check digital subtraction angiography (DSA) and angio-CT are performed in all cases (Fig. 13.9a–d). Angio-CT is helpful for detecting tumors by confirming the enhancement of the feeding area and for enabling the catheter to be placed at the appropriate position. Furthermore, weekly confirmation of the feeding artery by injection of a small amount of indigo carmine is important (Fig. 13.9e, f).

13.5 Radiotherapy

Radiotherapy is planned for all patients after appropriate immobilization using a thermoplastic mask and three-dimensional CT-based techniques. Conventional radiotherapy is performed with 4 or 6 MV at 2 Gy/fr/day. The irradiation field is changed according to lymph node status. In cases of N0 disease, the field contains the primary site and levels I–III of the neck on the ipsilateral side. The dose is delivered to 40 Gy/20fr. The portal is then reduced to only the primary site to spare the spinal cord. The total dose delivered to the primary tumor is 60 Gy/30fr. In cases of N1, N2a, and N2b diseases, the field contains the primary site and levels I–V of the neck on the ipsilateral side. The dose is delivered at 40 Gy/20fr. The portal is then reduced to the primary site and lymph node metastases. The dose for the spinal cord ranges from 40 Gy to 45 Gy. The total dose delivered to the primary tumor is 60 Gy/30fr and that to the metastatic lymph node sites is to 50 Gy/25fr. In cases of N2c disease, the field contains the primary site and levels I–V of the neck on bilateral sides. The dose is delivered at 40 Gy/20fr. The portal is then reduced to the primary site and lymph node metastases. The dose to the spinal cord ranges from 40 Gy to 45 Gy. The total dose delivered to the

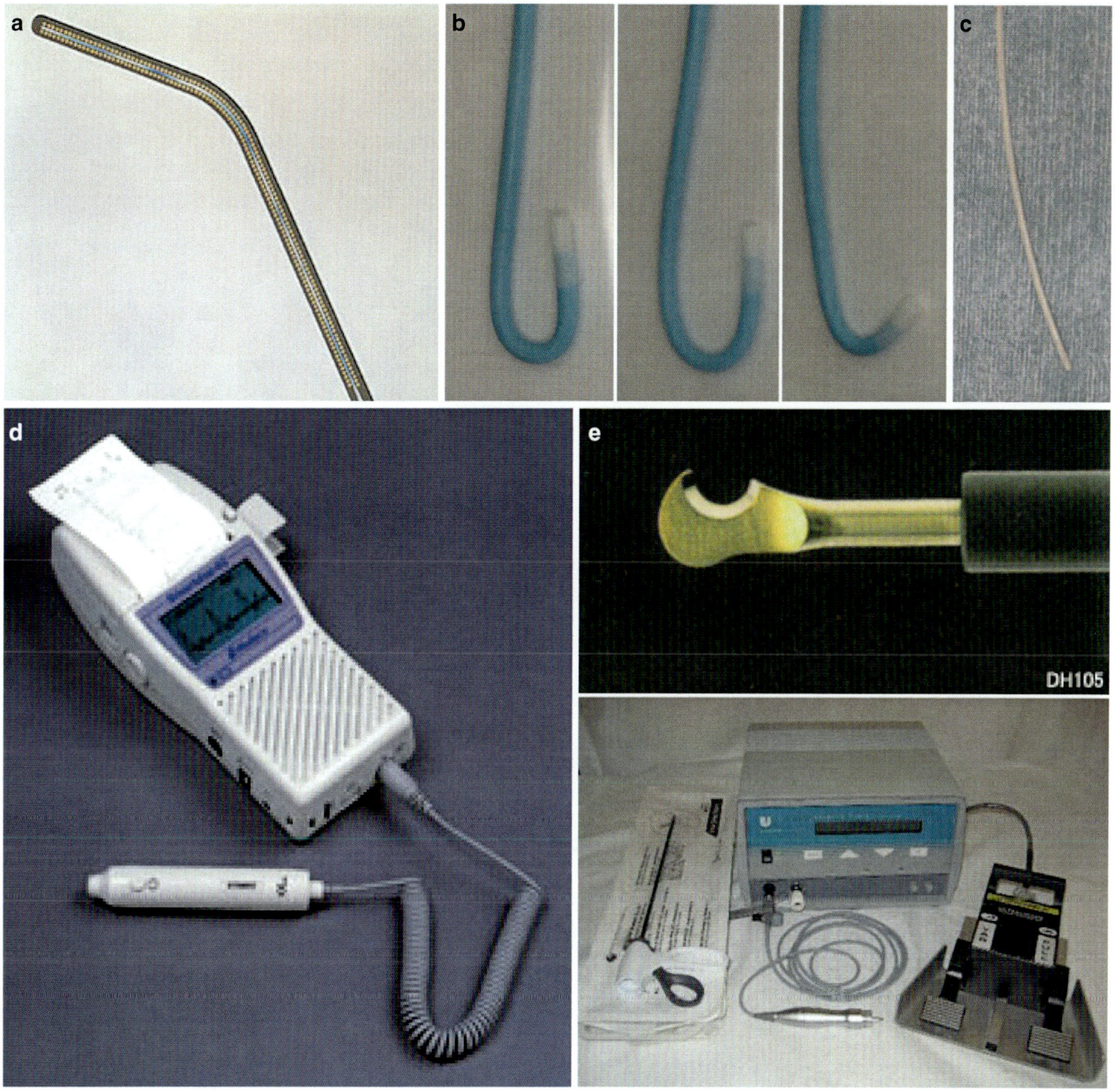

Fig. 13.6 (**a**) A 0.016-inch guidewire (Radifocus Guide Wire, Terumo Corp., Tokyo, Japan), (**b**) a hook-shaped catheter (Neck, Medikit Corp., Tokyo, Japan) (light, Neck 1G; *middle*, Neck 2G; *right*, Neck M), (**c**) a polyurethane straight catheter (Anthron P-U catheter, Toray Medical Co., Ltd., Tokyo, Japan), (**d**) ultrasonic blood flow detector (Smartdop 45, KDD Co, Ltd., Shiga, Japan), (**e**) electrosurgical diathermy (Harmonic scalpel, Johnson & Johnson K.K)

primary tumor is 60 Gy/30fr, and, if at all possible, the total dose delivered to the metastatic lymph node sites is 50 Gy/25fr.

13.6 Superselective Intra-arterial Chemoradiotherapy

The anticancer agent is injected in a bolus through the intra-arterial catheter when radiotherapy is performed. The total dose of docetaxel (DOC) is 60 mg/m^2 (10 mg/m^2/week) and that of CDDP is 150 mg/m^2 (5 mg/m^2/day) (Fig. 13.10). Sodium thiosulfate (1 g/m^2) is administered intravenously to provide effective CDDP neutralization after the anticancer agent is given. All patients are given a 5HT-3-receptor antagonist before administration of the anticancer agent.

13.7 Surgery

The purpose of this combined CRT using superselective intra-arterial infusion is to improve the local control rate and achieve good QOL without surgery. If there is residual primary tumor after this treatment or recurrence of the

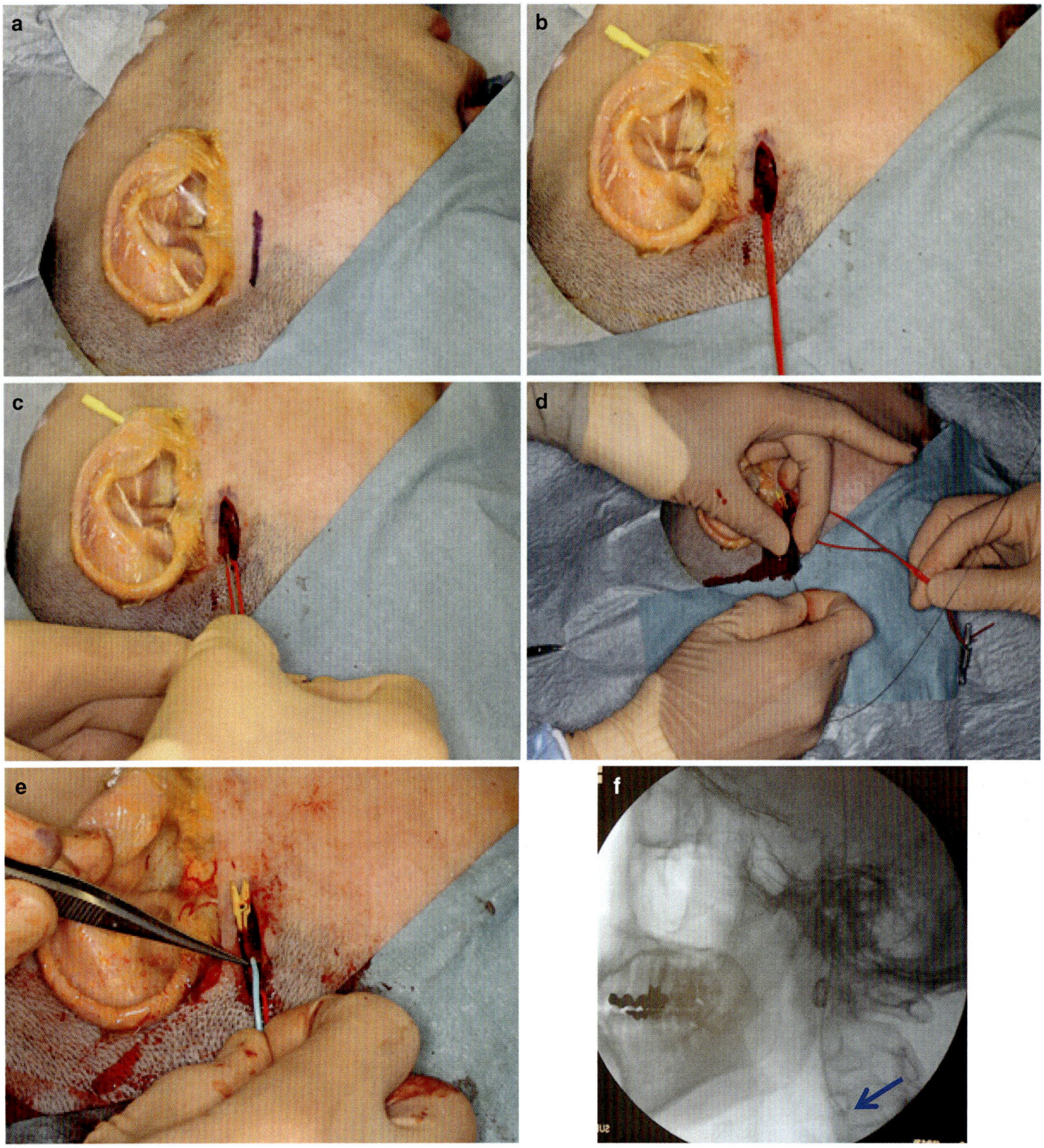

Fig. 13.7 STA is exposed by a 30-mm skin incision in the preauricular region (**a**, **b**). Indwelling needle is inserted into STA (**c**), and a guidewire is inserted into the common carotid artery (**d**). A hook-shaped catheter is inserted into STA along the guidewire (**e**) and placed below the bifurcation of the target artery (**f**, *arrowhead*). The tip of the catheter is then superselectively inserted into a target artery (**g**, facial artery, *arrowhead*) (**h**, maxillary artery, *arrowhead*). The position of the catheter is checked by injection of contrast medium and blue dye. Anterior and lower of the tumor is dyed from a facial artery (**i**, *arrowhead*), and posterior of the tumor is dyed from a maxillary artery (**j**, *arrowhead*).

primary lesion, salvage surgery is planned. In cases of cervical metastatic lymph nodes, the primary lesion is preserved and radical neck dissection is performed 5–6 weeks after the end of intra-arterial CRT.

13.8 Toxicity Assessment

Toxicities encountered during therapy are evaluated according to the National Cancer Institute—Common Terminology Criteria for Adverse Events v3.0.

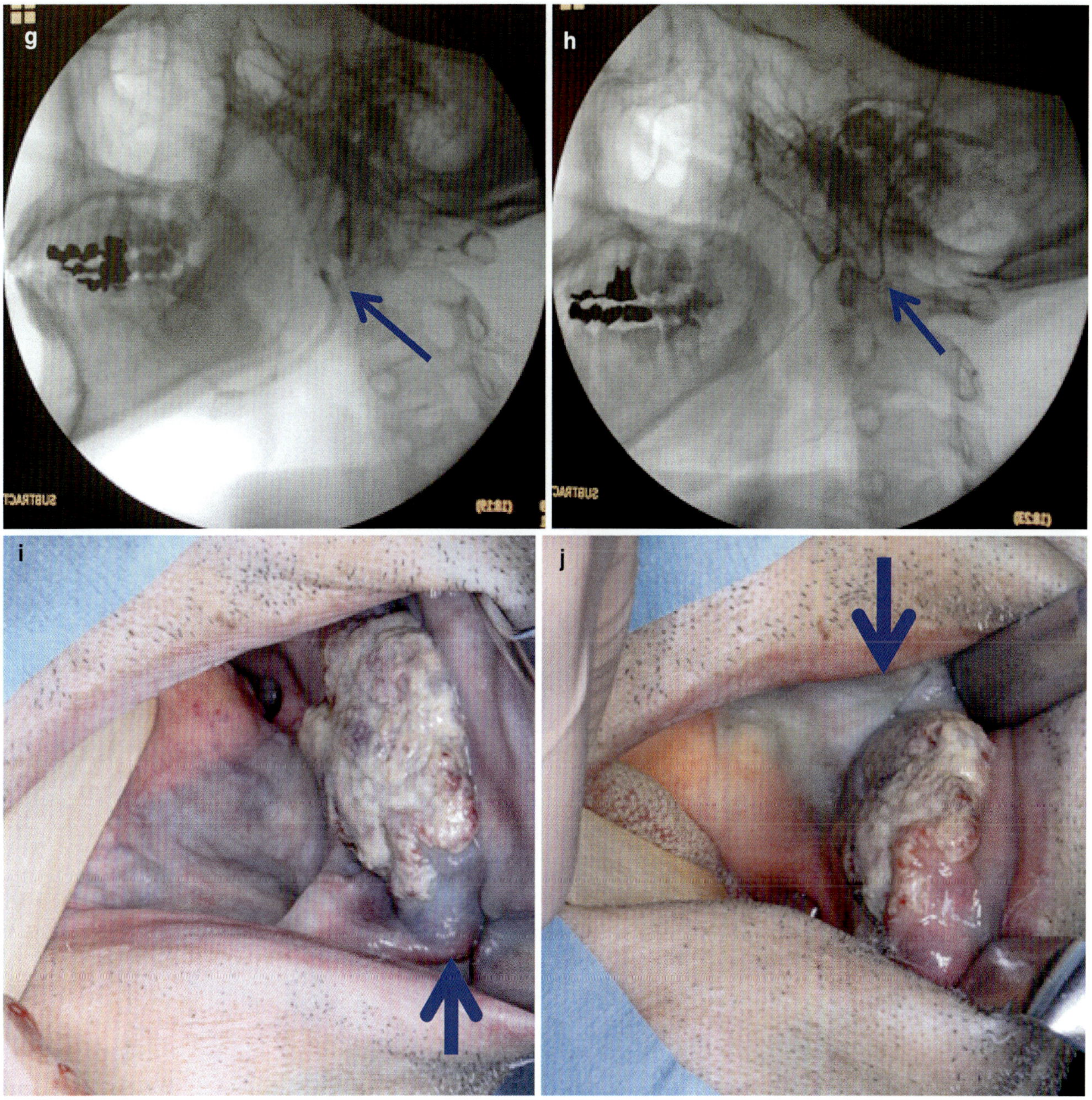

Fig. 13.7 (continued)

13.9 Results of Retrograde Superselective Intra-arterial CRT

One hundred and twelve patients with stages III and IV oral squamous cell carcinoma underwent retrograde intra-arterial chemoradiotherapy between August 2006 and July 2011. After intra-arterial CRT, the primary site complete response was achieved in 1998 (87.5 %) of 112 cases. Five-year survival and local control rates were 71.3 % and 79.3 %, respectively. Grade 3 or 4 toxicities included mucositis in 92.0 %, neutropenia in 30.4 %, dermatitis in 28.6 %, anemia in 26.8 %, and thrombocytopenia in 7.1 % of patients. Grade 3 toxicities included dysphagia in 72.3 %, nausea/vomiting in 21.4 %, fever in 8.0 %, and renal failure in 0.9 % of patients [31]. Retrograde superselective intra-arterial chemotherapy and daily concurrent radiotherapy for stages III and IV oral cancers provided good overall survival and local control. All patients had squamous cell carcinoma of the oral cavity in this study; this treatment has also been reported to be effective for sarcoma and adenoid cystic carcinoma of the head and neck [32, 33].

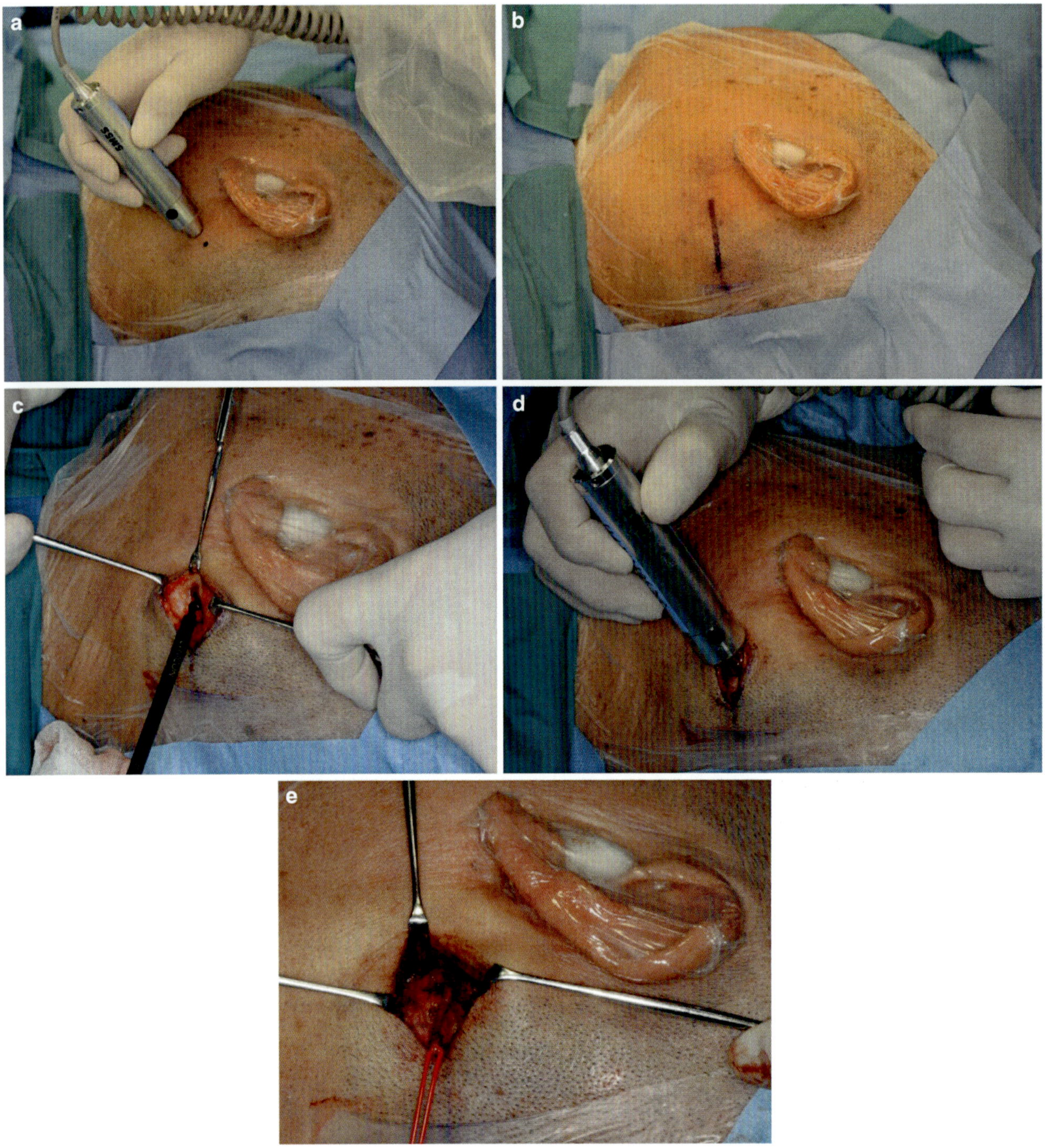

Fig. 13.8 OA is identified posterior of the mastoid process by an ultrasonic blood flow detector (**a**). A 35-mm skin incision is made (**b**), and the sternocleidomastoid muscle and splenius capitis muscle are safely transected using the ultrasonic scalpel (**c, d**), and OA is exposed (**e**). Then, the catheter is superselectively inserted into the target artery under fluoroscopic guidance

Case 1: Squamous cell carcinoma of the buccal mucosa (T3N0M0) (Fig. 13.11)

Superselective intra-arterial CRT (DOC total 60 mg/m^2; CDDP total 150 mg/m^2, total 60 Gy) was performed for 6 weeks. After completion of the treatment, pathological complete response was achieved at the primary site, and the patient has been free of disease for 5 years and 3 months.

13.10 Thermochemoradiotherapy

Patients with head and neck squamous cell carcinoma with advanced cervical metastases represent a treatment dilemma because their prognosis is generally considered to be poor. Especially when cervical lymph node metastases exceed 6 cm in their largest diameter (N3) or there are multiple

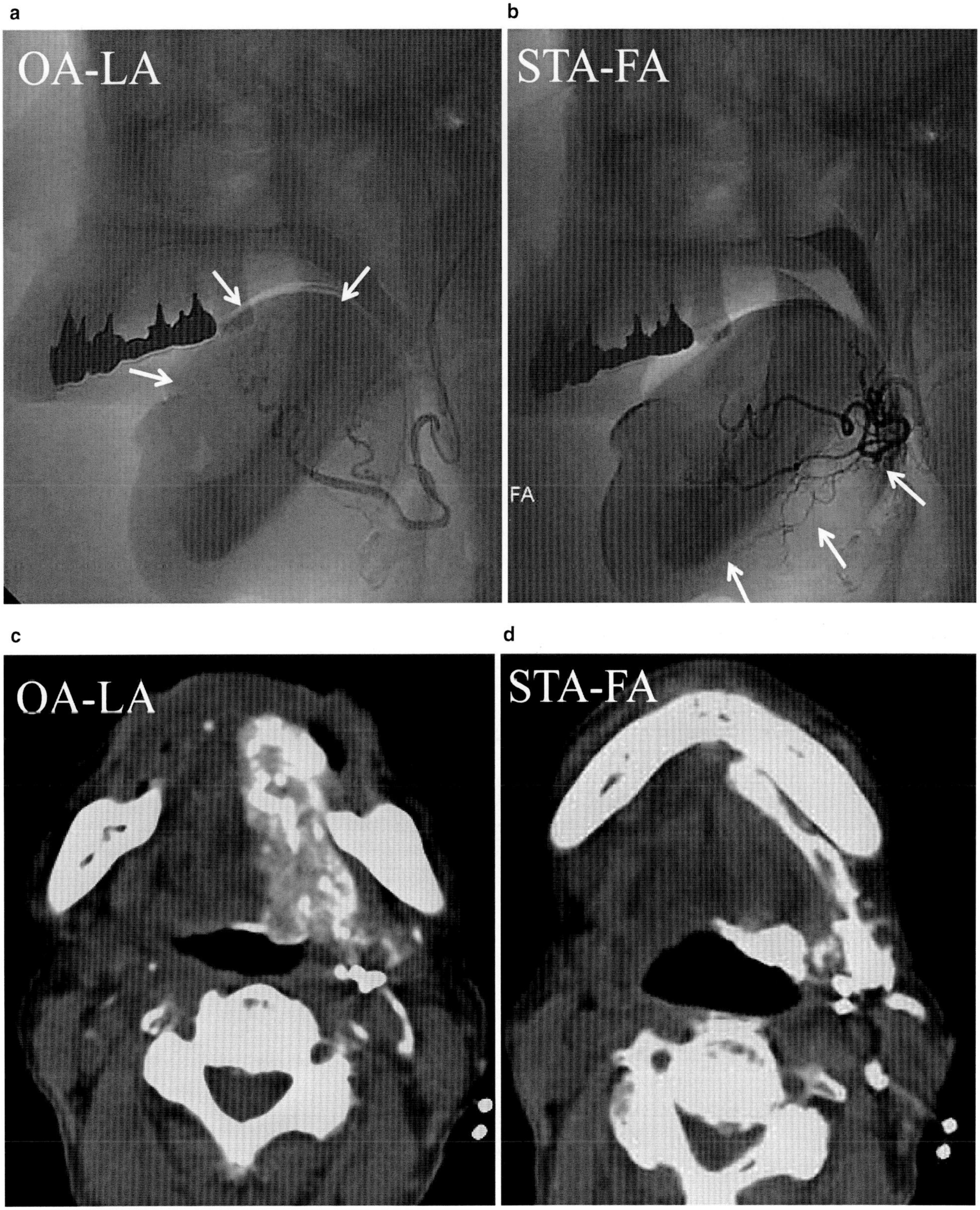

Fig. 13.9 Squamous cell carcinoma of the tongue (T3N1M0). (**a**, **b**) DSA of retrograde superselective intra-arterial infusion. Two catheters are superselectively inserted into left LA via OA (OA-LA) (**a**) and left FA via STA (STA-FA) (**b**). Tumor stain is seen with the use of contrast medium on flow-check DSA (*arrowhead*). (**c**, **d**) Axial views of angio-CT. Angio-CT images show that tumor staining of the left tongue from left LA (**c**) and the left mouth floor from left FA (**d**) can be seen with the use of contrast medium. (**e**, **f**) The left side of the tongue tumor extends to the floor of the mouth. The perfusion area from left LA is not visible to the floor of the mouth (**e**, *arrowhead*), and the perfusion area of the floor of the mouth and the inside of the mandible is seen from left FA (**f**, *arrowhead*)

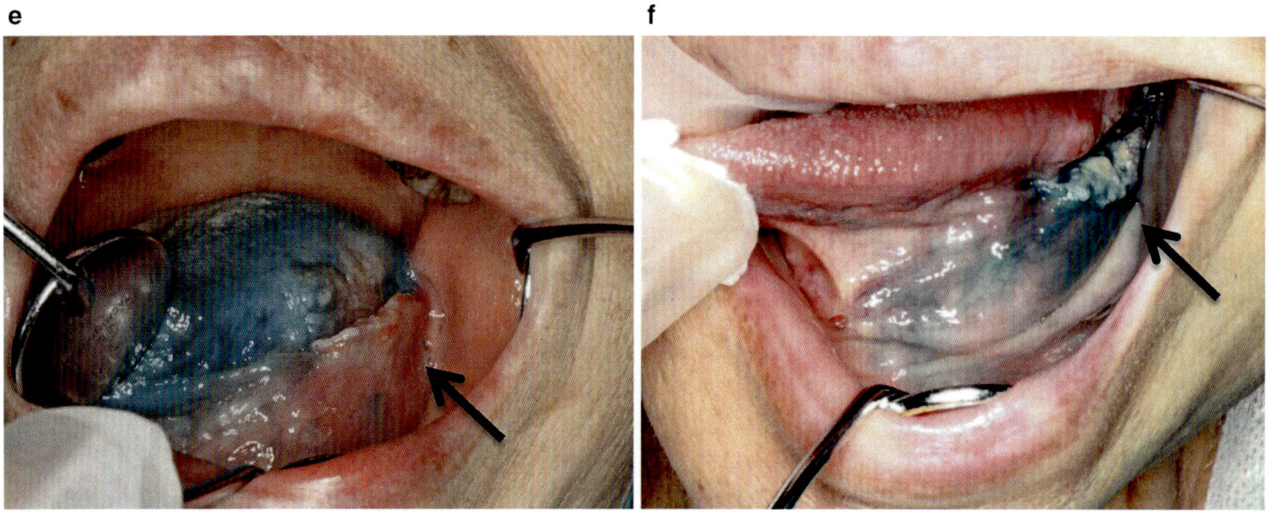

Fig. 13.9 (continued)

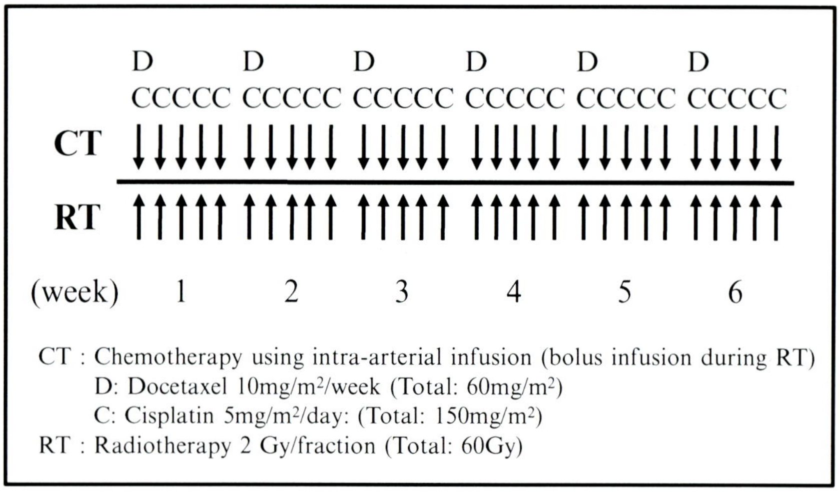

Fig. 13.10 Treatment schedule for chemoradiotherapy using intra-arterial infusion. External irradiation is performed 5 times a week at 2 Gy per fraction, to a total of 60 Gy, for 6 weeks. The anticancer agent is injected in a bolus through the intra-arterial catheter when radiotherapy is performed. The total dose of DOC is 60 mg/m^2 (15 mg/m^2/week), and that of CDDP is 150 mg/m^2 (5 mg/m^2/day)

lymph node metastases (N2b, 2c), treatment of these metastases is extremely difficult and is often associated with poor prognoses. The use of hyperthermia (HT) has generally been confined to cervical lymph node metastases accessible with a radiofrequency system employing external application and in combination with synergistic CRT.

13.11 Superselective Intra-arterial CRT Combined with HT

Our strategy for patients with advanced cervical metastases (N2 and N3) is to use thermochemoradiotherapy with retrograde superselective intra-arterial infusion. Treatment consists of superselective intra-arterial CRT (DOC total 60 mg/m^2; CDDP total 150 mg/m^2, total 60 Gy) and HT for 6 weeks. Radiofrequency capacitive heating equipment (8 MHz, maximum RF output of 60–1,500 W, Thermotron RF-8; Yamamoto Vinita Co. Ltd., Osaka, Japan) is used for HT. Two opposing 10-cm electrodes are generally used for heating the cervical lymph node metastases. The electrodes are covered with a water pad, and one is placed along the metastatic node, while the other is for the contralateral site (Fig. 13.12f). HT is applied once or twice per week and administered for 50 min within 30 min after each radiotherapy session.

13.12 Surgery After Thermochemoradiotherapy

The primary lesion and metastatic cervical lymph nodes are assessed 4 weeks after completion of all treatments. Patients are scheduled to undergo neck dissection 5–8 weeks after the end of thermochemoradiotherapy, unless distant

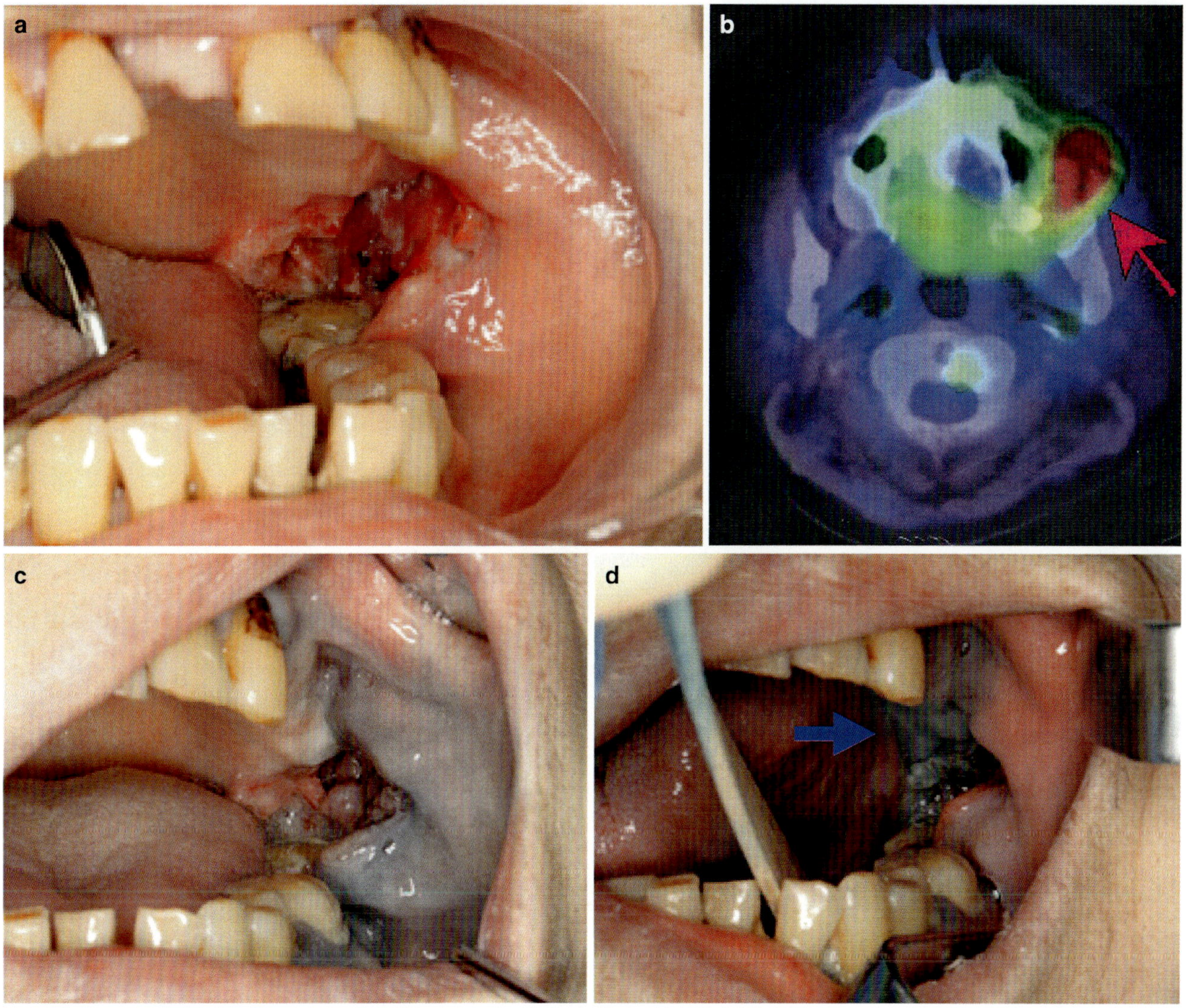

Fig. 13.11 Squamous cell carcinoma of the buccal mucosa (T3N0M0). Clinical findings reveal an ulcerated mass originating from the left buccal mucosa. The mass measures 42×32 mm and spreads to the upper and lower gingiva (**a**). Positron emission tomography–computed tomography (PET–CT) demonstrates high uptake of 18-fluorodeoxyglucose (FDG) at the left buccal mucosa (**b**, *arrowhead*). Two catheters are superselectively inserted into left FA and MA via left STA and OA. The perfusion area from the left FA is the buccal mucosa and the lower and upper gingiva (**c**). On the other hand, the perfusion area of the inside of the tumor, soft palate and anterior palatine arch, is seen from left MA (**d**, *arrowhead*). Tumor stain is seen with the use of contrast medium for the anterior side of the tumor (**e**, *arrowhead*) from FA and posterior side of the tumor (**f**, *arrowhead*) from MA. After the completion of treatment, the primary tumor has disappeared (**g**), and FDG uptake on PET–CT has disappeared (**h**)

metastases are found. If there is residual primary tumor after this treatment, salvage surgery involving both primary and cervical lymph nodes is performed.

13.13 Treatment Results of Thermochemoradiotherapy for Oral Cancer with N3 Cervical Lymph Node Metastases

We applied thermochemoradiotherapy using superselective intra-arterial infusion for patients with advanced cervical metastases and reported the treatment efficacy [34, 35, 36]. In our previous report, nine patients with N3 cervical lymph node metastases of oral squamous cell carcinoma underwent thermochemoradiotherapy using superselective intra-arterial infusion, and 5-year survival and locoregional control rates were 51 % and 88 %, respectively [34].

Case 2: Squamous cell carcinoma of the upper gingiva (T2N3M0) (Fig. 13.12)

Superselective intra-arterial CRT is combined with HT (DOC total 60 mg/m^2; CDDP total 150 mg/m^2, total 60 Gy, HT: 5 sessions) for 6 weeks. After the intra-arterial CRT is combined with HT, pathological complete response was achieved at the primary site. Radical neck dissection was carried out, and pathological complete response was recog-

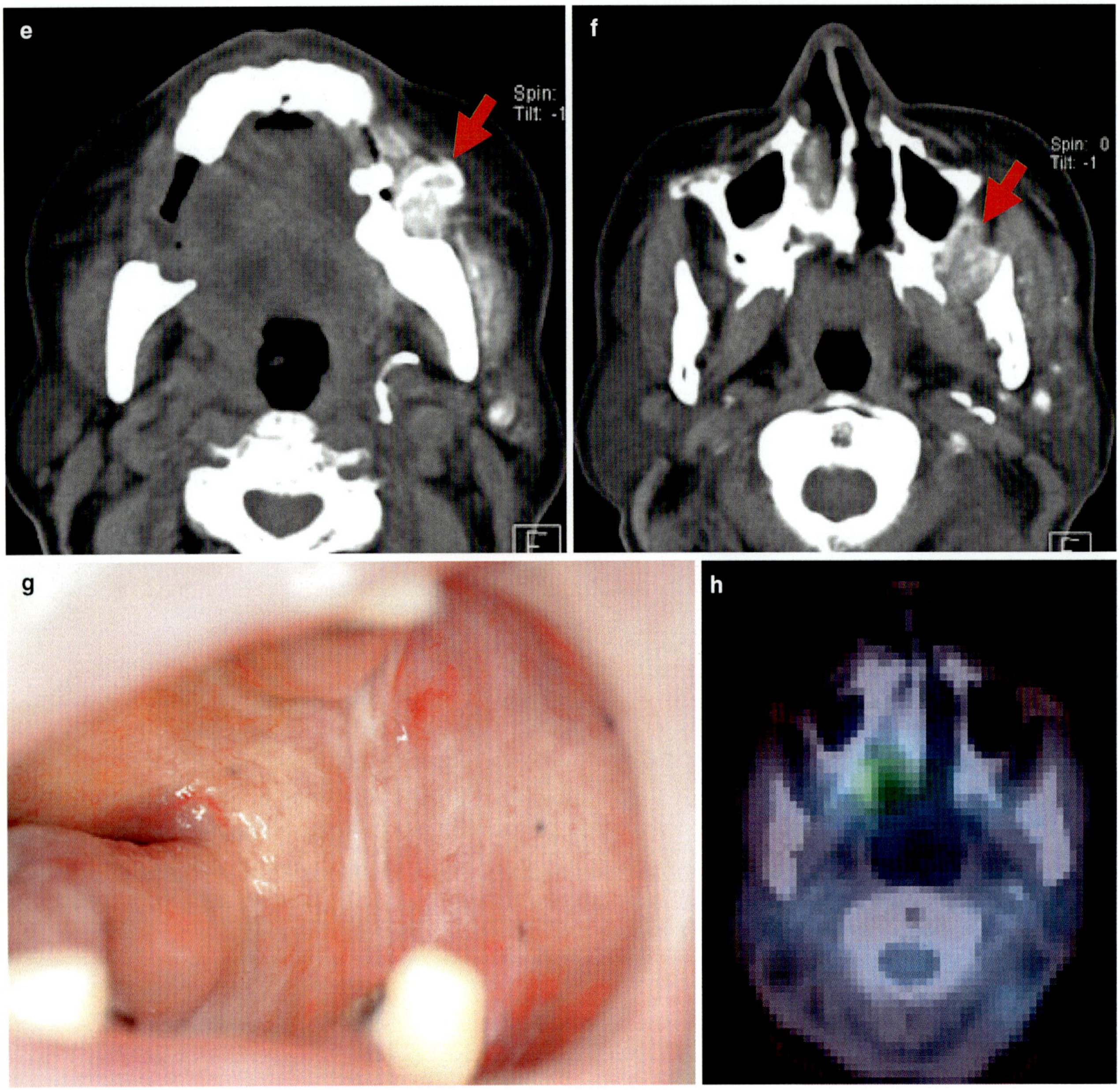

Fig. 13.11 (continued)

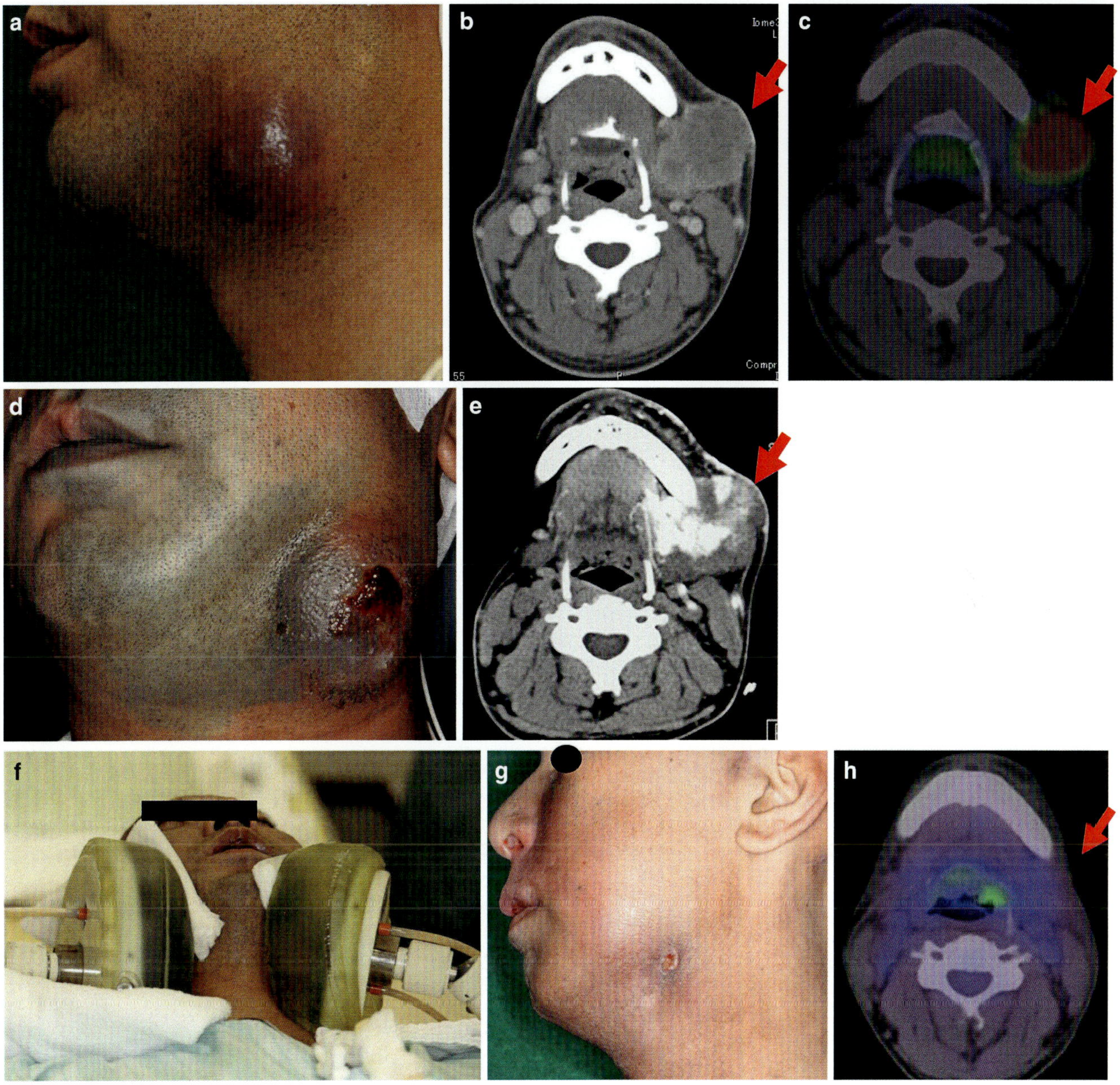

Fig. 13.12 Squamous cell carcinoma of the upper gingiva (T2N3M0). The patient has a large neck mass measured at 85×32 mm on the left side of the neck (**a**), and enhanced CT reveals a ring-enhanced mass in the left level II of the neck (**b**, *arrowhead*). PET–CT demonstrates high FDG uptake at the left cervical lymph nodes (SUV max: 13.2) (**c**, *arrowhead*). Two catheters are superselectively inserted into left FA and MA via left STA and OA. Dying of the skin surface of the N3 disease is confirmed by the injection of indigo carmine (**d**), and tumor stain is seen with the use of contrast medium via FA for the N3 cervical lymph node metastases on the flow-check angio-CT (**e**, *arrowhead*). Treatment consists of superselective intra-arterial CRT (DOC total 60 mg/m^2; CDDP total 150 mg/m^2, total 60 Gy) and HT (**f**) for 6 weeks. Five sessions of HT are given for cervical lymph node metastases. HT is administered for 50 min within 30 min after each session of CRT. The temperature of the central and peripheral skin surface of the neck tumor is over 42 °C. After the completion of treatment, N3 disease is much smaller than before treatment (**g**), and pathological complete response has been achieved at the primary site. FDG uptake on PET–CT of the N3 lymph node metastases has disappeared (**h**, *arrowhead*). Radical neck dissection has been carried out, and pathological complete response is recognized in the N3 cervical lymph node metastasis

nized at the N3 cervical lymph node metastasis. The patient has been free of disease for 5 years and 6 months.

13.14 Conclusion

Retrograde superselective intra-arterial infusion has become feasible for daily concurrent radiotherapy and chemotherapy. This combination CRT approach can preserve organs and minimize functional disturbances.

References

1. Klopp CT, Alford TC, Bateman J et al (1950) Fractionated intra-arterial cancer; chemotherapy with methyl bis amine hydrochloride; a preliminary report. Ann Surg 132:811–832
2. Sullivan RD, Miller E, Sikes MP (1959) Antimetabolite-metabolite combination cancer chemotherapy. Effects of intra-arterial methotrexate-intramuscular citrovorum factor therapy in human cancer. Cancer 12:1248–1262
3. Ramsden CH, Duff JK (1963) Continuous arterial infusion of head and neck tumors; improvements in technique by retrograde temporal artery catheterization. Cancer 16:133–135
4. Burn JI, Johnston ID, Davies AJ et al (1966) Cancer chemotherapy by continuous intra-arterial infusion of methotrexate. Br J Surg 53:329–336
5. Bertino JR, Mosher MB, DeConti RC (1973) Chemotherapy of cancer of the head and neck. Cancer 31:1141–1149
6. Auersperg M, Furlan L, Marolt F et al (1978) Intra-arterial chemotherapy and radiotherapy in locally advanced cancer of the oral cavity and oropharynx. Int J Radiat Oncol Biol Phys 4:273–277
7. Lee YY, Wallace S, Dimery I et al (1986) Intraarterial chemotherapy of head and neck tumors. Am J Neuroradiol 7:343–348
8. Lee YY, Dimery IW, Van Tassel P et al (1989) Superselective intra-arterial chemotherapy of advanced paranasal sinus tumors. Head Neck Surg 115:503–511
9. Robbins KT, Storniolo AM, Kerber C et al (1992) Rapid superselective high-dose cisplatin infusion for advanced head and neck malignancies. Head Neck 14:364–371
10. Robbins KT, Storniolo AM, Kerber C et al (1994) Phase I study of highly selective supradose cisplatin infusions for advanced head and neck cancer. J Clin Oncol 12:2113–2120
11. Robbins KT, Kumar PV, Regine WF et al (1997) Efficacy of target supradose cisplatin and concurrent radiation therapy for advanced head and neck cancer; the memphis experience. Int J Radiat Oncol Biol Phys 38:263–271
12. Ikushima I, Korogi Y, Ishii A et al (2007) Superselective arterial infusion chemotherapy for squamous cell carcinomas of the oral cavity: histopathologic effects on metastatic neck lymph nodes. Eur Arch Otorhinolaryngol 264:269–275
13. Sakashita T, Homma A, Oridate N et al (2012) Platinum concentration in sentinel lymph nodes after preoperative intra-arterial cisplatin chemotherapy targeting primary tongue cancer. Acta Otolaryngol 132:1121–1125
14. Ackerstaff AH, Tan IB, Rasch CR et al (2002) Quality-of-life assessment after supradose selective intra-arterial cisplatin and concomitant radiation (RADPLAT) for inoperable stage IV head and neck squamous cell carcinoma. Arch Otolaryngol Head Neck Surg 128:1185–1190
15. Valentino J, Spring PM, Shane M et al (2002) Interval pathologic assessments in patients treated with concurrent hyperfractionated radiation and intraarterial cisplatin (HYPERRADPLAT). Head Neck 24:539–544
16. Balm AJ, Rasch CR, Schornagel JH et al (2004) High-dose superselective intra-arterial cisplatin and concomitant radiation (RADPLAT) for advanced head and neck cancer. Head Neck 26: 485–493
17. Robbins KT, Kumar P, Harris J et al (2005) Supradose intra-arterial cisplatin and concurrent radiation therapy for the treatment of stage IV head and neck squamous cell carcinoma is feasible and efficacious in a multi-institutional setting: results of radiation therapy oncology group trial 9615. J Clin Oncol 23:1447–1454
18. Homma A, Oridate N, Suzuki F et al (2009) Superselective high-dose cisplatin infusion with concomitant radiotherapy in patients with advanced cancer of the nasal cavity and paranasal sinuses: a single institution experience. Cancer 115:4705–4714
19. Kobayashi W, Teh BG, Sakaki H et al (2010) Superselective intra-arterial chemoradiotherapy with docetaxel-nedaplatin for advanced oral cancer. Oral Oncol 46:860–863
20. Kano S, Homma A, Oridate N et al (2011) Superselective arterial cisplatin infusion with concomitant radiation therapy for base of tongue cancer. Oral Oncol 47:665–670
21. Rasch CR, Hauptmann M, Schornagel J et al (2010) Intra-arterial versus intravenous chemoradiation for advanced head and neck cancer: results of a randomized phase 3 trial. Cancer 116:2159–2165
22. Robbins KT, Howell SB, Williams JS (2010) Intra-arterial chemotherapy for head and neck cancer: is there a verdict? Cancer 116: 2068–2070
23. Hattori T, Hirano T, Toyoda S et al (1985) Superselective intra-arterial chemotherapy via the superficial temporal artery for head and neck tumor. Jpn J Radiol 45:1056–1058
24. Fuwa N, Ito Y, Kato E et al (1996) Superselective intra-arterial continuous chemotherapy with CBDCA for advanced head and neck cancer. Jpn J Head Neck Cancer 22:139–143
25. Tohnai I, Fuwa N, Hayashi Y et al (1998) New superselective intra-arterial infusion via superficial temporal artery for cancer of the tongue and tumour tissue platinum concentration after carboplatin (CBDCA) infusion. Oral Oncol 34:387–390
26. Fuwa N, Ito Y, Matsumoto A et al (2000) A combination therapy of continuous superselective intraarterial carboplatin infusion and radiation therapy for locally advanced head and neck carcinoma. Cancer 89:2099–2105
27. Tohnai I (2006) Chemotherapy using intra-arterial infusion for oral cancer. Nagoya J Med Sci 68:101–108
28. Mitsudo K, Shigetomi T, Fujimoto Y et al (2011) Organ preservation with daily concurrent chemoradiotherapy using superselective intra-arterial infusion via a superficial temporal artery for T3 and T4 head and neck cancer. Int J Radiat Oncol Biol Phys 79: 1428–1435
29. Fuwa N, Kodaira T, Furutani K et al (2008) A new method of selective intra-arterial infusion therapy via the superficial temporal artery for head and neck cancer. Oral Surg Oral Med Oral Pathol Oral Radiol Endod 105:783–789
30. Iwai T, Fuwa N, Hirota M, et al (2014) Secure surgical method for catheter placement via the occipital artery to achieve retrograde superselective intra-arterial chemotherapy for advanced oral cancer: Alternative to approach via the superficial temporal artery. Indian J Otolaryngol Head Neck Surg 66(2):205–207
31. Mitsudo K, Koizumi T, Iida M et al (2014) Retrograde superselective intra-arterial chemotherapy and daily concurrent radiotherapy for stage III and IV oral cancer: Analysis of therapeutic results in 112 cases. Radiother Oncol 111:306–310
32. Mitsudo K, Tohnai I, Fujimoto Y et al (2006) Leiomyosarcoma of the maxilla: effective chemotherapy with docetaxel (DOC) and cisplatin (CDDP) using superselective intra-arterial infusion via superficial temporary artery. Oral Oncol Extra 42:258–262

33. Adachi M, Mitsudo K, Yamamoto N et al (2013) Chemoradiotherapy for maxillary sinus adenoid cystic carcinoma using superselective intra-arterial infusion via a superficial temporal artery. Head Neck 35:e89–e93
34. Mitsudo K, Koizumi T, Iida M et al. (2012) Thermochemoradiation therapy using superselective intra-arterial infusion via superficial temporal and occipital arteries for oral cancer with N3 cervical lymph node metastases. Int J Radiat Oncol Biol Phys 83:e639-e645
35. Mitsudo K, Koizumi T, Iida M et al (2012) Thermochemoradiotherapy for Oral Cancer with N2, 3 Cervical Lymph Node Metastases using Retrograde Superselective Intra-Arterial Infusion. Themal Med. 28(2):23–28
36. Nishiguchi H, Mitsudo K, Yamamoto N et al (2013) Thermochemoradiotherapy using superselective intra-arterial infusion for N3 cervical lymph node metastases of tongue cancer. J Cancer Res Ther 9(4):718–720

Complication of Oral Cancer Treatment, Prevention, and Management

14

Satoru Ozeki

Abstract

Malignant lesions in the oral cavity are usually treated by surgical removal and several weeks of radiotherapy and/or chemotherapy. Oral cancer ablation results in the sacrifice of several functional and aesthetic organs. The latter modality can cause severe changes in the mucosal tissues, bone, salivary glands, and the teeth, most of which are irreversible. Proper management before, during, and after both modes of therapy will have a positive impact on the quality of life and decrease the morbidity associated with these treatment regimens.

This chapter will discuss the changes experienced within the oral environment during and after the treatment for oral cancer and discuss the early complications associated with oncologic treatments, surgery, radiotherapy, and chemotherapy for oral cancer and the potential long-term complications associated with treatments of oral cancer and their managements. The potential long-term complications are quite challenging for the oncologic team and the patient who survives oral cancer, primarily due to the highly specialized regional tissues involved in the surgical field.

Keywords

Mucositis • Oral complication • Oral functional disorder • Osteoradionecrosis • Xerostomia

14.1 Complications from Radiotherapy

14.1.1 Mucositis

The most common oral problems occurring after radiation and chemotherapy are mucositis that usually has an onset in the second week of therapy [1, 2]. As the mucous membranes of oral cavity are among the most radiation-sensitive tissue in the body, mucositis affects nearly 80 % of all patients who undergo head and neck radiotherapy and occurs in four phases [1, 3]. The inflammatory phase is begun as ionizing radiation causes the generation of free radicals. Mild erythema develops within the first week during a conventional course of 1.8–2.0 Gy/day. By the end of the second week, this reddened mucosal membrane develops small white patches called false membrane formation in the epithelial phase. The ulcerative phase features ulcerations of varied dimensions on any mucosal surface. At this point, most patients typically report the onset of sore throat and difficulty in swallowing. As therapy continues, these patchy areas become confluent by the third or fourth week. The consequent pain can be so intense that patients may have difficulty eating at times, complicating their ability to masticate and swallow; hence, adequate nutrition is necessary. The denuded mucosal surfaces also are a portal of entry for organisms of an altered oral microflora. This can lead to systemic bacterial or fungal infections together with the decline of host immunocompetence. Severe mucositis mandates that radiotherapy be postponed until adequate healing of the epithelium occurs. The healing phase may take several weeks after the last radiotherapy treatment [4].

S. Ozeki (✉)
Section of Oral Oncology, Department of Oral and Maxillofacial Surgery, Fukuoka Dental College,
2-15-1, Tamura, Sawara-ku, Fukuoka 814-0193, Japan
e-mail: ozekisat@college.fdcnet.ac.jp

T. Kirita and K. Omura (eds.), *Oral Cancer: Diagnosis and Therapy*,
DOI 10.1007/978-4-431-54938-3_14, © Springer Japan 2015

Accurate and reproducible evaluation of mucositis is important to monitor patient toxicity during therapy, to document the toxicity of conventional therapy, and to critically assess the effects of alternative therapies. Several oral toxicity scoring systems have been described, and the World Health Organization [5] and National Cancer Institute (NCI) [6] have developed a Mucositis Scale to allow for the basic categorization of the mucositis lesions according to severity (Tables 14.1 and 14.2) .

A sensitive, objective, and reproducible scoring system that can be widely applied is greatly needed (Fig. 14.1). Risk factors include the elderly, existing periodontal disease, poor diet, alcohol use, tobacco use, certain medications, oxygen therapy, and changes in breathing [7].

There is no universally accepted standard therapy for the prophylaxis or treatment of cancer therapy-induced oral mucositis. Numerous local and systemic approaches to the treatment of mucositis are available for the management of less severe grades of mucositis and consist of palliative relief of pain, an adequate nutrition level, and the monitoring and treatment of localized infections [8]. Liquid forms of systemic analgesics and antibiotics may be easier for the patient to swallow.

Topical coating agents can be most effective in promoting mucosal wound healing. Initially, the tissue must be cleansed of mucoid debris before the application of the agents. An oral liquid suspension can be used if the mouth is dry. All prostheses are to be removed during the oral-mucosal treatment. Topical liquid anesthetics such as 2 % viscous lidocaine may provide temporary analgesia. The suppressive effect on the gag-cough reflex leading to possible aspiration must be explained to the patient before using such topical anesthetic solutions. Prednisone, 40–80 mg per day prescribed for 1 week or less, may help to resolve some of the inflammation [9]. Varied rinses of sodium chloride and sodium bicarbonate may allow for tissue cleansing, moistening, and lubricating. These rinses, along with proper oral hygiene and hydration, are mainstays of prevention and treatment. Any oral medications that contain alcohol, thymol, eugenol, or phenol, which are part of most commercial mouthwashes, should be avoided because they can irritate and desiccate inflamed, compromised xerostomic tissues [10, 11].

Table 14.1 Methods available to assess for mucositis [5]

Grade	Clinical features
0	No signs and symptoms
1	Painless ulcers, edema, or mild soreness
2	Pain and ulcers, but can maintain ability to eat
3	Ulcers, unable to eat due to mucositis
4	Ulcers, need for parenteral or enteral support

14.1.2 Xerostomia

Xerostomia has been reported in association with radiotherapy (RT), chemotherapy, and some immunotherapies involving the major salivary glands. In radiotherapy, clinically, xerostomia has been reported with as little as two or three doses of 2 Gy, although many changes occurring with less than 60 Gy are reversible. However, doses greater than 30 Gy can cause permanent xerostomia [12]. The mean radiation doses that have been associated with permanent impairment of parotid gland saliva secretion are approximately 24 Gy for unstimulated saliva and 26 Gy for stimulated saliva [13]. Scoring systems that grade the severity of acute and late radiation-induced salivary hypofunction have been published by several organizations, including the NCI (Table 14.3) [14].

Xerostomia (dry mouth) changes the ability of the mouth to neutralize acid, clean the teeth and gums, and protect the mouth from infection. It is associated with an increased risk of radiation caries, which results from an increased number of caries-forming bacteria in the oral cavity, low salivary PH with loss of buffering capacity, decreased mechanical flushing, and decreased production of salivary proteins, immunoglobulins (i.e., IgA and IgG), lysozymes, and peroxidases [15]. Accumulation of plaque and other debris on teeth and periodontal tissues resulting from xerostomia may develop to a greatest risk of osteoradionecrosis [16]. Symptoms include dryness, a sore or burning feeling (especially on the tongue), cracked lips, cuts or cracks at the corners of the mouth, and changes in the surface of the tongue. As saliva is needed for taste, swallowing, and speech, xerostomia is associated with the development of dysgeusia or ageusia [11, 17].

Table 14.2 National cancer institute scoring criteria for mucositis [6]

Grade	Clinical examination	Functional/symptomatic
1	Erythema of the mucosa	Minimal symptoms, normal diet
2	Patchy ulceration or pseudomembranes	Symptomatic but can eat and swallow modified diet
3	Confluent ulcerations or pseudomembranes, bleeding with minor trauma	Symptomatic and unable to adequately aliment or hydrate orally
4	Tissue necrosis, significant spontaneous bleeding, life-threatening consequences	Symptoms associated with life-threatening consequences
5	Death	Death

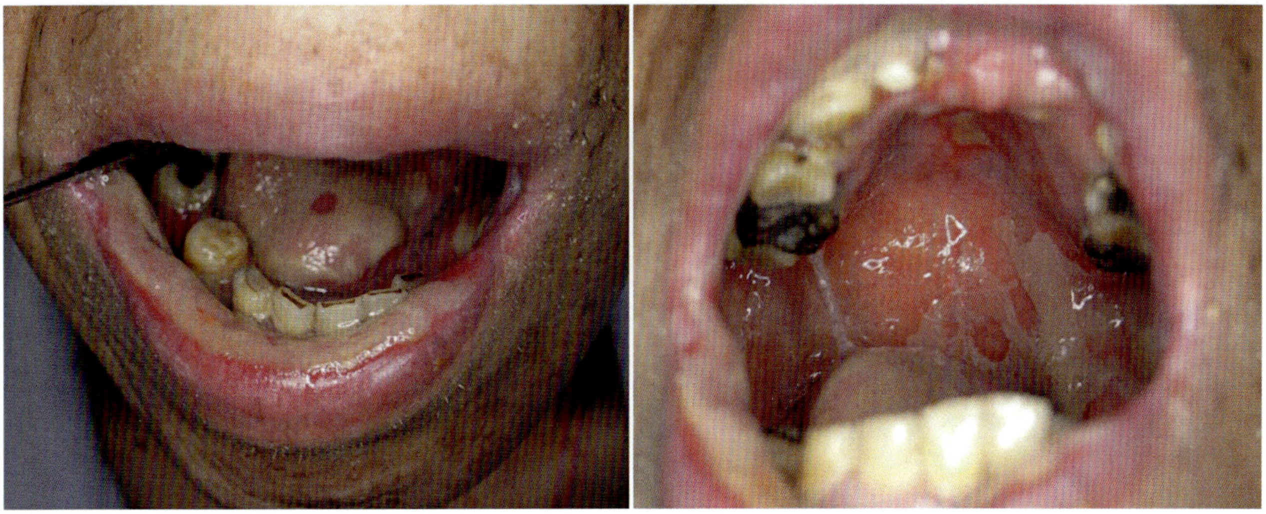

Fig. 14.1 Acute mucositis of the whole mucosa of the oral cavity and the oropharynx following postoperative chemoradiotherapy; 4 weeks of irradiation (approximately 40 Gy) combined with 5-Fu and CDDP for the tongue carcinoma. The mucositis scale of WHO and NCI is grade 3. The patient became dependent on feeding formulas through gastric tubes

Table 14.3 Radiation therapy oncology group (RTOG)—European Organization for Research and Treatment of Cancer (EORTC) scoring criteria for radiation-induced salivary gland morbidity [6]

Grade	Acute morbidity	Late morbidity
0	No change over baseline	None
1	Mild dryness, slightly thickened saliva, and slightly altered or metallic taste	Slight dryness of mouth with good response to stimulation
2	Moderate to complete dryness, thick sticky saliva, and markedly altered taste	Moderate dryness of mouth with poor response to stimulation
3	Not defined for acute xerostomia	Complete dryness of mouth with no response to stimulation
4	Acute salivary gland necrosis	Fibrosis

An extremely dry mouth will also impair proper speaking, wearing dentures, mastication, and the swallowing of foods.

To minimize the severity of xerostomia and oral complications, it is important to begin aggressive oral care before RT. Appropriate nutritional intake, effective oral hygiene, and early detection of oral lesions are important pretreatment practices. Evaluation in several weeks advance of therapy is essential to determine oral health status, perform necessary dental and oral interventions, and allow time for healing from any invasive procedures that are required. In particular, attention should be given to mucosal lesions, dental caries and endodontic disease, periodontal disease, ill-fitting dentures, orthodontic appliances, temporomandibular dysfunction, and salivary abnormalities. A stringent oral hygiene program is critical and should be continued before, during, and after therapy [11].

Frequent sips of water and water rinses are most commonly used and are essential for partial control of radiation-induced xerostomia. Patients are instructed to carry with them plastic bottles of water for constant use. Sugarless chewing gum and tart candy may be helpful. In some patients, pilocarpine hydrochloride solution (1 mg/mL) or Salagen tablets (5 mg) have been effective in stimulating saliva production [18]. Five milligrams, three or four times daily, has been an optimal dosage for most patients. The most common side effects include sweating, a "flushed" feeling, and stomach discomfort, but these usually occur only at higher dosages [19].

14.1.3 Osteoradionecrosis

Osteoradionecrosis (ORN), which is defined as necrosis of the bone in areas that have received radiotherapy, is one of the most serious complications of the postradiotherapy patient. Bone cells and vascularity may be irreversibly injured, and when ORN is progressive, it can lead to intolerable pain and interference with function or fracture.

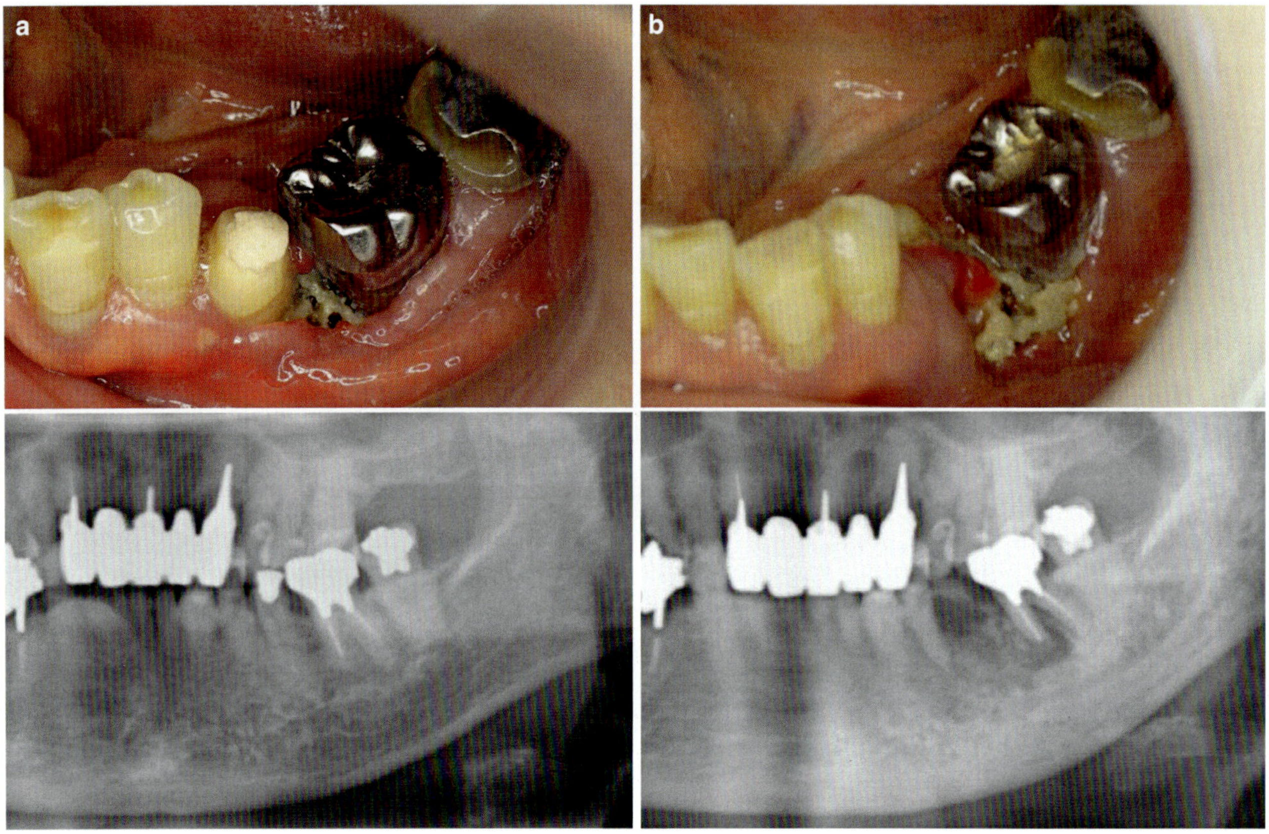

Fig. 14.2 Osteoradionecrosis following radiation therapy. (**a**) The mandible had been in the field of radiation for the floor of the mouth squamous cell carcinoma. One year after completion of radiation, the necrotic bone had developed. (**b**) At 3 years, the osteoradionecrosis continued to increase with frequent bouts of swelling, pain, and suppuration. The second premolar exfoliated. Antibiotics were ineffective, and a sequestrectomy was performed

The preventive and therapeutic use of antibiotics and hyperbaric oxygen (HBO) can be effective, but reproducible beneficial results remain uncertain [20]. The incidence of ORN varies from 4 % to 22 % depending on the reporting institution, aggressiveness of radiotherapy, and follow-up time [21–23].

The risk of developing spontaneous ORN is somewhat unpredictable but is related to the dose of radiation. Patients who have received doses of radiation in excess of 60 Gy have the highest risk of this pathological entity. Irradiated areas of bone supplied by damaged vessels with lack of oxygen and nutrients become ischemic and ultimately necrotic. The mandible is affected more frequently because it has less of a blood supply than the maxilla. Obviously, acute or chronic irritation or trauma to avascular mucosa and bone increases the risk of tissue breakdown and ORN. The risk seems to be increased in dentulous patients, even more so if the teeth within the treatment field are removed after therapy [21]. Spontaneous bone exposure usually occurs more than 1 year after radiation is completed. Any oral surgery procedure increases the risk of the development of spontaneous ORN, even if it is performed years after the last radiotherapy treatment (Fig. 14.2). The risk of ORN will be present for the remainder of the patient's life. Unfortunately, the passage of time does little to reverse the damage and the subsequent risk of ORN [24].

Certain facts emerge from UCSF (University of California, San Francisco) study [21, 24]:

1. Patients who were edentulous at the time of diagnosis of cancer had a relatively low risk of ORN.
2. Patients who were dentulous had a greater risk.
3. The increased risk in dentulous patients appeared to be associated with those who had tooth extractions after radiation therapy.
4. Dentulous patients with pretreatment extractions or no extractions appeared to have risks similar to those of the edentulous patients.
5. Spontaneous ORN occurred.
6. The most important risk factor for the development of osteonecrosis appeared to be the radiation dose to the bone, particularly in the mandible.
7. Clinical changes in skin and/or mucosa indicating radiation damage were a risk indicator for ORN.
8. The risk of ORN continued indefinitely following radiation therapy.

Treatment for ORN is variable. The risk of osteomyelitis, an infection of the bone, is increased in the postradiotherapy patient. Analgesic drugs can be taken depending on the severity of pain and patient response. The bony segments that perforate the mucosal tissues create a portal of entry for microbial organisms of the oral flora. If flares of swelling and suppuration occur only occasionally, antibiotics are usually effective. If pain and/or flares occur too frequently or present other difficulties for the patient, surgery must be considered. Aggressive surgical and antibiotic treatment is needed to debride the area and resolve the infection. Sequestrectomy must be done when sequestration develops. Small pieces of necrotic bone can be removed under local anesthesia; on the other hand, larger segments of bone may require hospitalization for their removal. Hyperbaric oxygen (HBO) treatments may help in the regeneration of new blood vessels with a resultant increase in the oxygen supply to the affected bone [25]. The only possible effectiveness is combining HBO with surgery and antibiotics. HBO involves sequential daily exposure to oxygen under pressure (2 h daily in hyperbaric chamber at 2 atmospheres of oxygen, 20–30 times) [19].

14.1.4 Other Oral Complications from Radiotherapy

14.1.4.1 *Candida* Infection

A resident oral fungal organism with pathogenic capabilities, *Candida albicans*, causes a common opportunistic infection in the oral tissues of radiotherapy patients. The normal competitive mechanisms among the microbial species of the oral environment and the immunocompetence of the host are usually sufficient to prevent infection of the mucosal tissues by this fungal organism. After radiotherapy, both of these protective mechanisms are altered, which can result in candidiasis in the oral tissues.

The most significant concern is that a Candida infection superimposed over an area of mucositis could be a source of a regional or systemic fungal infection, which could have fatal consequences in a patient already weakened by illness, surgery, radiotherapy, and/or chemotherapy. Treatments for these infections consist of antifungal oral suspensions, such as nystatin, that follow swish-and-swallow protocol [54]. Antifungal troches are difficult to use in patients whose salivary flow has diminished. Patients who wear complete or partial dentures, orthodontic retainers, or night guards must disinfect these appliances in accordance with the manufacturers' directions. The acrylic portions of these appliances have microscopic porosities in which *Candida albicans* organisms thrive and re-infect oral tissues that have been cleared of the infection. Systemic fungal infections in these patients have a high mortality rate and must be treated with intravenous antifungal agents in a hospital setting.

14.1.4.2 Loss of Taste

A loss of taste (dysgeusia) may also occur in almost all radiotherapy patients due to damage of the cells which occur primarily in the tongue papilla. There are essentially four tastes: sweet, sour, bitter, and salty. The four primary taste sensations are controlled by different locations on the tongue. For example, the anterior tongue and tip control sweet tastes, and the lateral sides control sour. Bitter tastes are picked up by the circumvallate papillae, and salty tastes can be detected throughout the tongue. The taste bud cells are very sensitive to radiation but usually are capable of repopulating within four months following treatment. Most patients report an alteration in their sense of taste. This is a direct result of the radiation's effect on taste buds. The extent of damage and the ability to regain the sensation of taste will depend on the cumulative dose of radiation and the number of taste buds involved. The degree to which taste returns is highly variable and varies from patient to patient. When the cumulative dose of 60 Gy has been reached, damage to the taste buds is usually permanent with the sensation of taste being lost [26]. Xerostomia and mucositis also contribute to dysgeusia.

14.1.4.3 Radiation Caries

One result of radiation xerostomia is a pronounced shift toward a highly acidogenic, highly cariogenic oral microflora. The decrease in pH levels, which is commensurate with the amount of damage to the salivary glands, begins the creation of a caries-prone oral environment. When the serous component of saliva decreases and the viscosity increases, adherence of cariogenic bacteria to tooth structure increases. These organisms thrive in the more acidic oral environment that develops after radiotherapy. These factors, coupled with the difficulty that patients have with their oral hygiene maintenance amidst sensitive teeth and soft tissues, create a problem known as "radiation caries" [24]. Radiation-induced dental effects primarily depend on salivary changes and occur when the glands are included in the field of treatment, not on direct irradiation of the teeth themselves. Direct irradiation of teeth may alter the organic or inorganic components in some manner, making them more susceptible to decalcification, but this has not been shown clearly [27].

To prevent or at least minimize radiation caries, oral hygiene must be maximal, including intensive home care and frequent office visits for examination and prophylaxis. Mouth rinsing is essential. Antiseptic mouth rinses, such as chlorhexidine, if tolerated, are helpful in eliminating debris and controlling microbial flora. In patients with hypersensitive mucosa, non-alcohol-containing and unflavored mouth rinses are available. Daily topical fluoride applications, as a rinsing solution, a gel delivered by means of a tray, or brushed on as a paste or gel, are all effective [28].

14.2 Complications from Chemotherapy

The toxic effects of chemotherapy are usually acute and add to the morbidity of treatment. Therefore, treatment must often balance between the adverse side effects of chemotherapy and the benefits of trying to increase response and survival. Adverse events of chemotherapy for oral cancer are described in Chap. 13, "Chemotherapy." Many chemotherapeutic agents exert their deleterious effect on normal cells as a result of the mitotic similarities between rapidly dividing malignant cells and those of normal cells. Because the cells of the oral mucosa undergo frequent turnover, they are subject to the nonspecific detrimental effects of chemotherapy. The oral tissues are also subject to other problems, such as bleeding and infection, caused by the effects of chemotherapy on the bone marrow cells. A review of these cells and their functions in the clotting mechanism and in appropriate immune function is necessary before the effects that chemotherapy has on these cellular elements, and ultimately, the host can be understood [24].

Because continued therapy further induces myelosuppression, leukopenia, thrombocytopenia, and erythrocytopenia, patients grow even more susceptible to infection, bleeding, and anemia, necessitating special care and precautions. Oral foci of infection can lead to bacteremias, fever, and pain. The reactivation of simplex and varicella zoster can cause significant mucosal breakdown, pain, and hemorrhage and can increase the risk of secondary infection. Fungal infection caused by *Candida* can spread systemically and cause serious infections. When using cytotoxic chemotherapeutic drugs, it is extremely important to keep patients free from the oral foci of infection and pain to minimize local infection and bacteremia and to enable patients to maintain a nutritious diet. Good oral hygiene is necessary [9].

Nausea is an added and significant problem. Maintaining hydration and adequate nutritional intake are often problems requiring special attention. Feeding tubes (nasogastric tube, gastrostomy) are frequently the best solution.

14.3 Complications from Surgery

The early complications from surgery for oral cancer which are described in Chaps. 7–9 are similar to other general surgical procedures. However, the potential long-term complications are quite challenging for the oncologic team as well as the patient who survives oral cancer, primarily due to the highly specialized regional tissues involved in the surgical field [29].

Over the last several decades, approach to treatment of oral cancer has changed very little with regard to primary tumor extirpation. On the contrary, the approach to cervical lymph nodes at risk for metastasis has been changed from radical neck dissection (RND) to more conservative ND – modified RND and supraomohyoid ND based on our better understanding of lymphatic drainage and accurate imaging diagnosis with US, CT, MRI, and PET. Also, the ability to offer a variety of reconstruction options with the available kinds of regional flaps, as well as composite free tissue transfer, has contributed to the overall significant improvements in functional and aesthetic outcomes. The head and neck cancer survivor today does not necessarily have to live with destructive disfigurement and speech and swallowing disturbances. Despite these surgical advances, the surgical process still results in the sacrifice of several functional and aesthetic organs during surgery for cancer of the oral cavity [30].

This chapter addresses long-term complications, issues with speech, and swallowing, chewing, and neurologic dysfunction.

14.3.1 Speech and Swallowing Difficulties

The impact of surgical resection of oral cancers on the two most important functions of oral cavity, speech and swallowing, can be significant. Swallowing can be divided into three phases: the voluntary oral phase and the involuntary pharyngeal and esophageal phases. In the voluntary oral phase of swallowing, the lips, jaw, tongue, and soft palate are involved in the preparation and holding of the bolus prior to propulsion into the oropharynx. The oral preparatory phase (formation of a bolus) and the oral phase of normal swallowing can be significantly impaired following resection of the lips, mandible, and maxilla including the teeth, tongue, and soft palate. Especially, loss of a significant portion of the tongue will limit the ability to transfer food into the appropriate position for grinding by dentition. Therefore, the first phase of swallowing is disrupted. The transfer of the bolus from the anterior portion of the oral cavity to the area of the tonsillar pillars, where the initiation of the swallowing reflex occurs, constitutes the second phase of swallowing. The harmonious coordination of the lips, tongue, buccal mucosa, and maxillomandibular complex is required for completion of these phases and progression to the pharyngeal phases of swallowing. Thus it can be seen that normal swallowing is achieved by a precise, well coordinated sequence of muscular activity involving all of those muscle groups. The same structures are associated with speech production and more specifically articulation. As a general rule, ablative surgery that involves the most anterior portion of the oral tongue is associated with significantly altered speech, while resections that incorporate the posterior tongue affect swallowing. As postsurgical time progresses, surgical site scarring and fibrosis, along with xerostomia from adjunctive radiotherapy, further impair speech and swallowing [31–33].

The complexity of the function of the oral cavity structures cannot always be restored to their presurgical status despite the use of swallowing maneuvers and free tissue transfer. Difficulties with articulation, chewing, and swallowing could become long-term problems for these patients, and adequate rehabilitation and support should be initiated early. Patients who develop functional impairment of speech and swallowing pose a variety of complex challenges to speech pathologists and other rehabilitation specialists, mandating the need to approach their issues from a multidisciplinary view. Early consultations with a speech pathologist with expertise in rehabilitation after treatment for oral cancer are critical to achieve a successful functional outcome. Patients should have the opportunity to meet with each member of the interdisciplinary team before head and neck cancer treatment is initiated [34, 35].

14.3.2 Masticatory Difficulties and Trismus

The tongue, floor of mouth, maxilla, and mandible with the adjacent tissues are vital structures used for mastication, and their anatomic and functional circumstances in the oral cavity are altered with cancer surgery. Mandibular or maxillary resection affects the grinding ability either due to loss of stable and reproducible stomatognathic system relationships or due to loss of tooth-to-tooth contacts and diminished biting forces. In addition, loss of soft tissue bulk and sensation causes difficulties with the patient's ability to manipulate the food bolus to the occlusal table, collect the bolus, and then combine it prior to swallowing [30].

Numerous studies have evaluated the limitations associated with mastication status post-cancer resection and the effects of reconstruction on masticatory function. Biting force testing, and those evaluating the tongue and cheek function, could be employed to evaluate the specific aspects of mastication. In addition questionnaires of the patients are used to access the overall efficiency in masticating food and the quality of life following mandibular resection with respect to success of reconstruction utilization. Unfortunately, significant variability in the testing instruments utilized in these studies has resulted in conflicting results and conclusions [36]. It is generally accepted that reconstruction of defects in the oral cavity at the minimum results in decreased scar formation and associated functional and cosmetic limitations. Soft tissue reconstruction with pedicle flaps and the use of reconstruction plates to bony continuity defects have been shown to be superior to simple closure techniques alone. With the availability of free tissue transfer, composite flaps can not only restore tissue bulk and facial aesthetics, but also provide masticatory function due to the potential for future dental rehabilitation [37, 38].

Trismus which is the inability to normally open the mouth is a common complaint following oral cancer surgery including the masseter/pterygoid muscles. Fibrosis and scar contraction of the muscles of mastication are the main reasons for the inability of the patient to open the mouth. Maxillary surgery and mandibulectomy involving the medial and lateral pterygoid muscles, the temporal muscle, and the masseter muscle result in trismus. It can also result from high-dose RT exposure to the TMJ region including the masseter/pterygoid muscles. Irradiation causes a thickening and scarring of the blood vessels that supply these muscles. The decreased oxygen and nutrient supply causes scars to form among the muscle fibers. Finally, disarticulation of the temporomandibular joint for tumor eradication will certainly lead to similar limited mouth opening.

Exercise regimens and mouth opening assisting devices, either active or passive, are regularly prescribed to assist these patients. Active/continuous motion devices have been shown to be effective and should be provided as preventive protocols because once established, trismus is difficult to manage. Unfortunately, if these steps are not incorporated early, before severe scarring has occurred, and maintained in the long term, only limited improvement in trismus can be expected. The presence of these difficulties with mastication, swallowing, and trismus results in limitations in food intake and compromises the nutritional status of patients. A significant number of these patients are forced to adapt specific diet modifications that may lead to nutritional deficits. Some patients become dependent on feeding formulas through gastric tubes. Although these formulations are appropriately balanced with adequate calories, issues of intolerance, diarrhea, dehydration, and electrolyte imbalance are very common. Nutritional education and support, along with close monitoring of the caloric and nutritional intake of these patients, will assist in preventing long-term deficits and frequent hospital admissions [39, 40].

14.3.3 Neurologic Complications from Oral Cancer Surgery

Several cranial nerves (CN) and the cervical plexus are sacrificed indispensably or accidentally during resection of primary tumors as well as neck dissection for removal of primary tumor and/or involved lymph nodes. Tumor size and location and the extent of neck disease if present often necessitate cranial nerves directly involved or in close proximity to be sacrificed. Furthermore the approaches often required to access and ensure adequate tumor resection can endanger the cranial nerves in the vicinity.

14.3.3.1 Lingual Nerve (CN V3)

The lingual nerve provides sensation and taste innervation, via the chorda tympani branch of the facial nerve, to the anterior 2/3 of the ipsilateral tongue. In the case of the cancer of the tongue and the floor of the mouth, the nerve should be cut during excision of the tongue and floor of mouth because of direct invasion of the primary tumor. However the nerve is usually preserved during neck dissection without resection of primary tumor; it may be injured accidentally during submandibular dissection. Ipsilateral loss of sensation to the tongue from lingual nerve injury can further impact on the difficulties with mastication, speech, and swallowing, and the patient may bite his or her tongue during speech and mastication. These injuries can occur from traction or dissection around the lingual nerve during surgery and may not always be recognized until later in the postoperative course. A compromised ability to taste foods due to chorda tympani nerve injury may also contribute to decreased food intake and malnutrition. Rehabilitation for speech and swallowing, using physical therapy, is usually beneficial for these patients [41].

14.3.3.2 Facial Nerve (CN VII): Marginal Mandibular Branch

Although the most common cause of facial nerve disorder is parotidectomy for the parotid gland tumors, the marginal mandibular branch of the facial nerve may be the most frequently damaged among the branches of facial nerve during oral cancer surgery with incision of submandibular region, elevation of the flaps for standard neck dissections, and access to the oral cavity for composite resections. The nerve runs at the undersurface of the platysma muscle and is superficial to the facial vein at the submandibular gland region. Injury to this nerve causes alteration of the mobility of the corner of the mouth due to the disruption of the innervation to the orbicularis oris and depressor anguli oris muscles. In addition to the functional disturbance, the damage of this branch has adverse cosmetic consequences. Inability to control the movement of the lower lip can interfere with liquid consumption.

Careful planning of the incisions, taking into consideration the route of the nerve and early identification during flap elevation, is the best way of preventing inadvertent injury to this branch of the facial nerve. Some functionality is normally restored if the neurologic injury is due to traction and not severance of the nerve, but it may take several months for spontaneous neurosensory recovery [41].

14.3.3.3 Vagus Nerve (CN X): Recurrent Laryngeal Nerve and Superior Laryngeal Nerve

Vagus nerve extends through the jugular foramen, then passes into the carotid sheath between the internal carotid artery and the internal jugular vein down to the neck, chest, and abdomen, where it contributes to the innervation of the viscera. Direct or indirect injury to the vagus nerve or its branches, specifically the recurrent and superior laryngeal nerves, can occur during dissection around the carotid sheath. This is mostly due to the traction on the main trunk of the nerve, or lack of identification of the nerve during neck dissection, or placement of hemostatic clips and use of electrocautery to control hemorrhage during surgery. Unilateral true vocal cord paralysis, in the median or paramedian position, is the result of injury to the recurrent laryngeal nerve and is generally well tolerated due to compensation from the intact contralateral vocal cord. However, mild to moderate hoarseness and diminished cough efforts are commonly experienced by patients. This problem becomes even more concerning in cases of bilateral injury when upper airway obstruction may result. Injury to the branches of the superior laryngeal nerve can occur during dissection around the superior thyroid branch of the external carotid artery. This may result in minor swallowing difficulties due to decreased sensation at the laryngeal inlet or decreased tensor capability of the true vocal cord. Early fatigability and decreased ability to phonate high-pitched sounds may seriously affect professional vocalists or public speakers. Direct laryngoscopy alone or in combination with motor speech evaluation and a high index of suspicion can all assist in the accurate diagnosis of these neurologic injuries. Prevention remains the best management, and patients who depend on their voice professionally require a detailed consultation and evaluation before and after surgery [30].

14.3.3.4 Spinal Accessory Nerve (CN XI)

Radical resection of the cervical lymph nodes, with adjacent muscles, vessels, and nerves including spinal accessory nerve, was advocated. This type of radical surgery was accompanied by serious postoperative functional and aesthetic complications, especially shoulder pain and spinal accessory nerve dysfunction. Pain, muscle weakness, shoulder movement restraint, deformity, and inability to lift up the upper extremity above 90° are the results of denervation of the trapezius muscle. Recently, the approach to cervical lymph nodes metastasis has been changed from radical neck dissection (RND) to modified RND to conserve the spinal accessory nerve and/or vein and muscle. However, nerve preservation is not synonymous with nerve function preservation, and "shoulder syndrome" can develop even when the spinal accessory nerve is not sacrificed. Some debate exists in the literature regarding the actual incidence of developing shoulder syndrome even after preserving the spinal accessory nerve. All studies have clearly demonstrated that when the nerve trunk and its anastomosis with the cervical plexus are preserved, patients have better postoperative function and significantly less pain and deformity. Careful dissection around the vicinity of the nerve, limited use of

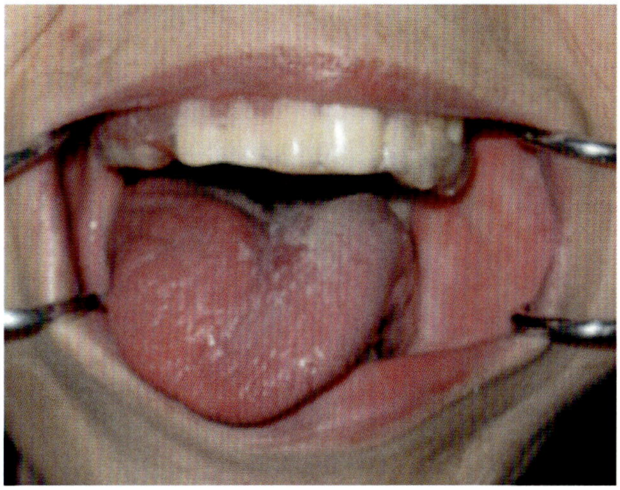

Fig. 14.3 Right hypoglossal nerve dysfunction with deviation of the tongue to the ipsilateral side following RND

electrocautery, and early identification based on known anatomical landmarks may help to limit surgically induced neural trauma [30].

14.3.3.5 Hypoglossal Nerve (CN XII)

The hypoglossal nerve provides motor innervation to the ipsilateral tongue. The nerve may be injured iatrogenically during neck dissection. Unless there is gross neural invasion by the cancer, the path of the nerve runs directly through the tumor, or when there is adhesion to metastatic lymph node with extranodal spread, the nerve is usually preserved. Hypoglossal nerve dysfunction can present with subclinical symptoms with deviation of the tongue to the ipsilateral side of injury (Fig. 14.3), accidental tongue biting, and dysarthria. Patients may also experience an amplification of their difficulties with mastication and swallowing that are already present following surgery. In cases of bilateral hypoglossal nerve injury, upper airway obstruction can occur when the patient is placed in a supine position. Additionally, atrophy of the muscles of the tongue can occur and add to the functional difficulties experienced by these patients.

14.3.3.6 Phrenic Nerve (C4)

The phrenic nerve is a nerve that originates in the neck (C3–C5) and passes down between the lung and heart to reach the diaphragm. It is important for breathing since the phrenic nerve is the motor innervation to this muscle. The injury to the phrenic nerve is another neurologic complication that may be encountered during neck dissection. This causes paralysis to the ipsilateral diaphragm as there are two phrenic nerves, the left and the right one. The diaphragm is responsible for 70 % of the respiratory movement and long-term pulmonary complications can originate from this type of injury. An attempt to limit the surgical dissection to a layer superficial to the pre-vertebral fascia, with identification of the nerve, may assist surgeons in preventing this complication [41].

14.3.3.7 Brachial Plexus (C5–C8, T1)

The brachial plexus is a network of nerve fibers, running from the spine, formed by the ventral rami of the lower fourth cervical and first thoracic nerve roots. It proceeds through the neck, the axilla (armpit region), and into the arm. An attempt to limit the surgical dissection to a layer superficial to the pre-vertebral fascia and careful use of electrocautery for hemostasis and dissection of fascia, with identification of the nerve, may assist surgeons in preventing this nerve injury.

14.3.3.8 Sympathetic Trunk

Disruption of the sympathetic trunk nerve fibers may cause ipsilateral Horner's syndrome. This is usually due to a surgical dissection that extends too far medially behind the carotid sheath. Horner's syndrome involves blepharoptosis (drooping of the upper eyelid) from loss of sympathetic innervation to the superior tarsal muscle, miosis (small pupils) or pupillary constriction, anhidrosis (decreased sweating on the affected side of the face), enophthalmos (the impression that the eye is sunk in), vascular dilation, and bloodshot conjunctiva. Since Horner's syndrome may reflect serious disease in the neck or chest (such as metastasis, tumor in the apex of the lung, thyrocervical venous dilatation, or vascular injuries), early recognition is of high importance.

References

1. Rubinstein EB, Peterson DE, Schubert M et al (2004) Clinical practice guidelines for the prevention and treatment of cancer therapy-induced oral and gastrointestinal mucositis. Cancer 100(S9): 2026–2046
2. Patni N, Patni S, Bapna N, Somani M, Gupta A, Ratnam BV (2004) The role amifostine in prophylaxis of radiotherapy induced mucositis and xerostomia in head and neck cancer. J Clin Oncol 22(14S):55–68
3. Sonis St, Eilers JP, Epstein JB et al (1999) Validation of a new scoring system for the assessment of clinical trial research of oral mucositis induced by radiation or chemotherapy. Mucositis Study Group. Cancer 85:2103–2113
4. Harrison JS, Dale RA, Haveman CW, Redding SW (2003) Oral complications in radiation therapy. Gen Dent 51(6):552–560
5. World Health Organization (1979) WHO handbook for reporting results of cancer treatment. World Health Organization, Geneva
6. Trotti A, Colevas AD, Setser A et al (2003) CTCAE v3.0: development of a comprehensive grading system for the adverse effects of cancer treatment. Semin Radiat Oncol 13:176–181
7. Eilers J (2004) Nursing interventions and supportive care for the prevention and treatment of oral mucositis associated with cancer treatment. Oncol Nurs Forum 31(Suppl 4):13–23
8. Kostler WJ, Hejna M, Wenzel C, Zielinski CC (2001) Oral mucositis complicating chemotherapy and/or radiotherapy: options for prevention and treatment. CA Cancer J Clin 51:290–315

9. Silverman S Jr (1999) Oral cancer : complications of therapy. Oral Surg Oral Med Oral Pathol Oral Radiol Endod 88(2):122–126
10. Kaminsky SB, Cillette WB, O'Lealy TJ (1978) Sodium absorption associated with oral hygiene procedures. J Am Dent Assoc 114: 644–646
11. Chambers MS, Garden AS et al (2007) Xerostomia and mucositis. In: Werning JW (ed) Oral cancer diagnosis, management, and rehabilitation. Thieme, New York
12. Eisbruch A, Kim HM et al (2001) Xerostomia and its predictors following parotid-sparing irradiation of head-and-neck cancer. Int J Radiat Oncol Biol Phys 50:695–704
13. Eisbruch A, Ten Haken RK et al (1999) Dose, volume, and function relationships in parotid salivary glands followirlg conformal and intensify-modulated irradiation of head and neck cancer. Int J Radiat Oncol Biol Phys 45:577–587
14. Cox JD, Stetz J, Pajak TF (1995) Toxicity criteria of the radiation therapy oncology group (RTOG) and the European organization for research and treatment of cancer (EORTC). Int J Radiat Oncol Biol Phys 31:1341–1346
15. Leek H, Albensson M (2002) Pilocarpine treatment of xerostomia in head and neck patients. Micron 33:153–1155
16. Berger AM, Kilroy T (1998) Oral complications of cancer therapy. In: Berger AM, Portenoy RK, Weissman DE (eds) Principles and practice of supportive oncology. Lippincott-Raven, Philadelphia, pp 223–236
17. Logemann JA, Smith CH, Paulos BR et al (2001) Effect of xerostomia on perception and performance of swallow function. Head Neck 23:317–321
18. Rode M, Smid L, Budihna M et al (2001) The influence of pilocarpine and biperiden on pH value and calcium, phosphate, and bicarbonate concentrations in saliva during and after radiotherapy for head and neck cancer. Oral Surg Oral Med Oral Pathol Oral Radiol Endod 92:509–514
19. Silverman S Jr (2003) Complications of treatment. In: Silverman S Jr (ed) Oral cancer, 5th edn. BC Decker, Hamilton
20. Tibbles PM, Edelsberg JS (1996) Hyperbaric-oxygen therapy. N Engl J Med 335:1642–1648
21. Morrish RB, Chan E, Silverman S Jr et al (1981) Osteonecrosis in patients irradiated for head and neck carcinoma. Cancer 47: 1980–1983
22. Beumer J, Silverman S Jr, Benak S (1972) Hard and soft tissue necroses following radiation therapy for oral cancer. J Pros Dent 27:640–644
23. Murray CG, Herson J, Daly TE et al (1980) Radiation necrosis of the mandible: a 10-year study. Int J Radiat Oncol Biol Phys 6:543–548
24. 9068: Oral Cancer and Complications of Cancer Therapies. http://www.netce.com/coursecontent.php?courseid=778. Accessed 21 Nov 2013
25. David LA, Sandor GKB, Evans AW, Brown DH (2001) Hyperbaric oxygen therapy and mandibular osteoradionecrosis: a retrospective study and analysis of treatment outcomes. J Can Dent Assoc 67:384
26. Rankin KV, Jones DL (eds) (1999) Oral health in cancer therapy: a guide for health care professionals. DOEP, Texas Cancer Council, Austin
27. Kielbassa AM, Munz I, Bruggmoser G, Schulte-Monting J (2002) Effect of demineralization and remineralization on microhardness of irradiated dentin. J Clin Dent 13:104–110
28. Epstein JB, Chin EA, Jacobson JJ et al (1998) The relationships among fluoride, cariogenic oral flora, and salivary flow rate during radiation therapy. Oral Surg Oral Med Oral Pathol Oral Radiol Endod 86:286–292
29. Kerawala CJ (2010) Complications of head and neck cancer surgery: prevention and management. Oral Oncol 46:433–435
30. Kolokythas A (2010) Long-term surgical complications in the oral cancer patient: comprehensive review. Part I. J Oral Maxillofac Res 1(3):e1/p1-10. http://www.ejomr.org/JOMR/archives/2010/3/e1/e1ht.pdfÄulnoneÄstrike0. Accessed 22 Nov 2013
31. LaBlance GR, Kraus K, Steckol KF (1991) Rehabilitation of swallowing and communication following glossectomy. Rehabil Nurs 16:266–270
32. Pauloski BR, Logemann JA, Colangelo LA, Rademaker AW et al (1998) Surgical variables affecting speech in treated patients with oral and oropharyngeal cancer. Laryngoscope 108:908–916
33. Pauloski BR, Logemann JA, Rademaker AW, McConnel FM et al (1993) Speech and swallowing function after anterior tongue and floor of mouth resection with distal flap reconstruction. J Speech Hear Res 36:267–276
34. Logemann JA (1988) The role of the speech language pathologist in the management of dysphagia. Otolaryngol Clin North Am 21:783–788, Review
35. Rentschler GJ, Mann MB (1980) The effects of glossectomy on intelligibility of speech and oral perceptual discrimination. J Oral Surg 38:348–354
36. Urken ML, Buchbinder D, Weinberg H, Vickery C et al (1991) Functional evaluation following microvascular oromandibular reconstruction of the oral cancer patient: a comparative study of reconstructed and nonreconstructed patients. Laryngoscope 101: 935–950
37. Vaughan ED (1982) An analysis of morbidity following major head and neck surgery with particular reference to mouth function. J Maxillofac Surg 10:129–134
38. Vaughan ED, Bainton R, Martin IC (1992) Improvements in morbidity of mouth cancer using microvascular free flap reconstructions. J Craniomaxillofac Surg 20:132–134
39. Hooley R, Levin H, Flores TC, Wheeler T, Steigeo E (1983) Predicting postoperative head and neck complications using nutritional assessment. Arch Otolaryngol 109:83–85
40. Picker H, Bichler E (1985) Nutritional and immunological investigations in head and neck cancer patients before and after therapy. Arch Otorhinolaryngol 242:149–153
41. Kim DD, Ord RA (2003) Complications in the treatment of head and neck cancer. Oral Maxillofac Surg Clin North Am 15:213–227

15 Oral and Dental Healthcare for Oral Cancer Patients: Planning, Management, and Dental Treatment

Kouji Katsura and Kumiko Aoki

Abstract

In recent years, the curability of oral cancers has increased because of improvements in cancer treatments, including radiotherapy, surgery, and chemotherapy. However, these treatments frequently cause dental and oral adverse events, including oral dysfunction, mucositis, salivary dysfunction, rampant dental caries, and osteonecrosis of jaws. Such dental and oral adverse events do not only lead to patient discomfort but also to decreased overall survival rate of patients owing to the required change of treatment regimen. Further, patients' quality of life is negatively influenced because of pain and oral dysfunction, along with concerns regarding adverse events and recurrence of cancer following cancer treatment. Therefore, the prevention and alleviation of such adverse events is paramount in maintaining oral health of patients with oral cancer. This chapter outlines planning and management procedures required to maintain an oral cancer patient's oral health.

Keywords

Chemotherapy • Dental management • Oral adverse event • Oral healthcare • Radiotherapy

15.1 Oral and Dental Healthcare for Oral Cancer Patients Receiving Head and Neck Radiotherapy

15.1.1 Oral and Dental Healthcare for Head and Neck Radiotherapy Patients

Representative oral adverse events associated with radiotherapy are shown in Table 15.1. Oral adverse events during radiotherapy do not only lead to patient discomfort but also to a reduced overall survival rate due to changes in treatment regimen. Oral adverse events after radiotherapy negatively influence the quality of a patient's life not only by causing discomfort but also through oral dysfunction. Furthermore, cancer patients are anxious about adverse events and recurrence after cancer treatments.

15.1.1.1 Radiation-Induced Oral Mucositis (Figs. 15.1 and 15.2)

Radiation-induced oral mucositis is a frequent and potentially dose-limiting acute adverse event that afflicts most radiation patients. Severe oral mucositis of grade 3 or 4 according to the Common Terminology Criteria for Adverse Events (CTCAE) v3.0 occurs in 35 % and 45 % of head and neck cancer patients undergoing radiotherapy alone and concurrent chemoradiotherapy, respectively. Radiation-induced oral mucositis directly affects patient prognosis given that half of the patients with such severe mucositis require a change in treatment regimen and/or a decrease in the total radiation dose. In addition, radiation-induced mucositis of the head and neck region may not only lead to pain but also

K. Katsura (✉)
Division of Oral and Maxillofacial Radiology, Niigata University Graduate School of Medical and Dental Sciences, 2-5274 Gakkocho-dori, Chuo-ku, Niigata 951-8514, Japan
e-mail: katsu@dent.niigata-u.ac.jp

K. Aoki
Department of Oral and Maxillofacial Surgery, Nara Medical University, School of Medicine, Nara, Japan
e-mail: kaoki@naramed-u.ac.jp

T. Kirita and K. Omura (eds.), *Oral Cancer: Diagnosis and Therapy*, DOI 10.1007/978-4-431-54938-3_15, © Springer Japan 2015

to aspiration pneumonia and malnutrition due to oral and pharyngeal dysfunction. The common sites where oral mucositis occurs are the buccal mucosa, tongue margin, and soft palate, although mucositis occurs on all mucosa included within the radiation field. The pathway of radiation- and chemotherapy-induced mucositis is described by Sonis [1]. Clinically, it occurs from day 7 of irradiation and becomes worse in a dose-dependent manner; it heals promptly within 2–3 weeks after the end of radiotherapy provided that there are no accompanying bacterial infections [1, 2].

The risk factors of radiation-induced oral mucositis are shown in Table 15.2. Accelerated hyperfractionation and concurrent chemotherapy are the most important treatment factors for oral mucositis. Since most of the patient-related factors of mucositis can be avoided by oral and dental management, such management before and during radiotherapy is of paramount importance. Recently, various clinical trials using sucralfate, chlorhexidine, or antimicrobial lozenges have been performed to prevent and treat radiation-induced oral mucositis; however, the Multinational Association of

Table 15.1 Representative oral adverse events associated with radiotherapy

During radiotherapy	After radiotherapy
Mucositis Salivary gland dysfunction Taste disturbance	Caries Periodontal disease Salivary gland dysfunction Trismus
	Osteoradionecrosis of jaws
	Hypoplasia of jaws Dental developmental abnormalities

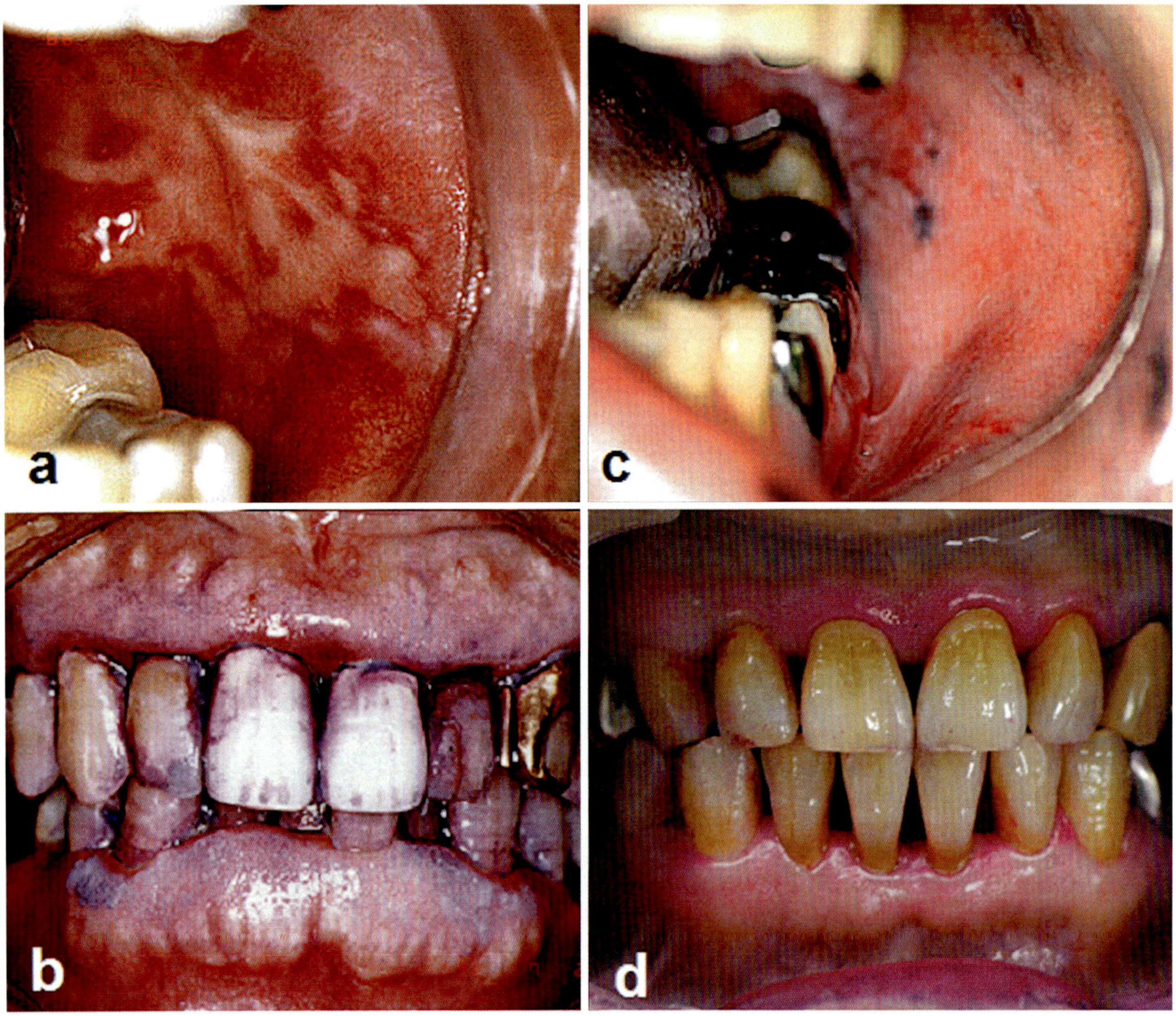

Fig. 15.1 Radiation-induced oral mucositis. Patients with tongue cancer receiving external beam radiotherapy with concurrent chemotherapy (radiation dose in the oral cavity: 56 Gy). *Intraoral photographs* indicate that the patient with poor oral hygiene (**a**, **b**) suffered from more severe oral mucositis compared with the patient with good oral hygiene (**c**, **d**) despite receiving the same radiation dose

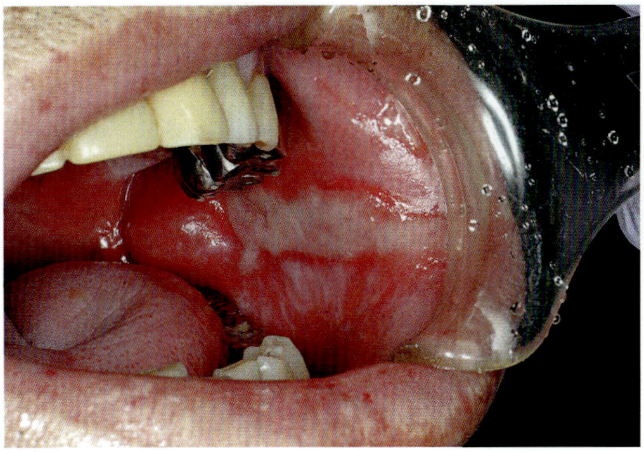

Fig. 15.2 Radiation-induced oral mucositis. A patient with nasopharyngeal cancer who received intensity-modulated radiation therapy (IMRT). *Intraoral photograph* at 36 Gy indicates an exaggerated mucositis along the dental arch by backscattered radiation

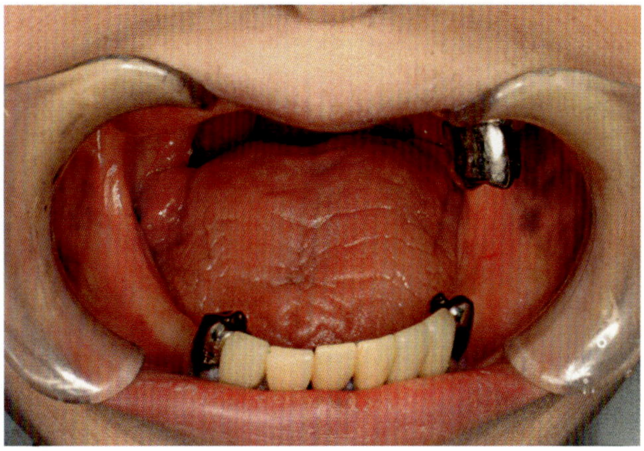

Fig. 15.3 Radiation-induced salivary gland dysfunction and taste disturbances. A patient with nasopharyngeal cancer who received external beam radiotherapy (70 Gy) with concurrent chemotherapy. *Intraoral photograph* indicates a dry mouth and a smooth tongue resulting from taste bud atrophy

Table 15.2 Risk factors for radiation-induced oral mucositis

Patient factors	Treatment factors
Age	Total radiation dose
Gender	Radiation dose rate
Europhile count	Radiation fraction size
Nutritional status	Radiation field size
Tobacco	Radiation site
Alcohol	Concurrent chemotherapy
Oral hygiene	
Amount of saliva	
Orthodontic appliance	
Dental metal	
Sharp tooth edge	

Supportive Care in Cancer (MASCC) clinical practice guidelines recommend oral care, midline radiation blocks, three dimensional radiation, and benzydamine [3].

15.1.1.2 Radiation-Induced Salivary Gland Dysfunction (Radiation Xerostomia) and Taste Disturbance (Fig. 15.3)

Radiation-induced salivary gland dysfunction and taste disturbance are highly frequent acute or late adverse events that afflict most radiation patients similarly to oral mucositis. Salivary gland dysfunction is caused by ischemia following vascular occlusion and atrophy of the acinous cells [4, 5]. The degree of dysfunction depends on the radiation dose and the irradiated volume of the parotid gland; the dysfunction is nonreversible when the irradiated volume exceeds 75 % and the radiation dose is between 30 Gy and 45 Gy. Therefore, most external irradiation patients with oral cancer cannot recover after treatment [6]. Salivary dysfunction leads to oral adverse events, such as dental caries, periodontitis, and oral infections, which decrease the buffering capacity and antibacterial effect of saliva. Clinically, most patients complain about the viscosity of their saliva from day 3 and dry mouth from day 14 of radiotherapy; treatment with pilocarpine hydrochloride, a salivation accelerant, is prescribed. If the effects of pilocarpine hydrochloride are insufficient, a moisturizer is co-prescribed. Finally, if symptoms do not improve, herbal medicines such as byakkokaninjinto or bakumondoto may be prescribed. In recent years, mitigation of radiation-induced salivary gland dysfunction by a dose reduction to the parotid gland using intensity-modulated radiation therapy (IMRT) has been studied [7].

Radiation-induced taste disturbance is caused by atrophy of the taste buds by radiation [8] and is also affected by tongue coating and hyposalivation. Clinically, most patients complain of hypogeusia from day 7 of radiotherapy and some patients progress to ageusia from approximately day 14; near-normal taste levels are recovered 90–180 days after the end of irradiation [9] and only a few patients continue to have dysgeusia for over a year. Taste disturbance during radiotherapy does not only impair the patients' quality of life but also their nutritional status and motivation for cancer treatment; appropriate supportive care, such as oral care instructions including tongue brushing and moisture retention of the oral cavity, is therefore required. Dietary modifications following the counseling of a nutritionist are also important. Finally, zinc sulfate, which aids taste bud cell regeneration, has been reported to accelerate the recovery from taste disturbance [10].

15.1.1.3 Radiation Caries and Periodontal Disease (Fig. 15.4)

Radiation caries and periodontal disease are highly frequent late adverse events and are a major risk factor for osteoradionecrosis. Therefore, periodic oral and dental management after radiotherapy for their prevention is essential. Radiation causes the following changes in tooth and periodontal tissues: (i) a decrease in the microhardness of the dentin; (ii) gap formation

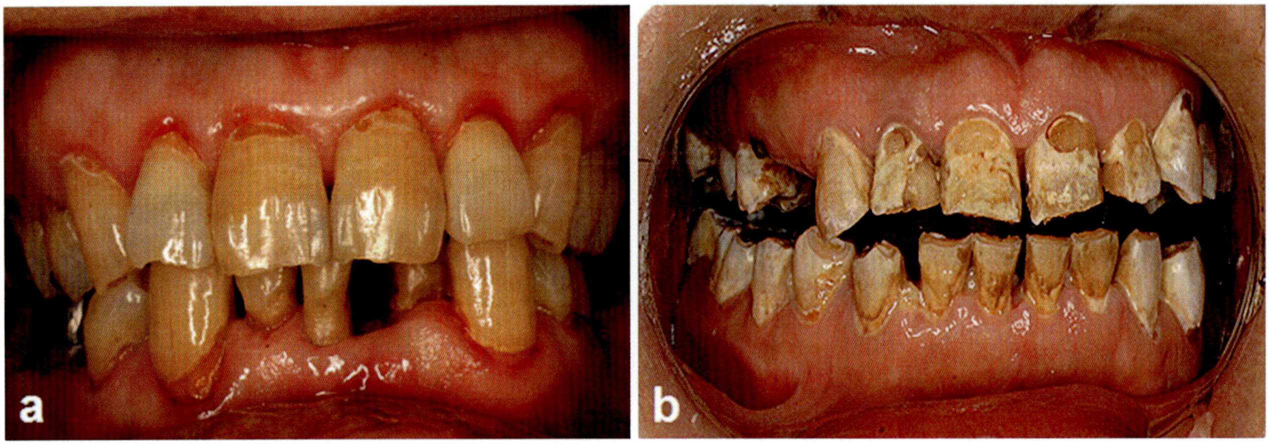

Fig. 15.4 Radiation caries and periodontitis. (**a**) A patient with tongue cancer who received postoperative external beam radiotherapy (60 Gy). *Intraoral photograph* 2 years after radiotherapy indicates multiple root surface caries, gingival swelling, and gingival redness. (**b**) Advanced case of radiation caries: a patient with floor of mouth cancer who received postoperative external beam radiotherapy (60 Gy). *Intraoral photograph* 6 months after radiotherapy indicates advanced multiple root surface caries

at the enamel–dentin junction; (iii) derangement of periodontal ligament fiber; and (iv) cytopenia, hypovascularization, and fibrosis of periodontal tissues [11–13]. However, the main factor influencing radiation caries and periodontitis is thought to be radiation-induced salivary dysfunction given that the above radiogenic damages are mild [14].

The preferred sites for radiation caries are the occlusal surface and cervical region of the tooth, indicating that they occur on the exposed dentin. Cervical caries, in particular, must be carefully monitored since an attachment loss of approximately 1–2 mm develops after radiotherapy [15]. Radiation caries progress rapidly; DMFT has been reported to increase to 7.7 within 4 years after radiotherapy [16]. Following strong hypersensitivity symptoms on a tooth, the radiation caries turns into pulpitis. In addition, oral radiotherapy patients often present with trismus.

The use of topical fluoride applications is recommended to prevent radiation caries following head and neck radiotherapy. However, Spak et al. described that 80 % of patients with an unstimulated salivary flow rate of <0.1 mL/min may develop at least 1 carious lesion per year, despite daily applications of a fluoride gel [17]. Topical fluoride applications may not be able to completely control dental caries in irradiated patients with severe hyposalivation for the following reasons: (i) extended meal times due to dysphagia caused by hyposalivation, causing demineralization of the root surface to progress more during meals, and (ii) the calcium and phosphate required for remineralization are insufficiently supplied due to the considerable decrease in saliva. Remineralizing agents have been added to topical fluoride applications with an aim to improve caries control in hyposalivation patients [18, 19].

Radiation periodontal disease progresses as rapidly as radiation caries and causes tooth loss by resorption of the alveolar bone; poor oral hygiene caused by hyposalivation and periodontal tissue atrophy caused by radiation are its main causes. Radiation periodontal disease can be stabilized through good oral hygiene. However, inflammatory symptoms such as the swelling and redness of the gingiva may often be unclear due to hypovascularization of periodontal tissue caused by radiation. Therefore, periodical evaluation of periodontal tissue through dental and/or panoramic radiography is necessary.

15.1.1.4 Trismus

Trismus, or limited jaw mobility, has been reported in 6–86 % patients who received radiation to the temporomandibular joint and/or the masseter/pterygoid muscles. The different incidence rates are attributed to a difference in the observation period and evaluation methods. The prevalence of trismus after conventional radiation, IMRT, and chemoradiotherapy has been reported to be approximately 25 %, 5 %, and 30 %, respectively. In addition, the prevalence increases following a higher radiation dose (over 60 Gy). The main cause of trismus is fibrosis of the soft tissue included within the radiation field. The early treatment of trismus aims to minimize the limitation of jaw mobility after radiotherapy; treatment should begin upon the first presentation of clinical signs of impaired jaw mobility. Treatment consists of a forced jaw opening exercise using various appliances. The US National Cancer Institute recommends opening of the jaw as wide as possible without causing pain 20 times, 3 times a day.

15.1.1.5 Osteoradionecrosis of the Jaws (Figs. 15.5 and 15.6)

Osteoradionecrosis of the jaws is a rare late adverse event. However, patients suffering from osteoradionecrosis of the jaws experience a substantial deterioration in their quality of life due to serious clinical symptoms such as chronic spontaneous pain, dysphagia, and facial deformation.

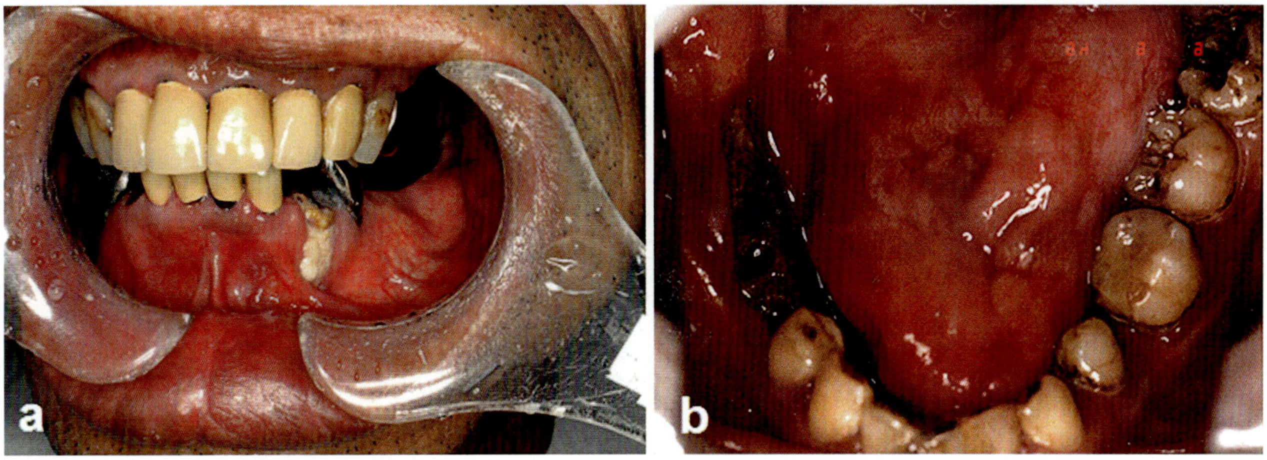

Fig. 15.5 Osteoradionecrosis of the jaw. (**a**) A patient with tongue cancer who received postoperative external beam radiotherapy (50 Gy). *Intraoral photograph* 5 years after radiotherapy indicates a severe gingival recession with bone exposure in the first premolar region. (**b**) A patient with tongue cancer who received interstitial radiotherapy (Cs-137, 75 Gy). *Intraoral photograph* 3 years after radiotherapy indicates bone exposure after extraction of the second premolar and first molar

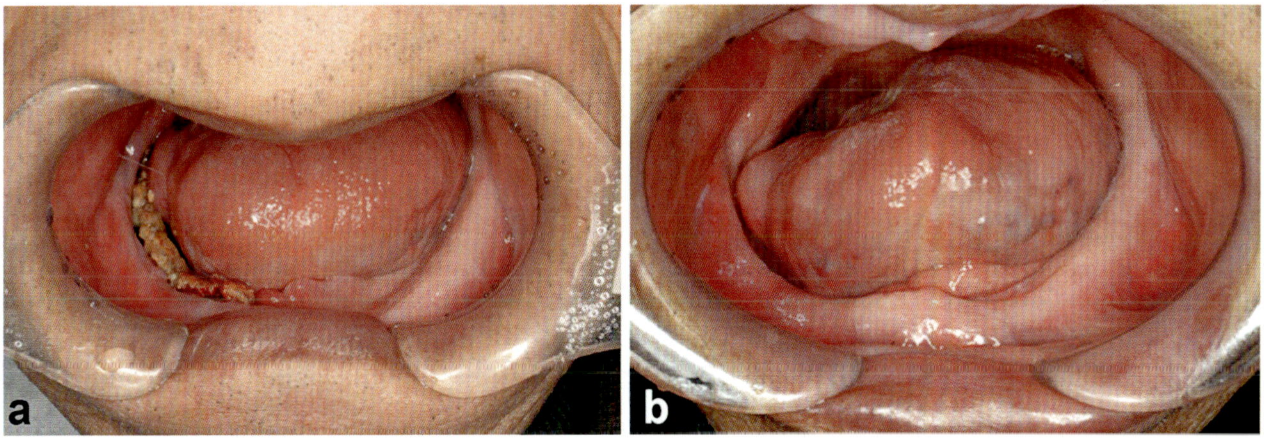

Fig. 15.6 Osteoradionecrosis of the jaw. A patient with tongue cancer who received interstitial radiotherapy (Cs-137, 75 Gy). (**a**) *Intraoral photograph* 5 years after radiotherapy indicates bone exposure induced because of the incompatibility of a complete denture. (**b**) Osteoradionecrosis healed by denture adjustment and conservative treatment without surgery 7 years after the onset of bone exposure

The risk factors for osteoradionecrosis of the jaws are the location of the primary tumor relative to the jaws, the radiation dose received by the jaws, and oral conditions such as dental caries with periapical lesion, periodontal disease, and poor oral hygiene [20–23]; predominant risk factors are shown in Table 15.3. In addition, osteoradionecrosis of the jaws is classified into spontaneous and traumatic osteoradionecrosis. Endarteritis, hyperemia, hyalinization, cellular loss, hypovascularization, thrombosis, and fibrosis are the most common histological findings in spontaneous osteoradionecrosis [24]; the pathogenesis is described as hypovascular, hypocellular, and hypoxic tissue formation [25]. These changes are the direct, dose-dependent, and irreversible effects of radiation. Traumatic osteoradionecrosis of the jaws occurs for a long period after radiotherapy and is caused by dental caries with periapical lesion, periodontal disease (Fig. 15.5a), teeth extraction (Fig. 15.5b), poor oral hygiene, and inadequate denture irritation (Fig. 15.6); tooth extraction

Table 15.3 Risk factors of osteoradionecrosis of jaws

Patient factors	Treatment factors
Tooth extraction	Total radiation dose
Teeth with periapical lesions	Radiation dose rate
Inadequate denture	Radiation fraction size
Oral hygiene	Radiation field size
Tobacco	Radiation site
Alcohol	Concurrent chemotherapy
Poor nutritional status	Mandibular resection
Tumor location	Neck dissection

is the greatest risk factor. The most common reasons for tooth extraction are untreatable dental caries and periodontitis. Therefore, periodical oral management is essential to decrease the risk of dental caries and periodontitis. In fact, the incidence rate of osteoradionecrosis of the jaws is decreased to less than 10 % by systematic oral management before and after radiotherapy [26].

There is no established cure for osteoradionecrosis of the jaws, although conservative treatments such as local irrigation and antimicrobial administration are considered to be the safest. Segmental or marginal mandibulectomy combined with hyperbaric oxygen therapy can be performed if conservative treatment is difficult to perform. In this case, the patient's quality of life is seriously impaired by dysfunction and deformity of the jaws.

15.1.1.6 Hypoplasia of the Jaws and Dental Development Abnormalities (Fig. 15.7)

Hypoplasia of the jaws and dental development abnormalities caused by radiation are limited to the radiation area. When patients receiving radiotherapy are younger, these abnormalities become more severe; the effects of radiation are stronger in patients aged 12 years or younger due to jaw growth and the formation of permanent teeth. Representative dental abnormalities caused by radiation are dental agenesis, microdontia, enamel hypoplasia, and shortened or tapering root. These adverse events do not only cause oral dysfunction and facial dysmorphic disorders but also mental distress in patients. Therefore, the long-term follow-up by a pediatrician, a psychiatrist, a plastic surgeon, and a dentist is required.

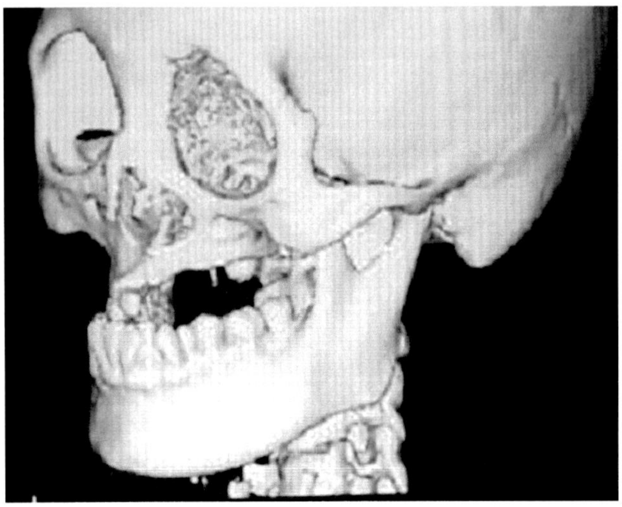

Fig. 15.7 A patient with osteosarcoma of the left maxilla who received external beam radiotherapy during childhood (details of radiotherapy are unclear). A three-dimensional reconstruction CT image indicates maxillary growth retardation and dental agenesis of the left side

15.1.2 Planning and Management for Head and Neck Radiotherapy Patients

Oral and dental management for head and neck radiotherapy patients aims to prevent and alleviate acute and late oral adverse events in order to improve the patient's overall survival rate and quality of life. Given that the treatments available for teeth included in the radiation field are limited, dentists and dental hygienists have to confirm or speculate the radiation field before dental treatment or management. Dental management for radiotherapy patients can be performed in three stages, namely before, during, and after radiotherapy. These stages aim to prepare the base for alleviation and prevention of acute and late oral adverse effects and improve the patient's quality of life. If the pre-radiotherapy stage is not conducted appropriately, subsequent stages cannot proceed smoothly. For reference, Table 15.4 shows the summary of our oral management protocol for radiotherapy patients. Considering the increasing number of cancer survivors, it is expected that dental management after radiotherapy will soon be provided in general dental clinics.

15.1.2.1 Oral and Dental Management Before Radiotherapy

The purpose of oral and dental management before radiotherapy is to lay the base for alleviation and prevention of acute and late oral adverse events. It consists of patient education and oral conditioning for head and neck radiotherapy. Ideally, oral and dental management including dental treatment should start within 2–3 weeks before radiotherapy.

Patient Education

Patient education aims to elucidate the oral adverse events caused by radiotherapy (appearance day, degree, duration, and negative effects on cancer treatment and patient's quality of life) and to instruct on their prevention and alleviation (oral self-care and interventional schedule of professional oral care). Since patient education is the most important factor in the prevention and alleviation of oral adverse events, the healthcare provider must take care to illustrate these comprehensibly. In addition, building a good rapport between medical care providers and patients is also an essential condition for a successful outcome.

Oral and Dental Conditioning

Oral and dental conditioning aims to remove the oral risk factor of radiation mucositis and osteoradionecrosis, as well as the oral sources of infection. Because the extraction of a tooth included within the radiation field is contraindicated after radiotherapy in principle, an untreatable tooth within the radiation field must be extracted before radiotherapy (Table. 15.4). In addition, when radiotherapy is started before the tooth extraction wound epithelializes, the immature

Table 15.4 Summary of our oral management protocol for patients receiving head and neck radiotherapy

Stage I	Stage II	Stage III
Before radiotherapy	During radiotherapy	After radiotherapy
Patient education	Self oral care	Preventive dental maintenance
Oral care instruction	Oral cleaning (3 times/day)	9,000 ppm fluoride application (every 3 months)
Removal of oral risk factors for radiation mucositis (refer Table 14.2)	Mouth rinsing and mouth moisture retention (8 times/day)	Periodontal examination and scaling (every 6 months)
Extraction of teeth with poor prognosis (particularly, teeth within the radiation field)	Denture cleaning (3 times/day)	Radiography examination (every 12 months)
Untreatable teeth	Professional oral care (once/week)	Resumption of dental treatment
Acute symptomatic teeth with apical lesions	Oral examination	
Teeth requiring surgical endodontics	Oral cleaning	
Advanced periodontal disease (>6 mm pocket depth and >60 % alveolar bone loss)	Symptomatic treatment	
Partially erupted third molar		
Temporary dental treatment		
Spacer production		

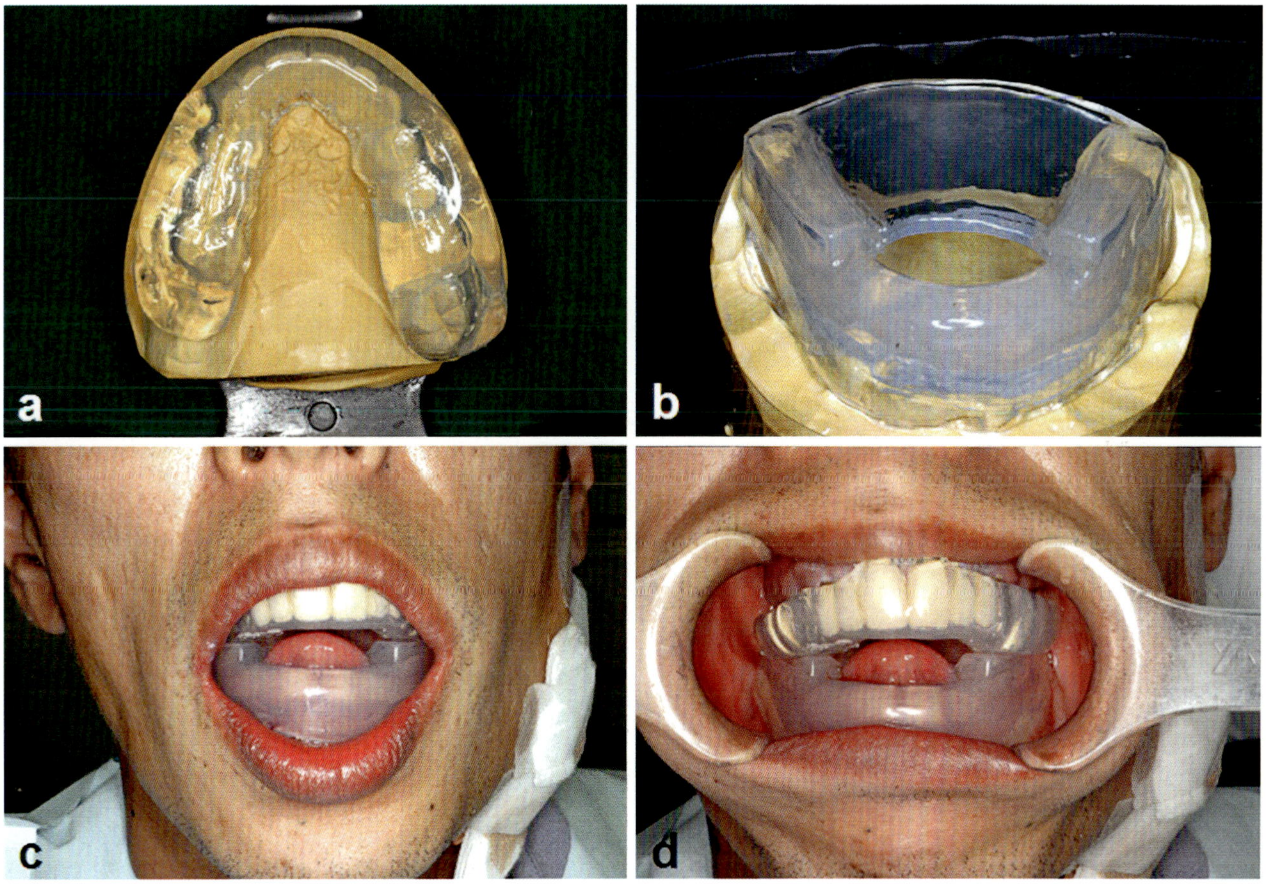

Fig. 15.8 Spacer provided to protect oral mucosa from the backscatter radiation. (**a**) Spacer for the upper jaw. (**b**) Spacer for the lower jaw with tongue-depressing plate. (**c**, **d**) Spacer in appropriate position. Note the anterior positioning of the tongue by the patient

granulation tissue will often slough off, causing osteoradionecrosis. Therefore, it is recommended that tooth extraction is performed at least 14 days before the start of radiotherapy and that the wound is fully closed.

Intraoral orthodontic appliances and metal dental restorations cause dose escalation at the surface of the oral mucosa due to backscattered radiation and are thus specific risk factors for radiation mucositis (Fig. 15.2). Therefore, an orthodontic appliance must be removed before the commencement of radiotherapy. Nevertheless, the removal of dental metal restorations such as full metal crowns incurs problems given that the time from their removal to the provisional restoration is limited as well as a financial burden due to the need of remanufacture after removal of the restoration is high. A spacer can be used to resolve these problems (Fig. 15.8), as it can eliminate the need for the removal of the metal dental restoration.

Since the influence of the backscatter radiation is within the range of 3–5 mm from the surface of the metal dental restoration, the spacer thickness should be more than 3 mm [27].

15.1.2.2 Oral and Dental Management During Radiotherapy

The main purpose of oral and dental management during radiotherapy is to prevent and alleviate radiation mucositis and radiation xerostomia, although there is no established treatment method for these. Therefore, supportive treatment such as preventive oral care and symptomatic treatment are mainly performed. Preventive oral care consists of self-care and professional care by a well-trained dental health provider. Self-care consists of toothbrushing, tongue and oral mucosa cleaning, mouth rinsing, and mouth moisture retention. Professional care consists of the examination of the oral status, oral care instructions, and professional oral cleaning. Since clinical changes in the oral conditions caused by radiation occur on a weekly basis, professional oral cleaning should be performed weekly from the start of radiotherapy to the disappearance of radiation mucositis. Symptomatic treatment consists of moisturizing instructions and pain management.

A regimen of oral and dental management during radiotherapy is shown in Table 15.4. If this regimen proceeds ideally, as in the case of conventional radiotherapy, most patients can avoid severe acute adverse events that would otherwise interrupt treatment.

15.1.2.3 Oral and Dental Management After Radiotherapy

The purpose of oral and dental management after radiotherapy is to prevent late adverse events such as radiation caries and osteoradionecrosis of the jaws. The risk factors of osteoradionecrosis of the jaws are non-restorable dental caries and severe periodontal disease. Therefore, periodical preventive dental maintenance is critical following radiotherapy. In fact, many studies have reported that the incidence rates of dental caries, periodontal disease, and osteoradionecrosis decrease by performing dental maintenance after radiotherapy [28, 29]. In addition, teeth with a temporary treatment before radiation therapy are treated.

Preventive Dental Maintenance

Preventive dental maintenance aims to prevent both dental caries and severe periodontitis, both of which have the potential to cause osteoradionecrosis of the jaws. Periodontal management and highly concentrated fluoride topical applications are essential to dental maintenance. A preventive dental maintenance regimen is shown in Table 15.4. If preventive dental maintenance is adequately provided, patients can maintain good oral conditions (Fig. 15.9).

The suggested regimen for preventive dental maintenance is as follows: (i) topical application of high-concentration fluoride once every 3 months; (ii) scaling and the topical application of high-concentration fluoride once every 6 months; (iii) measurement of the periodontal pocket depth and plaque index once every 6 months; and (iv) radiography examination once every 12 months. None of the patients should undergo any surgical dental treatment (such as tooth extraction or flap operation) after radiotherapy given that these considerably increase the probability of osteoradionecrosis. Most oral cancer patients are older than 40 years old and have many crown restorations; furthermore, a preferred site of radiation caries is the root surface. Therefore, the fluoride application methods showed in Fig. 15.10 or the custom tray is recommended. However, the type of fluoride gel or fluoride delivery system used does not significantly influence caries activity.

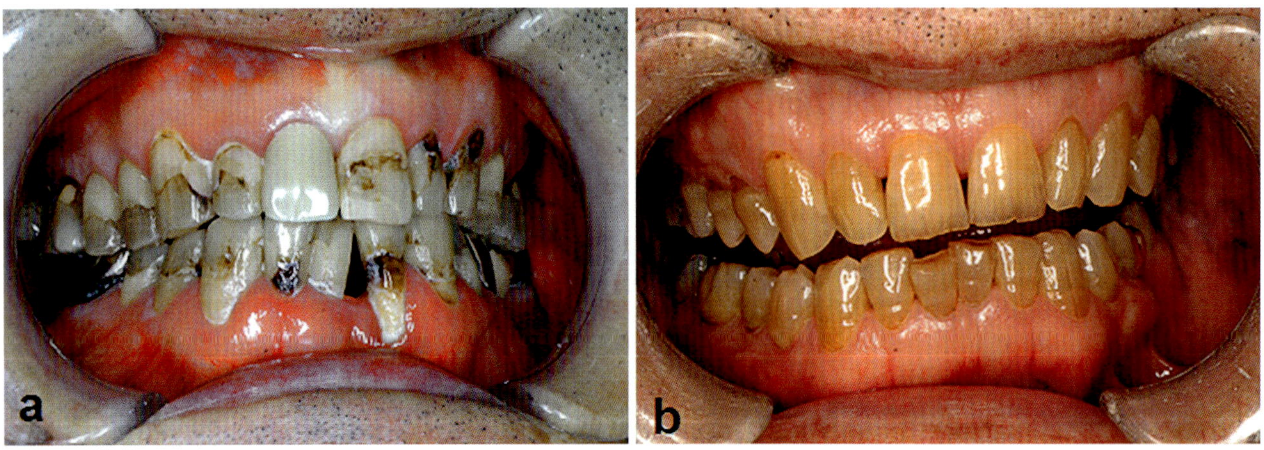

Fig. 15.9 The impact of preventive dental maintenance on patients receiving head and neck radiotherapy. (**a**) A patient without preventive dental maintenance 1 year after head and neck radiotherapy. (**b**) A patient with preventive dental maintenance 5 years after head and neck radiotherapy

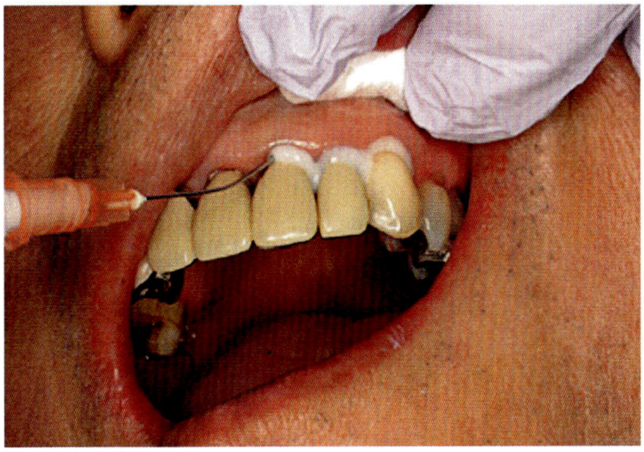

Fig. 15.10 Fluoride application method for patients receiving head and neck radiotherapy

15.1.3 Dental Treatment for Head and Neck Radiotherapy Patients

15.1.3.1 Dental Restoration

Some studies have reported that conventional glass ionomer restorations performed more poorly than resin-modified glass ionomer, composite resin, and amalgam restorations in radiotherapy-treated patients [30]. On the other hand, Hu et al. reported that glass ionomer restorations performed better compared with composite resin restorations in the long-term follow-up. Therefore, the restoration material for patients without periodical preventive dental management may have to use glass ionomer than other materials.

15.1.3.2 Endodontic Treatment (Fig. 15.11)

The success rate of endodontic treatment in the radiation field is more than 90 % [31], and no osteoradionecrosis caused by endodontic treatment has been reported to date. However, the endodontic treatment has to be performed with great attention in order to avoid bone infection. Furthermore, because formalin cresol causes bone necrosis when it leaks out from the root apex, its application must be performed carefully. If a calcium hydroxide water-based paste is available, it should be used instead of formalin cresol. Marx et al. reported that 6 months after radiation therapy there is less vascularity and thus less tissue perfusion and more fibrosis; these developments make the tissue more prone to osteoradionecrosis [24], indicating that the potential for adverse events increases gradually. Therefore, root canal treatment should be completed as quickly as possible after a diagnosis of pulpal and periapical pathology.

15.1.3.3 Periodontal Treatment

Because periodontal surgery such as a flap operation in the radiation field may cause osteoradionecrosis by the periosteal trauma, periodontal treatment should be confined to an initial intervention. On the other hand, the chlorhexidine gluconate solution should be used for irrigation of the periodontal pocket due to its positive effects on gingival inflammation.

15.1.3.4 Crown Prosthesis and Dentures

In order to prevent secondary caries, a dental crown and dental bridge should be the better cleaning shape and be set by a glass ionomer cement. Other than this, the special considerations are unnecessary. Since traumatic ulcers caused by dentures may induce osteoradionecrosis of the jaws (Fig. 15.6), their frequent adjustment is necessary. In addition, the acrylic resin lingual plate, which makes denture adjustment and denture repair easier than metal connectors such as lingual bar, should be designed for the mandibular major connector of partial denture (Fig. 15.12) because oral cancer patients often suffer from neck lymphedema with swelling of the oral mucosa after radiotherapy [32].

15.1.3.5 Dental Implantation

Because dental implantation may cause osteoradionecrosis and radiation soft tissue necrosis, dental implants in the radiation field are generally contraindicated. It has also been reported that irradiated bone has an up to 12-fold greater risk of dental implantation failure than non-irradiated bone [33]. On the other hand, some authors stated that dental implantation was safe in patients who have been irradiated at doses below 50–55 Gy [34, 35]. In any case, it is safer to place a dental implant outside of the radiation field. Hyperbaric oxygenation has a positive effect on osseointegration to improve angiogenesis, bone metabolism, and bone turnover of irradiated bone. It has been reported that hyperbaric oxygenation reduces the failure rate of dental implantation from 21.4 % to 13.5 % [36].

15.1.3.6 Tooth Extraction

A mandible irradiated at more than 60 Gy is at a high risk of osteoradionecrosis after tooth extraction [26]. On the other hand, a mandible irradiated at less than 50 Gy and the irradiated maxilla are at a low risk of osteoradionecrosis after tooth extraction. However, because they are not without the risk of the osteoradionecrosis, the extraction of a tooth within the radiation field should generally be considered as contraindicated. Furthermore, cellular loss and hypovascularization of the jaw bone progress gradually 6 months after the end of radiotherapy. Therefore, it should be considered that the risk of osteoradionecrosis induced by tooth extraction increases gradually.

When extraction of a tooth within the radiation field is required, the dentist must offer an explanation regarding the risk of osteoradionecrosis after tooth extraction, and the tooth extraction wound must be well sutured. In addition, prophylactic hyperbaric oxygen therapy (100 % oxygen, 2.4 atm absolute pressure, for 90 min, 20 times before extraction

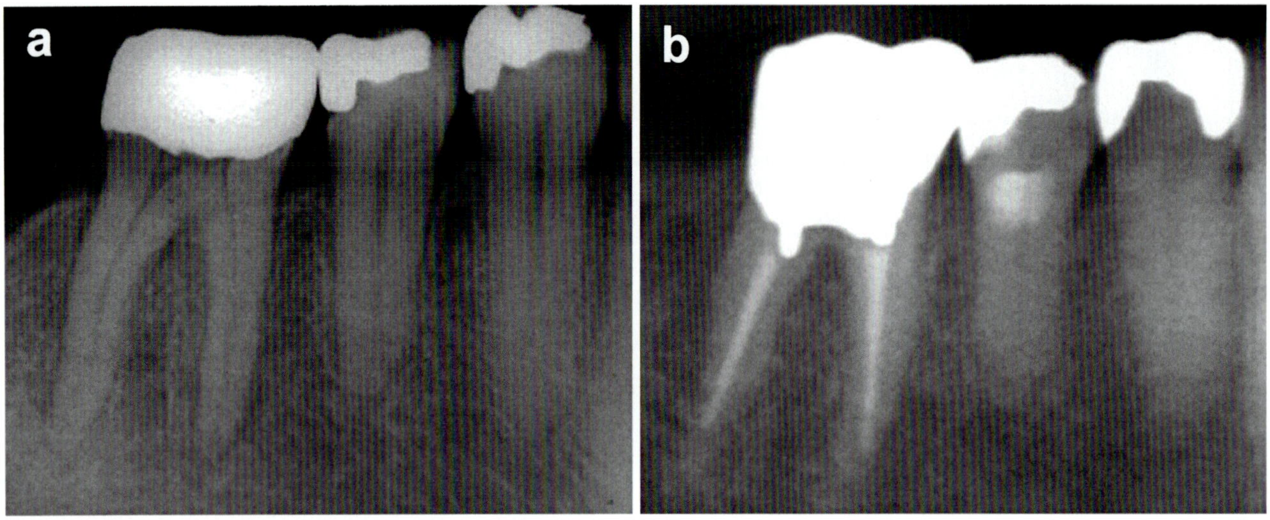

Fig. 15.11 A patient with right parotid cancer who received postoperative external beam radiotherapy (60 Gy). (**a**) Radiograph 3 years after radiotherapy indicates pulpitis with small periapical lesions of the first premolar. (**b**) On a radiograph 10 years after root canal treatment, periapical lesions had disappeared

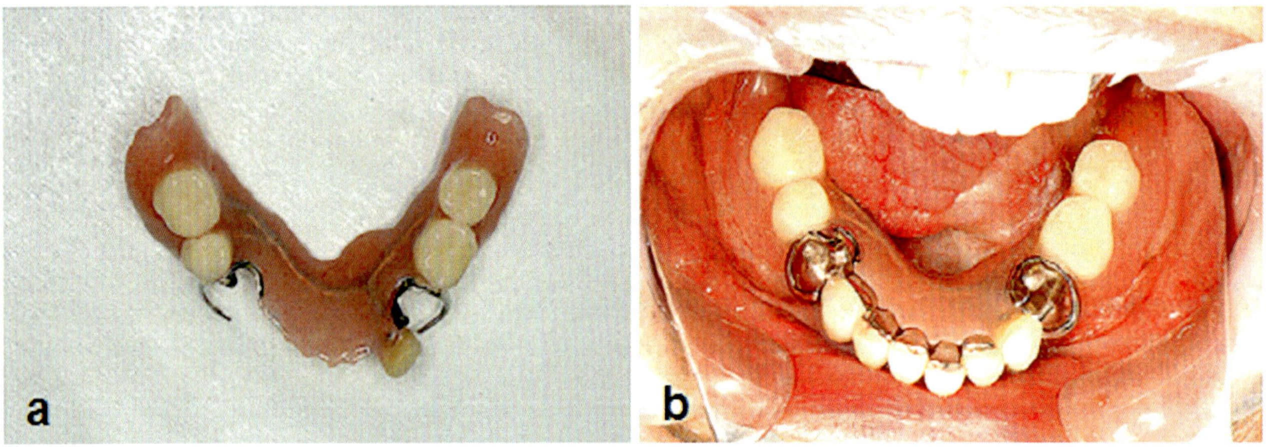

Fig. 15.12 Mandibular partial denture for patients receiving head and neck radiotherapy. (**a**) The acrylic resin lingual plate is designed for the mandibular major connector. (**b**) Denture worn by a patient with tongue cancer who received postoperative external beam radiotherapy (60 Gy)

and 10 times after extraction) is effective in reducing the risk of developing osteoradionecrosis after tooth extraction.

15.1.3.7 Osteoradionecrosis of the Jaws

When osteoradionecrosis of the jaws unfortunately occurs, the cause should initially be eliminated. Following this, conservative treatments such as the administration of antimicrobial agents, local irrigation, and debridement should be performed. If osteoradionecrosis cannot be controlled through conservative treatment, segmental or marginal mandibulectomy combined with hyperbaric oxygen therapy should be performed. However, the patient's quality of life will be negatively influenced by dysfunction and deformity of the jaw. A reference protocol for the treatment of osteoradionecrosis of the jaw, as described by Marx, is shown in Table 15.5.

Table 15.5 Marx protocol for the treatment of osteoradionecrosis

Stage I	The patient receives 30 dives (1 dive per day, Monday–Friday) to 2.4 atmospheres for 90 min. If the patient shows clinical improvement after reevaluation, hyperbaric oxygen therapy (HBO) is continued for a total 60 dives. If there is no improvement, the patient advances to stage II
Stage II	Sequestrectomy with primary mucosal closure is performed. The patient receives 30 more dives after surgery. If wound dehiscence and bone exposure occurs, the patient advances to stage III
Stage III	The patient undergoes resection of a bleeding healthy bone section after a minimum 30 dives. Hyperbaric dives are continued until a healthy closure is evident or until a total of 60 accumulated dives is reached. The patient is advanced to stage III-R
Stage III-R	The patient is administered an additional 20 dives in preparation for bone graft reconstruction 10 weeks after resection. The patient receives 10 more dives after reconstruction

15.2 Oral and Dental Healthcare: Planning and Management and Dental Treatment for Oral Cancer Patients Receiving Head and Neck Chemotherapy

15.2.1 Oral and Dental Healthcare for Head and Neck Chemotherapy Patients

Chemotherapy, an anticancer treatment, is associated with some adverse events. In the case of oral cancer patients, it is absolutely imperative to manage their oral health well in order to prevent severe complications. The major severe complications in the oral cavity include mucositis, dysgeusia, and oral infection.

15.2.1.1 Chemotherapy-Induced Oral Mucositis

Up to 40 % of oral cancer patients are at risk of developing chemotherapy-associated oral mucositis [2]. Although this proportion is less than that of direct radiotherapy to the mouth mucosa, upon development however, it may cause bleeding as well as acute and severe pain, resulting in an inability to eat. This is the primary reason for discontinuance of chemotherapy, and therefore it is important to control the development of oral mucositis and avoid serious nutritional disturbance.

There are two mechanisms in the development of oral mucositis from chemotherapy. The first is a direct effect of the anticancer agents, and the second is an indirect effect caused by a secondary infection of the oral cavity. In the first direct mechanism, anticancer medications causes free radical production in the oral mucosa and saliva that in turn leads to oxidative stress on the oral mucosa. The oxidative stress hinders regeneration of the oral mucosa, leading to the destruction and inflammation of the mucosal tissue. In the second indirect mechanism, anticancer treatment leads to leukocytopenia and a reduction of the innate immune response. This compromises the immune response of the oral mucosa, leading to secondary infection by normally harmless bacteria on the mucosal surface. This resultant oral mucositis is compounded by mechanical aggravation from mucosal contact with the sharp edges of teeth or ill-fitting denture.

The degree of oral mucositis is different depending on the route of administration of chemotherapy. In the case of intra-arterial chemotherapy that is administered to the primary tumor, severe mucositis occurs in the area of the administered anticancer agent (Fig. 15.13).

There are some risk factors which worsen symptoms of oral mucositis. These include the patient's age, poor oral hygiene, acute or chronic periodontal disease, bacterial, viral, or fungal infection secondary to periodontal disease, poor nutritional status, xerostomia (dry mouth) caused by radiotherapy or medication, and impaired salivary glands [37].

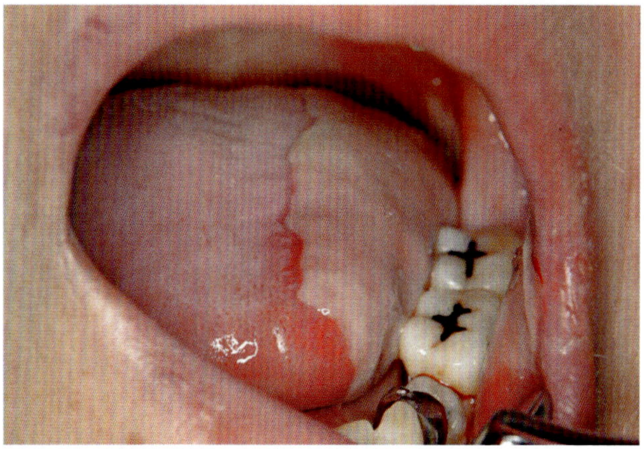

Fig. 15.13 Chemotherapy-induced oral mucositis. A patient with tongue cancer who received intra-arterial chemotherapy and developed mucositis in the area of the administered anticancer agent

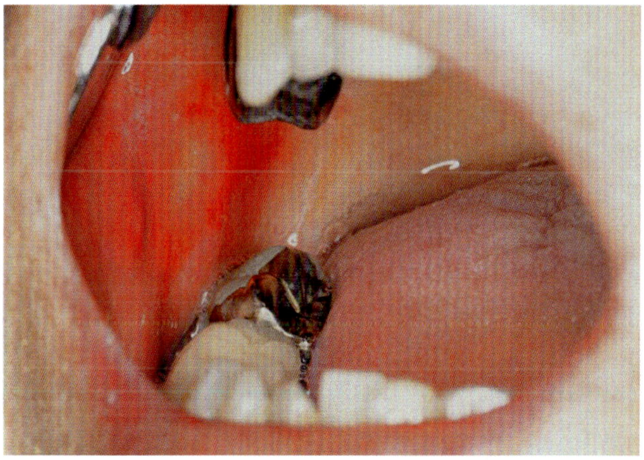

Fig. 15.14 Chemotherapy-induced oral mucositis. Partial mucositis can be found in the buccal mucosa especially in the region near the molars

Decrease in saliva due to impaired salivary glands affects restoration of epithelial tissue, the volume of germ, and the bacterial flora of the mouth.

Clinically, oral mucositis develops 7–10 days from the start of chemotherapy and recovers normally 14–21 days later [37]. There are several steps in the repair and the development of oral mucositis. Partial mucositis and oncogenesis can be found mostly on the lip (e.g., perleche), labial mucosa, lateral border of tongue, and buccal mucosa (especially the region near molars) (Fig. 15.14). The painful ulcers can seriously hinder eating and drinking [38].General ingestion would be hard due to the pain and also exacerbates the oral mucositis as the pain from toothbrushing leads to poor oral hygiene.

15.2.1.2 Chemotherapy-Induced Taste Disturbance

Taste disturbances are frequently observed in cancer patients undergoing chemotherapy and are serious adverse events.

The most common symptom during chemotherapy is a loss in taste, taste disturbances, and a bad taste in the mouth [39]. Taste disturbances affect the daily quality of life of these patients, leading to malnutrition, weight loss, and, in severe cases, difficulty in maintaining the chemotherapy regimen and possibly leading to significant morbidity. Although taste disturbance in patients undergoing cancer chemotherapy has been frequently observed, little is known about the underlying mechanisms. The etiology of these disturbances due to chemotherapy seems to be multifactorial and can include (1) alterations to the cell structure or receptor surface, (2) interruption in neural coding, (3) zinc deficiency, (4) lowered sensitivity of the taste buds for the taste component due to decreased salivary secretion, and (5) tongue coating. However, it is still unknown which mechanism(s) is(are) predominant or responsible.

A study reported the possibility that the taste disorder observed in rats administered S-1 was related to the degeneration of taste nerve fibers and intra-tongue ganglionic nerve cells, in contrast to the degeneration of mucosal epithelial basal cells and taste buds as seen in zinc-deficient rats [40].

15.2.1.3 Infection of the Oral Cavity

Myelosuppression such as leukopenia and neutropenia is the main adverse event associated with chemotherapy. The intraoral infection caused by oral bacteria is strongly correlated with immunocompetency. Therefore some dental problems (e.g., apical periodontitis, marginal periodontitis, pericoronitis of wisdom tooth) are effects consequent to myelosuppression.

In serious conditions, oral inflammation can lead to life-threatening sepsis. This inflammation can be caused by oral bacteria as well as herpes simplex virus and other viral or *Candida* species (Fig. 15.15).

15.2.2 Planning and Management for Oral Cancer Patients Receiving Chemotherapy

15.2.2.1 Oral and Dental Clinical Examination

Before commencing with chemotherapy, it is important to minimize the risk of adverse events through a thorough oral and dental clinical examination that includes x-ray examination. Preexisting problems identified through the examination should be resolved prior to chemotherapy. It is important to convince the patient of the necessity of the treatment before chemotherapy. In addition, the patient should be educated in the treatment planning with respect to oral hygiene maintenance, the dental treatment, and its management.

15.2.2.2 Oral Care

Oral care is fundamentally important to preventing adverse events. There are two types of oral care, one of which is self-performed by the patient and the other is professional dental care performed by dentists and dental hygienists that includes root planing and scaling performed after an appropriate dental examination. Maintaining good oral hygiene and cleaning by a professional oral caregiver that uses machine facilities make this procedure very simple for both the patient and nurse. The objective of a patient or a nurse is to keep the state of oral hygiene and cleanliness the same as that after professional oral care. The key to the patient's self-care is a perspicuous guidance by the dental hygienist. This is especially important in oral mucositis, where the methods of oral care are crucial to pain management and to prevent a secondary infection by oral bacteria. The objectives of the oral care are as follows: (1) removal of food particles retained in the oral cavity, (2) moisturization of the oral cavity, and (3) pain management. Basic oral self-care involves mouth cleaning at least three times in a day using a toothbrush that is soft with

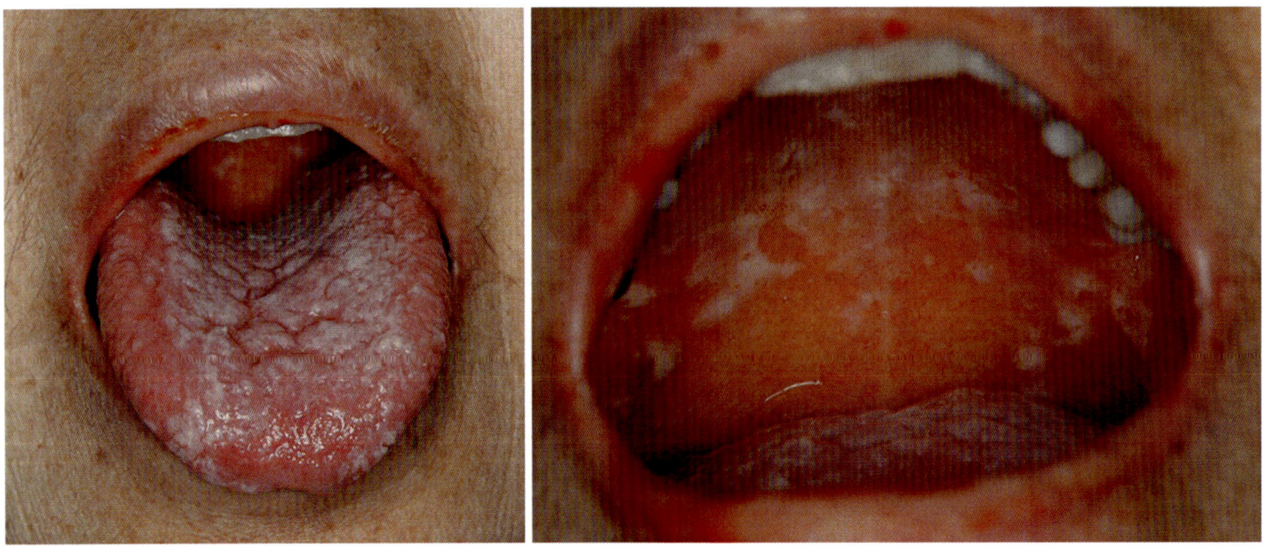

Fig. 15.15 Infection of the oral cavity by *Candida* species

a small head for reduced pain while brushing. In addition, fluoride containing alcohol-free toothpaste should be used as it is both useful for prevention of dental caries and better for sensitive conditions such as mucositis.

For efficient brushing, patients should be mindful of the plaque areas indicated by the dental hygienist. There are many studies reporting on the efficacy of mouthwashes in oral mucositis; however, a standard treatment has not been indicated. Although chlorhexidine, saline, and povidone–iodine are frequently provided, their effectiveness is variable [41].

For intraoral moisturizing, patients should increase the number of times of mouth rinsing, as well as use an accompanying moisturizing gel other than a mouthwash. This is necessary to prevent adhesion of oral bacteria to the teeth in addition to protecting the oral mucosa.

For pain mitigation, mouth rinsing can be performed with a mouthwash containing an anesthetic [42]. In cases where pain cannot be relieved by the aforementioned methods, an analgesic drug such as NSAIDs, acetaminophen, or opioids is recommended [43].

15.2.2.3 Team Approach

When ingestion is difficult due to pain, patients should focus primarily on their nutritional balance rather than improving their oral condition. In such instances, the meal should be easily digested and made palatable with seasoning, or in more extreme circumstances, nourishment may be supplied using an oral feeding tube or an intravenous transfusion. The team approach is important for preventing or managing chemotherapy-induced adverse events.

To support the patient's self care, the following matters are important: family care and support; assistance for oral self-care and evaluation of oral health by the nurses; guidance for self care by the dental hygienist; total management including prescribed medication by a dentist; control of the general physical condition including myelosuppression by their doctor; and supervision of their daily nutrition including the route of administration by the nutritionist. For patient education, psychological care is sometimes more helpful than the medical theory.

15.3 Oral and Dental Healthcare: Planning and Management and Dental Treatment for Oral Cancer Patients Receiving Ablative and Reconstructive Surgery

15.3.1 Planning and Management for Oral Cancer Patients Receiving Head Ablative and Reconstructive Surgery

15.3.1.1 Perioperative Dental Assessment

The general surgical field of oral cancer would be a place in the oral cavity where there are approximately several hundreds of millions to billions per 1 ml of intraoral saliva. In ablative and reconstructive surgery, a postoperative infection caused by oral bacteria is an inherent risk. Although there have been several different results reported for the rates of complications after oral cancer surgery, it is said that the incidence is about 40–60 % in general. The perioperative oral care is important to prevent an infection of the operation site as well as aspiration pneumonia.

Preoperative dental evaluation and appropriate dental care is very important for keeping an optimal status of intraoral hygiene prior to a surgical procedure. The scaling to scrape the tartar should be performed appropriately for preventing the occurrence of intraoral complications after the surgery [44]. All grossly septic teeth should be adequately assessed and considered for extraction in preoperative or intraoperative procedures. However, it is important to verify that the teeth is not buried or in an unmovable condition in the tumor. In such a situation the teeth should not be extracted prior to the definitive surgical resection.

The treatment of dental caries and defective prosthesis should be provided in advance of the surgery. Even in serious situations, all lesions that may cause difficulty in toothbrushing post-surgery should be treated immediately as it may increase the probability of an infection in the wounded area after surgery. These oral care procedures are necessary prior to surgery. After surgery, when oral care by the patient themselves would be impossible, care should then be performed by a dentist, a dental hygienist, or a nurse. In the case of dysphagia caused by a tissue deficit from surgery, special attention should be given to aspiration during oral care. When the patient is able to self-care, both the cleaning method(s) and the tool(s) they utilize should be under close supervision.

15.3.1.2 Prosthetic Rehabilitation

Dental prosthesis retentions correcting for functional disorder caused by an oral cancer surgery include obturators, maxillary prosthetics, and dental implants. In all cases, there are associated advantages and disadvantages. The maxillary prosthetics has a lower risk of surgical stress (Fig. 15.16). However, it is difficult to provide functional support to compensate for the defective area as it is unstable with respect to the mucous membrane and the remaining teeth and it also causes an irritating pressure to the remaining teeth. Discomfort that occurs at the time of attachment can sometimes cause a problem.

Dental implants require an increased number of operations as well as a longer treatment duration and this can cause greater physical and mental stress to the patient (Figs. 15.17 and 15.18). However it may increase masticatory efficiency, causes less stress for the remaining teeth, and is highly stable at the time of installation.

Current management of oral cancer following tumor resection includes reconstruction of the surgical defect

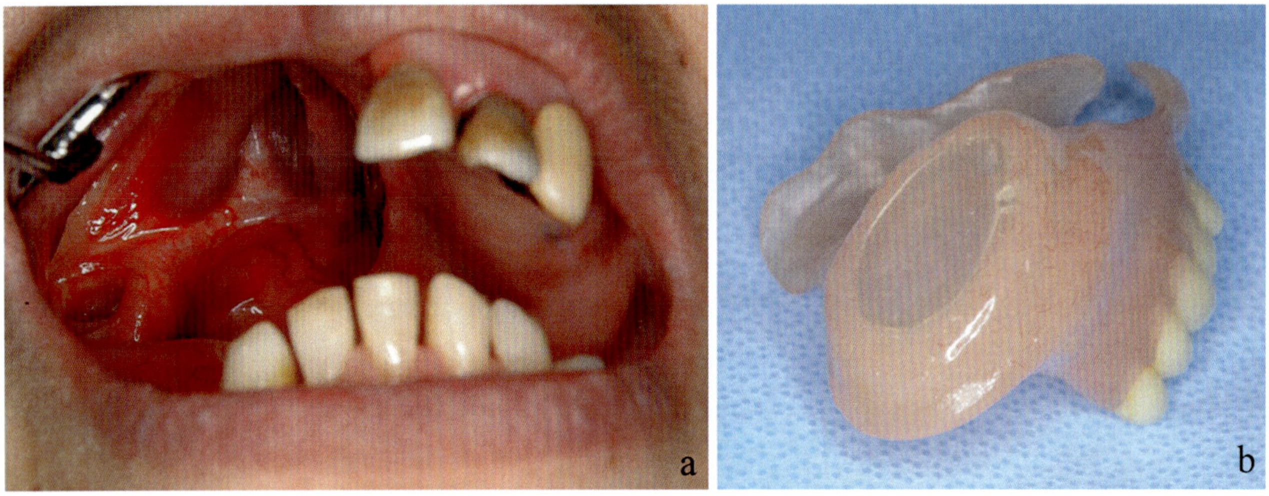

Fig. 15.16 A dental prosthesis retention correcting for functional disorder caused by a cancer surgery. (**a**) A patient with maxillary cancer postoperation. (**b**) The maxillary prosthetics

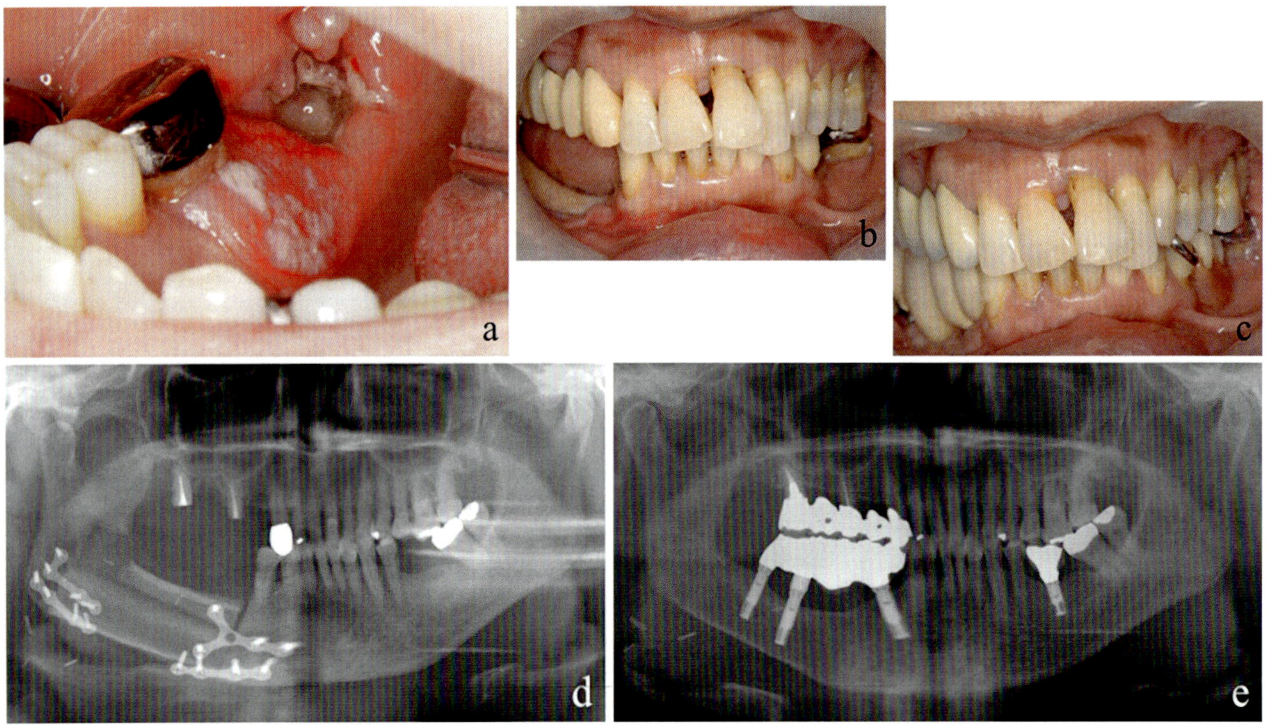

Fig. 15.17 The patient had carcinoma of the right lower gingiva. (**a**) Preoperative intraoral photograph. (**b**, **d**) Postoperative intraoral photograph and panorama x-ray of the mandibular reconstruction with free fibula flap. (**c**, **e**) Postoperative intraoral photograph and panorama x-ray of the surgery of dental implant

with free vascularized flaps and rehabilitation of orofacial form and function with the aid of endosteal implants. The choice of flap for reconstruction influences the use of implants, and further hard and soft tissue surgery is frequently required to enhance the success of oral rehabilitation [45]. When considering patients to be treated for oral cancer, the timing of implant installation is still subject to discussion [46].

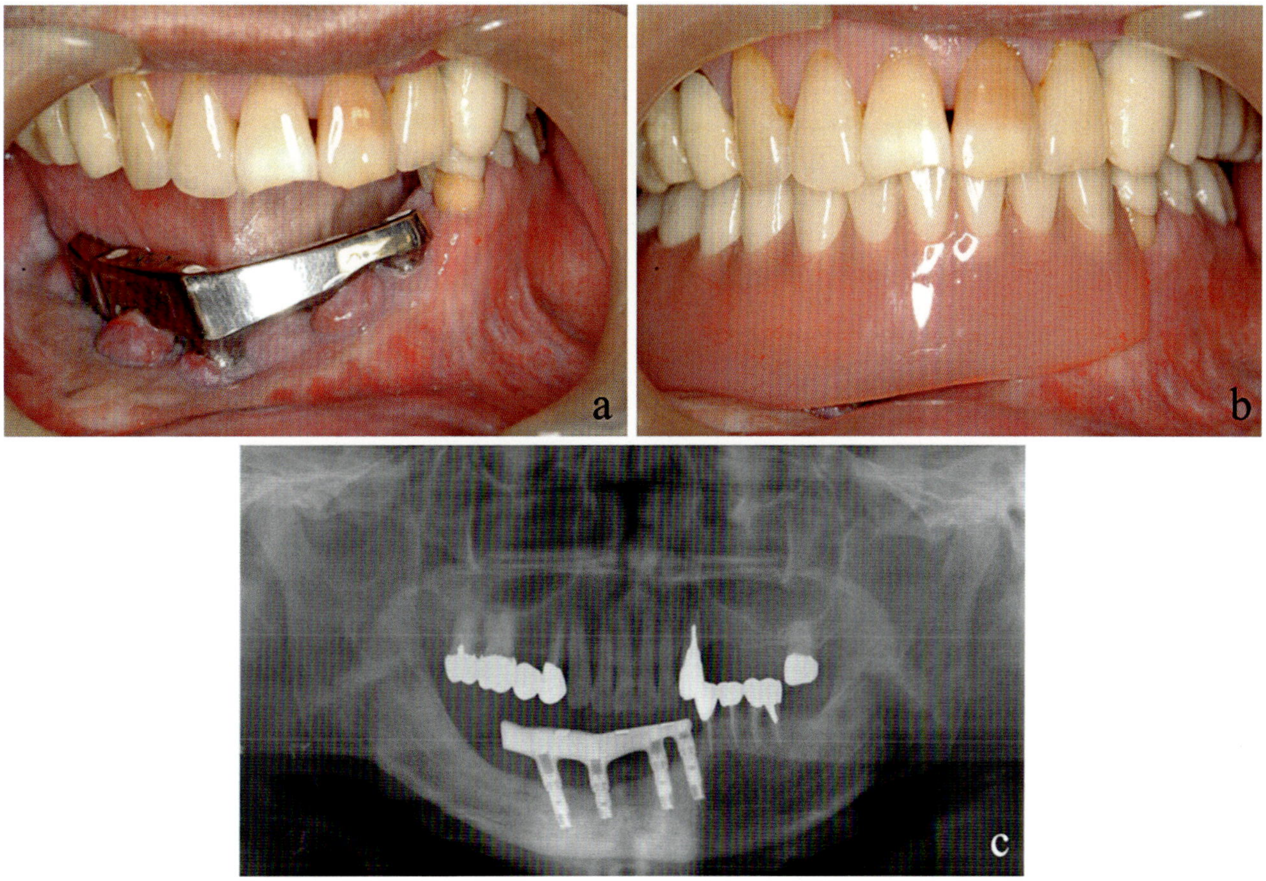

Fig. 15.18 The patient had carcinoma of the right lower gingiva. (**a**, **c**) Postoperative intraoral photograph and x-ray of the surgery of dental implant with magnetic attachment system. (**b**) Intraoral photograph of retaining mandibular denture

References

1. Sonis ST (2004) A biological approach to mucositis. J Support Oncol 2:21–36
2. Sonis ST, Elting LS, Keefe D et al (2004) Perspectives on cancer therapy-induced mucosal injury: pathogenesis, measurement, epidemiology, and consequences for patients. Cancer 100:1995–2025. doi:10.1002/cncr.20162
3. Keefe DM, Schubert MM, Elting LS et al (2007) Updated clinical practice guidelines for the prevention and treatment of mucositis. Cancer 109:820–831. doi:10.1002/cncr.224844
4. Stephens LC, Schultheiss TE, Price RE et al (1991) Radiation apoptosis of serous acinar cells of salivary and lacrimal glands. Cancer67:1539–1543.doi:10.1002/1097-0142(19910315)67:6<1539::AID-CNCR2820670613>3.0.CO;2-Q
5. Arsenian MA (1991) Cardiovascular sequelae of therapeutic thoracic radiation. Prog Cardiovasc Dis 33:299–311. doi:10.1016/0033-0620(91)90022-E
6. Möller P, Perrier M, Ozsahin M et al (2004) A prospective study of salivary gland function in patients undergoing radiotherapy for squamous cell carcinoma of the oropharynx. Oral Surg Oral Med Oral Pathol Oral Radiol Endod 97:173–189. doi:10.1016/S1079-2104(03)00473-6
7. Little M, Schipper M, Feng FY et al (2012) Reducing xerostomia after chemo-IMRT for head-and-neck cancer: beyond sparing the parotid glands. Int J Radiat Oncol Biol Phys 83:1007–1014. doi:10.1016/j.ijrobp.2011.09.004
8. Yamashita H, Nakagawa K, Tago M et al (2006) Taste dysfunction in patients receiving radiotherapy. Head Neck 28:508–516. doi:10.1002/hed.20347
9. Conger AD (1973) Loss and recovery of taste acuity in patients irradiated to the oral cavity. Radiat Res 53:338–347. doi:10.2307/3573539
10. Ripamonti C, Zecca E, Brunelli C et al (1998) A randomized, controlled clinical trial to evaluate the effects of zinc sulfate on cancer patients with taste alterations caused by head and neck irradiation. Cancer 82:1938–4195. doi:10.1002/(SICI)1097-0142(19980515)82:10<1938::AID-CNCR18>3.0.CO;2-U
11. Fujita M, Ogawa M, Furuki Y et al (1987) Changes of periodontal tissues followed by Co-60 irradiation. Dental Radiology 27:1–9. doi:org/10.11242/dentalradiology1960.27.1 (Japanese)
12. Kielbassa AM, Beetz I, Schendera A et al (1997) Irradiation effects on microhardness of fluoridated and non-fluoridated bovine dentin. Eur J Oral Sci 105:444–447. doi:10.1111/j.1600-0722.1997.tb02142.x
13. Pioch T (2004) Veränderungen der zahnhartsubstanzen. In: Kielbassa AM (ed) Trahlentherapie im kopf- und halsbereich: implikationen für zahnärzte, HNO-ärzte und radiotherapeuten. Schlütersche, Hannover
14. Kielbassa AM, Hinkelbein W, Hellwig E et al (2006) Radiation-related damage to dentition. Lancet Oncol 7:326–335. doi:10.1016/S1470-2045(06)70658-1
15. Epstein JB, Lunn R, Le N et al (1998) Periodontal attachment loss in patients after head and neck radiation therapy. Oral Surg Oral Med Oral Pathol Oral Radiol Endod 86:673–677. doi:10.1016/S1079-2104(98)90202-5

16. Pow EH, McMillan AS, Leung WK et al (2003) Oral health condition in southern Chinese after radiotherapy for nasopharyngeal carcinoma: extent and nature of the problem. Oral Dis 9:196–202. doi:10.1034/j.1601-0825.2003.02924.x
17. Spak CJ, Johnson G, Ekstrand J (1994) Caries incidence, salivary flow rate and efficacy of fluoride gel treatment in irradiated patients. Caries Res 28:388–393. doi:10.1159/000262007
18. Papas A, Russell D, Singh M et al (2008) Caries clinical trial of a remineralising toothpaste in radiation patients. Gerodontology 25:76–88. doi:10.1111/j.1741-2358.2007.00199.x
19. Hay KD, Thomson WM (2002) A clinical trial of the anticaries efficacy of casein derivatives complexed with calcium phosphate in patients with salivary gland dysfunction. Oral Surg Oral Med Oral Pathol Oral Radiol Endod 93:271–275. doi:10.1067/moe.2002.120521
20. Curi MM, Dib LL (1997) Osteoradionecrosis of the jaws: a retrospective study of the background factors and treatment in 104 cases. J Oral Maxillofac Surg 556:540–544. doi:10.1016/S0278-2391(97)90478-X
21. Kluth EV, Jain PR, Stuchell RN et al (1988) A study of factors contributing to the development of osteoradionecrosis of the jaws. J Prosthet Dent 592:194–201. doi:10.1016/0022-3913(88)90015-7
22. Murray CG, Daly TE, Zimmerman SO (1980) The relationship between dental disease and radiation necrosis of mandible. Oral Surg Oral Med Oral Pathol Oral Radiol Endod 492:99–104. doi:10.1016/0030-4220(80)90299-6
23. Katsura K, Sasai K, Sato K et al (2008) Relationship between oral health status and development of osteoradionecrosis of the mandible: a retrospective longitudinal study. Oral Surg Oral Med Oral Pathol Oral Radiol Endod 105:731–738. doi:10.1016/j.tripleo.2007.10.011
24. Marx RE, Johnson RP (1987) Studies in the radiobiology of osteoradionecrosis and their clinical significance. Oral Surg Oral Med Oral Pathol 64:379–390. doi:10.1016/0030-4220(87)90136-8
25. Marx RE (1983) Osteoradionecrosis: a new concept of its pathophysiology. J Oral Maxillofac Surg 41:283–288. doi:10.1016/0278-2391(83)90294-X
26. Nabil S, Samman N (2011) Risk factors for osteoradionecrosis after head and neck radiation: a systematic review. Oral Surg Oral Med Oral Pathol Oral Radiol 113:54–69. doi:10.1016/j.tripleo.2011.07.042
27. Reitemeier B, Reitemeier G, Schmidt A et al (2002) Evaluation of a device for attenuation of electron release from dental restorations in a therapeutic radiation field. J Prosthet Dent 87:323–327. doi:10.1067/mpr.2002.122506
28. Yamagishi K, Yamada T (2002) The effect of tooth brushing instruction for the high risk patients of dental caries and periodontitis after radiotherapy: the change of DMF incidence and bone resorption index. Meirin JDEOH 5:76–78 (Japanese)
29. Katsura K, Goto S, Sasai K et al (2009) The effect of dental management for maintaining dental health in patients with head and neck cancer after radiotherapy. Head Neck Cancer 35:266–272 (Japanese)
30. Hong CH, Napeñas JJ, Hodgson BD et al (2010) A systematic review of dental disease in patients undergoing cancer therapy. Support Care Cancer 18:1007–10021. doi:10.1007/s00520-010-0873-2
31. Lilly JP, Cox D, Arcuri M et al (1998) An evaluation of root canal treatment in patients who have received irradiation to the mandible and maxilla. Oral Surg Oral Med Oral Pathol Oral Radiol Endod 86:224–226
32. Katsura K, Hayashi T (2005) Non-neoplastic process after neck dissection demonstrated on enhanced CT in patients with head and neck cancer. Dentomaxillofac Radiol 34:297–303
33. Ihde S, Kopp S, Gundlach K et al (2009) Effects of radiation therapy on craniofacial and dental implants: a review of the literature. Oral Surg Oral Med Oral Pathol Oral Radiol Endod 107:56–65. doi:10.1016/j.tripleo.2008.06.014
34. Esposito M, Hirsch JM, Lekholm U et al (1998) Biological factors contributing to failures of osseointegrated oral implants. (II). Etiopathogenesis. Eur J Oral Sci 106:721–764. doi:10.1046/j.0909-8836.t01-2-.x
35. Keller EE, Tolman DE, Zuck SL et al (1997) Mandibular endosseous implants and autogenous bone grafting in irradiated tissue: a 10-year retrospective study. Int J Oral Maxillofac Implants 12:800–813
36. Granström G (2006) Placement of dental implants in irradiated bone: the case for using hyperbaric oxygen. J Oral Maxillofac Surg 64:812–818. doi:10.1016/j.joms.2006.01.012
37. Saadeh CE, Pharm D (2005) Chemotherapy- and radiotherapy-induced oral mucositis: review of preventive strategies and treatment. Pharmacotherapy 25(4):540–554
38. Rogers BB (2001) Mucositis in the oncology patient. Nurs Clin N Am 36:745–760
39. Sánchez-Lara K, Sosa-Sánchez R, Green-Renner D, Rodríguez C, Laviano A, Motola-Kuba D, Arrieta O (2010) Influence of taste disorders on dietary behaviors in cancer patients under chemotherapy. Nutr J 9:15. doi:10.1186/1475-2891-9-15
40. Aoki K, Obata K, Kurihara M, Kuniyasu H, Kirita T, Takaki M (2013) Possible peripheral mechanism for taste disorder in rats administered S-1. Int J Clin Oncol. doi:10.1007/s10147-013-0572-3
41. Potting CMJ, Uitterhoeve R, Op Reimer WS, Van Achterberg T (2006) The effectiveness of commonly used mouthwashes for the prevention of chemotherapy-induced oral mucositis: a systematic review. Eur J Cancer Care 15:431–439
42. Chandu A, Stulner C, Bridgeman AM, Smith AC (2002) Maintenance of mouth hygiene in patients with oral cancer in the immediate post-operative period. Aust Dent J 47:170–173
43. Zenda S, Matsuura K, Tachibana H, Homma A, Kirita T, Monden N, Iwae S (2011) Multicenter phase II study of an opioid-based pain control program for head and neck cancer patients receiving chemoradiotherapy. Radiother Oncol 101:410–414. doi:10.1016/j.radoncs
44. Carew JF, Singh B, Shah JP (2003) Work and staging. In: Jatin P (ed) Oral cancer, 1st edn. Mratin Dunitz, London
45. Hayter JP, Cawood JI (1996) Oral rehabilitation with endosteal implants and free flaps. Int J Oral Maxillofac Surg 25:3–12
46. Korfage A, Schoen PJ, Raghoebar GM, Roodenburg JL, Vissink A, Reintsema H (2010) Benefits of dental implants installed during ablative tumour surgery in oral cancer patients: a prospective 5-year clinical trial. Clin Oral Implants Res 21:971–979. doi:10.1111/j.1600-0501.2010.01930.x

Management of Speech Disorders Following Treatment for Oral Cancer

16

Koji Takahashi

Abstract

Speech and swallowing function might be affected directly by the treatment of cancer involving the oral structures. The primary goal of speech and swallowing rehabilitation in oral cancer patients is to optimize the potential for communication and eating as soon as possible. To reach this goal, treatment considerations need to focus on the ability to achieve complete tumor removal while minimizing the amount of functional deficit.

Changes in speech and swallow mechanism are common after ablative surgery and reconstruction of the oral structures. In addition, complications from reconstruction may adversely affect speech and swallowing.

This chapter focuses on articulation and resonance that are most frequently affected by treatment of oral cancer. Management of articulatory deficits and abnormal resonance is introduced in this chapter. Evaluation of speech in oral cancer patients is also introduced.

Keywords

Articulation • Resonance • Speech disorders • Speech therapy

16.1 Introduction

Speech function might be affected directly by the treatment of cancer involving the oral structures. The primary goal of speech rehabilitation in oral cancer patients is to optimize the potential for communication as soon as possible. To reach this goal, treatment considerations need to focus on the ability to achieve complete tumor removal while minimizing the amount of functional deficit.

Changes in the ability to produce intelligible speech are common after ablative surgery and reconstruction of the oral structures. In addition, complications from reconstruction may adversely affect articulation and resonance. Trismus may diminish vocal quality. However, the quality of articulation is not greatly influenced by trismus. Yokoyama and Takahashi et al. investigated the relationship between mouth-opening capacity and intelligibility of syllable and speech in 27 maxillectomized patients with/without maxillary prosthesis [1]. Intelligibilities of syllable and speech were almost same across three categories of mouth-opening capacity (≧40 mm, ≧30 mm, ≧20 mm) (Figs. 16.1 and 16.2).

Xerostomia is also a common side effect of radiation treatment secondary to inadequate salivation. Xerostomia may affect the resonance of sound through dry vocal tract and articulation produced by dry oral structures. An oral moisture-checking device (Mucus™) was developed in Japan (Fig. 16.3). Xerostomia can be quantitatively evaluated using this instrument. Future research using a sophisticated acoustic signal analyzer (Fig. 16.4) and an oral moisture-checking device will reveal the relationship between xerostomia and speech affected by xerostomia.

This chapter focuses on articulation and resonance that are most frequently affected by treatment of oral cancer. Evaluation of speech in oral cancer patients is also introduced.

K. Takahashi, D.D.S., Ph.D. (✉)
Division of Oral Rehabilitation Medicine, Department of Special Needs Oral medicine, School of Dentistry, Showa University, 2-1-1 Kitasenzoku Ohta-ku, Tokyo 145-8515, Japan
e-mail: tkouji@dent.showa-u.ac.jp

T. Kirita and K. Omura (eds.), *Oral Cancer: Diagnosis and Therapy*, DOI 10.1007/978-4-431-54938-3_16, © Springer Japan 2015

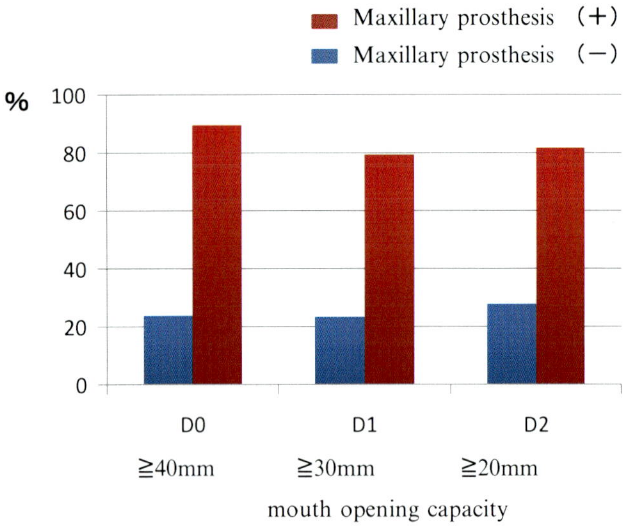

Fig. 16.1 Syllable intelligibility in 27 maxillectomized patients

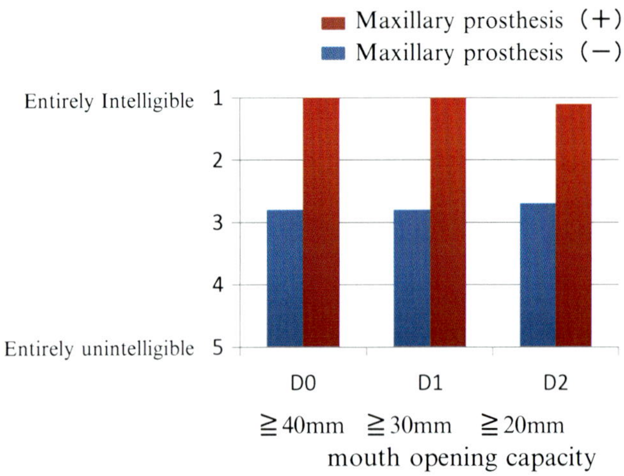

Fig. 16.2 Speech intelligibility in 27 maxillectomized patients

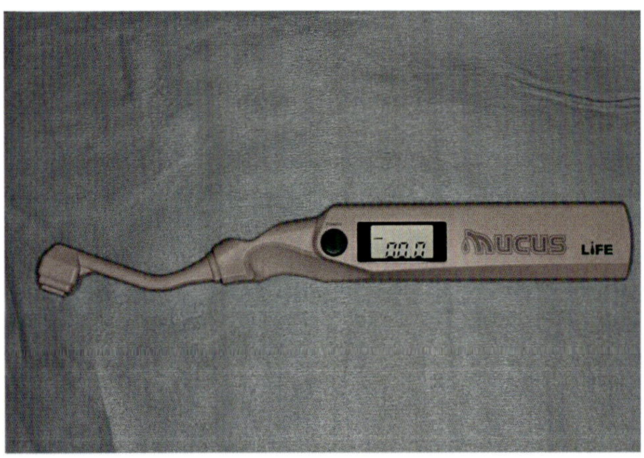

Fig. 16.3 Oral moisture-checking device (Mucus™)

16.2 Articulation

Adequate control of the lips, tongue, and soft palate is crucial for the production of intelligible speech. Any impairment in the range of motion, strength, and/or flexibility of these dynamic articulators may affect the ability to make the precise individual speech movements and coarticulations needed in connected speech. The resulting articulatory impairments typically cluster along placement, manner, and/or voicing parameters as opposed to misarticulation of an individual or isolated phoneme.

Management of articulatory deficits that may develop following oral cancer treatments typically follows five paradigms: oral facilitative exercise, directed articulation therapy, compensatory technique, surgical procedure, and prosthetic appliance.

16.2.1 Oral Facilitative Exercises

Oral facilitative exercises are generally prescribed exercises designed to increase strength, range of motion, and flexibility of the oral articulators. These exercises may also improve swallowing function, as adequate control of the oral musculature is necessary to prepare and propel a bolus from the oral cavity to the oropharynx. In a study of 102 patients who received range-of-motion exercises following surgical treatment for oral and oropharyngeal cancer, significant differences in global measures of swallowing and improvement in speech intelligibility were found at 3 months posttreatment [2].

Muscular strength and endurance can be improved through three basic types of exercises: isometric, isotonic, and isokinetic.

Isometric, or static, training involves resistance without movement [3]. An example of an isometric exercise to increase tongue strength would be to push the dorsum of the tongue against the palate as hard as possible. Clark has found that maximal isometric contractions of 6-s duration repeated 5–10 times daily produce the best results [4] (Figs. 16.5 and 16.6). Atha has studied the effects of isometric exercises and found that they should be performed at maximal effort, last long enough to involve all muscle fibers, and be repeated several times daily [5]. Isometric exercise can also be used to develop increased range of motion.

Isotonic, or dynamic, exercises use the principles of resistance with added motion. Lifting an object is an example of isotonic contractions. This exercise requires both a concentric or shortening contraction of the muscles and an eccentric or lengthening contraction. The advantage of this type of exercise is that it strengthens the targeted muscle through a range of motion as opposed to a static point.

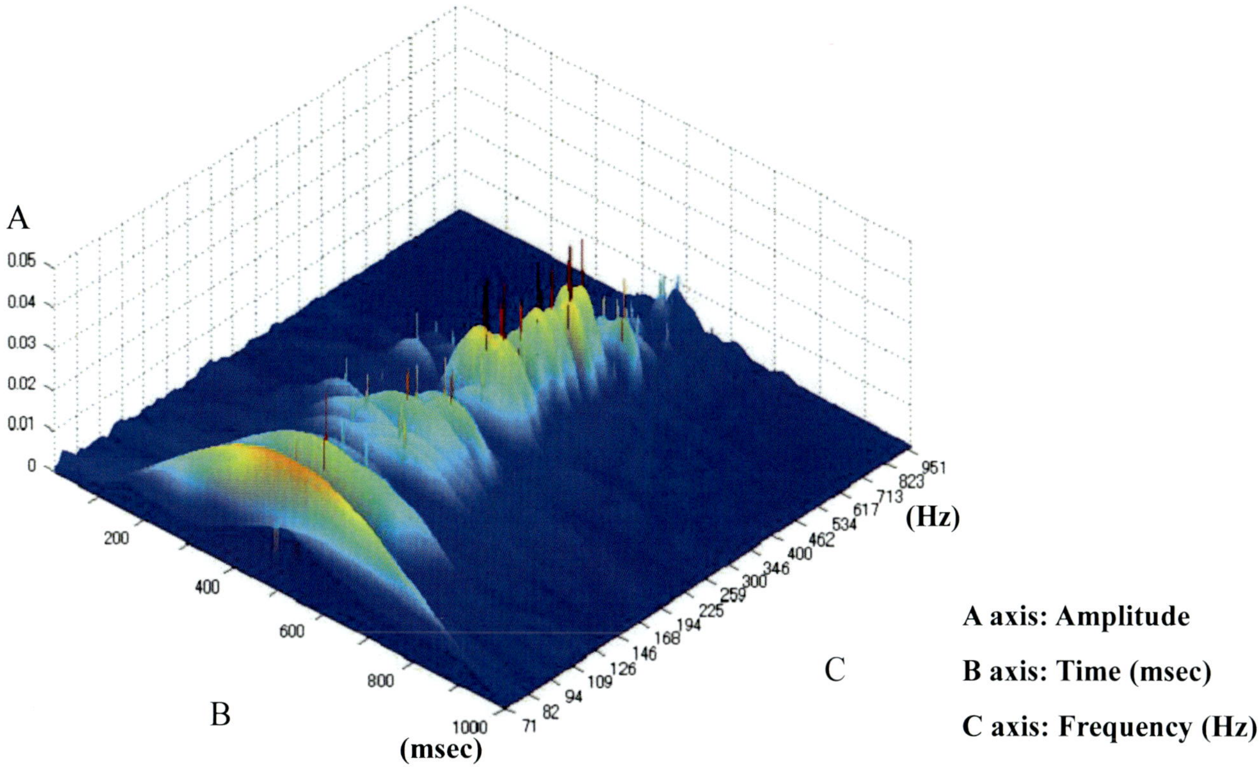

Fig. 16.4 An example of the three-dimensional display of speech sound analyzed using Hilbert transform

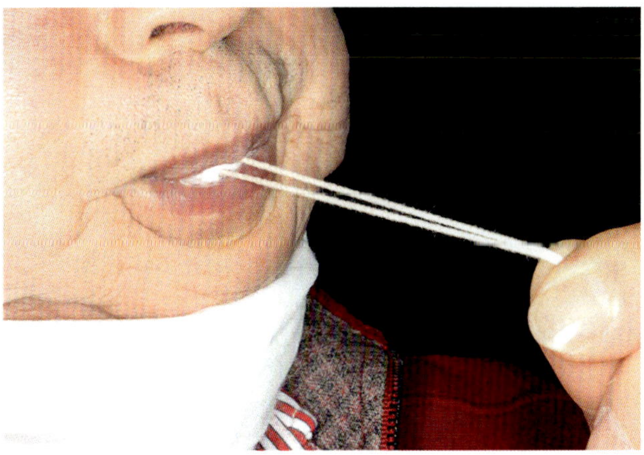

Fig. 16.5 Lip-strengthening exercise (button-pull exercise). Maximal effort for lip closure lasts 6 ~ 10 s. This exercise is repeated 6–10 times a day

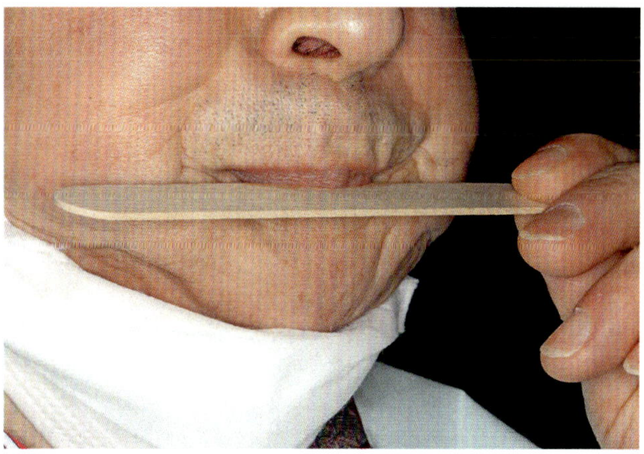

Fig. 16.6 Lip-strengthening exercise (blade-holding exercise). Maximal effort for lip closure lasts 6 ~ 10 s. This exercise is repeated 6–10 times a day

Isokinetic exercises combine resistance techniques at a constant speed of repetition. The target muscle shortens against an accommodating resistance that matches the force produced by the muscle throughout full range of motion [6]. An example of this type of exercise applied to improving tongue motion and strength might be to forcefully move the tongue laterally while applying a resisting pressure from the back of a metal spoon at a constant speed of repetition. Each of three basic types of exercises including isometric, isotonic, and isokinetic exercise is also very effective on the improvement of dysphagia following treatment for oral cancer.

A tongue pressure-measuring device consisting of a disposable probe and manometer was developed in Japan (Figs. 16.7 and 16.8). A labial closure strength device consisting of an indicator with a lip holder mounted to the sensor was also developed in Japan (Figs. 16.9 and 16.10). Using these measuring devices, the effectiveness of applied exercises can be evaluated quantitatively and easily.

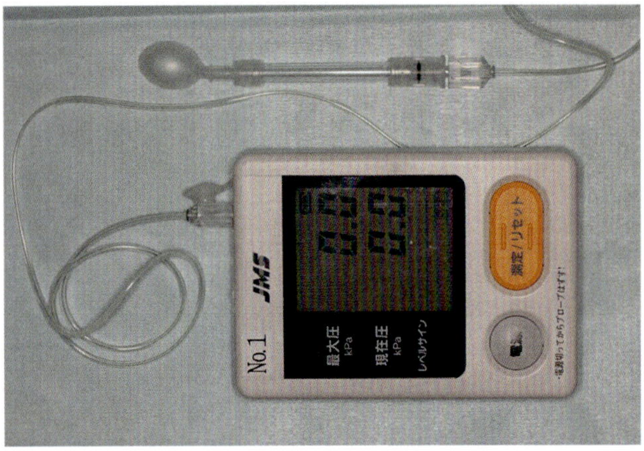

Fig. 16.7 A tongue pressure-measuring device (JMS tongue pressure measurement device™)

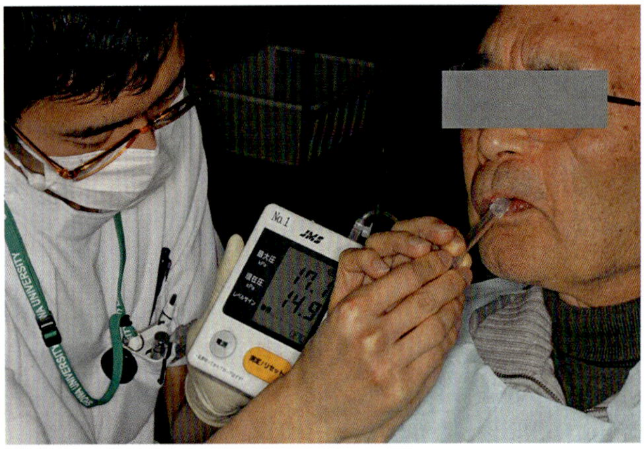

Fig. 16.8 Measurement of the maximal tongue pressure (JMS tongue pressure measurement device™)

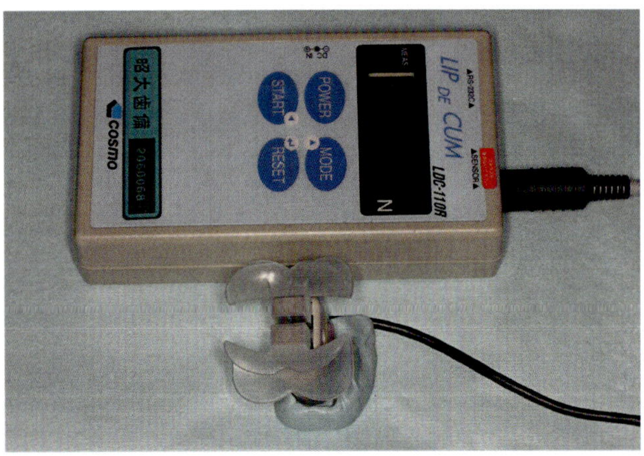

Fig. 16.9 A lip closure strength indicator [Lip De Cum®] with a lip holder [Ducklings®] mounted to the sensor

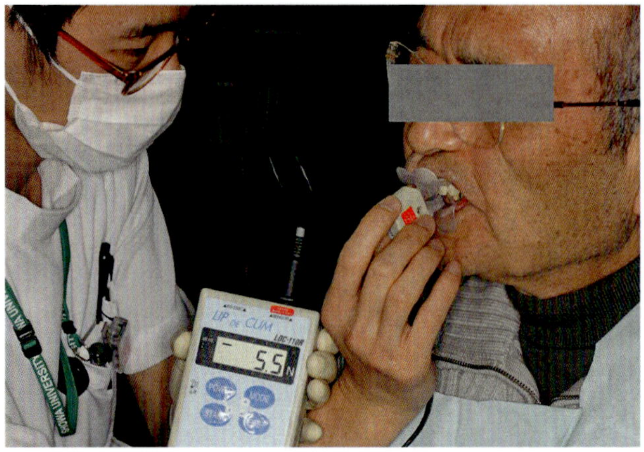

Fig. 16.10 Measurement of the maximal lip closure strength

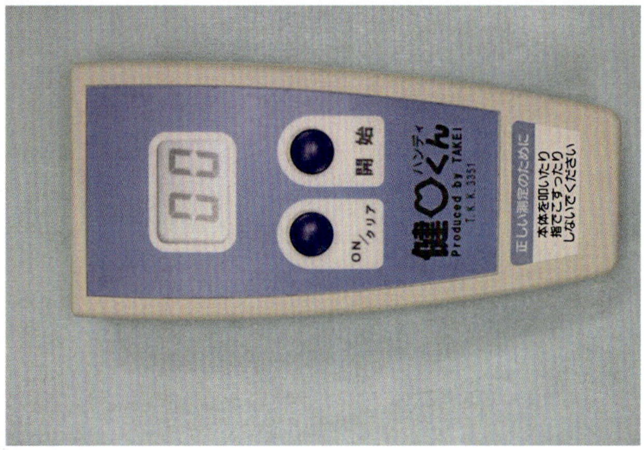

Fig. 16.11 An oral diadochokinetic rate-measuring device (Kenkokun™)

In addition to strength and range of motion, rapidity, flexibility, and motor skill exercises may be performed to improve the ability to quickly move from one articulatory position to another as accurately as possible. Rapid productions of consonant-vowel syllables may assist not only production of the targeted sound but also the ability to make the rapid adjustments needed for coarticulation. Oral diadochokinetic rate can be easily measured using a measuring device developed in Japan. Using this instrument, improvement in rapid oral motor skills can be assessed quantitatively and easily (Figs. 16.11 and 16.12).

16.2.2 Directed Articulation Therapy

Directed articulation therapy is frequently indicated to improve production of specific phonemes and phoneme groups. Patients who have undergone anterior or lateral tongue resections may have difficulty with sounds requiring tongue elevation and/or protrusion. The ability to generate adequate oral air pressure for production of fricatives and plosives may also be compromised in patients who have

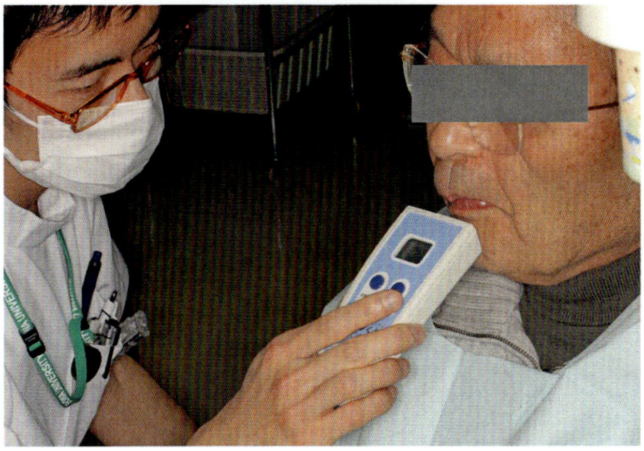

Fig. 16.12 Measurement of oral diadochokinetic rate

undergone base-of-tongue resections, as the remaining tongue tissue may not be able to produce adequate and controlled forceful movements. Patients with lip incompetence following lip resections or neural compromise to that area may experience difficulties with bilateral sounds and developing adequate lip plosion. Traditional articulation therapy with lip closure exercise may improve the production of these groups of sounds.

16.2.3 Compensatory Technique

Compensatory technique may need to be considered when the patient does not have the potential for correct placement of a targeted sound or group of sounds. For example, patients who have undergone extended tonsillar/palatal resections with base-of-tongue involvement may be unable to produce velar consonants even after directed articulation therapy; they may, however, be able to substitute a cough-like sound for the targeted /k/ sound, which facilitates adequate intelligibility. It is interesting to note that compensatory patterns differ between patients who have undergone total glossectomy versus those that have had a partial glossectomy. Partial glossectomees have been found to make use of the residual tongue stump in adaptive movements approximating the normal movement, whereas total glossectomees use true compensatory strategies.

The primary purpose of the compensatory strategy is to improve the intelligibility of speech in the most inconspicuous manner possible. Some compensatory strategies are developed unconsciously by the patient.

16.2.4 Surgical Procedures

Although complete tumor removal remains the prime objective during major oral cancer surgery, the emphasis is also on immediate functional restoration through primary reconstruction.

The type and extent of the surgical procedure have to be weighed against the patient's prognosis, extent of disease, and other comorbid factors influencing wound healing (e.g., history of radiation, chemotherapy, or diabetes).

The type of procedure used to reconstruct surgical defects in the oral and pharyngeal cavities may affect the strength, motion, and flexibility of the oral articulators as well as the shape of the resonating cavities. In general, the quality of life following radical surgery of the oral cavity is largely dependent on the adequacy of reconstruction. Small lesions can frequently be managed with primary suture or split-thickness skin graft. In larger lesions, local or distal flaps may be required. Secondary surgical procedures that may improve tongue mobility may also enhance the oropharyngeal resonating cavity (in the case of strictures) or improve velopharyngeal incompetence (VPI) and articulation after major oral surgery.

Patients who have undergone reconstruction with a split-thickness skin graft typically have better speech than those reconstructed with myocutaneous or hemitongue flaps [7]. Split-thickness flaps are thinner and provide less bulk. In contrast, a hemitongue flap may have reduced motion with tethering toward the defect and thus restrict articulation. Patients undergoing distal flap reconstructions may experience worse impairment in speech due to the adynamic nature of the flap and the lack of sensation and/or motor control.

The extent of involvement in adjacent structures may also affect the degree of speech impairment [8]. In addition, bulky distal flaps may interfere with the critical range, rate, and coordination necessary for good speech and swallowing function [9].

Increasing experience with microvascular techniques and better patient selection have led to the increased use of free flaps as the primary choice of reconstruction for many patients [10]. The type of free flap (musculocutaneous, osseomusculocutaneous, or cutaneous) may be designed to more closely, aesthetically and functionally, reconstitute the surgically ablated area. In cases where the mandible is reconstructed, immediate placement of osseointegrated dental implants may further enhance the patient's ability to masticate and articulate more clearly. Imai et al. investigated the relationship between the surgical procedure and speech intelligibility in 22 glossectomees (11 underwent direct suture, four received split-skin grafts, and seven received reconstruction with the free radial forearm flap) [11]. In this study, articulatory function after glossectomy was assessed mainly by using 100 Japanese syllable speech intelligibility test. The results were as follows: (1) Speech intelligibility after glossectomy is related to the extent of resected tongue tissue. (2) According to glossal sounds, subjects with more than half of the tongue resection showed low intelligibility scores for sounds produced with the rear portion of the tongue. (3) The glossectomees showed improvement in speech intelligibility about 6 months after their operation reaching a plateau thereafter. According to glossal sounds, speech intelligibility of the sounds produced with the rear portion of the tongue showed remarkable improvement. (4) Comparing the surgical methods among subjects with the same extent of resection, higher speech intelligibility was observed in those treated with split-skin graft and free radial forearm flap reconstruction than in those treated by direct suture. (5) Free radial forearm flap reconstruction has the advantage of high speech intelligibility scores for the sounds produced with the rear portion of the tongue and for plosive sounds. (6) Articulatory function after glossectomy was observed to be influenced more by flexibility of the remaining tongue tissue than by its volume.

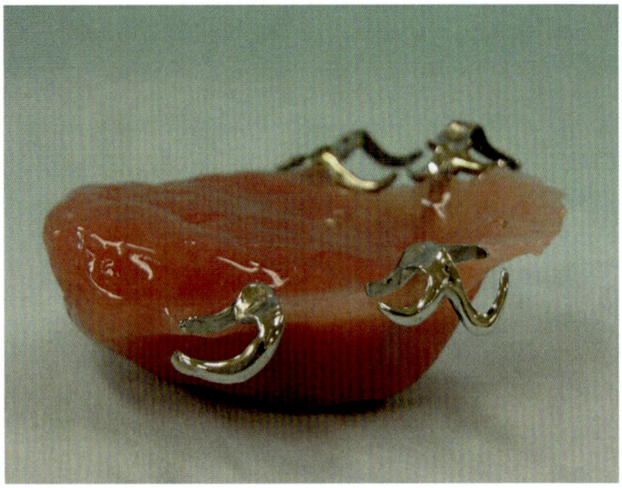

Fig. 16.14 Lateral view of a palatal augmentation prosthesis

16.2.5 Prosthetic Appliances

Prosthetic appliances to assist articulatory deficits include dentures and palatal augmentation prosthesis (PAP). For example, the edentulous patient may have difficulty achieving the correct placement for dentalized sounds. Furthermore, dentures that fit prior to surgical manipulation or irradiation may need to be adjusted due to alterations in the configuration of the oral cavity and the status of the mucosa during treatment.

Partially or totally glossectomized patients may experience difficulty making contact points between the residual tongue tissue and the palate. A PAP lowers the palatal vault to allow the palate to contact the remaining tongue tissue and improve the articulation, including palatolingual phonemes [12] (Figs. 16.13, 16.14, and 16.15). The palatal shape of PAP is adjusted using static palatograms recorded during pronunciation of glossal sounds (Fig. 16.16). PAP improves the swallowing function in addition to articulation (see Sect. 17.3.24(b) "Palatal augmentation prosthesis").

Imai S and Yamashita Y investigated the effects of palatal augmentation prostheses on speech intelligibility in 12 patients who underwent the resection of the tongue and the

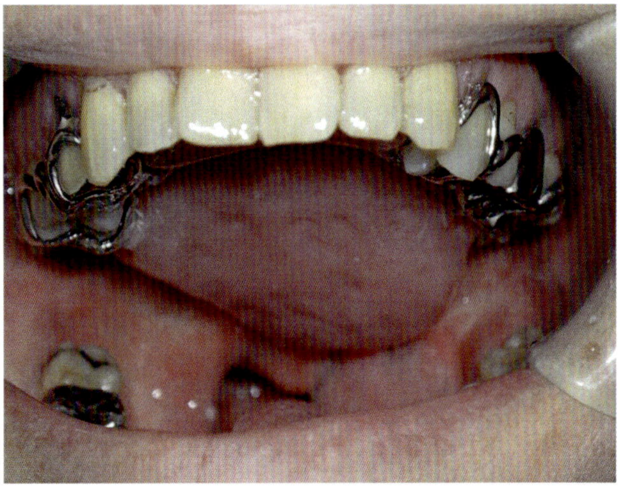

Fig. 16.15 Front view of palatal augmentation prosthesis in the mouth

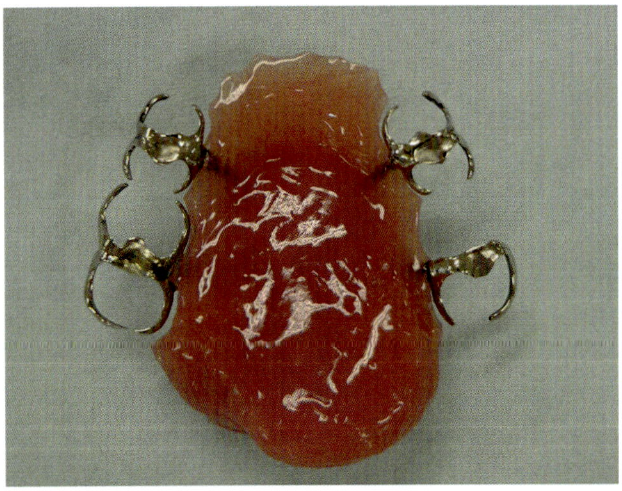

Fig. 16.13 Bottom view (*lingual view*) of a palatal augmentation prosthesis

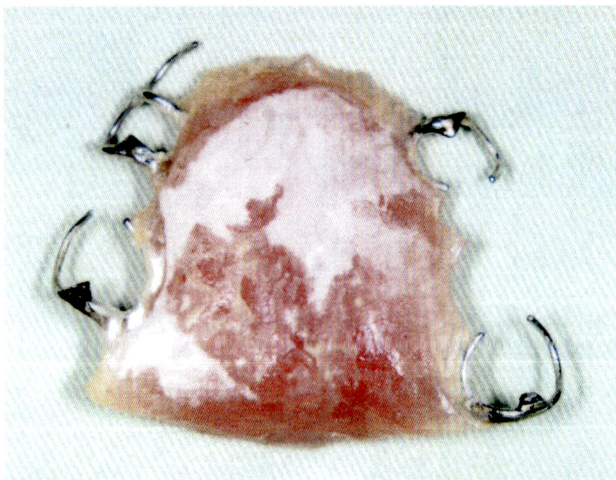

Fig. 16.16 An example of static palatogram recorded during pronunciation of /ki/

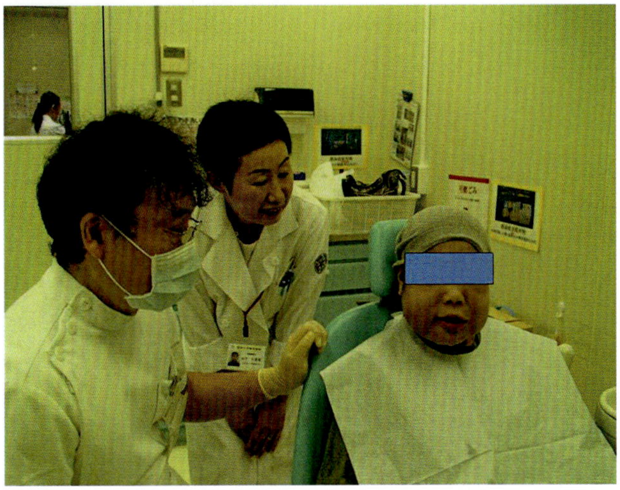

Fig. 16.17 A PAP is adjusted by the coordination between a dentist and a speech pathologist

floor of the mouth [13]. Speech improvement was evaluated by a standardized speech intelligibility test which consisted of 100 syllables.

Their results are summarized as follows: (1) Mean speech intelligibility on 79 glossal sounds improved from 42.3 %without PAP to 57.1 %with PAP. Nine of 12 patients showed remarkable improvement of more than 10 %. (2) According to the glossal sounds, speech intelligibility of the sounds produced with the blade and midportions of the tongue showed remarkable improvement. (3) According to the manner of articulation, speech intelligibility in fricatives, affricates, nasals, and taps was remarkably improved. These results clarify that the PAP is effective in improving speech intelligibility after the resection of the tongue and the floor of the mouth.

Rehabilitation using prosthetic appliances is best accomplished through coordinated efforts between the dentist and speech pathologist (Fig. 16.17). Modification in the shape and configuration of the palatal portion of the prosthesis frequently need to be made as the patient adjusts to the device. Specific needs are assessed by the speech pathologist and fabricated by the dentist.

16.3 Resonance

The primary function of the soft palate is to separate the oral and nasal cavities during swallowing to prevent nasal regurgitation and aerate and equalize pressures in the middle ear. The secondary objective of velopharyngeal closure is for speech purposes. Velopharyngeal closure is produced by sphincteric actions of the levator veli palatini and the superior pharyngeal constrictor muscles. Closure is selective during production for all vowels and consonants except for the nasal consonants.

VPI, even in small degrees, can lead to the perception of hypernasality. This may result from surgical resection of lesions extending to the palate with remaining insufficient bulk, secondary scarring, and/or inadequate tissue mobility. In addition, neurological denervation (cranial nerves IX and X) may temporarily or permanently interfere with palatal motion. This may result from direct tumor invasion, from radiation fibrosis with compression along the nerve roots, or from necessary sacrifice during surgical resection. VPI may result in nasal regurgitation of the bolus during swallow.

Hyponasality is typically perceived when there is blockage of nasal airflow during production of the nasal consonants. Nasal airflow can be impeded due to a space-occupying lesion in the nasopharynx, severe obstruction of the nasal cavities, or overcorrection of VPI.

Depending on the severity of blockage, nasal breathing may also be impaired. Treatment of hyponasality is most frequently directed to correcting the anatomic reason for obstructed nasal airflow.

Velopharyngeal closure is best assessed through videonasendoscopy in which dynamic images of the nasopharynx during production of specific speech tasks are viewed. In rare cases where nasendoscopy cannot be successfully performed, videofluoroscopic images can be obtained in lateral and basal views. Completeness of closure and analysis of any gap are essential to planning treatment. Small gap with minimal bubbling of secretions may be managed with speech therapy alone. More significant VPI may require a combined approach of prosthetics, surgical reconstruction, and speech intervention.

16.3.1 Speech Therapy

Speech rehabilitation is most effective in cases of mild VPI and for those that are neurologically based. Although structural defects may not improve with time or therapeutic exercise, patients may compensate for the lack of tissue bulk. Short-term therapy aimed at maximizing palatal and articulatory efforts may allow for improved velopharyngeal closure. Larger defects need either surgical reconstruction or prosthetic management.

VPI related to neurological compromise is more likely to respond to traditional speech therapy techniques aimed at increasing palatal and articulatory effort. Exercises designed to force the production of velar consonants may assist in increasing strength in the soft palate musculature while also improving the accuracy of these sounds, but the benefits of palatal exercises such as blowing have not been demonstrated to have a beneficial effect on speech production.

Individuals with VPI frequently develop compensatory measures to attempt to decrease some of the nasal airflow, which may include using increased respiratory effort, articulatory techniques, or high nasal airway resistance [14]. The use of increased vocal effort via greater respiratory support has recently received attention, particularly the Lee Silverman Voice Treatment program in its application in individuals with Parkinson's disease [15].

16.3.2 Surgical Procedures

Prosthetics are still preferred as the treatment of choice for most cases of VPI after major oral cancer surgery. However, primary palatal reconstruction with local, regional, or free flaps may be indicated in select patients undergoing significant mid-facial and/or palatal resections. Secondary procedures to improve VPI may also be indicated. The emphasis of flap design needs to be on reducing the abnormal nasal resonance while maintaining an adequate nasal airway. The flap design should allow for the maintenance of sufficient superior excursion of the soft palate remnant and closure at the nasopharyngeal inlet level. Smaller degrees of VPI may benefit palatopexy (surgically created adhesion of the soft palate to the posterior nasopharyngeal wall) and/or transnasal injection of autogenous materials into the nasopharyngeal wall (such as Teflon).

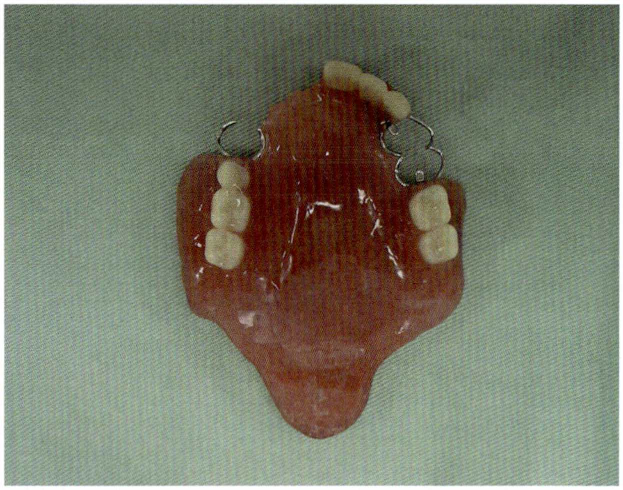

Fig. 16.19 Bottom view (*lingual view*) of a soft palate obturator

16.3.3 Prosthetic Appliances

Prosthetic management of VPI includes the use of palatal obturators, bulbs, and lifts. Defects in the hard palate following maxillectomy are more easily managed through obturation as the area is not dynamic and separation of the oral and nasal cavities is the only requirement. Management of VPI related to defects in the soft palate is more challenging due to the dynamic nature of posterosuperior palatal movement necessary for closure. Although the obturator may fill the surgical defect, its lack of dynamic motion may not result in complete and functional velopharyngeal closure. Typically, the obturator is individualized and designed to be larger than the original defect to allow the additional bulk to make contact with the posterior pharyngeal wall. A fine balance must be obtained to allow adequate closure while maintaining nasal breathing. Overclosure may result in hyponasality. Nasopharyngeal endoscopic examination is appropriate to meet these requirements (Figs. 16.18, 16.19, 16.20, 16.21,

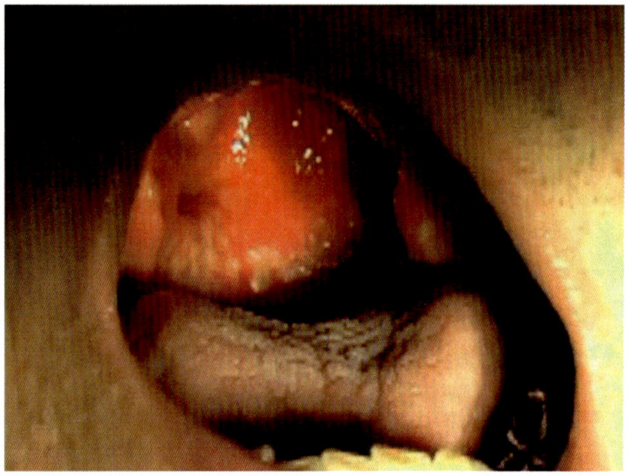

Fig. 16.20 Oral finding at rest in the soft palate-resected patient

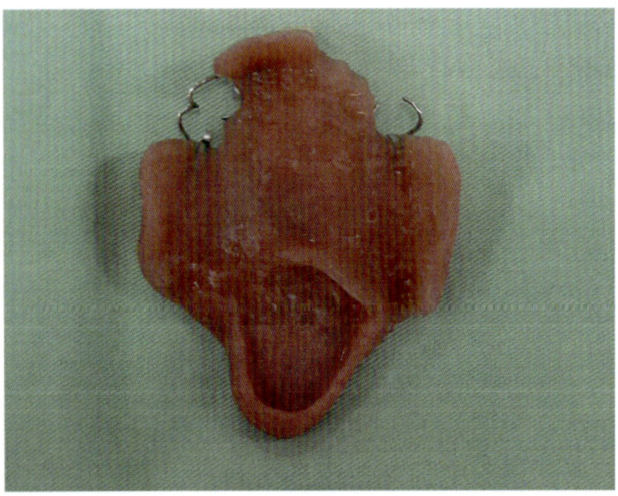

Fig. 16.18 Top view (*palatal view*) of a soft palate obturator

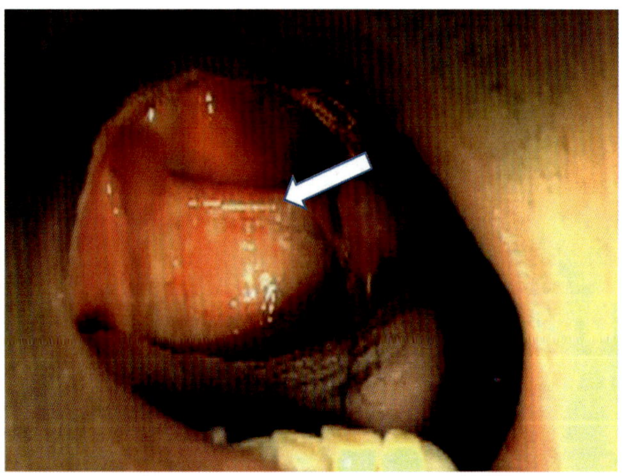

Fig. 16.21 Oral finding at production of /a/ in the soft palate-resected patient. A *white arrow* shows forward movement of the posterior pharyngeal wall

16.22, and 16.23) Nasal regurgitation during swallow is also drastically improved using these devices.

These devices may need to be altered as the patients adjust over time with therapy. In addition, pain related to radiation treatment may inhibit optimal use of the prosthesis, and the fit may need to be adjusted following its completion [12].

Palatal lift prostheses (PLP) are used more often where VPI is secondary to a neurological etiology. A dental appliance is attached to the upper dentition and conforms to the shape of hard palate. An extension is then created to conform to the area of incomplete closure (Figs. 16.24 and 16.25). In the case of a unilateral palatal paralysis, the extension would be fabricated on the affected side to permit closure when the uninvolved side actively closes. Patient tolerance is usually satisfactory, as a gag reflex is reduced or absent in many of these individuals. However, some individuals are not able to swallow at wearing PLP.

Speech bulb prosthesis is a prosthesis which closes the palatal and pharyngeal defects, improving the speech and swallow function (Figs. 16.26, 16.27, and 16.28).

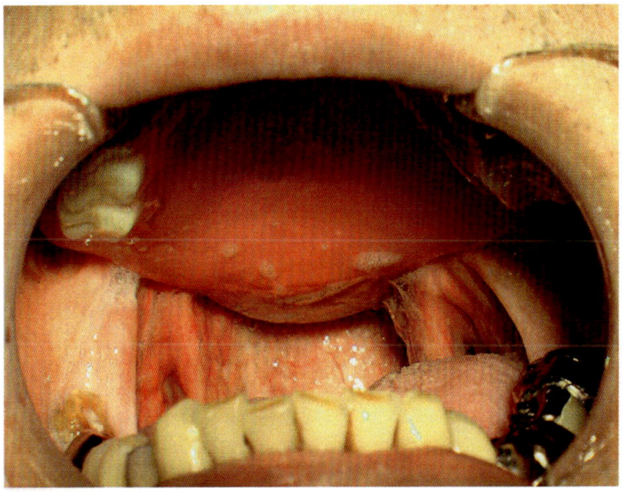

Fig. 16.22 Oral finding at wearing the soft palate obturator in the soft palate-resected patient

16.4 Evaluation of Speech in Oral Cancer Patients

Imai et al. investigated the effectiveness of a new method to measure sentence intelligibility for acquired articulation disorders in postsurgically oral and oropharyngeal cancer patients [16]. Nineteen oral and oropharyngeal cancer patients were assessed using a sentence intelligibility test developed for this investigation. A task was designed to measure success of communication. The test consists of 30 questions containing two or three key words for understanding. Each speech sample was judged by five naive listeners (dental school students). The results were as follows: (1) It was clarified that the sentence intelligibility test developed for this investigation has high validity. (2) Sentence intelligibility was found to be considerably high in postoperative oral and oropharyngeal cancer patients. (3) A significant correlation was found

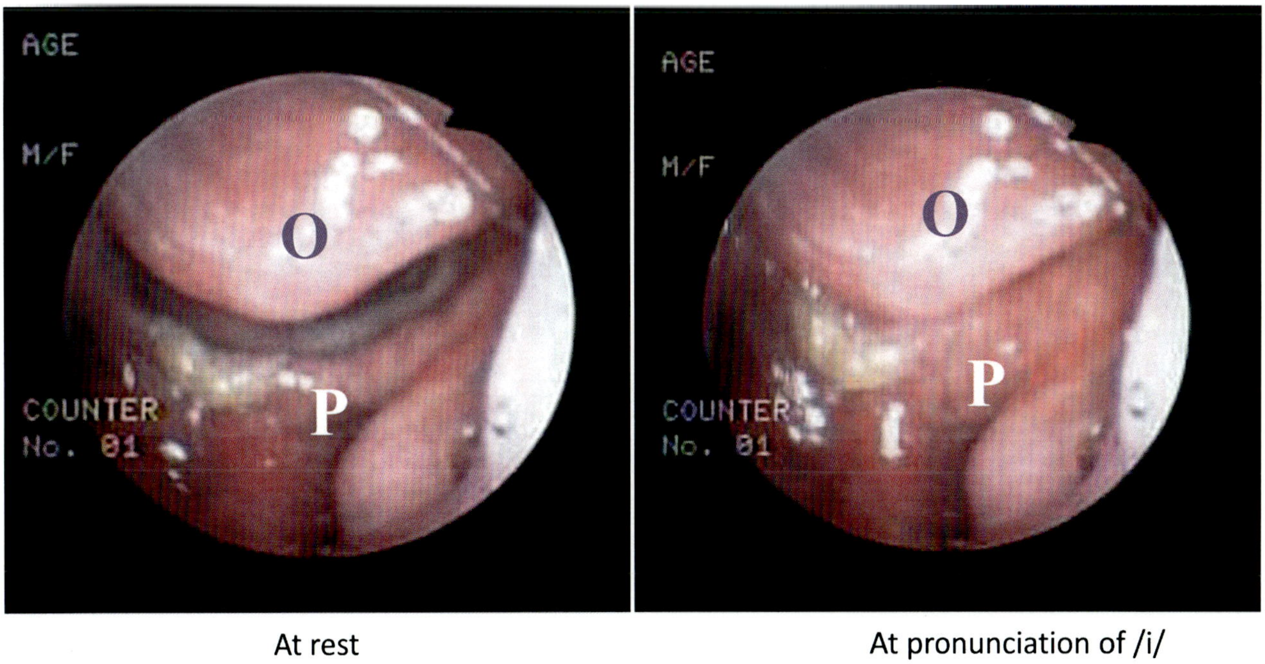

Fig. 16.23 Nasopharyngeal endoscopic images at wearing a soft palate obturator in the soft palate-resected patient. A gap between the posterior margin of soft palate obturator (*O*) and the posterior pharyngeal wall (*P*) found at rest vanished at pronunciation of /i/

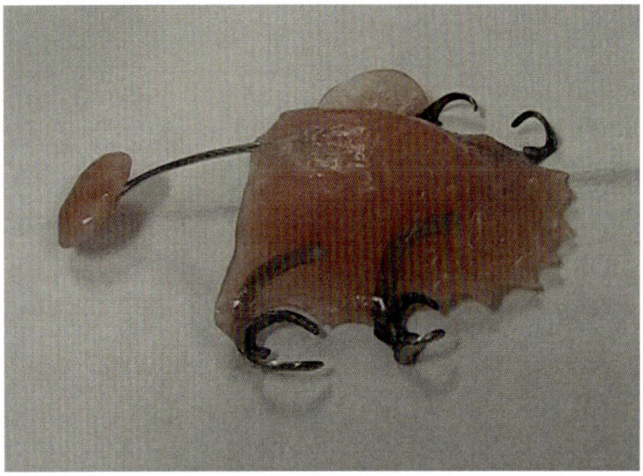

Fig. 16.24 Top view (*palatal view*) of a palatal lift prosthesis

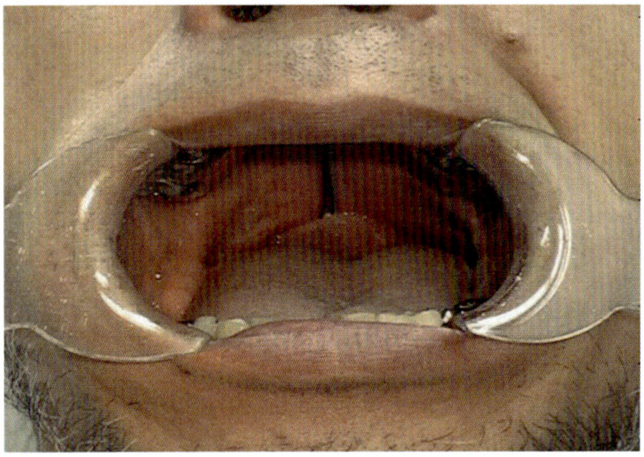

Fig. 16.25 Oral finding at wearing the palatal lift prosthesis in the stroke patient

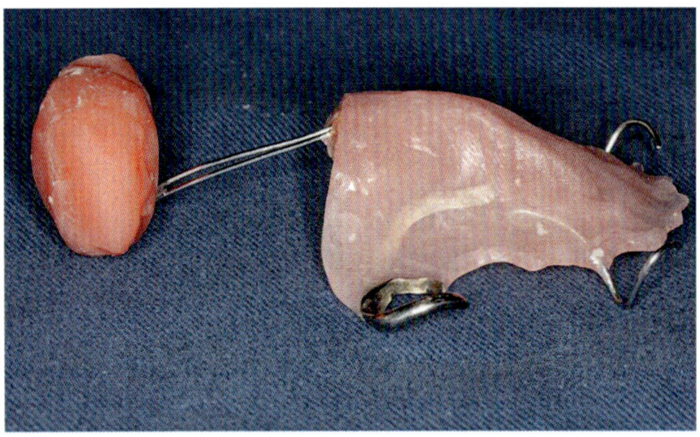

Fig. 16.26 Lateral view of a speech bulb prosthesis

between syllable and sentence intelligibility. The sentence intelligibility score was significantly higher than that of syllable intelligibility. Speech recognition is based on both bottom-up processing or acoustic data-driven processing and top-down processing or prediction-driven processing

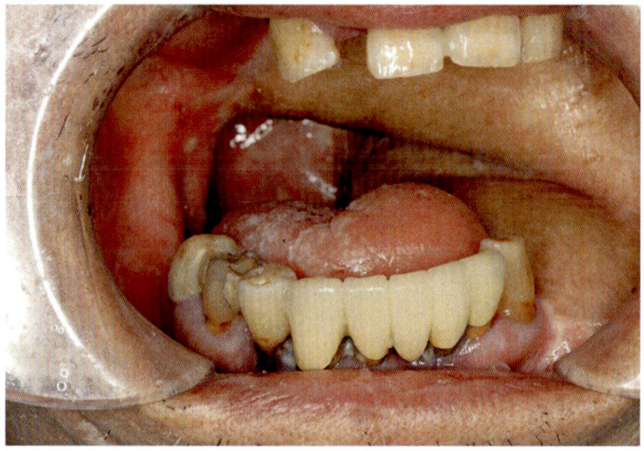

Fig. 16.27 Oral finding in the patient who underwent resection of maxilla, oropharynx, and mandible with reconstructive surgery using the rectus abdominis myocutaneous flap

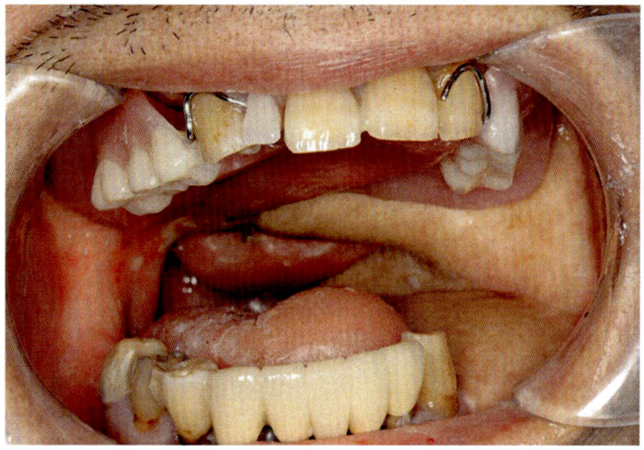

Fig. 16.28 Oral finding in the patient wearing a speech bulb prosthesis who underwent resection of maxilla, oropharynx, and mandible with reconstructive surgery using the rectus abdominis myocutaneous flap

based on linguistic knowledge. This is the reason why the sentence intelligibility was significantly higher than syllable intelligibility.

References

1. Yokoyama K, Takahashi K, Yamada H et al (2014) Speech disorders and nasal emissions of maxillary prosthetic patients in comparison of defects' patterns. In: Proceeding of the 32th annual meeting of Japan society for oral tumors, p 196
2. Logemann JA, Pauloski BR, Rademaker AW, Colangelo LA (1997) Speech and swallowing rehabilitation for head and neck cancer patients. Oncology 11(5):651–659
3. Fox EL, Kirby TE, Fox AR (1987) Bases of fitness. Macmillan, New York, pp 181–183
4. Clark DH (1973) Adaptations in strength and muscular endurance resulting from exercise. Exerc Sport Sci Rev 1:73–102
5. Atha J (1981) Strengthening muscle. Exerc Sport Sci Rev 9:1–78
6. Heyward VH (1991) Advanced fitness assessment and exercise prescription. Human Kinetics Books, Champaign

7. McConnell FM, Teichgraeber JF, Adler RK (1987) A comparison of three methods of oral reconstruction. Arch Otolaryngol Head Neck Surg 113:496–500
8. Leonard R, Goodrich S, McMenamin P, Donald P (1992) Differentiation of speakers with glossectomies by acoustic and perceptual measures. Am J Speech Lang Pathol 1:56–62
9. Pauloski BR, Logemann JA, Rademaker AW, McConnel FMS, Heiser MA et al (1993) Speech and swallowing function after anterior tongue and floor of mouth resection with distal flap reconstruction. J Speech Hear Res 36:267–276
10. Urken ML, Moscoso JF, Lawson W, Biller HF (1994) A systematic approach to functional reconstruction of the oral cavity following partial and total glossectomy. Arch Otolaryngol Head Neck Surg 120:589–601
11. Imai S, Michi K, Yamashita Y et al (1988) Speech intelligibility after resection of the tongue and floor of the mouth. The relation between the surgical excisions or operation methods and speech intelligibility. Jpn J Oral Maxillofac Surg 34:1567–1583
12. Pauloski BR, Logemann JA, Colangelo LA et al (1996) Effect of intraoral prostheses on swallowing function in postsurgical oral and oropharyngeal cancer patients. Am J Speech Lang Pathol 5:31–46
13. Imai S, Yamashita Y (1992) Effects of a palatal augmentation prosthesis on speech intelligibility in patients with glossectomy. Jpn J Commun Disorders 9:1–9
14. Warren DW (1986) Compensatory speech behaviors in individuals with cleft palate: a regulation/control phenomenon? Cleft Palate J 23:251–260
15. Ramig LO, Sapir S, Countryman S, Pawlas AA et al (2001) Intensive voice treatment (LSVT®) for patients with Parkinson's disease: a 2 year follow up. J Neurol Neurosurg Psychiatry 71: 493–498
16. Imai S, Yamashita Y et al (1997) Development of sentence intelligibility assessment method for patients with articulation disorders-application to postoperative oral and oropharyngeal cancer patients. Jpn J Logopedics Phoniatrics 38:357–365

Management of Dysphagia Following Treatment for Oral Cancer

17

Koji Takahashi

Abstract

This chapter is focusing on the management of dysphagia caused by the treatment of oral cancer. The causes, site-specific characteristics, evaluation, and treatment of dysphagia following oral cancer treatment are introduced in detail. The noninstrumental evaluating methods, the cervical auscultation, the videofluoroscopic swallow study, the videoendoscopic swallow study, and the ultrasound study are introduced in the section of the evaluation methods for dysphagia. The treatment methods for dysphagia include the airway clearance techniques, the compensatory techniques, and the swallow exercises. The short-term intensive dysphagia rehabilitation is also introduced. The sophisticated techniques and newly developed methods in both evaluation and treatment for dysphagia are introduced with a lot of clinical figures. Chapter 16 and this chapter provide the clinicians the way how to manage the oral and pharyngeal dysfunction caused after the treatment of oral cancer.

Keywords

Cervical auscultation • Evaluation of dysphagia • Management of dysphagia • Site specific characteristics • Treatment of dysphagia

17.1 Characteristics of Dysphagia After Treatment for Oral Cancer

17.1.1 Causes of Dysphagia in Oral Cancer

The causes of dysphagia in oral cancer patients are shown in Table 17.1. When cancers of the lips, maxilla, palate, tongue, floor of the mouth, mandible, and oropharynx are surgically treated, anatomical and physiological changes of each structure are inevitable because of the anatomic deficit and postoperative swelling and hence the flow of bolus and function of swallow-related structures are altered postsurgically [1, 2]. Patients may exhibit long-term effects as fibrosis, scar formation, and contracture of affected soft tissues that gradually worsen after the surgery. Related muscles that support swallow physiology such as the facial muscles, tongue muscles, suprahyoid muscles, masticatory muscles, palatine muscles, and pharyngeal muscles may be surgically invaded and cause functional disorders.

The progress of recent surgical reconstruction techniques has made it possible to perform various grafting techniques to surgically close the deficiency after the resection; however, morphological change and reduction of movement in remaining tissues are inevitable. Recently, the neurosurgical techniques (connecting the graft and host nerves) have been attempted to acquire movement and sensation in reconstructed structures. Results of these efforts still are not sufficient to restore total function.

Surgical invasion to the peripheral nerves also results in disordered movement and sensation. Damage to the hypoglossal nerve causes reduced movements in the tongue and hyoid bone, whereas damage to the facial nerve causes the labial closure insufficiency, hypogeusia, and decreased

K. Takahashi, D.D.S., Ph.D. (✉)
Division of Oral Rehabilitation Medicine, Department of Special Needs Oral medicine, School of Dentistry, Showa University, 2-1-1 Kitasenzoku Ohta-ku, Tokyo 145-8515, Japan
e-mail: tkouji@dent.showa-u.ac.jp

T. Kirita and K. Omura (eds.), *Oral Cancer: Diagnosis and Therapy*, DOI 10.1007/978-4-431-54938-3_17, © Springer Japan 2015

Table 17.1 Causes of dysphagia in oral cancer

I. Causes associated with surgical treatment
A. Structural change
1. Changes of soft tissue and hard tissue Anatomic deficit, postoperative swelling, scar formation, and contracture in the lips, maxilla, palate, tongue, floor of the mouth, mandible, and oropharynx
2. Changes of muscles Anatomic deficit, postoperative swelling, scar formation, and contracture in the facial muscles, tongue muscles, suprahyoid muscles, masticatory muscles, palatine muscles, and pharyngeal muscles
3. Reconstruction Morphological change and reduction of movements in remained tissues
B. Impaired motor and sensory neuron
1. Damage to the trigeminal nerve
2. Damage to the facial nerve
3. Damage to the glossopharyngeal nerve
4. Damage to the vagus nerve
5. Damage to the hypoglossal nerve
C. Complications after tracheostomy (C1 and C3 are due to the tracheostomy tube; C2 is due to the tracheostomy tube with inflated cuff)
1. Restricted laryngeal movement
2. Compression of the esophagus
3. Excess tracheal secretion and pooling of the secretion
4. Reduced subglottic pressure
5. Reduced laryngeal sensitivity and delayed glottic closure reflex
II. Causes associated with radiotherapy
A. Mucositis
B. Neuropathy
C. Fibrosis
D. Xerostomia

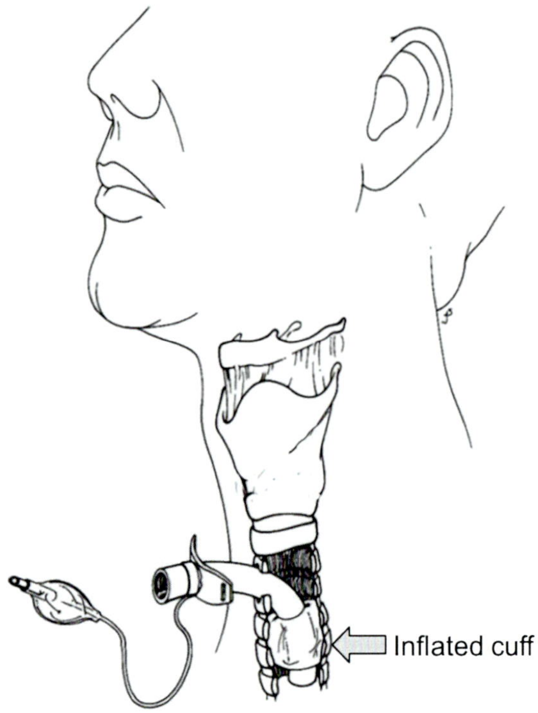

Fig. 17.1 Restricted laryngeal movement caused by the tracheostomy tube, indirect compression on the esophagus by the inflated cuff, excess tracheal secretions due to the constant irritation by the tracheostomy tube, and reduced subglottic pressure due to the expiratory air leakage through the tube

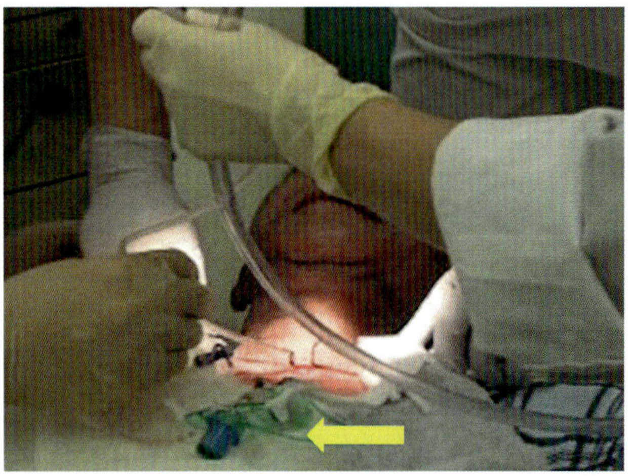

Fig. 17.2 The safe and effective weaning of a patient from a tracheostomy tube should be performed to facilitate decannulation. This glossectomized and mandibulectomized patient was transferred to our department from a different hospital where the patient wore tracheostomy tube with inflated cuff over 100 days after the surgery. A *yellow arrow* shows the tracheostomy tube with cuff

salivation from the submandibular and sublingual glands. When the glossopharyngeal nerve and vagus nerve are damaged, velopharyngeal insufficiency and motor and sensory disorders in pharynx and larynx are observed. Also, when the motor branches of the trigeminal nerve are damaged, movements of masticatory muscles are impaired. When the sensory branch of the trigeminal nerve is damaged, sensory paralysis of oral and facial regions are observed.

In addition, tracheostomy for airway control is not rare in oral cancer surgery. Patients with tracheostomy exhibit problems such as restricted laryngeal movement caused by the tracheostomy tube, indirect compression on the esophagus by the inflated cuff, excess tracheal secretions due to the constant irritation by the tracheostomy tube, and reduced subglottic pressure due to the expiratory air leakage through the tube (Fig. 17.1). These problems result in reduced laryngeal elevation, reduced bolus passage into the esophagus, diminished laryngeal reflex, penetration (bolus entering in the larynx above the vocal folds), and aspiration (bolus entering under the vocal folds), all of which complicate the dysphagia in tracheostomized patients [3–7]. The safe and effective weaning of a patient from a tracheostomy tube should be performed to facilitate decannulation (Figs. 17.2, 17.3, and 17.4).

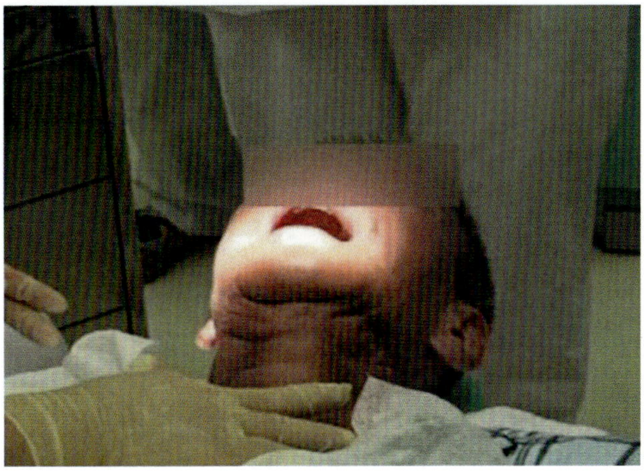

Fig. 17.3 Immediately after decannulation, the movement of vocal cord was very insufficient. The patient was encouraged to produce voicing as strongly as he can while the tracheostoma was occluded by my finger. During this procedure, suctioning from the mouth and tracheostoma was required

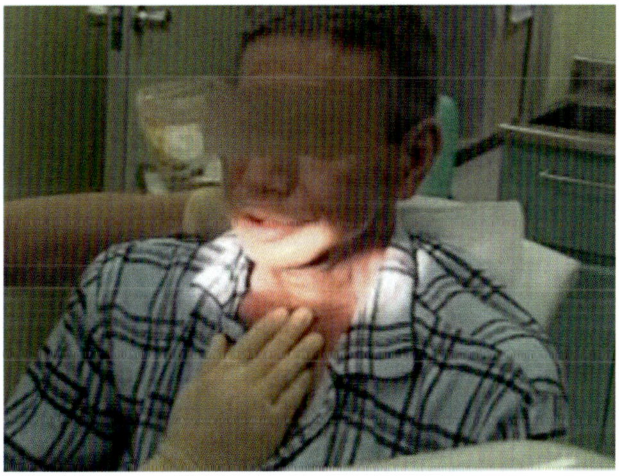

Fig. 17.4 The patient was encouraged to produce voicing and to expectorate secretions from the mouth as strongly as he can at the upright position, while the tracheostoma was occluded by my finger. After the safe breathing, voicing and strong huffing or coughing to expectorate secretions and sputa were verified; the retainer with peaking bulb was inserted into the tracheostoma instead of tracheostomy tube with cuff

Patients receiving radiotherapy in isolation or in combination with surgery or chemotherapy are at risk for swallowing difficulties as well. In the early stage of the therapy, pain from mucositis contributes directly to the patient's swallowing ability. During and following the therapy, as a result of neuropathy (peripheral nerve deficit), patients often complain of a reduced sense of taste, and in some cases, a delayed pharyngeal reflex is present. Furthermore, as fibrosis of the tissue advances over time, reduced oral and/or oropharyngeal movements and/or deficits in laryngeal elevation may develop dysphagia [8, 9]. Patients also experience reduced saliva flow or xerostomia after radiotherapy. Medications (pilocarpine, cevimeline, etc.) to stimulate saliva and pseudo-saliva products (mucin-containing spray, Xanthangum-containing liquid, Sodium carboxymethylcellulose-containing liquid, Sodium chloride-containing liquid, etc.) are often only partially effective. Chemoradiation treatment results in xerostomia and a significant increase in patient perception of swallowing difficulties [10]. Xerostomia primarily affects mastication and oral manipulation of a dry, absorbent food material [11]. However, xerostomia does not affect the physiologic aspects of bolus transport or pharyngeal swallow [10, 11]. Xerostomia affects the oropharyngeal sensory process and comfort of eating more than pharyngeal swallow [10].

In summary, the swallowing disorders result from the various treatments (surgery, radiotherapy, or combination of both) for the oral cancer. Dysphagia that occurs after cancer treatments result from altered movement and coordination of structures within the swallowing mechanism.

17.1.2 Site-Specific Characteristics

1. Labial Cancer
   When the lips or marginal mandibular branch of the facial nerve is surgically affected, labial movement insufficiency is observed. Also, when the mental nerve (inferior alveolar nerve) is surgically affected, lower lip paralysis (sensation loss) is observed. In each case, problems such as drooling and the extraoral leakage of bolus are recognized as a result of labial closure insufficiency.
2. Tongue Cancer and Oral Floor Cancer
   Surgeries involving the tongue and the oral floor often result in problems with taste, bolus formulation and containment, and bolus transport from the front to the back of the mouth. Also, problems in the pharyngeal phase are often recognized because oral and pharyngeal coordination is disordered [12]. In general, patients with tongue and oral floor cancer demonstrate problems such as (1) premature leakage of bolus into the pharynx, (2) bolus control and transport difficulties, (3) residue of bolus in the oral cavity, and (4) delayed onset of pharyngeal swallow.
3. Mandibular Gingival Cancer
   Problems shown by this group of patients include (1) limited mastication due to the loss of teeth and masticatory muscles, deviation of reconstructed mandible, and sensory loss, (2) residue of bolus in the oral vestibule due to the loss of the lower alveolar ridge, alterations of shape, tension, and sensitivity in buccal tissues, (3) trismus due to the scar formation and contracture of the affected tissues, and (4) drooling and extraoral leakage of bolus due to the labial closure insufficiency or lower lip paralysis.
4. Maxillary Gingival Cancer and Palatal Cancer (Maxillary Cancer)
   The swallowing problems in patients with the resected maxilla include (1) mastication difficulty due to the loss of teeth, (2)

entry of bolus into the nasal cavity due to the oronasal fistula or velopharyngeal insufficiency, (3) residue of bolus in the oral vestibule due to the loss of the upper alveolar ridge and alterations of shape in buccal tissues, (4) drooling and extraoral leakage of bolus due to the labial closure insufficiency or upper lip paralysis, and (5) trismus if the fauces or internal and external pterygoid muscles are surgically affected.

5. Oropharyngeal Cancer
   The oropharynx extends superiorly from the soft palate to the epiglottis inferiorly and anteriorly from the tongue base to the posterior pharyngeal wall posteriorly. Deficits of swallowing following oropharyngeal cancer include (1) nasal regurgitation due to velopharyngeal insufficiency, (2) bolus transport difficulty due to reduced tongue base mobility, (3) delayed onset of pharyngeal swallow due to reduced oropharyngeal sensation, (4) residue of bolus in the oral vestibule due to the alterations of shape and sensitivity in buccal tissues, and (5) trismus due to surgical invasion to the fauces or internal and external pterygoid muscles [13, 14].

17.2 Evaluation of Dysphagia

17.2.1 Noninstrumental Evaluations

1. Medical Interview
   A medical interview enables a clinician to help identify the onset, cause, site, and severity of dysphagia. From the symptoms described by the patients, a clinician is able to make assumptions of the disorders associated with swallowing such as insufficient labial closure, reduced tongue coordination for holding and transporting the bolus, cricopharyngeal dysfunction, reduced laryngeal elevation, weak pharyngeal contraction, and velopharyngeal incompetence (Table 17.1).
2. Inspection and Palpation
   The shape, function, and sensitivity of anatomical structures related to swallowing are investigated by inspection and palpation.
3. Ice Chip Swallow Test
   The ice chip swallow test is a test for patients who are highly suspect for aspiration. The examiner places ice chips in a patient's mouth and observes if the swallow reflex is delayed, for cough, or if voice alteration is present. In order to detect dysphagia, it is helpful to use cervical auscultation described below during this test. The cold stimulus of the ice chips is expected to trigger the pharyngeal swallow, and it is suitable not only as an assessment tool but also introductory swallowing material for direct swallow therapy.
4. Laryngeal Elevation Test
   Laryngeal elevation is one of the most essential components involved in swallowing. The extent and strength of the laryngeal elevation are assessed by placing the fingers at the thyroid cartilage of the patients when they swallow saliva. The extent of the laryngeal elevation in normal adults is about 1.5–2 cm (Fig. 17.5). Elevation under 1 cm is considered abnormal. The strength of the laryngeal elevation is considered normal when the index finger on the superior thyroid notch is flicked by the laryngeal elevation during the swallow (Fig. 17.6). For patients who have no signs of a pharyngeal swallow reflex, thermal–tactile stimulation to the anterior faucial pillars is given before performing the laryngeal elevation test.
5. Timed Water Swallow Test
   The timed water swallow test consists of the patient drinking 30 ml of water from a cup, with the examiner recording the time taken and number of swallows as well as noting the swallow-related episodes such as cough and wet/hoarse voice [15, 16]. Five seconds is considered as

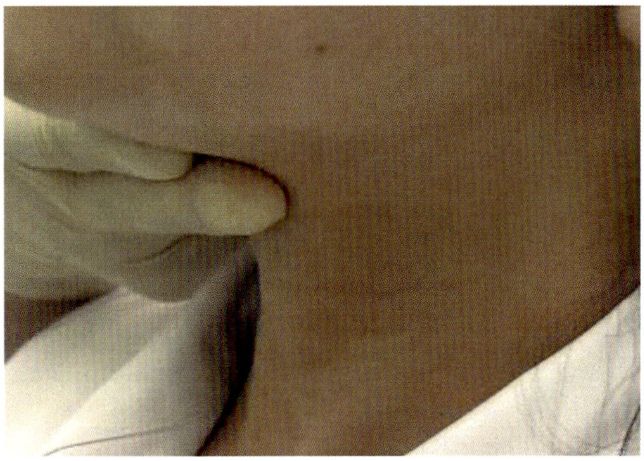

Fig. 17.5 The extent of the laryngeal elevation is assessed by placing the fingers just above the thyroid cartilage of the patient during saliva swallow

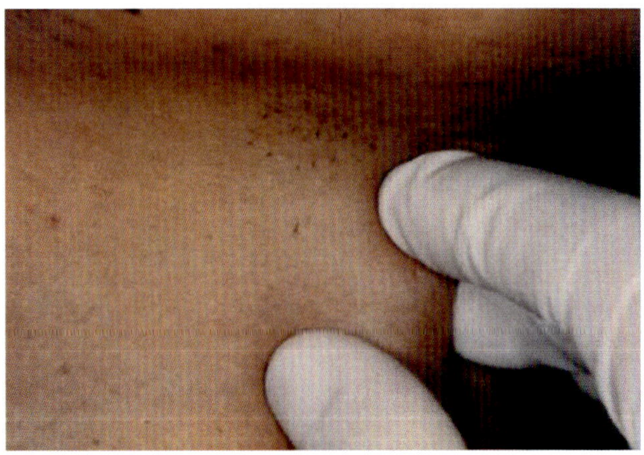

Fig. 17.6 The strength of the laryngeal elevation is assessed by placing the fingers just above the thyroid cartilage of the patient during saliva swallow

the threshold of dysphagia, and if a patient showed increase in duration and/or number of swallows, oral or pharyngeal swallow disorder is suspected. Because a large amount of water is swallowed in this test, it is not appropriate for patients who are suspected to have a severe swallowing disorder.

6. Modified Water Swallow Test (MWST)
   In the MWST, patients swallow 3 ml of cold water, and the presence of pharyngeal swallow reflex, cough, and respiratory change is recorded [17–19] (Table 17.2). This test is applicable for severe dysphagic patients. Combining this test with the cervical auscultation helps the examiner in detecting the occurrence of swallow.
7. Food Test (FT)
   In the food test, patients swallow each of 4 g of pudding and 4 g of rice porridge, and the presence of pharyngeal swallow reflex, cough, and respiratory change is recorded as with the MWST [19, 20] (Table 17.3). Using the cervical auscultation with this test also is helpful in detecting dysphagia.
8. Repetitive Saliva Swallowing Test (RSST)
   The RSST is a screening test to evaluate if patients have an ability to initiate volitional swallow. In this test, patients are asked to repeat dry swallows (swallowing saliva) for 30 s, and the number of swallows is recorded. For patients with dry mouth, artificial saliva may be used to moisten the oral cavity before performing the dry swallow. Three repetitive dry swallows within 30 s is the threshold for the elderly [21, 22]. Combining this test with the laryngeal elevation test helps the examiner in detecting the occurrence of swallow (Fig. 17.7).

Table 17.2 Scores and criteria of modified water swallow test (MWST)

Score	Criteria
Score 1	No swallow with/without dyspnea or cough
Score 2	Swallow with dyspnea (indication of silent aspiration)
Score 3	Swallow without dyspnea, but experienced cough or wet/hoarse voice
Score 4	Swallow without dyspnea nor cough
Score 5	Swallow without dyspnea nor cough, and perform two additional dry swallows within 30 s

Table 17.3 Scores and criteria of food test (FT)

Score	Criteria
Score 1	No swallow with/without dyspnea or cough
Score 2	Swallow with dyspnea (indication of silent aspiration)
SCORE 3	Swallow without dyspnea, but experienced cough or wet/hoarse voice <25 % retention in oral cavity
Score 4	Swallow without dyspnea nor cough >25 % retention in oral cavity
Score 5	Swallow without dyspnea nor cough and perform two additional dry swallows within 30 s

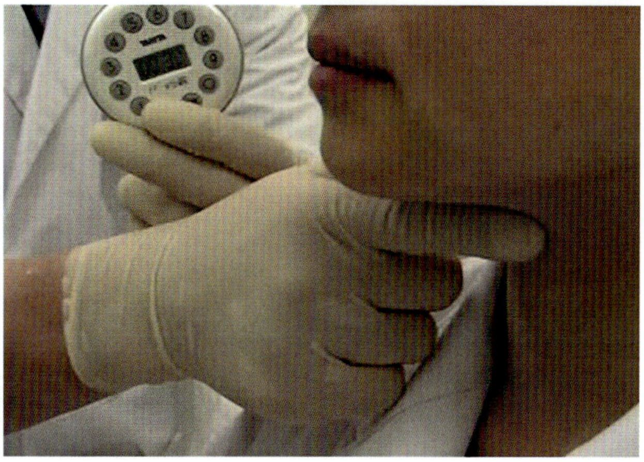

Fig. 17.7 The repetitive saliva swallowing test is a screening test to evaluate if patients have an ability to initiate volitional swallow. In this test, patients are asked to repeat dry swallows (swallowing saliva) for 30 s, and the number of swallows is recorded

17.2.2 Evaluation Using Simple Instruments: Cervical Auscultation

1. What Is Cervical Auscultation?
   Cervical auscultation is a technique used to evaluate the pharyngeal swallow by applying the stethoscope to the patient's neck and listening to the swallow and respiratory sounds [23] (Fig. 17.8). The clinician listens and evaluates the characteristics and duration of swallowing sounds and the characteristics and timing of respiratory sounds. Cervical auscultation is a noninvasive screening tool for assessing the aspiration and pharyngeal retention, and it has been used widely in the clinical setting dealing with dysphagia.
2. Supplies Needed for Cervical Auscultation
   (a) Stethoscope
   In cervical auscultation, a stethoscope is placed on a patient's neck to identify the sounds. The cervical area is a relatively small region compared to the chest or abdomen which is the usual region for auscultation. For cervical auscultation, a pediatric stethoscope is recommended (Fig. 17.9).
   (b) Swallow Materials
   For patients with severe swallowing disorders, a small amount of ice-cold water (1–2 ml) or few small ice chips are used. The movement of these ice-cold materials is easily noticed in the mouth and pharynx, and the cold stimulus is effective in triggering the pharyngeal swallow. Also, these materials can be cleared relatively easy, even if they are aspirated.
3. Procedures for Cervical Auscultation
   Before auscultation, the residual secretions in the oral cavity, pharynx, and larynx should be cleared in order to optimize the accuracy of the evaluation. Patients who are

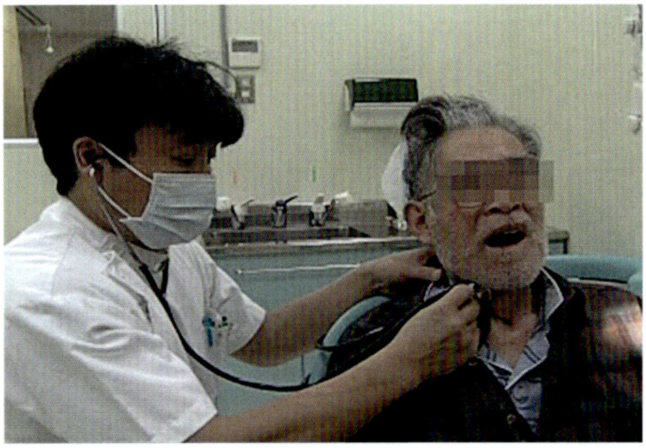

Fig. 17.8 Cervical auscultation is a technique used to evaluate the pharyngeal swallow by applying the stethoscope to the patient's neck and listening to the swallow and respiratory sounds

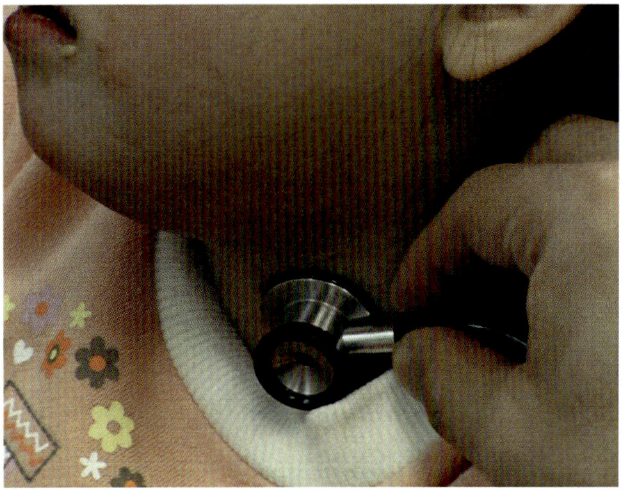

Fig. 17.9 The cervical area is a relatively small region compared to the chest or abdomen which is the usual region for auscultation. For cervical auscultation, a pediatric stethoscope is recommended

able to understand and follow the directions are instructed to clear the airway by strong voluntary cough or forced expiration (huffing). As the patient clears their secretions, they should bend forward with the trunk and neck lower than the horizontal angle of the body to get gravity assistance. If the airway is not cleared completely, suctioning is required. After airway clearance, the patient is asked to exhale, and the expiratory sound is auscultated. Then, as the swallowing material is given to the patient, the sounds produced during the swallow are evaluated. Finally, the patient is asked to exhale immediately after the swallow, and the expiratory sound is auscultated. Comparisons should be made between the pre-swallow expiratory sound and post-swallow expiratory sound to see if there is any alteration.

Table 17.4 Diagnosis and auditory characteristics of swallowing and expiratory sounds using cervical auscultation

Diagnosis		Diagnostic criteria (auditory characteristics)
Safe swallow[b]	1. Normal	Clear swallowing and expiratory sounds
	2. Acceptable	Clear expiratory sounds, repeated or weak swallowing sounds
Dysphagic swallow[b]	3. Residue[a]	Rough or gargling expiratory sounds after swallow, repeated or weak swallowing sounds
	4. Penetration[a]	Rough or gargling expiratory sounds after swallow, repeatedly weak swallowing sounds, breathing while swallowing
	5. Aspiration[a]	Rough or gargling expiratory sounds before/after swallow, repeatedly weak swallowing sounds, breathing while swallowing, uneven breathing, cough or slightly cough while/after swallow, liquid vibrating sound while expiration

[a]Auditory differentiation among residue, penetration, and aspiration is not clear

[b]Accuracy of auditory differentiation of dysphagic swallow from safe swallow is high (83.5 %)

For patients who are not able to follow the directions, the residual secretions are cleared by suctioning. After the airway clearance, spontaneous respiratory sounds, swallow sounds, and post-swallow respiratory sounds are auscultated and evaluated, respectively.

The postural adjustment and bolus volume modification may be implemented as the evaluation proceeds. However, if severe aspiration is suspected, stop the evaluation, and suction aspirated material immediately.

4. Interpreting the Sound Obtained by Cervical Auscultation
Prolonged or weak swallow sounds or multiple swallow sounds are associated with difficulties in bolus transport, pharyngeal contraction, laryngeal elevation, and cricopharyngeal opening. When a bubbling sound, throat clearing sound, or cough is heard during the swallow, aspiration is highly suspected. The presence of unexpected respiratory sounds during the swallow (respiratory sound during the apnea period) indicates laryngeal penetration (material enters the larynx, remains above the vocal folds), aspiration (material enters the airway, passes below the vocal folds), or swallow–respiration coordination (apnea–swallow–breathe sequence) disorder.

As for the respiratory (expiratory) sound after the swallow, a wet sound, gargling sound, or liquid vibrating sound (liquid vibration by the expiratory airflow at the airway actually witnessed in videofluoroscopic studies) is associated with laryngeal penetration, aspiration, or pharyngeal retention. Also, aspiration is suspected if wheezing sound, throat clearing, or cough is auscultated. In any case, it is important to clear the airway before the swallow to compare the respiratory (expiratory) sounds produced before and after the swallow (Table 17.4).

5. Accuracy of Cervical Auscultation for Detecting Dysphagia Evaluated by Acoustic Measurements and Auditory Assessment Takahashi et al. evaluated the accuracy of cervical auscultation for detecting dysphagic swallows in head and neck cancer patients [24]. In this study, swallowing and respiratory sounds were detected by accelerometer attached to the neck and recorded on VHS tape with videofluorographic (VF) images. In the first half of this study, acoustic signals of swallowing sounds and expiratory sounds were analyzed using the computed analyzing system. 0.79 s of the duration of swallowing sounds and 25.3 dB of the revised magnitude of the 0 to 250Hz band of expiratory sound signals were set as the critical values in order to differentiate dysphagic swallows from safe swallows. Comparison of these assessments with the VF findings showed significant agreement. Both percent agreements were 77.3 % (102/132, 150/194). In the latter half of this study, swallowing sounds during swallows and expiratory sounds before and after swallows were edited and presented to six examiners through headphones. Without videofluorographic images, each examiner auditorily assigned the sound samples to one of two categories: safe swallow or dysphagic swallow. The percent agreement of auditory judgements with VF images was assessed. The percent agreement of two categories (safe swallow or dysphagic swallow) judged auditorily with VF images averaged 83.5 % (441/528). These results revealed the effectiveness of cervical auscultation as a clinical tool for diagnosing a dysphagic swallow in head and neck cancer patients.

17.2.3 Evaluations Using Special Instruments

1. Videofluoroscopic Swallow Study (VFSS)
   (a) What is the videofluoroscopic swallow study?
   The VFSS is considered to be the most reliable evaluation technique for dysphagia. The videofluoroscopic (VF) image gives information on the anatomy and physiology of the swallow-related structures and movement patterns of the radiopaque bolus. The observation of the image helps a clinician to determine the impaired region and evaluate dysphagic symptoms such as retention, laryngeal penetration, and aspiration. Aspiration is generally classified into three types (before, during, or after the swallow) according to the time of its occurrence relative to the triggering of the pharyngeal swallow. Aspiration before the swallow occurs before the pharyngeal swallow is triggered while the airway is still open. It may result from reduced tongue control and delayed or absent pharyngeal reflex. Aspiration during the swallow occurs if the laryngeal closure is inadequate. Aspiration after the swallow occurs when the larynx lowers and opens for inhalation. It may result from restriction in pharyngeal contraction, tongue base posterior movement, laryngeal elevation, laryngeal closure, or cricopharyngeal opening.
   Normally, the lateral radiographic view is used to examine swallowing (Fig. 17.10). However, to evaluate the symmetry of the anatomical structures and bolus flow, the anterior–posterior view is used (Fig. 17.11). To evaluate the esophageal transit, the patient is imaged while standing obliquely (Fig. 17.12).
   Once the abnormalities in the patient's anatomy and/or physiology of swallowing mechanism have been identified, the clinician should introduce treatment strategies during the VFSS. Such strategies usually include compensatory techniques (changing head or body posture, modifying viscosity and volume of bolus), thermal–tactile stimulation prior to the swallow, and swallow maneuvers. These strategies are introduced during the VFSS so that the clinician is able to evaluate the impact of the intervention.
   (b) A new system combining clinical information of the patient during VFSS and the VF images
   VFSS is considered the gold standard examination for diagnosis of dysphagia. However, VFSS is the simple white and black silent movie lacking in important patient's clinical information including physique, level of alertness, motivation, facial expression,

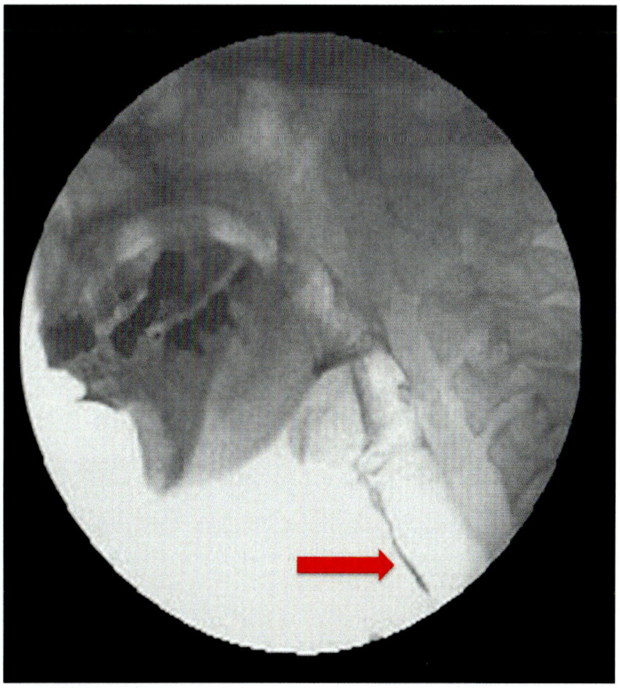

Fig. 17.10 An example of lateral view of the videofluoroscopic swallow study (*VFSS*). A *red arrow* shows aspiration of radiopaque material

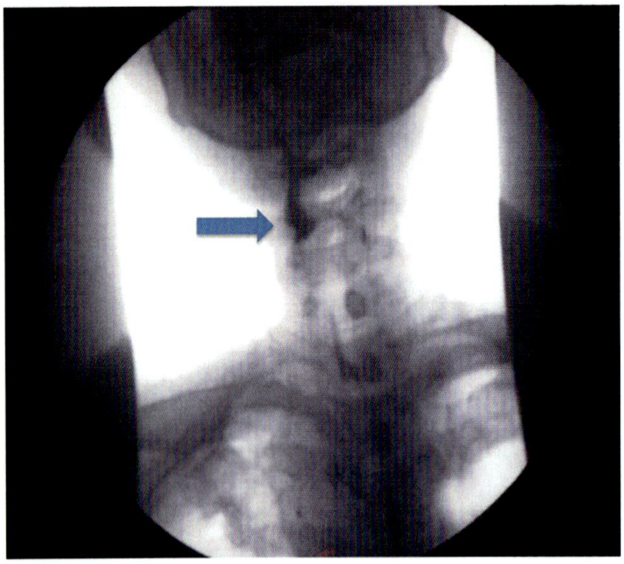

Fig. 17.11 The anterior–posterior view is used to evaluate the symmetry of the anatomical structures and bolus flow. A *blue arrow* shows radiopaque bolus entering the right pyriform sinus

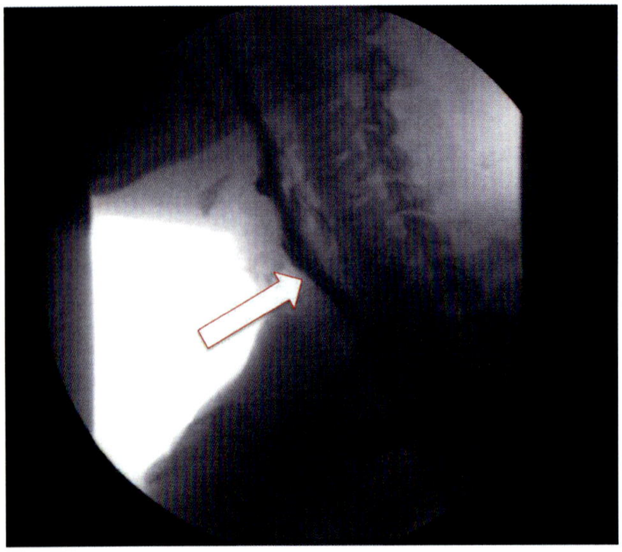

Fig. 17.12 The oblique view is used to evaluate the esophageal transit. A *white arrow* shows radiopaque bolus passing through the esophagus

posture, movement of swallow musculature, phonation, and respiratory, swallowing, and cough sounds.

We have built a new system to combine the important clinical information of dysphagic patient during the VFSS and VF images. Swallowing and respiratory sounds were detected and stored to the digital video recorder with VF images. By using another digital video recorder, subjects' outward appearance during VFSS was recorded. The two digital video data of the patients' outward appearance during VFSS and the VF images with the swallowing and respiratory sound signal were combined synchronously using the image editing system (Figs. 17.13 and 17.14). Our recent research indicates that the information acquired from VF images is insufficient to understand the clinical condition in the dysphagic patient. It is also revealed that additional information including the outward image of the patient during VFSS and detected swallowing and expiratory sounds plays an important role in realizing the dysphagic patient's condition. A team approach by many members of the medical community including medical doctor, dentist, speech–language pathologist, nurse, dental hygienist, physiotherapist, occupational therapist, and dietician is very efficient in the management of dysphagia. Using our system, sharing the accurate information obtained from the VF images with the outward image of the patient during VFSS and swallowing and expiratory sounds among the medical members could produce high efficiency in the management of dysphagia.

2. Videoendoscopic Swallow Study (VESS)

VESS is used to examine the anatomic structure of the nasopharynx, hypopharynx, and larynx, velopharyngeal function, glottal function, pooling of saliva or bolus, and presence of aspiration. Endoscopy is performed with a fiberoptic endoscope inserted into the nose, down to the level of the soft palate, or below.

Passage of the bolus and movement of the structures cannot be observed during the swallow because the velum, tongue base, posterior pharyngeal wall, or lateral pharyngeal wall close around the tip of the scope, blocking the image and causing a brief period referred to as "whiteout." When the endoscopic image returns to view, any residue of the bolus in the valleculae and pyriform sinus is noted. Then, the tip of the scope is advanced downward, and laryngeal penetration and/or tracheal aspiration is evaluated. The view of the moment of the aspiration is obliterated by the "whiteout." However, if aspiration is suspected, ask the patient to cough after the swallow. Aspirated material may be discharged from the subglottic region, and evidence of aspiration can be confirmed.

Once the impaired swallowing physiology is identified, compensatory techniques (changing head or body posture, modifying viscosity and volume of bolus) or swallow maneuvers may be implemented under endoscopic inspection to evaluate their impact on the patient's swallowing.

VESS is the pharyngeal local images lacking in important patient's clinical information including physique, level of alertness, motivation, facial expression, posture,

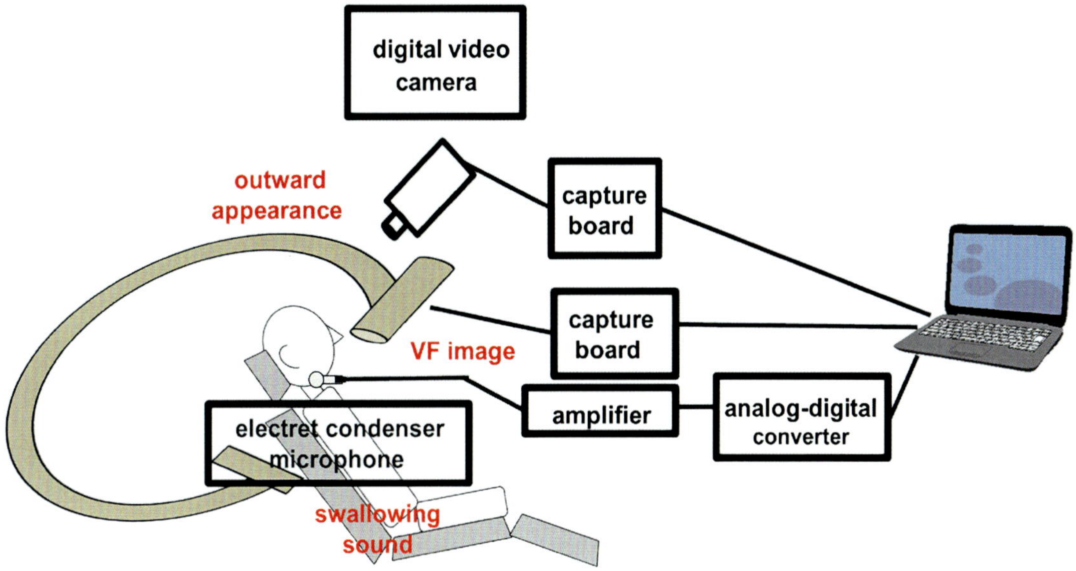

Fig. 17.13 A block diagram of a new system to combine clinical information of dysphagic patient during the VFSS and VF images. Outward appearance, VF images and sounds detected by an electret condenser microphone were fed to a computer and combined by image editing system

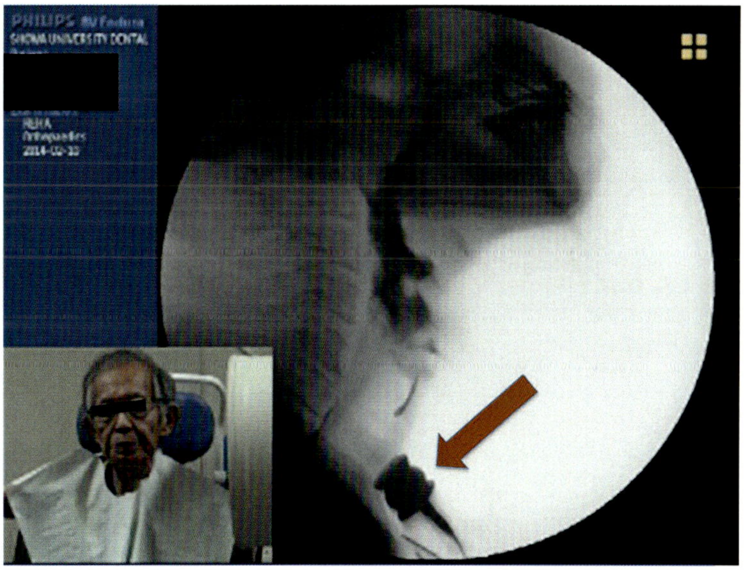

Fig. 17.14 An example of the monitor image of our system. A *red arrow* shows an acoustic probe loaded with an electret condenser microphone for detecting swallowing and respiratory sounds

movement of swallow musculature, phonation, and respiratory, swallowing, and cough sounds. For acquiring patient's clinical information during VESS, recording VE images and patients' outward appearance during VFSS with swallowing and respiratory sounds is recommended (Figs. 17.15 and 17.16).

VESS can be used as a visual biofeedback training method for the patient to learn swallow exercise faster (Fig. 17.17).

3. Ultrasound Study
   The ultrasound study of the oral cavity is a noninvasive imaging technique for detecting oral dysphagia, and it is used to observe tongue and hyoid bone movements, bolus manipulation, and bolus transport. B mode is used to study movements in sagittal or coronal section, and M mode is used to evaluate the chronological changes of a specific region (Figs. 17.18 and 17.19).

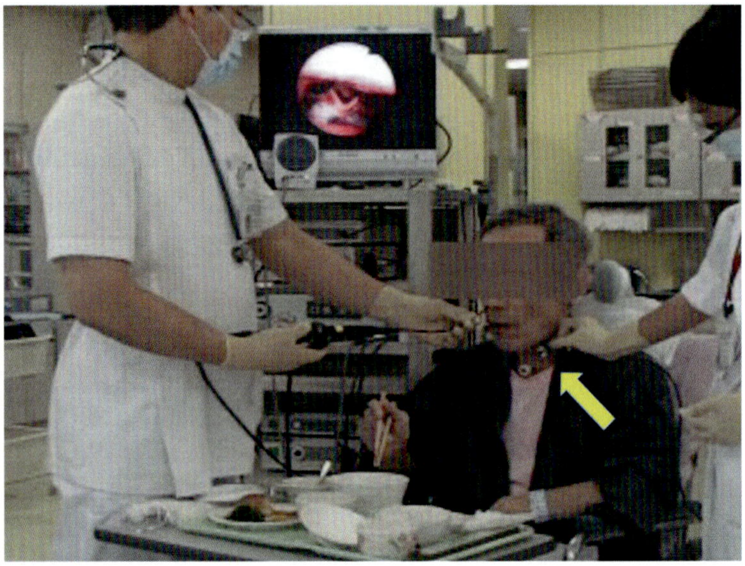

Fig. 17.15 For acquiring patient's clinical information during VESS, VE images and patients' outward appearance during VFSS are recorded with swallowing and respiratory sounds. A *yellow arrow* shows an acoustic probe loaded with an electret condenser microphone for detecting swallowing and respiratory sounds

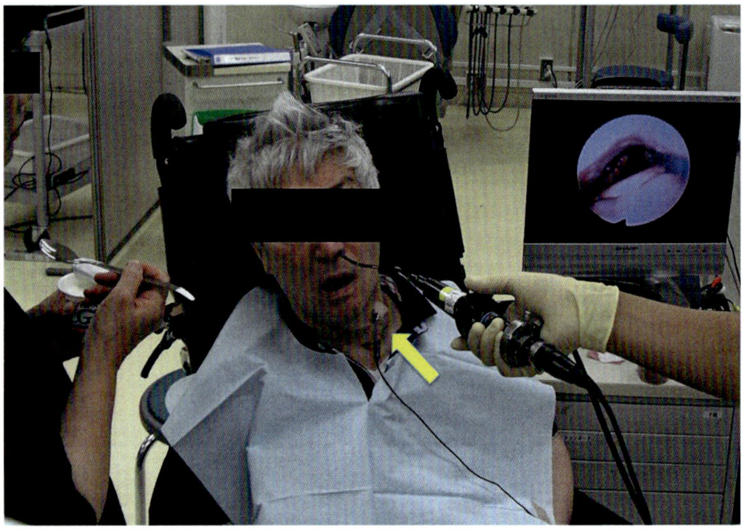

Fig. 17.16 VE images and patients' outward appearance during VFSS are recorded with swallowing and respiratory sounds. An acoustic probe loaded with an electret condenser microphone is attached to the neck for detecting swallowing and respiratory sounds (*yellow arrow*)

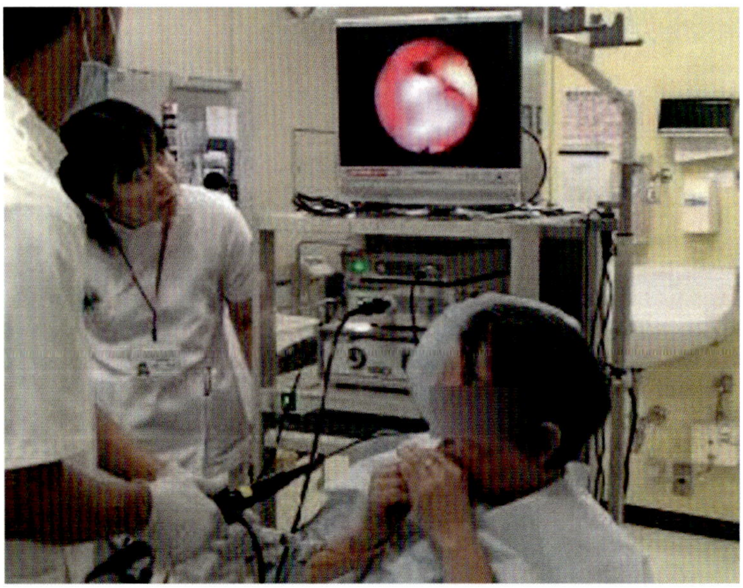

Fig. 17.17 VESS can be used as a visual biofeedback training method for the patient to learn swallow exercise faster. This patient tried balloon catheter dilatation while he saw the same monitor of VESS as behind

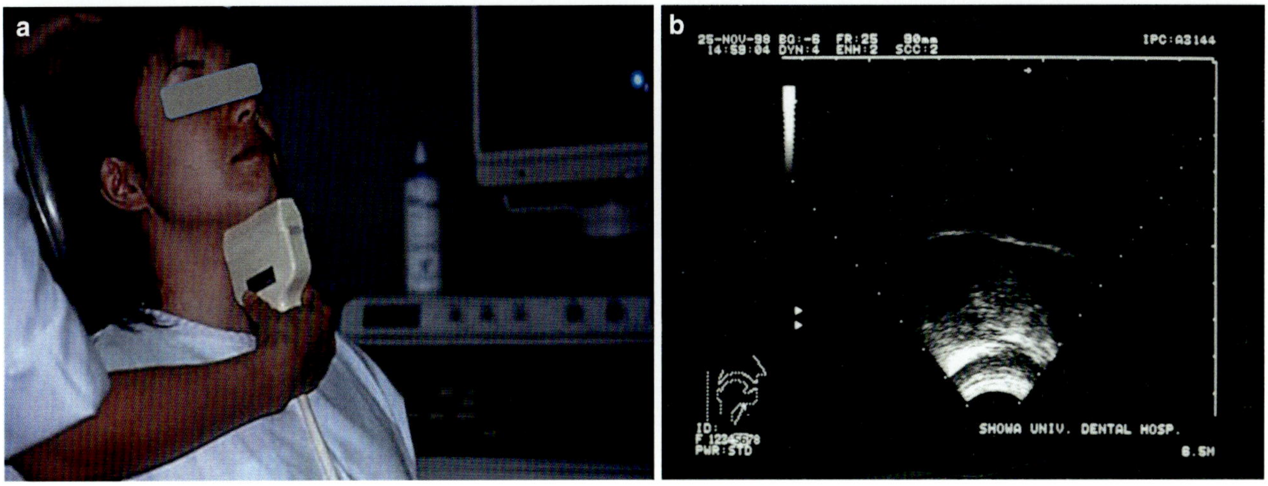

Fig. 17.18 (**a**) B mode of ultrasonography is used to examine movements in sagittal section. (**b**) Tongue movement during swallowing in one sagittal plane is visualized on the monitor

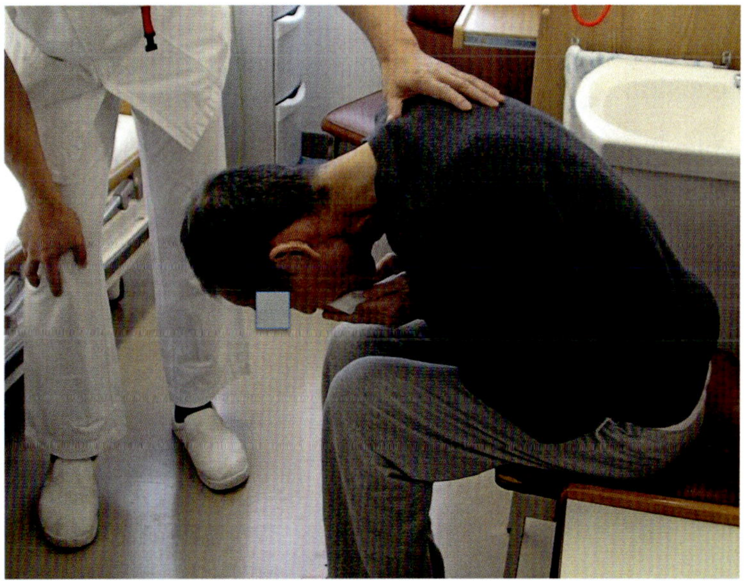

Fig. 17.19 Airway clearance technique to expectorate the secretion or bolus in the pharynx, larynx, and trachea

17.3 Treatment of Dysphagia in Oral Cancer

In order to improve swallowing in head and neck cancer patients, an individual treatment plan for each patient should be designed. Treatment techniques for dysphagia include airway clearance techniques, compensatory techniques, and swallow exercises. It is important to implement these techniques in combination to achieve maximum result [25–31].

17.3.1 Airway Clearance Techniques

When saliva, nasal mucus, and other secretions are not swallowed completely or accumulate in the oral cavity, pharynx, or larynx, the pharyngeal swallow reflex and/or cough reflex is often reduced secondary to the loss of sensory awareness of the secretions. For patients with excess secretion, deep respiration is introduced, and the expectoration method is introduced. To expectorate the secretion (or bolus), patients are asked first to inhale deeply, bend forward, and perform strong voluntary cough or forced expiration (huffing) (Fig. 17.19).

17.3.2 Compensatory Techniques

Compensatory techniques are those that control the flow of bolus and eliminate patient symptoms such as aspiration. Compensatory techniques include (1) postural adjustments, (2) modifying volume and speed of food presentation, (3) changing food and liquid consistency or viscosity, and (4) introducing an intraoral prosthesis. The following are the compensatory techniques that are often used in head and neck cancer patients with dysphagia:

1. Postural Adjustments

   Postural adjustment techniques improve swallowing disorders by changing the dimension and position of the pharynx, redirecting the bolus flow. There are a number of postural adjustment techniques. The clinician should correctly identify the patient's physiologic or anatomic disorder and decide the posture that is most effective [32]. Postural adjustment techniques are normally used temporarily until swallowing function improves.

   (a) The Chin-Up Posture

   The chin-up posture is used to drain the bolus from the oral cavity to the pharynx using gravity. This posture is effective for patients with bolus transport difficulties due to reduced tongue movement. However, this posture may have a negative impact on airway protection and increase the risk for the penetration or aspiration (Figs. 17.20 and 17.21). Thus the super-supraglottic swallow (explained below) should be taught in combination with this posture.

   (b) The Chin-Down Posture

   The chin-down posture involves touching one's chin to the neck. With this posture, the tongue base and epiglottis are pushed closer to the posterior pharyngeal wall, and the airway entrance (the superior laryngeal aperture) is narrowed. This posture is effective for patients who have a delayed pharyngeal swallow reflex, reduced tongue base retraction, and reduced airway entrance closure (Fig. 17.22) [33, 34].

   (c) Head Rotation to Weaker Side

   Rotating the head to the weaker side is the posture to narrow or close the weaker side of the hypopharynx and widen the stronger side of the hypopharynx so that the bolus flows down the stronger side (Fig. 17.23). Effectiveness of this posture is increased when it is combined with the head tilting posture explained next (Fig. 17.24).

   (d) Head Tilt to Stronger Side

   The head tilting posture uses the gravity to drain the bolus down the stronger side by tilting the head to the better or stronger side. The stronger side is usually better both in function and sensitivity. Oral and pharyngeal swallowing coordination is improved with this posture [35, 36].

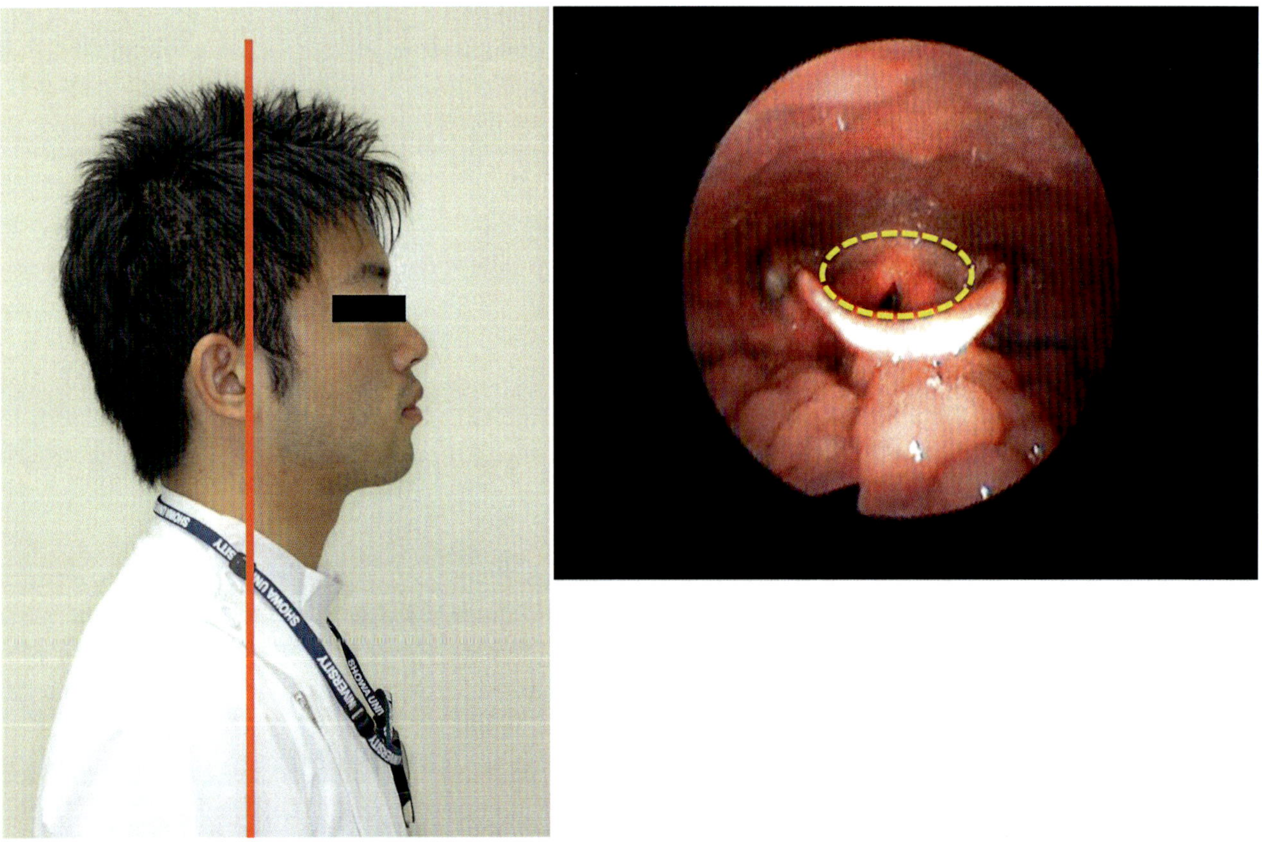

Fig. 17.20 Upright posture (*left*) and the superior laryngeal aperture (*yellow dot ellipse*) observed by VESS at this posture (*right*)

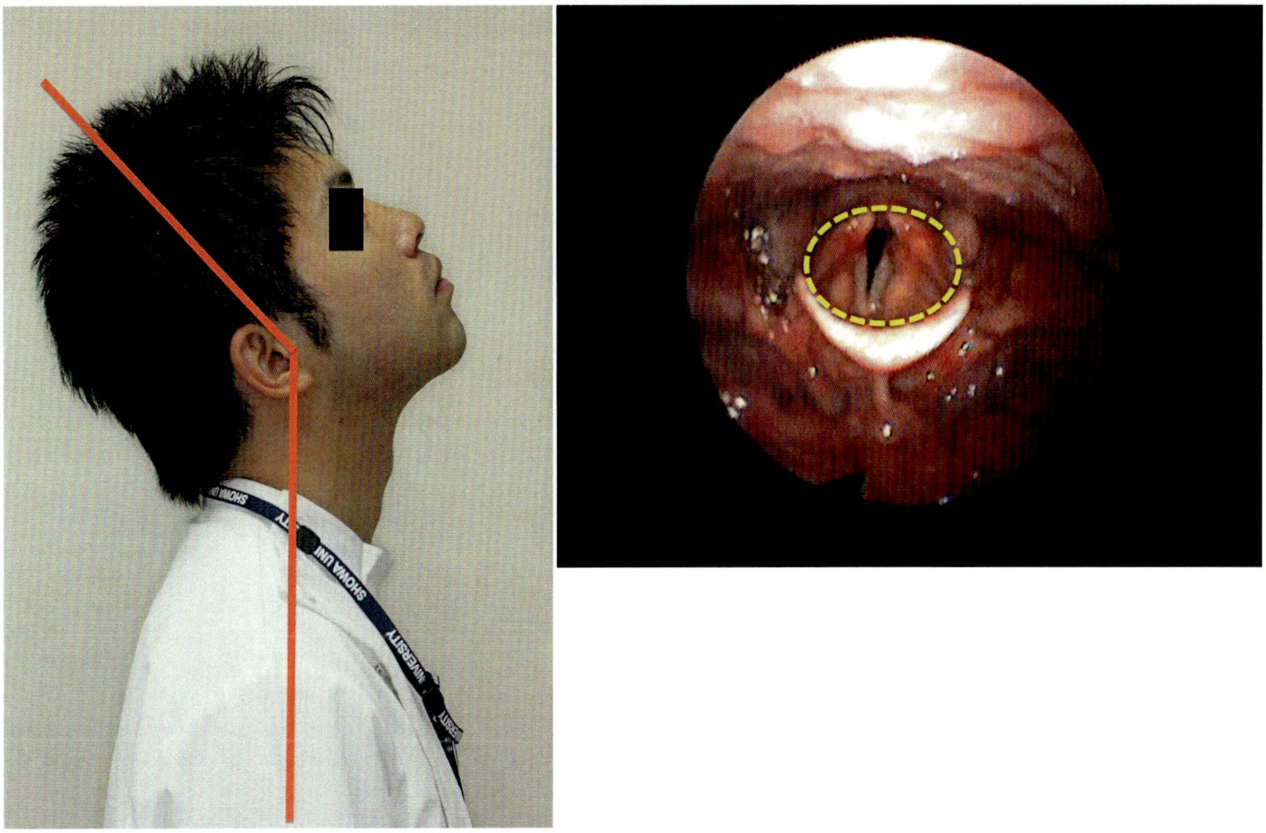

Fig. 17.21 Chin-up posture (*left*) and the superior laryngeal aperture (*yellow dot ellipse*) observed by VESS at this posture (*right*)

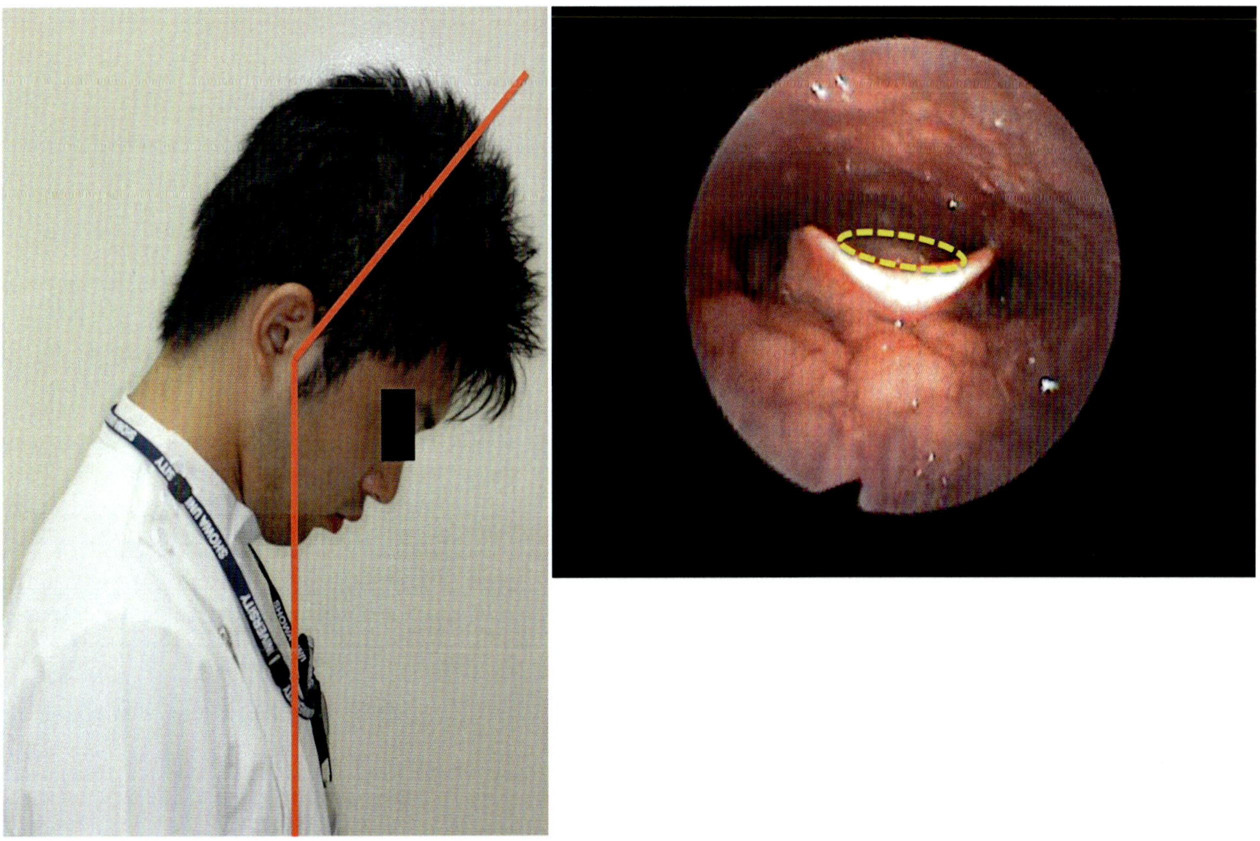

Fig. 17.22 Chin-down posture (*left*) and the superior laryngeal aperture (*yellow dot ellipse*) observed by VESS at this posture (*right*)

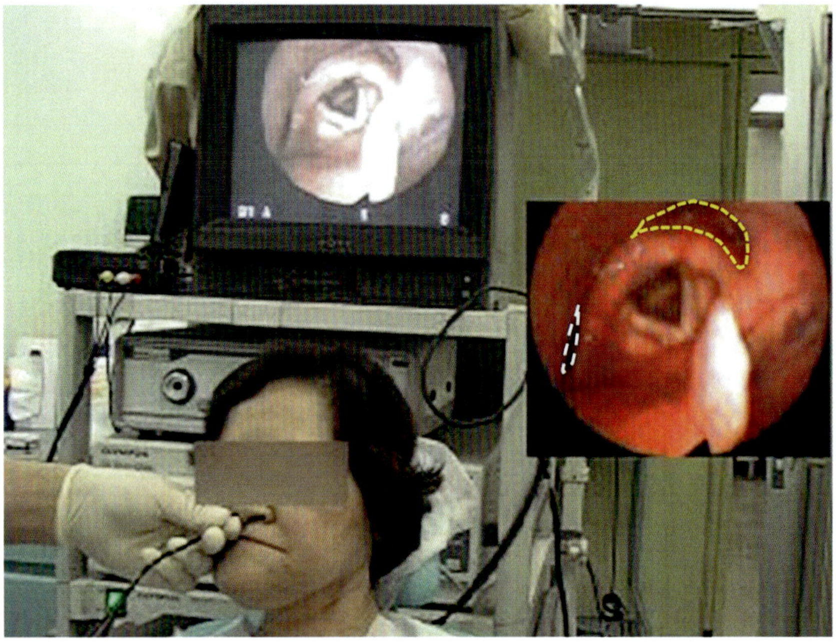

Fig. 17.23 Rotating the head to the weaker side (*the right side, white dot*) is the posture to narrow or close the weaker side (*the right side, white dot*) of the hypopharynx and widen the stronger side (*the left side, yellow dot*) of the hypopharynx

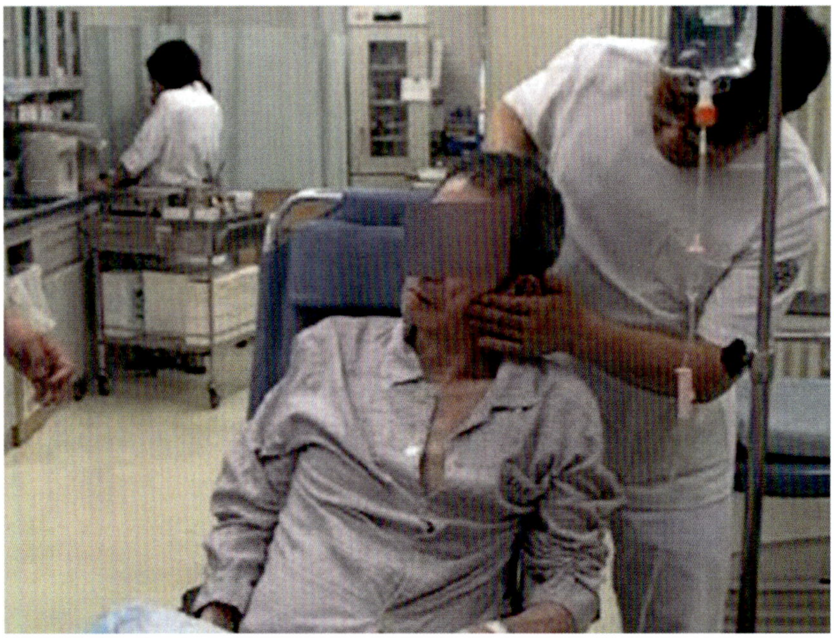

Fig. 17.24 Effectiveness of rotating the head to the weaker side is increased when it is combined with the head tilting posture

The result of the bolus movement analysis comparing the upright posture and the posture with head tilted to the stronger side is shown in Table 17.2. The swallow functions of twelve glossectomized patients were studied by videofluoroscopy. At the upright posture, aspiration is identified in these patients; however, aspiration is not identified when they tilted their head to the stronger side. The onset of laryngeal elevation (pharyngeal delay time, indicating the triggering of the pharyngeal swallow) and the pharyngeal transit time (indicating the bolus transport ability) were significantly shorter at the head tilt posture because the bolus flowed down the stronger side which was better in function and sensitivity than those of the weaker side.

2. Modifying Volume and Speed of Food Presentation
In patients with a weakened pharyngeal swallow, taking a large volume of bolus or taking a bolus too rapidly can result in a severe retention in the pharynx, which may lead to aspiration. Taking smaller boluses at a slower rate may eliminate any risk of aspiration in these patients.

3. Changing Food and Liquid Consistency or Viscosity
   This strategy is applied when other compensatory or therapy strategies are not successful. To avoid aspiration, the viscosity of food and liquid is modified, and the flow and cohesiveness of bolus is changed. The *National Dysphagia Diet* (NDD), published in 2002 by the American Dietetic Association, aims to establish standard terminology and practice applications of dietary texture modification in dysphagia management [37]. National Dysphagia Level I is a puree consistency diet (homogenous, very cohesive, pudding-like, requiring very little chewing ability). National Dysphagia Diet Level 2 is a mechanically altered diet (cohesive, moist, semisolid foods, requiring some chewing). National Dysphagia Diet Level 3 is a diet for advanced dysphagic patients (soft foods that require more chewing ability).
4. Introducing an Intraoral Prosthesis (see Sect. 16.2.5 Prosthetic Appliances)
   (a) Palatal Obturator and Maxillary Prosthesis
   The palatal obturator is a device that fills a defect created by surgical resection. This device is used mainly for patients with palatal resection. When the deficit extends to the soft palate, consideration in shaping the posterior edge of the device is needed to get palatal closure without obstructing the movement of the remaining soft palate. In such a case, the shape of the posterior edge is adjusted to the soft palate movement as patients swallow and speak.

   When the deficit extends to the upper alveolar ridge, a maxillary prosthesis is applied to close the oronasal (or maxillary sinus) fistula, fill the area of defect, and improve swallow function. If the deficit is fairly limited, the prosthesis is made in a similar shape to a normal denture. If the deficit is large, a hollow bulb prosthesis is created to reduce the weight of the prosthesis (Fig. 17.25). Because of the surgical invasion to the fauces or internal and external pterygoid muscles and postsurgical contracture, trismus is often seen in patients with large maxillary deficits. In this case, jaw-opening exercises are introduced before manufacturing the maxillary prosthesis. We developed the original jaw-opening exercise using the stacked dental thermoplastic sheets (Figs. 17.26a, b and 17.27a, b).
   (b) Palatal Augmentation Prosthesis (PAP)
   The PAP is introduced to patients with reduced tongue–palate contact during swallowing as a result of the surgical effect on the lingual, floor of the mouth, or suprahyoid muscle complex, postsurgical contracture, and/or hypoglossal nerve paralysis. This device is designed to lower the palatal vault to facilitate tongue–palate contact (Figs. 17.28, 17.29, and 17.30). Increased tongue–palate contact improves bolus transport [38–41]. The hollow-type PAP is contrived to decrease the weight of the prosthesis (Fig. 17.31).

The palatal area of the PAP is designed to achieve maximum tongue–palate contact during swallowing. A subsequent reshaping or reducing of the size of the prosthesis should be considered as the patient's tongue movement improves over time. To adjust the shape and thickness of the PAP, tongue–palate contact during swallowing is evaluated by the static palatogram. By applying this device, improvements in bolus control and transport are achieved (Fig. 17.32).

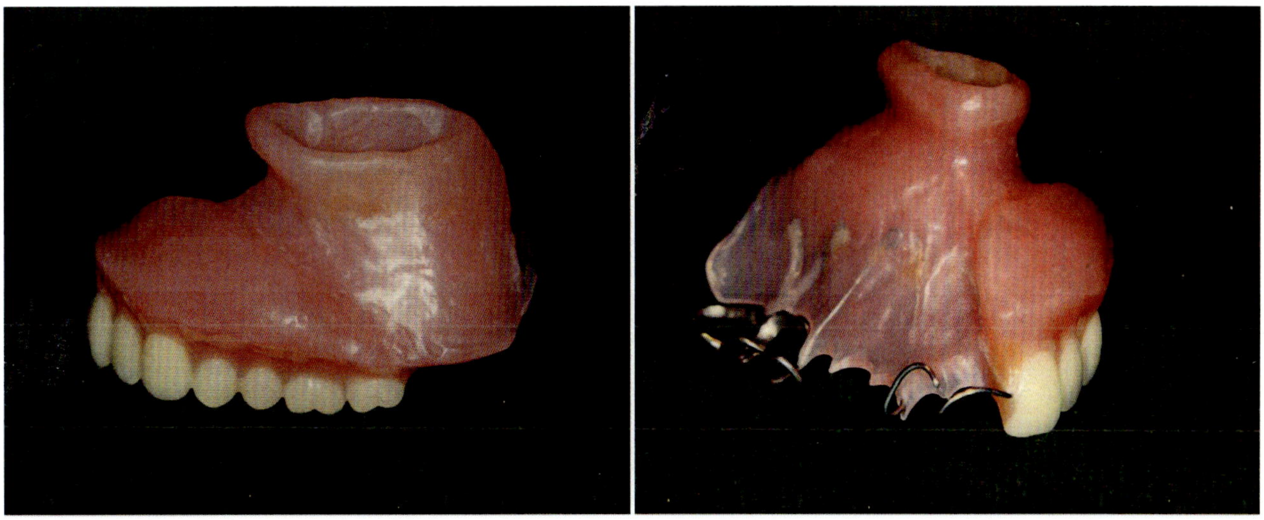

Fig. 17.25 A hollow bulb maxillary prosthesis. The hollow bulb is designed to reduce the weight of the prosthesis

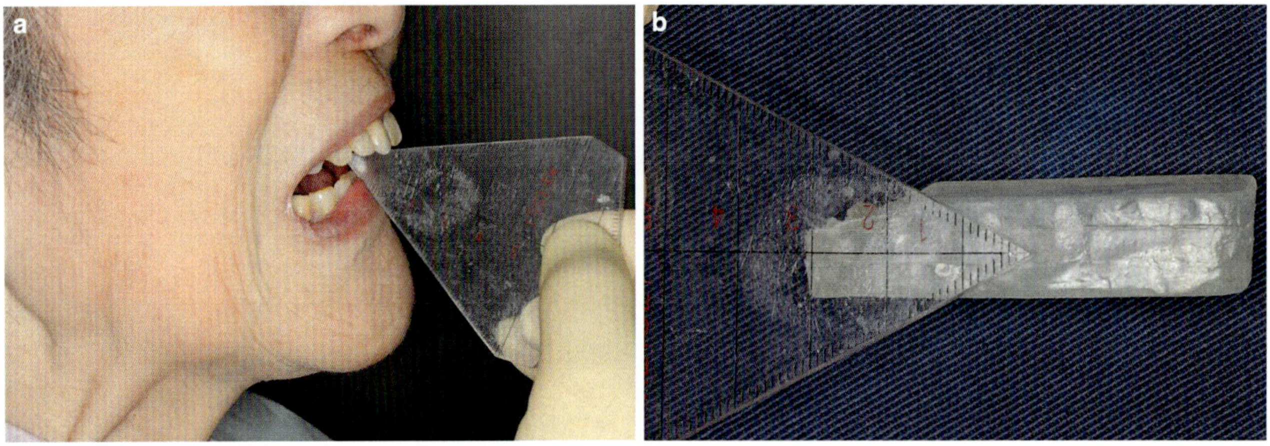

Fig. 17.26 (**a**) If trismus is severe, opening exercises are introduced before manufacturing the maxillary prosthesis. (**b**) Our original jaw-opening device is made by the stacked dental thermoplastic sheets. Thickness of the device is adjusted according to mouth opening capacity of the patient by the number of dental thermoplastic sheets stacked

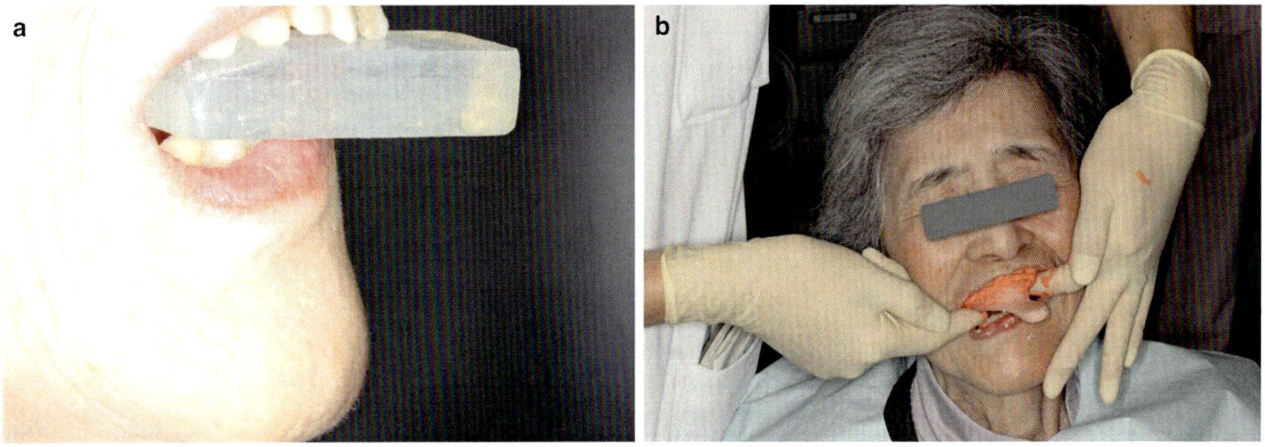

Fig. 17.27 (**a**) The patient bites the jaw-opening device as long as possible. (**b**) Impression is taken immediately after jaw-opening exercise

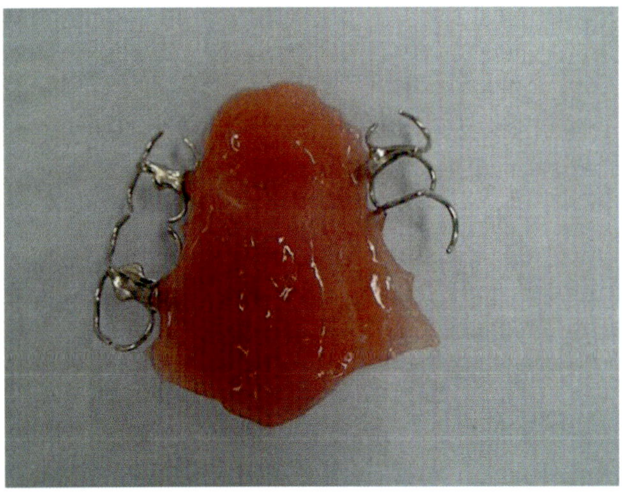

Fig. 17.28 Palatal view of palatal augmentation prosthesis

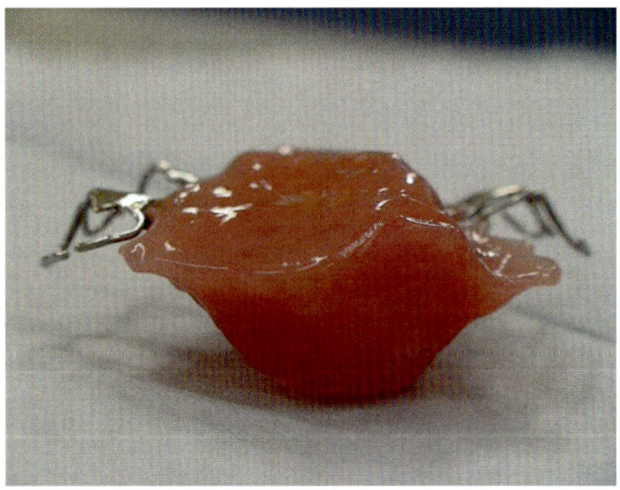

Fig. 17.29 Rear view of palatal augmentation prosthesis

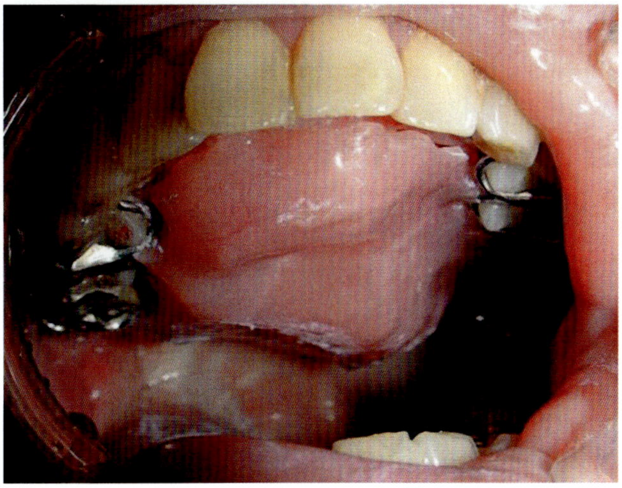

Fig. 17.30 Intraoral view of wearing a palatal augmentation prosthesis in the subtotally glossectomized patient

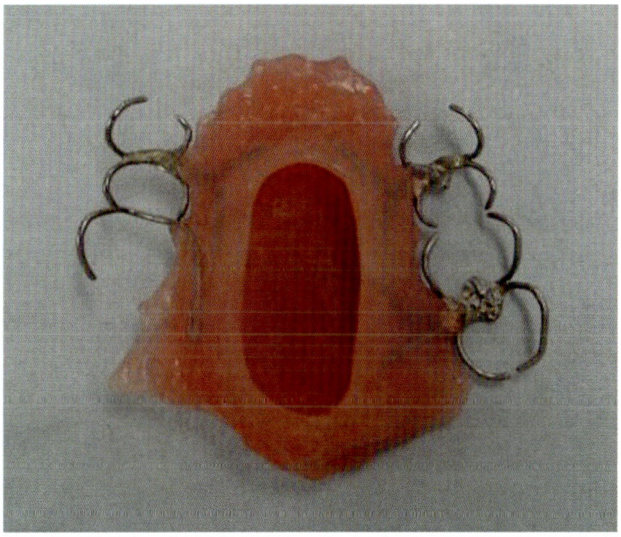

Fig. 17.31 The hollow-type PAP is contrived to decrease the weight of the prosthesis

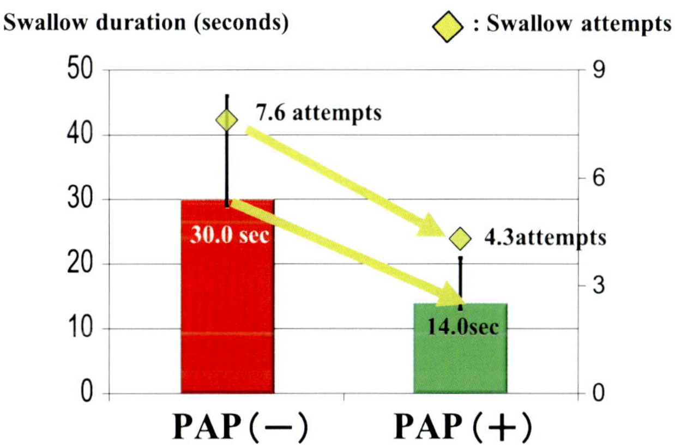

Fig. 17.32 Swallow duration and swallow attempts while swallowing 10 ml barium jelly without PAP and with PAP. Swallow duration and the number of swallow attempts are remarkably reduced using PAP

(c) Prosthetic Tongue
Prosthetic tongue is used for improvement of dysphagia following treatment of tongue and/or oral floor cancer. A prosthetic tongue is usually used for improving dysphagia rather than speech deficit (Fig. 17.33). The severe pooling at the resected oral floor is improved by wearing a prosthetic tongue (Fig. 17.34).

(d) Mandible Repositioning Appliances
Reconstructive techniques are used for fixation of a segmentally resected mandible using a mandibular titanium reconstructive plate with vascularized soft-tissue free flap or free vascularized bone flaps. However, reconstructive plates or free flaps should be removed if postoperative complications such as necrosis of the flap caused by loss of the venous outflow or the arterial supply, infection, plate exposure, and cancer recurrence occur.

In these cases, the remaining mandibular bone is pulled by insufficient soft tissue and scar tissue producing significant deviation of the mandible and loss of eating ability.

We developed a new technique for repositioning the mandibular deviation after segmental mandibulectomy in order to improve eating ability.

This technique requires mandible repositioning appliances (MRAs). MRAs include a maxillary and mandibular appliance. The patient's deviated mandible is moved manually toward its normal position by the dentist after the maxillary and mandible appliances are worn. The appliances are fixed using dental resin material. Patients wear the MRAs during sleep and for 3 h a day for 2–3 weeks to extend soft and scar tissue surrounding the mandible. MRAs are separated to the maxillary and mandible appliances and the same procedures are repeated for the deviated mandible to approximate to its normal position (Figs. 17.35 and 17.36). Using this technique, significant improvement in eating ability was verified by Fujishima's food intake level scale (FILS) (Fig. 17.37). The apnea–hypopnea index (AHI) was also significantly decreased by wearing the MRAs during sleep (Fig. 17.38).

17.3.3 Swallow Exercises (see Sect. 16.2.1 Oral Facilitative Exercises)

Objectives of swallow exercises include (1) improving range and/or elaboration of movements in oropharyngeal structures, (2) increasing sensory awareness for triggering the pharyngeal swallow, (3) improving the coordinated movements of the oral–pharyngeal structures, and (4) improving the function of the airway protection [42]. The following are the swallow exercises which are commonly applied to dysphagic patients with head and neck cancer:

1. Labial Closure Exercises
For patients who have difficulties with lip closure because of anatomic deficit or scar contracture, massage of the

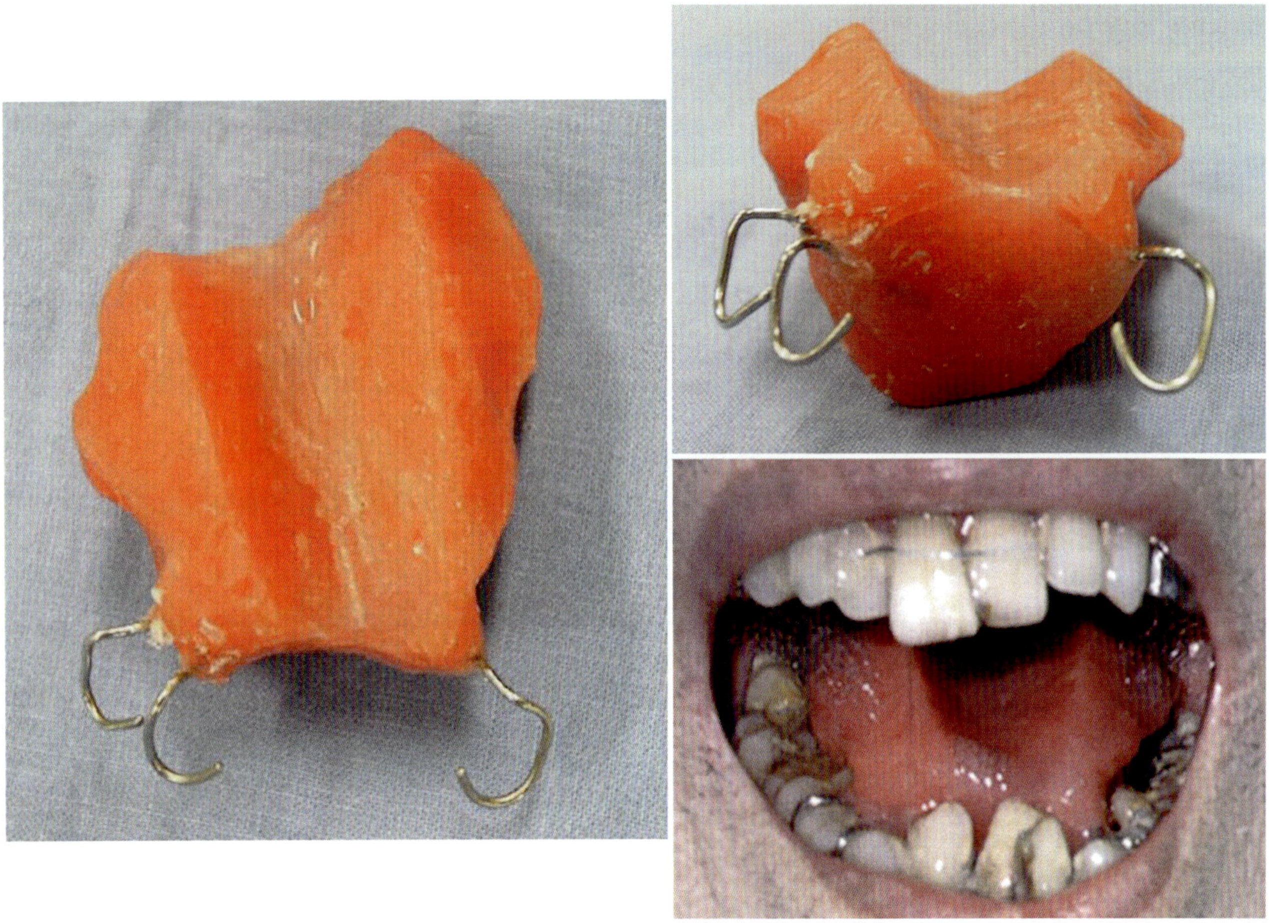

Fig. 17.33 An example of prosthetic tongue for a subtotal glossectomized patient. A prosthetic tongue is usually used for improving dysphagia rather than speech deficit

cheek and lips are done. Once the patient is able to maintain lip closure, resistance exercise is done to increase lip strength (Fig. 17.39).

2. Resistance Exercises for the Tongue
   Pushing the tongue against a tongue blade or fingers will improve both range of motion and strength (Fig. 17.40). This exercise is effective especially for patients with a reconstructed tongue whose range of movement is severely reduced. The exercise activates the movement of intrinsic tongue muscles (superior longitudinal muscle, inferior longitudinal muscle, verticalis muscle, and transverses muscle) as well as the suprahyoid muscles (digastric muscle, stylohyoid muscle, mylohyoid muscle, and geniohyoid muscle).
3. Swallow Maneuvers
   Swallow maneuvers are the techniques to improve dysphagia by bringing swallow physiology under voluntary control [43, 44]. The following maneuvers are the ones used in dysphagic patients with head and neck cancer.
   (a) Chin-Forward Swallow
   The chin-forward swallow is designed to widen the cricopharyngeal opening or the stenotic portion of hypopharynx and/or upper esophagus (Fig. 17.41). This method is often used for the patients who have undergone cricopharyngeal myotomy or laryngectomy.
   (b) Mendelsohn Maneuver
   The Mendelsohn maneuver is designed to increase the extent and duration of laryngeal elevation (Fig. 17.42). By prolonging the laryngeal elevation voluntarily during swallowing, duration and width of cricopharyngeal opening are increased. This maneuver is also effective in improving oral and oropharyngeal coordination of the swallow.
   (c) Super-Supraglottic Swallow
   The super-supraglottic swallow is designed to close the vocal folds, false vocal folds, and laryngeal vestibule voluntarily before and during the swallow. Patients are instructed to inhale first, hold their breath tightly as they swallow, cough immediately after the swallow, and re-swallow. During the maneuver, the arytenoid cartilages are tilted anteriorly to the base of the epiglottis, and the false vocal folds are closed tightly.

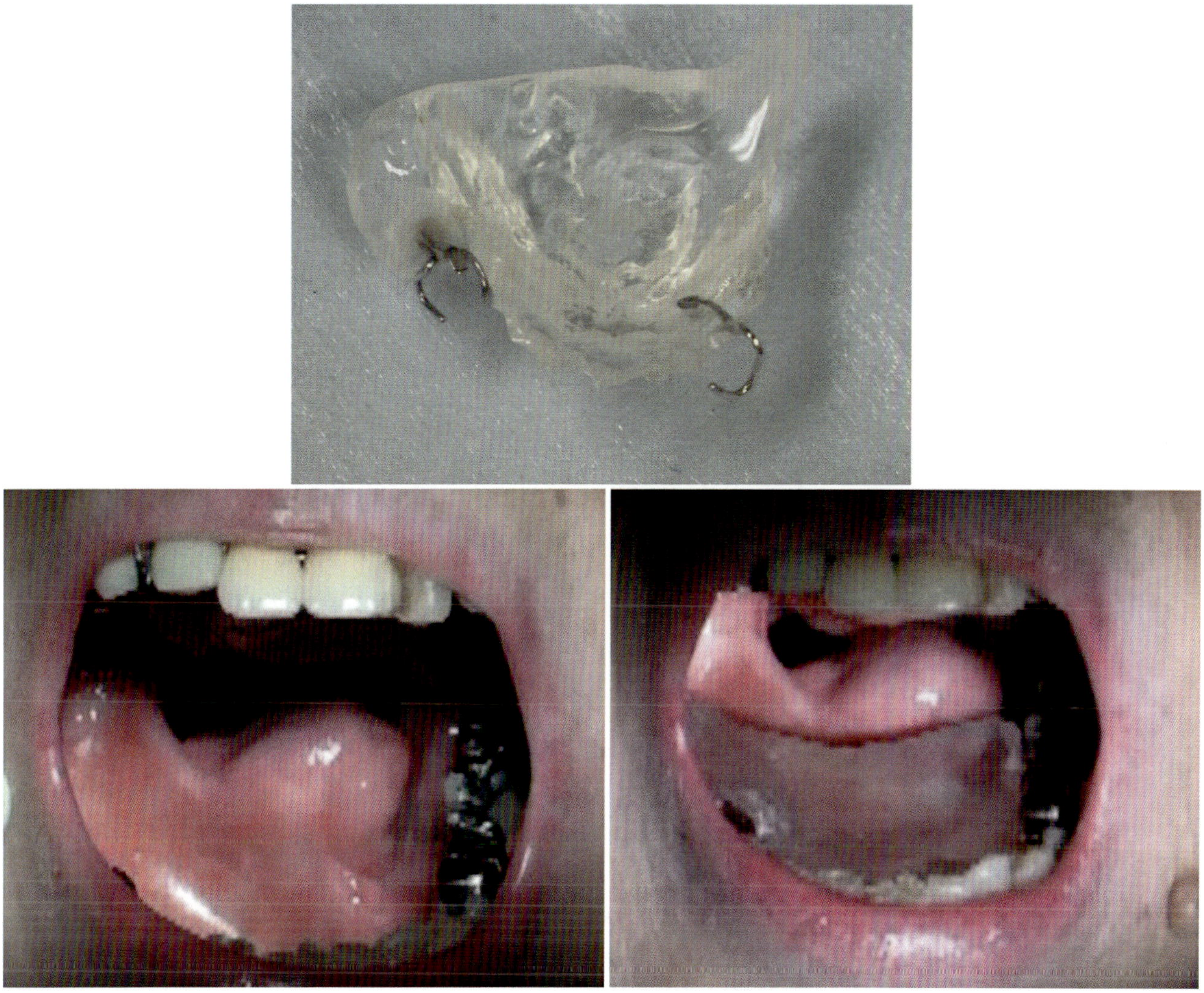

Fig. 17.34 An example of prosthetic tongue for an oral floor resected patient. The severe pooling at the resected oral floor is improved by wearing a prosthetic tongue

(d) Effortful Swallow

The effortful swallow is designed to increase the posterior motion of the tongue base during the pharyngeal swallow. Patients are asked to elevate the posterior tongue and push the posterior tongue against the palate during the swallow.

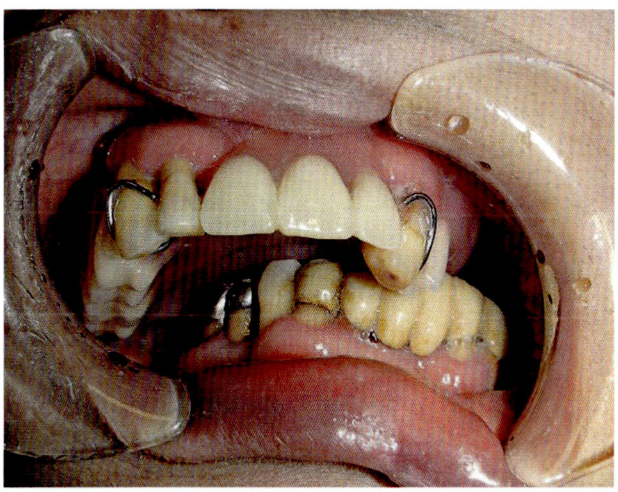

Fig. 17.35 This patient received left side segmental resection of the mandible and total neck dissection with reconstructive surgery using the rectus abdominis myocutaneous flap and titanium plates for the treatment of lower gingival carcinoma. Postoperatively, the RAMC flap and the titanium plates were removed because of vascular accidents of the flap. This is the oral view at the first visit of this patient to our clinic about 1 year after the surgery

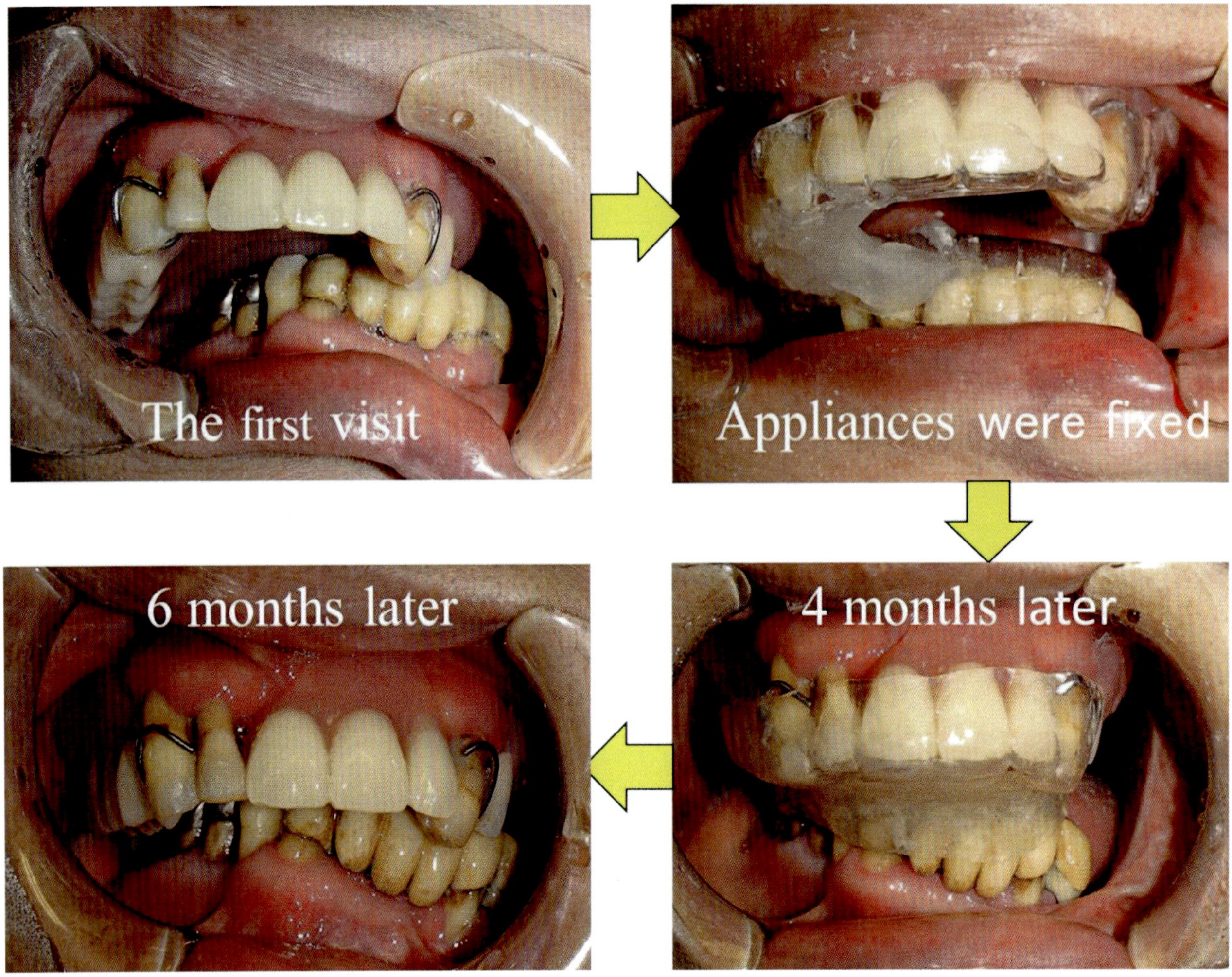

Fig. 17.36 MRAs include a maxillary and mandibular appliance. The deviated mandible is moved manually toward its normal position after the maxillary and mandible appliances are worn. The appliances are fixed using dental resin material. Patients wear the MRAs during sleep and for about 3 h a day for 2–3 weeks. MRAs are separated to the maxillary and mandible appliances and the same procedures are repeated to approximate the normal position

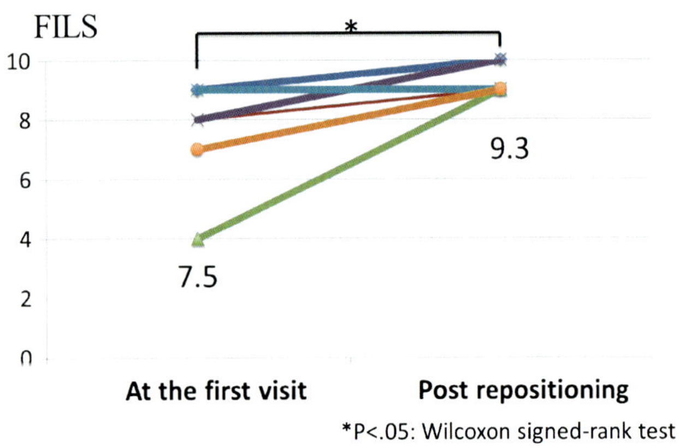

Fig. 17.37 Using mandibular repositioning technique, significant improvement in eating ability was verified by Fujishima's food intake level scale (*FILS*)

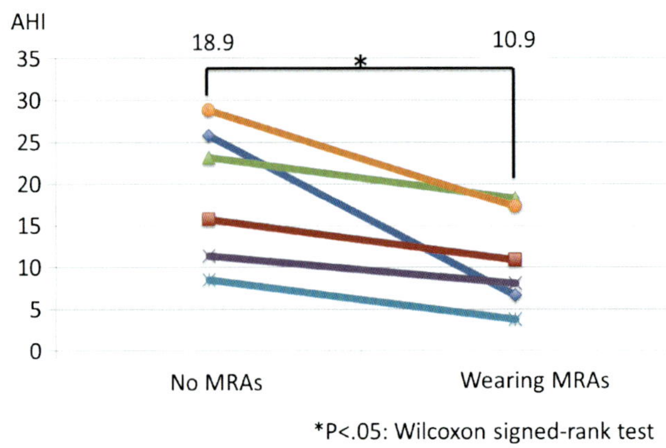

Fig. 17.38 The apnea–hypopnea index (*AHI*) was also significantly decreased by wearing the MRAs during sleep

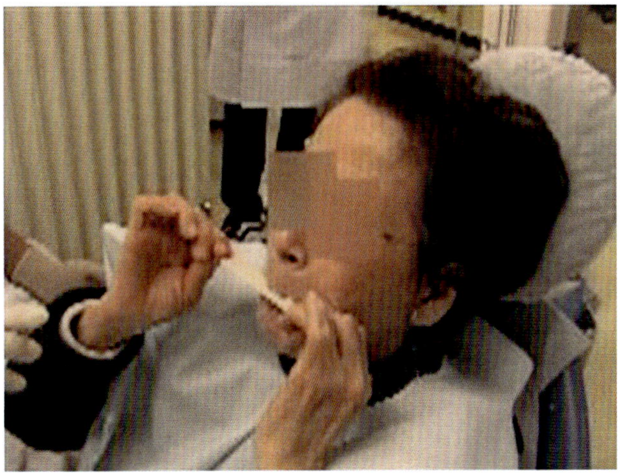

Fig. 17.39 Lip resistance exercise (blade holding exercise). Maximal effort for lip closure lasts 6 ~ 10 s. This exercise is repeated 6–10 times a day

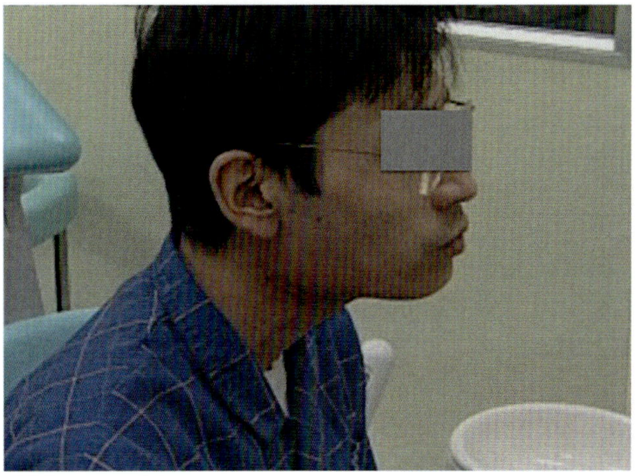

Fig. 17.41 The chin-forward swallow is designed to widen the crico-pharyngeal opening or the stenotic portion of hypopharynx and/or upper esophagus

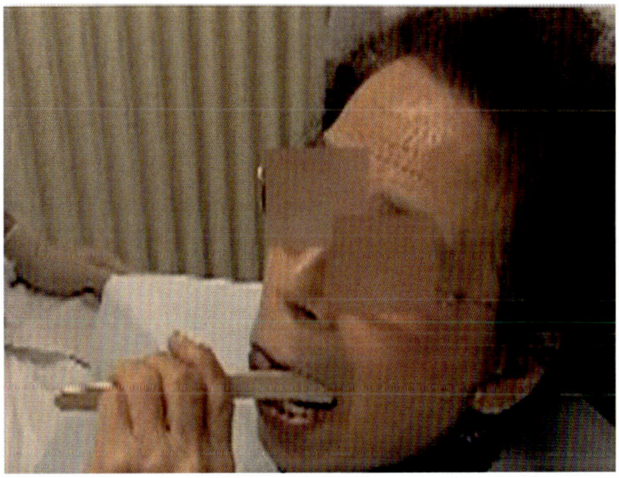

Fig. 17.40 Tongue resistance exercise (blade pushing exercise). Maximal effort for tongue pushing lasts 6 ~ 10 s. This exercise is repeated 6–10 times a day

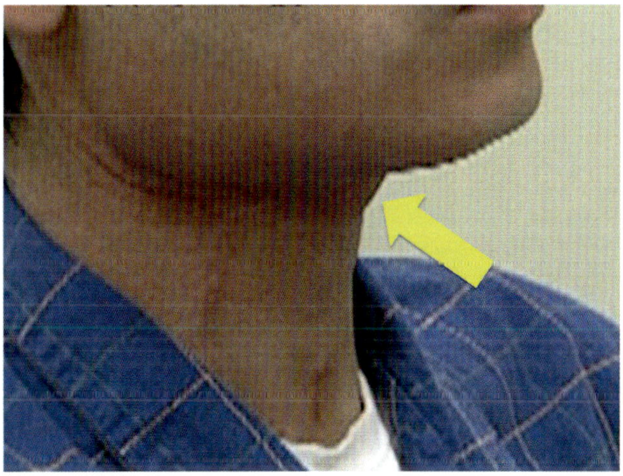

Fig. 17.42 The Mendelsohn maneuver is designed to increase the extent and duration of laryngeal elevation. A *yellow* allow shows the elevated larynx

(e) Showa Swallow Maneuver (Takahashi Maneuver)
The Showa swallow maneuver (Takahashi maneuver) was designed to improve airway protection, laryngeal elevation, and superior–posterior movement of the tongue base during swallowing. The Showa swallow maneuver (Takahashi maneuver) is equivalent to the combination of the Mendelsohn maneuver, the super-supraglottic maneuver, and the effortful swallow. To perform the Showa swallow maneuver, patients are instructed to "take in a deep breath and hold it, trying to push the posterior tongue against the roof of the mouth, squeeze the throat tightly, and swallow hard."

To evaluate the effectiveness of the Showa swallow maneuver, instrumental studies were done using CT, surface electromyography (sEMG), and video-fluoroscopic swallow study. The CT images showed that the airway was almost completely closed during the maneuver (Figs. 17.43 and 17.44). The muscle activity of suprahyoid muscle complex detected by sEMG during the Showa swallow maneuver was the greatest compared with the other swallow maneuvers (Figs. 17.45 and 17.46). Also, from the videofluoroscopic study, it was observed that the pharyngeal delay time (an indicator of the triggering of the pharyngeal swallow) and the pharyngeal transit time (an indicator of the bolus transport) were shortened at attempts of the Showa swallow maneuver.

4. Swallow Exercise Using a Nasogastric Tube
This exercise is an application of a so-called retrievable appliance. Patients swallow and pull back a nasogastric tube repeatedly to learn the actual swallowing movement. This exercise is especially effective for patients who have

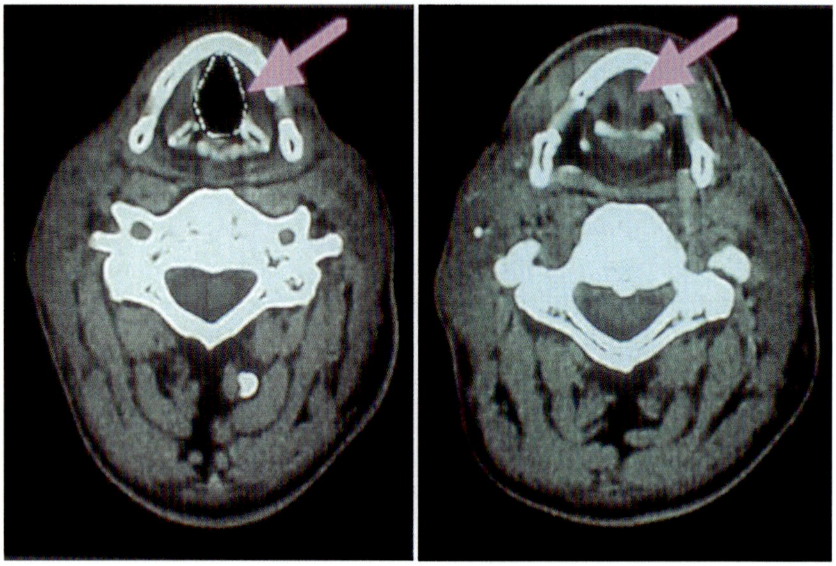

at rest
Normal: 1.22±0.39
Patient: 1.68±0.64

at Showa maneuver
Normal: 0.04±0.04
Patient: 0.06±0.09 (cm²)

Fig. 17.43 Orifice sizes were measured on 2-mm-sliced CT images at the levels of the true vocal folds. Six normal subjects and seven postsurgical oral cancer patients participated in CT examination

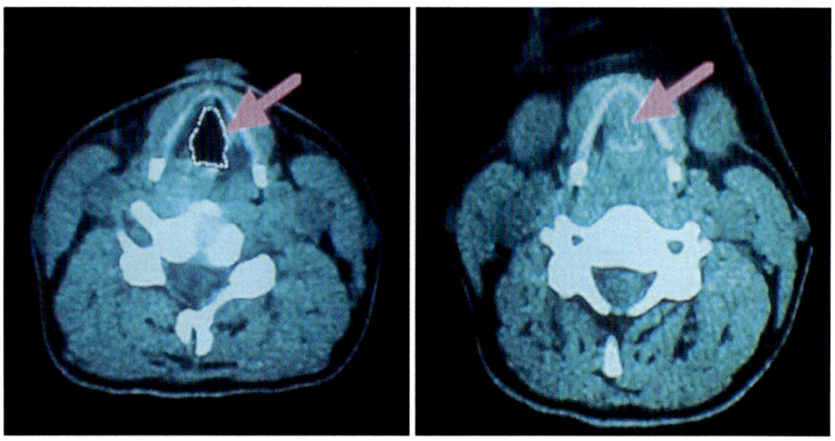

at rest
Normal: 1.8±0.9
Patient: 1.9±0.6

at Showa maneuver
Normal: 0.0±0.0
Patient: 0.3±0.6 (cm²)

Fig. 17.44 Orifice sizes were measured on 2-mm-sliced CT images at the levels of the false vocal folds. Six normal subjects and seven postsurgical oral cancer patients participated in CT examination

not had oral intake for a long time to relearn how to swallow and to improve the coordination of oral and pharyngeal function (Fig. 17.47a, b).

Swallowing maneuvers such as the Showa swallow maneuver may be practiced simultaneously during this exercise. Also, when a firm and thick tube is used, a stricture is expected to widen because of its bougie effect. Therefore, this technique can be applied to the patients with constricted cricopharyngeal opening or cricopharyngeal dysfunction.

5. Balloon Catheter Dilatation for Cricopharyngeal Opening
   The balloon catheter dilatation is a method applied to patients with constricted cricopharyngeal opening or cricopharyngeal dysfunction by mechanically stretching the contracted cricopharyngeal muscle [45]. Under VFSS, a balloon catheter is inserted through the mouth (or through the nose if there is an interference with pharyngeal reflex), liquid barium (contrast agent) is injected into the balloon, and the length of the catheter needed for the balloon to reach the cricopharyngeal opening is determined. Once the balloon is visualized in the appropriate position, it is inflated and pulled back to the level above the cricopharyngeal opening (Fig. 17.48a, b). Insertion of a balloon catheter into the esophagus and pulling back an inflated balloon catheter can also be verified using VESS (Fig. 17.49a–d).

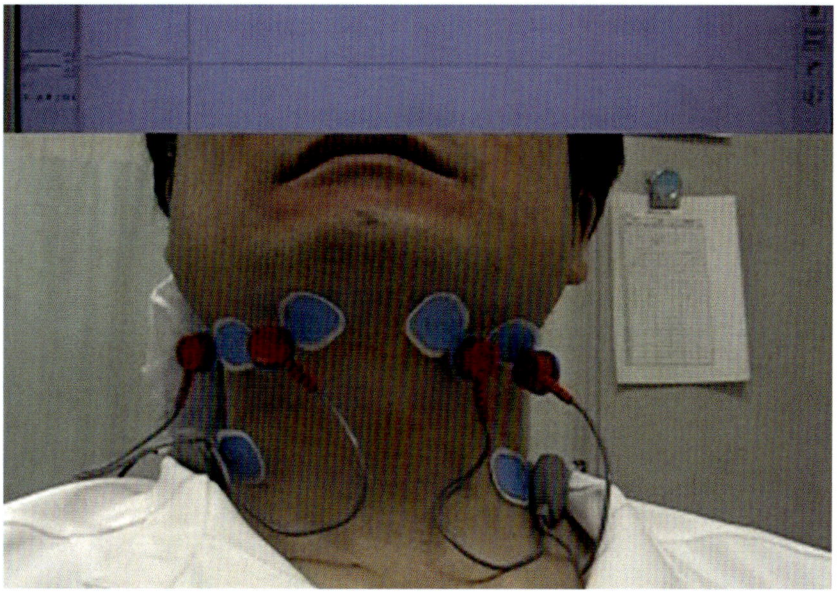

Fig. 17.45 The muscle activities of the suprahyoid muscle complex were detected by sEMG during the swallow maneuvers and dry swallows

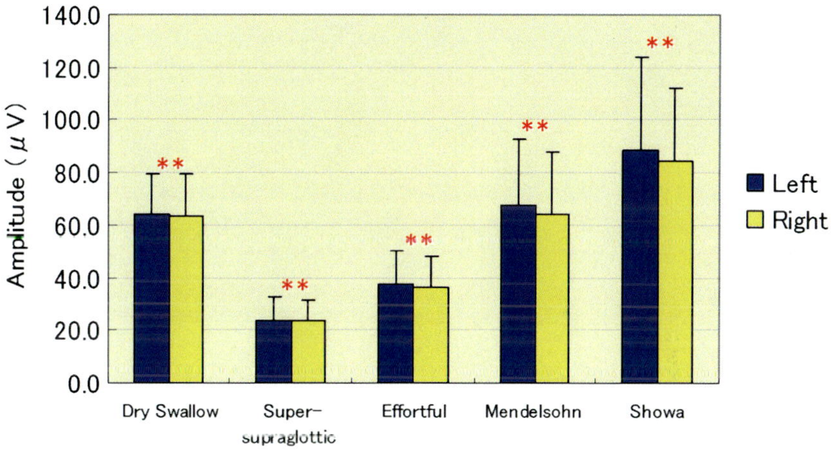

Fig. 17.46 Averaged peak amplitudes detected by sEMG. Activities at dry swallow and each of the swallow maneuvers were obtained from ten normal participants (** $p < 0.01$ by Kruskal–Wallis test)

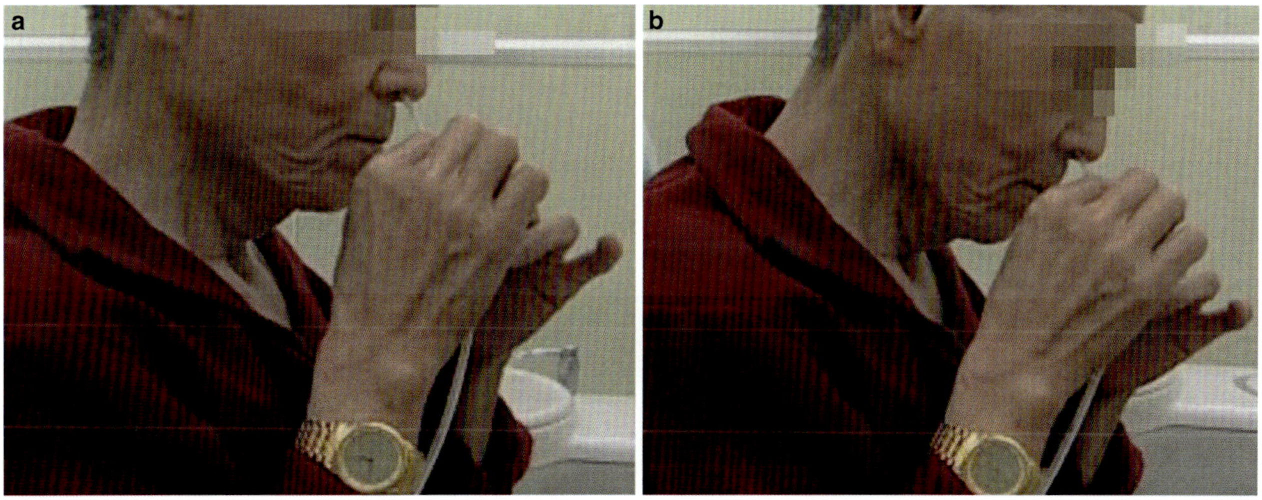

Fig. 17.47 Swallow exercise using a nasogastric tube. A patient swallows and pulls back a nasogastric tube repeatedly to learn the actual swallowing movement. This exercise is especially effective for patients who have not had oral intake for a long time to relearn how to swallow and to improve the coordination of oral and pharyngeal function

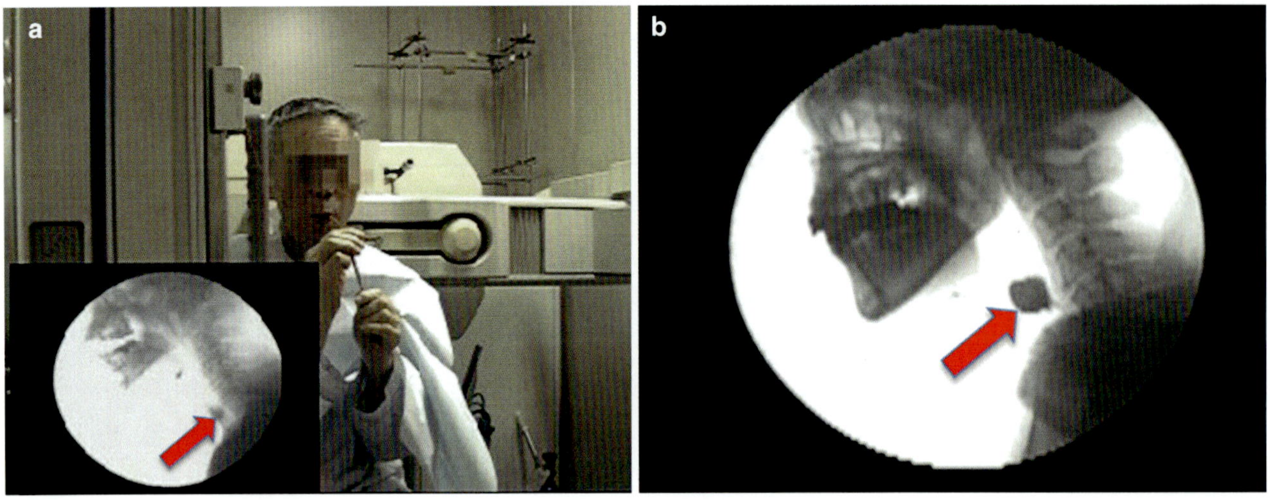

Fig. 17.48 Balloon catheter dilatation under VFSS. (**a**) The inflated balloon is just below the pharyngoesophageal segment (PE segment). (**b**) The inflated balloon is just above the PE segment. Once the balloon is visualized in the appropriate position, it is inflated and pulled back to the level above the cricopharyngeal opening. A *red arrow* shows an inflated balloon

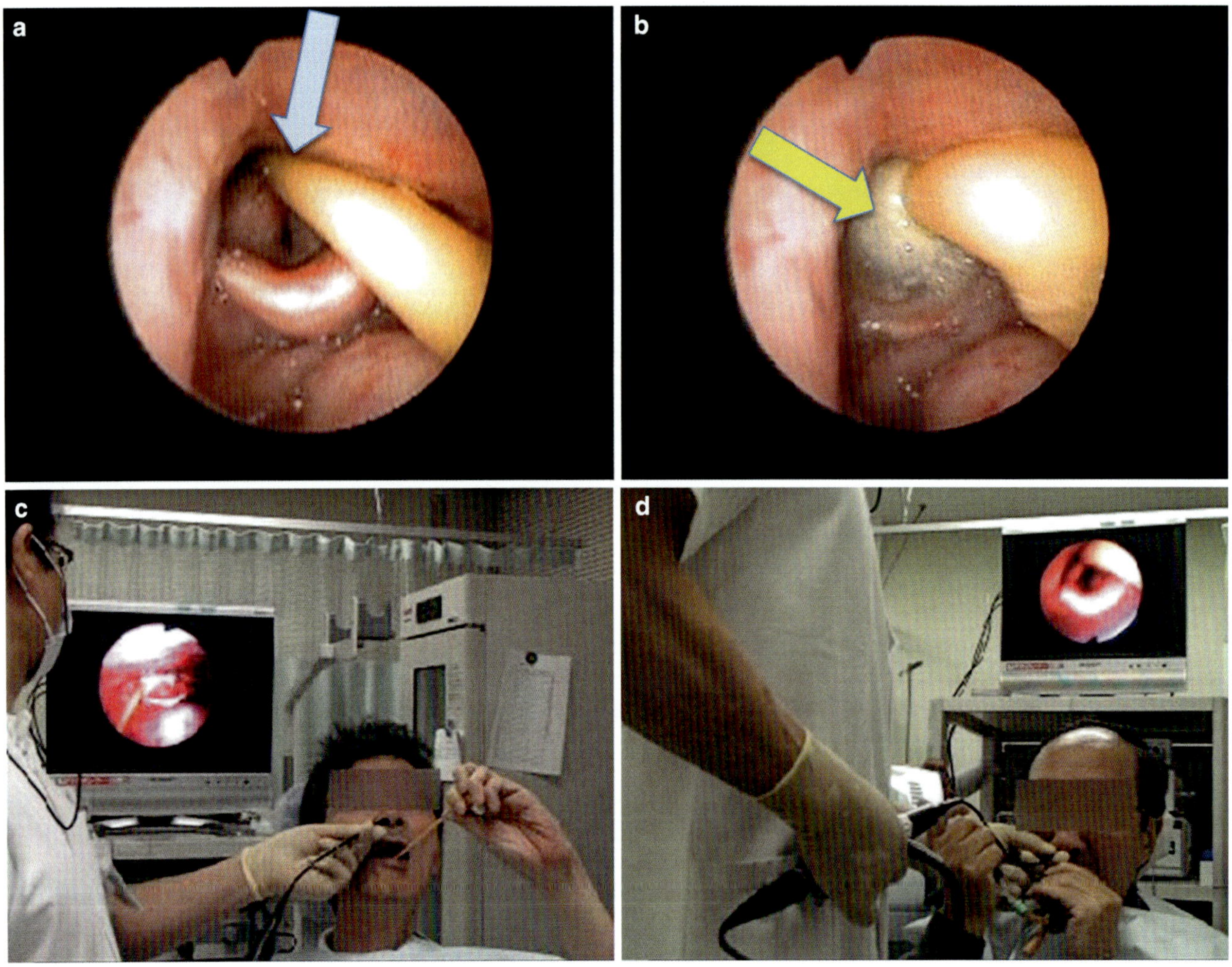

Fig. 17.49 Insertion of a balloon catheter into the esophagus and pulling back an inflated balloon catheter can be verified using VESS. (**a**) A *blue arrow* shows a deflated balloon catheter inserted into the esophagus, (**b**) a *yellow arrow* shows an inflated balloon, (**c**) transoral approach, (**d**) transnasal approach

6. Neck Stretching Exercises
   The postural adjustment techniques or swallowing maneuvers may not be performed sufficiently if the surgical effect extends to the neck (e.g., because of the neck dissection), and the movement of the neck is restricted by the postsurgical contracture. In such a case, neck stretching exercises are introduced to improve the neck mobility. Stretching exercises were divided to two major methods: the self-stretching method and the assisted stretching method (Fig. 17.50a–d). The assisted stretching method by the medical personnel or the professional physical trainer should be done first to learn the effective exercise.
7. The Shaker Exercise (Head-Raising Exercise)
   The Shaker exercise involves isometric and isokinetic neck exercises aimed at strengthening the suprahyoid muscles including the geniohyoid, thyrohyoid, and digastric muscles [46]. Patients are asked to lie flat on their back and raise the head enough to see the toes without raising the shoulders. The isometric strengthening portion involves three consecutive head lifts for 60 s, with a 60 s rest period between each head lift. The isometric exercise causes tension on the muscle without movement. The isokinetic strengthening portion involves 30 consecutive head lifts without holding. The velocity of the repetitive head lifts is kept constant; slower velocity produces greater strength gains. These exercises are the 6-week exercise program to be performed three times a day for 6 weeks for improving pharyngeal dysphagia.

   If the original head-raising exercise is too hard for the dysphagic patient to perform, modified head-raising exercises can be performed (Fig. 17.51a, b).
8. Biofeedback Training for Laryngeal Elevation Using sEMG
   sEMG, with the surface electrodes placed under the chin on the submandibular muscles, can be used to provide biofeedback regarding amount of effort utilized during swallow maneuvers [47]. In the case of the Showa swallow maneuver (Takahashi maneuver) and the Mendelsohn

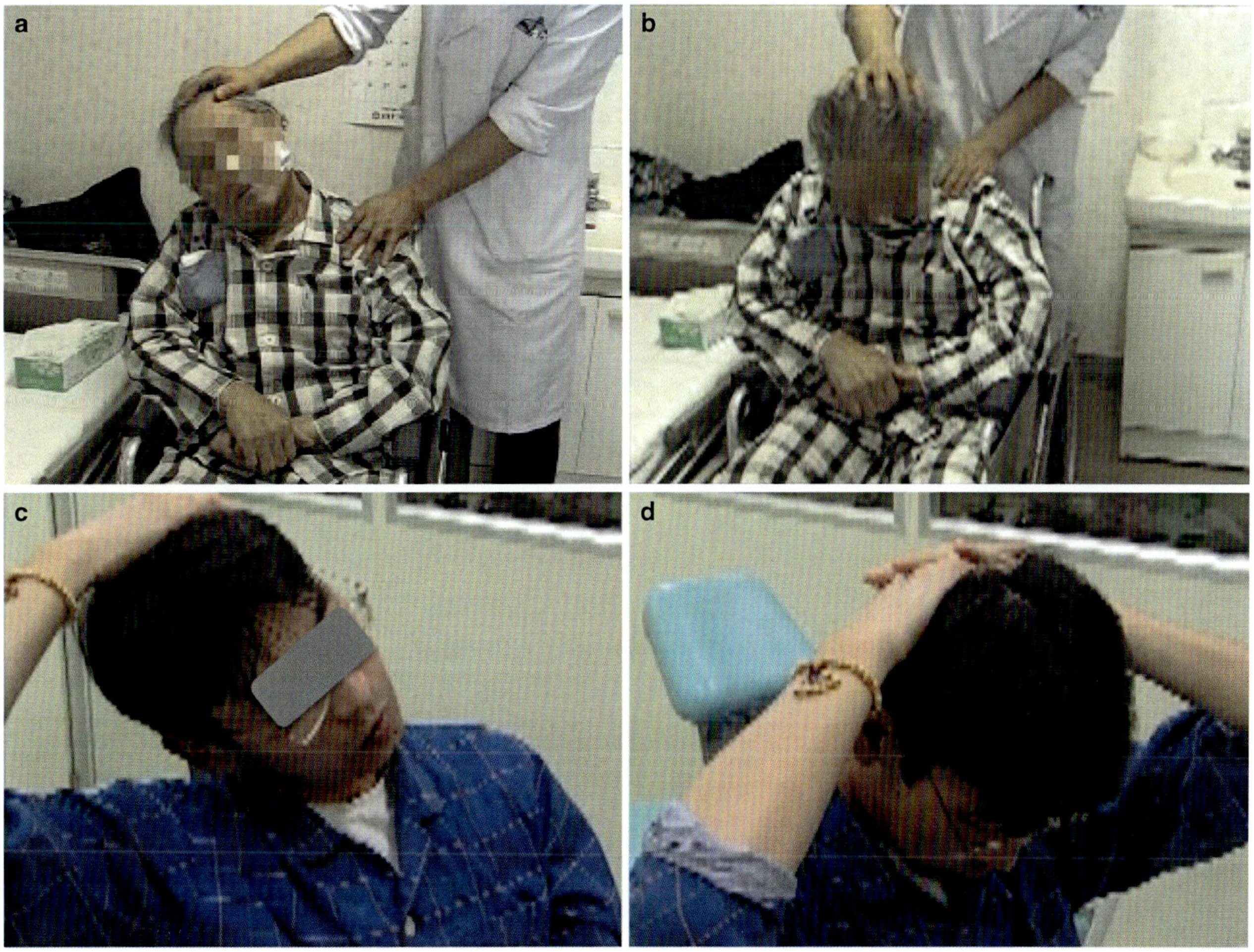

Fig. 17.50 Assisted stretching methods (**a** and **b**) and self-stretching methods (**c** and **d**) are shown. The assisted stretching methods by the medical personnel or the professional physical trainer should be done first to learn the effective exercise

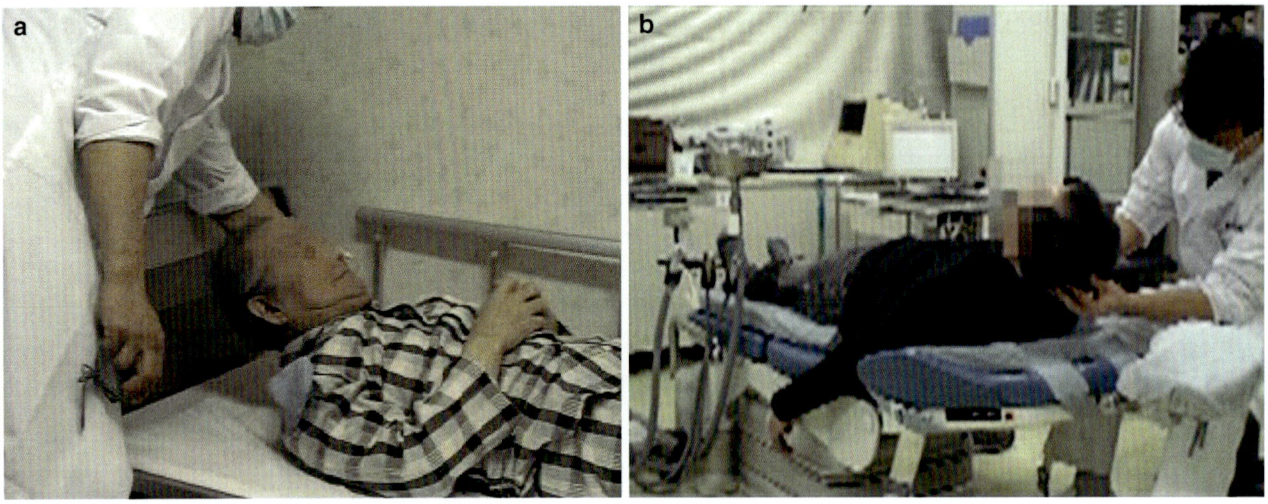

Fig. 17.51 The isometric strengthening portion of the Shaker exercise involves three consecutive head lifts for 60 s, with a 60 s rest period between each head lift. The isometric exercise causes tension on the muscle without movement. The isokinetic strengthening portion involves 30 consecutive head lifts without holding (**a**). If the original head-raising exercise is too hard for the dysphagic patient to perform, modified head-raising exercises can be performed (**b**). The head of this patient is supported by the hand of the medical practitioner

maneuver, the electrodes above the larynx would provide information on electrical activity in the laryngeal elevators during the maneuvers. Patients are able to look at both the amplitude and the duration of the signal, trying to increase both muscle effort (amplitude) and duration of muscle effort while performing the maneuvers (see Fig. 17.45).

9. Neuromuscular Electrical Stimulation to the Suprahyoid Muscles
   Neuromuscular electrical stimulation (NMES) is used as an adjunct modality in the treatment of dysphagia [48, 49]. VitalStim® therapy was approved by the US Food and Drug Administration in 2001 for the treatment of dysphagia through the application of NMES to the suprahyoid muscles (Fig. 17.52).
   NMES in conjunction with swallowing exercise (i.e., the Showa swallow maneuver) seems to be more effective than the swallow maneuver alone. VitalStim® therapy can also be applied to the patients who are not able to follow the therapist's instructions.

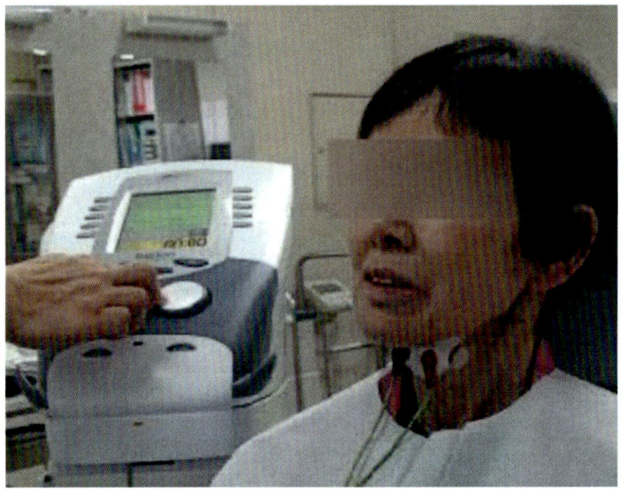

Fig. 17.52 Neuromuscular electrical stimulation (*NMES*) is used as an adjunct modality in the treatment of dysphagia. NMES is used to strengthen the suprahyoid muscles

17.3.3.1 Short-Term Hospitalized Intensive Dysphagia Rehabilitation for the Patients with Severe Dysphagia

In our department, the short-term hospitalized intensive dysphagia rehabilitation program with the aim of deciding on an appropriate rehabilitation plan and familiarization with rehabilitation techniques is provided to the patients with severe dysphagia [50–52] (Fig. 17.53).

The effectiveness of a short-term hospitalized intensive dysphagia rehabilitation program for posttreatment head and neck cancer patients with severe dysphagia was verified. Twenty-three patients with severe dysphagia following treatment for head and neck cancer served as subjects in our study 33).

After the swallowing assessment at admission, two (8.6 %) patients were upgraded and five (21.7 %) were downgraded than their pre-FOIS level. At admission, ten (43.5 %) patients were unable to take anything orally. During the hospitalization, ten (43.5 %) patients showed one or two levels of improvement on the FOIS, while one (4.3 %) showed decrease. Within 12 months after discharge, six (26.1 %) patients showed further improvement. Among them, four patients were no longer requiring tube feeding and returned to total oral intake (Figs. 17.54 and 17.55).

7:40am ～ 9:20am (1h40m)	Expectorating exercise, Respiratory training Neck stretching, Head-lift exercise (40s × 3set), Oral hygiene before and after meals, Eating training
11:30am ～ 1:20pm (1h50m)	Expectorating exercise, Respiratory training Neck stretching, Head -lift exercise (40s × 3set), Oral hygiene before and after meals, Eating training
5:30pm ～ 7:10pm (1h40m)	Expectorating exercise, Respiratory training Neck stretching, Head -lift exercise (40s × 3set), Oral hygiene before and after meals, Eating training

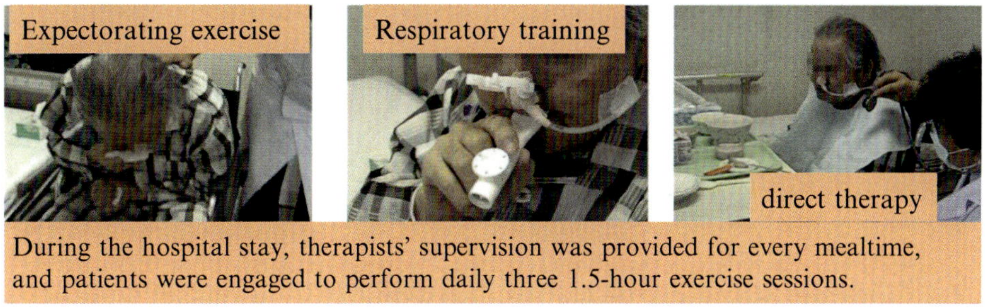

Fig. 17.53 An example of the intensive dysphagia rehabilitation

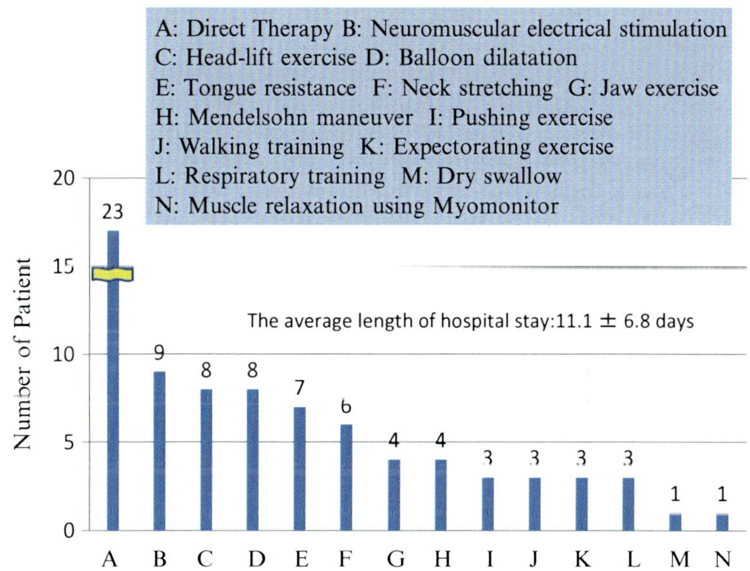

Fig. 17.54 Rehabilitation programs provided to patients

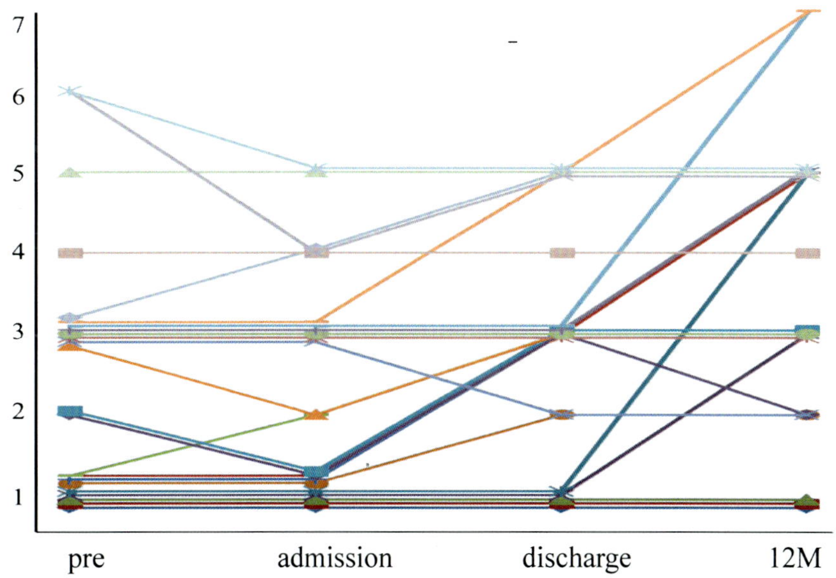

Fig. 17.55 Changes in patients' FOIS level over time

References

1. Pauloski BR, Logemann JA, Rademaker AW et al (1994) Speech and swallowing function after oral and oropharyngeal resections: one-year follow-up. Head Neck 16(4):313–322
2. McConnel FMS, McConnel FM, Logemann JA, Rademaker AW et al (1994) Surgical variables affecting postoperative swallowing efficiency in oral cancer patients: a pilot study. Laryngoscope 104(1):87–90
3. Bonanno PC (1971) Swallowing dysfunction after tracheotomy. Ann Surg 174:29–33
4. Cameron JL, Renolds J, Zuidema GD et al (1973) Aspiration in patients with tracheostomies. Surg Gynecol Obstetr 136:68–70
5. Bone DK, Davis JL, Zuidema GD, Cameron JL et al (1974) Aspiration pneumonia: prevention of aspiration in patients with tracheostomies. Ann Thoracic Surg 18:30–37
6. Nash M (1988) Swallowing problems in the tracheostomized patient. Otolaryngol Clin North Am 21(4):701–709
7. Muz J, Sandra H, Robert M, Ronnie F et al (1994) Scintigraphic assessment of aspiration in head and neck cancer patients with tracheostomy. Head Neck 16:17–20
8. Buchbinder D, Currivan RB, Kaplan AJ, Urken ML et al (1993) Mobilization regimens for the prevention of jaw hypomobility in the radiated patient: a comparison of three techniques. J Oral Maxillofac Surg 51:863–867
9. Pauloski BR, Rademaker AW, Logemann JA, Colangelo LA (1998) Speech and swallowing in irradiated and nonirradiated postsurgical oral cancer patients. Otolaryngol Head Neck Surg 118(5):616–624
10. Logemann JA, Smith CH, Pauloski BR, Rademaker AW, Lazarus CL et al (2001) Effects of xerostomia on perception and performance of swallow function. Head Neck 23(4):317–321
11. Hamlet S, Faull J, Klein B, Aref A et al (1997) Mastication and swallowing in patients with postirradiation xerostomia. Int J Radiat Oncol Biol Phys 37(4):789–796
12. Pauloski BR, Logemann JA, Joan CF, Colangelo LA et al (1995) Biomechanical analysis of the pharyngeal swallow in postsurgical patients with anterior tongue and floor of mouth resection and distal flap reconstruction. J Speech Hear Res 38:110–123
13. Ekberg O, Göran N et al (1983) Pharyngeal dysfunction after treatment for pharyngeal cancer with surgery and radiotherapy. Gastrointest Radiol 8:97–104
14. Logemann JA, Pauloski BR, Rademaker AW, McConnel FMS (1993) Speech and swallow function after tonsil/base of tongue resection with primary closure. J Speech Hear Res 36:918–926
15. Nishiwaki K, Tsuji T, Liu M, Hase K, Tanaka N, Fujiwara T (2005) Identification of a simple screening tool for dysphagia in patients with stroke using factor analysis of multiple dysphagia variables. J Rehabil Med 37(4):247–251
16. Okamoto N, Tomioka K, Saeki K, Iwamoto J et al (2012) Relationship between swallowing problems and tooth loss in community-dwelling independent elderly adults. J Am Geriatr Soc 60(5):849–853
17. Osawa A, Maeshima S, Tanahashi N (2013) Water-swallowing test: screening for aspiration in stroke patients. Cerebrovasc Dis 35(3):276–281
18. Wakasugi Y, Tohara H, Hattori F, Motohashi Y et al (2008) Screening test for silent aspiration at the bedside. Dysphagia 23(4).364–370
19. Saito E (2000) An integrated research on treatment and handling of dysphagia: general research report. In: Research project on aging and health, fiscal 1999 health and labour sciences research grant (Chief researcher: Saito E) (in Japanese) 3 ml food, Apr 2000, pp 1–18
20. Shinjo Y, Okitsu A, Ukeda I, Miyagi A, Domen K et al (2013) Effects of posture on subjective swallowing difficulty during screening tests for dysphagia. Int J Phys Med Rehabil 1(4):133
21. Oguchi K, Saitoh E, Baba M, Kusudo S et al (2000) The repetitive saliva swallowing test (RSST) as a screening test of functional dysphagia (2nd report)-validity of RSST (in Japanese). Jpn J Rehabil Med 37(6):383–388
22. Hongama S, Nagao K, Toko S et al (2012) MI sensor-aided screening system for assessing swallowing dysfunction: application to the repetitive saliva swallowing test. J Prosthodont Res 56(1): 53–57
23. Takahashi K (1998) Cervical auscultation. In: Kaneko Y (ed) Eating and swallowing rehabilitation. Ishiyaku Publishers, Tokyo, pp 171–175 (in Japanese)
24. Takahashi K, Uyama R, Hirano K, Yamashita Y et al (2001) Accuracy of cervical auscultation for detecting dysphagia in head and neck cancer patients (in Japanese). Head Neck Cancer 27(1):198–203
25. Logemann JA, Pauloski BR, Rademaker AW, McConnel FM, Heiser MA, Cardinale S et al (1997) Speech and swallowing rehabilitation in head and neck cancer patients. Oncology 11:651–659
26. Takahashi K (1998) Treatment strategies. In: Kaneko Y et al (eds) Dysphagia rehabilitation. Ishiyaku Publishing, Tokyo, pp 175–183 (in Japanese)
27. Takahashi K, Uyama R et al (1999) Swallow exercises in patients with head and neck cancer: objective assessment of swallow functions and subjective assessment by patients. Jpn J Head Neck Cancer 25(1):123–129
28. Takahashi K, Michi K (1999) Rehabilitation of dysphagia. In: Enomoto S et al (eds) Latest oral surgery (in Japanese), 4th edn. Ishiyaku Publishing, Tokyo, pp 422–426
29. Takahashi K (2000) Rehabilitation of dysphagia in patients with head and neck cancer (video). Tokyo, Ishiyaku Pub, in Japanese
30. Takahashi K (2003) Dysphagia rehabilitation: management of dysphagia in patients with head and neck cancer. In: Uematsu H et al (eds) Dental guidebook for the elderly. Ishiyaku Publishing, Tokyo, pp 265–273 (in Japanese)
31. Namba A, Yamashita Y, Takahashi K et al (2001) Application of a systematic manual for training swallowing disorders to postoperative oral cancer patients. J Jpn Stomatol Soc 50(2):122–129
32. Logemann JA, Ashford JR, McCullough G et al (1994) Effects of postural change on aspiration in head and neck surgical patients. Otolaryngol Head Neck Surg 110:222–227
33. Welch MV, Logemann JA, Rademaker AW, Kahrilas PJ et al (1993) Changes in pharyngeal dimensions effected by chin tuck. Arch Phys Med Rehabil 74:178–181
34. Shanahan TK, Logemann JA, Rademaker AW, Pauloski BR, Kahrilas PJ et al (1993) Chin-down posture effect on aspiration in dysphagic patients. Arch Phys Med Rehabil 74:736–739
35. Fukasawa M, Takahashi K et al (2004) Effects of postural adjustment techniques on dysphagia in head and neck surgical patients: videofluoroscopic comparison of the upright posture and the posture with head tilted to the stronger side. Jpn J Oral Maxillofac Surg 50(8):461–465, in Japanese
36. Fukasawa M, Takahashi K et al (2006) Effects of postural adjustment techniques on dysphagia in patients with tongue cancer: comparison of successful and unsuccessful cases with the head tilt posture. Jpn J Oral Maxillofac Surg 52:225–233, in Japanese
37. Felt P et al (2002) National dysphagia task force. In: The national dysphagia diet: standardization for optimal care. American Dietetic Association, Chicago
38. Wheeler R, Logemann JA, Rosen MS et al (1980) Maxillary reshaping prosthesis: effectiveness in improving speech and swallowing of post-surgical oral cancer patients. J Prosthet Dent 43:313–319
39. Davis J, Lazarus C, Logemann JA, Hurst PS et al (1987) Effect of maxillary glossectomy prosthesis on articulation and swallowing. J Prosthet Dent 57:715–719
40. Pauloski B et al (1996) Effect of intraoral prostheses on swallowing function in postsurgical oral and oropharyngeal cancer patients. Am J Speech Lang Pathol 5:31–46

41. Takahashi K (2006) Function recovering devices for disorders: devices for dysphagia. In: Mayazaki T et al (eds) Clinical dental engineering. Ishiyaku Publishing, Tokyo, pp 302–307 (in Japanese)
42. Michael A Crary (2010) Changing the swallow: active therapy techniques. Chapter 14 Treatment for Adults. pp285-296 Michael E. Groher and Michael A. Crary Dysphagia: Clinical Management in Adults and Children. 2010 Mosby Elsevier
43. Lazarus CL (1993) Effect of radiation therapy and voluntary maneuvers on swallow functioning in head and neck cancer patients. Clin Commun Disord 3(4):11–20
44. Lazarus CL, Logemann JA, Gibbons P (1993) Effect of maneuvers on swallowing function in a dysphagic oral cancer patient. Head Neck 15:419–424
45. Dou Z, Zu Y, Wen H, Wan G et al (2012) The effect of different catheter balloon dilatation modes on cricopharyngeal dysfunction in patients with dysphagia. Dysphagia 27(4):514–520
46. Shaker R, Easterling C, Kern M, Nitschke T et al (2002) Rehabilitation of swallowing by exercise in tube-fed patients with pharyngeal dysphagia secondary to abnormal UES opening. Gastroenterology 122(5):1314–1321
47. Crary MA, Groher ME (2000) Basic concepts of surface electromyographic biofeedback in the treatment of dysphagia. Am J Speech Lang Pathol 9:116–125
48. Beom J, Kim SJ, Han TR (2011) Electrical stimulation of the suprahyoid muscles in brain-injured patients with dysphagia: a pilot study. Ann Rehabil Med 35(3):322–327
49. Kim SR, Kwon KH, Cho BJ (2013) The effects of neuromuscular electrical stimulation on pharyngeal transit time. J Phys Ther Sci 25(7):849–851
50. Takahashi K (2009) Management of dysphagia in post-surgical head and neck cancer patients with intractable dysphagia-hospitalization for dysphagic patients who were told in other clinics that in would be impossible or extremely difficult to eat orally. J Jpn Soc Oral Tumors 21(4):245–254
51. Takahashi K, Uyama R, Yokoyama K, Nakamichi Y et al (2011) Management of dysphagia for patients being treated for head and neck cancer in our department. Head Neck Cancer 37(4):508–513
52. Yuasa K, Yokoyama K, Takei Y, Nakamichi Y et al (2013) Effectiveness of short-term intensive dysphagia rehabilitation in head and neck cancer patients with severe dysphagia. Dysphagia 28:647

QOL Management in Oral Cancer Patients

18

Yoshihide Ota and Takayuki Aoki

Abstract

In general, quality of life (QOL) in the broad sense refers to the well-being of individuals and societies. This concept covers not only physical/financial affluence, quantity of service, and individual self-care but also the spiritual aspect and self-actualization. In the medical care field, QOL influences not only the evaluation of treatment but also the treatment method. At present, concepts of values in life are diverse, and medical care considering both survival and QOL has become necessary. Therefore, QOL instruments using scales corresponding to the purpose in various areas have been developed. They have sometimes been revised because the concept of QOL varies across ages. Furthermore, QOL in oncology has characteristics different from that in other diseases. Cancer is a life-threatening disease, and many cancer patients have a mental shock when they are first notified to have cancer. QOL markedly varies before, during, and after treatment. For malignant tumors, it is significantly different depending on the stage of progression, onset site, extent of adverse events caused by treatment, and degree of residual disability. Even if a cancer survivor had a good course, QOL is often different from that before they develop cancer. Therefore, QOL evaluation in cancer patients is very difficult.

Keywords

Head and neck cancer • Oral cancer • QOL

18.1 QOL Definition

In general, quality of life (QOL) in the broad sense refers to the well-being of individuals and societies. This concept covers not only physical/financial affluence, quantity of service, and individual self-care but also the spiritual aspect and self-actualization. The 36th president of the United States, Lyndon Baines Johnson, declared national QOL improvement as part of his Great Society policy (1964) [1]. Since then, the term QOL has been generally used. In the medical care field, attention has been focused on improvement in QOL in the areas of terminal care of cancer and independent living of disabled persons since the 1970s. For elderly welfare, attention has been focused on seeking the reason for living or sensation of happiness for improvement in QOL. Thus, eventually, the concept of QOL became popular. At present, the World Health Organization (WHO) defines QOL as "an individual's perception of their position in life in the context of the culture and value systems in which they live and in relation to their goals, expectations, standards and concerns" [2].

18.1.1 QOL in Health Care

QOL is considered a multidimensional concept that is divided into health-related QOL (HRQOL) and non-health-related QOL (NHRQOL). The true impact of health and disease on

Y. Ota, D.D.S., Ph.D. (✉) • T. Aoki, D.D.S., Ph.D.
Department of Oral and Maxillofacial Surgery,
Tokai University School of Medicine, 143 Shimokasuya,
Isehara, Kanagawa 259-1193, Japan
e-mail: yotaorsg@ybb.ne.jp

T. Kirita and K. Omura (eds.), *Oral Cancer: Diagnosis and Therapy*,
DOI 10.1007/978-4-431-54938-3_18, © Springer Japan 2015

QOL is known as HRQOL [3, 4]. It is conceptualized as those aspects of QOL that are influenced directly by the health of a person. Development of tools to measure HRQOL in individuals over time has produced important benefits. On the other hand, NHQOL indirectly affects health and disease. Most QOL studies in the medical care field, including cancer treatment, focus on HRQOL [3, 4].

It is generally accepted that HRQOL includes numerous domains. There is a wide range of potential domains, but not all of them are relevant to all studies. However, wherever possible, relevant domains should be considered. For example, the following domains have been proposed: (1) physical status and functional abilities; (2) psychological status and well-being; (3) social interactions; (4) economic and/or vocational status and factors; and (5) religious and/or spiritual status. Among these, religious and/or spiritual status may be not so familiar to Japanese people [3–6].

Religion is a collection of cultural systems, belief systems, and worldviews that establishes symbols that relate humanity to spirituality and moral values. They tend to derive morality, ethics, religious laws, or a preferred lifestyle from their ideas about the cosmos and human nature. Spirituality has been defined in numerous ways, including a belief in a power operating in the universe that is greater than oneself, a sense of interconnectedness with all living creatures, and an awareness of the purpose and meaning of life and the development of absolute personal values. One can find meaning, hope, comfort, and inner peace in life through spirituality. Although spirituality is often associated with religious life, many believe that personal spirituality can be developed outside of religion. Acts of compassion and selflessness, altruism, and the experience of inner peace are all characteristics of spirituality. It is unclear how spirituality and religion are related to health. Some studies show that spiritual or religious beliefs and practices create a positive mental attitude that may help a patient feel better and improve the well-being of family caregivers [5, 6].

NHRQOL indirectly involves health and is classified into the following four domains: (1) personal–internal (including concepts of value/faith, hope/target, personality, and capabilities to cope); (2) personal–social (including social network, family structure, social group, economic conditions, and employment status); (3) external–natural environment (including air, water, land, climate, and geography); and (4) external–social environment [including cultural facilities, exposure to the culture, religious facilities, schools, commercial establishments, medical facilities and services, public policy, safety, traffic, communication, social amusement, characteristics (disposition), demographic composition, and commercial establishments]. NHRQOL is considered important in the public health field for health promotion rather than the medical care field [4].

HRQOL and NHRQOL are mutually influential and, as understood from above, there are common items between them. Depending on health status, the weight-to-volume ratio of HRQOL and NHRQOL varies. The healthier the person is the more important NHRQOL is compared with HRQOL. In the presence of disease or disability, HRQOL is more important than NHRQOL [4].

18.1.2 QOL in Oncology

Previously, outcome indices of cancer treatment included prolonged survival and reduced tumor load, based on the standpoint of medical providers. However, paternalism of cancer treatment has become unacceptable because of a shift in the health paradigm, which includes increased respect for the autonomy of patients, legal necessity for disclosure and informed consent, culture maturity, and health economics. Thus, the outcome of cancer treatment has changed. Specifically, QOL and cost performance of treatment have become new indices. From cancer treatment, patients tend to seek care rather than cure.

On the other hand, emphasis on the right of the patient to choose a medical treatment has often led to anxiety-provoking situations for patients. In modern society, extensive medical information can be obtained from the Internet or other sources. However, improper or incorrect information is also abundant. Therefore, cancer treatment according to evidence-based medicine (EBM) has been followed widely, leading to the creation of treatment guidelines by public institutions. In the future, although cancer treatment is performed according to EBM, it may become necessary to adapt with each patient's wishes and may become more complicated. In respecting the autonomy of patients, it is necessary to clarify EBM of QOL.

QOL in oncology has characteristics different from that in other diseases. Cancer is a life-threatening disease, and many cancer patients have a mental shock when they are first notified to have cancer. QOL markedly varies before, during, and after treatment. For malignant tumors, it is significantly different depending on the stage of progression, onset site, extent of adverse events caused by treatment, and degree of residual disability. Even in the same category of oral cancer, QOL is different between lingual cancer and gingival carcinoma. Furthermore, even if a cancer survivor had a benign course, QOL is often different from that before they develop cancer. Therefore, QOL evaluation in cancer patients is very difficult.

18.2 Quantitative Measurement

18.2.1 Purpose of Evaluation

QOL is basically a subjective concept consisting of multiple factors. Although qualitative research cannot be disregarded as a means to comprehend QOL, it is difficult to perform qualitative evaluation. In general, a study of QOL is conducted quantitatively, in principle, and the composing domains and items differ depending on the purpose.

As mentioned above, the concept of QOL was developed partly in a political aspect. In seeking for what is the most desirable life for people, it was necessary to develop useful instruments. In this context, the objective of QOL measurement to evaluate the life status of the citizens is necessary for public administration to plan a policy. As a concrete example, it is utilized for the planning of health promotion in the public health field [3, 4].

On the other hand, in the medical care field, QOL influences not only the evaluation of treatment but also the treatment method. At present, concepts of values in life are diverse, and medical care considering both survival and QOL has become necessary. Therefore, QOL instruments using scales corresponding to the purpose in various areas have been developed. Furthermore, they have sometimes been revised because the concept of QOL varies across ages.

18.2.2 Criteria for the Evaluation of QOL Questionnaires

At present, some excellent QOL measurement instruments have been authorized. However, QOL is subjective and heavily dependent on individual patients. Therefore, there are no questionnaires that can be used for all people. It is also difficult to evaluate whether an individual QOL measurement instrument is more valid. Several authors have suggested standards for the development and evaluation of instruments to measure health status. One of the most elaborate lists was proposed by the scientific advisory committee (SAC) of the Medical Outcomes Trust in 1994 [7, 8]. SAC defined a set of eight key attributes of instruments to measure health status and HRQOL: (1) conceptual and measurement model; (2) reliability; (3) validity; (4) responsiveness; (5) interpretability; (6) respondent and administrative burden; (7) alternate forms; and (8) cultural and language adaptations.

1. Conceptual and measurement model
   The concept to be measured needs to be defined properly and should match its intended use. There are two types of QOL measurement instruments: one evaluates using both subjective and objective indices and the other evaluates using only a subjective index.
2. Reliability
   Reliability is the degree to which the instrument is free of random error, which means free from errors in measurement caused by chance factors that influence measurement. The question of reliability arises as the function of scales is stretched to encompass the realm of prediction. One of the most popular reliability statistics in current use is Cronbach's alpha. Cronbach's alpha is a coefficient of internal consistency or average correlation of items in a survey instrument to gauge its reliability. In general, survey instruments are required to have a minimum Cronbach's alpha value of 0.7 and a correlation coefficient with another instrument of 0.75 [7, 8]. The reproducibility of these instruments should be determined using variance analysis. In Japan, WHO quality of life (WHOQOL) instrument is reported to have a Cronbach's alpha value between 0.87 and 0.97 and a correlation coefficient with general health questionnaire (GHQ) between −0.45 and −0.47 [9].
3. Validity
   Validity is the degree to which the instrument measures what it purports to measure. Validity of a measurement instrument does not refer to the instrument itself but to whether particular interpretations of its scores are well justified. It is inappropriate to speak of a measurement instrument as inherently valid or invalid. It is only meaningful to consider the validity of a specified purpose or interpretation of the resulting scores. Because multiple types of inferences may be entertained for scores from a given instrument, depending upon the situation in which it is to be used, the validity of each inference must be established. Several QOL measurement instruments in Japan are translated or somewhat revised from those developed in Europe and the United States [9, 10]. These partially include questionnaire entries not reflecting Japanese culture and way of life. Therefore, the responsive rate of these entries may be low; thus it is difficult to apply corresponding ones in foreign countries, without any modifications.
4. Responsiveness
   Responsiveness has been defined as the ability of a questionnaire to detect clinically important changes over time, even if these changes are small. An intervention study on the same specimen (sample, population) must describe changes in score over time. Where measurement instruments are used, the sample number for the study must enable statistical analysis. In clinically comparative studies, random sampling is expected, and the same treatment method is required including absence or presence of the control group.
5. Interpretability
   Interpretability is the degree to which one can assign easily understood meaning to an instrument's score. Investigators should provide information about what (change in) score would be clinically meaningful [7–10].
6. Respondent and administrative burden
   Burden refers to the time, effort, and other demands placed on those to whom the instrument is administered (respondent burden) or on those who administer the instrument (administrative burden) [7, 8].
7. Alternate forms
   Alternative means of administration include self-report, interviewer administered, computer assisted, etc. It is often important to know whether these modes of administration are comparable [7, 8].

8. Cultural and language adaptations or translations
   QOL measurement instruments repeatedly evaluate the expression of language/manner of speaking and understandability of questionnaire contents in each country to obtain equivalency in evaluation in different culture or language. Extremely complicated processes are required to develop a measurement instrument enabling comparison of QOL between different countries [7–10].

18.2.3 QOL in Oral Cancer

It is beyond controversy that the target of oral cancer treatment is permanent cure of the tumor, if there is a possibility of a permanent cure and the patient desires it. However, the evaluation of treatment for oral cancer must consider not only the survival rate of the patients but also their QOL. In addition, QOL should be evaluated taking survival into consideration [11].

QOL questionnaires used for oral cancer patients are divided into four groups: (1) general QOL questionnaire, (2) QOL questionnaire for general cancer, (3) specific QOL questionnaire for head and neck (oral) cancer, and (4) oral HRQOL (OHRQOL) (Table 18.1).

18.2.3.1 General QOL Questionnaire

1. WHOQOL instruments [2, 9, 11, 12]
   Several instruments have been developed to investigate QOL; however, most of them are developed by researchers in Europe and the United States. In these, the definition of QOL is different depending on the researcher, leading to different composition of each QOL instrument. Therefore, the WHO started to develop new QOL instruments in 1992, taking into consideration the international comparison in each country including developing countries. After meetings over a 2-year period by QOL experts and professionals in each medical institute in each country, QOL was defined as "an individual's perception of their position in life in the context of the culture and value systems in which they live and in relation to their goals, expectations, standards and concerns." The concept of QOL is composed of the following six domains:
   (a) Physical health
       Energy and fatigue; pain and discomfort; sleep and rest
   (b) Psychological
       Body image and appearance; negative feelings; positive feelings; self-esteem; thinking, learning, memory, and concentration
   (c) Level of independence
       Mobility; activities of daily living (ADL); dependence on medicinal substances and medical aids; work capacity
   (d) Social relationships
       Personal relationships; social support; sexual activity
   (e) Environment
       Financial resources; freedom; physical safety and security; health and social care: accessibility and quality; home environment; opportunities for acquiring new information and skills; participation in and opportunities for recreation/leisure; physical environment (pollution/noise/traffic/climate); transport
   (f) Spirituality/religion/personal beliefs
       In 1994, a pilot questionnaire was developed in English. It consisted of 300 standardized items, which were extracted from these six domains. This was verified by the administration of the WHOQOL Pilot Form in 15 field centers to 250 patients and 50 "healthy" respondents. These data were statistically analyzed, and the WHOQOL-100, composed of standardized and cross-nationality equivalent response scales of 100 common items, was completed. Furthermore, the WHOQOL-BREF (WHOQOL-26), an abbreviated 26-item version of the WHOQOL-100, was developed using data from the field trial version of the WHOQOL-100. The WHOQOL instruments can be used in particular cultural settings, but at the same time, results are comparable across cultures. The WHOQOL is now available in over 20 different languages, and its development in further languages is progressing. Their sensitivity to change is currently being assessed. Domain scores of the WHOQOL-BREF have been shown to correlate at approximately 0.9 with those of the WHOQOL-100. The WHOQOL-BREF has also been used in several studies in Japan [9].

Table 18.1 QOL questionnaires using for oral cancer patients

1. General QOL questionnaire
(a) WHOQOL instruments
(b) Medical outcomes study 36-item short form (SF-36)
(c) Karnofsky performance status (KPS)
2. QOL questionnaire for general cancer
(a) The European organization for research and treatment of cancer quality of life questionnaire (EORTC QLQ)-C30
(b) Functional assessment of cancer therapy scale general version (FACT-G)
(c) Quality of life questionnaire for cancer patients treated with anticancer drugs (QOL-ACD)
(d) Functional living index for cancer (FLIC)
3. Specific QOL questionnaire for head and neck cancer
(a) EORTC QLQ-H&N35
(b) The University of Washington quality of life questionnaire (UW-QOL)
(c) FACT H&N
4. Oral HRQOL (OHRQOL)
(a) The general oral health assessment index (GOHAI)
(b) Subjective oral health status indicators (SOHSI)
(c) Oral health impact profile (OHIP)

2. Medical outcomes study 36-item short form (SF-36) [11, 13, 14]
SF-36 is a questionnaire used to measure health status in general and was developed by Ware et al. In SF-36, one item is designed to assess perceived change in health status, and each of the remaining 35 items contributes to a score on one of the eight scales: physical functioning, role-physical, bodily pain, general health perception, vitality, social functioning, role-emotional, and mental health. Scores on these eight scales can be used to compute a summary index of physical health and a summary index of mental health. The Japanese version of SF-36 was developed, and Fukuhara et al. have verified its translation, adaptation, and validation.
3. Karnofsky performance status (KPS) [11, 15]
KPS is one of the earliest and most commonly used indices of patients' performance status. Recent papers still refer to the Karnofsky scale for validating a new measure. Administered by an observer, this 11-point rating system assesses symptoms, physical activities, self-care, and ability to work, with scores from 0 (dead) to 100 (normal). Although KPS is based on physical performance and dependency, it has been shown to be a valid, if crude, predictor of survival. The WHO has recommended an alternative five-point scale that is simple and easy to use. At present, KPS is used to confirm the validity of a new QOL instrument.

18.2.3.2 QOL Questionnaire for General Cancer

1. The European organization for research and treatment of cancer QOL questionnaire (EORTC QLQ) C30 [11, 16–20]
The EORTC QOL Study Group has developed a measurement strategy for the assessment of QOL in clinical trials. A core QOL questionnaire—the EORTC QLQ-C30—is used together with diagnosis-specific modules to increase the coverage, sensitivity, and specificity of the assessments in various patient and treatment groups.
It was designed to be cancer-specific, multidimensional in structure, appropriate for self-administration, applicable across a range of cultural settings, and suitable for use with additional site- or treatment-specific modules. The EORTC QLQ-C30 (version 3.0) consists of 30 questions. Of these, 24 questions form nine multi-item scales presenting various aspects of HRQOL, five functional scales (physical functioning, social functioning, emotional functioning, role functioning, and cognitive functioning), three symptom scales (fatigue, pain, nausea, and vomiting), and a global condition (health and QOL). The remaining six questions form single-item scales describing different cancer relevant symptoms. During the scoring procedure, raw EORTC QLQ-C30 scores are linearly transformed into 0 e100 scales. For global health status and the five functioning scales, a score of 100 corresponds to a high HRQOL. For financial difficulties and the eight symptoms, a score of100 implies maximum difficulty or symptom burden [16–18]. Subsequent versions were built on the same basic principles, culminating in the core 30-item EORTC QLQ-C30 (version 3.0) questionnaire, representing over 20 years of continuous development, refinement, and validation. It is a copyrighted instrument, which has been translated and validated into 81 languages and has been used in more than 3000 studies worldwide. At present, the QLQ-C30 (version 3.0) is the most recent version and should be used for all new studies [19].
While the EORTC QLQ-C30 is an important tool for assessing the generic aspects of QOL, it has limitations. Therefore, a modular approach was adopted for disease-specific treatment measurements. An essential aspect of the "modular" approach to QOL assessment adopted by the EORTC QLG (QOL Group) is the development of modules specific to tumor site, treatment modality, or a QOL dimension, to be administered in addition to the EORTC QLQ-C30. The modules, like the core questionnaire, are designed for use in cancer clinical trials. These modules include head and neck (QLQ-H&N35), bone metastases (QLQ-BM22), hepatocellular carcinoma (QLQ-HCC18), brain (QLQ-BN20), information (QLQ-INFO25), breast (QLQ-BR23), lung (QLQ-LC13), cervical cancer (QLQ-CX24), multiple myeloma (QLQ-MY20), colorectal (QLQ-CR29), neuroendocrine carcinoid (QLQ-GINET21), colorectal liver metastases (QLQ-LMC21), oesophageal (QLQ-OES18), endometrial (QLQ-EN24), oesophago gastric (QLQ OG25), gastric (QLQ STO22), ovarian (QLQ-OV28), prostate (QLQ-PR25), and elderly cancer patients (QLQ ELD14) [20].
The Japanese Version of the EORTC QLQ-C30 [17, 21]
The EORTC QLQ-C30 was developed in European countries. A Japanese version of the EORTC QLQ-C30 was also drawn up by EORTC itself. However, in Japan, where language and culture are different from European countries, is it possible to use the Japanese EORTC QLQ-C30 as a universally applicable instrument? To date, some cross-cultural validations have conducted. In evaluating psychometric testing, internal consistency by Cronbach's alpha, item discrimination by multitrait scaling analysis, and validity analysis with the ECOG performance score (PS) and the KPS scale were performed. These results show that the Japanese EORTC QLQ-C30 is potentially useful as an instrument and is universally applicable across cultures.
2. Functional assessment of cancer therapy scale general version (FACT-G) [11, 22–24]
The FACT-G is one of the most widely used cancer-specific QOL instruments that was developed by Cella et al [22, 23]. It has been validated across a wide range of

cancer patients, cultures, and languages and can be used to assess the impacts of cancer and its treatment on the physical and psychosocial well-being of patients. The fourth version of FACT-G consists of 27 Likert-type questions covering four domains: physical well-being (seven items), social/family well-being (seven items), emotional well-being (six items), and functional well-being (seven items). Scoring is on a 0–4 Likert-type scale, with higher scores representing better outcome. Summary scores can be calculated for each of these four domains, alongside a single overall score for the instrument. FACT-G meets all conditions such as ease of use (simplicity), credibility, validity, and responsiveness in clinical oncological studies.

The Japanese Version of the FACT-G [25]

FACT-G was translated and its usefulness was verified by Fukumoto et al. [25]. To determine if the FACT-G could be used in Japan, a cross-cultural validation was performed. The Japanese version was created through an iterative forward–backward translation sequence used throughout the FACT multilingual translation project. While evaluating psychometric testing, its construct validity was investigated by factor analysis and multitrait scaling analysis, and its clinical validity was estimated by known-groups comparison using stage, PS, and patient location and validated longitudinally by PS. The FACT-G (version 3.0) was administered to 180 patients with lung cancer. Analyses showed that the scales of physical well-being, functional well-being, emotional well-being, and relationship with doctors were constructively valid in Japan. Japanese patients felt that familial relationships were different than relationships with friends and neighbors, indicating that the social/family well-being scale needed cultural adaptation. Two items concerning coping with illness and acceptance of illness did not load predictably onto their respective scales and were considered cross-culturally problematic. However, clinical validity demonstrated its sensitivity. Japanese FACT-G (version 4.0) has been improved to address the weakness in an attempt to become an instrument that is applicable across cultures.

3. QOL questionnaire for cancer patients treated with anticancer drugs (QOL-ACD) [26–28]

   The EORTC QLQ-C30 and FACT-G are questionnaires developed in Europe and the United States, and the Japanese versions have been developed. However, there is a possibility that different QOL items are considered important in different nations or cultures. Therefore, development of a QOL scale fitting with the lifestyle of patients was sought in Japan. Thus, QOL-ACD was developed by the Japanese QOL Research Group as a generic questionnaire according to a multidimensional construct that could be used to assess QOL of Japanese patients undergoing chemotherapy for different types of cancer. The QOL-ACD is a 22-item, self-administered questionnaire, which consists of four domains evaluating functional well-being (items 1–6), physical well-being (items 7–11), mental well-being (items 12–16), and psychosocial well-being (items 17–21), as well as a face scale (item 22). The entire questionnaire is shown in Appendix A. The four domains were originally designated as daily activity, physical condition, psychological condition, and social attitude, respectively [26, 27]. For all items and domains, a higher score represents better QOL. QOL-ACD is also reported to be useful in patients with head and neck cancer [28].

4. Functional living index for cancer (FLIC) [11, 29, 30]

   The FLIC was developed at the Manitoba Cancer Treatment and Research Foundation Centre in Winnipeg. The questions were selected from a first-generation questionnaire consisting of approximately 250 questions. The FLIC contains 22 items to which the patient must respond by placing a slash mark on a linear analog scale that is divided into seven equal intervals. The score from each item is condensed to a composite score, and the higher the composite score, the better the QOL. Domains studied include physical well-being, emotional state, social ability, and family/situation factors. The FLIC has been translated into Japanese and used in several clinical studies; however, validity and reliability have not been confirmed.

18.2.3.3 Specific QOL Questionnaire for Head and Neck Cancer

1. EORTC QLQ-H&N35 [11, 20, 21, 31–39]

   The EORTC Quality of Life Group develops tumor site-specific modules to be used with a core questionnaire, the EORTC QLQ-C30. One of the first was the module for head and neck cancer patients, the EORTC QLQ-H&N37 [31], later revised and shortened to its final version with 35 items, the H&N35 [32]. This module consists of 7 multi-item scales measuring pain in the mouth, problems with swallowing, senses, speech, social eating, and social contact and 11 single-item scales assessing problems with teeth, mouth opening, dry mouth, sticky saliva, coughing, feeling ill, as well as use of analgesics, nutritional supplements, feeding tube, and finally weight gain and weight loss. The period of the QLQ-H&N35 module is "During the past week." Items from 1 to 30 are scored on a four-point Likert scale as follows: "not at all" (1), "a little" (2), "quite a bit" (3), and "very much" (4); items from 31 to 35 use a "no" (1) and "yes" (2) format as choices to answer [32]. The module has been translated into 53 languages [20] and is used worldwide as one of the standard instruments for measuring QOL in head and neck cancer patients [33–35]. Some issues have been raised that may hamper the use of the H&N35. One criticism is that patients may feel annoyed by some of the items, for example, those enquiring about problems with sexual functioning [36, 37]. A matter of debate is whether this presents difficulty for the researcher who feels uncomfortable in asking such questions or for the patient who feels embarrassed or irritated in answering. Another criticism concerns items that may not be applicable to some of the patients. For example, questions about swallowing solid food administered to patients who are tube fed or about hoarseness when the larynx has been removed [38, 39]. Little is known about the use of the H&N35 in research, the manner in which psychometric issues are reflected in different languages, and how well the multi-item scales are accepted by patients and investigators.

The Japanese Version of the EORTC QLQ-H&N35 [10, 21]

The Japanese version of the EORTC QLQ-H&N35 was developed by translating the original EU-English version, performing cultural adaptation, and further performing initial psychometric tests for use in Japanese head and neck cancer patients [10, 21]. Phase 1: The first intermediate Japanese version was produced according to the EORTC QOL Unit translation project guideline. The second intermediate version was the result of the backward translation project and two peer-to-peer discussion settings by health-care professionals related to the project. Phase 2: Focus group discussions with team members and semi-structured interviews with 108 participants were conducted to produce the final Japanese version. Cultural adaptation and validation yielded scores of the Japanese version of the QLQ-H&N35 module that are reliable by internal consistency (Cronbach's alpha) and the validation results showed acceptable correlation results by Pearson's product moment correlation coefficient (*r*). The questionnaire was well accepted, and the response rate was high (93.9 %). Convergent validity was moderate to high (from r=0.55–0.97, P<0.01), and discriminant validity was low; Cronbach's alpha coefficients of most scales had good reliability ($\alpha \geqq 0.70$), except that of the pain scale. In Japan, however, some correlation patterns between scales differed from that in the original European countries and cultures. The use of both qualitative and quantitative methods was important in developing the Japanese version of the QLQ-H&N35 module [10, 21].

2. The University of Washington quality of life questionnaire (UW-QOL) [11, 40–46]

The UW-QOL (version 4.0) is a patient self-completed questionnaire and currently tests 12 specific domains relating to the head and neck cancer patient. These are pain, appearance, activity, recreation, swallowing, chewing, speech, shoulder function, taste, saliva, mood, and anxiety. The brevity and simplicity of scoring in UW-QOL make it an easy measure in a busy clinical setting. A UW-QOL composite score from 0 to 100 was obtained by averaging the scores of the domains. When two or more domains were not answered, no composite score was calculated. Scoring is scaled, so that a score of 0 represents the worst QOL and a score of 100 represents the best QOL. The composite 12 (the average of the 12 domain scores) has been used by some investigators when describing HRQOL outcomes, although its psychometric properties have not been reported [11, 40–44].

Factor analysis is a useful method for understanding how items in a questionnaire relate to each other. It can be used to determine whether these data fit to a single construct (and, hence, a single composite-derived score) or whether multiple constructs are suggested. The derivation of multiple subscales, if appropriate, should improve sensitivity and responsiveness because more items of a similar construct are brought together. The UW-QOL has face, content, and construct validity [11, 40–44]. Although factor analysis has been reported for other head and neck cancer-specific questionnaires, to our knowledge, it has never been reported for the UW-QOL (version 4.0). The issue of interpreting clinically significant changes in patient-reported outcomes is important, especially when designing randomized trials. Such variables have been published for the Functional Assessment of Cancer Therapy–Head and Neck instrument [41, 45].

The UW-QOL domains and global scales have, at most, six discrete options and a skewed response, and these are difficult to handle in this context. Any composite or subscale score will have a wider numerical range and greater potential for being able to assess clinical effect in treatment evaluation studies and for calculating sample sizes.

The Japanese Version of the UW-QOL [46]

The UW-QOL was translated into Japanese with the consent of Professor Ernest Weymuller at the University of Washington. Then, after performing cultural adaptation, it was tested and has been used in Japanese head and neck cancer patients. However, the reliability and validity of the Japanese version have not been reviewed in detail [45].

3. FACT H&N [11, 47–52]

The FACT-G (version 4.0) consists of 27 items that yield scores in four domains (physical well-being, seven items; social/family well-being, seven items; emotional well-being, six items; and functional well-being, seven items). The FACT H&N contains 12 items (eating, swallowing, speaking, and aesthetics) that are specific to head and neck cancer patients. Each question consists of a declarative statement rated on a 0–4 Likert-type scale. Higher scores represent better QOL [11, 47–52].

The Japanese Version of the FACT H&N [51, 52]

Japanese patients felt that familial relationships were different than relationships with friends and neighbors, indicating that the social/family well-being scale needed cultural adaptation. Therefore, the social/family well-being scale in the Japanese version of FACT-G is composed of nine items: seven items of the FACT-G original and additional two items. Therefore, the Japanese version of FACT H&N is composed of 41 items: 29 items of the Japanese version of FACT-G and 12 added head and neck cancer-specific items. However, at present, the reliability and validity of the Japanese version have not been reviewed in detail.

18.2.3.4 OHRQOL

Oral state has significant influence on daily life including mastication, swallowing, articulation, and aesthetics. Thus, QOL questionnaires concerning not only oral cancer patients but also patients with oral diseases in general have been developed. OHRQOL is composed of items such as functioning, psychological aspects, pain/discomfort, and social aspect. Functioning includes mastication, swallowing, and articulation. Most OHRQOL instruments have no authoritative Japanese versions, and the validity and reliability of the Japanese version have been barely verified [53].

1. The general oral health assessment index (GOHAI) [53–55]
   GOHAI was developed for elderly people. However, it was demonstrated to be applicable for other age groups and has been used extensively. The GOHAI is a 12-item measure that assesses oral health-related problems affecting people in three hypothesized dimensions: physical function, psychosocial function, and pain or discomfort. The characteristic of GOHAI is that the number of questions is as small as 12 items, and thus, the burden on respondents is reduced. However, psychosocial aspects are reflected more heavily on evaluation than functioning compared with other OHRQOL instruments [53–55].
2. Subjective oral health status indicators (SOHSI) [53, 56, 57]
   SOHSI is a descriptive oral health survey of general populations developed by Locker et al. This instrument comprises the following scales: ability to chew, ability to speak, oral and facial pain symptoms, other oral symptoms, eating impact scale, communication/social relations impact scale, ADL scale, and worry/concern scale. The response format varies with each scale. The scales ability to chew, ability to speak, oral and facial pain symptoms, and other oral symptoms have a yes/no dichotomous response. The eating impact scale, ADL scale, and worry/concern scale have five-point rating scales of the frequency of occurrence of each item of the categories: all the time (scored 5),very often (scored 4), fairly often (scored 3), sometimes (scored 2), and never (scored 1). These indicators are useful for descriptive oral health surveys of general populations. All questions were administered as a self-completed questionnaire [53, 56, 57].
3. Oral health impact profile (OHIP) [53, 58, 59]
   The OHIP, developed by Slade et al., is one of the most commonly used measures of OHRQOL. This instrument contains 49 questions for seven dimensions, which has its foundation in the classification of impairments, disabilities, and handicaps developed by the WHO. These dimensions are hierarchically ordered so that the impacts described by the dimensions are considered gradually more disruptive to one's life. The dimensions are functional limitations, physical pain, psychological discomfort, physical disability, psychological disability, social disability, and handicap [53, 58, 59].

18.3 QOL in Cancer Clinical Trials [60]

Oncological research has a direct influence on the prognosis of patients. Therefore, QOL in cancer clinical trials should not be a primary endpoint but should be included as an exploratory secondary endpoint. QOL investigation is often conducted in Phase III trials. However, where the purpose is to investigate feasibility in QOL investigation, a trial with only a single arm is conducted in some cases. With regard to reconstructive therapy for head and neck cancer, QOL can be a primary endpoint.

18.4 QOL and Health Economics [53, 60]

Societal aging has advanced because of the change in social structure and the progression of medicine, and the rate of chronic diseases has become higher than that of acute diseases. Accordingly, medical care-related annual expenditure in the national budget has been ever increasing. Therefore, scientific evaluation of cost–benefit performance for treatment, diagnosis, and prevention of diseases has become critical. In medical checkups, contribution to survival tends to be regarded as more important than early discovery. Furthermore, the health paradigm has shifted from overcoming diseases to alleviation of symptoms, coexistence with diseases, and maintenance/promotion of health, and thus, QOL evaluation has been considered important.

Even in medical policy, it is necessary to analyze decreases in medical expenses from not only a macroeconomic viewpoint but also from a microeconomic viewpoint based on QOL evaluation of patients and to conduct efficient distribution of medical expenses. One of the analysis methods of health economics includes cost–utility analysis (CUA). This evaluates health from both aspects of quantity of life and QOL and indicates the satisfaction level of life. Utility expresses the severity of disease or symptom as a product of time and the QOL index during the time. Utility is indicated quantitatively using a scale from 0 (=death) to 1 (=health).

Representative time indices using QOL indices include quality adjusted life-year (QALY) and disability adjusted life-year (DALY). QALYs and DALYs are reciprocal, and CUA evaluation compares expense per 1 QALY unit (expense/QALY). At present, CUA is one of the most useful evaluation methods in health economics.

References

1. Baker F, Intagliata J (1982) Quality of life in the evaluation of community support systems. Eval Program Plann 5:69–79
2. World Health Organization (2014) The world health organization quality of life. NetPrints. http://www.who.int/mental_health/publications/whoqol/en/. Accessed 22 Mar 2014
3. Spilker B (1996) Introduction. In: Spilker B (ed) Quality of life and pharmacoeconomics in clinical trial. Lippincott Williams & Wilkins, New York, pp 1–10
4. Spikler B, Revicki DA (1996) Taxonomy of quality of life. In: Spilker B (ed) Quality of life and pharmacoeconomics in clinical trial. Lippincott Williams & Wilkins, New York, pp 25–31
5. Peterson M, Webb D (2006) Religion and spirituality in quality of life studies. Qual Life 1:107–116. doi:10.1007/s11482-006-9006-y
6. Balboni TA, Vanderwerker LC, Block SD, Paulk CS, Peteet JR, Prigerson HG (2007) Religiousness and spiritual support among advanced cancer patients and associations with end-of-life treatment preferences and quality of life. J Clin Oncol 25:555–560
7. Aaronson N, Alonso J, Burnam A, Lohr KN, Patrick DL, Perrin E, Stein RE (2002) Assessing health status and quality-of-life instruments: attributes and review criteria. Qual Life Res 11:193–205
8. Terwee CB, Bot SD, de Boer MR, van der Windt DA, Knol DL, Dekker J, Bouter LM, de Vet HC (2007) Quality criteria were proposed for measurement properties of health status questionnaires. J Clin Epidemiol 60:34–42
9. Tazaki M, Nakane Y, Endo T et al (1998) Results of a qualitative and field study using the WHOQOL instrument for cancer patients. Jpn J Clin Oncol 28:134–141
10. Toth G, Sakaguchi T, Mikami Y, Hirose H, Tsukud M (2005) A pilot study of the translation, cultural adaptation and validation of the EORTC head and neck cancer quality of life questionnaire module (QLQ-H&N35) for use in Japan. Auris Nasus Larynx 32:175–183
11. Rogers SN, Fisher SE, Woolgar JA (1999) A review of quality of life assessment in oral cancer. Int J Oral Maxillofac Surg 28(99):117. doi:10.1034/j.1399-0020.1999.282280204
12. Skevington SM, Lotfy M, O'Connell KA (2004) The World Health Organization's WHOQOL-BREF quality of life assessment: psychometric properties and results of the international field trial. A report from the WHOQOL Group. Qual Life Res 13:299–310
13. Ware JE Jr (1996) The SF-36 health survey. In: Spilker B (ed) Quality of life and pharmacoeconomics in clinical trial. Lippincott Williams & Wilkins, New York, pp 337–345
14. Fukuhara S, Bito S, Green J, Hsiao A, Kurokawa K (1998) Translation, adaptation, and validation of the SF-36 health survey for use in Japan. J Clin Epidemiol 51:1037–1044
15. Schag CC, Heinrich RL, Ganz PA (1984) Karnofsky. Performance status revisited: reliability, validity, and guidelines. J Clin Oncol 2:187–193
16. Fayers P, Bottomley A (2002) Quality of life research within the EORTC—the EORTC QLQ-C30. Eur J Cancer 38:S125–S133
17. Kobayashi K, Takeda F, Teramukai S et al (1998) A cross-validation of the European organization for research and treatment of cancer QLQ-C30 (EORTC QLQ-C30) for Japanese with Lung Cancer. Eur J Cancer 34:810–815
18. Silveira AP, Gonçalves J, Sequeira T, Ribeiro C, Lopes C, Monteiro E, Pimentel FL (2010) Patient reported outcomes in head and neck cancer: selecting instruments for quality of life integration in clinical protocols. Head Neck Oncol 2:32. doi:10.1186/1758-3284-2-32
19. EORTC QLQ-C30 (2014) NetPrints. http://groups.eortc.be/qol/eortc-qlq-c30. Accessed 22 Mar 2014
20. Why do we need modules? NetPrints. http://groups.eortc.be/qol/eortc-modules. Accessed 22 Mar 2014
21. Toth G, Tsukuda M (2004) The European organization for research and treatment of cancer (EORTC) quality of life questionnaire for Japanese patients with head and neck cancer: the Japanese version of QLQ-H&N35 (in Japanese). Gan To Kagaku Ryoho 31:461–467
22. Cella DF, Tulsky DS, Gray G et al (1993) The functional assessment of cancer therapy scale: development and validation of the general measure. J Clin Oncol 11:570–579
23. Cella DF (1993) Manual for the functional assessment of cancer therapy (FACT) measurement system (version 2). Rush Medical Center, Chicago
24. Weitzner MA, Meyers CA, Gelke CK, Byrne KS, Cella DF, Levin VA (1995) The functional assessment of cancer therapy (FACT) scale. Development of a brain subscale and revalidation of the general version (FACT-G) in patients with primary brain tumors. Cancer 75:1151–1161, 10.1002/1097-0142 (19950301)75:5<1151:AID-CNCR2820750515> 3.0.CO;2-Q
25. Fumimoto H, Kobayashi K, Chang CH, Eremenco S, Fujiki Y, Uemura S, Ohashi Y, Kudoh S (2001) Cross-cultural validation of an international questionnaire, the general measure of the functional assessment of cancer therapy scale (FACT-G), for Japanese. Qual Life Res 10:701–709. doi:10.1023/A.1013851216181
26. Kurihara M, Shimizu H, Tsuboi K, Kobayashi K, Murakami M, Eguchi K, Shimozuma K (1999) Development of quality of life questionnaire in Japan: quality of life assessment of cancer patients receiving chemotherapy. Psychooncology 8:355–363
27. Matsumoto M, Ohashi Y, Morita S et al (2002) The quality of life questionnaire for cancer patients treated with anticancer drugs (QOL-ACD): validity and reliability in Japanese patients with advanced non-small-cell lung cancer. Qual Life Res 11:483–493
28. Takumida M, Nishida I (1995) The quality of life for patients with cancer in the head and neck 2: time course observation of the quality of life (in Japanese). Jibi To Rinsho 41:766–773
29. Schipper H, Clinch J, McMurray A, Levitt M (1984) Measuring the quality of life of cancer patients: the functional living index-cancer Development and validation. J Clin Oncol 2:472–483
30. Laenen A, Alonso A (2010) The functional living index-cancer: estimating its reliability based on clinical trial data. Qual Life Res 19:103–109. doi:10.1007/s11136-009-9568-x
31. Bjordal K, Ahlner-Elmqvist M, Tollesson E, Jensen AB, Razavi D, Maher EJ, Kaasa S (1994) Development of a European organization for research and treatment of cancer (EORTC) questionnaire module to be used in quality of life assessments in head and neck cancer patients. EORTC quality of life study group. Acta Oncol 33:879–885
32. Bjordal K, de Graeff A, Fayers PM et al (2000) A 12 country field study of the EORTC QLQ-C30 (version 3.0) and the head and neck cancer specific module (EORTC QLQ-H&N35) in head and neck patients. EORTC quality of life group. Eur J Cancer 36:1796–1807
33. Mehanna HM, Morton RP (2006) Patients, views on the utility of quality of life questionnaires in head and neck cancer: a randomised trial. Clin Otolaryngol 31:310–316
34. Tschiesner U, Rogers SN, Harréus U, Berghaus A, Cieza A (2008) Content comparison of quality of life questionnaires used in head and neck cancer based on the international classification of functioning, disability and health: a systematic review. Eur Arch Otorhinolaryngol 265:627–637. doi:10.1007/s00405-008-0641-9

35. Singer S, Arraras JI, Chie WC et al (2013) Performance of the EORTC questionnaire for the assessment of quality of life in head and neck cancer patients EORTC QLQ-H&N35: a methodological review. Qual Life Res 22:1927–1941. doi:10.1007/s11136-012-0325-1
36. Jensen K, Jensen AB, Grau C (2007) Smoking has a negative impact upon health related quality of life after treatment for head and neck cancer. Oral Oncol 43:187–192
37. Bjordal K, Hammerlid E, Ahlner-Elmqvist M et al (1999) Quality of life in head and neck cancer patients: validation of the European organization for research and treatment of cancer quality of life questionnaire-H&N35. J Clin Oncol 17:1008–1019
38. Singer S, Wollbrück D, Wulke C et al (2009) Validation of the EORTC QLQ-C30 and EORTC QLQ-H&N35 in patients with laryngeal cancer after surgery. Head Neck 31:64–76. doi:10.1002/hed.20938
39. Sherman AC, Simonton S, Adams DC, Vural E, Owens B, Hanna E (2000) Assessing quality of life in patients with head and neck cancer: cross-validation of the European organization for research and treatment of cancer (EORTC) quality of life head and neck module (QLQ-H&N35). Arch Otolaryngol Head Neck Surg 126:459–467
40. Rogers SN, Gwanne S, Lowe D, Humphris G, Yueh B, Weymuller EA Jr (2002) The addition of mood and anxiety domains to the University of Washington quality of life scale. Head Neck 24:521–529
41. Rogers SN, Lowe D, Yueh B, Weymuller EA Jr (2010) The physical function and social-emotional function subscales of the University of Washington quality of life questionnaire. Arch Otolaryngol Head Neck Surg 136:352–357. doi:10.1001/archoto.2010.32
42. Rogers SN, Scott J, Chakrabati A, Lowe D (2008) The patients' account of outcome following primary surgery for oral and oropharyngeal cancer using a 'quality of life' questionnaire. Eur J Cancer Care 17:182–188. doi:10.1111/j.1365-2354.2007.00832.x
43. Rogers SN, Lowe D (2009) Screening for dysfunction to promote multidisciplinary intervention by using the University of Washington quality of life questionnaire. Arch Otolaryngol Head Neck Surg 135:369–375. doi:10.1001/archoto.2009.7
44. Rogers SN, Laher SH, Overend L, Lowe D (2002) Importance-rating using the University of Washington quality of life questionnaire in patients treated by primary surgery for oral and oro-pharyngeal cancer. J Craniomaxillofac Surg 30:125–132. doi:10.1054/jcms.2001.0273
45. Weymuller EA Jr, Yueh B, Deleyiannis FW, Kuntz AL, Alsarraf R, Coltrera MD (2000) Quality of life in head and neck cancer. Laryngoscope 110:4–7
46. Toth G, Tsukuda M (2003) The Importance of the assessment analysis and interpretation of quality of life (QOL) for persons with head and neck cancer possibilities and tools for the QOL measurement in Japan (in Japanese). Jibiinkoukatenbo 46:368–383
47. Silveira AP, Gonçalves J, Sequeira T, Ribeiro C, Lopes C, Monteiro E, Pimentel FL (2010) Patient reported outcomes in head and neck cancer: selecting instruments for quality of life integration in clinical protocols. Head Neck Oncol 31:2:32. doi:10.1186/1758-3284-2-32
48. Campbell BH, Marbella A, Layde PM (2000) Quality of life and recurrence concern in survivors of head and neck cancer. Laryngoscope 110:895–906
49. Ringash J, Bezjak A, O'Sullivan B, Redelmeier DA (2004) Interpreting differences in quality of life: the FACT-H&N in laryngeal cancer patients. Qual Life Res 13:725–733
50. Ringash J, O'Sullivan B, Bezjak A, Redelmeier DA (2007) Interpreting clinically significant changes in patient-reported outcomes. Cancer 110:196–202. doi:10.1002/cncr.22799
51. Mochizuki Y, Matsushima E, Omura K (2009) Perioperative assessment of psychological state and quality of life of head and neck cancer patients undergoing surgery. Int J Oral Maxillofac Surg 38:151–159. doi:10.1016/j.ijom.2008.11.007
52. Mochizuki Y, Omura K, Matsushima E (2009) Changing trend over time of psychological states and quality of life of oral cancer patients with surgery (in Japanese). Kokubyo Gakkai Zasshi 76:16–24
53. Hirano Y (2008) The significance of QOL evaluation in medical economics research (in Japanese). Osakafuritsudaigaku Keizai Kenkyu 53:139–155
54. Atchison KA, Dolan TA (1990) Development of the geriatric oral health assessment index. J Dent Educ 54:680–687
55. Enoki K, Ikebe K, Matsuda KI, Yoshida M, Maeda Y, Thomson WM (2013) Determinants of change in oral health-related quality of life over 7 years among older Japanese. J Oral Rehabil 40:252–257. doi:10.1111/joor.12031
56. Locker D, Miller Y (1994) Evaluation of subjective oral health status indicators. J Public Health Dent 54:167–176
57. Tajima M, Kohzuki M, Azuma S, Saeki S, Meguro M, Sugawara J (2007) Difference in quality of life according to the severity of malocclusion in Japanese orthodontic patients. Tohoku J Exp Med 212:71–80
58. Slade GD, Spencer AJ (1994) Development and evaluation of the oral health impact profile. Community Dent Health 11:3–11
59. Kieffer JM, Hoogstraten J (2008) Linking oral health, general health, and quality of life. Eur J Oral Sci 116:445–450. doi:10.1111/j.1600-0722.2008.00564.x
60. Sloan JA, Novotny PJ, Loprinzi CL Analyzing quality of life (QOL) endpoints in clinical trials via the SAS system. NetPrints. http://www2.sas.com/proceedings/sugi23/Stats/p225pt1.pdf

Palliative Care for Oral Cancer

19

Toshiya Koitabashi

Abstract

Palliative care is an approach that improves the quality of life of patients and their families facing the problems associated with life-threatening illness. For pain assessment, it is important to obtain not only the onset, duration, location, quality, pattern, character, and intensity of pain but also aggravating and relieving factors, associated symptoms and signs, and current pain management agents and their effectiveness. To treat cancer pain, this principles can be summarized in five steps (by the mouth, by the clock, by the ladder, for the individual, and attention to detail). The use of opioids should not be affected by unfounded fears such as respiratory depression, tolerance, or dependence. When satisfactory alleviation of cancer pain cannot be achieved as a result of regular assessment of the response to analgesics or therapy, opioid-resistant cancer pain should be assessed. Opioid-resistant cancer pain includes underdosing, poor absorption or intake of opioids, raised intracranial pressure, and neuropathic pain. In cases of neuropathic pain, adjuvant analgesics such as anticonvulsants or antidepressants should be considered. Both prevention and appropriate interventions for opioid-related adverse effects such as constipation, nausea and vomiting, and drowsiness are one of the key components to continue to treat cancer pain.

Keywords

Cancer pain • Neuropathic pain • Opioid • Palliative care

19.1 Etiology

Cancer is the most frequent cause of death (28.5 % of total death) in Japan, and this frequency is gradually increasing. Distressing symptoms are common with progressive life-limiting cancer, especially in their far-advanced stages [1]. Causes for suffering include disease-mediated symptoms such as pain, dyspnea, and fatigue. Moreover, psychological disorders, such as depression, anxiety, and loss of a sense of purpose in living; social demoralization, such as feelings of loss of previously held status and roles within society and family; and the existential or spiritual dimensions of suffering often accompany patients with end-stage diseases. Pain is one of the main and feared symptoms among far-advanced cancer patients (67 %) and also early-stage patients (33 %). Most of them experience continuous pain and almost half patients have severe pain. Causes of cancer pain consist of the cancer itself, complications of the cancer, treatment of the cancer, and comorbidities. The cancer itself makes bone, visceral, or soft tissue involvement, nerve compression or infiltration, muscle spasm, ulceration, raised intracranial pressure. Complications of the cancer involve pressure sores, constipation, postherpetic neuralgia, candidiasis, and lymphedema. The treatment of cancer induces neuropathy caused by chemotherapy, mucositis caused by radiotherapy, and surgery-related issues such as postoperative pain.

T. Koitabashi, M.D., Ph.D. (✉)
Department of Anesthesiology, Ichikawa General Hospital, Tokyo Dental College, Tokyo, Japan
e-mail: koitabas@tdc.ac.jp

T. Kirita and K. Omura (eds.), *Oral Cancer: Diagnosis and Therapy*,
DOI 10.1007/978-4-431-54938-3_19, © Springer Japan 2015

Comorbidities, which are shown in approximately 30 % of the patients, include non-cancer pain caused by decubitus or back pain, diabetic neuropathy, arthritis, and angina. The experience of pain can exacerbate physical conditions, depression, and anxiety, inducing the prevention of work and reduction of income.

19.2 Definition of Palliative Care

World Health Organization (WHO) has shown the definition of palliative care that it is an approach that improves the quality of life of patients and their families facing the problems associated with life-threatening illness, through the prevention and relief of suffering by means of early identification and impeccable assessment and treatment of pain and other problems, physical, psychological, and spiritual [2]. Pain includes not only physical but also psychological, social, and spiritual aspects; therefore palliative care integrates these four big issues. General palliative care is provided by the usual professional cares of the patient and family with low to moderate complexity of palliative care need. Specialist palliative care is provided for patients and their families with moderate to high complexity of palliative care need. Palliative care team offers a support to help patients live as actively as possible until death and the family cope during the patient's illness and in their own bereavement. Palliative care team consists of physicians to treat physical pain, psychologists, certified nurse in palliative care, pharmacists, nutritionists, and social workers and performs a team approach.

Palliative care was thought to be equal to the terminal care or end-of-life care. When the progressive state of the disease have not been able to regulate following the completion of appropriate anti-cancer treatments, the physicians have decided frequently to change the strategies from disease modifying treatment to supportive care or terminal care. Therefore, palliative care has traditionally been delivered to patients late in the course of the disease. However, late referrals to palliative care are inadequate to alter the quality and delivery of care provided to patients with cancer. To have a meaningful effect on patients' quality of life and end-of-life care, the current definition has changed that palliative care should be applied early in the course of illness, if applicable, in conjunction with other therapies that are intended to prolong life, such as chemotherapy or radiation (Fig. 19.1). As results of early initiation of palliative care, cancer survival days were reported to be prolonged. Temel et al. have shown that early palliative care led to significant improvements in both quality of life and mood among patients with metastatic non-small-cell lung cancer [3]. Survival rates in the early palliative care group were increased by approximately 3 months compared to that in the standard care group.

19.3 Physiology

Cancer pain is traditionally classified by either the origin or the location. Nociceptive, neuropathic, psychogenic, and mixed pain is usually used for the classification identified on the basis of the mechanism by which pain is produced. Somatic, visceral, or central pain is another definition classified by the location. Nociceptive cancer pain may result from the activation of the nociceptive receptor following damage to normal tissue or visceral structures. Neuropathic cancer pain is caused by a lesion or disease of the somatosensory nervous system. The underlying mechanisms of neuropathic

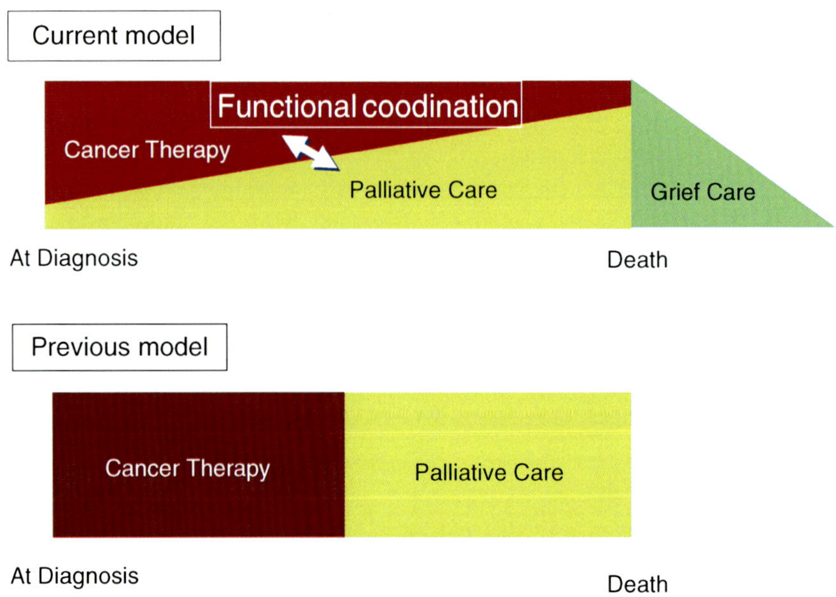

Fig. 19.1 Changes in the concept regarding palliative care model

pain are not understood fully, but it is recognized that pain occurs following reaction of the injured nerves abnormally. Patients may describe having a dull ache with a burning, shooting, or electric shock-like sensations. Psychogenic cancer pain is derived from psychological cause which is not accompanied with explicit physiological diseases.

Somatic cancer pain includes superficial and deep pain. The site of pain is usually localized or well recognized, and the proportion of pain is expressed as aching, throbbing, or tingling. Breakthrough pain is characterized as sudden onset, usually perceived by mobilization or coughing. Visceral cancer pain is caused by the irritation of the pleura or peritoneum and sudden contraction of luminal organs. The site of pain is often poorly localized, and the proportion of pain is described as gnawing or cramping pain.

19.4 Assessment of Pain

Pain assessment is a start point to treat pain. Therefore, failure to assess pain is a critical barrier to better pain management. Principles of pain assessment are follows: to begin with wide open questions before focusing on more specific problems, to watch the patient for clues regarding pain, and to avoid jumping to conclusions.

For pain assessment, it is important to obtain not only the onset, duration, location, quality, pattern, character, and intensity of pain but also aggravating and relieving factors, associated symptoms and signs, and current pain management agents and their effectiveness. Because pain intensity is dependent on each subject, patient self-report is the only gold standard for its assessment. As previously described, many patients have more than one type of pain, it is important that each pain should be assessed separately, and pain should be assessed at appropriate intervals. For example, both pain at rest and pain on mobilization or coughing should be assessed continuously and separately, and pain intensity for the previous 24 h should be evaluated every day following the initiation of treatment in order to change pain management regimen.

Unidimensional tools such as visual analogue scales, verbal rating scales, face scales, and numeric rating scales are employed to obtain information regarding the intensity of the pain experienced by the patient.

19.5 Principles of Pain Management [4]

Following obtaining patient pain information, identification of the patient's goals of treatment is necessary before the initiation of pain treatment. In 1986, the WHO published the book entitled *Cancer Pain Relief* and proposed the principles of cancer pain management. To treat cancer pain, these principles can be summarized in five steps (by the mouth, by the clock, by the ladder, for the individual, and attention to detail). By the mouth recommends the oral route in taking drugs into the body. But, in cases of oral cancer, the oral route may not be preferred, because of an inability to take drugs orally due to the invasion of cancer and its related treatments. By the clock indicates the necessity to administer analgesics at regular intervals and not as needed. For example, when slow-release morphine is prescribed after meals three times a day, the interval between dinner and breakfast may be more than 12 h, although the interval between breakfast and lunch would be only 5–6 h. The use of WHO ladder is a key component to treat cancer pain, which demonstrates the treatment process to select analgesics (Fig. 19.2). The analgesics should be selected based on an assessment of the intensity of pain experienced by the patient rather than physicians' clinical experiences. For the individual indicates analgesics needed by each patient vary

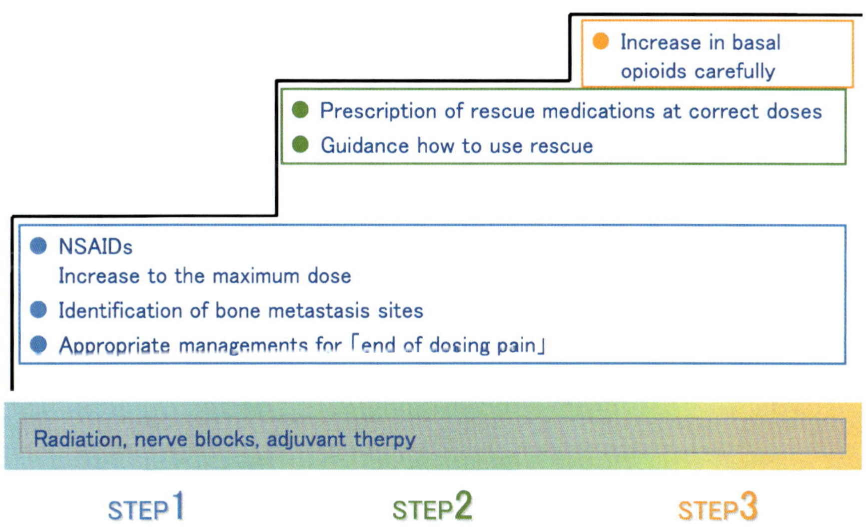

Fig. 19.2 The WHO ladder for cancer pain treatment

widely which is independent on an etiology of pain. In any cases, it is important to assess regularly to confirm not only the response to analgesics or therapy but also the maximum benefit with as few adverse effects as possible. Attention to detail expresses to ensure the patient's new treatment-induced pain such as opioid adverse events.

The use of opioids should not be affected by unfounded fears such as respiratory depression, tolerance, or dependence. In the palliative care area, psychological dependence rarely occurs, although high-dose fentanyl may cause ceiling effect. When opioid is prescribed, opioid titration is necessary. In the textbook, the concept of titration is described as a systematic process of incremental dose adjustment based on the patient's needs and responses. Titration includes either increment or decrement opioid dose, depending on the patient's needs and responses. The need for dose adjustment is based on reported severity of pain and frequency of need for breakthrough doses. The goal of titration is to use the smallest dose that provides satisfactory pain relief with the fewest adverse effects.

19.6 Classification of Analgesics and Typical Analgesics

The WHO ladder demonstrates the three steps when analgesics are prescribed for cancer pain. At step 1, non-opioids should be used. In Japan, nonsteroidal anti-inflammatory drugs (NSAIDs) and acetaminophen, which mediate their effect through mechanisms other than opioid receptors, are classified into step 1. In other countries, in addition to NSAIDs, both aspirin and paracetamol are used as step 1 agents. NSAIDs are of use in the treatment of pain mediated by prostaglandins, which serve to sensitize nociceptors. NSAIDs are recommended to use for the treatment of bone pain. NSAIDs suppress the production of prostaglandins through cyclooxygenase (COX) inhibition. COX includes COX-1 and COX-2. Nonspecific COX inhibitors have adverse effects such as gastrointestinal ulcer, asthma attack, and renal toxicity, although Cox-2-selective NSAIDs have reduced such effects.

Opioids are agents that act as an agonist at opioid receptor sites. Opioid receptors are identified at least in three types, mu, kappa, and delta. They are found in several areas of the brain including the spinal cord. Weak opioids such as tramadol and codeine are classified into step 2. They are used for the treatment of mild to moderate pain, which cannot be relieved by step 1 agents. When appropriate treatment cannot be achieved by step 2 agents and patients complain of moderate to severe pain, strong opioids (step 3) should be considered.

Tramadol has a dual analgesic effect. Tramadol is metabolized to an active metabolite by CYPs which has an affinity to opioid receptor, demonstrating weak opioid activity. Another tramadol analgesic effect is produced as serotonin-noradrenaline reuptake inhibitor effect. Therefore, tramadol has both weak opioid and adjuvant analgesic effects. In Japan, initial tramadol doses are between 50 and 100 mg a day, and maximum doses, 300 mg a day, although doses of 400 mg a day should not be exceeded in some countries. Adverse effects of tramadol include nausea, vomiting, dizziness, and drowsiness. A serious drug interaction, serotonin syndrome may develop when combined with some antidepressants (serotonergic drugs).

Most popular strong opioid is morphine which is extracted from opium poppy more than 200 years ago; therefore morphine is available to prescribe as starting opioid for moderate to severe cancer pain with low costs in many countries. Morphine has no ceiling effect to analgesia because of its full agonist activity to opioid receptors. Appropriate maintaining doses of morphine for cancer pain relief depend on individuals; therefore tailor-made titration for each individual is necessary. Morphine is metabolized in the liver into 2 main metabolites: morphine-6-glucuronide (M6G) and morphine-3-glucuronide (M3G). Patients with severe hepatic failure should be begun with a reduced dose of morphine. M6G has more potent analgesic effect than morphine itself. Morphine metabolites are eliminated by the kidney; therefore patients with renal dysfunction are at an increased risk of accumulation of metabolites, developing adverse effects such as somnolence or respiratory depression. Various morphine formulations are prepared. Oral route is described as the preferred route in WHO method, but if it becomes impossible for patients to take morphine orally, rectal, intravenous, or subcutaneous administration can be selected. Another option for the administration of morphine is epidural and intrathecal routes. The conversion ratio between routes is listed: oral morphine 60 mg = morphine suppositories 30 mg = iv morphine 20–30 mg.

Oxycodone is also a strong opioid analgesic similar to morphine. Commercially available oxycodone formulations are both 12 h modified-release oral preparation and intravenous solution in Japan. Oxycodone is metabolized in the liver into metabolites, which analgesic properties are negligible. The conversion ratio of morphine to oxycodone is approximately 3:2. The conversion ratio of oral to i.v. is approximately 4:3.

Fentanyl is a highly lipid-soluble strong opioid which is 100 times as potent as morphine. Fentanyl can be administered by intravenous, transdermal, and spinal routes. Fentanyl is metabolized in the liver into mainly inactive metabolites; therefore it can be prescribed for patients with renal failure. Constipation, one of the opioid-induced major adverse effects, occurred less frequently with fentanyl than with other opioids, because mu-1 selectivity is higher in fentanyl. Mu opioid receptor includes mu-1 and mu-2. Because bowel movement is mediated mainly through mu-2, higher mu-1 selectivity may be responsible for less constipation in fentanyl (Fig. 19.3). The transdermal administration is only

Fig. 19.3 Risk for the onset of constipation between fentanyl, oxycodone, and morphine. Revised from Southern Medical Journal 2004; 97: 129–134

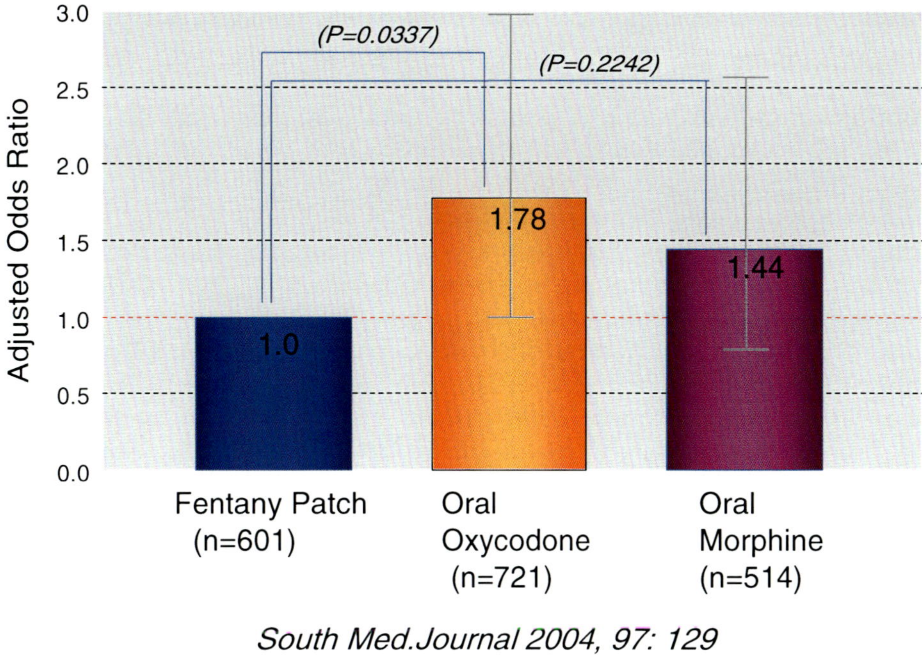

available with fentanyl. This route has apparent benefit to patients with nausea, vomiting, malabsorption, and dysphagia. In cases of oral cancer, transdermal fentanyl administration may be one of the most suitable methods, because dysphagia frequently occurred as a result of surgery, radiation, and tumor itself. The onset of analgesia following the application of the first fentanyl patch is approximately 12 h. The steady state of plasma fentanyl concentrations may be achieved for 48 and 96 h with a 3-day and 1 day patch, respectively. When the patch is removed, the plasma concentrations are halved approximately 17 h later. Therefore, transdermal fentanyl is not suitable for patients during opioid titration. In a 3-day patch, patients sometimes complain of dizziness and drowsiness, because the amount of fentanyl released in the first day is much more than that in the second and last days. On the other hand, there are some patients who have experienced pain on the third day following application of transdermal fentanyl, suggesting end-of-dose pain. End-of-dose pain is considered to be caused by a decrease in the mean plasma concentration of fentanyl even in the steady state between 24 and 72 h. Especially, the plasma fentanyl concentrations between 65 and 75 h are shown to be approximately one-half of that between 19 and 25 h following the application of fentanyl patch [5].

Patients frequently complain of breakthrough pain. This pain is characterized as a transient increase in pain intensity over background pain. Breakthrough pain which is rapid in onset and severe in intensity compared to the background pain is usually related to background pain. Breakthrough pain is classified into three types: incident pain, spontaneous pain, and end-of-dose pain. Incident pain is caused by movement or coughing. Spontaneous pain occurs with no identifiable cause, and its property is characterized as long-lasting pain which is compared to incident pain. End-of-dose pain causes gradual onset pain prior to scheduled analgesia. Treatment of breakthrough pain is divided into pharmacological and non-pharmacological management. Typical pharmacological intervention is the administration of short-acting opioid (rescue medication) at a dose of one-sixth of the total 24-h dose of opioid. However, the relationship between the basal opioid dose and rescue medication depends on patients, so that rescue medication should be titrated in each patient (for the individual). For incidental pain, preemptive use of a short-acting opioid at an appropriate interval before movement is good option. For spontaneous pain, short-acting opioid use just after the onset of pain is available. For end-of-dose pain, short-acting opioid can be used, but after that, physicians have to reassess the basal opioid regimen and alter it to increase the dose or shorten the dosing interval. Non-pharmacological management includes physical therapy and psychological therapy such as counseling to alleviate anxiety and education regarding limitations and exacerbating factors.

19.7 Neuropathic Pain

When satisfactory alleviation of cancer pain cannot be achieved as a result of regular assessment of the response to analgesics or therapy, we have to consider the possibilities regarding opioid-resistant cancer pain. Opioid-resistant cancer pain includes underdosing, poor absorption or intake of opioids, raised intracranial pressure, and neuropathic pain.

When opioid-resistant cancer pain is considered to be developed by the damage of central or peripheral nervous systems, neuropathic pain may be concerned. Neuropathic pain is caused by mainly direct tumor invasion to the nerve, bone metastasis, and antineoplastic agents. As an antineoplastic agent-related complication, a dose-dependent, predominantly sensory distal symmetric polyneuropathy which is caused by changes in the innervation territory corresponding to the involved part of the peripheral nervous system often occurs [6]. In Spain, the prevalence of neuropathic pain in cancer pain is reported as 33 % with above half the cases associated to nociceptive pain and 43 % treatment related following the recruitment of cancer patients more than 8,600 [7].

Adjuvant analgesics do not primarily act as analgesics, but their analgesic properties are widely recognized. When patients fail to achieve adequate relief following administration of either non-opioid or opioid analgesics, adjuvant analgesics should be considered. Anticonvulsants such as gabapentin or pregabalin are first-line agents for neuropathic pain, because neuronal hyperexcitability is thought to be of importance in the pathogenesis of neuropathic pain. Both agents cause a decrease in the release of excitatory neurotransmitters such as glutamate and substance P by binding to voltage-gated calcium channels in the dorsal horn. Gabapentin and pregabalin are GABA analogs, which have a more tolerable side effect profile and are easier to administer than carbamazepine. Pregabalin, in contrast to gabapentin, has a rapid absorption (T max, 1 h), and plasma concentration increases linearly with increasing dose. The higher bioavailability and rapid absorption allow for much lower doses to be used to achieve an equianalgesic effect to gabapentin. Being more potent than gabapentin, pregabalin achieved efficacy at lower doses and should lead to fewer dose-related adverse effects. In fact, pregabalin improved oxaliplatin-induced sensory neuropathy in almost half of the patients [8].

Tricyclic antidepressants (TCAs) such as amitriptyline and imipramine are also first-line agents for neuropathic pain. Both serotonin-selective reuptake inhibitors (SSRI) and serotonin-noradrenaline reuptake inhibitors (SNRI) are also used. TCAs have significant adverse effects such as anticholinergic effects (dry mouth, constipation, blurred vision, urinary retention) and arrhythmias. Therefore, up to 20 % of patients may give up continuing treatments. Duloxetine is one of the SNRIs and has the advantage over TCAs because of its less adverse effects. Analgesic action of TCAs often presents within a couple of days, although the onset of antidepressant effects takes a few weeks. Antiarrhythmic Na channel blockers such as lidocaine and mexiletine may be used for the treatment of pain caused by peritonitis or pleuritis. Corticosteroid is used for pain by reducing inflammatory sensitization of the nerves or the pressure effects of edema. Dexamethasone is popular because of the least mineral-corticoid effect and long duration of effect.

The use of opioids in combination with antiepileptic agents has been proposed by international guidelines to appropriately treat neuropathic pain [9]. Actually, bortezomib (a proteasome inhibitor drug)-induced neuropathic pain was alleviated by oxycodone [6].

19.8 Prevention and Treatment for Opioid-Related Adverse Effects

Both prevention and appropriate interventions for opioid-related adverse effects are one of the key components to continue to treat cancer pain. Because the degree of adverse effects has wide interindividual variation in sensitivity, "attention to detail" concept is a fundamental aspect to continue opioid therapy. The major opioid-related adverse effects are constipation, nausea and vomiting, and drowsiness. However, these symptoms are not opioid specific. For example, nausea is caused by increased intracranial pressure, mechanical obstruction of bowel, and constipation. Therefore, the first step to treat these symptoms is to exclude other reasons such as underlying disease and confirm the relationship between opioid and these adverse symptoms. Common management strategies for opioid-related adverse effects are mainly an employment of a specific therapy such as antiemetic drug administration or dose reduction of systemic opioid, but other options can be available. The first option is opioid switching, that is, the conversion to different opioids with the same potency. Another option is to reduce opioid requirements by the use of adjuvant analgesics and application of nerve blocks and anti-cancer therapies such as radiation and chemotherapy.

For opioid-related nausea and vomiting, either metoclopramide 10–20 mg/day p.o. or prochlorperazine 5–15 mg/day p.o. or continuous intravenous infusion is frequently prescribed. If nausea and vomiting persists, olanzapine 5–10 mg/day p.o. is considered when the patient is not suffering from diabetes mellitus. For opioid-related constipation, prophylactic laxative prescription is recommended. A combination of a bowel stimulant laxative and a stool softener may be used. For constipation, pharmacological tolerance cannot occur during opioid treatment; therefore opioid switching should be considered if this issue is severe. When opioid switching is considered, fentanyl is the most appropriate agent because higher mu-1 selectivity may be responsible for less constipation. Opioid-related drowsiness is related to relatively high opioid plasma concentrations. If drowsiness occurs without pain, a reduction of opioids should be considered. On the other hand, when drowsiness presents without alleviation of pain, physicians should evaluate the proportion of pain and consider using adjuvant drugs. In Japan, a psychostimulant such as methylphenidate is not allowed to be prescribed to alleviate drowsiness.

References

1. Fine PG (2005) The evolving and important role of anesthesiology in palliative care. Anesth Analg 100:183–188
2. World Health Organization (1990) Cancer Pain Relief and Palliative Care. WHO, Geneva
3. Temel JS, Greer JA, Muzikansky A, Gallagher ER, Admane S, Jackson VA, Dahlin CM, Blinderman CD, Jacobsen J, Pirl WF, Billings JA, Lynch TJ (2010) Early palliative care for patients with metastatic non-small-cell lung cancer. N Engl J Med 363:733–742
4. Watson M, Lucas C, Hoy A, Wells J (2009) Oxford handbook of palliative care, 2nd edn. Oxford University Press, New York
5. Kokubun H, Matoba M, Hoka S, Yamada Y, Yago K (2007) Relationship between serum fentanyl concentration and transdermal fentanyl dosage, and intra-individual variability in fentanyl concentration after application of fentanyl patches in patients with cancer pain. Jpn J Pharm Health Care Sci 33:200–205
6. Cartoni C, Brunetti GA, Federico V, Efficace F, Grammatico S, Tendas A, Scaramucci L, Cupelli L, D'Elia GM, Truini A, Niscola P, Petrucci MT (2012) Controlled-release oxycodone for the treatment of bortezomib-induced neuropathic pain in patients with multiple myeloma. Support Care Cancer 20:2621–2626
7. Gracia de Paredes ML, del Moral Gonzalez F, Martinez del Prado P, Marti Ciriquian JL, Enrech Frances S, Cobo Dols M, Esteban Gonzalez E, Ortega Granados AL, Majem Tarruella M, Cumplido Buron JD, Gasco Hernandez A, Lopez Miranda E, Ciria Santos JP, de Castro Carpeno FJ (2011) First evidence of oncologic neuropathic pain prevalence after screening 8615 cancer patients. Results of the on study. Ann Oncol 22:924–930
8. Saif MW, Syrigos K, Kaley K, Isufi I (2010) Role of pregabalin in treatment of oxaliplatin-induced sensory neuropathy. Anticancer Res 30:2927–2934
9. Attal N, Cruccu G, Haanpaa M, Hansson P, Jensen TS, Nurmikko T, Sampaio C, Sindrup S, Wiffen P, Task Force EFNS (2006) EFNS guidelines on pharmacological treatment of neuropathic pain. Eur J Neurol 13:1153–1169

Index

T. Kirita and K. Omura (eds.), *Oral Cancer: Diagnosis and Therapy*,
DOI 10.1007/978-4-431-54938-3, © Springer Japan 2015

Q

R

S